I0063827

Pancreatitis

Pancreatitis

Edited by

John A. Williams

Section Editors

Stephen J. Pandol
Markus M. Lerch
Julia Mayerle
Suresh T. Chari
Ashok K. Saluja
Marc G. Besselink
Pramod K. Garg
Philip A. Hart

Published in the United States of America by
Michigan Publishing
Manufactured in the United States of America

ISBN 978-1-60785-369-5 (hardcover), 978-1-60785-411-1 (e-book)

Cover image: Trypsin digestive enzyme molecule (human)
iStock.com/Molekuul

CONTENTS

CONTRIBUTORS

Ali A. Aghdassi, *Department of Medicine A, University Medicine Greifswald, Greifswald, Germany*

Hana Algül, *Department of Medicine 2, Technical University of Munich, Munich, Germany*

Dana K. Andersen, *Division of Digestive Diseases and Nutrition National Institute of Diabetes and Digestive and Kidney Diseases, National Institutes of Health, Bethesda, Maryland*

Minotti V. Apte, *Pancreatic Research Group, South Western Sydney Clinical School, University of New South Wales, Sydney, and Ingham Institute for Applied Medical Research, Liverpool, New South Wales, Australia*

Greg Beilman, *Departments of Surgery and Medicine, University of Minnesota, Minneapolis, MN, USA*

Maria Cristina Conti Bellocchi, *Department of Medicine, Pancreas Center, University of Verona, Verona, Italy*

Marc G. Besselink, *Department of Surgery, Academic Medical Center, Amsterdam, The Netherlands*

Georg Beyer, *Department of Medicine A, University Medicine Greifswald, Greifswald, Germany*

Yan Bi, *Department of Gastroenterology and Hepatology, Mayo Clinic, Rochester, MN, USA*

Thomas Bollen, *Department of Radiology, St. Antonius Hospital, Nieuwegein, The Netherlands*

Stefan A. Bouwense, *Department of Surgery, Radboud University Medical Center, Nijmegen, The Netherlands*

Joan M. Braganza, *Emeritus Reader, Manchester University, Manchester, UK*

Marco J. Bruno, *Dept. of Gastroenterology and Hepatology, Erasmus University Medical Center, Rotterdam, The Netherlands*

Djuna L. Cahen, *Dept. of Gastroenterology and Hepatology, Erasmus University Medical Center, Rotterdam, The Netherland / Dept. of Gastroenterology and Hepatology, Amstelland Medical Center, Amstelveen, The Netherlands*

Pietro Campagnola, *Department of Medicine, Pancreas Center, University of Verona, Verona, Italy*

C. Ross Carter, *West of Scotland Pancreatico-Biliary Unit, Glasgow Royal Infirmary, Glasgow, UK*

Güralp O. Ceyhan, *Department of Surgery, Technical University of Munich, Munich, Germany*

Suresh T. Chari, *Division of Gastroenterology and Hepatology, Mayo Clinic Rochester, MN, USA*

David N. Criddle, *Department of Cellular and Molecular Physiology, Institute of Translational Medicine and NIHR Liverpool Pancreas Biomedical Research Unit, University of Liverpool, UK*

David da Costa, *Department of Surgery, St. Antonius Hospital, Nieuwegein, The Netherlands*

Rajinder K. Dawra, *Department of Surgery, University of Miami Miller School of Medicine, Miami, FL, USA*

Jan De Waele, *Department of Critical Care Medicine, Ghent University Hospital De Pintelaan, Belgium*

Ihsan Ekin Demir, *Department of Surgery, Technical University of Munich, Munich, Germany*

Jan D'Haese, *Department of General, Visceral, Transplantation and Vascular Surgery, Ludwig Maximillians University, Munich, Germany*

Euan J. Dickson, *West of Scotland Pancreatico-Biliary Unit, Glasgow Royal Infirmary, Glasgow, UK*

Ajay Dixit, *Department of Surgery, University of Miami, Miller School of Medicine, Miami, Florida, USA*

Dana Dominguez, *University of California, San Francisco School of Medicine, San Francisco, CA, USA*

Asbjørn Mohr Drewes, *Department of Gastroenterology & Hepatology, Aalborg University Hospital, Aalborg, Denmark*

Vikas Dudeja, *Department of Surgery, University of Miami Miller School of Medicine, Miami, FL, USA*

Mouad Edderkaoui, *Cedars-Sinai Medical Center, VA-West Los Angeles & University of California, Los Angeles, CA, USA*

B. Joseph Elmunzer, *Division of Gastroenterology & Hepatology, Medical University of South Carolina, Charleston, SC, USA*

Martin L. Freeman, *Division of Gastroenterology, Department of Medicine and Departments of Surgery and Medicine, University of Minnesota, Minneapolis, MN, USA*

Helmut Friess, *Department of Surgery, Technical University of Munich, Munich, Germany*

Luca Frulloni, *Department of Medicine, Pancreas Center, University of Verona, Verona, Italy*

Larissa L. Fujii, *Division of Gastroenterology and Hepatology, Mayo Clinic, Rochester, MN, USA*

Pramod Kumar Garg, *Departments of Gastroenterology, All India Institute of Medical Sciences, New Delhi, India*

Simone Gärtner, *University Medicine Greifswald, Department of Medicine A, Greifswald, Germany*

Fred Gorelick, *Yale University School of Medicine, New Haven, CT, USA / VA HealthCare System, West Haven, CT, USA*

Guy Groblewski, *Department of Nutritional Sciences, University of Wisconsin, Madison, WI, USA*

Nalini M. Guda, *Aurora St.Luke's Medical Center, Milwaukee, WI, USA*

Ilya Gukovsky, *West Los Angele VA Medical center, Medicine, University of California at Los Angeles, CA, USA*

Jintao Guo, *Endoscopy Center, Shengjing Hospital of China Medical University, Shenyang, China*

Aida Habtezion, *Department of Medicine, Stanford University, Stanford, CA, USA*

Nora D.L. Hallensleben, *Dept. of Gastroenterology and Hepatology, Erasmus University Medical Center, Rotterdam, The Netherlands / Dept. of Surgery, St. Antonius Hospital, Nieuwegein, The Netherlands*

Shin Hamada, *Division of Gastroenterology, Tohoku University Graduate School of Medicine, Sendai, Japan*

Phil A. Hart, *Division of Gastroenterology and Hepatology, Mayo Clinic Rochester, MN, USA*

Péter Hegyi, *First Department of Medicine, University of Szeged, Szeged, Hungary / MTA-SZTE Translational Gastroenterology Research Group, Szeged, Hungary / Centre for Translational Medicine, Institute for Translational Medicine & First Department of Medicine, Department of Translational Medicine, University of Pécs*

Robbert A. Hollemans, *Dept. of Surgery, Academic Medical Center, Amsterdam, The Netherlands / Dept. of Surgery, St Antonius Hospital, Nieuwegein, The Netherlands*

Wei Huang, *NIHR Liverpool Pancreas Biomedical Research Unit, Royal Liverpool and Broadgreen University Hospitals NHS Trust and Institute of Translational Medicine, University of Liverpool, Liverpool, UK*

Sohail Z. Husain, *Department of Pediatrics, Children's Hospital of Pittsburgh of UPMC and the University of Pittsburgh School of Medicine, Pittsburgh, PA, USA*

Baoan Ji, *Department of Cancer Biology, Mayo Clinic, Jacksonville, FL, USA*

Terumi Kamisawa, *Department of Internal Medicine, Tokyo Metropolitan Komagome Hospital, Tokyo, Japan*

Devasenathipathy Kandasamy, *Department of Radiodiagnosis, All India Institute of Medical Science, New Delhi, India*

Shigeyuki Kawa, *Center for Health, Safety and Environmental Management, Shinshu University, Matsumoto, Japan*

Jutta Keller, *Department of Medicine, Israelitisches Krankenhaus, Hamburg, Germany*

Myung-Hwan Kim, *Department of Internal Medicine, University of Ulsan College of Medicine, Asan Medical Center, Seoul, South Korea*

Kimberly Kirkwood, *University of California, San Francisco School of Medicine, San Francisco, CA, USA*

Guenter Kloeppel, *Department of Pathology, Technical University of Munich, Germany*

Paul Georg Lankisch, *Department of General Internal Medicine and Gastroenterology, Clinical Center of Lüneburg, Lüneburg, Germany*

Peter Layer, *Department of Medicine, Israelitisches Krankenhaus, Hamburg, Germany*

Markus M. Lerch, *Department of Medicine A, University Medicine Greifswald, Greifswald, Germany*

Michael Levy, *Division of Gastroenterology and Hepatology, Mayo Clinic, Rochester, MN, USA*

J.-Matthias Löhr, *Gastrocentrum, Karolinska Institute & Karolinska University Hospital, Stockholm, Sweden*

Daniel Longnecker, *Department of Pathology, Geisel School of Medicine at Dartmouth, Lebanon, NH, USA*

Albert B. Lowenfels, *New York Medical College, Department of Surgery, Department Family and Community Medicine, Valhalla, NY, USA*

Aurelia Lugea, *Department of Medicine, Cedars-Sinai Medical Center, University of California and Department of Veterans Affairs, Los Angeles, CA, USA*

Jorge D. Machicado, *Division of Gastroenterology & Hepatology, University of Pittsburgh Medical Center, Pittsburgh, PA, USA*

József Maléth, *First Department of Medicine, University of Szeged, Szeged, Hungary / MTA-SZTE Translational Gastroenterology Research Group, Szeged, Hungary*

Olga A. Mareninova, *Veterans Affairs Greater Los Angeles Healthcare System and Department of Medicine, David Geffen School of Medicine, University of California at Los Angeles, CA, USA*

Masahiro Maruyama, *Department of Gastroenterology, Shinshu University School of Medicine, Matsumoto, Japan*

Atsushi Masamune, *Division of Gastroenterology, Tohoku University Graduate School of Medicine, Sendai, Japan*

Julia Mayerle, *Department of Medicine A, University of Greifswald, Greifswald, Germany*

Colin J. McKay, *West of Scotland Pancreatico-Biliary Unit, Glasgow Royal Infirmary, Glasgow, UK*

Joachim Mössner, *Division of Gastroenterology and Rheumatology, Department of Medicine, Neurology, and Dermatology University Hospitals of Leipzig, Leipzig, Germany*

Rajarshi Mukherjee, *NIHR Liverpool Pancreas Biomedical Research Unit, Royal Liverpool and Broadgreen University Hospitals NHS Trust and Institute of Translational Medicine, University of Liverpool, Liverpool, UK*

Sydne Muratore, *Departments of Surgery and Medicine, University of Minnesota, Minneapolis, MN, USA*

Sarah Navina, *Clin-Path Associates, Tempe, AZ, USA*

Camilla Nøjgaard, *Hvidovre University Hospital, Copenhagen, Denmark*

Kenji Notohara, *Kurashiki Central Hospital, 1-1-1 Miwa, Kurashiki, Japan*

Kazuichi Okazaki, *Department of Gastroenterology and Hepatology, Kansai Medical University, Osaka, Japan*

Søren Schou Olesen, *Department of Gastroenterology & Hepatology, Aalborg University Hospital*

Abrahim I. Orabi, *Department of Pediatrics, Children's Hospital of Pittsburgh of UPMC and the University of Pittsburgh School of Medicine, Pittsburgh, PA, USA*

Stephen Pandol, *Department of Medicine, Cedars-Sinai Medical Center, University of California and Department of Veterans Affairs, Los Angeles, CA, USA*

Krutika S. Patel, *Division of Gastroenterology and Hepatology, Mayo Clinic Scottsdale, AZ, USA*

George Perides, *Department of Surgery, Tufts Medical Center, Boston, MA, USA*

Romano C. Pirola, *Pancreatic Research Group, South Western Sydney Clinical School, University of New South Wales, Sydney, and Ingham Institute for Applied Medical Research, Liverpool, New South Wales, Australia*

Zoltán Rakonczay Jr., *First Department of Medicine and Department of Pathophysiology, University of Szeged, Szeged, Hungary*

Vinciane Rebours, *Pôle des Maladies de l'Appareil Digestif, Service de Pancréatologie, INSERM UMR1149. Hôpital Beaujon 100, Clichy, France / Pancreatology Unit, Beaujon Hospital, University Paris, Clichy, France*

Nageshwar Reddy, *Asian Institute of Gastroenterology, Hyderabad, India*

Anamika Reed, *Yale University School of Medicine, New Haven, CT, USA*

Ashok K. Saluja, *Department of Surgery, University of Miami Miller School of Medicine, Miami, FL, USA / University of Minnesota, Minneapolis, MN, USA*

Hjalmar C van Santvoort, *Dept. of Surgery, Academic Medical Center, Amsterdam, The Netherlands / Dept. of Surgery, St Antonius Hospital, Nieuwegein, The Netherlands*

Nicolien J. Schepers, *Dept. of Gastroenterology and Hepatology, Erasmus University Medical Center, Rotterdam, The Netherlands / Dept. of Gastroenterology and Hepatology, St. Antonius Hospital, Nieuwegein, The Netherlands*

Stephan Schorn, *Department of Surgery, Technical University of Munich, Munich, Germany*

Raju Sharma, *Department of Radiodiagnosis, All India Institute of Medical Science, New Delhi, India*

Celeste A. Shelton, *Departments of Medicine and Human Genetics, University of Pittsburgh, Pittsburgh PA, USA*

Tooru Shimosegawa, *Division of Gastroenterology, Tohoku University Graduate School of Medicine, Sendai, Japan*

Peter Simon, *University Medicine Greifswald, Department of Medicine A, Greifswald, Germany*

Vijay P. Singh, *Division of Gastroenterology and Hepatology, Mayo Clinic Scottsdale, AZ, USA*

Tae Jun Song, *Department of Internal Medicine, Inje University Ilsan Paik Hospital, Inje University College of Medicine, Koyang, South Korea*

Michael L. Steer, *Department of Surgery, Tufts Medical Center, Boston, MA, USA*

Antje Steveling, *University Medicine Greifswald, Department of Medicine A, Greifswald, Germany*

John H. Stone, *Rheumatology Unit, Massachusetts General Hospital, Boston, MA, USA*

Siyu Sun, *Endoscopy Center, Shengjing Hospital of China Medical University, Shenyang, China*

Robert Sutton, *NIHR Liverpool Pancreas Biomedical Research Unit, Royal Liverpool and Broadgreen University Hospitals NHS Trust and Institute of Translational Medicine, University of Liverpool, Liverpool, UK*

Naoki Takahashi, *Department of Radiology, Mayo Clinic, Rochester, MN, USA*

Rupjyoti Talukdar, *Asian Institute of Gastroenterology/ Asian Healthcare Foundation, Telangana, India*

Edwin Thrower, *Yale University & VA Healthcare, New Haven, CT, USA*

Elke Tieftrunk, *Department of Surgery, Technical University of Munich, Munich, Germany*

Kazushige Uchida, *Department of Gastroenterology and Hepatology, Kansai Medical University, Osaka, Japan*

Mark C. van Baal, *Department of Surgery, Tweesteden Hospital, Tilburg, The Netherlands*

Santhi Swaroop Vege, *Division of Gastroenterology and Hepatology, Mayo Clinic, Rochester, MN, USA*

Viktória Venglovecz, *Department of Pharmacology and Pharmacotherapy, University of Szeged, Szeged, Hungary*

Richard T. Waldron, *Department of Medicine, Cedars-Sinai Medical Center, University of California and Department of Veterans Affairs, Los Angeles, CA, USA*

Takayuki Watanabe, *Department of Gastroenterology, Shinshu University School of Medicine, Matsumoto Japan*

F. Ulrich Weiss, *Department of Medicine A, University Medicine Greifswald, Greifswald, Germany*

Li Wen, *NIHR Liverpool Pancreas Biomedical Research Unit, Royal Liverpool and Broadgreen University Hospitals NHS Trust and Institute of Translational Medicine, University of Liverpool, Liverpool, UK*

Jens Werner, *Department of General, Visceral, Transplantation and Vascular Surgery, Ludwig Maximillians University, Munich, Germany*

David C. Whitcomb, *Departments of Medicine, Human Genetics and Cell Biology and Physiology, University of Pittsburg Medical Center, Pittsburgh, PA, USA*

Jeremy S. Wilson, *Pancreatic Research Group, South Western Sydney Clinical School, University of New South Wales, Sydney, and Ingham Institute for Applied Medical Research, Liverpool, New South Wales, Australia*

Dhiraj Yadav, *Division of Gastroenterology & Hepatology, University of Pittsburgh Medical Center, Pittsburgh, PA, USA*

Lizhi Zhang, *Department of Laboratory and Anatomic Pathology, Mayo Clinic, Rochester, MN, USA*

PREFACE

This book is designed to summarize the current state of knowledge on the inflammatory disease pancreatitis. Acute pancreatitis is one of the most common reasons for hospitalization due to gastrointestinal disease, and there are no effective therapies beyond symptomatic treatments. Chronic pancreatitis reduces quality of life due to pain and inadequate digestion and predisposes patients to pancreatic cancer. Autoimmune pancreatitis is a more recently described entity and can respond to treatment.

This book describes the genesis, experimental animal models, and diagnosis and treatment of clinical disease. Chapters are relatively short and designed to be read in a sitting. This was accomplished by dividing topics into smaller units while maintaining depth of coverage. The pertinent literature is cited for both recent developments and comprehensive reviews. Overall there are 65 chapters presented in four sections: "Experimental Pancreatitis," "Acute Pancreatitis," "Chronic Pancreatitis," and "Autoimmune Pancreatitis." Each chapter is written by acknowledged experts from around the world reflecting the global nature of the Pancreas community. The book is directed primarily to pancreas researchers and clinical practitioners but will also appeal to an educated audience of individuals interested in the exocrine pancreas and its diseases.

This material was originally published as entries on the Pancreapedia site (www.pancreapedia.org). The Pancreapedia is an open-access knowledge base developed at the University of Michigan under the sponsorship of the American Pancreatic Association and with support from the National Library of Medicine. Topics were developed by the Editors of the Pancreapedia and Section Editors for different aspects of pancreatitis. Submitted manuscripts were subjected to peer review to ensure clarity and completeness, then edited and mounted within a month of receipt on the Pancreapedia website, thus avoiding the long delays of traditional reference books. For any Pancreapedia entry over 2 years old, the authors were given the opportunity to update their contribution. Book chapters were then further copyedited and type set. Illustrative material was included wherever possible. The book has been indexed and cross-referenced and is available in electronic and print formats. Future books are planned on other aspects of the exocrine pancreas and its diseases.

ACKNOWLEDGEMENTS

We thank all the authors who contributed their expertise and writing to a novel open access form of publishing, the Pancreapedia. This book could not have been realized without the advice and assistance of the Michigan Publishing arm of the University of Michigan Library, especially Charles Watkinson and Jason Colman. We especially thank the students both graduate and undergraduate from the University of Michigan School of Information who organized and formatted material and interacted with authors from the beginning of this enterprise including Gin Cordon, Rachel Leduc, Erin Zolkovsky, Emily Rinck, Ben Krawatz, Melissa Wu and Juliana Lam. We also thank the American Pancreatic Association and the National Library of Medicine for their invaluable support.

Experimental Pancreatitis

Section Editors: Stephen J. Pandol and Ashok K. Saluja

Chapter 1

Experimental acute pancreatitis: *In vitro* models

Olga A. Mareninova[1], Abrahim I. Orabi[2], and Sohail Z. Husain[2*]

[1]*Veterans Affairs Greater Los Angeles Healthcare System and Department of Medicine, David Geffen School of Medicine, University of California at Los Angeles, CA 90073 USA;*

[2]*Department of Pediatrics, Children's Hospital of Pittsburgh of UPMC and the University of Pittsburgh School of Medicine, Pittsburgh, PA 15224 USA.*

Introduction

Acute pancreatitis is an extremely painful and life-threatening inflammatory disease of the exocrine pancreas.[1,2] A sobering point for both clinicians and researchers is that treatment for acute pancreatitis remains largely supportive. Furthermore, there is a lack of therapies that target primary mechanisms underlying disease initiation or propagation. Reliable, relevant, and convenient experimental animal models that resemble the human disease are crucial to developing an understanding of pancreatitis pathobiology.[3-8] In this chapter, we will review the current *in vitro* (i.e., *ex vivo*) models that serve as surrogates for experimental acute pancreatitis. We will specifically discuss: (1) the standard process of preparing pancreatic acinar cells or pancreatic tissue components, (2) assays for assessing *in vitro* injury and inflammatory precursors, and (3) the array of nonalcoholic and alcoholic *in vitro* models of pancreatitis.

The pancreatic acinar cell is the main parenchymal cell of the pancreas. It comprises roughly 90% of the pancreatic parenchyma and synthesizes and secretes digestive enzymes in response to hormonal stimulation.[9-12] The acinar cell is considered the initial site of pancreatic injury that leads to pancreatitis; thus, acinar cell cultures have been used for decades to define the molecular events that occur during the early stages of the disease.[13-15] The advantage of these models is that they provide a high throughput (or at least rapid) system to examine whether cellular pathways or molecular targets modulate injurious *in vitro* corollaries to *in vivo* events including aberrant calcium (Ca^{2+}) signaling, activation of digestive proteases, nuclear factor (NF)-κB activation, mitochondrial dysfunction, and cell death through apoptosis or necrosis. A disadvantage is that they lack the full inflammatory or systemic components, so subsequent *in vivo* validation of *in vitro* findings is crucial.

Adenovirus-mediated gene transfer has enabled researchers to manipulate acinar cell function in the presence of pathological agents.[16,17] Another powerful genetic approach for studying pancreatitis *in vitro* is to isolate acinar cells from the pancreas of gene-targeted knockout or transgenic mice.[18-21]

Acinar Cell Preparations

Single, double, and large cluster acinar cell preparations

Isolated pancreatic acini and acinar cells can be prepared from rat, mouse, and guinea pig pancreas using a collagenase digestion protocol.[22-26] Depending on the stringency of the isolation protocol, single, double, and large cluster acinar cells are obtained (**Figure 1A-B**). The greatest determinant in acinar cell preparation stringency is the concentration and duration of collagenase digestion. Nonetheless, there are several collagenases to choose from, including Sigma Types II,[27] IV or V,[28] and Worthington type IV.[29] A newer collagenase P from Roche can be used to prepare smaller acini for electrophysiology;[30,31] Liberase (Roche) is another option. Some authorities use collagenase NB1 (Serva) to perform human islet cell isolation, which also yields acinar cells (and duct cells) for experimental use.[32,33] Acinar size and integrity are highly dependent on collagenase type and shearing force application.[34] After pancreatic tissue digestion, acinar cells can be purified away from ducts, islets, and blood vessels by filtration and bovine serum albumin (BSA) density sedimentation. Following this method, acini can be maintained in culture for 24-48 h, and after that time they start to lose their polarity and secretory capability.

Lobules

To assess the direct and indirect effects of agonists on acinar cell secretion, *in vitro* preparations should ideally contain nerves and islets in addition to acinar cells.

For this reason, pancreatic lobules are useful (**Figure 1C**). In the original description by Scheele and colleagues, pancreatic

*Corresponding author. Email: sohail.husain@chp.edu

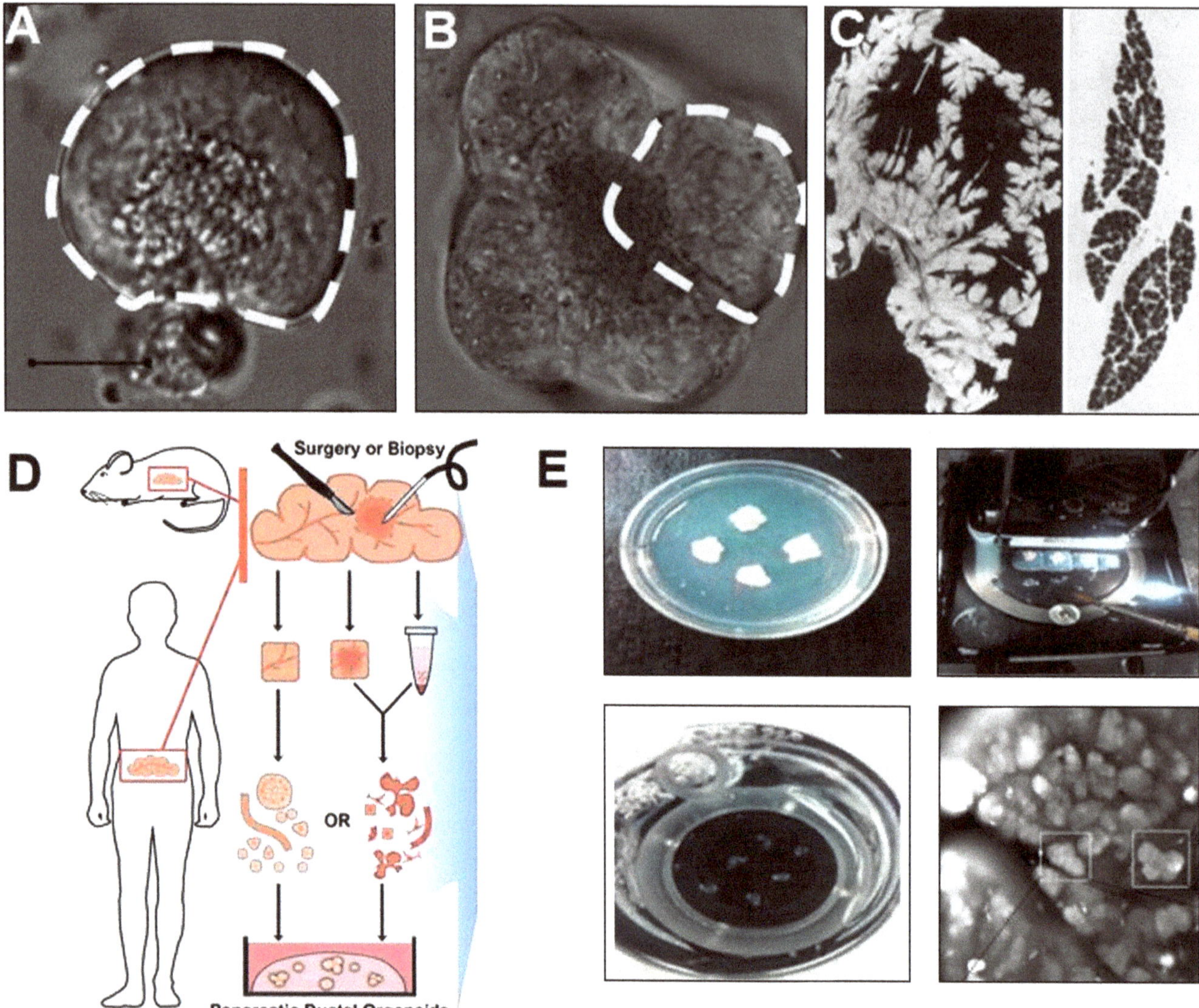

Figure 1. ***In vitro preparations of the pancreas*** **include (A) single acinar cell preparations,[22] (B) acini,[34] (C) pancreatic lobules,[35] (D) pancreatic organoids,[36] and (E) pancreatic slices.[37]** Republished with permission.

lobules were spread apart by injecting Krebs-Ringer bicarbonate (KRB) buffer into the loose connective tissue of the pancreas and then individually excised by micro-dissection under a stereomicroscope.[35,38] This procedure minimizes acinar cell damage since most of the surgical trauma is limited to ducts and vessels. The excised lobules preserve the overall acinar architecture of the tissue, and their small size allows for easy penetration of oxygen and solutes from the incubation medium. Following this method, lobules can be maintained for several hours in culture.[39-42]

Organoids

The most recent advance in studying pancreatic physiology *in vitro* involves the generation of pancreatic organoids (**Figure 1D**).[36-43] By definition, organoids are three-dimensional organ buds that arise from stem cells. With the use of growth factors, stem cell populations can be coaxed into forming balls of terminally differentiated cells that self-organize into distinctive layers. As described by Boj and colleagues, pancreatic organoids can be rapidly generated from resected pancreatic tumors and biopsies following manual digestion with collagenase II and seeded in growth factor-reduced Matrigel.[36] Conditioning the medium with the growth factor R-spondin promotes a predominantly duct cell population. These pancreatic organoids survive cryopreservation and exhibit ductal- and disease stage-specific characteristics. Further, pancreatic organoids from wild-type mice accurately recapitulate physiologically relevant aspects of disease progression *in vitro*. Following orthotopic transplantation, pancreatic organoids are capable of regenerating normal ductal architectures. This technique is particularly useful for studying duct cell phenotypes.[36]

Pancreas slice

The novel method of culturing pancreas slices is useful to preserve the integrity of the pancreatic milieu for at least 2 days (**Figure 1E**).[37,44] This technique allows for both *in situ* imaging of cellular events relevant to pancreatitis and genetic manipulation. To obtain a pancreas slice, Gaisano and colleagues gently infused a low melting agarose gel into the pancreatic duct of an anesthetized mouse via transduodenal puncture and common bile duct cannulation.[37,44] The pancreas was then excised and trimmed. The agarose renders the organ firm enough to slice it with a vibratome, at a thickness of 80-140 µm. Moreover, agarose is porous and thus provides free buffer exchange, ensuring optimal health in culture for up to 2 days. This technique permits both cell transfection and real-time imaging.

Acinar cell lines

The most commonly used cell line to study the exocrine pancreas is the rat pancreatic acinar cell line AR42J (**Figure 2**).

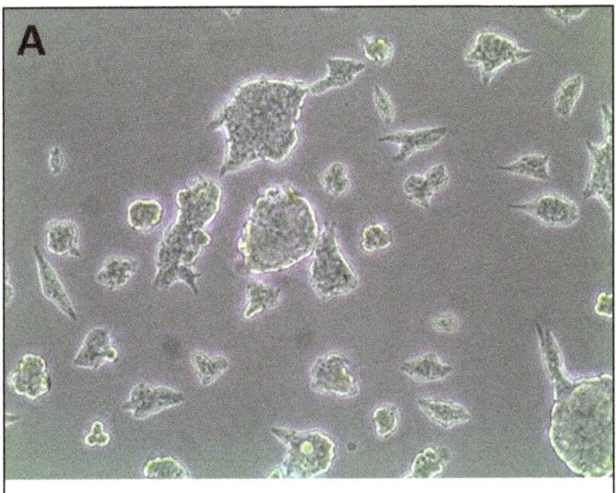

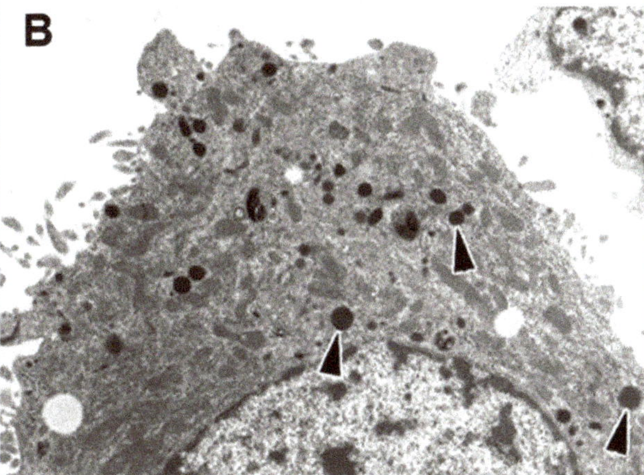

Figure 2. Morphological characteristics of the AR42J acinar cell line. AR42J cells primed with dexamethasone (100 nM) and visualized by (A)[45] light microscopy using a 20X objective or (B)[50] electron microscopy (arrowheads point to zymogen granules). Republished with permission.

These cells were derived from a transplantable tumor of the rat exocrine pancreas. They differ from primary pancreatic acinar cells in at least two ways: (1) they proliferate rapidly and (2), although they synthesize, store, and secrete digestive enzymes, they express atypical receptors and have atypical inositol phosphate metabolism and cytoskeleton rearrangement.[45] Dexamethasone favors their differentiation toward the acinar phenotype, including agonist-stimulated Ca^{2+} signaling.[46-49] AR42J cells are incubated for 48-72 h in culture medium supplemented with 100 nM dexamethasone prior to experimental treatment or induction. They are easily cultured in RPMI 1640 medium supplemented with glutamine, fetal bovine serum, and antibiotics at 37°C under humidified conditions of 95% air and 5% carbon dioxide. AR42J cells can be routinely plated at a density of 10^5 cells/mL in 75-cm^2 flasks and cultured for 7-10 days.

A less common acinar cell line is the 266-6 line derived from young adult mouse tumors that were induced with the elastase I/SV-40 T-antigen fusion gene. First described by Robert Hammer in 1985,[51] 266-6 cells retain a partially differentiated phenotype and express several digestive enzymes. They respond to carbachol and cholecystokinin (CCK) but not substance P, secretin, or vasoactive intestinal peptide (VIP). The culture method is the same as that described for AR42J cells except that there is no dexamethasone priming.

Assays for *In Vitro* Surrogates of Pancreatitis

Ca^{2+} signaling

Pancreatic acinar cells have served as an epithelial cell model for examining Ca^{2+} signaling for decades (**Figure 3**). Consistent with the polarized nature of acinar cells, Ca^{2+} signals in these cells exhibit highly organized spatial characteristics.[52] Most agonist-stimulated Ca^{2+} signals in acinar cells initiate in the apical region and propagate to the basolateral region.[10,53,54] Single-cell imaging of Ca^{2+} signals requires fluorescent dyes and confocal microscopy. A number of Ca^{2+}-sensing dyes are available, depending on the needs of the researcher.[55-58] The simplest dyes exhibit signature fluorescent properties upon binding Ca^{2+}; they are excited by a certain wavelength of light and emit photons at a certain emission wavelength (i.e., Fluo-3AM, Fluo-4AM). Conversely, ratiometric dyes (i.e., Fura-2) exhibit distinct spectral shifts upon Ca^{2+} binding, such that the Ca^{2+}-free form is excited maximally at 380 nm while the Ca^{2+}-bound form is excited maximally at 340 nm. Both states emit peak fluorescence at 510 nm.

Cells are loaded with the Ca^{2+} dye of choice, allowed to adhere to glass coverslips, and excited with the agonist of choice while collecting real-time images, usually with a laser scanning confocal microscope.[22]

Intra-acinar protease activation

Premature intracellular activation of digestive proteases has long been considered an early, initiating event in pancreatitis

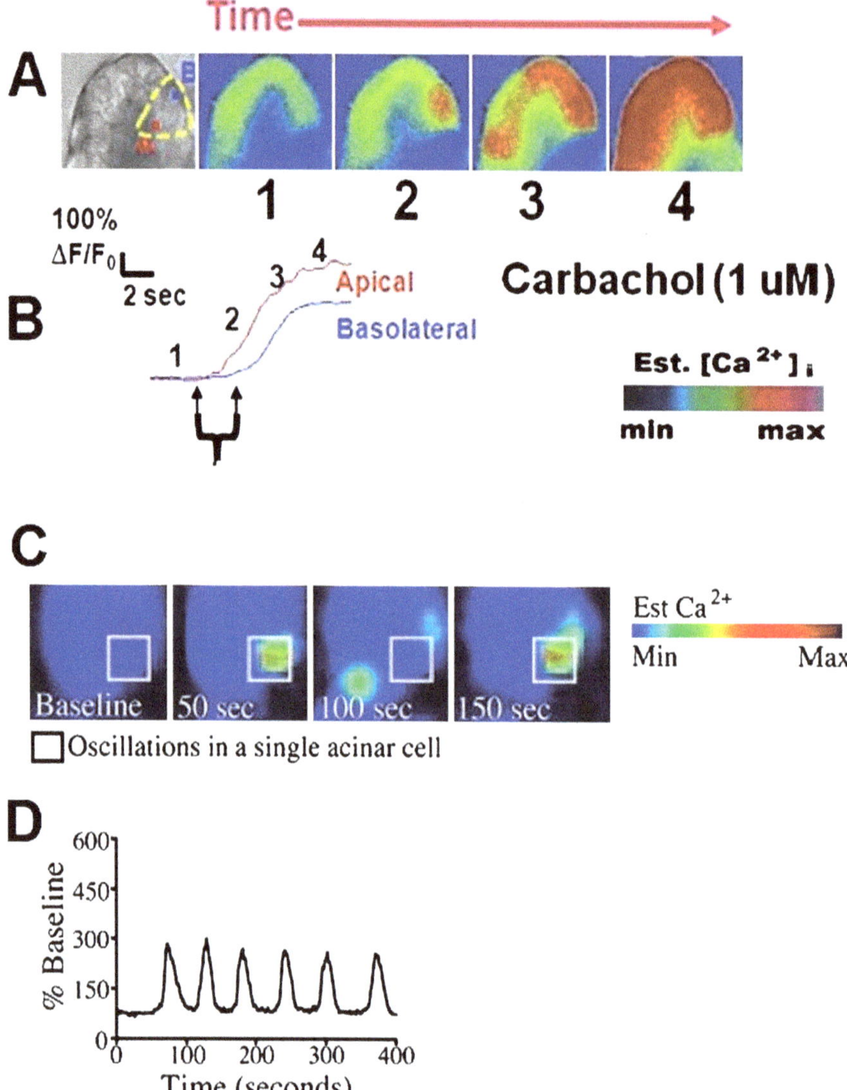

Figure 3. Typical Ca^{2+} transients upon stimulation with supraphysiologic concentrations of carbachol (1 μM) or physiologic concentrations of caerulein (10 pM). Changes in whole-cell Ca^{2+} were measured by time-lapse confocal microscopy using the Ca^{2+} dye Fluo-4AM (5 μM). Images are represented in pseudocolor with a color scale. (A) From left to right, bright field view of an acinus labeled at the apical and basolateral regions of interest. Upon stimulation with physiologic carbachol (1 μM, Ach analogue), subsequent images show the initiation of the Ca^{2+} signal in the apical region followed by propagation to the basal region. (B) Each paneled image (1-4) corresponds to a frame along a representative tracing of change in fluorescence over time for each region of interest. (C-D) Oscillating Ca^{2+} signals are observed in response to low-dose caerulein (10 pM, CCK analogue). Republished with permission.[59,60]

pathogenesis. The traditional method for examining intra-acinar protease activation involves probing pancreatic acinar cell lysates with a fluorogenic substrate for the protease of interest.[4,61,62] The readout is obtained from a fluorimeter (e.g., a fluorescent plate reader or cuvette system) in the form of a kinetic plot. These data can be normalized to total protein content or total DNA to control for cell loading. Since the initial description of these fluorogenic substrates in 1983,[63,64] bisamide derivatives of rhodamine 110 have been used as a sensitive and selective substrate for activated protease measurements. Proteolytic selectivity is achieved by using specific benzyloxycarbonyl-peptides. The tripeptide derivative bis-(CBZ-Ile-Pro-Arg)-R110 (BZiPAR) has been successfully used by some groups to measure trypsinogen activation by live microscopy.[3,65-67]

NF-κB translocation

NF-κB activation is thought to be an early and critical component of the inflammatory response during acute pancreatitis.[6] Traditional methods for examining NF-κB activity *in vitro* include protein determination of NF-κB

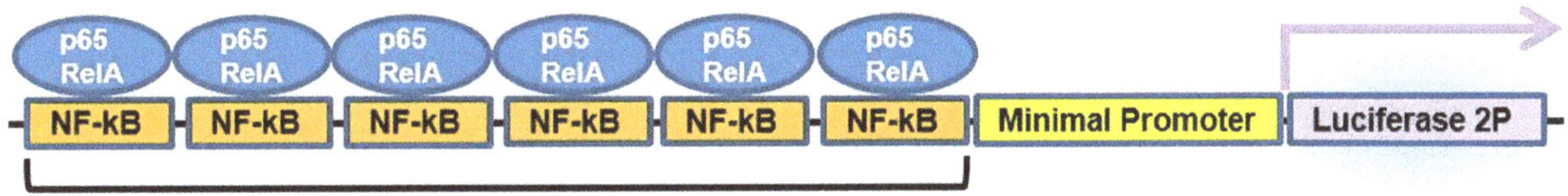

Figure 4. Schematic of the NF-κB-luciferase adenoviral construct. The construct contains six tandem-repeat transcription factor response elements, a minimal promoter, and a luciferase coding region. Binding of NF-κB subunits to a nuclear response element drives transcription of the luminescent protein luciferase. Republished with permission.[80]

pathway markers (i.e., phosphorylated IκB, p65 nuclear translocation, IKK upregulation), electromobility shift assay (EMSA), and immunohistochemistry for phosphorylated p65.[19,68] Newer techniques include the transfection (or usually infection via viral vectors in pancreatic cells) of NF-κB-luciferase reporters (**Figure 4**). With these techniques, binding of NF-κB subunits to a nuclear response element drives transcription of the gene encoding the luminescent luciferase protein. The most commonly used reporters are firefly[69] and renilla[70] luciferases. The development of secreted luciferases such as gaussia (Gluc), secreted alkaline phosphatase (SEAP), and cypridina allows for serial determination of NF-κB activity from the media over time.[71-74]

Mitochondrial damage

Mitochondrial dysfunction has been shown to play a critical role in the pathogenesis of pancreatic acinar cell injury, resulting in pancreatitis.[75] Manifestations of mitochondrial dysfunction in pancreatitis include loss of mitochondrial inner membrane potential ($\Delta\Psi m$), reactive oxygen species (ROS) production, release of the programmed cell death mediator cytochrome c into the cytosol, and failure of ATP production; these events lead to varying degrees of acinar cell necrosis or apoptosis.[76] Recent data show that preventing mitochondrial damage improves several aspects of pancreatitis and ameliorates disease severity.[77,78]

The effect of pancreatitis on $\Delta\Psi m$ can be measured in isolated acinar cells using the $\Delta\Psi m$-sensitive fluorescence probe tetramethylrhodamine methyl ester (TMRM), which is a lipophilic cation dye whose accumulation in mitochondria is proportional to the $\Delta\Psi m$. After preincubation with an agonist, cells are loaded with 1 μM TMRM for 10-20 min at 37°C and transferred to a fluorimeter to measure fluorescence intensity at 543 nm/570 nm.[77,79] $\Delta\Psi m$ can also be detected using another $\Delta\Psi m$-sensitive fluorescence probe JC-1, which exists as a green monomer at low $\Delta\Psi m$. Because JC-1 forms red fluorescent J-aggregates at higher potentials, the ratio between red (550 nm/600 nm) and green (485 nm/535 nm) fluorescence is used to monitor $\Delta\Psi m$. Decreased $\Delta\Psi m$ leads to depletion of intracellular ATP and subsequent necrosis. ATP levels in pancreatic acinar cells can be detected using a luciferin/luciferase luminescence-based assay that is normalized to protein content.

Permeabilization of the mitochondrial outer membrane occurs through opening of the mitochondrial permeability transition pore (MPTP), an event that is integral to apoptosis in pancreatitis. MPTP opening and subsequent mitochondrial outer membrane permeabilization result in the release of the mitochondrial resident protein cytochrome c into the cytosol. Cytochrome c release within acinar cells is assessed by immunoblotting against cytochrome c from cellular fractions of mitochondria-enriched membrane and cytosolic fractions.[81,82]

The mitochondria within acinar cells are highly susceptible to oxidative damage from ROS, and they also serve as primary generators of ROS when the electron transport chain within the inner mitochondrial membrane is perturbed (usually with $\Delta\Psi m$ loss). ROS can trigger cytochrome c release and death responses in pancreatic acinar cells, demonstrating the cross-talk between necrosis and apoptosis in the mitochondria.[78] Intracellular ROS levels are detected using 2,7-dichlorofluorescein (DCF).[81] ROS that is selectively generated by the mitochondria can be monitored by labeling the cells with the mitochondrial ROS-sensitive rhodamine-based fluorescent dye DHR123. Mitochondrial localization of DHR123 can be confirmed by co-staining the cells with the mitochondrial specific marker MitoTracker Red (CMXRos). Proper analysis of ROS production in living cells requires the combined use of several fluorescent ROS probes in parallel experiments, assessment of non-ROS related parameters that can induce artifacts (e.g., $\Delta\Psi$, pH), and the inclusion of adequate control conditions. For example, a common positive control known to stimulate the generation of mitochondrial ROS is rotenone, which inhibits complex I of the electron transport chain. A negative control is the mitochondrial uncoupler carbonyl cyanide m-chlorophenylhydrazone (CCCP), which blocks mitochondrial ROS production.

Cell injury

The three most common assays used to assess acinar cell injury include (1) lactate dehydrogenase (LDH) release; (2) propidium iodide (PI) uptake; and (3) reduction of MTT

(3-(4,5-dimethylthiazol-2-yl)-2,5-diphenyltetrazolium bromide). LDH catalyzes the interconversion of pyruvate to lactate and NADH to NAD^+.[83] Elevated levels of LDH are indicative of tissue injury and breakdown. LDH can be measured using colorimetric assays supplied by Promega (cat #G1780).[22] PI is a high-affinity DNA-binding dye that is effectively excluded from live cells.[84-86] Dead or dying cells have compromised plasma membranes and thereby allow PI to enter the nucleus and bind to DNA. MTT reduction is a measure of mitochondrial function and cell viability.[87-89] MTT is reduced to insoluble formazan by mitochondrial dehydrogenases. Water-insoluble formazan can be solubilized using isopropanol or other solvents. The dissolved material is measured spectrophotometrically, yielding absorbance as a function of the concentration of the converted dye.

Nonalcoholic Models

Secretagogues

The peptide hormone CCK and its analog caerulein has been used with *in vitro* models to reproducibly induce acute pancreatitis-like responses in acinar cells.[15,26,32,61,90-92] Pancreatic acinar cells express high- and low-affinity CCK receptors (CCKRs) that are activated by low and high concentrations of CCK, respectively.[93,94] Low concentrations in the picomolar range bind to high-affinity CCK receptors and maximally stimulate physiological acinar cell enzyme secretion.[95] High (supraphysiological) concentrations in the nanomolar range bind to low-affinity CCK receptors, which results in a relative reduction in the secretory response, a phenomenon that is thought to be pathological because it leads to the retention of prematurely activated proteases and their missorting.[65]

Digestive protease activation requires a rise in cytosolic Ca^{2+}, which occurs through release from intracellular Ca^{2+} pools (primarily the endoplasmic reticulum) that are gated by inositol trisphosphate receptors and ryanodine receptors.[3,4,10,96] Another consequence of supraphysiological CCK seen both *in vitro* and *in vivo* is the emergence of large intra-acinar vacuoles.[3,97,98]

There are other CCK analogues that do not lead to protease activation or pancreatitis even at high concentrations because they elicit distinct phenotypic responses and distinct cell signals. They include the O-phenyl-methyl-ester analogue of CCK (OPE) and JMV-180.[93,94] These agonists can serve as physiological controls to differentiate between pathological signals. The agonist bombesin (also known as gastrin-related peptide) causes intra-acinar protease activation but not acinar cell injury because, unlike CCK, bombesin does not cause activated proteases to be retained in acinar cells.[7] Other secretagogues that stimulate acinar cell enzyme secretion include secretin, VIP, and pituitary adenylate cyclase-activating peptide.[10,99,100]

Several investigations have questioned whether CCK hyperstimulation is relevant to human acinar cells.[92,101] Whereas CCK receptors are abundant on murine acinar cells, they have little to no expression in the human acinar cell.[102,103] Except for a notable recent report,[104] CCK failed to elicit a Ca^{2+} signal or a secretory response in isolated human acini.[102,105,106] By contrast, acetylcholine or its long-acting analog carbachol stimulates robust physiological and pathological (at high millimolar concentrations) responses in acinar cells from mouse, rat, and man.[107,108] Several clinical correlates of pancreatitis are associated with cholinergic overload, from exposure to scorpion toxin or organophosphates (which would prevent the degradation of acetylcholine by inhibiting endogenous acetylcholinesterases).[109-112]

Bile acids

The most common cause of acute pancreatitis is impaction of gallstones or sludge in the distal common bile duct, a situation called biliary pancreatitis.[113-116] There are two hotly debated and nonmutually exclusive theories for biliary pancreatitis: (1) increased pressure in the pancreatic duct and (2) reflux of bile into the pancreatic duct.[117] The latter can be recapitulated *in vitro* by exogenous administration of bile or its components. Bile is composed predominantly of the bile acids taurocholate (TC), taurochenodeoxycholate (TCDC), and taurodeoxycholate (TDC), while taurolithocholic acid 3-sulfate (TLCS) comprises a small fraction of bile.[118,119] However, TLCS is most commonly used *in vitro* because it is the least hydrophilic and therefore, the most potent of the naturally occurring bile acids. It induces Ca^{2+} signals at low micromolar concentrations that are below the critical micellar concentration.[120] Bile acids can be transported into pancreatic acinar cells through specific transporters, or they can bind to their cognate receptors including the transmembrane G-protein coupled receptor TGR5 (also known as the G-protein coupled bile acid receptor 1, or GPBAR1).[121,122] Bile acid administration triggers aberrant acinar cell Ca^{2+} signals leading to trypsinogen activation and cell death.[123-126] Rescuing ATP depletion by patching ATP into isolated acinar cells prevents necrotic cell death due to the bile acids.[123,127,128]

Fatty acids

Recent investigations into the role of obesity during acute pancreatitis have revealed that accumulation of intrapancreatic fat is associated with a greater tendency towards pancreatic necrosis during acute pancreatitis, which is associated with multisystem organ failure in obese individuals.[5,129,130] These findings provided a rationale to examine a direct role for fatty acids in acinar cell pathobiology *in vitro*. Unsaturated fatty acids in particular appear to play a proinflammatory role; they trigger pathological intracellular Ca^{2+}

signals, inhibit mitochondrial complexes I and V, and cause necrosis. Saturated fatty acids exert none of these effects.

Alcoholic Models

Alcohol is a major etiology of acute pancreatitis.[131,132] Chronic ethanol exposure appears to sensitize the pancreas to the pathologic effects of other concomitant stressors during disease development.[2,59,107,133]

The mechanism underlying alcohol's sensitizing effect is unclear. *In vitro* exposure to clinically relevant concentrations of ethanol (50-100 mM; for at least 1 h under sealed conditions) in combination with physiological concentrations of CCK or carbachol has been shown to trigger pathological pancreatitis responses in acinar cells, including protease activation, intracellular NF-κB activation, pro-inflammatory cytokine expression, vacuolization, and necrosis.[59,134-136] Some have found that using sealed conditions with minimal dead space is important in order to prevent evaporation of the ethanol.[59,134-136]

One mechanism of ethanol's toxic effects is through the actions of oxidative (acetaldehyde) and nonoxidative (fatty acid ethyl ester, FAEEs) metabolites.[137-142] Several studies have demonstrated that both pathways in ethanol metabolism are evident in the pancreas and that exposure of pancreatic acinar cells to ethanol alone results in accumulation of both acetaldehyde and FAEEs.[141,143,144] Nonoxidative FAEEs increase acinar cell lysosomal fragility and induce a rise in intracellular Ca^{2+},[145-147] along with premature intracellular digestive enzyme activation, acinar cell vacuolization, $\Delta\Psi m$ loss, ATP depletion, and cell necrosis.[127,141]

Summary

In summary, we have described methods for isolating pancreatic acinar cells, lobules, organoids, and slices. We also described *in vitro* assays for critical surrogates of pancreatitis. Lastly, we provided an overview of the various secretagogues and naturally occurring agonists that can be used to stimulate pancreatic acinar cells *in vitro* for the purpose of studying pathologic surrogates of pancreatitis. Such tools help researchers elucidate the molecular mechanisms mediating acute pancreatitis and allow them to test novel therapeutic agents that could reduce pancreatitis-mediated acinar cell damage.

References

1. Peery AF, Dellon ES, Lund J, Crockett SD, McGowan CE, Bulsiewicz WJ, et al. Burden of gastrointestinal disease in the United States: 2012 update. *Gastroenterology*. 2012; 143(5): 1179-1187. PMID: 22885331.
2. Lankisch PG, Apte M, Banks PA. Acute pancreatitis. *Lancet*. 2015; 386(9988): 85-96. PMID: 25616312.
3. Raraty M, Ward J, Erdemli G, Vaillant C, Neoptolemos JP, Sutton R, et al. Calcium-dependent enzyme activation and vacuole formation in the apical granular region of pancreatic acinar cells. *Proc Natl Acad Sci U S A*. 2000; 97(24): 13126-13131. PMID: 11087863.
4. Saluja AK, Bhagat L, Lee HS, Bhatia M, Frossard JL, Steer ML. Secretagogue-induced digestive enzyme activation and cell injury in rat pancreatic acini. *Am J Physiol Gastrointest Liver Physiol.* 1999; 276(4 Pt 1): G835-G842. PMID: 10198325.
5. Sah RP, Dawra RK, Saluja AK. New insights into the pathogenesis of pancreatitis. *Curr Opin Gastroenterol*. 2013; 29(5): 523-530. PMID: 23892538.
6. Rakonczay Z Jr, Hegyi P, Takács T, McCarroll J, Saluja AK. The role of NF-kappaB activation in the pathogenesis of acute pancreatitis. *Gut*. 2008; 57(2): 259-267. PMID: 17675325.
7. Grady T, Mah'Moud M, Otani T, Rhee S, Lerch MM, Gorelick FS. Zymogen proteolysis within the pancreatic acinar cell is associated with cellular injury. *Am J Physiol Gastrointest Liver Physiol.* 1998; 275(5 Pt 1): G1010-G1017. PMID: 9815031.
8. Grady T, Saluja A, Kaiser A, Steer M. Edema and intrapancreatic trypsinogen activation precede glutathione depletion during caerulein pancreatitis. *Am J Physiol Gastrointest Liver Physiol.* 1996; 271(1 Pt 1): G20-G26. PMID: 8760102.
9. Grossman A. An overview of pancreatic exocrine secretion. *Comp Biochem Physiol B*. 1984; 78(1): 1-13. PMID: 6378509.
10. Husain SZ, Prasad P, Grant WM, Kolodecik TR, Nathanson MH, Gorelick FS. The ryanodine receptor mediates early zymogen activation in pancreatitis. *Proc Natl Acad Sci U S A*. 2005; 102(40): 14386-14391. PMID: 16186498.
11. Frossard JL, Steer ML, Pastor CM. Acute pancreatitis. *Lancet*. 2008; 371(9607): 143-152. PMID: 18191686.
12. Eisses JF, Davis AW, Tosun AB, Dionise ZR, Chen C, Ozolek JA, et al. A computer-based automated algorithm for assessing acinar cell loss after experimental pancreatitis. *PLoS One*. 2014; 9(10): e110220. PMID: 25343460.
13. Amsterdam A, Jamieson JD. Structural and functional characterization of isolated pancreatic exocrine cells. *Proc Natl Acad Sci U S A*. 1972; 69(10): 3028-3032. PMID: 4342974.
14. Jamieson JD, Palade GE. Intracellular transport of secretory proteins in the pancreatic exocrine cell. II. Transport to condensing vacuoles and zymogen granules. *J Cell Biol*. 1967; 34(2): 597-615. PMID: 6035648.
15. Watanabe O, Baccino FM, Steer ML, and Meldolesi J. Supramaximal caerulein stimulation and ultrastructure of rat pancreatic acinar cell: early morphological changes during development of experimental pancreatitis. *Am J Physiol Gastrointest Liver Physiol.* 1984; 246(4 Pt 1): G457-G467. PMID: 6720895.
16. Nicke B, Tseng MJ, Fenrich M, and Logsdon CD. Adenovirus-mediated gene transfer of RasN17 inhibits specific CCK actions on pancreatic acinar cells. *Am J Physiol Gastrointest Liver Physiol.* 1999; 276(2 Pt 1): G499-G506. PMID: 9950825.
17. Zhang L, Graziano K, Pham T, Logsdon CD, Simeone DM. Adenovirus-mediated gene transfer of dominant-negative Smad4 blocks TGF-beta signaling in pancreatic acinar cells. *Am J Physiol Gastrointest Liver Physiol.* 2001; 280(6): G1247-G1253. PMID: 11352818.

18. Muili KA, Ahmad M, Orabi AI, Mahmood SM, Shah AU, Molkentin JD, et al. Pharmacological and genetic inhibition of calcineurin protects against carbachol-induced pathological zymogen activation and acinar cell injury. *Am J Physiol Gastrointest Liver Physiol.* 2012; 302(8): G898-G905. PMID: 22323127.
19. Kang R, Zhang Q, Hou W, Yan Z, Chen R, Bonaroti J, et al. Intracellular Hmgb1 inhibits inflammatory nucleosome release and limits acute pancreatitis in mice. *Gastroenterology.* 2014; 146(4): 1097-1107. PMID: 24361123.
20. Xiao X, Guo P, Prasadan K, Shiota C, Peirish L, Fischbach S, et al. Pancreatic cell tracing, lineage tagging and targeted genetic manipulations in multiple cell types using pancreatic ductal infusion of adeno-associated viral vectors and/or cell-tagging dyes. *Nat Protocol.* 2014; 9(12): 2719-2724. PMID: 25356582.
21. Hoque R, Farooq A, Ghani A, Gorelick F, Mehal WZ. Lactate reduces liver and pancreatic injury in Toll-like receptor- and inflammasome-mediated inflammation via GPR81-mediated suppression of innate immunity. *Gastroenterology.* 2014; 146(7): 1763-1774. PMID: 24657625.
22. Orabi AI, Muili KA, Wang D, Jin S, Perides G, Husain SZ. Preparation of pancreatic acinar cells for the purpose of calcium imaging, cell injury measurements, and adenoviral infection. *J Vis Exp.* 2013; 77: e50391. PMID: 23851390.
23. Burnham DB, McChesney DJ, Thurston KC, Williams JA. Interaction of cholecystokinin and vasoactive intestinal polypeptide on function of mouse pancreatic acini in vitro. *J Physiol.* 1984; 349: 475-482. PMID: 6204039.
24. Peikin SR, Rottman AJ, Batzri S, Gardner JD. Kinetics of amylase release by dispersed acini prepared from guinea pig pancreas. *Am J Physiol.* 1978; 235(6): E743-E749. PMID: 736135.
25. Schultz GS, Sarras MP Jr, Gunther GR, Hull BE, Alicea HA, Gorelick FS, et al. Guinea pig pancreatic acini prepared with purified collagenase. *Exp Cell Res.* 1980; 130(1): 49-62. PMID: 6256185.
26. Williams JA, Korc M, Dormer RL. Action of secretagogues on a new preparation of functionally intact, isolated pancreatic acini. *Am J Physiol.* 1978; 235(5): 517-524. PMID: 215042.
27. Won JH, Cottrell WJ, Foster TH, Yule DI. Ca^{2+} release dynamics in parotid and pancreatic exocrine acinar cells evoked by spatially limited flash photolysis. *Am J Physiol Gastrointest Liver Physiol.* 2007; 293(6): G1166-G1177. PMID: 17901163.
28. Mooren FC, Turi S, Gunzel D, Schlue WR, Domschke W, Singh J, et al. Calcium-magnesium interactions in pancreatic acinar cells. *FASEB J.* 2001; 15(3): 659-672. PMID: 11259384.
29. Frick TW, Fernandez-del-Castillo C, Bimmler D, Warshaw AL. Elevated calcium and activation of trypsinogen in rat pancreatic acini. *Gut.* 1997; 41(3): 339-343. PMID: 9378389.
30. Zhao H and Muallem S. Na^+, K^+, and Cl^- transport in resting pancreatic acinar cells. *J Gen Physiol.* 1995; 106(6): 1225-1242. PMID: 8786358.
31. Means AL, Meszoely IM, Suzuki K, Miyamoto Y, Rustgi AK, Coffey RJ Jr, et al. Pancreatic epithelial plasticity mediated by acinar cell transdifferentiation and generation of nestin-positive intermediates. *Development.* 2005; 132(16): 3767-3776. PMID: 16020518.
32. Lewarchik CM, Orabi AI, Jin S, Wang D, Muili KA, Shah AU, et al. The ryanodine receptor is expressed in human pancreatic acinar cells and contributes to acinar cell injury. *Am J Physiol Gastrointest Liver Physiol.* 2014; 307(5): G574-G581. PMID: 25012845.
33. Bottino R, Bertera S, Grupillo M, Melvin PR, Humar A, Mazariegos G, et al. Isolation of human islets for autologous islet transplantation in children and adolescents with chronic pancreatitis. *J Transplant.* 2012; 2012: 642787. PMID: 22461976.
34. Park MK, Lee M, Petersen OH. Morphological and functional changes of dissociated single pancreatic acinar cells: testing the suitability of the single cell as a model for exocytosis and calcium signaling. *Cell Calcium.* 2004; 35(4): 367-379. PMID: 15036953.
35. Scheele GA, Palade GE. Studies on the guinea pig pancreas. Parallel discharge of exocrine enzyme activities. *J Biol Chem.* 1975; 250(7): 2660-2670. PMID: 1123325.
36. Boj SF, Hwang CI, Baker LA, Chio, II, Engle DD, Corbo V, et al. Organoid models of human and mouse ductal pancreatic cancer. *Cell.* 2015; 160(1-2): 324-338. PMID: 25557080.
37. Huang YC, Rupnik M, Gaisano HY. Unperturbed islet alpha-cell function examined in mouse pancreas tissue slices. *J Physiol.* 2011; 589(Pt 2): 395-408. PMID: 21078586.
38. Flowe KM, Welling TH, Mulholland MW. Gastrin-releasing peptide stimulation of amylase release from rat pancreatic lobules involves intrapancreatic neurons. *Pancreas.* 1994; 9(4): 513-517. PMID: 7524066.
39. Barreto SG, Carati CJ, Toouli J, Saccone GT. The islet-acinar axis of the pancreas: more than just insulin. *Am J Physiol Gastrointest Liver Physiol.* 2010; 299(1): G10-G22. PMID: 20395539.
40. Barreto SG, Woods CM, Carati CJ, Schloithe AC, Jaya SR, Toouli J, et al. Galanin inhibits caerulein-stimulated pancreatic amylase secretion via cholinergic nerves and insulin. *Am J Physiol Gastrointest Liver Physiol.* 2009; 297(2): G333-G339. PMID: 19497960.
41. Schloithe AC, Sutherland K, Woods CM, Blackshaw LA, Davison JS, Toouli J, et al. A novel preparation to study rat pancreatic spinal and vagal mechanosensitive afferents in vitro. *Neurogastroenterol Motil.* 2008; 20(9): 1060-1069. PMID: 18482253.
42. Linari G, Nencini P, Nucerito V. Cadmium inhibits stimulated amylase secretion from isolated pancreatic lobules of the guinea-pig. *Pharmacol Res Society.* 2001; 43(3): 219-223. PMID: 11401412.
43. Huch M, Bonfanti P, Boj SF, Sato T, Loomans CJ, van de Wetering M, et al. Unlimited in vitro expansion of adult bi-potent pancreas progenitors through the Lgr5/R-spondin axis. *EMBO J.* 2013; 32(20): 2708-2721. PMID: 24045232.
44. Huang YC, Gaisano HY, Leung YM. Electrophysiological identification of mouse islet alpha-cells: from isolated single alpha-cells to in situ assessment within pancreas slices. *Islets.* 2011; 3(4): 139-143. PMID: 21623173.
45. Gonzalez A, Santofimia-Castaño, Salido GM. Culture of pancreatic AR42J cell for use as a model for acinar cell function. In: *The Pancreapedia: Exocrine Pancreas Knowledge*

Base. American Pancreatic Association; 2011. DOI: 10.3998/panc.2011.26.

46. Szmola R, Sahin-Toth M. Pancreatitis-associated chymotrypsinogen C (CTRC) mutant elicits endoplasmic reticulum stress in pancreatic acinar cells. *Gut*. 2010; 59(3): 365-372. PMID: 19951900.
47. Christophe J. Pancreatic tumoral cell line AR42J: an amphicrine model. *Am J Physiol Gastrointest Liver Physiol*. 1994; 266(6 Pt 1): G963-G971. PMID: 7517639.
48. Logsdon CD, Moessner J, Williams JA, Goldfine ID. Glucocorticoids increase amylase mRNA levels, secretory organelles, and secretion in pancreatic acinar AR42J cells. *J Cell Biol*. 1985; 100(4): 1200-1208. PMID: 2579957.
49. Barnhart DC, Sarosi GA Jr, Romanchuk G, Mulholland MW. Calcium signaling induced by angiotensin II in the pancreatic acinar cell line AR42J. *Pancreas*. 1999; 18(2): 189-196. PMID: 10090417.
50. De Lisle RC, Norkina O, Roach E, Ziemer D. Expression of pro-Muclin in pancreatic AR42J cells induces functional regulated secretory granules. *Am J Physiol Cell Physiol*. 2005; 289(5): C1169-C1178. PMID: 15987769.
51. Ornitz DM, Palmiter RD, Hammer RE, Brinster RL, Swift GH, MacDonald RJ. Specific expression of an elastase-human growth hormone fusion gene in pancreatic acinar cells of transgenic mice. *Nature*. 1985; 313(6003): 600-602. PMID: 3844051.
52. Petersen OH, Tepikin AV. Polarized calcium signaling in exocrine gland cells. *Annu Rev Physiol*. 2008; 70: 273-299. PMID: 17850212.
53. Kasai H, Augustine GJ. Cytosolic Ca^{2+} gradients triggering unidirectional fluid secretion from exocrine pancreas. *Nature*. 1990; 348(6303): 735-738. PMID: 1701852.
54. Giovannucci DR, Bruce JIE, Straub SV, Arreola J, Sneyd J, Shuttleworth TJ, et al. Cytosolic Ca^{2+} and Ca^{2+}-activated Cl^- current dynamics: insights from two functionally distinct mouse exocrine cells. *J Physiol*. 2002; 540(2): 469-484. PMID: 11956337.
55. Minta A, Kao JP, Tsien RY. Fluorescent indicators for cytosolic calcium based on rhodamine and fluorescein chromophores. *J Biol Chem*. 1989; 264(14): 8171-8178. PMID: 2498308.
56. Grynkiewicz G, Poenie M, Tsien RY. A new generation of Ca^{2+} indicators with greatly improved fluorescence properties. *J Biol Chem*. 1985; 260(6): 3440-3450. PMID: 3838314.
57. Thomas D, Tovey SC, Collins TJ, Bootman MD, Berridge MJ, Lipp P. A comparison of fluorescent Ca^{2+} indicator properties and their use in measuring elementary and global Ca^{2+} signals. *Cell Calcium*. 2000; 28(4): 213-223. PMID: 11032777.
58. Orabi AI, Nathanson MH, Husain SZ. Measuring Ca^{2+} dynamics in pancreatic acini using confocal microscopy. In: *The Pancreapedia: Exocrine Pancreas Knowledge Base*. American Pancreatic Association; 2011. DOI: 10.3998/panc.2011.30.
59. Orabi AI, Shah AU, Muili K, Luo Y, Mahmood SM, Ahmad A, et al. Ethanol enhances carbachol-induced protease activation and accelerates Ca^{2+} waves in isolated rat pancreatic acini. *J Biol Chem*. 2011; 286(16): 14090-14097. PMID: 21372126.
60. Reed AM, Husain SZ, Thrower E, Alexandre M, Shah A, Gorelick FS, et al. Low extracellular pH induces damage in the pancreatic acinar cell by enhancing calcium signaling. *J Biol Chem*. 2011; 286(3): 1919-1926. PMID: 21084290.
61. Leach SD, Modlin IM, Scheele GA, Gorelick FS. Intracellular activation of digestive zymogens in rat pancreatic acini. Stimulation by high doses of cholecystokinin. *J Clin Invest*. 1991; 87(1): 362-366. PMID: 1985109.
62. Shah AU, Sarwar A, Orabi AI, Gautam S, Grant WM, Park AJ, et al. Protease Activation during in vivo Pancreatitis is Dependent upon Calcineurin Activation. *Am J Physiol Gastrointest Liver Physiol*. 2009; 297(5): G967-G973. PMID: 19713471.
63. Leytus SP, Toledo DL, Mangel WF. Theory and experimental method for determining individual kinetic constants of fast-acting, irreversible proteinase inhibitors. *Biochim Biophys Acta*. 1984; 788(1): 74-86. PMID: 6204689.
64. Leytus SP, Patterson WL, Mangel WF. New class of sensitive and selective fluorogenic substrates for serine proteinases. Amino acid and dipeptide derivatives of rhodamine. *Biochem J*. 1983; 215(2): 253-260. PMID: 6228222.
65. Lerch MM, Gorelick FS. Early trypsinogen activation in acute pancreatitis. *Med Clin North Am*. 2000; 84(3): 549-563, viii. PMID: 10872413.
66. Kim MS, Lee KP, Yang D, Shin DM, Abramowitz J, Kiyonaka S, et al. Genetic and pharmacologic inhibition of the Ca^{2+} influx channel TRPC3 protects secretory epithelia from Ca^{2+}-dependent toxicity. *Gastroenterology*. 2011; 140(7): 2107-2115. PMID: 21354153.
67. Krüger B, Albrecht E, Lerch MM. The role of intracellular calcium signaling in premature protease activation and the onset of pancreatitis. *Am J Pathol*. 2000; 157(1): 43-50. PMID: 10880374.
68. Tando Y, Algül H, Schneider G, Weber CK, Weidenbach H, Adler G, et al. Induction of IkappaB-kinase by cholecystokinin is mediated by trypsinogen activation in rat pancreatic lobules. *Digestion*. 2002; 66(4): 237-245. PMID: 12592100.
69. de Wet JR, Wood KV, DeLuca M, Helinski DR, Subramani S. Firefly luciferase gene: structure and expression in mammalian cells. *Mol Cell Biol*. 1987; 7(2): 725-737. PMID: 3821727.
70. Lorenz WW, McCann RO, Longiaru M, Cormier MJ. Isolation and expression of a cDNA encoding Renilla reniformis luciferase. *Proc Natl Acad Sci U S A*. 1991; 88(10): 4438-4442. PMID: 1674607.
71. Badr CE, Niers JM, Tjon-Kon-Fat LA, Noske DP, Wurdinger T, Tannous BA. Real-time monitoring of nuclear factor kappaB activity in cultured cells and in animal models. *Mol Imaging*. 2009; 8(5): 278-290. PMID: 19796605.
72. Nakajima Y, Kobayashi K, Yamagishi K, Enomoto T, Ohmiya Y. cDNA cloning and characterization of a secreted luciferase from the luminous Japanese ostracod, Cypridina noctiluca. *Biosci Biotechnol Biochem*. 2004; 68(3): 565-570. PMID:15056888.
73. Haridas V, Shrivastava A, Su J, Yu GL, Ni J, Liu D, et al. VEGI, a new member of the TNF family activates nuclear factor-kappa B and c-Jun N-terminal kinase and modulates cell growth. *Oncogene*. 1999; 18(47): 6496-6504. PMID: 10597252.
74. Tannous BA, Kim DE, Fernandez JL, Weissleder R, Breakefield XO. Codon-optimized Gaussia luciferase cDNA

for mammalian gene expression in culture and in vivo. *Mol Ther*. 2005; 11(3): 435-443. PMID: 15727940.

75. Maléth J, Rakonczay Z, Jr., Venglovecz V, Dolman NJ, Hegyi P. Central role of mitochondrial injury in the pathogenesis of acute pancreatitis. *Acta Physiol*. 2013; 207(2): 226-235. PMID: 23167280.
76. Odinokova IV, Sung KF, Mareninova OA, Hermann K, Gukovsky I, Gukovskaya AS. Mitochondrial mechanisms of death responses in pancreatitis. *J Gastroenterol Hepatol*. 2008; 23 Suppl 1: S25-S30. PMID: 18336659.
77. Shalbueva N, Mareninova OA, Gerloff A, Yuan J, Waldron RT, Pandol SJ, et al. Effects of oxidative alcohol metabolism on the mitochondrial permeability transition pore and necrosis in a mouse model of alcoholic pancreatitis. *Gastroenterology*. 2013; 144(2): 437-446. PMID: 23103769.
78. Mukherjee R, Mareninova OA, Odinokova IV, Huang W, Murphy J, Chvanov M, et al. Mechanism of mitochondrial permeability transition pore induction and damage in the pancreas: inhibition prevents acute pancreatitis by protecting production of ATP. *Gut*. 2015 Jun 12. [Epub ahead of print] PMID: 26071131.
79. Odinokova IV, Shalbuyeva N, Gukovskaya AS, Mareninova OA. Isolation of pancreatic mitochondria and measurement of their functional parameters. In: *The Pancreapedia: Exocrine Pancreas Knowledge Base*. American Pancreatic Association; 2011. DOI: 10.3998/panc.2011.25.
80. Orabi AI, Sah S, Javed TA, Lemon KL, Good ML, Guo P, et al. Dynamic imaging of pancreatic nuclear factor κB (NF-κB) activation in live mice using adeno-associated virus (AAV) infusion and bioluminescence. *J Biol Chem*. 2015; 290(18): 11309-11320. PMID: 25802340.
81. Odinokova IV, Sung KF, Mareninova OA, Hermann K, Evtodienko Y, Andreyev A, et al. Mechanisms regulating cytochrome c release in pancreatic mitochondria. *Gut*. 2009; 58(3): 431-442. PMID: 18596195.
82. Mareninova OA, Sung KF, Hong P, Lugea A, Pandol SJ, Gukovsky I, et al. Cell death in pancreatitis: caspases protect from necrotizing pancreatitis. *J Biol Chem*. 2006; 281(6): 3370-3381. PMID: 16339139.
83. Madern D. Molecular evolution within the L-malate and L-lactate dehydrogenase super-family. *J Mol Evol*. 2002; 54(6): 825-840. PMID: 12029364.
84. Lecoeur H. Nuclear apoptosis detection by flow cytometry: influence of endogenous endonucleases. *Exp Cell Res*. 2002; 277(1): 1-14. PMID: 12061813.
85. Suzuki T, Fujikura K, Higashiyama T, Takata K. DNA staining for fluorescence and laser confocal microscopy. *J Histochem Cytochem*. 1997; 45(1): 49-53. PMID: 9010468.
86. Moore A, Donahue CJ, Bauer KD, Mather JP. Simultaneous measurement of cell cycle and apoptotic cell death. *Methods Cell Biol*. 1998; 57: 265-278. PMID: 9648110.
87. Berridge MV, Herst PM, Tan AS. Tetrazolium dyes as tools in cell biology: new insights into their cellular reduction. *Biotechnol Annu Rev*. 2005; 11: 127-152. PMID: 16216776.
88. Mosmann T. Rapid colorimetric assay for cellular growth and survival: application to proliferation and cytotoxicity assays. *J Immunol Methods*. 1983; 65(1-2): 55-63. PMID: 6606682.
89. Cory AH, Owen TC, Barltrop JA, Cory JG. Use of an aqueous soluble tetrazolium/formazan assay for cell growth assays in culture. *Cancer Commun*. 1991; 3(7): 207-212. PMID: 1867954.
90. Saluja AK, Donovan EA, Yamanaka K, Yamaguchi Y, Hofbauer B, Steer ML. Cerulein-induced in vitro activation of trypsinogen in rat pancreatic acini is mediated by cathepsin B. *Gastroenterology*. 1997; 113(1): 304-310. PMID: 9207291.
91. Burnham DB, Williams JA. Effects of high concentrations of secretagogues on the morphology and secretory activity of the pancreas: a role for microfilaments. *Cell Tissue Res*. 1982; 22(1): 201-212. PMID: 6174234.
92. Saluja AK, Lerch MM, Phillips PA, Dudeja V. Why does pancreatic overstimulation cause pancreatitis? *Annu Rev Physiol*. 2007; 69: 249-269. PMID: 17059357.
93. Miller LJ, Lybrand TP. Molecular basis of agonist binding to the type A cholecystokinin receptor. *Pharmacol Toxicol*. 2002; 91(6): 282-285. PMID: 12688369.
94. Williams JA. Receptor biology and intracellular regulatory mechanisms in pancreatic acinar cells. *Curr Opin Gastroenterol*. 2002; 18(5): 529-535. PMID: 17033329.
95. Williams JA. Intracellular signaling mechanisms activated by cholecystokinin-regulating synthesis and secretion of digestive enzymes in pancreatic acinar cells. *Annu Rev Physiol*. 2001; 63: 77-97. PMID: 11181949.
96. Leite MF, Burgstahler AD, Nathanson MH. Ca^{2+} waves require sequential activation of inositol trisphosphate receptors and ryanodine receptors in pancreatic acini. *Gastroenterology*. 2002; 122(2): 415-427. PMID: 11832456.
97. Gukovsky I, Pandol SJ, Gukovskaya AS. Organellar dysfunction in the pathogenesis of pancreatitis. *Antioxid Redox Signal*. 2011; 15(10): 2699-2710. PMID: 21834686.
98. Sherwood MW, Prior IA, Voronina SG, Barrow SL, Woodsmith JD, Gerasimenko OV, et al. Activation of trypsinogen in large endocytic vacuoles of pancreatic acinar cells. *Proc Natl Acad Sci U S A*. 2007; 104(13): 5674-5679. PMID: 17363470.
99. Shah AU, Grant WM, Latif SU, Mannan ZM, Park AJ, Husain SZ. Cyclic-AMP accelerates calcium waves in pancreatic acinar cells. *Am J Physiol Gastrointest Liver Physiol*. 2008; 294(6): G1328-G1334. PMID: 18388188.
100. Schmidt WE, Meyer-Alber A, Waschulewski IH, Fetz I, Höcker M, Kern HF, et al. Serine/threonine phosphatases play a role in stimulus-secretion coupling in pancreatic acinar cells. *Z Gastroenterol*. 1994; 32(4): 226-231. PMID: 7517088.
101. Saluja A, Logsdon C, Garg P. Direct versus indirect action of cholecystokinin on human pancreatic acinar cells: is it time for a judgment after a century of trial? *Gastroenterology*. 2008; 135(2): 357-360. PMID: 18616945.
102. Ji B, Bi Y, Simeone D, Mortensen RM, Logsdon CD. Human pancreatic acinar cells lack functional responses to cholecystokinin and gastrin. *Gastroenterology*. 2001; 121(6): 1380-1390. PMID: 11729117.
103. Wank SA, Pisegna JR, de Weerth A. Cholecystokinin receptor family. Molecular cloning, structure, and functional

expression in rat, guinea pig, and human. *Ann N Y Acad Sci.* 1994; 713: 49-66. PMID: 8185215.

104. Murphy JA, Criddle DN, Sherwood M, Chvanov M, Mukherjee R, McLaughlin E, et al. Direct activation of cytosolic Ca^{2+} signaling and enzyme secretion by cholecystokinin in human pancreatic acinar cells. *Gastroenterology.* 2008; 135(2): 632-641. PMID: 18555802.
105. Miyasaka K, Shinozaki H, Jimi A, Funakoshi A. Amylase secretion from dispersed human pancreatic acini: neither cholecystokinin a nor cholecystokinin B receptors mediate amylase secretion in vitro. *Pancreas.* 2002; 25(2): 161-165. PMID: 12142739.
106. Susini C, Estival A, Scemama JL, Ruellan C, Vaysse N, Clemente F, et al. Studies on human pancreatic acini: action of secretagogues on amylase release and cellular cyclic AMP accumulation. *Pancreas.* 1986; 1(2): 124-129. PMID: 2437561.
107. Lugea A, Gong J, Nguyen J, Nieto J, French SW, Pandol SJ. Cholinergic mediation of alcohol-induced experimental pancreatitis. *Alcohol Clin Exp Res.* 2010; 34(10): 1768-1781. PMID: 20626730.
108. Owyang C and Logsdon CD. New insights into neurohormonal regulation of pancreatic secretion. *Gastroenterology.* 2004; 127(3): 957-969. PMID: 15362050.
109. Roeyen G, Chapelle T, Jorens P, de Beeck BO, Ysebaert D. Necrotizing pancreatitis due to poisoning with organophosphate pesticides. *Acta Gastroenterol Belg.* 2008; 71(1): 27-29. PMID: 18396746.
110. Singh S, Bhardwaj U, Verma SK, Bhalla A, Gill K. Hyperamylasemia and acute pancreatitis following anticholinesterase poisoning. *Hum Exp Toxicol.* 2007; 26(6): 467-471. PMID: 17698941.
111. Tomiyama M, Arai A, Kimura T, Suzuki C, Watanabe M, Kawarabayashi T, et al. Exacerbation of chronic pancreatitis induced by anticholinesterase medications in myasthenia gravis. *Eur J Neurol.* 2008; 15(5): e40-e41. PMID: 18325026.
112. Votanopoulos KI, Lee TC, Dominguez EP, Choi YU, Sweeney JF. Propoxur induced pancreatitis after inhalation of baygon pesticide. *Pancreas.* 2007; 34(3): 379-380. PMID: 17414064.
113. Bai HX, Lowe ME, Husain SZ. What have we learned about acute pancreatitis in children? *J Pediatr Gastroenterol Nutr.* 2011; 52(3): 262-270. PMID: 21336157.
114. Lowenfels AB, Sullivan T, Fiorianti J, Maisonneuve P. The epidemiology and impact of pancreatic diseases in the United States. *Curr Gastroenterol Rep.* 2005; 7(2): 90-95. PMID: 15802095.
115. Ma MH, Bai HX, Park AJ, Latif SU, Mistry PK, Pashankar D, et al. Risk factors associated with biliary pancreatitis in children. *J Pediatr Gastroenterol Nutr.* 2012; 54(5): 651-656. PMID: 22002481.
116. van Geenen EJ, van der Peet DL, Bhagirath P, Mulder CJ, Bruno MJ. Etiology and diagnosis of acute biliary pancreatitis. *Nat Rev Gastroenterol Hepatol.* 2010; 7(9): 495-502. PMID: 20703238.
117. Lerch MM, Aghdassi AA. The role of bile acids in gallstone-induced pancreatitis. *Gastroenterology.* 2010; 138(2): 429-433. PMID: 20034603.
118. Fisher MM, Yousef IM. Sex differences in the bile acid composition of human bile: studies in patients with and without gallstones. *Can Med Assoc J.* 1973; 109(3): 190-193. PMID: 4728947.
119. Weinman SA, Jalil S. Bile Secretion and Cholestasis. Textbook of Gastroenterology 5th Ed. T. Yamada, Blackwell Publishing Ltd.: 401-428, 2008.
120. Hofmann AF, Roda A. Physicochemical properties of bile acids and their relationship to biological properties: an overview of the problem. *J Lipid Res* 1984; 25(13): 1477-1489. PMID: 6397555.
121. Perides G, Laukkarinen JM, Vassileva G, Steer ML. Biliary acute pancreatitis in mice is mediated by the G-protein-coupled cell surface bile acid receptor Gpbar1. *Gastroenterology.* 2010; 138(2): 715-725. PMID: 19900448.
122. Kim JY, Kim KH, Lee JA, Namkung W, Sun AQ, Ananthanarayanan M, et al. Transporter-mediated bile acid uptake causes Ca^{2+}-dependent cell death in rat pancreatic acinar cells. *Gastroenterology.* 2002; 122(7): 1941-1953. PMID: 12055600.
123. Voronina S, Longbottom R, Sutton R, Petersen OH, Tepikin A. Bile acids induce calcium signals in mouse pancreatic acinar cells: implications for bile-induced pancreatic pathology. *J Physiol.* 2002; 540(Pt 1): 49-55. PMID: 11927668.
124. Muili KA, Jin S, Orabi AI, Eisses JF, Javed TA, Le T, et al. Pancreatic acinar cell NF-kappaB activation due to bile acid exposure is dependent on calcineurin. *J Biol Chem.* 2013; 288(29): 21065-21073. PMID: 23744075.
125. Muili KA, Wang D, Orabi AI, Sarwar S, Luo Y, Javed TA, et al. Bile acids induce pancreatic acinar cell injury and pancreatitis by activating calcineurin. *J Biol Chem.* 2013; 288(1): 570-580. PMID: 23148215.
126. Husain SZ, Orabi AI, Muili KA, Luo Y, Sarwar S, Mahmood SM, et al. Ryanodine receptors contribute to bile acid-induced pathological calcium signaling and pancreatitis in mice. *Am J Physiol Gastrointest Liver Physiol.* 2012; 302(12): G1423-G1433. PMID: 22517774.
127. Voronina SG, Barrow SL, Simpson AW, Gerasimenko OV, da Silva Xavier G, Rutter GA, et al. Dynamic changes in cytosolic and mitochondrial ATP levels in pancreatic acinar cells. *Gastroenterology.* 2010; 138(5): 1976-1987. PMID: 20102715.
128. Booth DM MJ, Mukherjee R, Awais M, Neoptolemos JP, Gerasimenko OV, Tepikin AV, et al. Reactive oxygen species induced by bile acid induce apoptosis and protect against necrosis in pancreatic acinar cells. *Gastroenterology.* 2011; 140(7): 9. PMID: 21354148.
129. Durgampudi C, Noel P, Patel K, Cline R, Trivedi RN, DeLany JP, et al. Acute lipotoxicity regulates severity of biliary acute pancreatitis without affecting its initiation. *Am J Pathol.* 2014; 184(6): 1773-1784. PMID: 24854864.
130. Navina S, Acharya C, DeLany JP, Orlichenko LS, Baty CJ, Shiva SS, et al. Lipotoxicity causes multisystem organ failure and exacerbates acute pancreatitis in obesity. *Sci Transl Med.* 2011; 3(107): 107ra110. PMID: 22049070.
131. Frey CF, Zhou H, Harvey DJ, White RH. The incidence and case-fatality rates of acute biliary, alcoholic, and idiopathic pancreatitis in California, 1994-2001. *Pancreas.* 2006; 33(4): 336-344. PMID: 17079936.
132. Yadav D, Lowenfels AB. The epidemiology of pancreatitis and pancreatic cancer. *Gastroenterology.* 2013; 144(6): 1252-1261. PMID: 23622135.

133. Apte MV, Pirola RC, Wilson JS. Individual susceptibility to alcoholic pancreatitis. *J Gastroenterol Hepatol.* 2008; 23(s1): S63-S68. PMID: 18336667.
134. Fernández-Sánchez M, del Castillo-Vaquero A, Salido GM, González A. Ethanol exerts dual effects on calcium homeostasis in CCK-8-stimulated mouse pancreatic acinar cells. *BMC Cell Biol.* 2009; 10: 77. PMID: 19878551.
135. Lam PP, Cosen Binker LI, Lugea A, Pandol SJ, Gaisano HY. Alcohol redirects CCK-mediated apical exocytosis to the acinar basolateral membrane in alcoholic pancreatitis. *Traffic.* 2007; 8(5): 605-617. PMID: 17451559.
136. González A, Núñez AM, Granados MP, Pariente JA, Salido GM. Ethanol impairs CCK-8-evoked amylase secretion through Ca^{2+}-mediated ROS generation in mouse pancreatic acinar cells. *Alcohol.* 2006; 38(1): 51-57. PMID: 16762692.
137. Wu H, Bhopale KK, Ansari GAS, Kaphalia BS. Ethanol-induced cytotoxicity in rat pancreatic acinar AR42J cells: Role of fatty acid ethyl esters. *Alcohol Alcohol.* 2008; 43(1): 1-8. PMID: 17942438.
138. Best CA, Laposata M. Fatty acid ethyl esters: toxic non-oxidative metabolites of ethanol and markers of ethanol intake. *Front Biosci.* 2003; 8: e202-e217. PMID: 12456329.
139. Werner J, Laposata M, Fernández-del Castillo C, Saghir M, Iozzo RV, Lewandrowski KB, et al. Pancreatic injury in rats induced by fatty acid ethyl ester, a nonoxidative metabolite of alcohol. *Gastroenterology.* 1997; 113(1): 286-294. PMID: 9207289.
140. Werner J, Saghir M, Warshaw AL, Lewandrowski KB, Laposata M, Iozzo RV, et al. Alcoholic pancreatitis in rats: injury from nonoxidative metabolites of ethanol. *Am J Physiol Gastrointest Liver Physiol.* 2002; 283(1): G65-G73. PMID: 12065293.
141. Criddle DN, Murphy J, Fistetto G, Barrow S, Tepikin AV, Neoptolemos JP, et al. Fatty acid ethyl esters cause pancreatic calcium toxicity via inositol trisphosphate receptors and loss of ATP synthesis. *Gastroenterology.* 2006; 130(3): 781-793. PMID: 16530519.
142. Dolai S, Liang T, Lam PP, Fernandez NA, Chidambaram S, Gaisano HY. Effects of ethanol metabolites on exocytosis of pancreatic acinar cells in rats. *Gastroenterology.* 2012; 143(3): 832-843. PMID: 22710192.
143. Criddle DN, Raraty MG, Neoptolemos JP, Tepikin AV, Petersen OH, Sutton R. Ethanol toxicity in pancreatic acinar cells: mediation by nonoxidative fatty acid metabolites. *Proc Natl Acad Sci U S A* . 2004; 101(29): 10738-10743. PMID: 15247419.
144. Gukovskaya AS, Mouria M, Gukovsky I, Reyes CN, Kasho VN, Faller LD, et al. Ethanol metabolism and transcription factor activation in pancreatic acinar cells in rats. *Gastroenterology.* 2002; 122(1): 106-118. PMID: 11781286.
145. Haber PS, Wilson JS, Apte MV, and Pirola RC. Fatty acid ethyl esters increase rat pancreatic lysosomal fragility. *J Lab Clin Med.* 1993; 121(6): 759-764. PMID: 8505587.
146. Wilson JS, Korsten MA, Apte MV, Thomas MC, Haber PS, Pirola RC. Both ethanol consumption and protein deficiency increase the fragility of pancreatic lysosomes. *J Lab Clin Med.* 1990; 115(6): 749-755. PMID: 2366035.
147. Criddle DN, Sutton R, Petersen OH. Role of Ca^{2+} in pancreatic cell death induced by alcohol metabolites. *J Gastroenterol Hepatol.* 2006; 21 Suppl 3: S14-17. PMID: 16958662.

Chapter 2

Commonly employed rodent models of experimental acute pancreatitis: Their strengths and weaknesses, relevance to human disease, selection, and appropriate use

Péter Hegyi[1], George Perides[2], Michael L. Steer[2], and Zoltán Rakonczay Jr.[1*]

[1]*First Department of Medicine, University of Szeged, Szeged, Hungary;*
[2]*Department of Surgery, Tufts Medical Center, Boston, MA, USA.*

General Comments

Acute pancreatitis (AP) is a disorder with a sudden onset that can present in mild edematous and severe necrotizing forms.[1] Mild AP is usually self-limiting and is characterized by minimal or no distant organ dysfunction and an uncomplicated recovery. In contrast, severe necrotizing AP usually involves organ failure (pulmonary insufficiency, renal failure, shock, etc.), and local complications (e.g., infected necrosis, abscess, or pseudocyst formation). These complications of severe AP contribute to its high mortality and morbidity rates.

Despite intensive research, our understanding of AP pathophysiology is far from complete. Because it is generally not possible to obtain pancreatic tissue during the early stages of the clinical disease, most of our knowledge base comes from studies using *in vivo* animal models of AP.[2-6] Nowadays, *ex vivo* AP models are also becoming more widely used, especially for mechanistic studies. On the other hand, as AP is a systemic disease involving other organs besides the pancreas, the usefulness of *ex vivo* AP models is still limited, and the preferred use of *in vivo* models to investigate AP is more than justified.

About 80% of human AP cases are related to either ethanol abuse or gallstone disease. However, the disease will develop in only a minority (≤10%) of individuals who either harbor gall stones or consume alcohol, and there are no animal models of AP that can be induced by these conditions alone. Conversely, most of the agents commonly used to induce experimental AP in animals do not cause pancreatitis in humans.

Necrotizing clinical AP is usually characterized by large, patchy areas of hemorrhagic necrosis of pancreatic and peripancreatic tissues,[7-9] and it is not characterized by diffuse, homogeneous injury. The necrosis of severe clinical pancreatitis usually develops within the first 4 days after symptom onset in humans, whereas infection of the necrotic pancreas develops most frequently in 2 to 3 weeks after symptom onset.[10] Actually, many necrotizing AP deaths result from pancreatic infections, which are reported to occur in 30% to 70% of patients.[11] The incidence of infection correlates with the extent of intra- and extrapancreatic tissue necrosis. Rodents with necrotizing AP seem to be much more resistant to infections than humans, and considerable pancreatic infection rates are only reported for the invasive rodent AP models.[12]

With respect to disease treatment, researchers have often found that drugs that are beneficial in rodent models of experimental pancreatitis fail in clinical trials. This may be because most protocols in animals permit starting treatment before or very shortly after AP induction, which does not resemble the clinical situation where prophylactic therapy is only possible in cases of endoscopic retrograde cholangiopancreatography-induced AP.

It is likely that the rate of AP progression differs between experimental and clinical pancreatitis. Disease kinetics appear to depend on many parameters, including body mass. While many patients with severe pancreatitis are obese, most animal models of pancreatitis employ lean animals. At the time of emergency room presentation, which is usually 12 to 36 hours after symptom onset, the clinical disease is usually already quite developed.[3] In contrast, pronounced pathology requires many hours to develop in some models (i.e., choline-deficient ethionine-supplemented [CDE]-diet, L-arginine).

Despite these potentially important differences between clinical and experimental pancreatitis, we have come a long way since the first experimental AP model of retrograde injection of bile and olive oil into the dog pancreatic

*Corresponding author. Email: rakonczay.zoltan@med.u-szeged.hu

duct was described by Claude Bernard in 1856.[13] Since then, numerous AP models have been developed. In the past, large animals such as dogs and cats were commonly used in AP studies, but most modern investigations employ small animals, usually rats and mice. The latter species has become increasingly used, primarily due to the availability of genetically modified mouse strains. Although the use of larger animals may present fewer technical limitations related to the size of the subjects (such as surgical or therapeutic interventions including intravenous [i.v.] administration of drugs and fluids], rodents are also utilized more commonly because of financial, ethical, and practical reasons. Furthermore, inbred rodent strains are better standardized, and the utilization of larger numbers of animals per group can improve experimental statistical power. In this regard, the use of inbred rodent strains may offer distinct advantages over clinical studies, which are hampered by difficulties in recruiting and monitoring a sufficiently large and homogeneous population of patients.

Aims

The main aims of this review are to provide the reader with a general description of various commonly used *in vivo* rodent AP models, discuss their strengths and weaknesses, and explain how the various models relate to human disease. In addition to this summary, we will make a number of "opinion-based" comments regarding the use of these models and the interpretation of the results obtained. We will suggest (a) which models are most appropriate for addressing specific AP-related questions, (b) why we feel investigators should consider using more than one type of model for their studies, (c) how the severity of observed changes might best be quantitated, and (d) how discordant results from studies employing more than one type of model might best be interpreted. Our review will focus entirely on issues related to nonalcohol-related AP; we will not discuss models of alcohol-induced AP or chronic pancreatitis. In addition, we will not discuss issues related to hereditary pancreatitis, models of genetically induced AP, or those models that have only recently been described and have not been extensively used or validated. Our review will focus on *in vivo* models, but since most of the commonly used *in vivo* models can be replicated for *ex vivo* use, we will also briefly discuss some of these systems.

Types of Models

The ideal experimental AP model would be technically simple to create, minimally invasive, reproducible, well characterized, inexpensive, and resemble the human disease with respect to its triggering event, pathologic morphology, pathophysiology, disease course and response to treatment.[14] Needless to say, none of the existing AP models fulfill all of these criteria. Therefore, it is not surprising that none of the pancreatitis models is universally used and that AP pathophysiology remains poorly understood.

Noninvasive models of AP

In general, noninvasive AP models are relatively simple and inexpensive to create; therefore, their use has become quite popular. However, none of them are relevant to the human disease with respect to their etiology (i.e., their triggering event). This review will discuss the most commonly used noninvasive models induced by (a) supramaximal stimulation with secretagogues, (b) a CDE diet, and (c) administration of basic amino acids.

Secretagogue-induced models

Cerulein is a more stable analog of the gastrointestinal secretagogue hormone cholecystokinin (CCK). In maximally stimulating concentrations, cerulein or CCK causes digestive enzyme release from pancreatic acinar cells.[15] However, as initially shown by Lampel and Kern,[16] in higher, supramaximally stimulating concentrations, CCK or cerulein inhibit digestive enzyme secretion, cause premature intrapancreatic proteolytic enzyme activation, and induce AP. In rats, cerulein causes mild edematous AP,[16] but in mice, it causes more severe, necrotizing AP.[17] In both species, the disease is transient and self-limited. Therefore, it is not surprising that mortality in cerulein-induced pancreatitis is nonexistent in rats and negligible in mice. This may be due to a mild pulmonary injury in cerulein-induced AP that has been shown to resemble the early stages of adult respiratory distress syndrome in human AP.[18]

Cerulein can be administered parenterally via intraperitoneal (i.p.), i.v., or subcutaneous (s.c.) injections.[19] The i.v. route, which allows for continuous cerulein administration (at doses of 5-50 μg/kg/h), is considered the best way of administering the hormone to rats; however, it is not commonly used due to the requirement of central venous cannulation and anesthesia. For this reason, the cerulein-induced model is usually elicited by the i.p. or s.c. administration of several (4-12) hourly doses. In rats and mice, pancreatic injury (as manifested by trypsinogen activation, nuclear factor-κB activation, and vacuole formation) evolves within an hour of the start of cerulein administration, and the peak of histological changes (interstitial edema, inflammation, and acinar cell injury/death) occurs 3 to 6 hours after the start of secretagogue administration. By 24 hours after the start of supramaximal secretagogue stimulation, these changes begin to resolve, and 1 week later, the pancreas appears to be morphologically normal. Disease severity can be adjusted by varying the dose and number of cerulein injections. Similar to the clinical characteristics of human AP, cerulein-induced AP is more pronounced in aged mice, which exhibit higher mortality rates.[20] An advantage of using cerulein administration to elicit AP is the fact that isolated acini can also be exposed to supramaximally stimulating concentrations of cerulein; in this way, *in vivo* studies can be complemented by *ex vivo* studies under more controllable conditions.

A similar secretagogue-induced model has been developed to induce moderate AP in rats; it only requires a single i.p. injection of 25 to 250 μg/kg carbachol, a cholinergic agonist.[21,22] This model leads to edematous pancreatitis characterized by hyperamylasemia and cellular injury, as well as diarrhea and excessive lacrimation and salivation. Rats die at higher doses (250 μg/kg), presumably due to pulmonary edema. The pancreatitis induced by cholinergic agonists may be considered a model for the pancreatitis that results clinically from scorpion venom intoxication.[23,24]

The secretagogue-induced models are the most commonly used and best characterized AP rodent models, despite the questionable clinical relevance of their initiating event. In rodents, cerulein acts through the CCK receptors (in their low-affinity state) on acinar cells. However, it is debatable whether human acinar cells express any CCK receptors. Murphy *et al.* found that isolated human acinar cells respond to CCK by manifesting cytosolic calcium signaling, activating mitochondrial function, and stimulating digestive enzyme secretion.[25] In contrast, Ji *et al.*[26] and Miyasaka *et al.*[27] were unable to induce any functional responses. It is likely that even if human acinar cells express CCK receptors, their expression level is markedly lower than that in rodents.

CDE diet-induced model

This model was originally described by Lombardi *et al.*[28] It is the least invasive of the AP models because it requires no injections and no anesthesia or surgery. In this model, young female mice are fed a choline-deficient diet supplemented with 0.5% ethionine (CDE diet), and they develop acute hemorrhagic pancreatitis with fat necrosis throughout the peritoneal cavity. They also develop a poorly characterized but very prominent liver injury. Feeding only an ethionine-supplemented diet can lead to edematous pancreatitis.[29] CDE diet-induced AP onset is variable, but it usually takes 2 to 3 days of diet administration for the disease to develop. Systemic effects such as acidosis, hypoxia, and hypovolemia can also be observed. If the diet is fed *ad libitum*, it is usually lethal after 4 or 5 days. Consumption of the CDE diet (and, thus, the severity of diet-induced pancreatitis) can vary considerably between groups of animals. Some mice would rather die than eat the CDE diet, and this possible variability in CDE diet consumption can severely complicate experimental design. Careful record keeping and the use of large numbers of animals in each experimental group are important. Control and experimental groups of animals should only include young, age-matched female mice given aliquots of the same CDE diet preparation, and diet consumption should be controlled so that each animal consumes 3 g/day. Because mice are frequently cannibalistic, animal mortality should be determined by counting the number of living mice instead of dead mice. The mortality of the model can be varied by changing the duration of CDE diet administration.[30] Gilliland and Steer were able to reduce AP severity by modifying the feeding protocol.[31] The homogeneity and reproducibility of CDE diet-induced AP depend on controlling the sex, age, weight, and food intake of the mice. According to the most commonly used protocol, CD-1 female mice (11-13 g) are starved for 1 day (to promote subsequent CDE diet consumption), then fed 3 g/mouse of the CDE diet on each of the subsequent 3 days, then fasted for another day before being placed back on a regular laboratory diet. Young mice are more severely affected than adult mice, and females more than males.[32] Estradiol treatment of male mice sensitizes the animals to CDE diet-induced AP, so estrogens are likely to play an important role in the sex-specific nature of this model.[33] Systemic signs such as ascites, hypovolemia, acidosis, and hypoxia accompany the local pancreatic inflammation.[30] Unfortunately, the diet affects the liver as well as the central nervous system, and these nonpancreatic effects contribute to multiple organ failure and eventually death. Therefore, this model is not ideal for studying multiple organ distress syndromes because it can trigger those syndromes by mechanisms hat are unrelated to AP severity. Another drawback of this model is that it elicits a severe disturbance of glucose metabolism (i.e., hypoglycemia).[34] Also, despite severe acinar necrosis, the incidence of pancreatic infection is low (i.e., 3% and 8% in survivor and nonsurvivor mice, respectively).[12,35]

AP induced by basic amino acids

Whereas amino acids are essential components of the body, large i.p. doses of L-arginine,[36-38] L-ornithine,[39] and L-lysine[40] but not L-histidine[41] have been shown to induce severe acute necrotizing pancreatitis. L-arginine doses of 2.5 to 5.0 g/kg are most commonly used to induce experimental AP in rats. Two i.p. doses of 2.5 g/kg given at an interval of 1 hour do not produce as severe AP as a single 5 g/kg dose. For a long time, it was thought that this model of experimental pancreatitis could only be elicited in rats, but Dawra *et al.* recently showed that using even higher L-arginine doses (2 × 4 g/kg) can also induce AP in mice.[42,43] In the case of L-lysine, the disease evolves with the formation of vesicular structures, recently identified as damaged mitochondria,[40] within pancreatic acinar cells. Pancreatic edema and necrosis followed by inflammation has been observed in this model, and both peripancreatic necrosis and ascites can occur, but hemorrhage is not a typical feature of this model.

Basic amino acids induce selective acinar cell damage without any apparent effect on duct and islet cells. Thus, the basic amino acid-induced models seem to morphologically resemble human necrotizing pancreatitis in which nerves, major ducts, and islets are not markedly affected.[44] One important drawback of the basic amino acid-induced models is that extrapancreatic complications (e.g., pulmonary insufficiency) due to AP are mild in these models.[46] For this reason, these models are not suitable for studies focused on the pathophysiology of extrapancreatic AP-associated events. This may also explain the low mortality in this model. In mice, the effective and toxic/lethal doses of basic amino acids are very close to each other, and toxicity, which is frequently lethal, is most likely due to metabolic effects of the basic amino acids themselves rather than associated AP. Rats and mice become lethargic soon after receiving an i.p. injection of amino acids, and it takes several hours for the animals to recover from this phase. The mortality associated with the L-arginine mouse model has been reported to be 5% to 7%.[43] Administration of more than 5 g/kg L-arginine, 3 g/kg L-ornithine, or 2 g/kg L-lysine causes high mortality that occurs very shortly after the i.p. injection in rats, independent of AP. Notably, the sensitivity of rats to basic amino acids seems to be strain and age specific, and it is difficult to obtain a graded response (with the exception of L-arginine). Bohus *et al.* found a subset of Sprague Dawley rats that responded weakly to the injection of 4 g/kg L-arginine.[45] Similarly, we found that this occurred with i.p. administration of 2 g/kg L-lysine.[40]

As with many AP models, the clinical relevance of basic amino acid-induced pancreatic injury remains questionable. Saka *et al.* reported a 16-year-old male patient who was suspected to have arginine-induced AP after taking 500 mg arginine a day for 5 months.[47] However, this is not a very high dose, and the route of intake was oral, not i.p. Rats that (accidentally) receive the L-arginine injection into their bowels do not develop AP. Therefore, it is unlikely that arginine intake was the cause of AP in this patient.

Invasive AP models

The most commonly used invasive AP models build upon the "common channel theory" first proposed by Opie in 1901.[48] According to Opie's theory, when a gallstone is impacted in the papilla of Vater (at the end of the common biliopancreatic channel), it can create a common channel upstream to the impacted stone, allowing bile to retrogradely flow into the pancreatic duct and initiate AP. However, there are numerous arguments against this theory.[49] Among these objections is that in many individuals, the common channel is so short that a gallstone (or the edema around a stone) impacted in the papilla of Vater would also obstruct the pancreatic duct, which would prevent the outflow of pancreatic juice. However, it would also prevent bile reflux into the pancreatic duct. Another challenge to the common channel theory is that pancreatic duct pressure normally exceeds bile duct pressure, so in cases of stone-induced distal obstruction, pancreatic juice would be expected to reflux into the bile duct, while bile reflux into the pancreatic duct would likely be prevented. However, perhaps the most compelling of the objections is the fact that perfusion of the pancreatic duct with bile under normal pressures does not cause pancreatic damage unless ductal pressure is also increased. In spite of these various objections, the so-called "common channel theory" continues to be an attractive explanation for the frequently noted association between biliary tract stone passage and the onset of acute biliary pancreatitis.

Besides their attractive feature of possibly mimicking the triggering event of human biliary pancreatitis, the invasive AP models require anesthetizing animals, which by itself can be challenging. Furthermore, postoperative problems such as infections and difficulties in maintaining nutrition can make result interpretation difficult.

Retrograde ductal infusion

The retrograde infusion of substances (e.g., bile acids, enterokinase, trypsin) into the pancreatic duct of an animal via the ampulla of Vater is known to induce pancreatic inflammation. In fact, AP is also observed in about 5% of cases after retrograde infusion of an X-ray contrast material used for endoscopic retrograde cholangiopancreatography in humans.[50]

One of the most commonly used retrograde ductal infusion protocols was described by Aho *et al.* in rats.[51] Their model uses 3% to 5% sodium taurocholate (1 mL/kg) infused at a rate of 0.1 mL/min. Sodium bile salts used by others include glycodeoxycholate, taurodeoxycholate, chenodeoxycholate, and taurolithocholic acid 3-sulfate. Recently, the retrograde ductal infusion technique has been adapted for mice.[52-56] In either species, disease severity can be controlled by altering the concentration, volume, and infusion pressure of the injected bile acid. Administration of 3% sodium taurocholate causes mild pancreatitis with no mortality over 72 hours, while 5% sodium taurocholate causes more severe disease and a higher mortality rate. The disease induced by retrograde ductal bile acid infusion is also associated with extrapancreatic organ involvement, but the creation of the model unfortunately requires both anesthesia and a surgical procedure, which may make interpretation of the extrapancreatic effects very difficult. This is particularly true when studies are designed to evaluate acute lung injury after induction of pancreatitis by retrograde bile acid infusion into the pancreatic duct. Unlike the noninvasive necrotizing AP models, secondary pancreatic infections are more common following retrograde duct infusion. However, this higher infection rate may at least partly be the result of exogenously introduced organisms.

Technically, it is difficult to control for constant infusion pressure to produce a standard degree of pancreatic injury. The use of pumps makes the procedure more standardized. Uncontrolled pressure-related pancreatic damage should be avoided as it causes variation in AP severity. The retrograde ductal injection of substances such as bile acids will result in AP with a focal distribution mainly affecting the pancreatic head but not the tail.[52] This must always be kept in mind when sampling the pancreatic tissue for analysis. On the other hand, the disease that does develop in this model tends to have a patchy, nonhomogeneous distribution throughout the affected portion of the gland, which is similar to that seen in humans with AP.

In general, retrograde ductal infusion-induced pancreatitis is elicited in anesthetized rodents via a small laparotomy and transduodenal, transpapillary, cannulation of the pancreaticobiliary ductal system. After low-pressure infusion of a solution containing selected bile acids or other suspected pancreaticotoxic agents, the cannula is removed, and the animal allowed to recover. Control animals undergo infusion with only saline, which elicits only mild and transient pancreatic edema that fully resolves within 24 hours. Pancreatitis that develops following bile acid infusion usually evolves slowly and reaches its peak severity over the initial 12 to 24 hours. It is characterized by patchy pancreatic injury/necrosis, pancreatic inflammation, pancreatic edema, and intrapancreatic activation of digestive enzyme zymogens. Left untreated, bile acid infusion-induced pancreatitis in rodents spontaneously resolves over the subsequent week and the pancreas appears morphologically normal thereafter.

Schmidt *et al.* modified the rat duct infusion model by combining the short-term pressure and volume-controlled retrograde injection of low concentrations (5-10 mM) of sodium glycodeoxycholic acid with i.v. infusion of cerulein (5 μg/kg/h for 6 h).[57] This so-called "Boston Model" is thought to resemble human necrotizing AP in many ways including the fact that it triggers both local and systemic changes.[14] However, the triggering event does not resemble human AP.

Recent advances in the research of biliary AP models was reviewed by Wan *et al.*[54] One potentially important study in this field demonstrated that biliary AP may be a receptor-mediated disease.[58] The G protein-coupled bile acid receptor-1 (Gpbar1) is expressed in the apical membrane of acinar cells. Its genetic deletion significantly reduces biliary but not secretagogue-induced experimental AP.[58]

Closed duodenal loop

The closed duodenal loop model was originally described by Pfeffer *et al.* in dogs.[59] In this model, the duodenum is obstructed by the placement of two ligatures: one just beyond the pylorus and the second just beyond the point of biliopancreatic inflow. This creates a closed intestinal segment that communicates with the biliopancreatic duct. Bile is excluded by ligating the biliary duct, and gastric outflow is re-established by constructing a gastrojejunostomy. Closing the duodenal lumen both proximal and distal to the papilla of Vater will result in the reflux of duodenal contents into the biliopancreatic duct, and this will cause AP. The condition induced with this approach is quite variable and difficult to control. Most investigators note that inflammation is mild given the level of pancreatic necrosis.

The closed duodenal loop technique has also been adapted for rats by Nevalainen and Seppä.[60] In their model, an intraduodenal tube was placed into the intestinal lumen prior to its ligation to maintain duodenal continuity. Within 24 hours, a variable degree of hemorrhagic AP is observed. Increased serum amylase activity, pancreatic edema, acinar cell necrosis, hemorrhage, intra-abdominal fat necrosis, and the accumulation of ascitic fluid with high amylase activity are detected. Chetty *et al.* modified the latter model by instilling infected bile into the closed duodenal loop under pressure, and this resulted in a more reproducible AP.[61] Orda *et al.* injected a combination of sodium taurocholate and trypsin into the permanently occluded duodenal loop, and this resulted in a mortality of 45% within 1 week.[62] Dickson *et al.* histologically and bacteriologically analyzed three closed duodenal loop model variants.[63] Histological studies showed that the resulting AP is usually mild to moderate; it is severe only in association with sepsis. Bacteriological studies revealed gross infection as a major complication. Interestingly, pancreatic necrosis is not necessary for infection to occur in the closed duodenal loop model.[12] This and other observations made with the closed duodenal loop model suggest that the major cause of injury in this model may be ischemic necrosis of the duodenum rather that primary AP, and the closed duodenal loop model is rarely used by investigators.

Duct obstruction/ligation

Interestingly, simple ligation of the pancreatic duct does not usually induce severe AP in most animals. The major exception to this generalization seems to be the American opossum.[64] Short-term obstruction of the rat pancreatic duct results in mild interstitial pancreatic edema and hyperamylasemia,[65] while longer exposure to ligation results in atrophy of the rat exocrine pancreas with very mild or no inflammation.[66] However, combining duct obstruction with stimulation of pancreatic secretion can induce AP in rats.

The biliopancreatic ductal system of the opossum resembles that of humans in that the biliary and pancreatic ducts merge several centimeters before the combined duct

Table 1. Comparison of Rodent Acute Pancreatitis Models (the good and the bad).

Model type (animal)	CDE diet (mouse)	Amino acid arginine (mouse/rat)	Secretagogue cerulein (mouse/rat)	Bile acid duct infusion (mouse/rat)
Relevant induction event	No	No	No	?Yes
Lobular & patchy pathology	No	No	No	Yes
Controllable severity	No	Yes in rats	Yes	Yes
Systemic toxicity	Yes	Yes	No	No
Uncontrollable lethality	Yes	Yes in mice	No	No
Knock-out animals	Yes	Yes	Yes	Yes
In vitro correlate	No	Yes	Yes	Yes
Need for surgery and anesthesia	No	No	No	Yes

opens into the duodenum. Duct ligation in the opossum causes severe necrotizing hemorrhagic AP that evolves over a period of several days. This pancreatitis is also associated with lung injury.[64,67] All of the animals die within 14 days after ligation. Experiments performed in American opossums suggest that bile may not be necessary to induce AP since the obstruction of the separate pancreatic duct produces pancreatitis that is similar in severity compared to that seen after simple ligation of the combined biliopancreatic duct.[67] Unfortunately, the opossum model has several limitations which are mainly species related.[68] The opossums used for these experiments are wild and therefore collected from the wilderness. Besides being difficult to maintain and handle, this also means that the animals are not inbred, so there are large interanimal variations. The animals also need to be preconditioned prior to their use for experiments since they are under considerable stress in the early days of captivity. Opossums are often infected with parasites and thus require anti-helminthic treatment. Furthermore, since they frequently acquire acute bacterial endocarditis in captivity, they should be given prophylactic antibiotics before use. Because of the difficulties involved in obtaining, handling, and caring for opossums, as well as the considerable animal-to-animal variations in results, the opossum model of duct ligation-induced pancreatitis is currently only infrequently used.

Choosing the "Best" AP Model

Basic requirements: cost and severity

Clinical material including pancreatic tissue is rarely available for study during the early phases of AP. Therefore, most investigations focused on mechanistic issues related to AP must be performed using animal as well as *ex-vivo* models of the disease. The two basic requirements of a useful animal model of AP are both pragmatically based; most of the commonly used pancreatitis models are (a) induced in rodents (rats and mice), which are cheap, easy to handle, readily available, and subject to genetic manipulation and (b) characterized by moderate to severe degrees of pancreatic injury. As noted earlier in this review, the severe form of clinical AP is responsible for almost all of the clinical pancreatitis-related morbidity and mortality, while mild clinical pancreatitis is largely a transient and self-limited disease with little or no morbidity or mortality.

The good and the bad about rodent models of AP

The four most frequently utilized types of rodent AP models are the (a) CDE diet-induced model, (b) basic amino acid-induced models, (c) secretagogue (cerulein)-induced models, and (d) retrograde duct infusion models. We will discuss their relative merits and identify those best suited for use in studies probing basic AP-related issues. In this discussion, we will evaluate these models in terms of eight separate criteria that each has an important impact on the overall value and utility of the models. These criteria **(Table 1)** are as follows:

1. Is the pancreatitis-triggering event in the model similar to the event(s) believed to trigger clinical AP (i.e., passage of biliary tract stones, ethanol abuse, exposure to certain drugs, expression of certain mutated genes, performance of endoscopic retrograde cholangiopancreatography, etc.)?
2. Do the pathologic changes elicited in the model replicate those noted in clinical pancreatitis (i.e., is the distribution of pancreatic injury lobular and patchy as in clinical AP or is it diffuse and homogeneous throughout the gland)?
3. Is pancreatic injury/inflammation severity controllable by the investigator and is the magnitude of

pancreatic injury significant so that increases or decreases in response to experimental interventions can be identified?

4. Is the model associated with significant systemic toxicity caused by the eliciting event(s) that could confound the interpretation of specific intrapancreatic and systemic changes associated with the model?
5. Is the magnitude of lethality in the model controllable by the investigator so that changes resulting from specific interventions can be detected and statistically evaluated?
6. Can the model be elicited in mice so that the many knock-out or otherwise genetically modified strains can be used in mechanistic studies?
7. Is there an *ex vivo* correlate of the model so that *in vitro* studies can be performed under conditions that are more controllable than those present when only *in vivo* studies are possible?
8. Does the model require surgery (which may be difficult) or anesthesia that may itself, trigger a variety of nonspecific systemic changes, thus complicating data interpretation and limiting the types of studies.

Strengths and weaknesses of individual models

The results of our "model comparison" in terms of these criteria can be summarized as follows (see **Table 1**):

CDE diet model in mice

The major strengths of this model are its utility in mice, thus enabling the use of genetically modified mouse strains, and the fact that it is a noninvasive model that requires neither anesthesia nor surgery. Unfortunately, these attractive features are more than offset by a number of weaknesses. These include the fact that (a) ingestion of the CDE diet is not associated with clinical AP, (b) CDE diet-induced pancreatic injury in mice is diffuse rather than lobular or patchy as is the case in clinical pancreatitis, and (c) there is no *ex vivo* correlate for this *in vivo* model. An even more critical flaw is the fact that CDE diet-induced pancreatitis severity in mice is highly dependent upon the age, sex, and size of the mouse and closely related to the amount of the CDE ingested and diet duration. To adjust for these animal-to-animal causes of varied pancreatitis severity, the investigator is forced to use large numbers of age- and sex-matched mice, each simultaneously exposed to a standard amount of the same CDE diet preparation. This can be extremely cumbersome even when only wild-type animals are being used and can represent an insurmountable obstacle when also employing genetically modified mice. Another critical flaw of the CDE diet-induced model stems from the fact that the diet is associated with the induction of severe and uncontrollable nonpancreatic injury (primarily central nervous system injury and severe liver toxicity), which probably account for most of the diet-induced mortality of this model. These nonpancreatic injuries also preclude the use of this model for studies focused on quantitation of pancreatitis-associated systemic phenomena such as pancreatitis-associated lung and/or renal injury.

Basic amino acid-induced model in mice and rats

Like the CDE diet-induced model, the AP models induced by administration of basic amino acids such as arginine are attractive because they are noninvasive and therefore do not require anesthesia or surgery. At least in the case of L-arginine, this form of pancreatitis can be elicited in mice, thus enabling the use of genetically modified animals. However, in mice there is a very narrow margin of error when arginine is used (i.e., the dose required to elicit pancreatic injury is only slightly less than the toxic dose for mice). As a result, control arginine-treated groups of animals are needed to demonstrate that otherwise untreated animals do in fact manifest nonlethal pancreatic injury. Other possible flaws in the L-arginine-induced models include the generalized, as opposed to patchy, distribution of pancreatic injury and the systemic toxicity of pancreatitis-eliciting doses of the basic amino acid. These shortcomings may preclude the use of this model in studies designed to explore issues related to systemic AP events (e.g., lung injury). Clearly, although exposure of acini to toxic concentrations of L-arginine results in cell damage,[69] this is not a likely triggering event in clinical pancreatitis. However, recent *in vitro* studies by our group indicate that basic amino acids such as L-lysine can elicit mitochondrial injury in acinar cells, and this is a known early event in secretagogue-induced and bile acid-induced pancreatitis.[40] In this regard, the basic amino acid-induced model may in fact be triggered by a clinically relevant mechanism (i.e., mitochondrial injury), but further studies are needed to confirm this.

Cerulein models in rats and mice

Rodent models are generated by administering supramaximally stimulating doses of the pancreatic secretagogue CCK or its analog cerulein. They are attractive models for a number of reasons including the fact that they are associated with easily controllable and reproducible AP severity without systemic toxicity or uncontrollable lethality. In addition, they are noninvasive in the sense that they require no anesthesia or surgical procedures, making them ideally suited to explore systemic events that occur during or after pancreatitis onset. Genetically engineered mice can be used, and *ex vivo* studies exploring the effects of supramaximal secretagogue stimulation on isolated acinar cells are easily performed. The major flaws of these models are (a) they are elicited by an event (supramaximal secretagogue stimulation) that is unlikely to contribute to clinical pancreatitis onset and (b) the observation that CCK or cerulein-induced pancreatitis is characterized by diffuse, homogeneous pancreatic injury rather than the patchy pancreatic injury that typifies clinical pancreatitis.

Retrograde bile acid infusion into the rodent pancreatic duct

These models have been extensively used with rats or larger animals, but our group recently showed that they can also be modified for use with mice.[52] The most attractive features of these models are (a) that their induction mimics an event (i.e., bile acid reflux into the pancreatic duct) that has been proposed to be the mechanism underlying the most common form of clinical, nonalcohol-related AP (i.e., biliary pancreatitis) and (b) the pancreatic injury that occurs in these models has a patchy or lobular distribution that closely resembles the injury distribution noted in clinical pancreatitis. Other attractive features of these models include their easily controllable and reproducible severity (especially in mice) and the fact that they are not associated with systemic toxicity or uncontrollable lethality. In addition, *ex vivo* studies in which isolated acini are exposed to bile acids can easily be performed, making it easier to explore the potential mechanisms by which bile acids trigger pancreatic injury and pancreatitis. The major weakness of these models stems from the fact that they require anesthesia and a laparotomy for their induction. First, in mice these procedures may be technically difficult. Second, in both mice and rats the pulmonary and other systemic effects of anesthesia and a laparotomy make it difficult, if not impossible, to isolate the effects of AP from those of surgery.

Quantitating the severity of rodent experimental AP

It is often critical that the experimentalist be able to reliably quantitate both the severity of the model and the response to experimental manipulation. Each of the models is characterized by hyperamylasemia/hyperlipasemia, pancreatic edema, intrapancreatic activation of digestive enzyme zymogens, pancreatic inflammation, and morphological changes suggestive of acinar cell injury/death. Hyperenzymemia is easily quantitated by measuring the activity of amylase and/or lipase in circulating blood. While it is standard practice to demonstrate that the model exhibits elevated serum amylase and/or lipase activity, the magnitude of that hyperenzymemia is not considered an indicator of pancreatitis severity.

The other characteristics of AP mentioned above are believed to be individual and separable indicators of pancreatitis severity, although they may be interobserver dependent to some degree. In our opinion, they should be separately measured and reported. Grading them on a 1 to 4+ scale and combining those scores to calculate a so-called "pancreatitis severity score" may be misleading because it presumes that the individual parameters of AP severity are interchangeable (e.g., that 1≈unit of pancreatic inflammation is equal to 1 unit of pancreatic edema or 1 unit of acinar cell injury/death). Pancreatic edema can be objectively quantitated by measuring pancreatic water content ([wet weight – dry weight]/wet weight),[70] although some investigators choose to morphologically quantitate edema by grading it as being 1 to 4+.

We favor the former method because it is more objective. Intrapancreatic zymogen activation can be fluorimetrically quantitated by measuring trypsin and/or chymotrypsin activity in pancreas homogenates using enzyme-specific fluorescent substrates,[70,71] while pancreatic inflammation can be quantitated by measuring the myeloperoxidase activity in pancreas homogenates.[72] Some investigators have preferred to monitor inflammation morphologically by quantitating inflammatory cells within pancreas tissue samples. Because of its ease and, in our opinion, greater reliability, we prefer the former method. Acinar cell injury/death is conventionally monitored morphometrically in tissue samples of unknown identity (i.e., in a "blinded" fashion) by quantitating the fraction of acinar cells which appear to be injured or dead,[71] but it is important to recognize that morphological distinction between injured and dead acinar cells is usually not possible.

The best model to use may depend upon the questions being asked

None of the AP rodent models is perfect; each has its own strengths/weaknesses. In our opinion, the best models to probe the very early pancreatic cell biological mechanisms underlying AP are those elicited by retrograde ductal infusion of bile acids in mice or rats. This judgment is based on the fact that those models are (a) triggered by a mechanism that may also be relevant to clinical pancreatitis and (b) characterized by a distribution of pancreatic changes that resembles that observed in clinical pancreatitis (i.e., patchy rather than homogeneous and diffuse). On the other hand, for studies focused on the more downstream events that might be expected to be similar regardless of the initial, triggering events, it would be appropriate to also employ the cerulein-induced models and/or basic amino acid-induced models. Because of their ease of use, noninvasive induction, and lack of systemic toxicity, the cerulein-induced models are most appropriate for studies focused on nonpancreas-related events associated with AP such as acute lung injury or the systemic inflammatory response syndrome.[73,74] For either mild (rat) or severe (mouse) pancreatitis, these cerulein-induced models avoid the need for anesthesia and a surgical procedure that could confound the results by causing pulmonary and systemic changes even in the absence of AP. In our opinion, there is little or no ongoing justification for the use of (a) the CDE diet-induced model, (b) pancreatic duct obstruction models, or (c) the closed duodenal loop model.

The value of performing studies using multiple rodent models of acute pancreatitis and interpreting discordant results

Many but certainly not all of the AP-related studies reported to date have been performed using two or more experimental models. The results with multiple models have been consistent in that identical interventions in different models have resulted in similar changes in pancreatitis severity. This has generally been interpreted as indicating that the phenomena being studied are relevant to the general issue of AP rather than idiosyncratic manifestations of model-specific phenomena. Recently, however, a series of studies using cerulein-induced and duct infusion-induced mice models performed genetic deletion and pharmacological inhibition of protease-activated receptor-2 (PAR2) and assessed their effects on pancreatitis severity. The studies showed that genetic deletion or pharmacological inhibition of PAR2 had dramatically different effects in the two models; they worsened the severity of cerulein-induced pancreatitis but lessened the severity of duct infusion-induced pancreatitis.[75,76] These unexpected and surprising results indicating that PAR2 exerts model-specific effects on AP severity were interpreted to indicate that the severities of the two models are differentially regulated by one or more PAR2-sensitive mechanisms. In addition to demonstrating the value of performing pancreatitis studies using two or more dissimilar disease models, these studies also raised an additional important question: how should the investigator interpret the relevance of results to the clinical situation when studies using multiple models yield discordant results? When and if this should occur, we propose that the guide to clinical relevance should be the model that most closely resembles clinical pancreatitis. In this case, the duct infusion-induced model because (a) in contrast to cerulein-induced pancreatitis, it is triggered by a mechanism that may replicate the events that trigger clinical pancreatitis and (b) it is characterized by a distribution of pancreatic injury similar to the clinical pathology (i.e., variable and patchy), while cerulein-induced AP yields diffuse and homogeneous injury.

Acknowledgements

Our research is supported by the Hungarian Scientific Research Fund (K116634 to P.H.) and the Momentum Grant of the Hungarian Academy of Sciences (LP2014-10/2014 to P.H.) and the National Institutes of Health (DK091327 to M.L.S.).

References

1. Pandol SJ, Saluja AK, Imrie CW, Banks PA. Acute pancreatitis: bench to the bedside. *Gastroenterology*. 2007; 132: 1127-1151. PMID: 17383433.
2. Banerjee AK, Galloway SW, Kingsnorth AN. Experimental models of acute pancreatitis. *Br J Surg*. 1994; 81: 1096-1103. PMID: 7953329.
3. Büchler M, Friess H, Uhl W, Beger HG. Clinical relevance of experimental acute pancreatitis. *Eur Surg Res*. 1992; 24 Suppl 1: 85-88. PMID: 1601028.
4. Rattner DW. Experimental models of acute pancreatitis and their relevance to human disease. *Scand J Gastroenterol Suppl*. 1996; 219: 6-9. PMID: 8865463.
5. Schmid SW, Uhl W, Kid M, Modlin IM, Buchler MW. Experimental models of acute pancreatitis and their clinical relevance. In: Buechler MW, Uhl W, Friess H, Malfertheiner P eds. *Acute Pancreatitis. Novel Concepts in Biology and Therapy.* Berlin: Blackwell Science; 1999.
6. Su KH, Cuthbertson C, Christophi C. Review of experimental animal models of acute pancreatitis. *HPB (Oxford)*. 2006; 8: 264-286. PMID: 18333137.
7. Klöppel G. Acute pancreatitis. *Semin Diagn Pathol*. 2004; 21: 221-226. PMID: 16273940.
8. Klöppel G, Maillet B. Pathology of acute and chronic pancreatitis. *Pancreas*. 1993; 8: 659-670. PMID: 8255882.
9. Nordback I, Lauslahti K. Clinical pathology of acute necrotising pancreatitis. *J Clin Pathol*. 1986; 39: 68-74. PMID: 3950033.
10. Beger HG, Bittner R, Block S, Büchler M. Bacterial contamination of pancreatic necrosis. A prospective clinical study. *Gastroenterology*. 1986; 91: 433-438. PMID: 3522342.
11. Beger HG, Rau B, Mayer J, Pralle U. Natural course of acute pancreatitis. *World J Surg*. 1997; 21: 130-135. PMID: 8995067.
12. van Minnen LP, Blom M, Timmerman HM, Visser MR, Gooszen HG, Akkermans LM. The use of animal models to study bacterial translocation during acute pancreatitis. *J Gastrointest Surg*. 2007; 11: 682-689. PMID: 17468930.
13. Bernard C. Leçons de Physiologie Expérimentale Appliquée a la Médecine, Vol. 2. Paris: Bailliere; 1856: 230-252.
14. Foitzik T, Hotz HG, Eibl G, Buhr HJ. Experimental models of acute pancreatitis: are they suitable for evaluating therapy? *Int J Colorectal Dis*. 2000; 15: 127-135. PMID: 10954184.
15. Saluja AK, Lerch MM, Phillips PA, Dudeja V. Why does pancreatic overstimulation cause pancreatitis? *Annu Rev Physiol*. 2007; 69: 249-269. PMID: 17059357.
16. Lampel M, Kern HF. Acute interstitial pancreatitis in the rat induced by excessive doses of a pancreatic secretagogue. *Virchows Arch A Pathol Anat Histol*. 1977; 373: 97-117. PMID: 139754.
17. Niederau C, Ferrell LD, Grendell JH. Caerulein-induced acute necrotizing pancreatitis in mice: protective effects of proglumide, benzotript, and secretin. *Gastroenterology*. 1985; 88: 1192-1204. PMID: 2984080.
18. Willemer S, Feddersen CO, Karges W, Adler G. Lung injury in acute experimental pancreatitis in rats. I. Morphological studies. *Int J Pancreatol*. 1991; 8: 305-321. PMID: 1791317.

19. Mayerle J, Sendler M, Lerch MM. Secretagogue (caerulein) induced pancreatitis in rodents. In: *The Pancreapedia: Exocrine Pancreas Knowledge Base*. American Pancreatic Association; 2011. DOI: 10.3998/panc.2013.2
20. Okamura D, Starr ME, Lee EY, Stromberg AJ, Evers BM, Saito H. Age-dependent vulnerability to experimental acute pancreatitis is associated with increased systemic inflammation and thrombosis. *Aging Cell*. 2012; 11: 760-769. PMID: 22672542.
21. Bilchik AJ, Zucker KA, Adrian TE, Modlin IM. Amelioration of cholinergic-induced pancreatitis with a selective cholecystokinin receptor antagonist. *Arch Surg*. 1990; 125: 1546-1549. PMID: 2244806
22. Grönroos JM, Laine J, Kaila T, Nevalainen TJ. Chronic alcohol intake and carbachol-induced acute pancreatitis in the rat. *Exp Toxicol Pathol*. 1994; 46: 163-167. PMID: 7987075.
23. Bartholomew C. Acute scorpion pancreatitis in Trinidad. *Br Med J*. 1970; 14: 666-668. PMID: 5443968.
24. Sofer S, Shalev H, Weizman Z, Shahak E, Gueron M. Acute pancreatitis in children following envenomation by the yellow scorpion *Leiurus quinquestriatus*. *Toxicon*. 1991; 29: 125-128. PMID: 2028471.
25. Murphy JA, Criddle DN, Sherwood M, Chvanov M, Mukherjee R, McLaughlin E, et al. Direct activation of cytosolic Ca^{2+} signaling and enzyme secretion by cholecystokinin in human pancreatic acinar cells. *Gastroenterology*. 2008; 135: 632-641. PMID: 18555802.
26. Ji B, Bi Y, Simeone D, Mortensen RM, Logsdon CD. Human pancreatic acinar cells lack functional responses to cholecystokinin and gastrin. *Gastroenterology*. 2001; 121: 1380-1390. PMID: 11729117.
27. Miyasaka K, Shinozaki H, Jimi A, Funakoshi A. Amylase secretion from dispersed human pancreatic acini: neither cholecystokinin a nor cholecystokinin B receptors mediate amylase secretion in vitro. *Pancreas*. 2002; 25: 161-165. PMID: 12142739.
28. Lombardi B, Estes LW, Longnecker DS. Acute hemorrhagic pancreatitis (massive necrosis) with fat necrosis induced in mice by DL-ethionine fed with a choline-deficient diet. *Am J Pathol*. 1975; 79: 465-480. PMID: 1094837.
29. De Almeida AL, Grossman MI. Experimental production of pancreatitis with ethionine. *Gastroenterology*. 1952; 20: 554-577. PMID: 14917176.
30. Niederau C, Lüthen R, Niederau MC, Grendell JH, Ferrell LD. Acute experimental hemorrhagic-necrotizing pancreatitis induced by feeding a choline-deficient, ethionine-supplemented diet. Methodology and standards. *Eur Surg Res*. 1992; 24 Suppl 1: 40-54. PMID: 1601023.
31. Gilliland L, Steer ML. Effects of ethionine on digestive enzyme synthesis and discharge by mouse pancreas. *Am J Physiol Gastrointest Liver Physiol*. 1980; 239: G418-G426. PMID: 6159794.
32. Lombardi B, Rao NK. Acute hemorrhagic pancreatic necrosis in mice. Influence of the age and sex of the animals and of dietary ethionine, choline, methionine, and adenine sulfate. *Am J Pathol*. 1975; 81: 87-100. PMID: 1180334.
33. Rao KN, Eagon PK, Okamura K, Van Thiel DH, Gavaler JS, Kelly RH, et al. Acute hemorrhagic pancreatic necrosis in mice. Induction in male mice treated with estradiol. *Am J Pathol*. 1982; 109: 8-14. PMID: 6181693.
34. Virji MA, Rao KN. Acute hemorrhagic pancreatitis in mice: A study of glucoregulatory hormones and glucose metabolism. *Am J Pathol*. 1985; 118: 162-167. PMID: 3881038.
35. Rattner DW, Compton CC, Gu ZY, Wilkinson R, Warshaw AL. Bacterial infection is not necessary for lethal necrotizing pancreatitis in mice. *Int J Pancreatol*. 1989; 5: 99-105. PMID: 2664023.
36. Hegyi P, Rakonczay Z Jr, Sári R, Góg C, Lonovics J, Takács T, et al. Larginine-induced experimental pancreatitis. *World J Gastroenterol*. 2004; 10: 2003-2009. PMID: 15237423.
37. Mizunuma T, Kawamura S, Kishino Y. Effects of injecting excess arginine on rat pancreas. *J Nutr*. 1984; 114: 467-471. PMID: 6199486.
38. Tani S, Itoh H, Okabayashi Y, Nakamura T, Fujii M, Fujisawa T, Koide M, Otsuki M. New model of acute necrotizing pancreatitis induced by excessive doses of arginine in rats. *Dig Dis Sci*. 1990; 35: 367-374. PMID: 2307082.
39. Rakonczay Z Jr, Hegyi P, Dósa S, Iványi B, Jármay K, Biczó G, et al. A new severe acute necrotizing pancreatitis model induced by L-ornithine in rats. *Crit Care Med*. 2008; 36: 2117-2127. PMID: 18594222.
40. Biczó G, Hegyi P, Dósa S, Shalbuyeva N, Berczi S, Sinervirta R, et al. The crucial role of early mitochondrial injury in L-lysine-induced acute pancreatitis. *Antioxid Redox Signal*. 2011; 15: 2669-2681. PMID: 21644850.
41. Biczó G, Hegyi P, Dósa S, Balla Z, Venglovecz V, Iványi B, et al. Aliphatic, but not imidazole, basic amino acids cause severe acute necrotizing pancreatitis in rats. *Pancreas*. 2011; 40: 486-487. PMID: 21412124.
42. Dawra R, Sharif R, Phillips P, Dudeja V, Dhaulakhandi D, Saluja AK. Development of a new mouse model of acute pancreatitis induced by administration of L-arginine. *Am J Physiol Gastrointest Liver Physiol*. 2007; 292: G1009-G1018. PMID: 17170029.
43. Dawra R, Saluja AK. L-arginine-induced experimental acute pancreatitis. In: *The Pancreapedia: Exocrine Pancreas Knowledge Base*. American Pancreatic Association; 2011. DOI: 10.3998/panc.2012.6
44. Kovalska I, Dronov O, Zemskov S, Deneka E, Zemskova M. Patterns of pathomorphological changes in acute necrotizing pancreatitis. *Int J Inflam*. 2012; 2012: 508915. PMID: 22611517.
45. Bohus E, Coen M, Keun HC, Ebbels TM, Beckonert O, Lindon JC, et al. Temporal metabonomic modeling of L-arginine-induced exocrine pancreatitis. *J Proteome Res*. 2008; 7: 4435-4445. PMID: 18710274.
46. Elder AS, Saccone GT, Bersten AD, Dixon DL. L-arginine-induced acute pancreatitis results in mild lung inflammation without altered respiratory mechanics. *Exp Lung Res*. 2011; 37: 1-9. PMID: 21077777.
47. Saka M, Tüzün A, Ateş Y, Bağci S, Karaeren N, Dağalp K. Acute pancreatitis possibly due to arginine use: a case report. *Turk J Gastroenterol*. 2004; 15: 56-58. PMID: 15264124.
48. Opie EL. The etiology of acute hemorrhagic pancreatitis. *Bull Johns Hopkins Hosp*. 1901; 12: 182-188.

49. Steer ML, Perides G. Pathogenesis: How does acute pancreatitis develop? In: Domínguez-Muñoz JE ed. *Clinical Pancreatology: For Practising Gastroenterologists and Surgeons*. Oxford, UK: Blackwell Publishing Ltd.; 2007: 10-26.
50. Sherman S, Lehman GA. ERCP- and endoscopic sphincterotomy-induced pancreatitis. *Pancreas*. 1991; 6: 350-367. PMID: 1713676.
51. Aho HJ, Koskensalo SM, Nevalainen TJ. Experimental pancreatitis in the rat. Sodium taurocholate-induced acute haemorrhagic pancreatitis. *Scand J Gastroenterol*. 1980; 15: 411-416. PMID: 7433903.
52. Laukkarinen JM, van Acker GJ, Weiss ER, Steer ML, Perides G. A mouse model of acute biliary pancreatitis induced by retrograde pancreatic duct infusion of Na-taurocholate. *Gut*. 2007; 56: 1590-1598. PMID: 17591621.
53. Perides G, van Acker GJ, Laukkarinen JM, Steer ML. Experimental acute biliary pancreatitis induced by retrograde infusion of bile acids into the mouse pancreatic duct. *Nat Protocol*. 2010; 5: 335-341. PMID: 20134432.
54. Wan MH, Huang W, Latawiec D, Jiang K, Booth DM, Elliott V, et al. Review of experimental animal models of biliary acute pancreatitis and recent advances in basic research. *HPB (Oxford)*. 2012; 14: 73-81. PMID: 22221567.
55. Wittel UA, Wiech T, Chakraborty S, Boss B, Lauch R, Batra SK, et al. Taurocholate-induced pancreatitis: a model of severe necrotizing pancreatitis in mice. *Pancreas*. 2008; 36: e9-e21. PMID: 18376298.
56. Ziegler KM, Wade TE, Wang S, Swartz-Basile DA, Pitt HA, Zyromski NJ. Validation of a novel, physiologic model of experimental acute pancreatitis in the mouse. *Am J Transl Res*. 2011; 3: 159-165. PMID: 21416058.
57. Schmidt J, Rattner DW, Lewandrowski K, Compton CC, Mandavilli U, Knoefel WT, et al. A better model of acute pancreatitis for evaluating therapy. *Ann Surg*. 1992; 215: 44-56. PMID: 1731649.
58. Perides G, Laukkarinen JM, Vassileva G, Steer ML. Biliary acute pancreatitis in mice is mediated by the G-protein-coupled cell surface bile acid receptor Gpbar1. *Gastroenterology*. 2010; 138: 715-725. PMID: 19900448.
59. Pfeffer RB, Stasior O, Hilton JW. The clinical picture of the sequential development of acute hemorrhagic pancreatitis in the dog. *Surg Forum*. 1957; 8: 248-251. PMID: 13529599.
60. Nevalainen TJ, Seppä A. Acute pancreatitis caused by closed duodenal loop in the rat. *Scand J Gastroenterol*. 1975; 10: 521-527. PMID: 1153948.
61. Chetty U, Gilmour HM, Taylor TV. Experimental acute pancreatitis in the rat—a new model. *Gut*. 1980; 21: 115-117. PMID: 6155312.
62. Orda R, Hadas N, Orda S, Wiznitzer T. Experimental acute pancreatitis. Inducement by taurocholate sodium-trypsin injection into a temporarily closed duodenal loop in the rat. *Arch Surg*. 1980; 115: 327-329. PMID: 6153522.
63. Dickson AP, Foulis AK, Imrie CW. Histology and bacteriology of closed duodenal loop models of experimental acute pancreatitis in the rat. *Digestion*. 1986; 34: 15-21. PMID: 3709998.
64. Senninger N, Moody FG, Coelho JC, Van Buren DH. The role of biliary obstruction in the pathogenesis of acute pancreatitis in the opossum. *Surgery*. 1986; 99: 688-693. PMID: 2424109.
65. Ohshio G, Saluja A, Steer ML. Effects of short-term pancreatic duct obstruction in rats. *Gastroenterology*. 1991; 100: 196-202. PMID: 1700960.
66. Churg A, Richter WR. Early changes in the exocrine pancreas of the dog and rat after ligation of the pancreatic duct. A light and electron microscopic study. *Am J Pathol*. 1971; 63: 521-546. PMID: 5581235.
67. Lerch MM, Saluja AK, Rünzi M, Dawra R, Saluja M, Steer ML. Pancreatic duct obstruction triggers acute necrotizing pancreatitis in the opossum. *Gastroenterology*. 1993; 104: 853-861. PMID: 7680018.
68. Steer ML. Models for the study of pancreatitis. In: Souba WW, Wilmore DW, eds. *Surgical Research*. San Diego, CA: Academic Press; 2001: 733-746.
69. Hu G, Shen J, Cheng L, Guo C, Xu X, Wang F, et al. Reg4 protects against acinar cell necrosis in experimental pancreatitis. *Gut*. 2011; 60: 820-828. PMID: 21193457.
70. Grady T, Salja A, Kaiser A, Steer M. Edema and intrapancreatic trypsinogen activation preced glutathione depletion druing caerulein pancreatitis. *Am J Physiol Gastrointest Liver Physiol*. 1996; 271: G20-G26. PMID 8760102.
71. Kaiser AM, Saluja AK, Sengupta A, Saluja M, Steer ML. Relationship between severity, necrosis, and apoptosis in five models of experimental acute pancreatitis *Am J Physiol*. 1995; 269: C1295-C1304. PMID: 7491921.
72. Dawra R, Ku YS, Sharif R, Dhaulakhandi D, Phillips P, Dudeja V, Saluja AK. An improved method for extracting myeloperoxidase and determining its activity in the pancreas and lungs during pancreatitis. *Pancreas*. 2009; 37: 62-68. PMID: 18580446
73. Severgnini M Takahashi S, Rozo LM, Homer RJ, Kuhn C, Jhung JW, et al. Activation of the STAT pathway in acute lung injury. *Am J Physiol Lung Cell Mol* Physiol. 2004; 286: L1282-L1292. PMID: 14729509
74. Zhang H, Neuhöfer P, Song L, Rabe B, Lesina M, Kurkowski MU, et al. IL-6 trans-signaling promotes pancreatitis-associated lung injury and lethality. *J Clin Invest*. 2013; 123: 1019-1031. PMID: 23426178.
75. Laukkarinen JM, Weiss ER, van Acker GJ, Steer ML, Perides G. Proetase-activated receptor-2 exerts contrasting model-specific effects on acute experimental pancreatitits. *J Biol Chem*. 2008; 283: 20703-20712. PMID: 18511423.
76. Michael ES, Kuliopulos A, Covic L, Steer ML, Perides G. Pharmacologic inhibition of PAR2 with the pepducin P2pal-18S protects mice against acute experimental biliary pancreatitis. *Am J Physiol Gastrointest Liver Physiol*. 2013; 304: G516-G526. PMID: 23275617

Chapter 3

Calcium signaling, mitochondria, and acute pancreatitis: Avenues for therapy

Li Wen, Rajarshi Mukherjee, Wei Huang, and Robert Sutton*

NIHR Liverpool Pancreas Biomedical Research Unit, Royal Liverpool and Broadgreen University Hospitals NHS Trust and Institute of Translational Medicine, University of Liverpool, Liverpool, UK.

The role of the pancreatic acinar cell in acute pancreatitis

Pancreatic necrosis, systemic inflammatory response syndrome, multiple organ failure, and sepsis are characteristic of severe acute pancreatitis (AP), which results in the death of one in four patients and does not have a specific drug therapy.[1,2] As the pancreatic acinar cell is an initial site of injury,[1,3] commonly initiated by bile or ethanol excess, investigation of its behavior in response to toxins that induce AP may determine critical mechanisms and importantly identify new drug targets. In view of the critical roles of calcium (Ca^{2+}) signaling in normal stimulus-secretion and stimulus-metabolism coupling, and the long known toxicity of raised intracellular Ca^{2+}, we proposed the hypothesis that prolonged elevations of cytosolic Ca^{2+} is the key trigger of AP.[4] Since that proposal over 20 years ago, increasing evidence has confirmed that sustained elevation of the cytosolic Ca^{2+} concentration ($[Ca^{2+}]_C$) is a critical trigger for pancreatic acinar cell injury and necrosis that depends on store-operated Ca^{2+} entry (SOCE).[5-10]

The critical role of Ca^{2+} entry in acinar cell injury

Intracellular Ca^{2+} signals control normal secretion from pancreatic acinar cells but can become a critical trigger in pathogenesis. Physiological concentrations of acetylcholine (ACh) and cholecystokinin (CCK) generate repetitive elevations in $[Ca^{2+}]_C$ within the cellular apical pole that elicit stimulus-metabolism coupling to generate adenosine triphosphate (ATP) from the mitochondria and stimulus-secretion coupling to initiate exocytosis.[11] Intermittently, global extension of short-lived signals throughout the cell are necessary for nuclear signaling contributing to transcription and translation.[11] Elevations of $[Ca^{2+}]_C$ are buffered in the mitochondria, notably those surrounding the apical pole, with subsequent reuptake into the endoplasmic reticulum (ER) by sarcoER Ca^{2+} ATPase (SERCA) pumps and extrusion by plasma membrane Ca^{2+} pump (PMCA) (**Figure 1**). In contrast, toxins such as bile acids[12] and oxidative[13] and nonoxidative metabolites[5,14] of ethanol and CCK hyperstimulation[15,16] each elicit abnormal elevations of $[Ca^{2+}]_C$ that are global and sustained. The abnormal elevations induce premature intracellular enzyme activation, mitochondrial dysfunction, impaired autophagy, vacuolization, and necrosis, all of which contribute to AP pathogenesis.[17] Maintenance of these abnormal elevations depends on continued emptying of the ER Ca^{2+} store and activation of SOCE and Ca^{2+}-release activated Ca^{2+} currents (CRAC) to replenish the ER store.[6,10] Ca^{2+} chelation prevents zymogen activation and vacuolization through attenuation of Ca^{2+} overload in acinar cells in vitro[9,18] and ameliorates AP severity in vivo.[19]

Excessive Ca^{2+} release from intracellular stores occurs predominantly via inositol 1,4,5-trisphosphate receptor (IP_3R) Ca^{2+} channels.[20] Pancreatic acinar cells express all three IP_3R subtypes in the apical region, close to the luminal membrane,[21-23] but IP_3R types 2 and 3 are predominantly responsible for physiological Ca^{2+} signaling and enzyme secretion.[21] Stimuli such as CCK,[24] the bile acid taurolithocholic acid 3-sulphate (TLCS),[25,26] alcohol,[27] and fatty acid ethyl esters (FAEEs)[5,20] cause intracellular Ca^{2+} release in pancreatic acinar cells primarily via IP_3Rs, an effect inhibited by double knockout of IP_3R types 2 and 3[21] or by caffeine.[16,20]

Since the discovery of the Ca^{2+} entry channel ORAI1, ORAI1 has been shown to be the principal SOCE channel in the pancreatic acinar cell,[23] opening of which is coordinated by stromal interaction molecules (STIM1 and STIM2), following decreases in ER Ca^{2+} store concentrations.[6,23,28,29]

GSK-7975A and CM_128 have been developed independently by GlaxoSmithKline[6,28,30] and CalciMedica,[10] respectively, to block ORAI1 channels, although only CM_128 continues towards clinical

*Corresponding author. Email: R.Sutton@liverpool.ac.uk

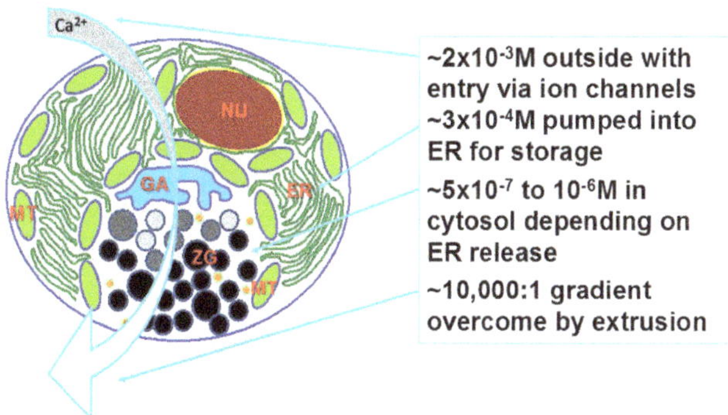

Figure 1. Ca^{2+} signaling in the pancreatic acinar cell depends on tight control of concentrations across the plasma membrane and within subcellular organelles. In resting conditions $[Ca^{2+}]_c$ is ~10,000 fold lower than outside the cell, with Ca^{2+} stored mainly in the ER. Stimulus-secretion coupling operates by secretagogue-elicited GPCR activation to release second messengers that bind to inositol trisphosphate and ryanodine receptors on the ER, through which Ca^{2+} is released into the cytosol and mitochondria, initiating ATP production that provides energy for secretion. Ca^{2+} is cleared by reuptake into the ER and extrusion from the cell; the Ca^{2+} extruded is replenished via puncta that form between the ER and plasma membrane in response to low ER Ca^{2+} levels, allowing entry via ORAI channels. Pancreatitis toxins induce excessive ER Ca^{2+} release, initiating a vicious circle that overwhelms the cell (ER: endoplasmic reticulum; GA: Golgi apparatus; MT: mitochondria; NU: nucleus; ZG: zymogen granules).

development. GSK-7975A inhibits SOCE induced by thapsigargin in isolated murine pancreatic acinar cells over the range 1-50 μM (half-maximal inhibitory concentration $[IC_{50}]$ ~3.4 μM)[6] inhibits endocytic vacuole formation[31] and reduces necrosis induced by toxins that cause AP.[6,10,31] CM_128 is a new molecular entity, the effects of which we have recently confirmed to be similar.[10] We have also shown that ORAI inhibition inhibits SOCE and necrosis in human pancreatic acinar cells, and ORAI inhibition can markedly reduce the severity of multiple models of experimental AP.

Genetic knockout of the transient receptor potential canonical (TRPC) 3 channel,[32] a nonselective cation channel regulated in part by STIM1 via TRPC1,[33] results in a ~50% reduction of in vivo serum amylase elevation and edema formation induced by four cerulein injections.[32] These results supported a role for SOCE in AP, but in a single, mild model with few parameters of response.

As indicated, we have defined the concentration-dependent inhibitory effects of GSK-7975A and CM_128 on SOCE and necrosis in murine and human pancreatic acinar cells induced by TLCS[26,34] or CCK-8.[9,32] The effects of CM_128 on ORAI1 were confirmed by examination of its effect on Ca^{2+} release-activated Ca^{2+} currents (I_{CRAC}),[6,28,29] in ORAI1/STIM1-transfected HEK 293 cells.[28] GSK-7975A was given at selected doses in vivo after induction of AP with TLCS (TLCS-AP),[35] seven injections of cerulein (CER-AP),[36] or ethanol and palmitoleic acid (FAEE-AP).[14] Since GSK-7975A markedly reduced all parameters of pathobiologic response in a dose-dependent manner, a high dose of GSK-7975A and separately CM_128 were begun at two different time points after disease induction to clarify the effects of early versus late drug administration. In all models, drug administration started 1 h after disease induction was highly effective in reducing parameters of the pathobiologic response,[10] significantly more so than when begun 6 hours after disease induction, in all models. These data provide thorough preclinical validation for ORAI channel inhibition as a potential early treatment for AP.

We found that GSK-7975A and the new molecular entity CM_128 could inhibit toxin-induced SOCE in murine and human pancreatic acinar cells in a concentration-dependent manner, exceeding a >90% block of relative control values in some protocols.[10] We also found both GSK-7975A and CM_128 to significantly reduce necrotic cell death pathway activation in murine and human pancreatic acinar cells exposed to TLCS, which induces AP in vivo.[35,36] While effects of GSK-7975A have been described for thapsigargin- and FAEE-induced murine pancreatic acinar SOCE,[6] we found GSK-7975A to have a similarly critical effect on TLCS- and CCK-induced murine pancreatic acinar SOCE, as well as thapsigargin-induced human pancreatic acinar SOCE and TLCS-induced human pancreatic acinar necrotic cell death pathway activation.[10] CM_128 showed higher potency (IC_{50} ~0.1 μM from ORAI1/STIM1-transfected HEK 293 cell patch clamp data), and unlike GSK-7975A, no loss of efficacy at high doses. Comprehensive in vivo evaluation using three diverse, clinically representative AP models[10] with prior pharmacokinetic assessment demonstrated the validity of SOCE inhibition as a therapeutic approach. Thus, administration of either compound within an hour following disease induction was markedly effective across a representative range of local and systemic biochemical, immunological, and histological disease responses. These data provide robust confirmation of the hypothesis that cytosolic Ca^{2+} overload is a critical trigger of AP.[4]

Further confirmation of the role of cytosolic Ca^{2+} overload in AP has come from our work with xanthines.[37] We defined the inhibitory effects of methylxanthines on IP_3R-mediated Ca^{2+} release from the pancreatic acinar ER store into the cytosol and potential application in AP. It has been shown that caffeine inhibits IP_3Rs, as well as IP_3 production in a concentration-dependent manner.[38] We found that inhibition of IP_3R-mediated Ca^{2+} release is attributable at least in part to an action on the IP_3R, since xanthines inhibited IP_3R-mediated Ca^{2+} release elicited by uncaged IP_3.[37] Caffeine, theophylline, and paraxanthine prevented physiological Ca^{2+} signaling and toxic elevations of $[Ca^{2+}]_C$ induced by agents (CCK and TLCS) that cause AP in a concentration-dependent manner (500 μM to 10 mM), also inhibiting falls in mitochondrial membrane potential ($\Delta\Psi_M$) and necrotic cell death pathway activation. An inhibitory action on phosphodiesterase (PDE) preventing cAMP/cGMP degradation could not account for the effects on toxic $[Ca^{2+}]_C$ overload, since additional cAMP/cGMP did not prevent these. Extending these findings in vivo, caffeine significantly reduced the severity of multiple, diverse models of AP.[37] The combined concentrations of di- and trimethylxanthines after the 25 mg/kg caffeine protocol were within the range over which effects on both IP_3R-mediated Ca^{2+} release and toxic elevations of $[Ca^{2+}]_C$ were identified. Despite the half-life of caffeine in mice of ~60 min,[39] the combined peak concentrations of di- and trimethylxanthines with 25 mg/kg caffeine regimen (seven injections) were >2 mM, and serum caffeine was >400 µM 6 h after the last caffeine injection. Following similar protocols of 25 mg/kg theophylline or paraxanthine, concentrations were far below the effective range on IP_3Rs but within the effective range on PDE (approaching 100 µM 10 min after the last dimethylxanthine injection),[40] and no protective effects on in vivo AP were seen. Since pancreatic cellular injury initiates and determines AP severity, the protective effect of caffeine on AP is likely to have been mediated by inhibition of IP_3R-mediated Ca^{2+} release.

The effects of Ca^{2+} elevation in mitochondria

The pancreatic acinar cell typifies nonexcitable exocrine cells with a high secretory turnover that is heavily dependent on mitochondrial production of ATP.[11] While zymogen activation has long been considered the principle mechanism of injury,[1,3] mitochondrial dysfunction has been increasingly implicated,[5,13,14,41-44] presumed consequent upon intracellular Ca^{2+} overload induced by toxins that include bile acids and ethanol metabolites.[5,14,45] Mitochondrial uptake of Ca^{2+} drives normal cellular bioenergetics, but high Ca^{2+} loads induce increasingly drastic responses culminating in necrosis.[46] Mitochondrial matrix Ca^{2+} overload leads to opening of the mitochondrial permeability transition pore (MPTP), a nonspecific channel that forms in the inner mitochondrial membrane allowing passage of particles <1,500 Da, causing loss of $\Delta\psi_m$ essential to ATP production.[46] Recent evidence implicates F_0F_1 ATP synthase in MPTP formation.[47,48] MPTP opening is physiological in low conductance mode, releasing Ca^{2+} and reactive oxygen species (ROS) to match metabolism with workload,[49,50] but pathological in high conductance mode compromising ATP production and inducing cell death.[46] Both functions are regulated by the mitochondrial matrix protein peptidyl-prolyl *cis-trans* isomerase (PPI) cyclophilin D (also known as cyclophilin F).[51]

Our work has demonstrated that MPTP opening is critical to experimental AP, mediating impaired ATP production, defective autophagy, zymogen activation, inflammatory responses and necrosis,[52] all features of AP at molecular, cellular, and whole organism levels.[1] We have established the general significance of MPTP opening as a central mechanism in the pathogenesis of AP, and the primary role in this process of Ca^{2+} overload. Patch clamp data show how tight control of cytosolic Ca^{2+} elevation is essential to normal stimulus-secretion coupling by IP_3Rs and ryanodine receptors (RyRs)[11] is lost in wild-type but maintained in *Ppif*$^{-/-}$ pancreatic acinar cells, which lack functional MPTP; these cells preserve their ATP supply and clear Ca^{2+} more effectively. Coupling of ER IP_3Rs and RyRs with outer mitochondrial membranes tightly localizes high Ca^{2+} concentrations[53] but may expose mitochondria to abnormal Ca^{2+} release despite modulation by Bcl-2 family proteins.[43] We have shown that pancreatitis toxins cause abnormal release of Ca^{2+} via IP_3Rs and RyRs that overload pancreatic acinar mitochondria[52] that are markedly sensitive to Ca^{2+} signals.[54] The mitochondrial Ca^{2+} overload induces high conductance MPTP opening and dissipates $\Delta\psi_m$, initiating collapse of ATP production, diminished Ca^{2+} clearance, activation of PGAM5 (phosphoglycerate mutase family member 5, a mitochondrial protein phosphatase), and subsequent necrosis.[52] Importantly for a disease without specific treatment, pharmacological MPTP inhibition[10,55] administered after AP induction came close to preventing all injury, notably in the clinically relevant TLCS-AP.

For more than a century following an original postulate by Chiari,[56] AP has been viewed as an autodigestive disease consequent on pathological zymogen activation.[3,7,57-59] In experimental AP, zymogens are activated inside acinar cells within minutes of toxin exposure,[1,3,9,60] which we have shown to result from induction of the MPTP, caused by and contributing to Ca^{2+} overload. Sustained Ca^{2+} overload may activate degradative calpains, phospholipases, or other enzymes[51] and damage zymogen granules, inducing autophagic[60] and/or endolysosomal[61] responses that activate digestive enzymes. Such activation was not completely prevented by MPTP inhibition; however, this was likely from global cytosolic Ca^{2+} overload that was seen to be more effectively cleared in *Ppif*$^{-/-}$ cells, without which overload no enzyme activation occurs.[9] Nevertheless, intracellular expression of trypsin per se without mitochondrial injury leads to apoptotic not necrotic pathway activation.[57] Trypsinogen activation does not appear necessary for either local or systemic inflammation;[62] knockout of cathepsin B greatly reduces trypsinogen activation with little effect on serum interleukin-6 or lung injury.[58] Hereditary pancreatitis caused by cationic trypsinogen gene mutations rarely features clinically significant pancreatic necrosis;[63,64] further, systemic protease inhibition has had little success as a clinical strategy,[1] suggesting that while zymogen activation contributes, it is not the critical driver of AP. Our work, however, shows that MPTP opening triggers defective autophagy, while inhibition of MPTP opening preserves ATP supply, increasing the efficiency of autophagy and decreasing zymogen activation. Together with major effects of MPTP opening on PGAM5 activation that implements necrosis,[65,66] and on local and systemic inflammatory responses, these findings now centrally place mitochondrial injury in AP.

Our data show that IP_3Rs and RyRs in pancreatic acinar cells are vulnerable to specific toxins that markedly increase their Ca^{2+} channel open-state probabilities.[52] Toxic transformation of Ca^{2+} channel function induced pancreatic acinar cell necrosis through Ca^{2+}-dependent formation of the MPTP, with diminished ATP production the critical consequence. Toxic transformation by different toxins was specific to different second messengers, identifying the potential for a variety of deleterious effects. ATP deficiency may be further exacerbated by fatty acids released on hydrolysis of FAEEs or triglycerides,[67] which may inhibit beta-oxidation.[5] Without sufficient ATP, cytosolic Ca^{2+} overload produces a vicious circle in which high affinity, low capacity SERCA and PMCA pump clearance of cytosolic Ca^{2+} is impaired, further mitochondrial injury sustained, and necrotic cell death accelerated.[5,45] Although the toxicity of cytosolic Ca^{2+} overload depends on Ca^{2+} store refilling from outside the cell,[9,32] specific second messenger receptor blockade demonstrated Ca^{2+} overload to be due completely to release from their Ca^{2+} channels,[52] not direct effects of toxins on Ca^{2+} entry or extrusion.

Whereas the vast majority of previous studies undertaken to determine mechanisms and/or new targets in AP have used only one model, we have used four models[52] that are broadly representative of a range of etiologies including biliary (TLCS-AP), hyperstimulation (CER-AP), ethanolic (FAEE-AP), and amino acid-induced (CDE-AP).[1,68] Our experimental AP findings are entirely consistent with those made in isolated mitochondria and cells, identifying a generalized mechanism of pancreatic injury and necrosis, confirmed in murine and human pancreatic acinar cells, pancreas lobules, and tissue slices. Pancreatic necrosis drives the inflammasome,[69] which can be induced by MPTP opening[70] and is part of the systemic inflammatory response contributing to multiple organ failure.[2] Further pancreatic injury is driven through tumor necrosis factor receptor activation that also promotes MPTP opening[71] and Ca^{2+} deregulation, activating calcineurin and calcineurin-dependent transcription factor nuclear factor of activated T cells.[72]

Therapeutic avenues for AP

Our novel human data support the potential applicability of SOCE inhibition as a treatment for clinical AP (**Figure 2**). Both GSK-7975A and CM_128 blocked SOCE promptly, shown to result in complete block of human ORAI1 by CM_128.[10] While an action on other ORAI channels cannot be excluded and could be desirable, ORAI1 is the primary channel for SOCE into pancreatic acinar cells[6,23] and is blocked by both compounds. ORAI channels also contribute to inflammatory cell responses including neutrophil migration and activation.[73] Inhibition of innate immune responses significantly reduces the severity of experimental AP,[74] thus, there may be a contribution from ORAI inhibition of immune cells. Nevertheless while knockout of ORAI1/STIM1 SOCE inhibits neutrophil functions, it does not prevent all,[73] so the primary contribution of ORAI blockade in our experiments is likely to have been in the pancreas. Further, since SOCE inhibition for clinical AP would necessarily be short-term, inhibition of the adaptive immune system[73] would also be short term. ORAI blockade has less effect on other cell types in which ORAI channels have a less prominent role, such as electrically excitable cells in which other ion channels (e.g., nonselective cation channels) have a larger role in Ca^{2+} entry.[75] However, nonselective cation channels permit limited SOCE into pancreatic acinar cells[6,32] that could sustain essential Ca^{2+} entry.[75] Without such Ca^{2+} entry, continued activation of the plasma membrane Ca^{2+}-ATPase pump upon secretagogue- or toxin-mediated release of Ca^{2+} from intracellular stores could deplete these stores to deleterious levels, inducing or exacerbating ER stress.[76]

Both ORAI inhibitory compounds were administered after disease induction to model treatment of clinical AP, but delay in administration of either compound to 6 h after

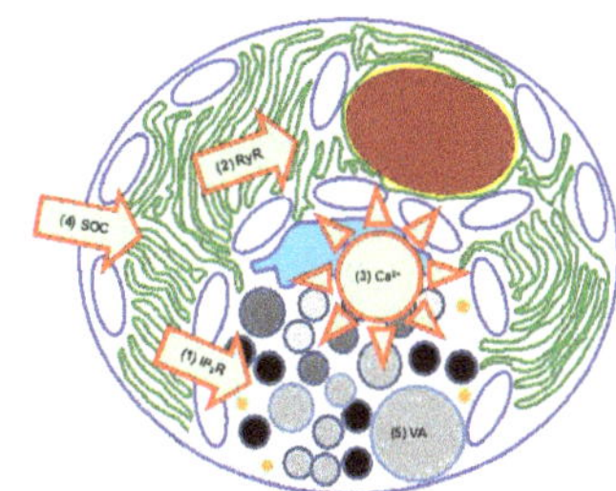

(1) Pancreatitis toxins open IP_3Rs and (2) RyRs causing (3) Ca^{2+} release; (4) ER Ca^{2+} depletion results in STIM1- and STIM2-mediated entry through ORAI channels; (5) Mitochondrial Ca^{2+} overload impairs ATP production, disorders autophagy, inducing vacuole (VA) formation

Figure 2. Abnormal Ca^{2+} signaling in the pancreatic acinar cell initiated by pancreatitis toxins (e.g., bile acids, FAEEs, hyperstimulation) causes injury dependent on continued store-operated Ca^{2+} (SOC) entry via ORAI channels. As a consequence, mitochondria are overloaded with Ca^{2+}, failing to produce adequate ATP to clear the Ca^{2+} and protect the cell. Autophagy is defective, and vacuoles develop presaging cell death. Ca^{2+} entry blockade prevents these events, avoiding prolonged, global cytosolic Ca^{2+} overload. This was first demonstrated by removal of Ca^{2+} from the external medium surrounding isolated cells and has since been shown using ORAI blockers applied to isolated human and murine pancreatic acinar cells. These findings have since been extended into three murine models of experimental AP, in which this strategy of Ca^{2+} entry inhibition with ORAI blockers has been demonstrated to be highly effective.

disease induction resulted in diminished efficacy, dependent on the endpoint measured and the model employed.[10] While biological time courses including that of AP are longer in humans than mice,[1,2,36,77] with pancreatic necrosis typically detected within days rather than hours,[78] human pancreatic acinar necrotic cell death pathway activation may begin soon after clinical AP onset, shown here in mouse models within 6 h. Door-to-needle times of less than 60 min are established guidelines for patients with acute myocardial infarction (30 min)[79] and acute ischemic stroke (60 min),[80] making every second count, with national and international quality improvement initiatives underway towards fully achieving these.[81]

Although pancreatic necrosis has a less rapid time course and is characteristically not the result of major arterial occlusion,[1] the translational implication of our work is that door-to-needle time is an important issue in administration of any treatment for AP that targets the pathogenesis of pancreatic injury, which drives the disease. Previously clinical trials of treatments for AP have "enriched" recruitment with patients predicted to have severe disease (often with recruitment up to 72 h after admission),[82] which delays therapy initiation. Furthermore, the expansion of disease categories from the original Atlanta Classification (mild and severe)[83] into the revised Atlanta (mild, moderate, and severe)[84] and Determinant-Based (mild, moderate, severe, critical)[85] classification, further complicates patient selection from among these potentially overlapping subgroups. To minimize door-to-needle time, a quicker and more accurate approach to patient selection is required for trials of any therapy, such as that offered here with ORAI inhibition by CM_128, a novel molecular entity currently undergoing preclinical toxicological evaluation prior to phase I trials.

With respect to inhibition of Ca^{2+} release within the pancreatic acinar cell rather than Ca^{2+} entry into the cell, it is important to note that in our studies, high doses of caffeine were required to reduce experimental AP severity. The most effective 25 mg/kg regimen extended into toxicity, indicative of a very narrow therapeutic index. At this dose, the number of hourly injections had to be reduced from seven to two in FAEE-AP to avoid mortality; in CER-AP, 50 mg/kg resulted in caffeine intoxication syndrome, although no visible side effects were observed at 25 mg/kg. In humans even 10 mg/kg caffeine would be likely to induce caffeine intoxication, with florid neuro-excitotoxic and other undesirable side effects.[40] There is marked individual variability in caffeine metabolism and pharmacokinetics.[40] Since the half-life in humans typically ranges from 3 to 7 hours, repeated high doses would be hazardous unless rapid therapeutic monitoring were possible. Nevertheless, our study has demonstrated proof of principle that caffeine causes marked amelioration of experimental AP, largely through inhibition of IP_3R-mediated signaling. Medicinal chemistry starting with the template of caffeine and/or other compounds that inhibit IP_3R-mediated signaling could lead to more potent, selective, and safer drug candidates for AP. This approach, however, might have effects on IP_3R-mediated signaling in other cells, tissues, and organs including the brain and other solid organs.

Our data from the cyclophilin D knockout and pharmacotherapy with Debio-025 (nonimmunosuppressive derivative of cyclosporin A) or TRO40303 (in clinical development for other indications) show the potential for MPTP inhibition as an alternative strategy to ORAI inhibition (**Figure 3**).

The effect of this approach was remarkably effective in both isolated human and murine pancreatic acinar cells as well as in four models of experimental AP.[52] The attractions of this approach are made stronger by the relatively modest phenotype of the cyclophilin D knockout that is able to grow, develop, and breed normally; there is an extensive range of pathologies that cyclophilin D knockout protects against, although capacity for exercise is reduced and there is some impact on memory in later life.[49,50] These effects are unlikely to be important for short-term administration as would be required in AP and has not proven a problem in long-term cyclosporin A administration.

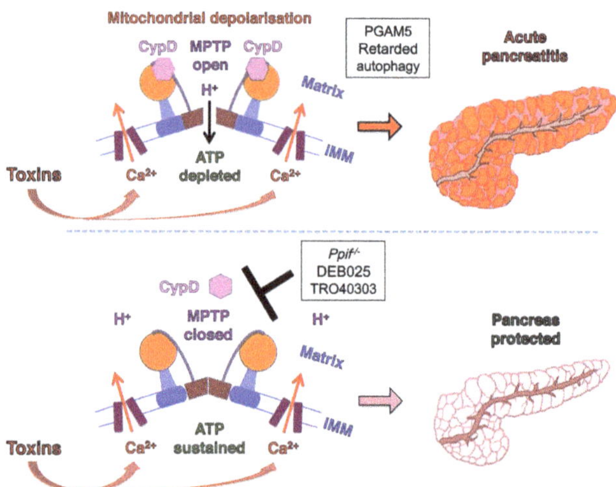

Figure 3. The MPTP plays a critical role in AP development. Pancreatitis toxins induce a sustained rise in $[Ca^{2+}]_C$ that crosses the inner mitochondrial membrane (IMM) via the mitochondrial uniporter to enter the mitochondrial matrix. Consequent Ca^{2+}-cyclophilin D (CypD) activation promotes MPTP opening, causing mitochondrial depolarization and impaired ATP production, failure of Ca^{2+} clearance and cell injury. When MPTP opening is inhibited by genetic ($Ppif^{-/-}$) or pharmacological means (DEB025 or TR040303), mitochondrial membrane potential is preserved and ATP production sustained. This maintains cellular integrity to clear Ca^{2+} more effectively and prevents the development of AP (lower panel) (Copyright © BMJ Publishing Group Ltd and British Society of Gastroenterology. All rights reserved: http://gut.bmj.com/content/65/8/1333.full).

Acknowledgement

The findings described in this review are in part derived from three recent original open access articles ([35,52]: Copyright

See [35]: http://gut.bmj.com/content/65/8/1333.full; [52]: http://gut.bmj.com/content/early/2015/12/07/gutjnl-2015-309363.full [85]: http://www.gastrojournal.org/article/S0016-5085(15)00571-5/fulltext).

We acknowledge funding support from Liverpool China Scholarship Council, CORE, the UK Medical Research Council, CalciMedica, and the Biomedical Research Unit Funding scheme of the UK National Institute for Health Research. Robert Sutton is an NIHR Senior Investigator.

References

1. Pandol SJ, Saluja AK, Imrie CW, Banks PA. Acute pancreatitis: bench to the bedside. *Gastroenterology*. 2007; 132: 1127-1151. PMID: 17383433.
2. Petrov MS, Shanbhag S, Chakraborty M, Phillips AR, Windsor JA. Organ failure and infection of pancreatic necrosis as determinants of mortality in patients with acute pancreatitis. *Gastroenterology*. 2010; 139: 813-820. PMID: 20540942.
3. Leach SD, Modlin IM, Scheele GA, Gorelick FS. Intracellular activation of digestive zymogens in rat pancreatic acini. Stimulation by high doses of cholecystokinin. *J Clin Invest*. 1991; 87: 362-366. PMID: 1985109.
4. Ward JB, Petersen OH, Jenkins SA, Sutton R. Is an elevated concentration of acinar cytosolic free ionised calcium the trigger for acute pancreatitis? *Lancet* 1995; 346: 1016-1019. PMID: 7475553.
5. Criddle DN, Murphy J, Fistetto G, Barrow S, Tepikin AV, Neoptolemos JP, et al. Fatty acid ethyl esters cause pancreatic calcium toxicity via inositol trisphosphate receptors and loss of ATP synthesis. *Gastroenterology*. 2006; 130: 781-793. PMID: 16530519.
6. Gerasimenko JV, Gryshchenko O, Ferdek PE, Stapleton E, Hebert TO, Bychkova S, et al. Ca^{2+} release-activated Ca^{2+} channel blockade as a potential tool in antipancreatitis therapy. *Proc Natl Acad Sci U S A*. 2013; 110: 13186-13191. PMID: 23878235.
7. Husain SZ, Prasad P, Grant WM, Kolodecik TR, Nathanson MH, Gorelick FS. The ryanodine receptor mediates early zymogen activation in pancreatitis. *Proc Natl Acad Sci U S A*. 2005; 102: 14386-14391. PMID: 16186498.
8. Kruger B, Albrecht E, Lerch MM. The role of intracellular calcium signaling in premature protease activation and the onset of pancreatitis. *Am J Pathol*. 2000; 157: 43-50. PMID: 10880374.
9. Raraty M, Ward J, Erdemli G, Vaillant C, Neoptolemos JP, Sutton R, et al. Calcium-dependent enzyme activation and vacuole formation in the apical granular region of pancreatic acinar cells. *Proc Natl Acad Sci U S A*. 2000; 97: 13126-13131. PMID: 11087863.
10. Wen L, Voronina S, Javed MA, Awais M, Szatmary P, Latawiec D, et al. Inhibitors of ORAI1 prevent cytosolic calcium-associated injury of human pancreatic acinar cells and acute pancreatitis in 3 mouse models. *Gastroenterology*. 2015; 149: 481-492. PMID: 25917787.
11. Petersen OH, Tepikin AV. Polarized calcium signaling in exocrine gland cells. *Annu Rev Physiol*. 2008; 70: 273-299. PMID: 17850212.
12. Voronina SG, Gryshchenko OV, Gerasimenko OV, Green AK, Petersen OH, Tepikin AV. Bile acids induce a cationic current, depolarizing pancreatic acinar cells and increasing the intracellular Na^+ concentration. *J Biol Chem*. 2005; 280: 1764-1770. PMID: 15536077.
13. Shalbueva N, Mareninova OA, Gerloff A, Yuan J, Waldron RT, Pandol SJ, et al. Effects of oxidative alcohol metabolism on the mitochondrial permeability transition pore and necrosis in a mouse model of alcoholic pancreatitis. *Gastroenterology*. 2013; 144: 437-446. PMID: 23103769.
14. Huang W, Booth DM, Cane MC, Chvanov M, Javed MA, Elliott VL, et al. Fatty acid ethyl ester synthase inhibition ameliorates ethanol-induced Ca^{2+}-dependent mitochondrial dysfunction and acute pancreatitis. *Gut*. 2014; 63: 1313-1324. PMID: 24162590.
15. Criddle DN, Booth DM, Mukherjee R, McLaughlin E, Green GM, Sutton R, et al. Cholecystokinin-58 and cholecystokinin-8 exhibit similar actions on calcium signaling, zymogen secretion, and cell fate in murine pancreatic acinar cells. *Am J Physiol Gastrointest Liver Physiol*. 2009; 297: G1085-G1092. PMID: 19815626.
16. Murphy JA, Criddle DN, Sherwood M, Chvanov M, Mukherjee R, McLaughlin E, et al. Direct activation of cytosolic Ca^{2+} signaling and enzyme secretion by cholecystokinin in human pancreatic acinar cells. *Gastroenterology*. 2008; 135: 632-641. PMID: 18555802.
17. Criddle DN, McLaughlin E, Murphy JA, Petersen OH, Sutton R. The pancreas misled: signals to pancreatitis. *Pancreatology*. 2007; 7: 436-446. PMID: 17898533.
18. Saluja AK, Bhagat L, Lee HS, Bhatia M, Frossard JL, Steer ML. Secretagogue-induced digestive enzyme activation and cell injury in rat pancreatic acini. *Am J Physiol Gastrointest Liver Physiol*. 1999; 276 4 Pt 1: G835-G842. PMID: 10198325.
19. Mooren F, Hlouschek V, Finkes T, Turi S, Weber IA, Singh J, et al. Early changes in pancreatic acinar cell calcium signaling after pancreatic duct obstruction. *J Biol Chem*. 2003; 278: 9361-9369. PMID: 12522141.
20. Gerasimenko JV, Lur G, Sherwood MW, Ebisui E, Tepikin AV, Mikoshiba K, et al. Pancreatic protease activation by alcohol metabolite depends on Ca^{2+} release via acid store IP3 receptors. *Proc Natl Acad Sci U S A* 106(26): 10758-10763, 2009. PMID: 19528657.
21. Futatsugi A, Nakamura T, Yamada MK, Ebisui E, Nakamura K, Uchida K, et al. IP3 receptor types 2 and 3 mediate exocrine secretion underlying energy metabolism. *Science*. 2005; 309: 2232-2234. PMID: 16195467.
22. Lur G, Sherwood MW, Ebisui E, Haynes L, Feske S, Sutton R, et al. InsP(3)receptors and Orai channels in pancreatic acinar cells: co-localization and its consequences. *Biochem J*. 2011; 436: 231-239. PMID: 21568942.

23. Lur G, Haynes LP, Prior IA, Gerasimenko OV, Feske S, Petersen OH, et al. Ribosome-free terminals of rough ER allow formation of STIM1 puncta and segregation of STIM1 from IP(3) receptors. *Curr Biol.* 2009; 19: 1648-1653. PMID: 19765991.
24. Cancela JM, Van Coppenolle F, Galione A, Tepikin AV, Petersen OH. Transformation of local Ca^{2+} spikes to global Ca^{2+} transients: the combinatorial roles of multiple Ca^{2+} releasing messengers. *EMBO J.* 2002; 21: 909-919. PMID: 11867519.
25. Gerasimenko JV, Flowerdew SE, Voronina SG, Sukhomlin TK, Tepikin AV, Petersen OH, et al. Bile acids induce Ca^{2+} release from both the endoplasmic reticulum and acidic intracellular calcium stores through activation of inositol trisphosphate receptors and ryanodine receptors. *J Biol Chem.* 2006; 281: 40154-40163. PMID: 17074764.
26. Voronina S, Longbottom R, Sutton R, Petersen OH, Tepikin A. Bile acids induce calcium signals in mouse pancreatic acinar cells: implications for bile-induced pancreatic pathology. *J Physiol.* 2002; 540 Pt 1: 49-55. PMID: 11927668.
27. Gerasimenko JV, Lur G, Ferdek P, Sherwood MW, Ebisui E, Tepikin AV, et al. Calmodulin protects against alcohol-induced pancreatic trypsinogen activation elicited via Ca^{2+} release through IP3 receptors. *Proc Natl Acad Sci U S A.* 2011; 108: 5873-5878. PMID: 21436055.
28. Derler I, Schindl R, Fritsch R, Heftberger P, Riedl MC, Begg M, et al. The action of selective CRAC channel blockers is affected by the Orai pore geometry. *Cell Calcium.* 2013; 53: 139-151. PMID: 23218667.
29. Muik M, Schindl R, Fahrner M, Romanin C. Ca^{2+} release-activated Ca^{2+} (CRAC) current, structure, and function. *Cell Mol Life Sci.* 2012; 69: 4163-4176. PMID: 22802126.
30. Rice LV, Bax HJ, Russell LJ, Barrett VJ, Walton SE, Deakin AM, et al. Characterization of selective Calcium-Release Activated Calcium channel blockers in mast cells and T-cells from human, rat, mouse and guinea-pig preparations. *Eur J Pharmacol.* 2013; 704: 49-57. PMID: 23454522.
31. Voronina S, Collier D, Chvanov M, Middlehurst B, Beckett AJ, Prior IA, et al. The role of Ca^{2+} influx in endocytic vacuole formation in pancreatic acinar cells. *Biochem J.* 2015; 465: 405-412. PMID: 25370603.
32. Kim MS, Hong JH, Li Q, Shin DM, Abramowitz J, Birnbaumer L, et al. Deletion of TRPC3 in mice reduces store-operated Ca^{2+} influx and the severity of acute pancreatitis. *Gastroenterology.* 2009; 137: 1509-1517. PMID: 19622358.
33. Lee KP, Choi S, Hong JH, Ahuja M, Graham S, Ma R, et al. Molecular determinants mediating gating of Transient Receptor Potential Canonical (TRPC) channels by stromal interaction molecule 1 (STIM1). *J Biol Chem.* 2014; 289: 6372-6382. PMID: 24464579.
34. Petersen OH, Sutton R. Ca^{2+} signalling and pancreatitis: effects of alcohol, bile and coffee. *Trends Pharmacol Sci.* 2006; 27: 113-120. PMID: 16406087.
35. Laukkarinen JM, Van Acker GJ, Weiss ER, Steer ML, Perides G. A mouse model of acute biliary pancreatitis induced by retrograde pancreatic duct infusion of Na-taurocholate. *Gut.* 2007; 56: 1590-1598. PMID: 17591621.
36. Lerch MM, Gorelick FS. Models of acute and chronic pancreatitis. *Gastroenterology.* 2013; 144: 1180-1193. PMID: 23622127.
37. Huang W, Cane MC, Mukherjee R, Szatmary P, Zhang X, Elliott V, et al. Caffeine protects against experimental acute pancreatitis by inhibition of inositol 1,4,5-trisphosphate receptor-mediated Ca^{2+} release. *Gut.* 2015. In press. PMID: 26642860.
38. Toescu EC, O'Neill SC, Petersen OH, Eisner DA. Caffeine inhibits the agonist-evoked cytosolic Ca^{2+} signal in mouse pancreatic acinar cells by blocking inositol trisphosphate production. *J Biol Chem.* 1992; 267: 23467-23470. PMID: 1429689.
39. Bonati M, Latini R, Tognoni G, Young JF, Garattini S. Interspecies comparison of in vivo caffeine pharmacokinetics in man, monkey, rabbit, rat, and mouse. *Drug Metab Rev.* 1984; 15: 1355-1383. PMID: 6543526.
40. Fredholm BB, Battig K, Holmen J, Nehlig A, Zvartau EE. Actions of caffeine in the brain with special reference to factors that contribute to its widespread use. *Pharmacol Rev.* 1999; 51: 83-133. PMID: 10049999.
41. Lerch MM, Halangk W, Mayerle J. Preventing pancreatitis by protecting the mitochondrial permeability transition pore. *Gastroenterology.* 2013; 144: 265-269. PMID: 23260493.
42. Schild L, Matthias R, Stanarius A, Wolf G, Augustin W, Halangk W. Induction of permeability transition in pancreatic mitochondria by cerulein in rats. *Mol Cell Biochem.* 1999; 195: 191-197. PMID: 10395083.
43. Sung KF, Odinokova IV, Mareninova OA, Rakonczay Z Jr, Hegyi P, Pandol SJ, et al. Prosurvival Bcl-2 proteins stabilize pancreatic mitochondria and protect against necrosis in experimental pancreatitis. *Exp Cell Res.* 2009; 315: 1975-1989. PMID: 19331832.
44. Voronina SG, Barrow SL, Simpson AW, Gerasimenko OV, da Silva Xavier G, Rutter GA, et al. Dynamic changes in cytosolic and mitochondrial ATP levels in pancreatic acinar cells. *Gastroenterology.* 2010; 138: 1976-1987. PMID: 20102715.
45. Booth DM, Murphy JA, Mukherjee R, Awais M, Neoptolemos JP, Gerasimenko OV, et al. Reactive oxygen species induced by bile acid induce apoptosis and protect against necrosis in pancreatic acinar cells. *Gastroenterology.* 2011; 140: 2116-2125. PMID: 21354148.
46. Halestrap AP, Richardson AP. The mitochondrial permeability transition: a current perspective on its identity and role in ischaemia/reperfusion injury. *J Mol Cell Cardiol.* 2015; 78: 129-141. PMID: 25179911.
47. Alavian KN, Beutner G, Lazrove E, Sacchetti S, Park HA, Licznerski P, et al. An uncoupling channel within the c-subunit ring of the F1FO ATP synthase is the mitochondrial permeability transition pore. *Proc Natl Acad Sci U S A.* 2014; 111: 10580-10585. PMID: 24979777.
48. Giorgio V, von Stockum S, Antoniel M, Fabbro A, Fogolari F, Forte M, et al. Dimers of mitochondrial ATP synthase form the permeability transition pore. *Proc Natl Acad Sci U S A.* 2013; 110: 5887-5892. PMID: 23530243.
49. Elrod JW, Molkentin JD. Physiologic functions of cyclophilin D and the mitochondrial permeability transition pore. *Circ J.* 2013; 77: 1111-1122. PMID: 23538482.

50. Elrod JW, Wong R, Mishra S, Vagnozzi RJ, Sakthievel B, Goonasekera SA, et al. Cyclophilin D controls mitochondrial pore-dependent Ca^{2+} exchange, metabolic flexibility, and propensity for heart failure in mice. *J Clin Invest*. 2010; 120: 3680-3687. PMID: 20890047.
51. Vandenabeele P, Galluzzi L, Vanden Berghe T, Kroemer G. Molecular mechanisms of necroptosis: an ordered cellular explosion. *Nat Rev Mol Cell Biol*. 2010; 11: 700-714. PMID: 20823910.
52. Mukherjee R, Mareninova OA, Odinokova IV, Huang W, Murphy J, Chvanov M, et al. Mechanism of mitochondrial permeability transition pore induction and damage in the pancreas: inhibition prevents acute pancreatitis by protecting production of ATP. *Gut*. 2016; 65: 1333-1346. PMID: 26071131.
53. Rizzuto R, Pinton P, Carrington W, Fay FS, Fogarty KE, Lifshitz LM, et al. Close contacts with the endoplasmic reticulum as determinants of mitochondrial Ca^{2+} responses. *Science*. 1998; 280: 1763-1766. PMID: 9624056.
54. O'Gara PT, Kushner FG, Ascheim DD, Casey DE Jr, Chung MK, de Lemos JA, et al. 2013 ACCF/AHA guideline for the management of ST-elevation myocardial infarction: a report of the American College of Cardiology Foundation/American Heart Association Task Force on Practice Guidelines. *Circulation*. 2013; 127: e362-425. PMID: 23247304.
55. Naoumov NV. Cyclophilin inhibition as potential therapy for liver diseases. *J Hepatol*. 2014; 6: 1166-1174. PMID: 25048953.
56. Chiari H. Uber die Selbstverdauung des menschlichen Pankreas. *Z Heilk*. 1896; 17: 69-96.
57. Gaiser S, Daniluk J, Liu Y, Tsou L, Chu J, Lee W, et al. Intracellular activation of trypsinogen in transgenic mice induces acute but not chronic pancreatitis. *Gut*. 2011; 60: 1379-1388. PMID: 21471572.
58. Halangk W, Lerch MM, Brandt-Nedelev B, Roth W, Ruthenbuerger M, Reinheckel T, et al. Role of cathepsin B in intracellular trypsinogen activation and the onset of acute pancreatitis. *J Clin Invest*. 2000; 106: 773-781. PMID: 10995788.
59. Saluja A, Saluja M, Villa A, Leli U, Rutledge P, Meldolesi J, et al. Pancreatic duct obstruction in rabbits causes digestive zymogen and lysosomal enzyme colocalization. *J Clin Invest*. 1989; 84: 1260-1266. PMID: 2477393.
60. Mareninova OA, Hermann K, French SW, O'Konski MS, Pandol SJ, Webster P, et al. Impaired autophagic flux mediates acinar cell vacuole formation and trypsinogen activation in rodent models of acute pancreatitis. *J Clin Invest*. 2009; 119: 3340-3355. PMID: 19805911.
61. Sherwood MW, Prior IA, Voronina SG, Barrow SL, Woodsmith JD, Gerasimenko OV, et al. Activation of trypsinogen in large endocytic vacuoles of pancreatic acinar cells. *Proc Natl Acad Sci U S A*. 2007; 104: 5674-5679. PMID: 17363470.
62. Dawra R, Sah RP, Dudeja V, Rishi L, Talukdar R, Garg P, et al. Intra-acinar trypsinogen activation mediates early stages of pancreatic injury but not inflammation in mice with acute pancreatitis. *Gastroenterology*. 2011; 141: 2210-2217. PMID: 21875495.
63. Howes N, Lerch MM, Greenhalf W, Stocken DD, Ellis I, Simon P, et al. Clinical and genetic characteristics of hereditary pancreatitis in Europe. *Clin Gastroenterol Hepatol*. 2004; 2: 252-261. PMID: 15017610.
64. Whitcomb DC, Gorry MC, Preston RA, Furey W, Sossenheimer MJ, Ulrich CD, et al. Hereditary pancreatitis is caused by a mutation in the cationic trypsinogen gene. *Nat Genet*. 1996; 14: 141-145. PMID: 8841182.
65. Sekine S, Kanamaru Y, Koike M, Nishihara A, Okada M, Kinoshita H, et al. Rhomboid protease PARL mediates the mitochondrial membrane potential loss-induced cleavage of PGAM5. *J Biol Chem*. 2012; 287: 34635-34645. PMID: 22915595.
66. Wang Z, Jiang H, Chen S, Du F, Wang X. The mitochondrial phosphatase PGAM5 functions at the convergence point of multiple necrotic death pathways. *Cell*. 2012; 148: 228-243. PMID: 22265414.
67. Navina S, Acharya C, DeLany JP, Orlichenko LS, Baty CJ, Shiva SS, et al. Lipotoxicity causes multisystem organ failure and exacerbates acute pancreatitis in obesity. *Sci Transl Med*. 2011; 3: 107ra110. PMID: 22049070.
68. Simon P, Weiss FU, Zimmer KP, Koch HG, Lerch MM. Acute and chronic pancreatitis in patients with inborn errors of metabolism. *Pancreatology*. 2001; 1: 448-456. PMID: 12120223.
69. Hoque R, Sohail M, Malik A, Sarwar S, Luo Y, Shah A, et al. TLR9 and the NLRP3 inflammasome link acinar cell death with inflammation in acute pancreatitis. *Gastroenterology*. 2011; 141: 358-369. PMID: 21439959.
70. Nakahira K, Haspel JA, Rathinam VA, Lee SJ, Dolinay T, Lam HC, et al. Autophagy proteins regulate innate immune responses by inhibiting the release of mitochondrial DNA mediated by the NALP3 inflammasome. *Nat Immunol*. 2011; 12: 222-230. PMID: 21151103.
71. He S, Wang L, Miao L, Wang T, Du F, Zhao L, et al. Receptor interacting protein kinase-3 determines cellular necrotic response to TNF-alpha. *Cell*. 2009; 137: 1100-1111. PMID: 19524512.
72. Muili KA, Wang D, Orabi AI, Sarwar S, Luo Y, Javed TA, et al. Bile acids induce pancreatic acinar cell injury and pancreatitis by activating calcineurin. *J Biol Chem* 2013; 288: 570-580. PMID: 23148215.
73. Bergmeier W, Weidinger C, Zee I, Feske S. Emerging roles of store-operated Ca^{2+} entry through STIM and ORAI proteins in immunity, hemostasis and cancer. *Channels (Austin)*. 2013; 7: 379-391. PMID: 23511024.
74. Gukovskaya AS, Vaquero E, Zaninovic V, Gorelick FS, Lusis AJ, Brennan ML, et al. Neutrophils and NADPH oxidase mediate intrapancreatic trypsin activation in murine experimental acute pancreatitis. *Gastroenterology*. 2002; 122: 974-984. PMID: 11910350.
75. Choi S, Maleth J, Jha A, Lee KP, Kim MS, So I, et al. The TRPCs-STIM1-Orai interaction. *Handb Exp Pharmacol*. 2014; 223: 1035-1054. PMID: 24961979.
76. Mekahli D, Bultynck G, Parys JB, De Smedt H, Missiaen L. Endoplasmic-reticulum calcium depletion and disease. *Cold Spring Harb Perspect Biol*. 2011; 3. PMID: 21441595.
77. Demetrius L, Legendre S, Harremoes P. Evolutionary entropy: a predictor of body size, metabolic rate and

maximal life span. *Bull Math Biol*. 2009; 71: 800-818. PMID: 19172360.

78. Spanier BW, Nio Y, van der Hulst RW, Tuynman HA, Dijkgraaf MG, Bruno MJ. Practice and yield of early CT scan in acute pancreatitis: a Dutch Observational Multicenter Study. *Pancreatology*. 2010; 10: 222-228. PMID: 20484959.
79. Odinokova IV, Sung KF, Mareninova OA, Hermann K, Evtodienko Y, Andreyev A, et al. Mechanisms regulating cytochrome c release in pancreatic mitochondria. *Gut*. 2009; 58: 431-442. PMID: 18596195.
80. Jauch EC, Saver JL, Adams HP, Jr., Bruno A, Connors JJ, Demaerschalk BM, et al. Guidelines for the early management of patients with acute ischemic stroke: a guideline for healthcare professionals from the American Heart Association/American Stroke Association. *Stroke*. 2013; 44: 870-947. PMID: 23370205.
81. Fonarow GC, Zhao X, Smith EE, Saver JL, Reeves MJ, Bhatt DL, et al. Door-to-needle times for tissue plasminogen activator administration and clinical outcomes in acute ischemic stroke before and after a quality improvement initiative. *JAMA*. 2014; 311: 1632-1640. PMID: 24756513.
82. Villatoro E, Mulla M, Larvin M. Antibiotic therapy for prophylaxis against infection of pancreatic necrosis in acute pancreatitis. *Cochrane Database Syst Rev*. 2010; 5: CD002941. PMID: 20464721.
83. Bradley EL, 3rd. A clinically based classification system for acute pancreatitis. Summary of the International Symposium on Acute Pancreatitis, Atlanta, Ga, September 11 through 13, 1992. *Arch Surg*. 1993; 128: 586-590. PMID: 8489394.
84. Banks PA, Bollen TL, Dervenis C, Gooszen HG, Johnson CD, Sarr MG, et al. Classification of acute pancreatitis–2012: revision of the Atlanta classification and definitions by international consensus. *Gut*. 2013; 62: 102-111. PMID: 23100216.
85. Dellinger EP, Forsmark CE, Layer P, Levy P, Maravi-Poma E, Petrov MS, et al. Determinant-based classification of acute pancreatitis severity: an international multidisciplinary consultation. *Ann Surg*. 2012; 256: 875-880. PMID: 22735715.

Chapter 4

Role of trypsinogen activation in genesis of pancreatitis

Ajay Dixit, Rajinder K. Dawra, Vikas Dudeja, and Ashok K. Saluja*

Department of Surgery, Miller School of Medicine, University of Miami, Miami FL.

Introduction

Pancreatitis is an inflammatory disease of the pancreas that starts in pancreatic acinar cells and results in significant morbidity and mortality.[1] More than a century ago, the pathologist Dr. Hans Chiari proposed that the acute pancreatitis (AP) is a disease rather than an infection, in which the pancreas destroys itself through autodigestion.[2] Since then, elucidating the mechanism, site, and importance of premature activation of digestive enzymes, especially trypsin, have become major areas of investigation in AP pathobiology. Premature activation of trypsin has been observed both *in vitro* hyperstimulation and in animal models of AP.[3-7] In this review, we discuss our current understanding of the role of trypsin in the pancreatitis pathophysiology.

Physiology of trypsinogen in health

Trypsin is synthesized as trypsinogen, an inactive precursor, in the rough endoplasmic reticulum (ER) and transported to the Golgi apparatus for sorting. Trypsinogen is always cosynthesized and packed with a pancreatic secretory trypsin inhibitor (PSTI) that inhibits its premature activation. Once, it reaches the Golgi system, trypsinogen and other digestive enzymes condense into core particles and are packed in zymogen granules. The condensed enzymes are stable, and minimal activation happens within the zymogen granules. Once acini receive secretory stimuli, these zymogen granules are released in to the lumen of the pancreatic duct, which carries the digestive enzymes into the duodenum. Once there, enteropeptidase activates trypsinogen by removing 7-10 amino acid from the N-terminal region known as trypsinogen activation peptide (TAP). Removal of TAP induces a conformational change that results in active trypsin. TAP is immunologically distinct from the same sequence within trypsinogen, thereby allowing detection of trypsinogen activation in situ.[8,9]

Intra-acinar location of trypsin activation during AP

While it is clear that intra-acinar trypsin activation occurs, the exact intracellular location where trypsin is activated is a hotly debated area in pancreatitis research. Subcellular fractionation and analysis of pancreatic homogenate shortly after pancreatitis induction have provided insight about the location of trypsinogen activation. *In vitro* studies of acinar cells showed that within 30 min of hyperstimulation, most of the active trypsin localizes to a heavy, zymogen-rich pellet; after 60 min of hyperstimulation, trypsin activity shifts to the supernatant. This shift is paralleled by appearance of immunoreactive TAP and cathepsin B, a lysosomal enzyme capable of activating trypsinogen, in the soluble fraction.[10] This experimental evidence led to development of the "colocalization hypothesis," which purports that lysosomal enzymes and zymogens fuse to form structures termed "colocalization organelles" during AP. It has been proposed that lysosomal enzyme cathepsin B activates trypsinogen to trypsin inside these colocalization organelles. Studies have shown that premature trypsinogen activation occurs in membrane-bound compartments resembling autophagic vesicles formed in association with the colocalization of zymogen and lysosomes.[5] In these colocalized vacuoles, the lysosomal protease cathepsin B activates trypsinogen. Hypothetically, active trypsin further activates other digestive enzymes within acinar cells, presumably in the same manner as normally occurs in the duodenum. These colocalization vacuoles have been observed in all models of experimental pancreatitis, as well as in pathological specimens of human pancreatitis. Studies that have demonstrated that cathepsin B can activate trypsinogen *in vitro* further support this theory.[11,12] It seems that <1% of the trypsinogen peptide is hydrolyzed in the absence of cathepsin B, but after incubation with cathepsin B for 30 min at pH 5, 96% of trypsinogen peptide was hydrolyzed.[11] Interestingly, cathepsin B-mediated trypsinogen activation does not seem to be a crucial pathogenic step in hereditary

*Corresponding author. Email: asaluja@miami.edu

pancreatitis patients with the D22G and K23R trypsinogen mutations.[11]

Role of trypsin during AP

For decades, intra-acinar trypsin activation has been considered to be the key event in AP, and this trypsin-centric hypothesis is supported by various observations. Inhibition of trypsin, by somewhat nonspecific protease inhibitors, provides protection against injury during AP.[13,14] Furthermore, limiting trypsinogen activation by inhibiting the activity of cathepsin B or deleting the cathepsin B gene also decreases pancreatic injury during AP, again suggesting that trypsinogen activation is important for pancreatic damage.[13,15] Halangk et al. showed that cathepsin B knock out (KO) mice have less necrosis compared to wild-type (WT) mice.[15] However, the degree of leukocyte infiltration in the pancreas or lungs during pancreatitis was not affected by the absence of cathepsin B, indicating that cathepsin B, and thus trypsin act independent of local and systemic inflammation.

The strongest support for the trypsin-centric theory is the identification of mutations in the cationic trypsinogen gene *PRSS1* in hereditary pancreatitis, an uncommon form of pancreatitis with autosomal dominant inheritance.[16] *In vitro* biochemical studies of pancreatitis-associated p.R122H mutations of human cationic trypsinogen showed that this trypsinogen variant has an increased propensity for auto-activation and is resistant to degradation by chymotrypsin C.[17] However, this mutation is not exclusively activating; it has pleiotropic effects, and there is no direct evidence for increased intracellular trypsin activity in patients with hereditary pancreatitis due to this mutation.[18] Furthermore, these patients experience episodic attacks rather than continuous disease. In a mouse model of hereditary pancreatitis generated by transgenic expression of R122H trypsinogen, no increased trypsinogen activation was observed, again indicating the involvement of other factors. The R122H mutation has been shown to increase the frequency of trypsin auto-activation.[18-20] An investigation of another *PRSS1* mutant (p.R116C) revealed an entirely novel mechanism of acinar cell injury that is unrelated to trypsinogen activation. The mutation induces proenzyme misfolding, leading to ER stress and unfolded protein response (UPR) activation.[20] The trypsinogen activation hypothesis of hereditary pancreatitis also does not explain incomplete penetrance, the intermittent nature of the disease, and lack of progression to chronic pancreatitis (CP) in some individuals despite recurrent episodes. While emerging epidemiologic and genetic data continue to link pancreatitis to trypsinogen activation, it is becoming increasingly clear that with the exception of hereditary pancreatitis and cystic fibrosis, a direct simplistic genetic mechanism for AP may not exist. Rather, it is likely that a complex interplay between genetic, environmental, and developmental factors influences pancreatitis susceptibility and severity.

Evaluating the role of trypsin activation, Gaiser et al. showed that expression of active trypsin in pancreas was sufficient for AP induction.[19] Indeed, moderate to low constitutive expression of rat anionic trypsinogen *PRSS2* in acini was sufficient to induce pancreatitis. Though the study diverged from the known pattern of transient to high-level trypsin activation, which is an important limitation of this model, the conclusions provide additional support for the role of trypsin activation in pancreatitis pathogenesis.[19] However, this overexpression model is somewhat artificial and lacks the stimuli and other intra-acinar processes observed during AP. Contrary to these findings, a study by Wartmann et al. reported that cathepsin L KO mice have much higher trypsinogen activation but significantly reduced pancreatic injury, suggesting that trypsinogen activation may even have a protective role during pancreatitis by degrading trypsinogen and other proteases.[21]

To obtain further insight into the role of trypsin in AP, we generated a novel KO mouse lacking trypsinogen isoform-7 (T7, mouse paralog of human cationic trypsinogen, *PRSS1*).[22] In this mouse strain, we do not observe intra-acinar pathologic trypsin activation during AP, suggesting that T7 is responsible for pathologic trypsin activation. Intriguingly, in these novel KO mice ($T^{-/-}$), we observed that acinar cell necrosis during caerulein- (**Figure 1A**) and L-arginine-induced AP is reduced to about half of that observed in mice with intact T7.[22] *In vitro*, we noted that acini lacking T7 do not undergo necrosis (as measured by lactate dehydrogenase [LDH] release) when stimulated by a supramaximal dose of caerulein. Furthermore, we observed that nuclear factor (NF)-κB activation and local or systemic inflammation are not altered by the absence of trypsin (**Figure 1B-C**).[22] Collectively, these data suggest that trypsin is only partly responsible for acinar cell necrosis observed during AP, and local and systemic inflammation is independent of trypsin. One could also extrapolate this to suggest that inflammatory cells and mediators are responsible for acinar cell injury observed in the absence of trypsin. The fact that markers of local and systemic injury during pancreatitis were not affected by the absence of trypsinogen activation underscores the importance of under-appreciated trypsin-independent events in AP.[23]

Therefore, it is likely that trypsin is only required to initiate injury and trypsin-independent inflammatory pathways (importantly NF-κB) that determine disease progression and severity.

Mechanism by which trypsin leads to acinar cell injury

We recently evaluated the mechanism by which trypsin induces cell death in acinar cells and observed that trypsin makes colocalized vesicles fragile, which causes cathepsin

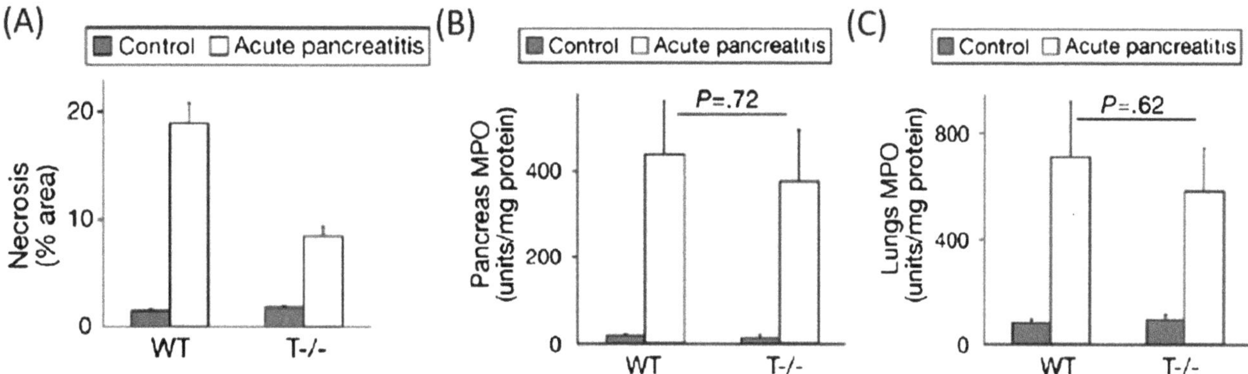

Figure 1. Trypsin contributes partially to acinar cell necrosis during AP. Local and systemic inflammation during AP are independent of trypsin activation. AP was induced by repeated injections caerulein (50 μg/kg intraperitoneally. every hour for 10 h). A) Quantification of necrosis by morphometry. B) Quantification of neutrophil infiltration (MPO) as a measure of inflammation in the pancreas and C) lung MPO as a measure of lung inflammation. Modified from Dawra et al.[22]

B to escape into the cytosol, which in turn causes cell death during pancreatitis.[24] Supramaximal stimulation by caerulein causes cathepsin B leakage into the cytoplasm (**Figure 2A**). This release is dependent on trypsin, as in its absence either in $T^{-/-}$ mice or by pharmacologic inhibition of trypsin (**Figure 2B**), cathepsin B release into the cytosol during AP was prevented. These data suggest that active trypsin within the colocalized organelles plays a role in making the membranes fragile and thus prone to leakage. Furthermore, only small amounts of cathepsin B, amylase, active trypsin, and arylsulfatase are released from the colocalized organelles into the cytosol. This suggests, as we previously observed, that only a portion of lysosomes and zymogen granules come together and colocalize. The factors that determine which colocalized organelles become leaky and release their contents into the cytosol are not known and will be studied in future investigations.

Supramaximal caerulein stimulation leads to apoptosis that can be prevented by pretreatment with cathepsin B and trypsin inhibitors, suggesting roles of both cathepsin B and trypsin in acinar cell apoptosis (**Figure 2C**). However, when cathepsin B or trypsin was added to permeabilized acini to simulate the presence of cathepsin B or trypsin in the cytosol, dose-dependent activation of apoptosis was seen in the presence of cytosolic cathepsin B but not trypsin (**Figure 2D**).[24] This suggests a role of cytosolic cathepsin B but not trypsin in acinar cell apoptosis induction. These observations are supported by similar findings from experiments using $T^{-/-}$ and cathepsin B KO animals.[24] The most logical inference from these studies is that active trypsin within the colocalized organelles is involved in making the organelles "leaky," causing cathepsin B to enter the cytosol where the newly released cathepsin B activates apoptotic pathways. Inhibition of trypsin prevents the colocalized organelles from becoming fragile, thereby preventing cathepsin B release into the cytosol. Exogenous trypsin failed to activate caspase when incubated with streptolysin-O-permeabilized acinar cells, suggesting that trypsin does not directly cause acinar cell death.

Extrinsic and intrinsic pathways are two major routes through which apoptosis occurs. The extrinsic pathway involves death receptors and is activated in response to external signals, whereas the intrinsic pathway involves mitochondria and occurs in response to internal signals. Lysosomal disruption has been implicated in initiating the intrinsic apoptotic pathway involving cleavage of the pro-apoptotic Bcl-2 family member Bid. Upon apoptotic stimuli, Bcl-2 apoptosis-promoting protein Bax undergoes a conformational change and translocates to mitochondria, where it oligomerizes and forms pores that allow cytochrome c release into cytoplasm. It has also been shown that in early stages of experimental AP, there is a release of cytochrome c into the cytosol that in turn activates caspase-9, which subsequently leads to caspase-3 activation. Caspase-3 then executes intracellular apoptotic events via different downstream mediators.[25]

Our studies suggest that during acinar cell death, cathepsin B is released into the cytosol and induces apoptosis predominantly via the intrinsic pathway by inducing Bid cleavage and Bax activation. Truncated Bid and activated Bax cause release of cytochrome c from mitochondria, which leads to caspase-3 activation and acinar cell apoptosis. This cathepsin B-induced apoptosis was fully inhibited in acini pretreated with CA074-me (**Figure 2C**). Moreover, the reduction of cytosolic cytochrome c after pretreatment with a cytochrome c antibody reduced cathepsin B-triggered acinar cell apoptosis, again indicating apoptosis via the intrinsic pathway.[24]

Interestingly, the amount of cathepsin B in the cytosol determines whether acinar cell die via apoptosis or necrosis. A small amount of cathepsin B activates apoptosis, whereas larger amounts shift the cell toward the necrotic

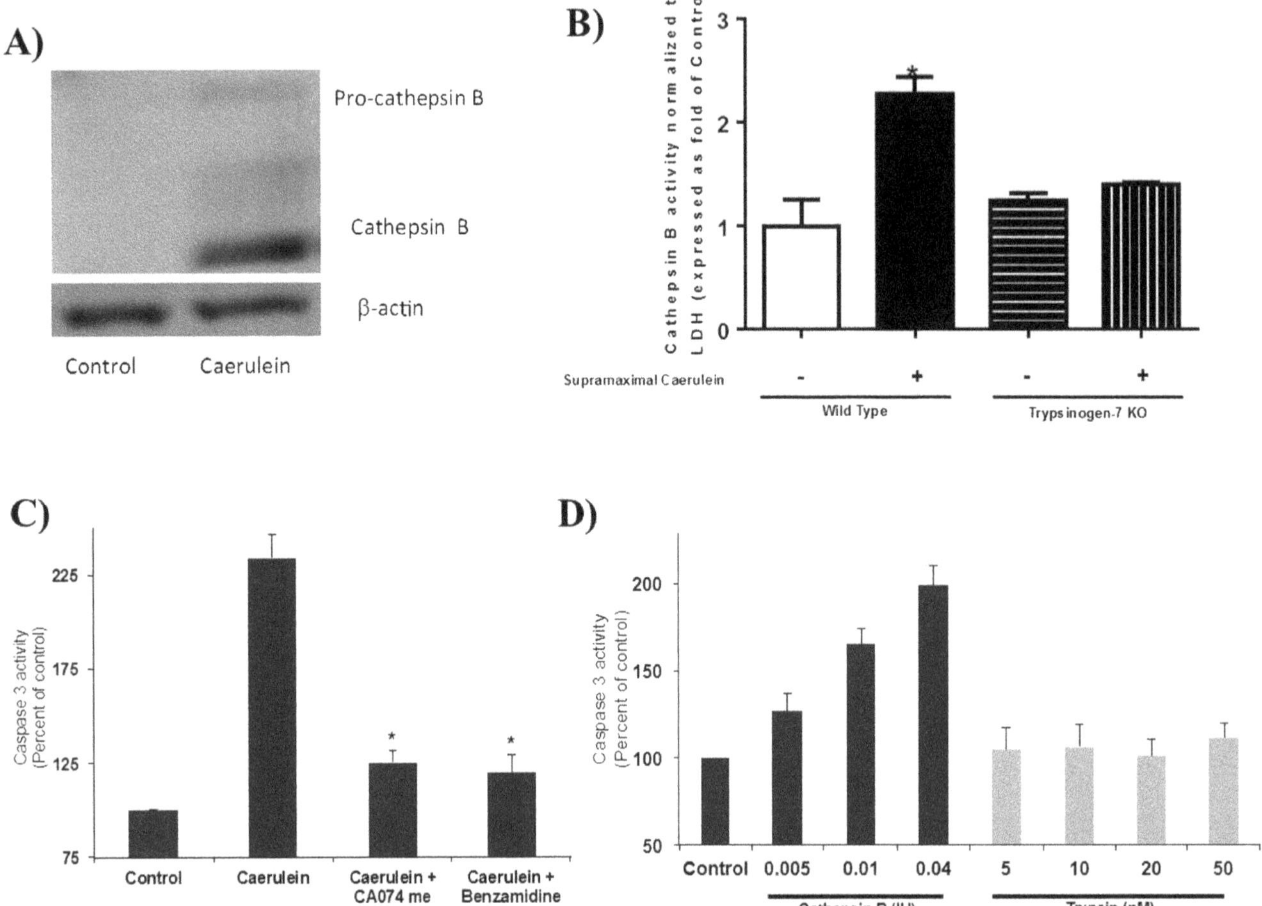

Figure 2. (A) Supramaximal caerulein stimulation increases cytosolic cathepsin B levels in acinar cells. (B) Cytosolic cathepsin B activity normalized to LDH is increased in pancreatic acinar cell treated with supramaximal caerulein. A similar increase was not observed in $T^{-/-}$ mice, suggesting that trypsin activity is required for cathepsin B release into the cytosol. (C) Caspase-3 activity in control acinar cells and those treated with supramaximal caerulein alone or with CA047 or benzamidine. (D) Addition of exogenous cathepsin B but not trypsin to SLO permeabilized normal rat pancreatic acinar cells and led to caspase-3 activation. Caspase-3 activity was induced by cathepsin B in a concentration-dependent manner, and no activity was seen with any trypsin dose. Values are expressed as percent of total and normalized to per mg protein. Modified from Talukdar et al.[24]

pathway. Necrosis is a form of cell death involving organelle swelling and plasma membrane rupture. Necrosis was once considered accidental cell death caused by overwhelming physical or chemical trauma. However, we now know that specific genes can induce necrosis in a regulated manner. The terms programmed necrosis, necroptosis, and regulated necrosis have been used to distinguish these types of cell death from accidental necrosis. Receptor-interacting protein 3 (RIP-3) is an important regulator of necroptosis. Upon activation, RIP-3 forms a complex with receptor activating kinase 1 (RIP-1). This complex activates a cascade of events that eventually lead to cell necrosis.[26] The leakage of a large amount of cathepsin B following acinar cell hyperstimulation leads to RIP-1/RIP-3 complex formation, which shifts the form of death from apoptosis to necrosis. In the future, studies designed to elucidate the key molecules favoring RIP-1/RIP-3 complex formation and downstream events in AP pathogenesis may help clarify what determines apoptosis versus necrosis during AP.

Besides premature trypsinogen activation, intra-acinar NF-κB activation was previously shown to result in local pancreatic damage and systemic inflammation.[27,28] NF-κB-related injury was persistent in acinar cells even in the absence of trypsin in $T^{-/-}$ mice, suggesting its trypsin-independent role in acinar cell injury. Although activation of other inflammatory cascades has been described in AP and may theoretically lead to trypsin- and NF-κB-independent injury, which need to explored in further studies, these pathways are generally known to be minor players compared to NF-κB signaling.

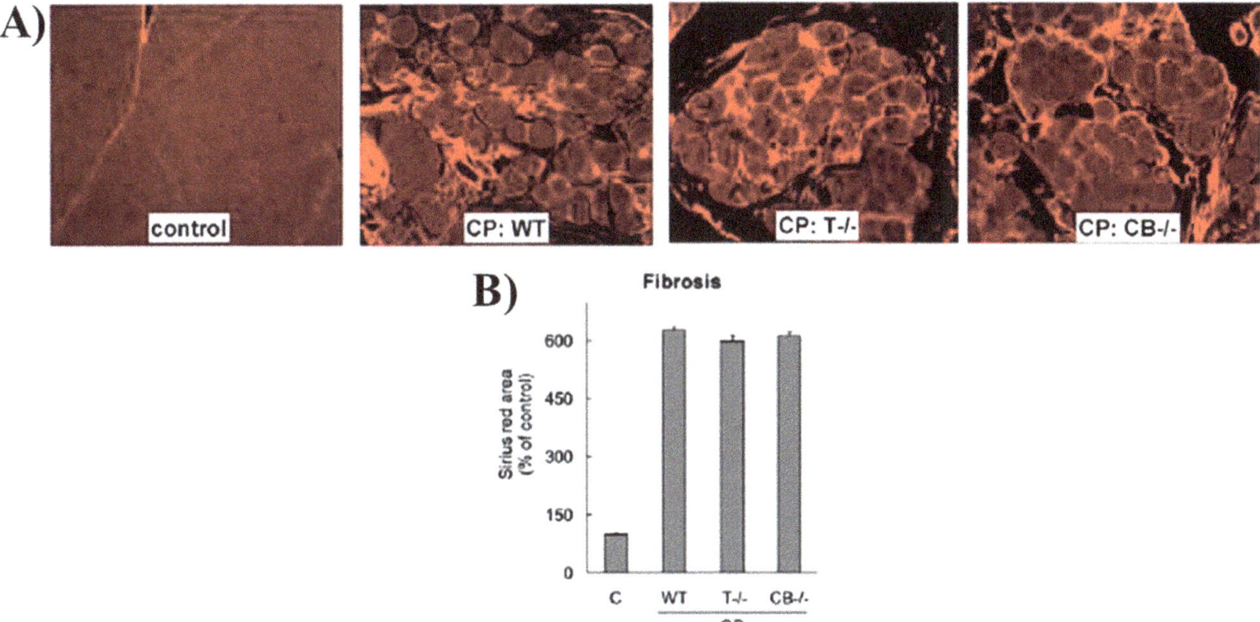

Figure 3. CP severity is not modulated by absence of trypsin. (A) Representative pictures of CP showing acinar fibrosis in WT, $T^{-/-}$, and $CB^{-/-}$ CP groups. Fibrosis was detected by Sirius red staining. (B) Quantification of Sirius red staining indicates comparable fibrosis in WT, $T^{-/-}$, and $CB^{-/-}$ CP groups. Modified from Sah et al.[32]

Soluble inflammatory cell mediators like tumor necrosis factor-α, which is a product of the activated NF-κB pathway, were shown to directly induce premature trypsinogen activation and necrosis in pancreatic acinar cells, suggesting a contribution of inflammatory signaling in disease initiation and progression.[29] Thus, NF-κB activation may also be the key early event responsible for progression of systemic injury. This supposition was further supported by another important study that demonstrated a partial reduction in acinar necrosis during pancreatitis in mice lacking the p50 unit of NF-κB ($p50^{-/-}$).[30] Gukovskaya et al. observed that neutrophils recruited during inflammation were able to activate trypsin in acinar cell, and this was dependent on neutrophil NAPDH oxidase,[31] suggesting involvement of immune cells like neutrophils in further promoting acinar cell injury.

Role of trypsin in CP

Using our $T^{-/-}$ mice we have also explored the role of trypsin in CP.[32] Using the caerulein model of CP we found comparable levels of acinar cell damage and fibrosis (**Figure 3**)

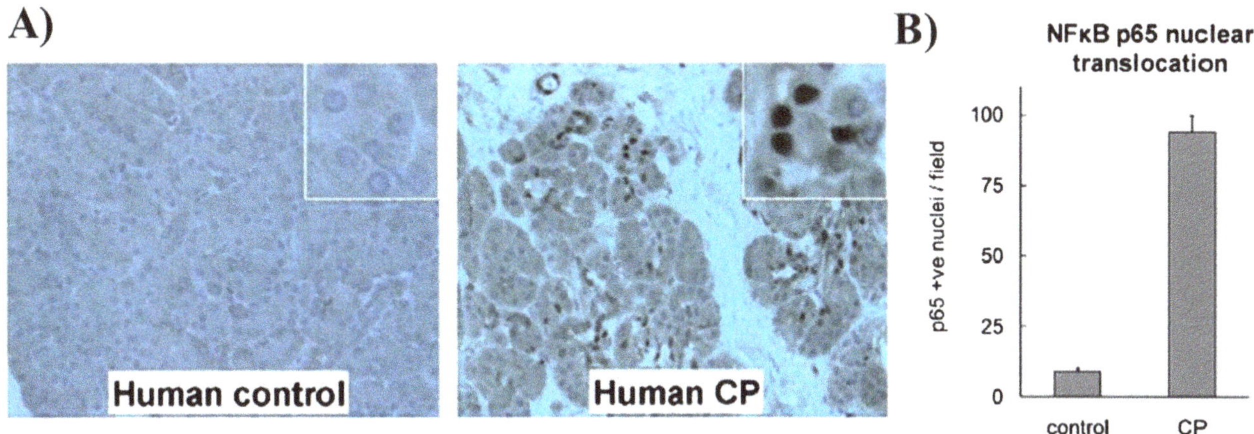

Figure 4. NF-kB activation in human CP samples. (A) Persistent NF-κB activation is observed in human CP. NF-κB component protein p65 immunostaining shows its nuclear localization in acinar cells in human CP sections (200×) (insets: zoomed-in views showing nucleus from acinar cells showing positive stain for p65). (B) The nuclear stain was quantified and represented here. Pancreas sections from seven CP patients and seven controls were analyzed. Modified from Sah et al.[32]

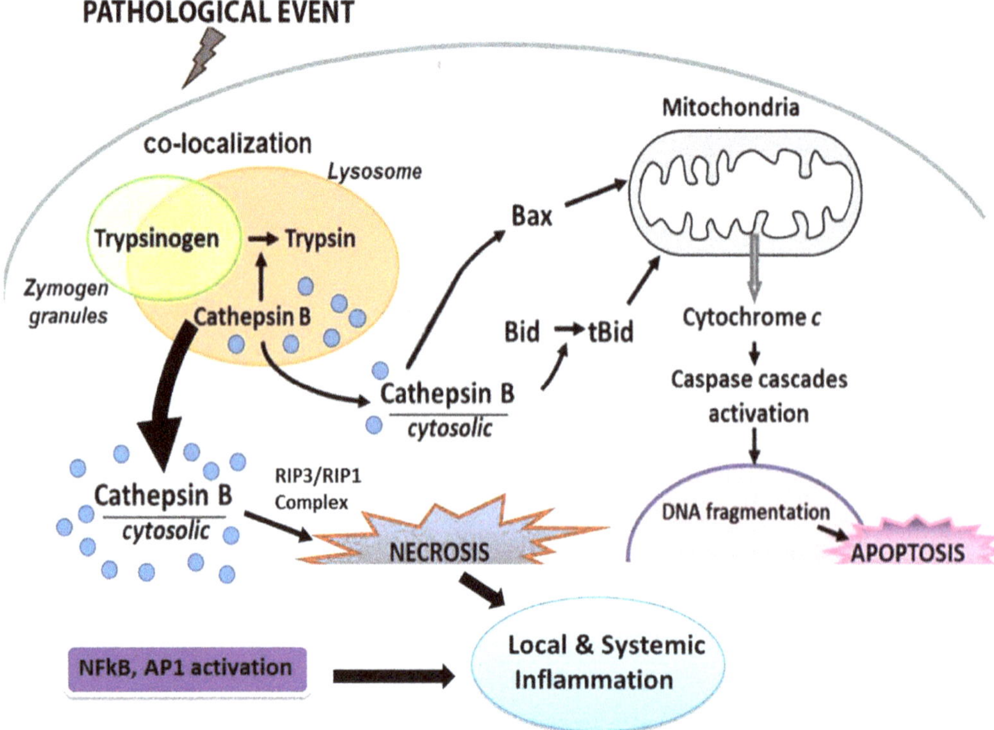

Figure 5. Schematic representation of major pathophysiologic events in pancreatitis.

in $T^{-/-}$ and WT C57BL/6 mice, suggesting trypsin-independent activation of acinar necrosis and stellate cell activation in CP. We further looked at T cell infiltration and NF-κB activation and found that it was comparable in both $T^{-/-}$ and WT. [32] Taken together, these findings support the hypothesis that persistent inflammation, possibly driven by NF-κB-dependent pathways, can lead to CP even in absence of trypsin. We further verified this in human CP samples, and all tested samples had high NF-κB activity (**Figure 4**).

Pancreatic acinar cells contain protein-synthesizing machinery for secretory proteins, and any stress leading to disturbance in cellular homeostasis can cause ER stress which can then activate evolutionarily conserved UPR pathways. A study from our group showed that during acinar cell injury there is ER stress and UPR activation as evidenced by upregulation of UPR components like CHOP, ATF-4, GRP-78, and XBP-1 during caerulein-induced CP. However, $T^{-/-}$ that lack intra-acinar trypsinogen activation show comparable levels of ER stress and activation of UPR, suggesting a minimal role of trypsin in causing ER stress during CP.[33]

In conclusion, different genetic mouse models of trypsin overexpression or lacking trypsinogen activation have produced exciting results that challenge the century-old trypsin-centered theory of pancreatitis. Our current understanding of AP pathogenesis is depicted in **Figure 5**. No doubt trypsin is important for disease initiation, however, its contribution to the disease mechanism has been overestimated. The use of trypsin protease inhibitors in clinical practice fails to provide any resolution for SAP patients.[34] It is becoming increasingly clear that cathepsin B release, NF-κB signaling, and ER stress in acinar cells are all crucial to pancreatitis pathogenesis and could be important drug targets for pancreatitis.

References

1. Pandol SJ, Saluja AK, Imrie CW, Banks PA. Acute pancreatitis: bench to the bedside. *Gastroenterology*. 2007; 132: 1127-1151. PMID: 17383433.
2. Chiari H. Über die Selbstverdauung des menschlichen Pankreas. *Zeitschrift für Heilkunde*. 1896; 17: 69-96.
3. Lerch MM, Gorelick FS. Early trypsinogen activation in acute pancreatitis. *Med Clin North Am*. 2000; 84: 549-563, viii. PMID: 10872413.
4. Mithöfer K, Fernández-del Castillo C, Rattner D, Warshaw AL. Subcellular kinetics of early trypsinogen activation in acute rodent pancreatitis. *Am J Physiol*. 1998; 274: G71-G79. PMID: 9458775.
5. Saluja A, Hashimoto S, Saluja M, Powers RE, Meldolesi J, Steer ML. Subcellular redistribution of lysosomal enzymes during caerulein-induced pancreatitis. *Am J Physiol*. 1987; 253: G508-G516. PMID: 2821825.
6. Saluja A, Saluja M, Villa A, Leli U, Rutledge P, Meldolesi J, et al. Pancreatic duct obstruction in rabbits causes digestive

zymogen and lysosomal enzyme colocalization. *J Clin Invest.* 1989; 84: 1260-1266. PMID: 2477393.

7. Saluja AK, Bhagat L, Lee HS, Bhatia M, Frossard JL, Steer ML. Secretagogue-induced digestive enzyme activation and cell injury in rat pancreatic acini. *Am J Physiol Gastrointest Liver Physiol.* 1999; 276: G835-G842. PMID: 10198325.
8. Abita JP, Delaage M, Lazdunski M. The mechanism of activation of trypsinogen. The role of the four N-terminal aspartyl residues. *Eur J Biochem.* 1969; 8: 314-324. PMID: 5816755.
9. Go VLW, DiMagno EP, Gardner JD, Lebenthal E, Reber HA, Scheele GA, eds. *The Pancreas: Biology, Pathobiology, and Disease*. New York, NY: Raven Press; 1993.
10. Hofbauer B, Saluja AK, Lerch MM, Bhagat L, Bhatia M, Lee HS, et al. Intra-acinar cell activation of trypsinogen during caerulein-induced pancreatitis in rats. *Am J Physiol Gastrointest Liver Physiol.* 1998; 275: G352-G362. PMID: 9688663.
11. Teich N, Bodeker H, Keim V. Cathepsin B cleavage of the trypsinogen activation peptide. *BMC Gastroenterol.* 2002; 2: 16. PMID: 12102727.
12. Saluja AK, Donovan EA, Yamanaka K, Yamaguchi Y, Hofbauer B, Steer ML. Caerulein-induced in vitro activation of trypsinogen in rat pancreatic acini is mediated by cathepsin B. *Gastroenterology.* 1997; 113: 304-310. PMID: 9207291.
13. Van Acker GJ, Saluja AK, Bhagat L, Singh VP, Song AM, Steer ML. Cathepsin B inhibition prevents trypsinogen activation and reduces pancreatitis severity. *Am J Physiol Gastrointest Liver Physiol.* 2002; 283: G794-G800. PMID: 12181196.
14. Van Acker GJ, Weiss E, Steer ML, Perides G. Cause-effect relationships between zymogen activation and other early events in secretagogue-induced acute pancreatitis. *Am J Physiol Gastrointest Liver Physiol.* 2007; 292: G1738-G1746. PMID: 17332471.
15. Halangk W, Lerch MM, Brandt-Nedelev B, Roth W, Ruthenbuerger M, Reinheckel T, et al. Role of cathepsin B in intracellular trypsinogen activation and the onset of acute pancreatitis. *J Clin Invest.* 2000; 106: 773-781. PMID: 10995788.
16. Whitcomb DC, Gorry MC, Preston RA, Furey W, Sossenheimer MJ, Ulrich CD, et al. Hereditary pancreatitis is caused by a mutation in the cationic trypsinogen gene. *Nat Genet.* 1996; 14: 141-145. PMID: 8841182.
17. Teich N, Rosendahl J, Tóth M, Mössner J, Sahin-Tóth M. Mutations of human cationic trypsinogen (PRSS1) and chronic pancreatitis. *Hum Mutat.* 2006; 27: 721-730. PMID: 16791840.
18. Archer H, Jura N, Keller J, Jacobson M, Bar-Sagi D. A mouse model of hereditary pancreatitis generated by transgenic expression of R122H trypsinogen. *Gastroenterology.* 2006; 131: 1844-1855. PMID: 17087933.
19. Gaiser S, Daniluk J, Liu Y, Tsou L, Chu J, Lee W, et al. Intracellular activation of trypsinogen in transgenic mice induces acute but not chronic pancreatitis. *Gut.* 2011; 60: 1379-1388. PMID: 21471572.
20. Kereszturi E, Szmola R, Kukor Z, Simon P, Weiss FU, Lerch MM, et al. Hereditary pancreatitis caused by mutation-induced misfolding of human cationic trypsinogen: a novel disease mechanism. *Hum Mutat.* 2009; 30(4): 575-582. PMID: 19191323.
21. Wartmann T, Mayerle J, Kähne T, Sahin-Tóth M, Ruthenbürger M, Matthias R, et al. Cathepsin L inactivates human trypsinogen, whereas cathepsin L-deletion reduces the severity of pancreatitis in mice. *Gastroenterology.* 2010; 138: 726-737. PMID: 19900452.
22. Dawra R, Sah RP, Dudeja V, Rishi L, Talukdar R, Garg P, et al. Intra-acinar trypsinogen activation mediates early stages of pancreatic injury but not inflammation in mice with acute pancreatitis. *Gastroenterology.* 2011; 141: 2210-2217. PMID: 21875495.
23. Hietaranta AJ, Saluja AK, Bhagat L, Singh VP, Song AM, Steer ML. Relationship between NF-kappaB and trypsinogen activation in rat pancreas after supramaximal caerulein stimulation. *Biochem Biophys Res Commun.* 2001; 280: 388-395. PMID: 11162528.
24. Talukdar R, Sareen A, Zhu H, Yuan Z, Dixit A, Cheema H, et al. Release of cathepsin-B in cytosol causes cell death in acute pancreatitis. *Gastroenterology.* 2016 Aug 9. [Epub ahead of print] PMID: 27519471.
25. Elmore S. Apoptosis: a review of programmed cell death. *Toxicol Pathol.* 2007; 35: 495-516. PMID: 17562483.
26. Moriwaki K, Chan FK. RIP3: a molecular switch for necrosis and inflammation. *Genes Dev.* 2013; 27: 1640-1649. PMID: 23913919.
27. Baumann B, Wagner M, Aleksic T, von Wichert G, Weber CK, Adler G, et al. Constitutive IKK2 activation in acinar cells is sufficient to induce pancreatitis in vivo. *J Clin Invest.* 2007; 117: 1502-1513. PMID: 17525799.
28. Chen X, Ji B, Han B, Ernst SA, Simeone D, Logsdon CD. NF-kappaB activation in pancreas induces pancreatic and systemic inflammatory response. *Gastroenterology.* 2002; 122: 448-457. PMID: 11832459.
29. Sendler M, Dummer A, Weiss FU, Kruger B, Wartmann T, Scharffetter-Kochanek K, et al. Tumour necrosis factor alpha secretion induces protease activation and acinar cell necrosis in acute experimental pancreatitis in mice. *Gut.* 2013; 62: 430-439. PMID: 22490516.
30. Altavilla D, Famulari C, Passaniti M, Galeano M, Macri A, Seminara P, et al. Attenuated caerulein-induced pancreatitis in nuclear factor-kappaB-deficient mice. *Lab Invest.* 2003; 83: 1723-1732. PMID: 14691290.
31. Gukovskaya AS, Vaquero E, Zaninovic V, Gorelick FS, Lusis AJ, Brennan ML, et al. Neutrophils and NADPH oxidase mediate intrapancreatic trypsin activation in murine experimental acute pancreatitis. *Gastroenterology.* 2002; 122: 974-984. PMID: 11910350.
32. Sah RP, Dudeja V, Dawra RK, Saluja AK. Caerulein-induced chronic pancreatitis does not require intra-acinar activation of trypsinogen in mice. *Gastroenterology.* 2013; 144: 1076-1085. PMID: 23354015.
33. Sah RP, Garg SK, Dixit AK, Dudeja V, Dawra RK, Saluja AK. Endoplasmic reticulum stress is chronically activated in chronic pancreatitis. *J Biol Chem.* 2014; 289: 27551-27561. PMID: 25077966.
34. Singh VP, Chari ST. Protease inhibitors in acute pancreatitis: lessons from the bench and failed clinical trials. *Gastroenterology.* 2005; 128: 2172-2174. PMID: 15940654.

Chapter 5

The role of cytokines and inflammation in the genesis of experimental pancreatitis

Peter Szatmary[1*] and Ilya Gukovsky[2*]

[1]*NIHR Liverpool Pancreas Biomedical Research Unit and Department of Cellular and Molecular Physiology, University of Liverpool, UK;* [2]*David Geffen School of Medicine, University of California at Los Angeles and VA Greater Los Angeles, CA, USA.*

Introduction

Pancreatic acinar cell injury triggers the synthesis and release of pro-inflammatory cytokines and chemokines.[1-5] Together with damage-associated molecular patterns (DAMPs) such as histones, high-mobility group box1 protein (HMGB1) and ATP[6] released by acinar cell death, this initiates an acute, sterile inflammatory response,[7] in a manner that shares similarities with the molecular/signaling events observed in sepsis.[8] The resulting early cellular response, consisting of glandular infiltration by neutrophils and monocytes, appears to exacerbate pancreatic injury and is at least in part responsible for early onset organ failure seen in some cases of acute pancreatitis (AP).[9,10] The clinical significance of these events is highlighted by the utility of cytokine measurements in predicting outcome in human AP.[11] Inflammation is either self-limiting or self-perpetuating resulting in significant organ necrosis. Several days to weeks into the disease, development of immune anergy—or compensatory anti-inflammatory response syndrome—has been described in patients,[12] associated with infection of pancreatic necrosis and multisystem organ failure. There are important differences in the immunological response to pancreatitis observed in humans and in experimental models[13]; however, animal and cell models remain critical in furthering our understanding of molecular mechanisms, signaling pathways, and new drug targets. This review describes the roles of key cytokines and chemokines in commonly used experimental models of pancreatitis and how the cytokine profile is affected by model choice. Where relevant, we present and compare quantitative data reported in various models.

Tissue injury and inflammatory cell recruitment

Tissue injury caused by pancreatitis toxins leads to the release of DAMPs: nuclear proteins (e.g., histones and HMGB1), nuclear and mitochondrial DNA, heat shock proteins, and ATP.[6,14] Nuclear proteins in particular can be measured in plasma as early as 4 h after induction of experimental AP.[15,16] These act via common immune sensors and mediators to initiate sterile inflammation.[17] Other mechanisms whereby injured pancreatic acinar cells trigger the inflammatory response is through synthesis and release of cytokines[1] and chemokines,[18] and upregulation of adhesion molecules such as the intercellular adhesion molecule-1 (ICAM-1),[19] which together promote neutrophil and monocyte infiltration[20,21] and exacerbate tissue injury.[5,21-23]

Chemokines that recruit innate immune cells in pancreatitis

Chemokines (chemotactic cytokines) are positively charged polypeptides with highly conserved cysteine (C) residues within the N-terminal sequence, classifying them as "C," "CC," "CXC," or "CX3C" types.[24,25] The presence or absence of a glutamate-leucine-arginine sequence further divides chemokines into "ELR" and "non-ELR" chemokines, with ELR-chemokines exhibiting highest activity in chemotaxis assays.[26,27]

In the context of AP, the most extensively investigated chemokines are CC-ligand 2 (CCL2, also known as monocyte chemoattractant protein-1 or MCP-1), CXC-ligand 1 (CXCL1, also known as cytokine-induced neutrophil chemoattractant or CINC in rat and keratinocyte cytokine or KC in mouse), and CXC-ligand 2 (CXCL2, also known as macrophage inflammatory protein 2-alpha or MIP2a). CCL2 acts predominantly via the CC-receptor CCR2, although it also binds to CCR4[28], whereas CXCL1 and CXCL2 both act via CXCR2.[29]

CXC ligands

In response to cerulein (a CCK-8 orthologue widely used to elicit early pancreatitis responses in isolated acini, an

*Corresponding authors. Email: P.Szatmary@liverpool.ac.uk, igukovsk@ucla.edu

ex vivo pancreatitis model), murine pancreatic acinar cells upregulate CXCL1 and CXCL2 mRNA levels within 90 min, with a supramaximally stimulating cerulein concentration of 0.1 μM producing an 8-fold increase in CXCL1 and 10-fold increase in CXCL2 expression.[30] In a mouse model of cerulein-induced AP (CER-AP), 10 hourly doses of 50 μg/kg cerulein results in an increase in CXCL2 concentration from <10 to 110 pg/mL in serum, 190 pg/mL in the pancreas, and 240 pg/mL in lung homogenate.[31] A >40-fold increase in pancreatic CXCL2 mRNA expression was measured in rat CER-AP.[32] Pretreatment with an anti-CXCL2 antibody was shown to reduce pancreatic edema, inflammatory cell infiltration, and necrosis, as well as reduce pancreatic and lung myeloperoxidase.[31] Antibodies against CXCL1 elicit similar protection for pancreatic and lung injury in rats.[33] Inhibition of CXCR2 with antileukinate,[34] evasin-3,[35] or AZD8309[36] improves the above parameters, as does CXCR2 knockout in the context of cerulein-induced acute and chronic pancreatitis.[37] Glycyrrhizin, a licorice extract, reduces the ability of isolated pancreatic acinar cells to produce CCL2 and CXCL2 in response to cerulein,[38] and treatment with glycyrrhizin was shown to attenuate pancreatic injury in response to cerulein in vivo.[39] Taken together, these data convincingly demonstrate the crucial role of the CXCL2/CXCR2 axis in the genesis of experimental AP.

A chemokine that has gained recent prominence is CX3CL1, or fractalkine. CX3CL1 uniquely acts as both a chemoattractant and surface adhesion molecule; induced by other cytokines (in particular tumor necrosis factor [TNF]α), it is expressed on the surface of vascular endothelium and enhances leukocyte adhesion by increasing integrin binding avidity.[40] In the rat bile-acid model of AP, serum CX3CL1 has been shown to rise from 150 pg/mL at baseline to peak at 1,400 pg/ml 16 h following intraductal taurocholate infusion.[41] AR42J cells (a rat cell line retaining some acinar cell characteristics) are able to synthesize and release CX3CL1 in response to cerulein, and they express the CX3CR1 receptor, which on stimulation triggers TNFα synthesis and release.[42] More recently, acinar cell CX3CR1 expression has been reported in normal rat pancreas; it is upregulated in models of acute and chronic pancreatitis in which it induces pancreatic stellate cell proliferation.[43] To date, no specific CX3CL1 inhibitors have been tested in AP; however, CX3CL1 siRNA has been shown to reduce pro-inflammatory cytokine release in the context of taurocholate-induced AP (TC-AP).[44]

CC ligands

CCL2 expression increases in CER-AP by about 30% in the lung, 60% in blood, and 140-fold in the pancreas.[45] Knockout of CCL2[45] or inhibition with evasin-3[35] reduced pancreatic leukocyte infiltration and necrosis and decreased hyperamylasemia in murine CER-AP, while evasin-4 treatment only ameliorated lung injury. Inhibition of CCL2 production with the relatively specific inhibitor bindarit reduced serum amylase and histopathologic scores in rat TC-AP.[46] Antibody-mediated inhibition of CCL2 in this model had similar effects on the pancreas and also dramatically reduced other serum cytokines including TNFα and interleukin (IL)-6, and -10.[47] This effect, however, was only partially reproduced by genetic ablation of its known receptors, CCR2 or CCR4, suggesting alternatives and redundancies in CCL2 signaling pathways. Interestingly, CCR2 knockout exacerbated chronic pancreatitis in the repetitive cerulein model.[48] Together, these findings highlight a key role of CCL2 in early inflammation.

Mediators of early cellular infiltration and systemic inflammatory response

Neutrophils are among the earliest innate immune cells to respond to tissue injury and the chemokines released in response to tissue injury in AP; with infiltration of the pancreas by neutrophils observed as early as 1 h after induction of experimental pancreatitis and lung infiltration after 3 h.[49] The severity of human AP correlates with circulating levels of IL-8, a major neutrophil-activating chemokine, as well as with neutrophil elastase.[50] Antibody-mediated depletion of neutrophils ameliorates experimental AP (especially the lung injury),[23,51-53] as does the genetic ablation of ICAM-1[21] or neutrophil NADPH oxidase.[22] Interestingly, the latter knockout reduced the pathologic, intrapancreatic increase in trypsin activity in CER-AP,[22] which was previously considered acinar cell autonomous. Inhibitors of neutrophil elastase have also shown promise in the treatment of pancreatitis-associated lung injury.[54,55]

Neutrophils and monocytes contribute to further cytokine release, which is amplified by activated peritoneal macrophages and hepatic Kupffer cells to enhance levels in the systemic circulation,[56-58] manifesting clinically as systemic inflammatory response syndrome (SIRS). The amplification links pancreatic injury to organ dysfunction associated with severe AP. In this context, the most relevant cytokines for discussion are IL-6, IL-1β, and TNFα.

IL-6

IL-6 is a key cytokine involved in early inflammation in AP. It belongs to a family of nine IL-6 type cytokines and has unusual signaling properties. Although IL-6 is produced and secreted by many cell types, very few (predominately hepatocytes, neutrophils and macrophages) express IL-6 receptors, leading to the assumption of a very specific pro-inflammatory role for this cytokine.[59] However, in complex with a soluble form of its receptor (sIL-6R) IL-6 can induce signals in cells not expressing the IL-6R—a phenomenon termed trans-signaling.[60-62]

IL-6 expression is upregulated in AR42J cells,[63,64] rodent pancreatic acinar cells,[65] and indeed murine salivary gland[66] following stimulation. In vivo models of experimental AP show the rise of serum IL-6 levels correlating with model severity, from less than 10 pg/mL to 50-100 pg/mL (24 h) and 200 pg/mL (72 h) in mouse CER-AP,[67,68] to 400 pg/mL following intraductal taurolithocholate-sulfate infusion.[69] Intraductal infusion of taurocholate leads to the highest levels of serum IL-6: 2,000 pg/mL 24-48 h after AP induction.[70] Interestingly, the increase in pancreatic IL-6 mRNA expression in this model (as well as other injury parameters) is much greater in the head than in the tail of the pancreas.[71] A ~100-fold increase in pancreatic IL-6 mRNA expression has been reported in rat CER-AP.[32]

Administering IL-6 together with cerulein caused total lethality in mice after 4 days, and IL-6 trans-signaling has been demonstrated to link experimental pancreatitis to acute lung injury.[72] Furthermore, even though acinar cells are clearly able to secrete IL-6, pancreatic IL-6 in CER-AP appears to derive predominantly from invading myeloid cells.[72] As may be expected, inhibition of IL-6 signaling, either with neutralizing antibody[73,74] or by genetic modification of an upstream signaling pathway,[75] ameliorates cerulein- and bile acid-induced AP. A very pronounced effect of IL-6 genetic ablation on CER-AP occurs in the context of diet-induced obesity; in this setting, IL-6 is responsible for delayed clearance of neutrophilic infiltrate and associated pancreatic necrosis.[76]

TNFα

TNFα was initially identified as a serum factor able to induce necrosis in solid tumors.[77] Since then, anti-TNF signaling strategies have been successfully employed in a number of inflammatory diseases resulting in a deeper understanding of its therapeutic manipulation.[78] TNFα is synthesized in membrane-bound form in many tissues in experimental AP[79] and requires cleavage by TNFα-converting enzyme (TACE or ADAM17) to be released in soluble form.[80] TNFα activity is dependent on its binding to one of two receptors: TNFR1 or TNFR2. TNFR1 is ubiquitously expressed and linked to TNFR1-associated death domain protein, with activation of this pathway resulting in the induction of programmed cell death.[81] TNFR2 is predominantly expressed on immune and endothelial cells, lacks a death domain, and responds primarily to the membrane-bound form of TNFα[82] to promote cell survival, proliferation, and inflammation. Both receptors can be shed following inflammatory stimuli, rendering them soluble and able to bind and inactivate circulating TNFα.[83]

Due to this complex binding pattern, measuring TNFα with commercial kits can be difficult, as some kits only measure free TNFα. In rat bile-acid induced AP, for example, free TNFα increased from 3 to 7.5 pg/mL within 1 h, only to return to baseline after 3 h.[84] Total TNFα increased from 2.5 to 7.5 ng/mL in the same time period and remained at the higher level for 9 h. Levels of soluble TNFR1 and 2 similarly increased within 1 h and remained elevated for at least 9 h. Plasma levels in rats with bile-acid induced AP rise from 20 to 80 pg/mL within 24 h.[85]

TNFα was one of the first cytokines whose mRNA expression was found to be induced in experimental AP.[86] Pancreatic acinar cells can themselves synthesize TNFα,[1] and gene expression is upregulated in response to cerulein and lipopolysaccharide as rapidly as within 30 min, with maximal expression after 6 h.[87] Vascular endothelial cells are also able to synthesize and release TNFα in response to DAMPs such as double-stranded DNA,[88] which are abundant in AP due to cellular necrosis and actively released from neutrophils in the form of neutrophil extracellular traps.[89] While neutrophil recruitment can be sustained via TNFR1 alone, monocyte recruitment is dependent on TNFR2, and upregulation of this receptor on the vascular endothelium contributes to selective recruitment of inflammatory monocytes.[90] TNFα was the first cytokine (together with IL-1) implicated by genetic means in the pathogenic mechanism of pancreatitis.[91] Genetic deletion of TNFα, or use of neutralizing antibodies prevents leukocyte-induced trypsin activation and necrosis in isolated acini.[92] TNFα also regulates acinar cell apoptosis in AP.[1] In rat TC-AP, infliximab (a monoclonal anti-TNFα antibody) attenuated pancreas and lung injury,[93] an effect seemingly enhanced by concomitant octreotide therapy.[94] Furthermore, the use of infliximab alone or in combination was proposed to limit intestinal dysfunction in this model.[95]

The complex roles of TNFα in both pro- and anti-inflammatory processes make it a difficult target for translation into clinical practice in AP.

IL-1

The IL-1 family of cytokines, which includes pro-inflammatory IL-1α/β, -18, -33, and -36, as well as anti-inflammatory IL-1 receptor antagonist (IL-1ra), -36ra, and IL-38, are another group of cytokines mediating sterile inflammation in AP. IL-1 (α and β) are produced as pro-enzymes and require proteolytic cleavage by caspase-1 (also known as IL-1 converting enzyme or ICE) or by neutrophil proteases to develop maximal biological activity.[96] IL-1α/β both act via the same receptor and are inactivated by competitive binding to soluble IL-1ra, a naturally occurring IL-1 inhibitor regulated through many of the same pathways as IL-1 itself.[96] IL-1 blockade is proving particularly effective in rheumatologic diseases, with a number of agents approved for clinical use.[97]

IL-1β, ICE, and IL-1ra mRNA are all expressed at low levels in mouse pancreas but increase rapidly on cerulein stimulation or on a choline deficient, ethionine-supplemented (CDE) diet.[98] Serum levels of IL-1β rise from a <10 pg/mL baseline to 150 pg/mL after 6 h in CER-AP, or to 200 pg/mL after 48 h in CDE-AP. Similar levels of IL-1ra could be detected in serum over the same time scales.[98] Using glycodeoxycholic acid ductal infusion in rats, levels as high as 5,000 pg/mL have been reported 12 h after AP induction.[16]

Targeted IL-1β overexpression in murine pancreas produced inflammatory changes consistent with chronic pancreatitis in animals as young as 6 weeks,[99] and co-administration of IL-1β exacerbated pancreatic and lung injury in rat CER-AP.[100] Accordingly, recombinant IL-1ra effectively attenuated damage in mouse[101] and rat[102] chronic pancreatitis models. The synthetic IL-1ra Anakinra (a modification of recombinant IL-1ra licensed for the treatment of rheumatoid arthritis) also attenuated pancreatic injury in rat CER-AP.[103] Reduction of biologically active IL-1β through inhibition of caspase-1 has also been shown to have some end-organ protective effects, for example by reducing renal injury,[104] lung injury,[105] and mortality[106] associated with rat TC-AP. It should be remembered, however, that IL-1β can be activated in other ways—for example, by neutrophil proteases. Another member of the IL-1 family, IL-33, links these signaling pathways by stimulating IL-6, CCL2, and CXCL2 release, as demonstrated in isolated murine pancreatic acinar cells.[107]

MIF

Activated T lymphocytes, inflammatory monocytes, and resident macrophages release macrophage migration inhibitory factor (MIF),[108] a pro-inflammatory cytokine that acts to further stimulate other macrophages[109] and T lymphocytes.[110] In experimental AP in rats, MIF reaches peak concentrations of around 120 ng/mL (ascites and plasma) within 2-4 h in CER-AP and 280 ng/mL (ascites) within 1 h or 200 ng/mL (plasma) 10 h following TC-AP induction. Pretreatment with anti-MIF antibody decreased plasma TNFα levels and reduced the lethality of TCA-AP and CDE-AP.[111]

Resolution of inflammation and delayed immune anergy

The interplay of inflammatory cells aims to control and clear the site of injury of cellular debris (and pathogens) quickly and effectively, then repair and restore function to the surrounding tissue. Cessation of inflammation thus requires anti-inflammatory signals to overpower the pro-inflammatory ones. For example, monocyte/macrophage subsets encountering apoptotic cells including neutrophils respond by releasing anti-inflammatory cytokines and are critical to resolution of inflammation.[112] Dysfunction of these regulatory systems together with ongoing injury can lead to nonresolving inflammation, progression to chronic pancreatitis, or even pancreatic neoplasia.[5] Many of these anti-inflammatory cytokines are released alongside their pro-inflammatory counterparts and have been discussed above (IL-1ra and soluble TNF receptors); the two other cytokines central to resolution of acute inflammation in AP are IL-10 and transforming growth factor beta (TGF-β).

IL-10

IL-10 is the foremost member of class-II cytokines, a family of anti-inflammatory cytokines that includes IL-19, -20, -22, -24, -26, -28, and -29. It is produced by a wide range of leukocytes including B cells, T cells, monocyte/macrophages, and dendritic cells, and it was initially described as a cytokine synthesis inhibitory factor due to its ability to inhibit interferon gamma release by Th1 cells.[113] In fact, IL-10 inhibits release of many pro-inflammatory cytokines on a transcriptional level via signal transducer and activator of transcription 3 (STAT3).[114] IL-10 also directly inhibits T cell expansion through downregulation of class II major histocompatibility complex and costimulatory molecules such as CD80/CD86.[115]

As with many other cytokines discussed in this review, pancreatic acinar cells also produce and secrete IL-10 and upregulate its production in response to pancreatitis toxins.[116] Levels in systemic circulation, however, are likely to derive from infiltrating leukocytes, as well as splenocytes[117] and hepatic Kupffer cells.[118,119] Knockout of B cells, another source of IL-10, exacerbates murine CER-AP in a manner that can be rescued by adoptive transfer of B cells.[120]

In rat bile-acid infusion AP model, IL-10 rises from a baseline of 10 pg/mL to 5,000 pg/mL after 6 h, earlier than the pro-inflammatory cytokines IL-1β and IL-6, and then drops to a new baseline of 2,000 pg/mL for the next 6 h. Rats administered exogenous IL-10 either before or after CER-AP induction had lower serum amylase and pro-inflammatory cytokine levels, as well as less histologic pancreatic damage.[121] Although there are currently no licensed IL-10 analogues in clinical use, agents shown to increase pancreatic IL-10, such as insulin-like growth factor 1 (IGF-1), have been tried in the context of experimental AP. Given during the course of rat CER-AP, IGF-1 ameliorated pancreatic damage and reduced pro-inflammatory cytokine levels (although other explanations are possible for such an effect).[122] Other strategies to enhance IL-10 secretion include administering IL-4 to cultured liver macrophages, which effectively reverses their polarization from a pro-inflammatory M1-type to an anti-inflammatory,

IL-10-producing M2-type in vitro.[123] Adenoviral transfer of the IL-4 gene into pancreatic stellate cells similarly increased endogenous IL-10 expression.[124] Injection of such an IL-4 gene-carrying vector into the rat gastric artery led to a transient increase in pancreatic IL-10 after 2 weeks.[125] While these methods are clearly not ready for translation into clinical trials, they are important proof-of-principle studies and add to our understanding of this particular cytokine signaling axis. As could be expected, knockout of IL-10 greatly exacerbated pancreas injury in repetitive-cerulein mouse model of chronic pancreatitis.[126]

TGF-β

TGF-β is a member of a family of about 40 related factors promoting growth and cellular differentiation. Of the three mammalian isoforms, TGF-β1, -β2 and -β3, TGF-β1 is the most extensively studied.[127] Its overall effects are strongly cytostatic and anti-inflammatory (through inhibition of pro-inflammatory M1-type macrophages and Th1-type lymphocytes, as well as promotion of anti-inflammatory M2-type macrophages, Th2-type lymphocytes, and regulatory T cells).[128] TGF-β1 production is upregulated early in the course of mouse CER-AP, and expression of a non-functional, dominant negative TGF receptor type II ameliorated pancreatic injury in this model.[129] Interestingly, acini isolated from these mice did not exhibit restricted stimulation at high cerulein concentrations.[129] In rat CER-AP, increased TGF-β1 mRNA expression was detectable by the end of the first hour.[130] As early as 5 h following ductal infusion with sodium deoxycholate, rat TGF-β plasma levels were as high as 10 ng/mL (twice as high as following macrophage depletion).[131] Hepatic injury in this model was reduced by both depletion of liver macrophages and the use a TGF-β neutralizing antibody.[131] Notably, TGF-β mRNA expression is upregulated much later in rat L-arginine-induced AP (not until 2 days after induction) ,[132] in accord with slower development of pancreatitis in this model. In a comprehensive time-course analysis of TGF-β mRNA expression, increased TGF-β1 mRNA was detectable within 4 h of cerulein injection in rats; however, there was a clear peak in expression between 2 and 3 days after AP induction.[133] Peak TGF-β1 expression correlated well with collagen mRNA levels in that study, supporting a role for this cytokine in pancreatic repair. Administration of recombinant TGF-β1 was reported to have little effect on a single course of cerulein AP, whereas it led to increased collagen deposition and scarring after six courses of cerulein treatment.[134] As such, this cytokine may be critical in the transition from recurrent acute to chronic pancreatitis.[134] Inhibition of TGF-β activity via a viral vector expressing a soluble TGF-β receptor reduced fibrosis in a repetitive cerulein model of chronic pancreaititis.[135] Similarly, use of neutralizing TGF-β1 antibody reduced fibrosis and extracellular matrix deposition in rat CER-AP, demonstrating a key role of TGF-β in regulating pancreas repair/regeneration.[136] In a recent study,[137] TGF-β1 was shown to cause abdominal hyperalgesia in a rat model of bile-acid induced AP. TGF receptors were upregulated in the dorsal root ganglion of rats in this model; administration of recombinant TGF-β1 enhanced while inhibition of TGF-β1 attenuated abdominal hyperalgesia, suggesting a major contribution of this cytokine to pain, a key response of human chronic pancreatitis.[137]

Compensatory anti-inflammatory response syndrome

Prolonged disease activity is associated with immune anergy in AP. The concept of a compensatory anti-inflammatory response syndrome (CARS) was first raised in an attempt to understand the failure of anti-endotoxin strategies in sepsis.[138] Mediators of CARS (predominantly TGF-β, IL-4, IL-10, and CCL2) are released by neutrophils and monocytes[139,140] and contribute to immunoparalysis by promoting a Th2-type adaptive immune response and predisposing to superinfection.[141] The time scale of pro- and anti-inflammatory cytokine release is similar in patients,[142] with peak cytokine concentration within 48 h of disease onset; thus, anti-inflammatory cytokines presumably limit the extent of systemic response. A significant subset of patients, however, develop considerable immune anergy, predisposing to superinfection.[142] In CER-AP, myeloid-derived suppressor cells producing IL-10 acting via the MyD88 pathway appear to contribute significantly to the development of immune anergy; targeting of this pathway and/or the involved cell types present untapped opportunities for novel AP management therapies.[143]

Conclusion

In AP, injured and dying acinar cells release DAMPs and cytokines to attract and recruit innate immune cells, rapidly initiating the inflammatory response (which can develop within 1 h). Infiltrating cells augment cytokine signaling to encourage further immune cell recruitment and modulate inflammation. Cytokines and chemokines released in this way (**Table 1**) are responded to by resident hepatic macrophages, which further amplify the signals leading to detectable plasma cytokines and SIRS. Anti-inflammatory cytokines are produced and released on the same time scale as their pro-inflammatory counterparts; however, as long as there is ongoing tissue injury and DAMP release, the balance of cytokines promotes further inflammation. Excessive release of anti-inflammatory cytokines drives immune anergy, which contributes to late mortality by reducing immunity to opportunistic infections.

Table 1. Key cytokines and chemokines mediating the inflammatory response of pancreatitis

Signaling molecule	Source in AP	Receptors and targets	Function	References
Cytokines				
TNFα	Acinar cells, endothelium, monocytes, Kupffer cells	TNFR1: widely expressed; TNFR2: immune and endothelial cells	Pro-inflammatory; regulates apoptosis, mediates trypsin activation in acinar cells	1, 18, 71, 79-92, 140
IL-1β	Pancreas (beta cells, stellate cells), lung, liver, spleen, monocytes	Secreted as a pro-enzyme, converted by ICE or neutrophil proteases to its active form; acts on IL-1R (widely expressed)	Pro-inflammatory; increases vascular permeability Soluble IL-1ra inhibits IL-1β activity	79, 91, 96, 98-106
IL-6	Ubiquitous expression	IL-6R: hepatocytes, neutrophils, macrophages; soluble sIL-6R mediates trans-signaling	Pro-inflammatory; contributes to lung injury in AP; lethal if administered in the context of experimental AP	18, 32, 59, 63-65, 70-76
IL-10	Lymphocytes (B- and T-), monocytes/macrophages, dendritic cells, Kupffer cells	IL-10R: widely expressed	Anti-inflammatory; inhibits pro-inflammatory cytokine release from lymphocytes via STAT3; downregulates MHCII costimulatory molecules CD80/CD86, reducing clonal expansion of T-lymphocytes.	16, 113-121, 124-126, 140
Chemokines				
CCL2	Acinar cells and possibly other cell types in the pancreas	CCR2, CCR4	Pro-inflammatory, monocyte chemoattractant, mediates pancreas and lung injury in experimental AP	2, 18, 35, 38, 45-48, 71, 139
CXCL1/2	Acinar cells, macrophages	CXCR2: neutrophils and myeloid derived suppressor cells	Pro-inflammatory, strong neutrophil chemoattractants	18, 30-38, 71

The overlap and redundancy of cytokine activities and signaling pathways, together with differences in responses depending on local factors, largely account for the limited success with which cytokine antagonists have been translated from bench to bedside. Any successful immune-therapy for pancreatitis will likely require detailed cytokine profiling and/or immune phenotyping to establish personalized responses to disease and therapy.

References

1. Gukovskaya AS, Gukovsky I, Zaninovic V, Song M, Sandoval D, Gukovsky S, et al. Pancreatic acinar cells produce, release, and respond to tumor necrosis factor-alpha. Role in regulating cell death and pancreatitis. *J Clin Invest.* 1997; 100: 1853-1862. PMID: 9312187.
2. Grady T, Liang P, Ernst SA, Logsdon CD. Chemokine gene expression in rat pancreatic acinar cells is an early event associated with acute pancreatitis. *Gastroenterology.* 1997; 113: 1966-1975. PMID: 9394737.
3. Norman J. The role of cytokines in the pathogenesis of acute pancreatitis. *Am J Surg.* 1998; 175: 76-83. PMID: 9445247.
4. Habtezion A. Inflammation in acute and chronic pancreatitis. *Curr Opin Gastroenterol.* 2015; 31: 395-399. PMID: 26107390.
5. Gukovsky I, Li N, Todoric J, Gukovskaya A, Karin M. Inflammation, autophagy, and obesity: common features in the pathogenesis of pancreatitis and pancreatic cancer. *Gastroenterology.* 2013; 144: 1199-1209. PMID: 23622129.
6. Kang R, Lotze MT, Zeh HJ, Billiar TR, Tang D. Cell death and DAMPs in acute pancreatitis. *Mol Med.* 2014; 20: 466-477. PMID: 25105302.
7. Hoque R, Malik AF, Gorelick F, Mehal WZ. Sterile inflammatory response in acute pancreatitis. *Pancreas.* 2012; 41: 353-357. PMID: 22415665.
8. Shanmugam MK, Bhatia M. The role of pro-inflammatory molecules and pharmacological agents in acute pancreatitis and sepsis. *Inflamm Allergy Drug Targets.* 2010; 9: 20-31. PMID: 19663805.
9. Oiva J, Mustonen H, Kylanpaa ML, Kuuliala K, Siitonen S, Kemppainen E, et al. Patients with acute pancreatitis complicated by organ dysfunction show abnormal peripheral blood polymorphonuclear leukocyte signaling. *Pancreatology.* 2013; 13: 118-124. PMID: 23561969.

10. Oiva J, Mustonen H, Kylanpaa ML, Kyhala L, Alanara T, Aittomaki S, et al. Patients with acute pancreatitis complicated by organ failure show highly aberrant monocyte signaling profiles assessed by phospho-specific flow cytometry. *Crit Care Med.* 2010; 38: 1702-1708. PMID: 20512034.
11. Staubli SM,Oertli D, Nebiker CA. Laboratory markers predicting severity of acute pancreatitis. *Crit Rev Clin Lab Sci.* 2015; 52: 273-283. PMID: 26173077.
12. Mayerle J, Dummer A, Sendler M, Malla SR, van den Brandt C, Teller S, et al. Differential roles of inflammatory cells in pancreatitis. *J Gastroenterol Hepatol.* 2012; 27 Suppl 2: 47-51. PMID: 22320916.
13. Xue J, Sharma V, Habtezion A. Immune cells and immune-based therapy in pancreatitis. *Immunol Res.* 2014; 58: 378-386. PMID: 24710635.
14. Yu G, Wan R, Hu Y, Ni J, Yin G, Xing M, et al. Pancreatic acinar cells-derived cyclophilin A promotes pancreatic damage by activating NF-kappaB pathway in experimental pancreatitis. *Biochem Biophys Res Commun.* 2014; 444: 75-80. PMID: 24434144.
15. Ou X, Cheng Z, Liu T, Tang Z, Huang W, Szatmary P, et al. Circulating histone levels reflect disease severity in animal models of acute pancreatitis. *Pancreas.* 2015; 44: 1089-1095. PMID: 26335015.
16. Schneider L, Jabrailova B, Strobel O, Hackert T, Werner J. Inflammatory profiling of early experimental necrotizing pancreatitis. *Life Sci.* 2015; 126: 76-80. PMID: 25711429.
17. Chen GY, Nunez G. Sterile inflammation: sensing and reacting to damage. *Nat Rev Immunol.* 2010; 10: 826-837. PMID: 21088683.
18. Blinman TA, Gukovsky I, Mouria M, Zaninovic V, Livingston E, Pandol SJ, et al. Activation of pancreatic acinar cells on isolation from tissue: cytokine upregulation via p38 MAP kinase. *Am J Physiol Cell Physiol.* 2000; 279: C1993-C2003. PMID: 11078716.
19. Zaninovic V, Gukovskaya AS, Gukovsky I, Mouria M, Pandol SJ. Cerulein upregulates ICAM-1 in pancreatic acinar cells, which mediates neutrophil adhesion to these cells. *Am J Physiol Gastrointest Liver Physiol.* 2000; 279: G666-G676. PMID: 11005752.
20. Lundberg AH, Granger N, Russell J, Callicutt S, Gaber LW, Kotb M, et al. Temporal correlation of tumor necrosis factor-alpha release, upregulation of pulmonary ICAM-1 and VCAM-1, neutrophil sequestration, and lung injury in diet-induced pancreatitis. *J Gastrointest Surg.* 2000; 4: 248-257. PMID: 10769087.
21. Frossard JL, Saluja A, Bhagat L, Lee HS, Bhatia M, Hofbauer B, et al. The role of intercellular adhesion molecule 1 and neutrophils in acute pancreatitis and pancreatitis-associated lung injury. *Gastroenterology.* 1999; 116: 694-701. PMID: 10029629.
22. Gukovskaya AS, Vaquero E, Zaninovic V, Gorelick FS, Lusis AJ, Brennan ML, et al. Neutrophils and NADPH oxidase mediate intrapancreatic trypsin activation in murine experimental acute pancreatitis. *Gastroenterology.* 2002; 122: 974-984. PMID: 11910350.
23. Bhatia M, Saluja AK, Hofbauer B, Lee HS, Frossard JL, Steer ML. The effects of neutrophil depletion on a completely noninvasive model of acute pancreatitis-associated lung injury. *Int J Pancreatol.* 1998; 24: 77-83. PMID: 9816540.
24. Repnik U, Starr AE, Overall CM, Turk B. Cysteine cathepsins activate ELR chemokines and inactivate non-ELR chemokines. *J Biol Chem.* 2015; 290: 13800-13811. PMID: 25833952.
25. Zlotnik A, Yoshie O. The chemokine superfamily revisited. *Immunity.* 2012; 36: 705-716. PMID: 22633458.
26. Wuyts A, Govaerts C, Struyf S, Lenaerts JP, Put W, Conings R, et al. Isolation of the CXC chemokines ENA-78, GRO alpha and GRO gamma from tumor cells and leukocytes reveals NH2-terminal heterogeneity. Functional comparison of different natural isoforms. *Eur J Biochem.* 1999; 260: 421-429. PMID: 10095777.
27. King AG, Johanson K, Frey CL, DeMarsh PL, White JR, McDevitt P, et al. Identification of unique truncated KC/GRO beta chemokines with potent hematopoietic and anti-infective activities. *J Immunol.* 2000; 164: 3774-3782. PMID: 10725737.
28. Zhang J, Patel L, Pienta KJ. Targeting chemokine (C-C motif) ligand 2 (CCL2) as an example of translation of cancer molecular biology to the clinic. *Prog Mol Biol Transl Sci.* 2010; 95: 31-53. PMID: 21075328.
29. Veenstra M, Ransohoff RM. Chemokine receptor CXCR2: physiology regulator and neuroinflammation controller? *J Neuroimmunol.* 2012; 246: 1-9. PMID: 22445294.
30. Orlichenko LS, Behari J, Yeh TH, Liu S, Stolz DB, Saluja AK, et al. Transcriptional regulation of CXC-ELR chemokines KC and MIP-2 in mouse pancreatic acini. *Am J Physiol Gastrointest Liver Physiol.* 2010; 299: G867-G876. PMID: 20671197.
31. Pastor CM, Rubbia-Brandt L, Hadengue A, Jordan M, Morel P, Frossard JL. Role of macrophage inflammatory peptide-2 in cerulein-induced acute pancreatitis and pancreatitis-associated lung injury. *Lab Invest.* 2003; 83: 471-478. PMID: 12695550.
32. Gukovsky I, Gukovskaya AS, Blinman TA, Zaninovic V, Pandol SJ. Early NF-kappaB activation is associated with hormone-induced pancreatitis. *Am J Physiol Gastrointest Liver Physiol.* 1998; 275: G1402-G1414. PMID: 9843778.
33. Bhatia M, Brady M, Zagorski J, Christmas SE, Campbell F, Neoptolemos JP, et al. Treatment with neutralising antibody against cytokine induced neutrophil chemoattractant (CINC) protects rats against acute pancreatitis associated lung injury. *Gut.* 2000; 47: 838-844. PMID: 11076884.
34. Bhatia M, Hegde A. Treatment with antileukinate, a CXCR2 chemokine receptor antagonist, protects mice against acute pancreatitis and associated lung injury. *Regul Pept.* 2007; 138: 40-48. PMID: 17014919.
35. Montecucco F, Mach F, Lenglet S, Vonlaufen A, Gomes Quindere AL, Pelli G, et al. Treatment with Evasin-3 abrogates neutrophil-mediated inflammation in mouse acute pancreatitis. *Eur J Clin Invest.* 2014; 44: 940-950. PMID: 25132144.
36. Malla SR, Kärrman Mårdh C, Günther A, Mahajan UM, Sendler M, D'Haese J, et al. Effect of oral administration of AZD8309, a CXCR2 antagonist, on the severity of experimental pancreatitis. *Pancreatology.* 2016 Jul 14. [Epub ahead of print]. PMID: 27450968.

37. Steele CW, Karim SA, Foth M, Rishi L, Leach JD, Porter RJ, et al. CXCR2 inhibition suppresses acute and chronic pancreatic inflammation. *J Pathol.* 2015; 237: 85-97. PMID: 25950520.
38. Panahi Y, Fakhari S, Mohammadi M, Rahmani MR, Hakhamaneshi MS, Jalili A. Glycyrrhizin down-regulates CCL2 and CXCL2 expression in cerulein-stimulated pancreatic acinar cells. *Am J Clin Exp Immunol.* 2015; 4: 1-6. PMID: 26155433.
39. Fakhari S, Abdolmohammadi K, Panahi Y, Nikkhoo B, Peirmohammadi H, Rahmani MR, et al. Glycyrrhizin attenuates tissue injury and reduces neutrophil accumulation in experimental acute pancreatitis. *Int J Clin Exp Pathol.* 2014; 7: 101-109. PMID: 24427330.
40. Umehara H, Bloom ET, Okazaki T, Nagano Y, Yoshie O and Imai T. Fractalkine in vascular biology: from basic research to clinical disease. *Arterioscler Thromb Vasc Biol* 24(1): 34-40, 2004. PMID: 12969992.
41. Huang LY, Chen P, Xu LX, Zhou YF, Li WG, Yuan YZ. Fractalkine as a marker for assessment of severe acute pancreatitis. *J Dig Dis.* 2012; 13: 225-231. PMID: 22435508.
42. Huang LY, Chen P, Xu LX, Zhou YF, Zhang YP, Yuan YZ. Fractalkine upregulates inflammation through CX3CR1 and the Jak-Stat pathway in severe acute pancreatitis rat model. *Inflammation.* 2012; 35: 1023-1030. PMID: 22213034.
43. Uchida M, Ito T, Nakamura T, Hijioka M, Igarashi H, Oono T, et al. Pancreatic stellate cells and CX3CR1: occurrence in normal pancreas and acute and chronic pancreatitis and effect of their activation by a CX3CR1 agonist. *Pancreas.* 2014; 43: 708-719. PMID: 24681877.
44. Huang L, Ma J, Tang Y, Chen P, Zhang S, Zhang Y, et al. siRNA-based targeting of fractalkine overexpression suppresses inflammation development in a severe acute pancreatitis rat model. *Int J Mol Med.* 2012; 30: 514-520. PMID: 22751862.
45. Frossard JL, Lenglet S, Montecucco F, Steffens S, Galan K, Pelli G, et al. Role of CCL-2, CCR-2 and CCR-4 in cerulein-induced acute pancreatitis and pancreatitis-associated lung injury. *J Clin Pathol.* 2011; 64: 387-393. PMID: 21345872.
46. Zhou GX, Zhu XJ, Ding XL, Zhang H, Chen JP, Qiang H, et al. Protective effects of MCP-1 inhibitor on a rat model of severe acute pancreatitis. *Hepatobiliary Pancreat Dis Int.* 2010; 9: 201-207. PMID: 20382594.
47. Ishibashi T, Zhao H, Kawabe K, Oono T, Egashira K, Suzuki K, et al. Blocking of monocyte chemoattractant protein-1 (MCP-1) activity attenuates the severity of acute pancreatitis in rats. *J Gastroenterol.* 2008; 43: 79-85. PMID: 18297440.
48. Nakamura Y, Kanai T, Saeki K, Takabe M, Irie J, Miyoshi J, et al. CCR2 knockout exacerbates cerulein-induced chronic pancreatitis with hyperglycemia via decreased GLP-1 receptor expression and insulin secretion. *Am J Physiol Gastrointest Liver Physiol.* 2013; 304: G700-G707. PMID: 23449669.
49. Folch E, Closa D, Prats N, Gelpi E, Rosello-Catafau J. Leukotriene generation and neutrophil infiltration after experimental acute pancreatitis. *Inflammation.* 1998; 22: 83-93. PMID: 9484652.
50. Gross V, Andreesen R, Leser HG, Ceska M, Liehl E, Lausen M, et al. Interleukin-8 and neutrophil activation in acute pancreatitis. *Eur J Clin Invest.* 1992; 22: 200-203. PMID: 1582445.
51. Inoue S, Nakao A, Kishimoto W, Murakami H, Itoh K, Itoh T, et al. Anti-neutrophil antibody attenuates the severity of acute lung injury in rats with experimental acute pancreatitis. *Arch Surg.* 1995; 130: 93-98. PMID: 7802585.
52. Murakami H, Nakao A, Kishimoto W, Nakano M, Takagi H. Detection of O2- generation and neutrophil accumulation in rat lungs after acute necrotizing pancreatitis. *Surgery.* 1995; 118: 547-554. PMID: 7652692.
53. Sandoval D, Gukovskaya A, Reavey P, Gukovsky S, Sisk A, Braquet P, et al. The role of neutrophils and platelet-activating factor in mediating experimental pancreatitis. *Gastroenterology.* 1996; 111: 1081-1091. PMID: 8831604.
54. Imamura M, Mikami Y, Takahashi H, Yamauchi H. Effect of a specific synthetic inhibitor of neutrophil elastase (ONO-5046) on the course of acute hemorrhagic pancreatitis in dogs. *J Hepatobiliary Pancreat Surg.* 1998; 5: 422-428. PMID: 9931392.
55. Wang HH, Tang AM, Chen L, Zhou MT. Potential of sivelestat in protection against severe acute pancreatitis-associated lung injury in rats. *Exp Lung Res.* 2012; 38: 445-452. PMID: 23005337.
56. Lundberg AH, Eubanks JW 3rd, Henry J, Sabek O, Kotb M, Gaber L, et al. Trypsin stimulates production of cytokines from peritoneal macrophages in vitro and in vivo. *Pancreas.* 2000; 21: 41-51. PMID: 10881931.
57. Gloor B, Todd KE, Lane JS, Lewis MP, Reber HA. Hepatic Kupffer cell blockade reduces mortality of acute hemorrhagic pancreatitis in mice. *J Gastrointest Surg.* 1998; 2: 430-435. PMID: 9843602.
58. Gloor B, Blinman TA, Rigberg DA, Todd KE, Lane JS, Hines OJ, et al. Kupffer cell blockade reduces hepatic and systemic cytokine levels and lung injury in hemorrhagic pancreatitis in rats. *Pancreas.* 2000; 21: 414-420. PMID: 11075997.
59. Scheller J, Garbers C, Rose-John S. Interleukin-6: from basic biology to selective blockade of pro-inflammatory activities. *Semin Immunol.* 2014; 26: 2-12. PMID: 24325804.
60. Garbers C, Scheller J. Interleukin-6 and interleukin-11: same same but different. *Biol Chem.* 2013; 394: 1145-1161. PMID: 23740659.
61. Rose-John S, Heinrich PC. Soluble receptors for cytokines and growth factors: generation and biological function. *Biochem J.* 1994; 300: 281-290. PMID: 8002928.
62. Rabe B, Chalaris A, May U, Waetzig GH, Seegert D, Williams AS, et al. Transgenic blockade of interleukin 6 transsignaling abrogates inflammation. *Blood.* 2008; 111: 1021-1028. PMID: 17989316.
63. Chan YC, Leung PS. Involvement of redox-sensitive extracellular-regulated kinases in angiotensin II-induced interleukin-6 expression in pancreatic acinar cells. *J Pharmacol Exp Ther.* 2009; 329: 450-458. PMID: 19211919.
64. Jiang CY, Wang W, Tang JX, Yuan ZR. The adipocytokine resistin stimulates the production of proinflammatory cytokines TNF-alpha and IL-6 in pancreatic acinar cells via

NF-kappaB activation. *J Endocrinol Invest.* 2013; 36: 986-992. PMID: 23765438.

65. Kang M, Park KS, Seo JY, Kim H. Lycopene inhibits IL-6 expression in cerulein-stimulated pancreatic acinar cells. *Genes Nutr.* 2011; 6: 117-123. PMID: 21484151.
66. Purwanti N, Azlina A, Karabasil MR, Hasegawa T, Yao C, Akamatsu T, et al. Involvement of the IL-6/STAT3/Sca-1 system in proliferation of duct cells following duct ligation in the submandibular gland of mice. *J Med Invest.* 2009; 56 Suppl: 253-254. PMID: 20224192.
67. Yu JH, Kim KH, Kim H. SOCS 3 and PPAR-gamma ligands inhibit the expression of IL-6 and TGF-beta1 by regulating JAK2/STAT3 signaling in pancreas. *Int J Biochem Cell Biol.* 2008; 40: 677-688. PMID: 18035585.
68. Huang W, Cash N, Wen L, Szatmary P, Mukherjee R, Armstrong J, et al. Effects of the mitochondria-targeted antioxidant mitoquinone in murine acute pancreatitis. *Mediators Inflamm.* 2015; 2015: 901780. PMID: 25878403.
69. Huang W, Cane MC, Mukherjee R, Szatmary P, Zhang X, Elliott V, et al. Caffeine protects against experimental acute pancreatitis by inhibition of inositol 1,4,5-trisphosphate receptor-mediated Ca^{2+} release. *Gut.* 2015 Dec 7. [Epub ahead of print]. PMID: 26642860.
70. Schmidt AI, Seifert GJ, Lauch R, Wolff-Vorbeck G, Chikhladze S, Hopt UT, et al. Organ-specific monocyte activation in necrotizing pancreatitis in mice. *J Surg Res.* 2015; 197: 374-381. PMID: 25982373.
71. Vaquero E, Gukovsky I, Zaninovic V, Gukovskaya AS, Pandol SJ. Localized pancreatic NF-kappaB activation and inflammatory response in taurocholate-induced pancreatitis. *Am J Physiol Gastrointest Liver Physiol.* 2001; 280: G1197-G1208. PMID: 11352813.
72. Zhang H, Neuhofer P, Song L, Rabe B, Lesina M, Kurkowski MU, et al. IL-6 trans-signaling promotes pancreatitis-associated lung injury and lethality. *J Clin Invest.* 2013; 123: 1019-1031. PMID: 23426178.
73. Chao KC, Chao KF, Chuang CC, Liu SH. Blockade of interleukin 6 accelerates acinar cell apoptosis and attenuates experimental acute pancreatitis in vivo. *Br J Surg.* 2006; 93: 332-338. PMID: 16392107.
74. Chen KL, Lv ZY, Yang HW, Liu Y, Long FW, Zhou B, et al. Effects of tocilizumab on experimental severe acute pancreatitis and associated acute lung injury. *Crit Care Med.* 2016; 44: e664-e677. PMID: 26963319.
75. Tietz AB, Malo A, Diebold J, Kotlyarov A, Herbst A, Kolligs FT, et al. Gene deletion of MK2 inhibits TNF-alpha and IL-6 and protects against cerulein-induced pancreatitis. *Am J Physiol Gastrointest Liver Physiol.* 2006; 290: G1298-G1306. PMID: 16423921.
76. Pini M, Rhodes DH, Castellanos KJ, Hall AR, Cabay RJ, Chennuri R, et al. Role of IL-6 in the resolution of pancreatitis in obese mice. *J Leukoc Biol.* 2012; 91: 957-966. PMID: 22427681.
77. Aggarwal BB, Gupta SC, Kim JH. Historical perspectives on tumor necrosis factor and its superfamily: 25 years later, a golden journey. *Blood.* 2012; 119: 651-665. PMID: 22053109.
78. Kalliolias GD, Ivashkiv LB. TNF biology, pathogenic mechanisms and emerging therapeutic strategies. *Nat Rev Rheumatol.* 2016; 12: 49-62. PMID: 26656660.
79. Norman JG, Fink GW, Denham W, Yang J, Carter G, Sexton C, et al. Tissue-specific cytokine production during experimental acute pancreatitis. A probable mechanism for distant organ dysfunction. *Dig Dis Sci.* 1997; 42: 1783-1788. PMID: 9286248.
80. Issuree PD, Maretzky T, McIlwain DR, Monette S, Qing X, Lang PA, et al. iRHOM2 is a critical pathogenic mediator of inflammatory arthritis. *J Clin Invest.* 2013; 123: 928-932. PMID: 23348744.
81. Brenner D, Blaser H, Mak TW. Regulation of tumour necrosis factor signalling: live or let die. *Nat Rev Immunol.* 2015; 15: 362-374. PMID: 26008591.
82. Grell M, Douni E, Wajant H, Lohden M, Clauss M, Maxeiner B, et al. The transmembrane form of tumor necrosis factor is the prime activating ligand of the 80 kDa tumor necrosis factor receptor. *Cell.* 1995; 83: 793-802. PMID: 8521496.
83. Porteu F, Hieblot C. Tumor necrosis factor induces a selective shedding of its p75 receptor from human neutrophils. *J Biol Chem.* 1994; 269: 2834-2840. PMID: 8300617.
84. Granell S, Pereda J, Gomez-Cambronero L, Cassinello N, Sabater L, Closa D, et al. Circulating TNF-alpha and its soluble receptors during experimental acute pancreatitis. *Cytokine.* 2004; 25: 187-191. PMID: 15164724.
85. Ramudo L, Manso MA, Sevillano S, de Dios I. Kinetic study of TNF-alpha production and its regulatory mechanisms in acinar cells during acute pancreatitis induced by bile-pancreatic duct obstruction. *J Pathol.* 2005; 206: 9-16. PMID: 15761843.
86. Norman JG, Fink GW, Franz MG. Acute pancreatitis induces intrapancreatic tumor necrosis factor gene expression. *Arch Surg.* 1995; 130: 966-970. PMID: 7661681.
87. Vaccaro MI, Ropolo A, Grasso D, Calvo EL, Ferreria M, Iovanna JL, et al. Pancreatic acinar cells submitted to stress activate TNF-alpha gene expression. *Biochem Biophys Res Commun.* 2000; 268: 485-490. PMID: 10679231.
88. Patel SJ, Jindal R, King KR, Tilles AW, Yarmush ML. The inflammatory response to double stranded DNA in endothelial cells is mediated by NFkappaB and TNFalpha. *PLoS One.* 2011; 6: e19910. PMID: 21611132.
89. Merza M, Hartman H, Rahman M, Hwaiz R, Zhang E, Renstrom E, et al. Neutrophil extracellular traps induce trypsin activation, inflammation, and tissue damage in mice with severe acute pancreatitis. *Gastroenterology.* 2015; 149: 1920-1931. PMID: 26302488.
90. Venkatesh D, Ernandez T, Rosetti F, Batal I, Cullere X, Luscinskas FW, et al. Endothelial TNF receptor 2 induces IRF1 transcription factor-dependent interferon-beta autocrine signaling to promote monocyte recruitment. *Immunity.* 2013; 38: 1025-1037. PMID: 23623383.
91. Denham W, Yang J, Fink G, Denham D, Carter G, Ward K, et al. Gene targeting demonstrates additive detrimental effects of interleukin 1 and tumor necrosis factor during pancreatitis. *Gastroenterology.* 1997; 113: 1741-1746. PMID: 9352880.
92. Sendler M, Dummer A, Weiss FU, Kruger B, Wartmann T, Scharffetter-Kochanek K, et al. Tumour necrosis factor alpha secretion induces protease activation and acinar cell necrosis in acute experimental pancreatitis in mice. *Gut.* 2013; 62: 430-439. PMID: 22490516.

93. Luo S, Wang R, Jiang W, Lin X, Qiu P, Yan G. A novel recombinant snake venom metalloproteinase from Agkistrodon acutus protects against taurocholate-induced severe acute pancreatitis in rats. *Biochimie*. 2010; 92: 1354-1361. PMID: 20600562.
94. Huang YX, Li WD, Jia L, Qiu JH, Jiang SM, Ou Y, et al. Infliximab enhances the therapeutic effectiveness of octreotide on acute necrotizing pancreatitis in rat model. *Pancreas*. 2012; 41: 849-854. PMID: 22450369.
95. Li WD, Jia L, Ou Y, Jiang SM, Qiu JH, Huang YX, et al. Infliximab: protective effect to intestinal barrier function of rat with acute necrosis pancreatitis at early stage. *Pancreas*. 2013; 42: 366-367. PMID: 23407490.
96. Afonina IS, Muller C, Martin SJ, Beyaert R. Proteolytic processing of interleukin-1 family cytokines: variations on a common theme. *Immunity*. 2015; 42: 991-1004. PMID: 26084020.
97. Kahlenberg JM. Anti-inflammatory panacea? The expanding therapeutics of interleukin-1 blockade. *Curr Opin Rheumatol*. 2016; 28: 197-203. PMID: 26859478.
98. Fink GW, Norman JG. Specific changes in the pancreatic expression of the interleukin 1 family of genes during experimental acute pancreatitis. *Cytokine*. 1997; 9: 1023-1027. PMID: 9417814.
99. Romac JM, Shahid RA, Choi SS, Karaca GF, Westphalen CB, Wang TC, et al. Pancreatic secretory trypsin inhibitor I reduces the severity of chronic pancreatitis in mice overexpressing interleukin-1beta in the pancreas. *Am J Physiol Gastrointest Liver Physiol*. 2012; 302: G535-G541. PMID: 22173919.
100. Noel P, Patel K, Durgampudi C, Trivedi RN, de Oliveira C, Crowell MD, et al. Peripancreatic fat necrosis worsens acute pancreatitis independent of pancreatic necrosis via unsaturated fatty acids increased in human pancreatic necrosis collections. *Gut*. 2016; 65: 100-111. PMID: 25500204.
101. Shen J, Gao J, Zhang J, Xiang D, Wang X, Qian L, et al. Recombinant human interleukin-1 receptor antagonist (rhIL-1Ra) attenuates caerulein-induced chronic pancreatitis in mice. *Biomed Pharmacother*. 2012; 66: 83-88. PMID: 22281291.
102. Xu C, Shen J, Zhang J, Jia Z, He Z, Zhuang X, et al. Recombinant interleukin-1 receptor antagonist attenuates the severity of chronic pancreatitis induced by TNBS in rats. *Biochem Pharmacol*. 2015; 93: 449-460. PMID: 25559498.
103. Kaplan M, Yazgan Y, Tanoglu A, Berber U, Oncu K, Kara M, et al. Effectiveness of interleukin-1 receptor antagonist (Anakinra) on cerulein-induced experimental acute pancreatitis in rats. *Scand J Gastroenterol*. 2014; 49: 1124-1130. PMID: 24912987.
104. Zhang XH, Li ML, Wang B, Guo MX, Zhu RM. Caspase-1 inhibition alleviates acute renal injury in rats with severe acute pancreatitis. *World J Gastroenterol*. 2014; 20: 10457-10463. PMID: 25132762.
105. Zhang XH, Zhu RM, Xu WA, Wan HJ, Lu H. Therapeutic effects of caspase-1 inhibitors on acute lung injury in experimental severe acute pancreatitis. *World J Gastroenterol*. 2007; 13: 623-627. PMID: 17278232.
106. Paszkowski AS, Rau B, Mayer JM, Moller P, Beger HG. Therapeutic application of caspase 1/interleukin-1beta-converting enzyme inhibitor decreases the death rate in severe acute experimental pancreatitis. *Ann Surg*. 2002; 235: 68-76. PMID: 11753044.
107. Kempuraj D, Twait EC, Williard DE, Yuan Z, Meyerholz DK, Samuel I. The novel cytokine interleukin-33 activates acinar cell proinflammatory pathways and induces acute pancreatic inflammation in mice. *PLoS One*. 2013; 8: e56866. PMID: 23418608.
108. Bernhagen J, Calandra T, Mitchell RA, Martin SB, Tracey KJ, Voelter W, et al. MIF is a pituitary-derived cytokine that potentiates lethal endotoxaemia. *Nature*. 1993; 365: 756-759. PMID: 8413654.
109. Bernhagen J, Mitchell RA, Calandra T, Voelter W, Cerami A, Bucala R. Purification, bioactivity, and secondary structure analysis of mouse and human macrophage migration inhibitory factor (MIF). *Biochemistry*. 1994; 33: 14144-14155. PMID: 7947826.
110. Bacher M, Metz CN, Calandra T, Mayer K, Chesney J, Lohoff M, et al. An essential regulatory role for macrophage migration inhibitory factor in T-cell activation. *Proc Natl Acad Sci U S A*. 1996; 93: 7849-7854. PMID: 8755565.
111. Sakai Y, Masamune A, Satoh A, Nishihira J, Yamagiwa T, Shimosegawa T. Macrophage migration inhibitory factor is a critical mediator of severe acute pancreatitis. *Gastroenterology*. 2003; 124: 725-736. PMID: 12612911.
112. Devitt A, Marshall LJ. The innate immune system and the clearance of apoptotic cells. *J Leukoc Biol*. 2011; 90: 447-457. PMID: 21562053.
113. Shouval DS, Ouahed J, Biswas A, Goettel JA, Horwitz BH, Klein C, et al. Interleukin 10 receptor signaling: master regulator of intestinal mucosal homeostasis in mice and humans. *Adv Immunol*. 2014; 122: 177-210. PMID: 24507158.
114. Hutchins AP, Diez D, Miranda-Saavedra D. The IL-10/STAT3-mediated anti-inflammatory response: recent developments and future challenges. *Brief Funct Genomics*. 2013; 12: 489-498. PMID: 23943603.
115. Palomares O, Martin-Fontecha M, Lauener R, Traidl-Hoffmann C, Cavkaytar O, Akdis M, et al. Regulatory T cells and immune regulation of allergic diseases: roles of IL-10 and TGF-beta. *Genes Immun*. 2014; 15: 511-520. PMID: 25056447.
116. Ramudo L, Manso MA, Vicente S, De Dios I. Pro- and anti-inflammatory response of acinar cells during acute pancreatitis. Effect of N-acetyl cysteine. *Cytokine*. 2005; 32: 125-131. PMID: 16263306.
117. Gotoh K, Inoue M, Shiraishi K, Masaki T, Chiba S, Mitsutomi K, et al. Spleen-derived interleukin-10 down-regulates the severity of high-fat diet-induced non-alcoholic fatty pancreas disease. *PLoS One*. 2012; 7: e53154. PMID: 23285260.
118. Badger SA, Jones C, McCaigue M, Clements BW, Parks RW, Diamond T, et al. Cytokine response to portal endotoxaemia and neutrophil stimulation in obstructive jaundice. *Eur J Gastroenterol Hepatol*. 2012; 24: 25-32. PMID: 22027701.
119. Pastor CM, Vonlaufen A, Georgi F, Hadengue A, Morel P, Frossard JL. Neutrophil depletion–but not prevention of

Kupffer cell activation–decreases the severity of cerulein-induced acute pancreatitis. *World J Gastroenterol.* 2006; 12: 1219-1224. PMID: 16534874.

120. Qiu Z, Yu P, Bai B, Hao Y, Wang S, Zhao Z, et al. Regulatory B10 cells play a protective role in severe acute pancreatitis. *Inflamm Res.* 2016; 65: 647-654. PMID: 27085321.
121. Rongione AJ, Kusske AM, Kwan K, Ashley SW, Reber HA, McFadden DW. Interleukin 10 reduces the severity of acute pancreatitis in rats. *Gastroenterology.* 1997; 112: 960-967. PMID: 9041259.
122. Warzecha Z, Dembinski A, Ceranowicz P, Konturek SJ, Tomaszewska R, Stachura J, et al. IGF-1 stimulates production of interleukin-10 and inhibits development of caerulein-induced pancreatitis. *J Physiol Pharmacol.* 2003; 54: 575-590. PMID: 14726612.
123. Xu L, Yang F, Lin R, Han C, Liu J, Ding Z. Induction of m2 polarization in primary culture liver macrophages from rats with acute pancreatitis. *PLoS One.* 2014; 9: e108014. PMID: 25259888.
124. Brock P, Sparmann G, Ritter T, Jaster R, Liebe S, Emmrich J. Adenovirus-mediated gene transfer of interleukin-4 into pancreatic stellate cells promotes interleukin-10 expression. *J Cell Mol Med.* 2006; 10: 884-895. PMID: 17125592.
125. Brock P, Sparmann G, Ritter T, Jaster R, Liebe S, Emmrich J. Interleukin-4 gene transfer into rat pancreas by recombinant adenovirus. *Scand J Gastroenterol.* 2005; 40: 1109-1117. PMID: 16165721.
126. Demols A, Van Laethem JL, Quertinmont E, Degraef C, Delhaye M, Geerts A, et al. Endogenous interleukin-10 modulates fibrosis and regeneration in experimental chronic pancreatitis. *Am J Physiol Gastrointest Liver Physiol.* 2002; 282: G1105-G1112. PMID: 12016137.
127. Katz LH, Likhter M, Jogunoori W, Belkin M, Ohshiro K, Mishra L. TGF-beta signaling in liver and gastrointestinal cancers. *Cancer Lett.* 2016; 379: 166-172. PMID: 27039259.
128. Achyut BR, Yang L. Transforming growth factor-beta in the gastrointestinal and hepatic tumor microenvironment. *Gastroenterology.* 2011; 141: 1167-1178. PMID: 21839702.
129. Wildi S, Kleeff J, Mayerle J, Zimmermann A, Bottinger EP, Wakefield L, et al. Suppression of transforming growth factor beta signalling aborts caerulein induced pancreatitis and eliminates restricted stimulation at high caerulein concentrations. *Gut.* 2007; 56: 685-692. PMID: 17135311.
130. Konturek PC, Dembinski A, Warzecha Z, Ceranowicz P, Konturek SJ, Stachura J, et al. Expression of transforming growth factor-beta 1 and epidermal growth factor in caerulein-induced pancreatitis in rat. *J Physiol Pharmacol.* 1997; 48: 59-72. PMID: 9098826.
131. Hori Y, Takeyama Y, Ueda T, Shinkai M, Takase K, Kuroda Y. Macrophage-derived transforming growth factor-beta1 induces hepatocellular injury via apoptosis in rat severe acute pancreatitis. *Surgery.* 2000; 127: 641-649. PMID: 10840359.
132. Kihara Y, Tashiro M, Nakamura H, Yamaguchi T, Yoshikawa H, Otsuki M. Role of TGF-beta1, extracellular matrix, and matrix metalloproteinase in the healing process of the pancreas after induction of acute necrotizing pancreatitis using arginine in rats. *Pancreas.* 2001; 23: 288-295. PMID: 11590325.
133. Riesle E, Friess H, Zhao L, Wagner M, Uhl W, Baczako K, et al. Increased expression of transforming growth factor beta s after acute oedematous pancreatitis in rats suggests a role in pancreatic repair. *Gut.* 1997; 40: 73-79. PMID: 9155579.
134. Van Laethem JL, Robberecht P, Resibois A, Deviere J. Transforming growth factor beta promotes development of fibrosis after repeated courses of acute pancreatitis in mice. *Gastroenterology.* 1996; 110: 576-582. PMID: 8566606.
135. Nagashio Y, Ueno H, Imamura M, Asaumi H, Watanabe S, Yamaguchi T, et al. Inhibition of transforming growth factor beta decreases pancreatic fibrosis and protects the pancreas against chronic injury in mice. *Lab Invest.* 2004; 84: 1610-1618. PMID: 15502860.
136. Menke A, Yamaguchi H, Gress TM, Adler G. Extracellular matrix is reduced by inhibition of transforming growth factor beta1 in pancreatitis in the rat. *Gastroenterology.* 1997; 113: 295-303. PMID: 9207290.
137. Zhang X, Zheng H, Zhu HY, Hu S, Wang S, Jiang X, et al. Acute effects of transforming growth factor-beta1 on neuronal excitability and involvement in the pain of rats with chronic pancreatitis. *J Neurogastroenterol Motil.* 2016; 22: 333-343. PMID: 26645248.
138. Bone RC. Sir Isaac Newton, sepsis, SIRS, and CARS. *Crit Care Med.* 1996; 24: 1125-1128. PMID: 8674323.
139. Takahashi H, Tsuda Y, Kobayashi M, Herndon DN, Suzuki F. CCL2 as a trigger of manifestations of compensatory anti-inflammatory response syndrome in mice with severe systemic inflammatory response syndrome. *J Leukoc Biol.* 2006; 79: 789-796. PMID: 16434696.
140. Ho YP, Chiu CT, Sheen IS, Tseng SC, Lai PC, Ho SY, et al. Tumor necrosis factor-alpha and interleukin-10 contribute to immunoparalysis in patients with acute pancreatitis. *Hum Immunol.* 2011; 72: 18-23. PMID: 20937337.
141. Kobayashi M, Kobayashi H, Herndon DN, Pollard RB, Suzuki F. Burn-associated Candida albicans infection caused by CD30+ type 2 T cells. *J Leukoc Biol.* 1998; 63: 723-731. PMID: 9620665.
142. Gunjaca I, Zunic J, Gunjaca M, Kovac Z. Circulating cytokine levels in acute pancreatitis-model of SIRS/CARS can help in the clinical assessment of disease severity. *Inflammation.* 2012; 35: 758-763. PMID: 21826480.
143. Koike Y, Kanai T, Saeki K, Nakamura Y, Nakano M, Mikami Y, et al. MyD88-dependent interleukin-10 production from regulatory CD11b(+)Gr-1(high) cells suppresses development of acute cerulein pancreatitis in mice. *Immunol Lett.* 2012; 148: 172-177. PMID: 23022387.

Chapter 6

Animal models of chronic pancreatitis

Anamika M. Reed[1] and Fred S. Gorelick[1,2*]

[1]*Yale University School of Medicine, New Haven, Connecticut;*
[2]*VA HealthCare System, West Haven, Connecticut.*

Introduction

Chronic pancreatitis is a progressive, inflammatory disease of the pancreas that leads to inflammation and fibrosis, with the potential for exocrine and endocrine insufficiency. The prevalence of the disease is estimated to be 42 per 1,00,000 and rising.[1,2] The pathogenesis of chronic pancreatitis is incompletely understood and complex, involving the interplay of environmental, metabolic, and genetic factors that modulate inflammatory and fibrotic pathways. Although alcohol is the leading cause of chronic pancreatitis, other toxic, hereditary, and obstructive insults can lead to similar histologic and clinical manifestations. Studying the cellular mechanisms responsible for chronic pancreatitis in human subjects is difficult for a number of reasons including the undefined natural history of the disease, a lack of reliable tests for early chronic pancreatitis, and inaccessibility of human tissue. Therefore, animal models are essential to advancing our understanding of the pathophysiologic processes responsible for chronic pancreatitis.

Though chronic alcohol abuse is the leading cause of chronic pancreatitis, a number of other etiologies including toxins, obstructive lesions, and genetic disorders can cause chronic pancreatitis. There is no consensus as to how these diverse etiologic factors lead to a common histological endpoint. Theories of pathogenesis fall into two broad categories: those in which repeated episodes of acute pancreatitis (AP) lead to chronic pancreatitis and those in which an initiating injurious event is perpetuated and progresses to irreversible injury in the appropriate environment (**Figure 1**).

A prominent model of the latter is the sentinel acute pancreatitis event (SAPE) hypothesis, which posits that a single AP episode can progress to chronic pancreatitis in a conducive environment. If the sentinel episode is severe enough to attract monocytes and activate stellate cells, fibrosis can develop in the presence of continued injurious stimuli.[3] Although some theories of injury focus on acinar cell injury, others focus on duct cells as the initial target of damage.[4,5] Finally, some hypothesize that that multiple different pathways can lead to chronic pancreatitis using different mechanisms. All models of chronic pancreatitis, except autoimmune models, share the same histologic endpoints (**Figure 2**) and can lead to similar disease severity. These include some or all of the following features: chronic inflammation, stellate cell proliferation/activation, acinar cell dropout, ductal dilatation, intraductal calcifications, and nerve enlargement.

Animal models can be classified according to the mechanism of disease and species used, though in some cases various mechanisms are combined to capture the multiple factors that lead to disease (**Figure 3**). Although most animal models result in histopathologic disease, clinically relevant parameters listed in **Table 1**, such as pain, exocrine and endocrine insufficiency, and predisposition to malignancy are frequently not addressed. This review summarizes the most widely used models of chronic pancreatitis, discusses their strengths and weaknesses, and highlights particularly clinically relevant aspects of various models.

Features of chronic pancreatitis in human patients include multiple structural and functional characteristics that can be reproduced in animal models. No available animal model of chronic pancreatitis is known to replicate all of these features.

Chemical Models

Cerulein pancreatitis

Various agents can be administered systemically or locally to produce chronic pancreatitis (**Table 2**).

Treatment with supraphysiologic doses of the cholecystokinin (CCK) analogue cerulein is employed in a widely used animal model of AP. At low doses, cerulein provides physiologic stimulation to CCK receptors and enhances secretion from the acinar cell. However, animals treated with high-dose cerulein (10-100×physiologic doses; 20-50 μg/kg, intravenously or intraperitoneally) develop mild to moderate acute interstitial pancreatitis. The cerulein model of AP is

*Corresponding author. Email: fred.gorelick@yale.edu

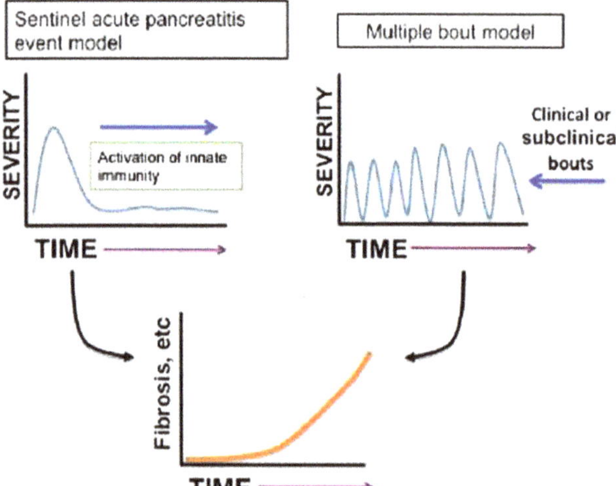

Figure 1. Models of evolution to chronic pancreatitis. In the traditional model, repeated bouts of AP lead to fibrosis. An example of this model is the induction of chronic pancreatitis through repetitive cerulein injections. The Sentinal Acute Pancreatitis Event (SAPE) model proposes that an initiating event like an AP episode activates the immune system allowing risk factors to drive profibrotic, anti-inflammatory pathways that lead to chronic pancreatitis. Ethanol sensitization models such as the ethanol/lipopolysaccharide (LPS) model conform to this hypothesis. Both models can result in similar severity of final pancreatic injury.

characterized by aberrant zymogen activation in the acinar cell, inhibition of secretion, increased inflammation, and cellular damage. Exocrine pancreatic structure and function recover within 24 to 48 hours in this model.

The cerulein model of chronic pancreatitis requires repeated cerulein injections over time and is the most

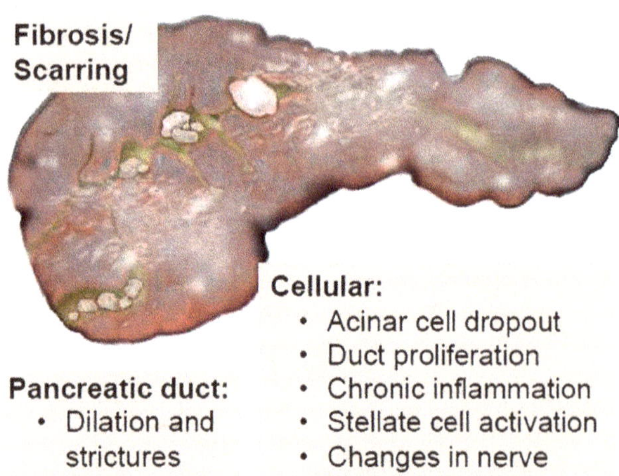

Figure 2. Histopathologic features of chronic pancreatitis. Animal models of chronic pancreatitis share histological endpoints including fibrosis, pancreatic duct abnormalities, and cellular changes.

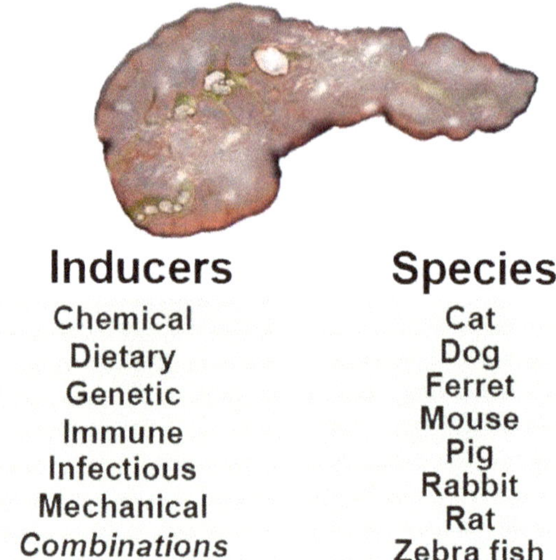

Figure 3. Animal models of chronic pancreatitis vary in mechanism and species used. A variety of different trigger mechanisms and animal species have been used in animal models of chronic pancreatitis.

commonly used, reproducible model of chronic pancreatitis. There are a number of protocols that vary in dose, interval, and duration of cerulein injections.[6-8] This model produces morphohistologic findings compatible with chronic pancreatitis in humans, including fibrosis, chronic inflammation, atrophy, transdifferentiation of acini into duct-like cells, and ductal dilatation[7] as seen in **Figure 4**.

Interestingly, these findings can occur even in the absence of zymogen activation.[9] This model is widely used because of its reproducibility and technical ease in rodents, making it an attractive technique for use in transgenic mice. The cerulein model mirrors chronic pancreatitis in humans because it involves repetitive injurious stimulation, paralleling the progression from recurrent AP to chronic pancreatitis that occurs in some patients.[10] However, human pancreatitis is not associated with elevated CCK levels. Furthermore, it remains controversial whether human acinar cells express CCK receptors like rodent acinar cells.[11,12] Therefore, it is appropriate to question the relevance of the cerulein model to human disease with respect to CCK's role, even though it may fully reflect other aspects of disease.

Table 1. Chronic pancreatitis characteristics studied in animal models.

- Fibrosis
- Inflammation
- Exocrine function
- Endocrine function
- Pain
- Predisposition to cancer

Table 2. Chemical models of chronic pancreatitis.

- Cerulein
  - Repeated dosing
  - Combined with:
    - Lipopolysaccride (LPS)
    - Chronic ethanol
    - Cyclosporine A
    - Dibutyltin dichloride (DBTC)
- Ethanol/LPS
- Arginine
- Choline-deficient ethionine supplemented (CDE) diet
- Trinitrobenzene sulfonic acid (TNBS)

Repetitive administration of cerulein, sometimes in the presence of sensitizing agents, is the most commonly used model of chronic pancreatitis. Ethanol can be combined with cerulein or LPS to produce chronic pancreatitis. Other toxic compounds can be administered systemically or by retrograde infusion into the pancreatic duct.

The cerulein model of chronic pancreatitis serves as the basis for studying the sensitizing effects of other agents. The bacterial endotoxin LPS is a particularly relevant agent because chronic alcohol consumption leads to increased gut permeability, predisposing to bacterial translocation and increased serum LPS levels.[13] LPS has been shown activate pancreatic stellate cells and stimulate inflammatory cytokines through activation of toll-like receptor 4 (TLR4) and nuclear factor-κB (NF-κB).[14] The addition of LPS to the repeated cerulein injection model accelerates disease progression and worsens its severity as measured by acinar cell atrophy, fibrosis, and the development of tubular complexes.[15]

Cyclosporine A (CsA) has also been used a sensitizing agent in cerulein-induced chronic pancreatitis. In this model, rats received just two doses of intraperitoneal cerulein during a 15-day treatment with intraperitoneal CsA. Rats treated with cerulein alone fully recover from AP, while those cotreated with cyclosporine exhibit chronic pancreatitis with atrophy, mononuclear inflammatory infiltrate, and enhanced collagen deposition.[16] Increases in transforming growth factor (TGF)-β are thought to mediate the effects of cyclosporine by activating pancreatic stellate cells, increasing collagenase inhibitor production, and inhibiting matrix degrading proteases. Due to reportedly high toxicity rates by some investigators, the use of this model is limited.

Other toxins

Feeding of a choline-deficient ethionine-supplemented (CDE) diet induces acute hemorrhagic pancreatitis in mice.[17,18] The mechanism responsible for CDE-induced pancreatic damage is not known. Long-term administration of the CDE diet intermittently over 24 weeks leads to histologic changes consistent with chronic pancreatitis, including acinar atrophy, fibrosis, and the development of tubular complexes. Additionally, increased expression of epidermal growth factor receptor, serine protease inhibitor Kazal type 3 (SPINK3), and TGF-α, which are all implicated in the progression from chronic pancreatitis to pancreatic adenocarcinoma, were observed in this model. However, malignant lesions did not form even after 54 weeks of CDE feeding.[19]

L-arginine, an essential amino acids, administered intraperitoneally in high doses has been shown to cause severe, necrotizing AP in animal models.[20] The mechanisms responsible for the effects of L-arginine on the pancreas are unknown, though reactive oxygen species production and direct activation of the immune system have been postulated. Repeated injections of lower doses

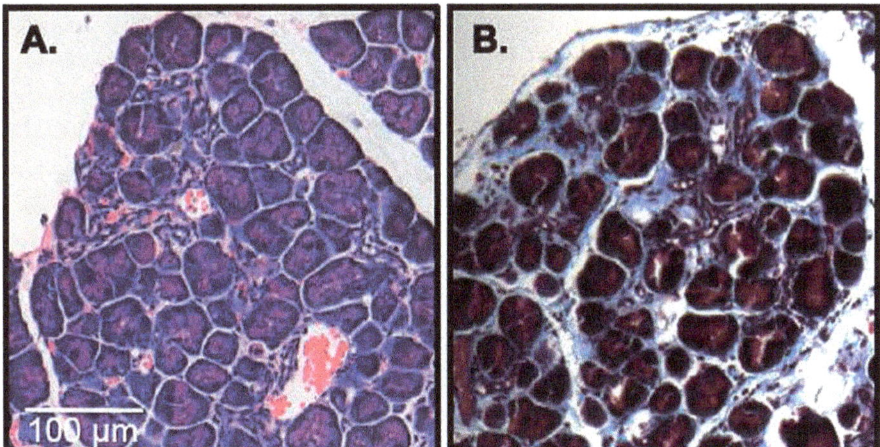

Figure 4. Repeated cerulein injections lead to chronic pancreatitis in mice. After a 2-week cerulein injection protocol, hematoxylin and eosin staining shows (A) significant inflammation, and trichrome staining (B) reveals fibrosis in the exocrine pancreas. Images provided by Chuhan Chung, Yale University.

of L-arginine given over several weeks produce necrosis followed by chronic inflammation and fibrosis with impaired glucose tolerance in rats.[21,22] Unlike most human chronic pancreatitis, fibrotic tissue is replaced by adipose tissue over time, limiting its usefulness as a histologic model of chronic pancreatitis.

Intravenous or intraperitoneal injection of dibutyltin dichloride (DBTC), a compound used in polyvinyl chloride production, leads to acute interstitial pancreatitis through direct toxicity on acinar cells and by causing chronic biliary obstruction through the formation of obstructing plugs in the distal common bile duct.[23,24] With repeated DBTC injections, rats develop chronic inflammation and fibrosis.[25,26] However, this model is not highly reproducible, as only one-third of animals display histologic changes consistent with chronic pancreatitis. The CDE, L-arginine, and DBTC models are limited by the fact that none of these compounds cause pancreatitis in humans, their mechanisms of actions are unknown, and they each produce nonspecific extrapancreatic injury.

Alcohol

Alcohol is the leading cause of chronic pancreatitis. However, less than 10% of alcoholics develop chronic pancreatitis.[27] The lack of a homogeneous, dose-dependent effect of alcohol on the human exocrine pancreas is reflected in ethanol animal models. Ethanol feeding alone does not produce chronic pancreatitis in animal models. The most informative use of this model has been its use in studies of sensitization to other injurious agents.

The Lieber-DeCarli method of chronic alcohol feeding involves supplementing liquid feed with 36% ethanol and is useful in overcoming rodents' natural aversion to alcohol.[28] Pancreata from chronically alcohol fed animals appear histologically normal without significant gross inflammation or fibrosis. More intense alcohol feeding by continuous gavage, which produces sustained blood alcohol levels of 250-500 mg/dL, also fails to produce significant histologic changes consistent with chronic pancreatitis.[29] Other models of repeated ethanol feeding including the ethanol agar block feeding model and supplementing drinking water with ethanol fail to achieve consistently elevated levels of blood ethanol.[30,31] Therefore, chronic ethanol feeding cannot be used on its own as an experimental model of chronic pancreatitis. However, despite the lack of histologic changes, chronic ethanol feeding has pronounced biochemical effects including increased production of fatty acid esters, mitochondrial injury, and pancreatic stellate cell activation. Therefore, the model still provides insight into the pathogenesis of alcohol-induced chronic pancreatitis.[32-34]

Combining chronic alcohol feeding with other injurious stimuli creates histologic damage and provides a reliable model of chronic pancreatitis. Rats fed the Lieber-DeCarli diet challenged with repeated high-dose cerulein injections show changes consistent with human alcoholic chronic pancreatitis. While animals treated only with cerulein recovered, those sensitized with ethanol developed fibrosis, calcifications, and necrosis. Furthermore, the immune cell profile at each stage of injury was markedly different in ethanol-sensitized rats compared to cerulein-only controls.[35,36] Similar results were seen in a mouse version of the same model.[36]

In another model, rats fed Lieber-DiCarli diets were challenged with LPS. In this model ethanol-fed rats but not those on the control diet developed fibrosis and displayed stellate cell activation.[37] This model has direct clinical relevance because alcoholics are known to have increased gut permeability, which encourages higher circulating LPS levels.[13,38] The LPS/alcohol model has been used to study the effects of alcohol abstinence on chronic pancreatitis progression and has shown that alcohol withdrawal leads to fibrosis regression and increased pancreatic stellate cell apoptosis.[16] Of the chronic pancreatitis summarized in this review, the combined use of ethanol feeding and LPS appears to have the most relevance to disease etiology encountered in clinical disease. The histologic responses are also very similar to those that develop in human disease (**Figure 5**).

These alcohol sensitization models conform to the SAPE hypothesis of chronic pancreatitis (**Figure 1**). Even in the presence of important risk factors like heavy alcohol intake, a sentinel inflammatory event, like an episode of AP, is required to activate the immune system and prime the pancreas for chronic inflammation. Then fibrosis may develop depending on the presence of continued risk factors that modulate the immune response.[3]

Retrograde infusion of toxic substances

Several models involving the retrograde infusion of toxic substances have been attempted. These models deliver toxins only to the pancreas, unlike the models that require systemic toxin administration described above. Retrograde infusion of the cytotoxic unsaturated fatty acid oleic acid destroys acinar cells and causes acute inflammation.[39] Because the exocrine pancreatic parenchyma undergoes fatty replacement rather than fibrosis over time, this model is not ideal for studying human chronic pancreatitis. Infusion of trinitrobenzene sulfonic acid into the pancreatic duct leads to acute necrotizing pancreatitis at 48 hours and fibrosis, inflammation, and atrophy consistent with chronic pancreatitis at later time points.[40] Retrograde infusion of bile acids provides an attractive model to study AP because gallstone obstruction is a common cause of AP.[41] This method is thought to elicit pancreatitis through direct toxic effects on the acinar cell that is mediated by G

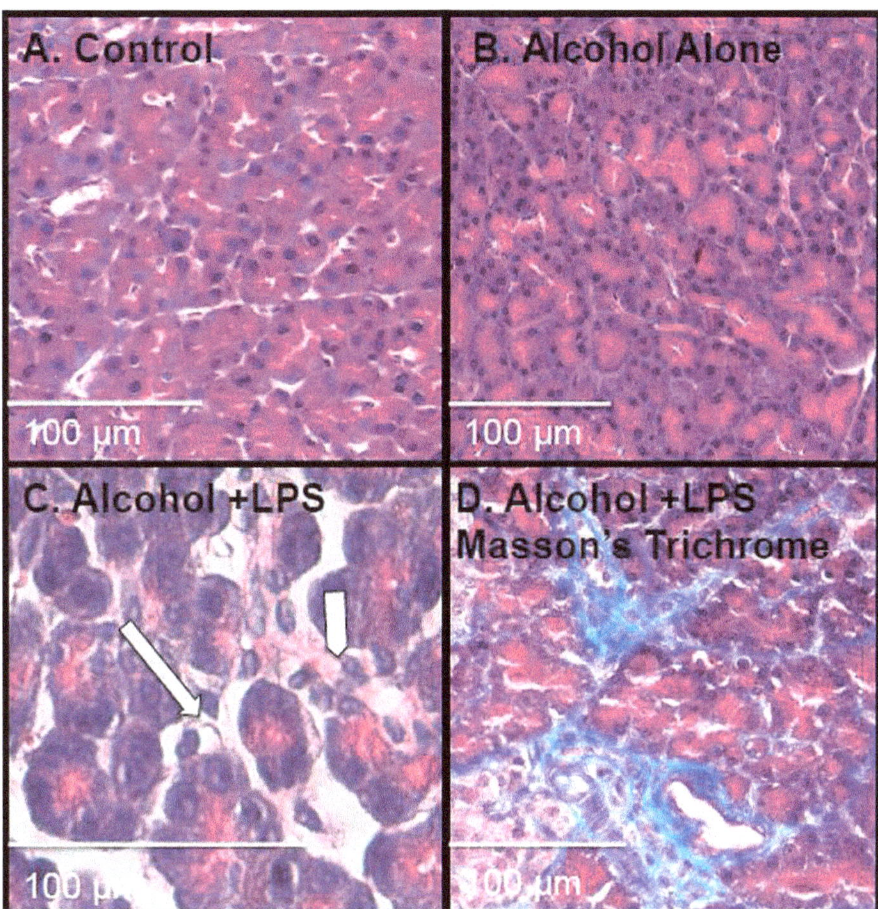

Figure 5. Alcohol/LPS leads to chronic pancreatitis in rats. In untreated rats (A) and rats treated with alcohol alone, acinar architecture is well preserved, and morphohistologic features of chronic pancreatitis are absent. Rats treated with alcohol in the presence of LPS (C-D) show findings consistent with chronic pancreatitis including vacuolization (arrow), inflammatory infiltrate (arrowhead), acinar cell dropout, and fibrosis (blue staining in D). Images provided by Minoti Apte, University of New South Wales.

protein-coupled bile acid receptor 1 (Gpbar1). Chronic pancreatitis caused by obstructive lesions may also be mediated by bile reflux into the pancreatic duct. While retrograde infusion of high doses of sodium taurocholate leads to the death of most rats by 72 hours, some survivors display atrophy and fibrosis.[42] Retrograde infusion of lower doses of sodium taurocholate produces milder acute injury with return to normal histopathology at 14 days.[6] Drawbacks of this model include its technical difficulty and the finding that injury is often localized to the pancreatic head.

Obstructive Models

Obstructive lesions such as tumors and trauma are rare causes of chronic pancreatitis. In humans with chronic pancreatitis from any cause, protein plugs form in small pancreatic ducts, and pancreatic ductal pressure is elevated.[43,44] Therefore, obstruction of the pancreatic duct provides a rational model for studying chronic pancreatitis (**Table 3**). One week after dogs or rats undergo ductal ligation, their pancreata display ductal dilatation, disorganized acinar cell arrangement, fibrosis with collagen deposition, and inflammatory infiltrate in interstitial spaces.[45] Pancreatic duct ligation in rabbits and dogs also results in significantly impaired glucose tolerance.[46] Pancreatic ductal ligation in the mouse is technically challenging because of the small size of the pancreatic duct. Furthermore, the redundant duct anatomy of the

Table 3. Mechanical models of chronic pancreatitis.

- Duct obstruction
  - Entire duct or segmental
  - Partial obstruction or complete obstruction
- Duct hypertension

Obstructive chronic pancreatitis has been produced in several different species by complete or partial pancreatic duct ligation or through inducing pancreatic ductal hypertension.

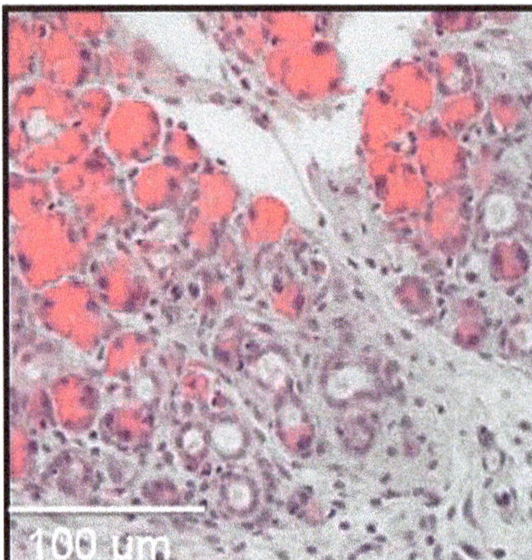

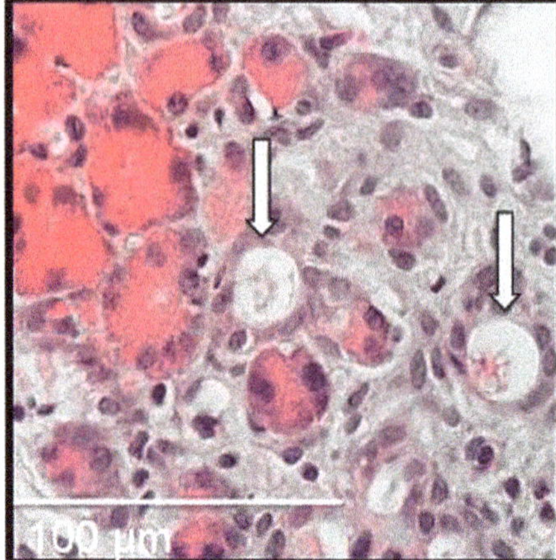

Figure 6. Pancreatic ductal ligation in mice leads to histology consistent with chronic pancreatitis. Characteristic histologic features including loss of normal acinar architecture, inflammation, and the formation of duct-like structures (arrows) are seen soon after pancreatic duct ligation in the mouse. Images provided by Howard Crawford, Mayo Clinic (Jacksonville, Florida).

mouse leads to histopathologic changes in some but not all pancreatic lobes. Edema, increased inflammatory infiltrate, enhanced apoptosis, and acinar cell dropout are seen 3 days after pancreatic duct ligation.[47] By 5 days after pancreatic ductal ligation, there few remaining normal acinar cells and abundant proliferation of duct-like cells with fibrosis. Seven days after ligation, metaplastic ducts, which are resistant to apoptosis are observed. **Figure 6** demonstrates the early histologic changes after pancreatic duct ligation. After several months there is intralobular fatty replacement of the exocrine pancreas.[48] Partial pancreatic obstruction in dogs can be accomplished by inserting a small plastic tube into the pancreatic duct to produce pancreatic acinar atrophy, fibrosis, and inflammation.[49]

Given that pancreatic duct ligation leads to eventual complete acinar cell loss rather than fibrosis, a model that causes pancreatic ductal hypertension without pancreatic ductal obstruction was developed. In this technically challenging model, pancreatic ductal hypertension was induced by implanting pancreatic, biliary, and duodenal cannulas in rats. The free end of the pancreatic duct cannula was then vertically raised to create increased hydrostatic pressure for 2 weeks.[6] Rats with pancreatic ductal hypertension showed significant fibrosis with collagen deposition, lymphocytic inflammatory infiltrate, and plug formation in the main pancreatic duct.

Genetic Models

Several transgenic models based on known susceptibility genes in humans have been developed (**Table 4**). These animal models have direct clinical relevance to human disease. The fidelity with which the transgenic animal phenotype mimics human disease varies widely.

CFTR

Cystic fibrosis is a common autosomal recessive disease among Caucasian populations that affects multiple organ systems including the respiratory tract and gastrointestinal (GI) organs. It is caused by mutations in the *CFTR* gene located on chromosome 7, which encodes a regulated chloride channel. Most patients with cystic fibrosis develop pancreatic insufficiency, and these individuals are at high risk for chronic pancreatitis.[50] Patients who are not homozygotes or compound heterozygotes for the classical, severe CFTR mutations and, therefore, do not have cystic fibrosis, can express other milder phenotypic variants. Patients who are homozygotes or compound heterozygotes, with at least one

Table 4. Genetic models of chronic pancreatitis.

- **A. General** (including pancreatic development)
  - CFTR deficient mice, pigs, and ferrets
  - SPINK3 $^{-/-}$ mice
  - Kif3a $^{-/-}$ mice (PDX-1)
  - Wistar Bonn/Kobori (WBN/Kob) rats
  - Hedgehog (zebra fish)
  - Cytokeratin 8 (human) in mice
  - E2F1/E2F2 double-deficient (DKO) mice
  - IKKa $^{-/-}$ mice (PDX-1)
  - PEDF null mice
- **B. Acinar cell**
  - PRSSI (cationic trypsinogen) R122H mice
  - Ras activity (K-Ras)
  - PERK $^{-/-}$ (elastase)
  - IL-1b mice (elastase)
- **C. Duct Cells**
  - COX2 overexpression duct cells (BK5)
  - LXRβ deletion

Genetic models of chronic pancreatitis can target genes that are generally or specifically expressed in acinar or duct cells.

allele encoding a mild variant have a 40%-80% increased risk of developing chronic pancreatitis.[51] Heterozygotes for CFTR mutations have a 3-4-fold increased risk of developing chronic pancreatitis, with the subset of patients who coexpress mutated SPINK1 at the highest risk.[21]

Several transgenic animal models have been used to study the relationship between CFTR mutations and chronic pancreatitis. Mice homozygous for the S489X mutation, which encodes a truncated protein, display a phenotype that has many features of human cystic fibrosis.[52] In particular, these mice fail to thrive and develop meconium ileus and alterations in mucous and serous glands. The mice have modest exocrine insufficiency with lower trypsin and lipase activities than controls, an abnormally acidic duodenum because of decreased pancreatic bicarbonate secretion, and blunted secretory responses to CCK.[53] CFTR mutant mice develop more severe acute cerulein-induced pancreatitis with a more exuberant inflammatory response and decreased apoptosis than controls.[53] Although these transgenic mice have enhanced expression of proinflammatory cytokine genes at baseline, they do not develop chronic pancreatitis. Death from intestinal obstruction occurs during weaning by 40 days of age in nearly all CFTR-/- mice, limiting the usefulness of this murine model for studying CFTR-related chronic pancreatitis.

A porcine model of cystic fibrosis was developed to more closely replicate human disease. CFTR-/- pigs appear normal at birth but soon develop meconium ileus and failure to thrive.[54] The piglets require surgery to relieve intestinal obstruction from meconium ileus and prevent perforation. They also eventually develop infertility and focal biliary cirrhosis. Porcine CFTR-/- pancreata appear small, with increased adiposity and inflammation. Centroacinar spaces and ducts are dilated and obstructed by eosinophilic material. CF pigs also have significantly lower levels of pancreatic amylase, lipase, and trypsin.[55] The baseline volume and pH of pancreatic fluid are depressed in CF pigs, and they do not respond to secretin stimulation with increased pancreatic secretions like wild-type pigs. Newborn CF piglet pancreata display a mixed inflammatory infiltrate with neutrophils, macrophages, effector and cytotoxic T cells, activated T helper cells, and natural killer (NK) T cells.[56] Additionally, fetal CF pig acinar cells display increased expression of proinflammatory, complement cascade, and profibrotic genes. Furthermore, increased apoptosis, α-smooth muscle actin, and TGFβ-1 are observed in newborn and fetal CF pigs. These findings suggest upregulation of fibrotic pathways, providing a superior model for CF-related pancreatic disease.[57] Although the CF pig model appears to very closely resemble human disease, the high cost of the animals limits the opportunities for studying this model.

A ferret model of CF has also been developed. Newborn CFTR-/- animals display dilated pancreatic ducts with inspissated zymogen secretions, and 75% of animals maintain this phenotype during infancy. A small minority of cases develop more severe lesions including fibrosis and loss of pancreatic parenchyma. Because these animals have high early mortality because of meconium ileus and GI malabsorption, a gut-corrected transgenic CFTR knockout (KO) that only expresses CFTR in the intestines and does not suffer from meconium ileus was created.[58] Although the latter model is more amenable to study, its use has been limited.

PRSS1

Mutations in cationic trypsinogen are responsible for 80% of cases of hereditary pancreatitis that are not caused by CF. These mutations affect the regulatory regions of trypsinogen, rendering it more vulnerable to inappropriate activation. The R122H missense mutation of the cationic trypsinogen gene (*PRSS1*) was the first identified mutation responsible for hereditary pancreatitis and is an attractive target for manipulation in mouse models.[59] In one model, transgenic mice with the R122H mutation in murine trypsin 4 targeted to pancreatic acinar cells were produced. These mice develop inflammation, fibrosis, and acinar cell dedifferentiation. There is activation of acinar cell-specific inflammatory signaling pathways and c-Jun-N-terminal kinase, which mediates TNF-α-induced cell death.[60] Unfortunately, this model is no longer available. Another model created mice transgenic for human R122H cationic trypsinogen targeted to the pancreas. These animals have elevated lipase levels, but no spontaneous alterations in pancreatic histology.[61] Cerulein-induced chronic pancreatitis is more severe in both models.

SPINK3

The serine protease inhibitor Kazal type 1 (*SPINK1*) encodes for a protease inhibitor that is upregulated in inflammatory states and safeguards against aberrant intracellular zymogen activation. SPINK mutations are common in humans, though the vast majority of those with even "high-risk" mutations do not develop pancreatitis.[62] Deficiency of SPINK3, a homologue of SPINK1, is lethal by 2 weeks in KO mice. Analysis of acinar cells isolated from neonatal mice revealed enhanced trypsin activation.[63] Embryonic pancreatic specimens revealed autophagic degeneration of acinar cells, which progressed to rapid cell death after birth.[64] SPINK3 heterozygotes have reduced trypsin inhibitor capacity compared to wild-type mice because they express less SPINK3 protein. However, SPINK3 heterozygotes do demonstrate increased susceptibility to cerulein-induced pancreatitis, suggesting that a threshold level of SPINK3 is sufficient to protect against pancreatitis.[65] Although these animals do not manifest spontaneous chronic pancreatitis, the model highlights the important role of SPINK in exocrine pancreas maintenance and regeneration.

KRAS

The oncogene *KRAS* is the most common gene mutated in pancreatic ductal adenocarcinoma (PDAC) and is also mutated in about 40% of patients with chronic pancreatitis.[66] Transgenic mice that overexpress activated KRAS in acinar cells demonstrate fibrosis and inflammation that mimics the histologic findings of human chronic pancreatitis.[67] Elevated levels of Ras activity in this model leads to the spontaneous development of PDAC, making it an attractive model for the progression from chronic pancreatitis to pancreatic cancer. Inflammatory stimuli that produce transient Ras signaling in wild-type animals induced prolonged Ras, NF-κB, and COX-2 activity in mice expressing oncogenic KRAS, leading to chronic inflammation and precancerous lesions.[68] Thus, the KRAS model likely reflects a mechanism seen in human chronic pancreatitis with respect to chronic inflammation and fibrosis.

Other genetic models

Several other genetic models do not have an obvious correlate in human disease, but can be useful in understanding the pathways that lead to chronic pancreatitis. Acinar cells have an extensive endoplasmic reticulum (ER) network with associated chaperones and foldases to manage the production and secretion of digestive enzymes. Regulatory mechanisms direct misfolded proteins to ER-associated degradation pathways. Stressors such as oxidative damage, overloading the protein-folding capacity of the ER, or the presence of mutant proteins lead to ER stress and trigger the unfolded protein response, which is an important mediator of acinar cell damage in alcohol-induced pancreatitis.[69] The ER sensor PERK (protein kinase RNA-like ER kinase) responds to ER stress by decreasing overall protein translation while enhancing regulators of redox status and glutathione production. Pancreas-specific PERK KO mice develop pancreatic exocrine and endocrine dysfunction rapidly after birth.[70] Acinar cell death in this model occurs through ischemia, which then triggers an inflammatory response consisting of neutrophils and macrophages.[71] This model highlights the importance of the ER stress response in maintaining acinar cell function and may be relevant to the rare human disease Wolcott-Rallison syndrome, which is caused by a mutation in the *PERK* gene and characterized by early onset diabetes, skeletal dysplasia, and exocrine pancreatic insufficiency.

Defects in primary cilia have been implicated in polycystic kidney disease (PKD). Pancreatic lesions, especially pancreatic cysts and occasionally chronic pancreatitis, are more common in patients in PKD. To study this disease, a mouse model with pancreas-specific inactivation of *Kif3a*, which encodes kinesin-2, was developed. Kinesin-2 is a protein that is required for cilia assembly. The pancreata of these mice display acinoductular metaplasia, fibrosis, eventual pancreatic lipomatosis, and cyst formation.[72] These findings provide a model for the pancreatic diseases associated with PKD and primary ciliary dyskinesia (Kartagener's syndrome).

Another model focuses on the role of the inflammatory cytokine IL-1β by employing transgenic mice that selectively overexpress human IL-1β in the pancreas. These elastase sshIL-1β mice develop acinar cell atrophy, pancreatic ductal dilatation, mixed inflammatory infiltrate, acinar-ductal metaplasia, and fibrosis.[73] The mice are susceptible to more severe chronic pancreatitis after 20 weeks of cerulein treatment. There are also increased expression levels of tumor necrosis factor-alpha (TNF-α); chemokine (C-X-C motif) ligand 1; stromal cell-derived factor 1, TGF-β1; matrix metallopeptidases 2, 7, and 9; inhibitor of metalloproteinase 1; and cyclooxygenase 2 (COX-2). Given this profile, IL-1β likely induces acinar cell damage by recruiting and activating inflammatory cells and pancreatic stellate cells.

WBN/Kob rats, initially developed as a model for gastric tumors, also spontaneously develop pancreatic fibrosis and diabetes mellitus.[74] By 3 months of age, the mice develop focal pancreatic necrosis and inflammation that slowly encompasses the entire pancreas. By 4 months, fibrosis is seen in the exocrine pancreas, with eventual expansion to the endocrine pancreas. The rats become diabetic at 60-90 months. These findings are only seen in sexually mature, male mice, suggesting a role for androgen in the pathogenesis of the pancreatic lesions. A limitation of this model is that exact nature of the genetic alterations responsible for the phenotype of this mouse strain is unknown. Chromosomal mapping identified polymorphisms in three candidate genes: *Rac2*, *Grap2*, and *Xpnpep3*.[75] Rac2 is a GTPase member of the Rho family, which plays a role in apoptosis, phagocytosis, and cytoskeletal reorganization. Grap2 is an adaptor protein that participates in leukocyte specific protein-tyrosine kinase signaling. Finally, Xpnpep3, localizes to mitochondria and is involved in ciliary function. Which of these candidate genes is responsible for the pancreatic phenotype of WBN/Kob mice requires further study.

The hedgehog signaling pathway plays a key role in patterning events in normal mammalian development. Indian hedgehog (Ihh), a member of this family, is upregulated in human chronic pancreatitis.[76] To explore the contribution of the Hedgehog pathway in the pathogenesis of chronic pancreatitis, transgenic zebrafish that overexpress Ihh and Sonic hedgehog (Shh) along with green fluorescent protein were developed.[77] Both mutants have similar phenotypes. Neither form of transgenic zebrafish develop derangements in acinar differentiation, but both develop fibrosis over time with increased expression of matrix metalloproteinase and TGF-β.

Keratins are epithelia-specific intermediate filament proteins involved in pancreatic acinar cell homeostasis.

Some human studies suggest that mutations in the keratin 8 gene are associated with chronic pancreatitis,[78] but others did not find an association between keratin 8 mutations and chronic pancreatitis.[79] When human keratin K8 is overexpressed in HK8 transgenic mice, acinar cells display inflammation, fibrosis, dysplasia, and parenchymal replacement by adipose tissue.[80]

The E2F family of DNA-binding transcriptional activators is comprised of six members (E2F1-6)that heterodimerize with the transcription factor DP to regulate the expression of genes involved in cell growth and differentiation. E2F1/E2F2 double KO mice lose acinar cells and develop fibrosis and fat replacement without significant inflammation after 2 weeks. The endocrine pancreas also becomes progressively atrophic. The mice have a shortened lifespan, in part, because of the development of frank diabetes with decreased insulin levels and hyperglycemia and exocrine insufficiency with steatorrhea. These studies suggest that E2F1 and E2F2 play critical roles in pancreatic homeostasis.[81]

IκB kinase α (IKKα), a subunit of the IKK complex, regulates the activation of the NF-κB transcription factor and is critical for epidermal differentiation, keratinocyte differentiation, and skeletal patterning. Conditional IKKα KO mice, with IKKα deficiency in acinar, ductal, and islet cells develop spontaneous and progressive acinar cell damage, fibrosis, and inflammation, as well as endocrine insufficiency. The pathway underlying these defects was shown to be impaired autophagic protein degradation, leading to ER stress and elevated expression of CHOP (C/EBP homologous protein), a proapoptotic transcription factor.[82]

Pigment epithelial-derived factor (PEDF) is involved in maintaining a normal extracellular matrix and regulating intracellular lipid metabolism. At baseline, PEDF-null mice express markers suggestive of pancreatic stellate cell activation, but there are no changes in acinar cell morphology. However, there is sensitization to cerulein-induced chronic injury. PEDF KO animals display more pronounced fibrotic changes than wild-type mice with greater weight loss, suggestive of exocrine insufficiency. Surprisingly, PEDF-deficient mice recover from fibrotic injury similarly to wild-type controls, suggesting that PEDF is not required for the compensatory mechanisms involved in the resolution of pancreatic tissue fibrosis.[83]

Pancreatic duct cell

Cyclooxygenase-2 (COX-2) is a rate-limiting enzyme for the production of prostaglandin, which is a critical mediator of chronic inflammation. Mice with overexpression of COX-2 driven by a BK5 promoter (BK5 mice) have high levels of COX-2 in ductal cells. High prostaglandin levels drive the development of chronic pancreatitis with histologic features including inflammation, fibrosis, and ductal metaplasia foci. Older mice spontaneously develop lesions consistent with pancreatic ductal adenocarcinoma.[84]

Liver X receptor β (LXRβ) is a nuclear receptor with a key role in cholesterol, triglyceride, and glucose metabolism and is expressed in pancreatic duct epithelial cells. LXRβ-null mice display periductal inflammation with increased cell death of ductal epithelial cells. Additionally, pancreatic cells have enlarged Golgi cisternae, and the ducts are dilated with markedly dense secretory fluid. The KO mice develop pancreatic exocrine insufficiency with weight loss and decreased fat stores. The secretory defect in LXRβ null mice is likely mediated by loss of aquaporin-1, a membrane water channel protein that regulates transcellular fluid transport.[85]

Viral Models

Infection with group B coxsackieviruses has been implicated in a number of diseases including acute and chronic pancreatitis, making it a clinically relevant model of disease.[86] This model of pancreatitis involves infection with one of two coxsackie B4 virus strains. The CVB4-P strain produces mild AP, which completely resolves after 10 days. The more virulent CVB4-V strain produces more severe, necrotizing AP, followed by a chronic phase of disease characterized by acinar-ductal metaplasia, an inflammatory infiltrate, fibrosis, and fatty replacement of the pancreas. Microarray data analysis was employed to determine which genes correlated with disease resolution versus progression to chronic disease. In mild, reversible CVB4-P disease, there is enhanced expression of embryonic markers, which are likely involved in pancreatic regeneration. The gene expression map for the chronic CVB4-V model emphasized genes involved in apoptosis and fibrosis. Markers of innate and adaptive immunity also varied in the two models. While the CVB4-P infection is associated with alternatively activated (M2) macrophages and T helper 2 (Th2) cells, the progressive CVB4-V model is characterized by increased expression of classically activated (M1) macrophages and T helper 1 (Th1). The differences between CVB4-P and CVB4-V infection provide a useful approach to study why some injurious stimuli lead to reversible pancreatic injury in humans, while others progress to chronic pancreatitis.[87]

Models of Autoimmune Pancreatitis

Autoimmune pancreatitis (AIP) is a distinct fibro-inflammatory pancreatic disorder with two subtypes. Type 1 AIP is associated with elevated serum immunoglobulin G (IgG)4 and IgG4-positive lesions in other tissues. Additionally, the pancreas of patients affected by type 1 is often diffusely enlarged with characteristic lymphoplasmacytic sclerosing histology. In contrast, type 2 AIP is not associated with IgG4. Instead, the exocrine pancreas develops focal granulocyte-epithelial lesions. Type 2 AIP is associated with inflammatory bowel disease (IBD) in more that 15% of cases.

MRL-Mp mice spontaneously develop a number of autoimmune diseases including glomerulonephritis, arteritis, and arthritis. Chronic pancreatitis develops in 75% of female MRL-Mp mice at 34-38 weeks with mononuclear inflammatory infiltrate, destruction and fatty replacement of pancreatic acini.[88] The injection of polyinosinic:polycytidylic acid (poly I:C), which is structurally similar to double-stranded viral RNA and proinflammatory, leads to activation of macrophages and NK and B cells, and increased cytokine production, thus accelerating and improving disease penetrance. All female MRL-Mp mice treated with poly I:C develop chronic pancreatitis with infiltration of $CD4^+$ T cells and activated macrophages by 18 weeks. In this model, the mice do not develop other overt autoimmune conditions.[89]

Interleukin 10 (IL-10) KO mice spontaneously develop colitis and are a widely used model of IBD. When IL-10 KO mice are treated with poly I:C, they develop pancreatitis with a mononuclear inflammatory infiltrate, acini destruction, fibrosis, and fatty changes.[90] This histology, like that of the MRL-Mp model, resembles that seen with type I AIP. This finding is unexpected because type 2 but not type 1 is associated with IBD.

One theory of AIP pathogenesis implicates immune responses to microorganisms in the environmental etiology of AIP. To explore this hypothesis, mice were injected with heat-killed *Escherichia coli*. Shortly after inoculation, these mice develop acinar inflammatory infiltrate composed mainly of granulocytes and periductal fibrosis. Months after the final inoculation, lesions similar to granulocyte epithelial lesions of type 2 AIP form. There is also marked, periductal fibrosis and acinar to ductal metaplasia. *E. coli*- treated mice also have increased serum IgG levels and extrapancreatic disease with salivary gland involvement. This model mixes features of type I (extrapancreatic involvement, elevated IgG) and type 2 (histology) AIP.[91]

A lesser used model immunizes neonatally thymectomized mice with carbonic anhydrase and lactoferrin. These agents were chosen because autoantibodies against carbonic anhydrase II and lactoferrin have been identified in patients with AIP. These mice develop pancreatic inflammation mediated by Th1 $CD4^+$ T cells.[92] They also show extrapancreatic involvement with salivary gland inflammation and cholangitis.

Though each of these models employs an autoimmune pathogenic mechanism, none of them accurately reproduce the constellation of clinical and histologic features of either type 1 or 2 AIP. Therefore, the relevance to human disease is unclear. Another issue complicating this and all murine models of inflammatory disease is the lack of congruence of genomic responses to inflammatory stimuli in humans and mice.[93]

Clinical Relevance of Pancreatitis Models

Selecting the appropriate animal model of chronic pancreatitis depends on the experimental question being investigated. **Table 5** summarizes the most relevant features of the various models. The most widely used animal model of chronic pancreatitis is repetitive cerulein injection. This nonsurgical model allows for a relatively technically simple, inexpensive, flexible, and highly reproducible mechanism of replicating the histopathologic findings seen in human pancreatitis. However, given that hyperstimulation is not involved in the pathogenesis of human disease, the relevance of the cerulein model with respect to disease initiation is questionable, though it does accurately represent later events in human disease. The LPS/ethanol model of pancreatitis is a clinically relevant model of the events that lead to alcoholic chronic pancreatitis. It is also unique in its ability to address early disease durability/reversibility. However, chronic alcohol feeding of rodents can be challenging. Additionally, it is a rat model and is therefore not optimized for genetically modified mice. Another complicating factor in all mice models is that recent studies comparing acute inflammatory responses between mice and humans have shown dramatic differences in cytokine responses between these two species.[93] The types of inflammatory cells and cytokines expressed in animal models of chronic pancreatitis, their levels, and time dependence are being defined. Studies to date have been performed in only a few models and underscore the complexity of these responses.[54,87] It will be a challenge to determine whether these responses, which are likely central to the pathogenesis of chronic pancreatitis, are conserved between species. Another issue with animal models of pancreatitis is that although they provide an accurate morphohistologic model of pancreatitis, they do not fully address other clinically relevant aspects of human disease, including endocrine and exocrine insufficiency, pain, and increased susceptibility to pancreatic adenocarcinoma.

Exocrine and endocrine insufficiency occur late in the course of chronic pancreatitis. The extent of exocrine insufficiency produced by the cerulein model of chronic pancreatitis is not well characterized, though the significant decrease in acinar cell protein content at 6 weeks may indicate reduced exocrine function.[94] The cerulein model does not produce endocrine insufficiency on its own;however, it can occur when combined another insult. In one rat model, repetitive cerulein injection model is combined with the stress of water immersion.[95,96] This model results in histologic endocrine cellular damage, hyperglycemia, and decreased insulin levels. The L-arginine model results in

Table 5. Summary of animal models of chronic pancreatitis.

	Inflammation	Fibrosis	Exocrine Dysfunction	Endocrine Dysfunction	Predisposition To Cancer	Pain	Notes
Toxic Models							
Cerulein[7-9,13,15,65,98]	X	X					Highly reproducible, technically simple. Can be combined with other agents (LPS, CsA). Addition of water stress produces endocrine insufficiency. Exocrine insufficiency not well studied.
CDE diet[19]	X	X					Choline-deficient ethionine-supplemented diet. Nonspecific effects.
L-arginine[20-22]	X	X	X	X			Nonspecific effects, fatty replacement of pancreas.
DBTC[23-25]	X	X				X	Nonspecific effects, not highly reproducible.
Ethanol alone[5,29-33,109]							Several methods of alcohol feeding (Lieber-DeCarli, gavage, agar block, supplemented drinking water) do not cause histological changes.
Ethanol + cerulein[35,36]	X	X					Ethanol sensitization prevents recovery from repetitive cerulein.
Ethanol + LPS[38,37,107]	X	X					Physiologically relevant. Used to study pancreatitis durability.
Retrograde infusion of TNBS[40,104]	X	X				X	Technically challenging. Used to study pain pathways.
Retrograde infusion of oleic acid[39]	X						Technically challenging. Fatty replacement of pancreas.
Obstructive Models							
Duct ligation[45-48]	X	X		X			Mice, rats, canines, rabbits. Complete ligation or partial obstruction of part or all of the PD. Technically challenging.
Duct hypertension[6]	X	X					Technically challenging.
Genetic Models							
CFTR[52-58,108]	X		X				KO of CFTR chloride channel in mice, pigs, or ferrets. Porcine model most closely models human pancreatic disease.

(*Continued*)

Table 5. Continued

	Inflammation	Fibrosis	Exocrine Dysfunction	Endocrine Dysfunction	Predisposition To Cancer	Pain	Notes
PRSS1[60,61]	X	X					Pancreas-specific mouse or human R122H mutation in cationic trypsinogen. Model for common form of human hereditary pancreatitis.
SPINK3[63-65]							KO of serine protease inhibitor Kazal type 3 (mouse homologue of SPINK1). Rapid cell death after birth. Lethal at 2 weeks.
KRAS[62,68]	X	X			X		Overexpression of oncogenic KRAS. Most useful model in studying progression to PDAC.
PERK[70,71]	X		X	X			Pancreas-specific KO of ER sensor protein kinase RNA-like ER kinase, a mediator of the ER stress response.
Kif3a[72]		X					Pancreas-specific Kif3a inactivation. Kif3a encodes kinesin-2 (cilia assembly). Causes metaplasia, lipomatosis, cyst formation.
IL-1β[73]	X	X					Pancreas-specific IL-1β (inflammatory cytokine) overexpression. More susceptible to cerulein-induced chronic pancreatitis.
WBN/Kob[74,75]	X	X		X			Genetic alterations unknown. Mature, male rats only.
Hedgehog[77]		X					Overexpression of Indian hedgehog and Sonic hedgehog in zebrafish.
Keratin[80]	X	X					Human keratin K8 overexpression. Metaplasia, dysplasia, lipomatosis.
E2F1/E2F2 DKO[81]		X	X	X			KO of transcriptional activators cause fibrosis without inflammation.
IKKα[42]	X	X		X			Pancreas-specific KO of NF-κβ kinase. Also develops AP.

(Continued)

Table 5. Continued

	Inflammation	Fibrosis	Exocrine Dysfunction	Endocrine Dysfunction	Predisposition To Cancer	Pain	Notes
PEDF[83]							KO of pigment-derived epithelial factor. No spontaneous injury. Increased susceptibility to cerulein-induced chronic injury.
Cox-2[84]	X	X			X		Overexpression of COX-2, the rate-limiting enzyme in prostaglandin synthesis, in pancreatic duct cells.
LXRβ[85]	X		X				KO of liver X receptor β in duct cells reduces aquaporin-1 levels.
Viral Model							
Coxsackievirus[87]	X	X					Severe (CVB4-P) and mild (CVB4-P) strains.
Autoimmune Models							
MRL-Mp[89,110]							Treatment with poly I:C accelerates and worsens disease. Histology similar to type I AIP.
IL-10KO[110]	X	X					Histology of type I AIP, but develop IBD like type 2 AIP.
E. coli innoculation[91]	X	X					Histology of type 2 AIP, but increased IgG and extrapancreatic involvement similar to type 1 AIP.
Carbonic anhydrase II, lactoferrin[92]	X						Extrapancreatic involvement of salivary glands, bile ducts

Models of pancreatitis are classified by their mechanism of injury and clinically relevant features.

exocrine and endocrine insufficiency coinciding with pancreatic atrophy.[48] The WBN/Kob mouse model also produces endocrine insufficiency, with diabetes occurring spontaneously at 60-90 weeks. PERK-/- mice exhibit decreased endocrine function between 4 and 8 weeks.[70,74] Both WBN/Kob and PERK-/- mice also exhibit exocrine insufficiency. Additionally, the surgical pancreatic duct ligation models produce exocrine and endocrine insufficiency.[49,97]

Chronic pancreatitis is an important risk factor for the development of pancreatic adenocarcinoma, increasing the risk of cancer tenfold. The potential for progression from pancreatitis to cancer is not addressed in the most commonly used animal models. Mice that overexpress oncogenic KRAS provide a useful, clinically relevant model of the development of pancreatic adenocarcinoma from chronic pancreatitis. In these experimental models, healthy cells are resistant to malignant transformation, while a background of chronic pancreatitis encourages high penetrance of oncogenic KRAS with the development of pancreatic intraepithelial neoplasiaand PDAC.[98,99] It is likely that chronic pancreatic injury induces acinar cell proliferation for tissue repair, either by mature acinar cell dedifferentiation or progenitor cell recruitment.[100] These cells, which have increased embryonic markers, may be key in the progression from pancreatitis to cancer.

Abdominal pain in AP can be severe, impacts patient quality of life, and is the most frequent reason for hospitalization.[101] Given that there are no targeted therapies for chronic pancreatitis pain, characterization of pain pathways could be helpful in developing potential therapies. In the DBTC mouse model of pancreatitis, pain measured by behavioral responses to visceral stimuli was mediated by bradykinin and IL-6.[102,103] The IL-6 trinitrobenzene sulfonic acid infusion model identified nerve growth factor as a mediator of pancreatic nociceptor excitability and pain behaviors in rats.[104-106]

Conclusion

Animal models provide a reproducible method for examining the pathogenesis of chronic pancreatitis. Repetitive cerulein injection is the most widely used model because it is technically straightforward, reproducible, and flexible. However, while the histopathologic findings reproduce those seen in humans with chronic pancreatitis, the relevance of cerulein as a triggering mechanism in the pathogenesis of human disease is questionable. Other models, like the alcohol/LPS model, mechanical injury, and genetic and viral models employ triggers with direct correlates to known risk factors for chronic pancreatitis in humans. Ultimately, the choice of animal model depends upon the hypothesis being tested. A central concern in unraveling the mechanisms of chronic pancreatitis is understanding how genetic and environmental risk factors interact to initiate and advance disease in some patients but not others. This issue presents a particular challenge in the development of animal models, which must be highly reproducible to be practically useful. Furthermore, no currently available models reproduce all relevant aspects of disease: histopathology, endocrine/exocrine insufficiency, pain, and increased risk of progression to cancer. The development of new models or combining known models in new ways may provide further insight into the complex pathogenesis of chronic pancreatitis.

Funding

Supported by a National Institutes of Health K08 (DK090104 to A.M.R.) and a Merit Award from the Veterans Administration, a National Institutes of Health R01 (DK54021) from the NIDDK, and a National Institutes of Health R21 from the NIAAA to (AA020847) to F.S.G.

References

1. Jupp J, Fine D, Johnson CD. The epidemiology and socioeconomic impact of chronic pancreatitis. *Best Pract Res Clin Gastroenterol.* 2010; 24: 219-231. PMID: 20510824
2. Yadav D, Timmons L, Benson JT, Dierkhising RA, Chari ST. Incidence, prevalence, and survival of chronic pancreatitis: a population-based study. *Am J Gastroenterol.* 2011; 106: 2192-2199. PMID: 21946280
3. Whitcomb DC. Value of genetic testing in the management of pancreatitis. *Gut.* 2004; 53: 1710-1717. PMID: 15479696
4. Sarles H. Etiopathogenesis and definition of chronic pancreatitis. *Dig Dis Sci.* 1986; 31: 91S-107S. PMID: 3525051
5. Witt H, Apte MV, Keim V, Wilson JS. Chronic pancreatitis: challenges and advances in pathogenesis, genetics, diagnosis, and therapy. *Gastroenterology.* 2007; 132: 1557-1573. PMID: 17466744
6. Yamamoto M, Otani M, Otsuki M. A new model of chronic pancreatitis in rats. *Am J Physiol Gastrointest Liver Physiol.* 2006; 291: G700-G708. PMID: 16959955
7. Neuschwander-Tetri BA, Burton FR, Presti ME, Britton RS, Janney CG, Garvin PR, et al. Repetitive self-limited acute pancreatitis induces pancreatic fibrogenesis in the mouse. *Dig Dis Sci.* 2000; 45: 665-674. PMID: 10759232
8. Feng D, Park O, Radaeva S, Wang H, Yin S, Kong X, et al. Interleukin-22 ameliorates cerulein-induced pancreatitis in mice by inhibiting the autophagic pathway. *Int J Biol Sci.* 2012; 8: 249-257. PMID: 22253568
9. Sah RP, Dudeja V, Dawra RK, Saluja AK. Cerulein-induced chronic pancreatitis does not require intra-acinar activation of trypsinogen in mice. *Gastroenterology.* 2013; 144: 1076-1085. PMID: 23354015
10. Lara LF, Levy MJ. Idiopathic recurrent acute pancreatitis. *MedGenMed.* 2004; 6: 10. PMID: 15775837
11. Ji B, Bi Y, Simeone D, Mortensen RM, Logsdon CD. Human pancreatic acinar cells lack functional responses to

cholecystokinin and gastrin. *Gastroenterology*. 2001; 121: 1380-1390. PMID: 11729117
12. Murphy JA, Criddle DN, Sherwood M, Chvanov M, Mukherjee R, McLaughlin E, et al. Direct activation of cytosolic Ca^{2+} signaling and enzyme secretion by cholecystokinin in human pancreatic acinar cells. *Gastroenterology*. 2008; 135: 632-641. PMID: 18555802
13. Bode C, Kugler V, Bode JC. Endotoxemia in patients with alcoholic and non-alcoholic cirrhosis and in subjects with no evidence of chronic liver disease following acute alcohol excess. *J Hepatol*. 1987; 4: 8-14. PMID: 3571935
14. Masamune A, Kikuta K, Watanabe T, Satoh K, Satoh A, Shimosegawa T. Pancreatic stellate cells express Toll-like receptors. *J Gastroenterol*. 2008; 43: 352-362. PMID: 18592153
15. Ohashi S, Nishio A, Nakmura H, Kido M, Ueno S, Uza N, et al. Protective roles of redox-active protein thioredoxin-1 for severe acute pancreatitis. *Am J Physiol Gastrointest Liver Physiol*. 2006; 290: G772-G781. PMID: 163222089
16. Vaquero E, Molero X, Tian X, Salas A, Malagelada JR. Myofibroblast proliferation, fibrosis, and defective pancreatic repair induced by cyclosporin in rats. *Gut*. 1999; 45: 269-277. PMID: 10403741
17. Gilliland L, Steer ML. Effects of ethionine on digestive enzyme synthesis and discharge by mouse pancreas. *Am J Physiol Gastrointest Liver Physiol*. 1980; 239: G418-G426. PMID: 6159794
18. Niederau C, Luthen R, Niederau MC, Grendell JH, Ferrell LD. Acute experimental hemorrhagic-necrotizing pancreatitis induced by feeding a choline-deficient, ethionine-supplemented diet. Methodology and standards. *Eur Surg Res*. 1992; 24: 40-54. PMID: 1601023
19. Ida S, Ohmuraya M, Hirota M, Ozaki N, Hiramatsu S, Uehara H, et al. Chronic pancreatitis in mice by treatment with choline-deficient ethionine-supplemented diet. *Exp Anim*. 2010; 59: 421-429. PMID: 20660988
20. Mizunuma T, Kawamura S, Kishino Y. Effects of injecting excess arginine on rat pancreas. *J Nutr*. 1984; 114: 467-471. PMID: 6199486
21. Weaver C, Bishop AE, Polak JM. Pancreatic changes elicited by chronic administration of excess L-arginine. *Exp Mol Pathol*. 1994; 60: 71-87. PMID: 8070543
22. Delaney CP, McGeeney KF, Dervan P, Fitzpatrick JM. Pancreatic atrophy: a new model using serial intra-peritoneal injections of L-arginine. *Scand J Gastroenterol*. 1993; 28: 1086-1090. PMID: 8303212
23. Merkord J, Hennighausen G. Acute pancreatitis and bile duct lesions in rat induced by dibutyltin dichloride. *Exp Pathol*. 1989; 36: 59-62. PMID: 2731591
24. Merkord J, Jonas L, Weber H, Kroning G, Nizze H, Hennighausen G. Acute interstitial pancreatitis in rats induced by dibutyltin dichloride (DBTC): pathogenesis and natural course of lesions. *Pancreas*. 1997; 15: 392-401. PMID: 9361094
25. Sparmann G, Merkord J, Jaschke A, Nizze HH, Jonas L, Lohr M, et al. Pancreatic fibrosis in experimental pancreatitis induced by dibutyltin dichloride. *Gastroenterology*. 1997; 112: 1664-1672. PMID: 9136846
26. Merkord J, Weber H, Kroning G, Hennighausen G. Repeated administration of a mild acute toxic dose of di-n-butyltin dichloride at intervals of 3 weeks induces severe lesions in pancreas and liver of rats. *Hum Exp Toxicol*. 2001; 20: 386-392. PMID: 11727788
27. Ammann RW. The natural history of alcoholic chronic pancreatitis. *Intern Med*. 2001; 40: 368-375. PMID: 11393404
28. Lieber CS, DeCarli LM. The feeding of ethanol in liquid diets. *Alcohol Clin Exp Res*. 1986; 10: 550-553. PMID: 3026198
29. Tsukamoto H, Sankaran H, Delgado G, Reidelberger RD, Deveney CW, Largman C. Increased pancreatic acinar content and secretion of cationic trypsinogen following 30-day continuous ethanol intoxication in rats. *Biochem Pharmacol*. 1986; 35: 3623-3629. PMID: 3768045
30. Coleman RA, Young BM, Turner LE, Cook RT. A practical method of chronic ethanol administration in mice. *Methods Mol Biol*. 2008; 447: 49-59. PMID: 18369910
31. Bautista AP. Chronic alcohol intoxication induces hepatic injury through enhanced macrophage inflammatory protein-2 production and intercellular adhesion molecule-1 expression in the liver. *Hepatology*. 1997; 25: 335-342. PMID: 9021944
32. Winston JH, He ZJ, Shenoy M, Xiao SY, Pasricha PJ. Molecular and behavioral changes in nociception in a novel rat model of chronic pancreatitis for the study of pain. *Pain*. 2005; 117: 214-222. PMID: 16098667
33. Pfutzer RH, Tadic SD, Thompson BS, Zhang JY, Ford ME, Eagon PK, et al. Pancreatic cholesterol esterase, ES-10, and fatty acid ethyl ester synthase III gene expression are increased in the pancreas and liver but not in the brain or heart with long-term ethanol feeding in rats. *Pancreas*. 2002; 25: 101-106. PMID: 12131779
34. Li HS, Zhang JY, Thompson BS, Deng XY, Ford ME, Wood PG, et al. Rat mitochondrial ATP synthase ATP5G3: cloning and upregulation in pancreas after chronic ethanol feeding. *Physiol Genomics*. 2001; 6: 91-98. PMID: 11459924
35. Deng X, Wang L, Elm MS, Gabazadeh D, Diorio GJ, Eagon PK, et al. Chronic alcohol consumption accelerates fibrosis in response to cerulein-induced pancreatitis in rats. *Am J Pathol*. 2005; 166: 93-106. PMID: 15632003
36. Perides G, Tao X, West N, Sharma A, Steer ML. A mouse model of ethanol dependent pancreatic fibrosis. *Gut*. 2005; 54: 1461-1467. PMID: 15870229
37. Vonlaufen A, Phillips PA, Xu Z, Zhang X, Yang L, Pirola RC, et al. Withdrawal of alcohol promotes regression while continued alcohol intake promotes persistence of LPS-induced pancreatic injury in alcohol-fed rats. *Gut*. 2011; 60: 238-246. PMID: 20870739
38. Swanson G, Forsyth CB, Tang Y, Shaikh M, Zhang L, Turek FW, et al. Role of intestinal circadian genes in alcohol-induced gut leakiness. *Alcohol Clin Exp Res*. 2011; 35: 1305-1314. PMID: 21463335
39. Mundlos S, Adler G, Schaar M, Koop I, Arnold R. Exocrine pancreatic function in oleic acid-induced pancreatic insufficiency in rats. *Pancreas*. 1986; 1: 29-36. PMID: 2437560
40. Puig-Divi V, Molero X, Salas A, Guarner F, Guarner L, Malagelada JR. Induction of chronic pancreatic disease by trinitrobenzene sulfonic acid infusion into rat pancreatic ducts. *Pancreas*. 1996; 13: 417-424. PMID: 8899803
41. Perides G, Laukkarinen JM, Vassileva G, Steer ML. Biliary acute pancreatitis in mice is mediated by the G-protein-coupled cell surface bile acid receptor Gpbar1. *Gastroenterology*. 2010; 138: 715-725. PMID: 19900448

42. Aho HJ, Koskensalo SM, Nevalainen TJ. Experimental pancreatitis in the rat. Sodium taurocholate-induced acute haemorrhagic pancreatitis. *Scand J Gastroenterol.* 1980; 15: 411-416. PMID: 7433903
43. Sarles H, Sahel J. Pathology of chronic calcifying pancreatitis. *Am J Gastroenterol.* 1976; 66: 117-139. PMID: 788498
44. Bradley EL 3rd. Pancreatic duct pressure in chronic pancreatitis. *Am J Surg.* 1982; 144: 313-316. PMID: 7114368
45. Churg A, Richter WR. Early changes in the exocrine pancreas of the dog and rat after ligation of the pancreatic duct. A light and electron microscopic study. *Am J Pathol.* 1971; 63: 521-546. PMID: 5581235
46. Heptner W, Neubauer HP, Schleyerbach R. Glucose tolerance and insulin secretion in rabbits and dogs after ligation of the pancreatic ducts. *Diabetologia.* 1974; 10: 193-196. PMID: 4602674
47. Scoggins CR, Meszoely IM, Wada M, Means AL, Yang L, Leach SD. p53-dependent acinar cell apoptosis triggers epithelial proliferation in duct-ligated murine pancreas. *Am J Physiol Gastrointest Liver Physiol.* 2000; 279: G827-G836. PMID: 11005771
48. Watanabe S, Abe K, Anbo Y, Katoh H. Changes in the mouse exocrine pancreas after pancreatic duct ligation: a qualitative and quantitative histological study. *Arch Histol Cytol.* 1995; 58: 365-374. PMID: 8527243
49. Tanaka T, Ichiba Y, Fujoo Y, Itoh H, Kodama O, Dohi K. New canine model of chronic pancreatitis due to chronic ischemia with incomplete pancreatic duct obstruction. *Digestion.* 1988; 41: 149-155. PMID: 3224767
50. De Boeck K, Weren M, Proesmans M, Kerem E. Pancreatitis among patients with cystic fibrosis: correlation with pancreatic status and genotype. *Pediatrics.* 2005; 115: e463-e469. PMID: 15772171
51. Ooi CY, Dorfman R, Cipolli M, Gonska T, Castellani C, Keenan K, et al. Type of CFTR mutation determines risk of pancreatitis in patients with cystic fibrosis. *Gastroenterology.* 2011; 140: 153-161. PMID: 20923678
52. Snouwaert JN, Brigman KK, Latour AM, Malouf NN, Boucher RC, Smithies O, et al. An animal model for cystic fibrosis made by gene targeting. *Science.* 1992; 257: 1083-1088. PMID: 1380723
53. Dimagno MJ, Lee SH, Hao Y, Zhou SY, McKenna BJ, Owyang C. A proinflammatory, antiapoptotic phenotype underlies the susceptibility to acute pancreatitis in cystic fibrosis transmembrane regulator (-/-) mice. *Gastroenterology.* 2005; 129: 665-681. PMID: 16083720
54. Rogers CS, Stoltz DA, Meyerolz DK, Ostedgaard LS, Rokhlina T, Taft PJ, et al. Disruption of the CFTR gene produces a model of cystic fibrosis in newborn pigs. *Science.* 2008; 321: 1837-1841. PMID: 18818360
55. Uc A, Giriyappa R, Meyerholz DK, Griffin M, Ostedgaard LS, Tang XX, et al. Pancreatic and biliary secretion are both altered in cystic fibrosis pigs. *Am J Physiol Gastrointest Liver Physiol.* 2012; 303: G961-G968. PMID: 22936270
56. Abu-El-Haija M, Sinkora M, Meyerholz DK, Welsh MJ, McCray PB. Jr, Butler J, et al. An activated immune and inflammatory response targets the pancreas of newborn pigs with cystic fibrosis. *Pancreatology.* 2011; 11: 506-515.
57. Abu-El-Haija M, Ramachandran S, Meyerholz DK, Abu-El-Haija M, Griffin M, Giriyappa RL, et al. Pancreatic damage in fetal and newborn cystic fibrosis pigs involves the activation of inflammatory and remodeling pathways. *Am J Pathol.* 2012; 181: 499-507. PMID: 22683312
58. Sun X, Sui H, Fisher JT, Yan Z, Liu X, Cho HJ, et al. Disease phenotype of a ferret CFTR-knockout model of cystic fibrosis. *J Clin Invest.* 2010; 120: 3149-3160. PMID: 20739752
59. Whitcomb DC. Hereditary pancreatitis: new insights into acute and chronic pancreatitis. *Gut.* 1999; 45: 317-322. PMID: 10446089
60. Archer H, Jura N, Keller J, Jacobson M, Bar-Sagi D. A mouse model of hereditary pancreatitis generated by transgenic expression of R122H trypsinogen. *Gastroenterology.* 2006; 131: 1844-1855. PMID: 17087933
61. Selig L, Sack U, Gaiser S, Kloppel G, Savkovic V, Mossner K, et al. Characterisation of a transgenic mouse expressing R122H human cationic trypsinogen. *BMC Gastroenterol.* 2006; 6: 30. PMID: 17069643
62. Pfutzer RH, Barmada MM, Brunskill AP, Finch R, Hart PS, Neoptolemos J, et al. SPINK1/PSTI polymorphisms act as disease modifiers in familial and idiopathic chronic pancreatitis. *Gastroenterology.* 2000; 119: 615-623. PMID: 10982753
63. Ohmuraya M, Hirota M, Araki K, Baba H, Yamamura K. Enhanced trypsin activity in pancreatic acinar cells deficient for serine protease inhibitor kazal type 3. *Pancreas.* 2006; 33: 104-106. PMID: 16804421
64. Ohmuraya M, Hirota M, Araki M, Mizushima N, Matsui M, Mizumoto T, et al. Autophagic cell death of pancreatic acinar cells in serine protease inhibitor Kazal type 3-deficient mice. *Gastroenterology.* 2005; 129: 696-705. PMID: 16083722
65. Romac JM, Ohmuraya M, Bittner C, Majeed MF, Vigna SR, Que J, et al. Transgenic expression of pancreatic secretory trypsin inhibitor-1 rescues SPINK3-deficient mice and restores a normal pancreatic phenotype. *Am J Physiol Gastrointest Liver Physiol.* 2010; 298: G518-G524. PMID: 20110462
66. Lohr M, Maisonneuve P, Lowenfels AB. K-Ras mutations and benign pancreatic disease. *Int J Pancreatol.* 2000; 27: 93-103. PMID: 10862508
67. Ji B, Tsou L, Wang H, Gaiser S, Chang DZ, Daniluk J, et al. Ras activity levels control the development of pancreatic diseases. *Gastroenterology.* 2009; 137: 1072-1082. PMID: 19501586
68. Daniluk J, Liu Y, Deng D, Chu J, Huang H, Gaiser S, et al. An NF-kappaB pathway-mediated positive feedback loop amplifies Ras activity to pathological levels in mice. *J Clin Invest.* 2012; 122: 1519-1528. PMID: 22406536
69. Lugea A, Tischler D, Nguyen J, Gong J, Gukovsky I, French SW, et al. Adaptive unfolded protein response attenuates alcohol-induced pancreatic damage. *Gastroenterology.* 2011; 140: 987-997. PMID: 21111739
70. Harding HP, Zeng H, Zhang Y, Jungries R, Chung P, Plesken H, et al. Diabetes mellitus and exocrine pancreatic dysfunction in perk-/- mice reveals a role for translational control in secretory cell survival. *Mol Cell.* 2001; 7: 1153-1163. PMID: 11430819

71. Iida K, Li Y, McGrath BC, Frank A, Cavener DR. PERK eIF2 alpha kinase is required to regulate the viability of the exocrine pancreas in mice. *BMC Cell Biol.* 2007; 8: 38. PMID: 17727724
72. Cano DA, Sekine S, Hebrok M. Primary cilia deletion in pancreatic epithelial cells results in cyst formation and pancreatitis. *Gastroenterology.* 2006; 131: 1856-1869. PMID: 17123526
73. Marrache F, Tu SP, Bhagat G, Pendyala S, Osterreicher CH, Gordon S, et al. Overexpression of interleukin-1beta in the murine pancreas results in chronic pancreatitis. *Gastroenterology.* 2008; 135: 1277-1287. PMID: 18789941
74. Ohashi K, Kim JH, Hara H, Aso R, Akimoto T, Nakama K. WBN/Kob rats. A new spontaneously occurring model of chronic pancreatitis. *Int J Pancreatol.* 1990; 6: 231-247. PMID: 1698893
75. Mori M, Fu X, Chen L, Zhang G, Higuchi K. Hereditary pancreatitis model WBN/Kob rat strain has a unique haplotype in the Pdwk1 region on chromosome 7. *Exp Anim.* 2009; 58: 409-413. PMID: 19654439
76. Kayed H, Kleeff J, Keleg S, Buchler MW, Friess H. Distribution of Indian hedgehog and its receptors patched and smoothened in human chronic pancreatitis. *J Endocrinol.* 2003; 178: 467-478. PMID: 12967338
77. Jung IH, Jung DE, Park YN, Song SY, Park SW. Aberrant Hedgehog ligands induce progressive pancreatic fibrosis by paracrine activation of myofibroblasts and ductular cells in transgenic zebrafish. *PLoS One.* 2011; 6: e27941. PMID: 22164219
78. Cavestro GM, Frulloni L, Nouvenne A, Neri TM, Calore B, Ferri B, et al. Association of keratin 8 gene mutation with chronic pancreatitis. *Dig Liver Dis.* 2003; 35: 416-420. PMID: 12868678
79. Treiber M, Schulz HU, Landt O, Drenth JP, Castellani C, Real FX, et al. Keratin 8 sequence variants in patients with pancreatitis and pancreatic cancer. *J Mol Med (Berl).* 2006; 84: 1015-1022. PMID: 17039343
80. Casanova ML, Bravo A, Ramírez A, Morreale de Escobar G, Were F, Merlino G, et al. Exocrine pancreatic disorders in transsgenic mice expressing human keratin 8. *J Clin Invest.* 1999; 103: 1587-1595. PMID: 10359568
81. Iglesias A, Murga M, Laresgoiti U, Skoudy A, Bernales I, Fullaondo A, et al. Diabetes and exocrine pancreatic insufficiency in E2F1/E2F2 double-mutant mice. *J Clin Invest.* 2004; 113: 1398-1407. PMID: 15146237
82. Li N, Wu X, Holzer RG, Lee JH, Todoric J, Park EJ, et al. Loss of acinar cell IKKalpha triggers spontaneous pancreatitis in mice. *J Clin Invest.* 2013; 123: 2231-2243. PMID: 23563314
83. Schmitz JC, Protiva P, Gattu AK, Utsumi T, Iwakiri Y, Neto AG, et al. Pigment epithelium-derived factor regulates early pancreatic fibrotic responses and suppresses the profibrotic cytokine thrombospondin-1. *Am J Pathol.* 2011; 179: 2990-2999. PMID: 21964188
84. Colby JK, Klein RD, McArthur MJ, Conti CJ, Kiquchi K, Kawamoto T, et al. Progressive metaplastic and dysplastic changes in mouse pancreas induced by cyclooxygenase-2 overexpression. *Neoplasia.* 2008; 10: 782-796. PMID: 18670639
85. Gabbi C, Kim HJ, Hultenby K, Bouton D, Toresson G, Warner M, et al. Pancreatic exocrine insufficiency in LXRbeta-/- mice is associated with a reduction in aquaporin-1 expression. *Proc Natl Acad Sci U S A.* 2008; 105: 15052-15057. PMID: 18806227
86. Ramsingh AI, Lee WT, Collins DN, Armstrong LE. Differential recruitment of B and T cells in coxsackievirus B4-induced pancreatitis is influenced by a capsid protein. *J Virol.* 1997; 71: 8690-8697. PMID: 9343227
87. Ostrowski SE, Reilly AA, Collins DN, Ramsingh AL. Progression or resolution of coxsackievirus B4-induced pancreatitis: a genomic analysis. *J Virol.* 2004; 78: 8229-8237. PMID: 15254194
88. Kanno H, Nose M, Itoh J, Taniquchi Y, Kyogoku M. Spontaneous development of pancreatitis in the MRL/Mp strain of mice in autoimmune mechanism. *Clin Exp Immunol.* 1992; 89: 68-73. PMID: 1352748
89. Qu WM, Miyazaki T, Terada M, Okada K, Mori S, Kanno H, et al. A novel autoimmune pancreatitis model in MRL mice treated with polyinosinic:polycytidylic acid. *Clin Exp Immunol.* 2002; 129: 27-34. PMID: 12100019
90. Yamaguchi T, Kihara Y, Taquchi M, Naqashio Y, Tashiro M, Nakamura H, et al. Persistent destruction of the basement membrane of the pancreatic duct contributes to progressive acinar atrophy in rats with experimentally induced pancreatitis. *Pancreas.* 2005; 31: 365-372. PMID: 16258372
91. Haruta I, Yanagisawa N, Kawamura S, Furukawa T, Shimizu K, Kato H, et al. A mouse model of autoimmune pancreatitis with salivary gland involvement triggered by innate immunity via persistent exposure to avirulent bacteria. *Lab Invest.* 2010; 90: 1757-1769. PMID: 20733561
92. Uchida K, Okazaki K, Nishi T, Uose S, Nakase H, Ohana M, et al. Experimental immune-mediated pancreatitis in neonatally thymectomized mice immunized with carbonic anhydrase II and lactoferrin. *Lab Invest.* 2002; 82: 411-424. PMID: 11950899
93. Seok J, Warren HS, Cuenca AG, Mindrinos MN, Baker HV, Xu W, et al. Genomic responses in mouse models poorly mimic human inflammatory diseases. *Proc Natl Acad Sci U S A.* 2013; 110: 3507-3512. PMID: 23401516
94. Ohashi S, Nishio A, Nakamura H, Asada M, Tamaki H, Kawasaki K, et al. Overexpression of redox-active protein thioredoxin-1 prevents development of chronic pancreatitis in mice. *Antioxid Redox Signal.* 2006; 8: 1835-1845. PMID: 16987036
95. Miyahara T, Kawabuchi M, Goto M, Nakano I, Nada O, Nawata H. Morphological study of pancreatic endocrine in an experimental chronic pancreatitis with diabetes induced by stress and cerulein. *Ultrastruct Pathol.* 1999; 23: 171-180. PMID: 10445284
96. Goto M, Nakano I, Kimura T, Miyahara T, Kinjo M, Nawata H. New chronic pancreatitis model with diabetes induced by cerulein plus stress in rats. *Dig Dis Sci.* 1995; 40: 2356-2363. PMID: 7587814
97. Boerma D, Straatsburg IH, Offerhaus GJ, Gouma DJ, Van Gulik TM. Experimental model of obstructive, chronic pancreatitis in pigs. *Dig Surg.* 2003; 20: 520-526. PMID: 14534374

98. Guerra C, Schumacher AJ, Canamero M, Grippo PJ, Verdaguer L, Dubus P, et al. Chronic pancreatitis is essential for induction of pancreatic ductal adenocarcinoma by K-Ras oncogenes in adult mice. *Cancer Cell*. 2007; 11: 291-302. PMID: 17349585
99. Guerra C, Collado M, Navas C, Schuhmacher AJ, Hernandez-Porras I, Canamero M, et al. Pancreatitis-induced inflammation contributes to pancreatic cancer by inhibiting oncogene-induced senescence. *Cancer Cell*. 2011; 19: 728-739. PMID: 21665147
100. Guerra C, Barbacid M. Genetically engineered mouse models of pancreatic adenocarcinoma. *Mol Oncol*. 2013; 7: 232-247. PMID: 23506980
101. Gardner TB, Kennedy AT, Gelrud A, Banks PA, Vege SS, Gordon SR, et al. Chronic pancreatitis and its effect on employment and health care experience: results of a prospective American multicenter study. *Pancreas* 2010; 39: 498-501. PMID: 20118821
102. Chen Q, Vera-Portocarrero LP, Ossipov MH, Vardanyan M, Lai J, Porreca F. Attenuation of persistent experimental pancreatitis pain by a bradykinin b2 receptor antagonist. *Pancreas*. 2010; 39: 1220-1225. PMID: 20531238
103. Vardanyan M, Melemedjian OK, Price TJ, Ossipov MH, Lai J, Roberts E, et al. Reversal of pancreatitis-induced pain by an orally available, small molecule interleukin-6 receptor antagonist. *Pain*. 2010; 151: 257-265. PMID: 20599324
104. Zhu Y, Mehta K, Li C, Xu GY, Liu L, Colak T, et al. Systemic administration of anti-NGF increases A-type potassium currents and decreases pancreatic nociceptor excitability in a rat model of chronic pancreatitis. *Am J Physiol Gastrointest Liver Physiol*. 2012; 302: G176-G181. PMID: 22038828
105. Whitcomb DC, Gorry MC, Preston RA, Furey W, Sossenheimer MJ, Ulrich CD, et al. Hereditary pancreatitis is caused by a mutation in the cationic trypsinogen gene. *Nat Genet*. 1996; 14: 141-145. PMID: 8841182
106. Zhu Y, Colak T, Shenoy M, Liu L, Pai R, Li C, Mehta K, et al. Nerve growth factor modulates TRPV1 expression and function and mediates pain in chronic pancreatitis. *Gastroenterology*. 2011; 141: 370-377. PMID: 21473865
107. Vonlaufen A, Xu Z, Daniel B, Kumar RK, Pirola R, Wilson J, et al. Bacterial endotoxin: a trigger factor for alcoholic pancreatitis? Evidence from a novel, physiologically relevant animal model. *Gastroenterology*. 2007; 133: 1293-1303. PMID: 17919500
108. De Lisle RC, Isom KS, Ziemer D, Cotton CU. Changes in the exocrine pancreas secondary to altered small intestinal function in the CF mouse. *Am J Physiol Gastrointest Liver Physiol*. 2001; 281: G899-G906. PMID: 11557509
109. Wilson JS, Apte MV. Role of alcohol metabolism in alcoholic pancreatitis. *Pancreas*. 2003; 27: 311-315. PMID: 14576493
110. Yamashina M, Nishio A, Nakayama S, Okazaki T, Uchida K, Fukui T, et al. Comparative study on experimental autoimmune pancreatitis and its extrapancreatic involvement in mice. *Pancreas*. 2012; 41: 1255-1262. PMID: 22836854

Chapter 7

Immune modulation in acute and chronic pancreatitis

Aida Habtezion[1*] and Hana Algül[2]

[1]*Division of Gastroenterology and Hepatology, Stanford University School of Medicine, Stanford, California, USA;*
[2]*II. Medizinische Klinik, Klinikum rechts der Isar, Technische Universität München, Munich, Germany.*

Introduction

Acute pancreatitis

Acute pancreatitis (AP) is one of the most common gastrointestinal causes for hospital admission. AP can develop in response to various factors (e.g., gallstones, excessive alcohol consumption, viral infections, and strong reactions to certain medications). Initiating events for acinar cell injury take place locally. Premature enzyme activation and abnormal exocytosis of zymogens are potent triggers of inflammation, edema, and tissue damage. In the beginning, inflammation, edema, and tissue damage are localized. However, these events can progress to systemic complications (e.g., multiple organ dysfunction [MOD] primarily affecting lung, liver, and kidney).

Based on physiological findings and laboratory values, AP can be classified as mild, moderate, or severe. In most cases, patients are suffering from mild AP, which is reflected in upper abdominal pain that can radiate into the back, often accompanied by a swollen and tender abdomen, and in 85% of cases, followed by nausea and vomiting. In contrast to this, less than 25% of patients develop moderate to severe pancreatitis.[1,2] Severe pancreatitis is characterized by pancreatic dysfunction, local and systemic complications (e.g., MOD), followed by a difficult and long recovery, and in some cases, death.

Immune cells are crucial mediators that determine the complex pathophysiology of this disease. The balance between pro- and anti-inflammatory events in AP is key to disease severity.[3]

Chronic pancreatitis

Recurrent AP can result in chronic pancreatitis (CP), which is a progressive inflammatory and fibrotic disease that can lead to exocrine and endocrine insufficiency.[4] Although less common than AP, CP is associated with significant morbidity and health care cost. CP is commonly associated with excessive alcohol consumption and remains an important risk factor for developing pancreatic cancer.[5] Other factors such as the genetic mutations causing hereditary pancreatitis also contribute to the development of this chronic, debilitating disease. Immune responses associated with CP are increasingly appreciated, although the role of immune cells is not as well studied as in AP. More recently, manipulations of immune pathways have challenged the notion of the "irreversible" nature of this disease.

In this review, we focus on the role of immune cells, pathways, and immune mediators associated with AP and CP. Autoimmune pancreatitis is covered elsewhere.

Immune cells in pancreatitis

Neutrophils

Neutrophils are not typically present in the normal, healthy pancreas.[6] However, AP involves the release of inflammatory mediators by acinar cells, in response to the damage, triggering innate immune mechanisms that recruit immune cells to the site of inflammation. Initially, neutrophils and monocytes are recruited, followed by dendritic cells (DCs), mast cells, T cells, and platelets. Migration of immune cells is a multistep process that engages diverse adhesion molecules.[7] A prominent protein required for neutrophil adhesion to the endothelium and epithelium is intercellular adhesion molecule-1 (ICAM-1),[8] which is constitutively expressed at a low level on the endothelium and some epithelium sites. At inflammation sites (e.g., damaged acinar cells), ICAM-1 is produced in higher amounts, thus leading to increased neutrophil adhesion. Furthermore, the cholecystokinin analogue cerulein upregulates ICAM-1 mRNA and protein expression in cerulein-induced pancreatitis.[9,10] Interestingly, ICAM-1 knockout mice were protected compared to control mice.[11] The study using the same mouse model demonstrated that serum, pancreatic, and lung levels of ICAM-1 increased during AP.[11]

*Corresponding author. Email: aidah@stanford.edu

Oxidative stress is one of the mechanisms by which infiltrated neutrophils induce damage in AP. Nicotinamide adenine dinucleotide phosphate (NADPH) oxidase is an important oxidative stress protein.[12] In AP, NADPH oxidase expression and activity are increased.[13] Through oxidative stress, infiltrating neutrophils substantially contribute to trypsin activation in acinar cells during AP.[14,15] In a rat model of cerulein-induced pancreatitis, it was demonstrated that trypsin activation was supported through a mechanism involving NADPH oxidase.[13] Furthermore, immunohistochemical analysis and measurement of reactive oxygen species (ROS) production indicated that NADPH oxidase was present in infiltrated neutrophils but not pancreatic acinar cells. Consistent with this finding, neutrophil depletion and NADPH oxidase deficiency both inhibit trypsin activation and cerulein-induced damage in the pancreas.[14]

Monocytes/macrophages

Monocytes are another major mediator of AP.[16] Similar to neutrophils, the recruiting mechanisms involve signals deriving from damaged pancreatic acinar cells.[17] It is believed that activation of primary monocytes is influenced by chemokine (C-C motif) ligands 2 (CCL2), CCL3, and CCL5.[6] Signals originally sent by acinar cells are multiplied by activated monocytes.[18] As a result, tumor necrosis factor (TNF)-α, interleukin-1 (IL-1), IL-6, and ICAM-1 are produced at higher levels, which assists disease progression. This signal amplification specifically affects lung, liver, and kidney tissues, leading to systemic inflammation.[19] Interestingly, a recent study addressing the role of myeloid RelA/p65 in IL-6 regulation in cerulein-induced AP unequivocally demonstrated that myeloid cells, namely macrophages, play the central role and are the major source of IL-6.[20] Macrophages and IL-6, through IL-6 trans-signaling were responsible for AP-associated acute lung injury.

Interestingly, several macrophage populations are responsible for systemic organ inflammation. In severe pancreatitis, peritoneal macrophages are rapidly activated due to excessive production of pancreatic enzymes and cytokines. Consequently, this leads to release of mediators including pro-inflammatory cytokines such as TNF-α, IL-1β, IL-6, and enzymes such as nitric oxide (NO) synthase (iNOS) that easily reach the bloodstream, thus contributing to the inflammatory responses in severe pancreatitis.[21,22] Association of these macrophages with the complications of severe pancreatitis was clearly demonstrated in several studies.[23] Peritoneal lavage in rats suffering from AP significantly reduced the cytotoxic effect of ascitic fluid. Then investigators concluded that this was a consequence of a reduced number of peritoneal macrophages, thus there was a milder response to activating mediators from ascitic fluid.

A second population that significantly contributes to the secondary complications in AP is alveolar macrophages. Upon activation, these cells have great capability to produce cytokines and NO, and attract large numbers of leukocytes to the lungs. Lung injury, as a secondary effect of AP, is largely related to high iNOS activity and high NO levels.[24] Another population of macrophages involved in AP are Kupffer cells, which normally respond to toxic substances in the blood, thus participating in the acute liver response. However, during the AP, inflammatory mediators released into the bloodstream by a damaged pancreas can activate Kupffer cells and induce systemic inflammation.[25] In vitro analysis of Kupffer cell activity demonstrated that pancreatic enzymes could activate these cells.[26] Nonetheless, hepatic damage is only evident in late stages of pancreatitis. Interestingly, another study raised doubt regarding the possibility that acute liver responses in AP could be induced by inflammatory mediators released by the pancreas.[27] The authors provided evidence of endotoxin contamination of porcine pancreatic elastase responsible for activating Kupffer cells in AP. Pancreatic elastase, free of contamination, failed to activate murine macrophages to release TNF-α and exert a pro-inflammatory effect in vivo. Nonetheless, the authors could not exclude that other fragments might activate Kupffer cells.

Significant macrophage infitration has been observed in experimental models of CP. Notably, the macrophages are found in proximity to fibrotic areas.[28,29] Lipopolysaccharide (LPS)-activated macrophages stimulate PSC activation and promote collagen and fibronectin synthesis in cultured pancreatic stellate cells (PSCs).[30] Toll-like receptor 4 (TLR4) binds LPS, and TLR4+ monocyte/macrophages play an important role in the pathogenesis of AP.[31,32] However, a role for macrophage TLR4 in CP remains to be defined. Unlike in AP, alternatively activated macrophages predominate in CP, and inhibiting macrophage IL-4Rα signalling decreases PSC activation, fibrosis, and disease progression in cerulein-induced mouse model of CP.[29] Alcohol feeding and cerulein treatment in mice have an additive effect in increasing arginase-expressing macrophages in the pancreas,[33] suggesting a role for alternatively activated macrophages. The contribution of myeloid cells, especially macrophages, is highlighted by the fact that myeloid and not acinar nuclear factor kappa B (NF-κB) activation (RelA/p65) is necessary for promoting fibroisis in cerulein-mediated expermental CP.[34]

Dendritic Cells (DCs)

As active participants of inflammation, through mentoring T-cell responses, DCs emerge as both potent promoters and suppressors of inflammation.[35] Numerous publications highlight their importance in a number of organ-specific inflammatory diseases. It was demonstrated that DC depletion in a mouse model of cerulein-induced AP massively increased pancreatic damage and pancreatic exocrine cell death, followed by consequent mortality.[36] Interestingly, it seems that DCs have dual roles in AP. They galvanize the inflammatory response to damage via production of different inflammatory mediators (e.g., IL-6, TNF-α, and CCL2), but on the other hand, protect the pancreas following cellular stress. The same group demonstrated that DCs are required for pancreatic viability in AP, as the they are the major cell type clearing byproducts of injury.

DCs also increase in cerulein-induced CP.[37] Moreover, adoptive transfer of bone marrow-derived DCs and in vivo expansion of DCs, using Fms-like tyrosine kinase-3 ligand (FLT3L), resulted in PSC activation and worsened CP. These effects seem to be mediated via DC-CD4+ T cell activation, since CD4+ T cell-deficient mice were protected from the effects of the DCs. TLR4 can signal in MyD88-dependent and -independent pathways; interestingly, in this study MyD88-deficient DC transfer further worsened CP, suggesting opposing roles of TLR4 downstream signalling in DCs during pancreatic inflammation. More studies are likely to reveal the role of different subsets of DCs in pancreatitis.

T cells

Initial studies that demonstrated the involvement of CD4+ T cells were performed in nude mice and in vivo CD4(+) or CD8(+) T cell-depleted mice. These experiments revealed a pivotal role in the development of tissue injury during experimental AP in mice. Indeed, the reduction of peripheral blood $CD4^+$ T lymphocytes is associated with persistent organ failure during AP.[38] In contrast, an increase in immune cell infiltration, mainly T cells and macrophages, is observed in CP.[29,39,40] In the dibutyltin dichloride (DBTC) rat model of CP, increases in both CD4+ and CD8+ T cells were observed, and over time there was a decrease in the CD4+/CD8+ T cell ratio due to a continuous rise in infiltrating CD8+ T cells.[41] Moreover, increases in IFNγ, IL-2, and IL-2 receptor transcripts during the chronic phase suggested a role for lymphocyte activation in disease pathogenesis.

Increases in mononuclear cell (lymphocytes and macrophages) infiltrates in pancreatic tissues are observed in patients with CP.[40,42] Among the infiltrating lymphocytes, T cells were predominant with higher CD8+ relative to CD4+ T cells, and they were localized between the parenchyma and fibrotic areas. Interestingly, a significant increase in perforin mRNA-expressing CD8+ and CD56+ cells were observed in pancreatic tissue sections from patients with alcoholic CP, suggesting a possible role for cytotoxic CD8+ and/or NK T cells in this disease.[43] In contrast, amongst circulating leukocytes, CD8+ and CD56+ were reportedly lower in a handful number of CP patients compared to healthy controls.[44] In addition, unlike the decreased CD4+/CD8+ T cell ratio reported by Hunger et al in pancreatic tissue, an increased CD4+/CD8+ T cell ratio was found in the circulation of patients with CP,[44] suggesting differences in both T cell activation and recruitment. However, another study found that CD4+ but not CD8+ was the predominant tissue infiltrating T cells in CP patients.[45] This study found the CD4+ T cell to be localized in the fibrous area, whereas CD8+ T cells expressing the αE integrin (CD103), implicated in mediating T cell adhesion to intestine epithelium E-cadherin, were scattered between ductal cells, suggesting possible microenvironment-dependent functional differences among infiltrating T cell subsets.

An interesting study comparing bone marrow and blood mononuclear cells from healthy, CP, and pancreatic cancer patients, as well as infiltrating lymphocytes from CP lesions found that only CP patients had a strong IL-10-producing Foxp3+ regulatory T cell responses against pancreatitis-associated antigens.[46] Moreover, increased circulating memory T cells and persistence of dysregulated immune responses, even long after the removal of CP lesions,[47] support the hypothesis of ongoing CP-specific T cell responses.

Mediators for immune cell recruitment

Examples of cytokines/chemokines involved

Under inflammatory and noninflammatory conditions, cytokines and in particular chemokines play an important role in leukocyte recruitment.[48-50] Distinct and differential expression of cytokines and chemokines have been described in AP and CP.[51-53] Based on overexpression of chemokines and chemokine receptors observed, several investigators employed blockade approaches to modulate and show protective effects against experimental pancreatitis.

Protective effects of inhibiting the chemokine CCL2/MCP-1 (CCR2 ligand) have been shown by multiple investigators using different rodent models of AP.[54-57] Results form CCR2-deficient mice were also consistent with these findings.[58] CCR5-deficient mice on the other hand had exacerbated cerulein-induced AP, and may have been due to the fact that CCR5 knockout mice had increased CCL2/MCP-1 and other monocyte/macrophage chemoattractant production that may have accounted for the pronounced pancreatic inflammation.[59] Inhibition of other chemokines or chemokine receptors such as cytokine-induced neutrophil chemoattractant (CINC), serum chemokine (C-X3-C motif) ligand 1 (CX3CL1)/fractalkine, CXCR2, and CCR1 were also shown to ameliorate pancreatic and/or its associated lung inflammation.[60-65] Leukocyte migration is a multistep process involving trafficking receptors and adhesion molecules.[66,67] Consistent with the significance of leukocyte migration in pancreatitis, a pathogenic role was also demonstrated for ICAM-1 in various experimental AP models.[68-72]

CCR2 ligands are also elevated in experimental CP, and competitive bone marrow studies show a role for CCR2 in monocyte/macrophage accumulation in the chronically inflamed pancreas.[29] However, a worse disease outcome was reported in cerulein-induced CP in CCR2 knockout mice compared to their wild-type counterparts.[58] Thus, further studies are needed to clarify the role for CCR2 in CP. Similar to AP, CXCR2 inhibition had a protective effect in experimental CP.[65] Significant mRNA increases for CCR5 and its chemokine ligands CCL5 and CCL3 in the pancreas were evident in patients with CP.[73] Moreover, the majority of the CCR5-positive cells by immunostaining were also CD68-positive, suggesting a role for CCR5 in monocyte/macrophage recruitment in CP. Overall, there are fewer experimental studies on chemokine and chemokine receptor blockade in CP compared to AP models. Nevertheless, modulations of chemokine and chemokine receptors appear to impact immune cell infiltration and disease outcomes, at least in experimental models of both AP and CP.

Transcription factors in pancreatitis

NF-κB is one of the central transcription factors, and a main mediator responsible for pancreatitis pathophysiology. The most prominent regulatory functions of NF-κB are inflammatory responses, cell proliferation, and apoptosis. NF-κB is formed by different homo- and heterodimers of members of the NF-κB/Rel family and can be activated by different stimuli (e.g., cytokines, LPS, oxidative stress, and activators of protein kinase C).[74-77]

The earliest study to demonstrate early activation of NF-κB in AP was presented by Stephen Pandol's group and confirmed by another group 1 year later.[78,79] However, both studies presented different conclusions with respect to the role of NF-κB in AP. Since then, NF-κB activation has been reported in numerous publications.[80-82]

In most studies, pharmacologic NF-κB inhibition ameliorated the inflammatory response, necrosis, and other parameters of pancreatitis severity. However, the pharmacologic agents were largely nonspecific, such as antioxidants and proteasomal inhibitors. Thus, it was expected that the new tool of genetically engineered mouse models would help to clarify the role of NF-κB in AP. But surprisingly, the controversies were perpetuated with evidence that the I kappa B kinase (IKK)/NF-κB/RelA pathway leads to both aggravation[34,79,83,84] and amelioration[78,85-88] of pancreatitis. However, this paradox can be resolved, at least in part, by realizing that acinar cell NF-κB activation triggers both pro- and anti-inflammatory pathways. Even more, this system is strikingly context dependent, and its fine-tuning will require exhaustive characterization of the underlying mechanisms. A recent study demonstrated that fine-tuning of this pathway via the IκB protein Bcl-3 determines AP severity.[89] These studies underscore both the complexity and gaps in our understanding of this pathway. And yet, it is expected that with more clarification of its role in pancreatitis pathogenesis, the therapeutic potential of this system for treatment of pancreatitis will become clearer.

Although, intra-acinar NF-κB activation was shown to be highly present in human CP,[90] its pathophysiological role is less understood. While loss of IKKβ has no impact on pancreatic integrity,[91] deletion of IKKα in the pancreas induces spontaneous chronic inflammation. IKKα was shown to potentially control autophagic protein degradation and maintain pancreatic acinar cell homeostasis. Further, other studies revealed the critical role for NF-κB in myeloid cells in inducing fibrosis during CP.[34]

Signal transducer and activator of transcription 3

Signal transducer and activator of transcription 3 (STAT3) is among the most promising new cancer therapy targets. It is generally considered to be a direct transcription factor, and IL-6 is a well known traditional activator of STAT3.[92] STAT3 is highly involved in several pathologic processes in the pancreas (e.g., acinar-to-ductal metaplasia and AP/CP progression). It is highly associated with cell survival, proliferation, and differentiation, as well as tissue inflammation.[93] Using a model of cerulein-induced AP, it was demonstrated that conditional STAT3 knockout mice showed more damage with higher levels of serum amylase and lipase, as well as significantly higher infiltration of inflammatory cells in the pancreas.[94]

Interestingly, STAT3 activation in the pancreas emerged as highly responsible for the secondary effect of severe AP: acute lung injury.[20] Furthermore, the authors demonstrated different STAT3 phosphorylation sites, namely $STAT3^{S727}$ and $STAT3^{Y705}$. Additionally, genetic inhibition of IL-6 signaling (in IL-$6^{-/-}$ mice) where $STAT3^{S727}$ emerged, unlike blocking IL-6 trans-signaling (in opt_sgp130Fc mice) where $STAT3^{S727}$ did not emerge, eliminates protective mechanisms during inflammation. Nonetheless, the authors could not explain whether STAT3 phosphorylation status could account for the differences in local tissue damage.

Therapeutic approaches targeting inflammation in the pancreas

AP

Given the profound and increasing understanding of pathology and regulatory mechanisms of AP, numerous studies have evaluated mediators and different pathways with the aim to provide evidence for the development of pharmaceutical therapies. Unfortunately, several facts have contributed to treatment limitations. Firstly, AP can be multifactorial with unidentified causes. Secondly, it is accepted that disease initiation is followed by common inflammatory mechanisms, but this might not be the case in all patients. Thirdly, disease initiation and duration are individual, so the time of treatment initiation is not uniform. This makes it difficult to predict the final outcome as to whether a patient develops mild or severe pancreatitis.[95] Conservative management, such as antibiotics and bowel rest have been insufficient treatment for AP. Many agents beneficial for AP in animal studies failed to achieve the same success in early clinical trials.

One of the first attempts to influence immune system mediators was with lexipafant.[96] This drug is one of the most potent platelet-activating factor (PAF) receptor antagonists. Disappointingly, a clinical study in patients with severe AP failed to demonstrate an effect on new organ failure during treatment.[97] Thus, this study demonstrated that an antagonist of PAF activity on its own is not sufficient to ameliorate systemic inflammatory response syndrome in severe AP. The latest reviews summarized recent therapeutics and experimental approaches that target immune responses in AP.[95,98] Several therapeutic agents, depleting or regulating immune cells via various mechanisms of action, demonstrated protective roles against AP in animal models:

- **Glycyrrhizin** is a therapeutic agent that reduces serum levels of CCL2 and amylase and lipase activity by inhibiting the recruitment of inflammatory cells into the pancreas[99]
- **Sivelestat** demonstrated strong anti-inflammatory potential; it interferes with regulatory mechanisms of immune cells and reduces expression of lipase, amylase, IL-1β, TNF-α, and NF-αB; its administration increases antioxidant power and IL-4 serum levels[100]
- **Flavocoxid** reduces levels of TNF-α, serum levels of prostaglandin E2 (PGE2) and leukotriene B4 (LTB4), and lessens histological damage. It influences neutrophil and macrophage action via cyclooxygenase-2 (COX-2) and 5-lipoxygenase (5-LOX) blockade[101]
- **Rofecoxib** and lisinopril decrease levels of CCL2, CCL3, TNF-α, and IL-6, influencing macrophage infiltration via COX-2 pathway inhibition[102]

It is essential to mention IL-6 inhibitors as highly promising drug targets for AP. Tocilizumab has emerged as remarkably efficient for treating several inflammatory diseases. Recent reports demonstrated positive effects of tocilizumab on experimental severe AP and associated acute lung injury in rats.[103] Severe AP was induced by retrograde injection of sodium taurocholate into the biliopancreatic duct. Following the administration of tocilizumab, pancreatic and lung histopathological scores were reduced; serum amylase, C-reactive protein, and lung surfactant protein levels were decreased; and myeloperoxidase activity was attenuated. In line with these findings, pancreatic NF-κB and STAT3 were decreased, and the serum chemokine (C-X-C motif) ligand 1 (CXCL1) was down regulated in rats after tocilizumab administration.

In an interesting and novel approach proposed only recently, treatment with CO-releasing molecule-2 (CORM-2) decreased mortality, pancreatic damage, and lung injury in a mouse model of AP.[32] This treatment decreased systemic inflammatory cytokines and suppressed systemic and pancreatic macrophage activation. Such cellular therapeutic approaches, therefore, offers an alternative treatment route.

CP

As mentioned previously, increases in mononuclear cell (particularly T cells and macrophages) infiltrates in pancreatic tissues are observed in patients with CP as compared to the normal pancreas.[40] Alternatively activated macrophages are abundant in CP, especially in the vicinity of the fibrosis and activated PSCs.[29,73] Differences in inflammatory infiltrates with increases in lymphocytes and macrophages, as well as DCs around the ducts, were reported in nonalcohol- versus alcohol-related CP pathologies.[104] However the nonalcoholic group comprised a heterogeneous group of patients (including 4/12 patients with associated nonpancreatic immune disease manifestations), although no major histologic differences were noted between the patients. Thus, whether functional and immune response differences exist between alcohol- and nonalcohol-mediated CP remains to be defined in studies with large numbers of patients. In addition, immune cell infiltration and responses are likely dynamic processes that vary with stage and disease progression. In agreement with this, early disease is associated with moderate inflammatory cell collections or dispersed in the fibrous tissue; later disease stages are characterized by scant lymphocyte infiltration around the ducts and neurons.[39] Recent experimental data show that macrophages can influence fibrosis and CP progression.[29] More importantly, immune mediated pathways targeting IL-4Rα signaling could alter established CP-associated fibrosis and slow disease progression. Thus immune targets might offer novel future therapies in CP, although the dilemma of diagnosing early clinical CP remains.

Conclusion

To date, experimental therapies used for AP treatment have demonstrated some success, but have given more challenges and unanswered questions from the clinical side. Numerous preclinical studies often gave diverse, and in some cases, contradictory results. Unfortunately, inconsistency in conclusions after drug testing does not give us an open window for translating these drugs into clinical trials. Turning our direction and changing our approach from classic, standard AP drug treatments, towards targeting immune response might bring more promising results and significantly better disease outcomes. Also, it might be rewarding to try combinational therapies targeting immune cells together with classic approaches. These questions and assumptions need to be answered in the near future. CP adds another challenge where immune responses are quite different from AP responses. In addition, translating experimental findings will require better diagnostic criteria that can identify patients with early and late disease.

References

1. Whitcomb DC. Clinical practice. Acute pancreatitis. *N Engl J Med.* 2006;354:2142-2150. PMID: 16707751.
2. Lankisch PG, Apte M, Banks PA. Acute pancreatitis. *Lancet.* 2015;386:85-96. PMID: 25616312.
3. Habtezion A. Inflammation in acute and chronic pancreatitis. *Curr Opin Gastroenterol.* 2015;31:395-399. PMID: 26107390.
4. Majumder S, Chari ST. Chronic pancreatitis. *Lancet.* 2016;387:1957-1966. PMID: 26948434.
5. Yadav D, Lowenfels AB. The epidemiology of pancreatitis and pancreatic cancer. *Gastroenterology.* 2013;144:1252-1261. PMID: 23622135.
6. Sandoval D, Gukovskaya A, Reavey P, Gukovsky S, Sisk A, Braquet P, et al. The role of neutrophils and platelet-activating factor in mediating experimental pancreatitis. *Gastroenterology.* 1996;111:1081-1091. PMID: 8831604.
7. Rinderknecht H. Fatal pancreatitis, a consequence of excessive leukocyte stimulation? *Int J Pancreatol.* 1988;3:105-112. PMID: 2834471.
8. Granger DN. Cell adhesion and migration. II. Leukocyte-endothelial cell adhesion in the digestive system. *Am J Physiol Gastrointest Liver Physiol.* 1997;273:G982-G986. PMID: 9374693.
9. Gorelick FS, Adler G, Kern HF. Cerulein-induced pancreatitis. In: Go VLW, DiMagno EP, Gardner JD, Lebenthal E, Reber HA, GA Scheele, eds. *The Pancreas: Biology, Pathobiology, and Disease.* New York, NY: Raven Press; 1993:501-526.
10. Zaninovic V, Gukovskaya AS, Gukovsky I, Mouria M, Pandol SJ. Cerulein upregulates ICAM-1 in pancreatic acinar cells, which mediates neutrophil adhesion to these cells. *Am J Physiol Gastrointest Liver Physiol.* 2000;279:G666-G676. PMID: 11005752.
11. Frossard JL, Saluja A, Bhagat L, Lee HS, Bhatia M, Hofbauer B, et al. The role of intercellular adhesion molecule 1 and neutrophils in acute pancreatitis and pancreatitis-associated lung injury. *Gastroenterology.* 1999;116:694-701. PMID: 10029629.
12. Ushio-Fukai M. Compartmentalization of redox signaling through NADPH oxidase-derived ROS. *Antioxid Redox Signal.* 2009;11:1289-1299. PMID: 18999986.
13. Chan YC, Leung PS. Angiotensin II type 1 receptor-dependent nuclear factor-kappaB activation-mediated proinflammatory actions in a rat model of obstructive acute pancreatitis. *J Pharmacol Exp Ther.* 2007;323:10-18. PMID: 17616560.
14. Gukovskaya AS, Vaquero E, Zaninovic V, Gorelick FS, Lusis AJ, Brennan ML, et al. Neutrophils and NADPH oxidase mediate intrapancreatic trypsin activation in murine experimental acute pancreatitis. *Gastroenterology.* 2002;122:974-984. PMID: 11910350.
15. Sendler M, Dummer A, Weiss FU, Krüger B, Wartmann T, Scharffetter-Kochanek K, et al. Tumour necrosis factor alpha secretion induces protease activation and acinar cell necrosis in acute experimental pancreatitis in mice. *Gut.* 2013;62:430-439. PMID: 22490516.
16. Perides G, Weiss ER, Michael ES, Laukkarinen JM, Duffield JS, Steer ML. TNF-alpha-dependent regulation of acute pancreatitis severity by Ly-6C(hi) monocytes in mice. *J Biol Chem.* 2011;286:13327-13335. PMID: 21343291.
17. Gukovskaya AS, Gukovsky I, Zaninovic V, Song M, Sandoval D, Gukovsky S, et al. Pancreatic acinar cells produce, release, and respond to tumor necrosis factor-alpha. Role in regulating cell death and pancreatitis. *J Clin Invest.* 1997;100:1853-1862. PMID: 9312187.
18. Bhatia M, Brady M, Shokuhi S, Christmas S, Neoptolemos JP, Slavin J. Inflammatory mediators in acute pancreatitis. *J Pathol.* 2000;190:117-125. PMID: 10657008.
19. McKay C, Imrie CW, Baxter JN. Mononuclear phagocyte activation and acute pancreatitis. *Scand J Gastroenterol Suppl.* 1996;219:32-36. PMID: 8865469.
20. Zhang H, Neuhöfer P, Song L, Rabe B, Lesina M, Kurkowski MU, et al. IL-6 trans-signaling promotes pancreatitis-associated lung injury and lethality. *J Clin Invest.* 2013;123:1019-1031. PMID: 23426178.
21. Dugernier T, Laterre PF, Reynaert MS. Ascites fluid in severe acute pancreatitis: from pathophysiology to therapy. *Acta Gastroenterol Belg.* 2000;63:264-268. PMID: 11189983.
22. Gea-Sorli S, Closa D. In vitro, but not in vivo, reversibility of peritoneal macrophages activation during experimental acute pancreatitis. *BMC Immunol.* 2009;10:42. PMID: 19646232.
23. Takeyama Y, Nishikawa J, Ueda T, Hori Y, Yamamoto M, Kuroda Y. Involvement of peritoneal macrophage in the induction of cytotoxicity due to apoptosis in ascitic fluid associated with severe acute pancreatitis. *J Surg Res.* 1999;82:163-171. PMID: 10090825.
24. Closa D, Sabater L, Fernández-Cruz L, Prats N, Gelpí E, Roselló-Catafau J. Activation of alveolar macrophages in lung injury associated with experimental acute pancreatitis is mediated by the liver. *Ann Surg.* 1999;229:230-236. PMID: 10024105.
25. Li HG, Zhou ZG, Li Y, Zheng XL, Lei S, Zhu L, et al. Alterations of Toll-like receptor 4 expression on peripheral blood monocytes during the early stage of human acute pancreatitis. *Dig Dis Sci.* 2007;52:1973-1978. PMID: 17415654.
26. Folch-Puy E. Importance of the liver in systemic complications associated with acute pancreatitis: the role of Kupffer cells. *J Pathol.* 2007;211:383-388. PMID: 17212343.
27. Geisler F, Algul H, Riemann M, Schmid RM. Questioning current concepts in acute pancreatitis: endotoxin contamination of porcine pancreatic elastase is responsible for experimental pancreatitis-associated distant organ failure. *J Immunol.* 2005;174:6431-6439. PMID: 15879145.

28. Deng X, Wang L, Elm MS, Gabazadeh D, Diorio GJ, Eagon PK, et al. Chronic alcohol consumption accelerates fibrosis in response to cerulein-induced pancreatitis in rats. *Am J Pathol.* 2005;166:93-106. PMID: 15632003.
29. Xue J, Sharma V, Hsieh MH, Chawla A, Murali R, Pandol SJ, et al. Alternatively activated macrophages promote pancreatic fibrosis in chronic pancreatitis. *Nat Commun.* 2015;6:7158. PMID: 25981357.
30. Schmid-Kotsas A, Gross HJ, Menke A, Weidenbach H, Adler G, Siech M, et al. Lipopolysaccharide-activated macrophages stimulate the synthesis of collagen type I and C-fibronectin in cultured pancreatic stellate cells. *Am J Pathol.* 1999;155:1749-1758. PMID: 10550331.
31. Sharif R, Dawra R, Wasiluk K, Phillips P, Dudeja V, Kurt-Jones E, et al. Impact of toll-like receptor 4 on the severity of acute pancreatitis and pancreatitis-associated lung injury in mice. *Gut.* 2009;58:813-819. PMID: 19201771.
32. Xue J, Habtezion A. Carbon monoxide-based therapy ameliorates acute pancreatitis via TLR4 inhibition. *J Clin Invest.* 2014;124:437-447. PMID: 24334457.
33. Xu S, Chheda C, Ouhaddi Y, Benhaddou H, Bourhim M, Grippo PJ, et al. Characterization of Mouse Models of Early Pancreatic Lesions Induced by Alcohol and Chronic Pancreatitis. *Pancreas.* 2015;44:882-887. PMID: 26166469.
34. Treiber M, Neuhöfer P, Anetsberger E, Einwächter H, Lesina M, Rickmann M, et al. Myeloid, but not pancreatic, RelA/p65 is required for fibrosis in a mouse model of chronic pancreatitis. *Gastroenterology.* 2011;141:1473-1485. PMID: 21763242.
35. Xue J, Sharma V, Habtezion A. Immune cells and immune-based therapy in pancreatitis. *Immunol Res.* 2014;58:378-386. PMID: 24710635.
36. Bedrosian AS, Nguyen AH, Hackman M, Connolly MK, Malhotra A, Ibrahim J, et al. Dendritic cells promote pancreatic viability in mice with acute pancreatitis. *Gastroenterology.* 2011;141:1915-1926. PMID: 21801698.
37. Ochi A, Nguyen AH, Bedrosian AS, Mushlin HM, Zarbakhsh S, Barilla R, et al. MyD88 inhibition amplifies dendritic cell capacity to promote pancreatic carcinogenesis via Th2 cells. *J Exp Med.* 2012;209:1671-1687. PMID: 22908323.
38. Yang Z, Zhang Y, Dong L, Yang C, Gou S, Yin T, et al. The Reduction of Peripheral Blood CD4+ T Cell Indicates Persistent Organ Failure in Acute Pancreatitis. *PLoS One.* 2015;10:e0125529. PMID: 25938229.
39. Kloppel G, Maillet B. Pathology of acute and chronic pancreatitis. *Pancreas.* 1993;8:659-670. PMID: 8255882.
40. Emmrich J, Weber I, Nausch M, Sparmann G, Koch K, Seyfarth M, et al. Immunohistochemical characterization of the pancreatic cellular infiltrate in normal pancreas, chronic pancreatitis and pancreatic carcinoma. *Digestion.* 1998;59:192-198. PMID: 9643678.
41. Sparmann G, Behrend S, Merkord J, Kleine HD, Graser E, Ritter T, et al. Cytokine mRNA levels and lymphocyte infiltration in pancreatic tissue during experimental chronic pancreatitis induced by dibutyltin dichloride. *Dig Dis Sci.* 2001;46:1647-1656. PMID: 11508663.
42. Jaskiewicz K, Nalecz A, Rzepko R, Sledzinski Z. Immunocytes and activated stellate cells in pancreatic fibrogenesis. *Pancreas.* 2003;26:239-242. PMID: 12657949.
43. Hunger RE, Mueller C, Z'Graggen K, Friess H, Büchler MW. Cytotoxic cells are activated in cellular infiltrates of alcoholic chronic pancreatitis. *Gastroenterology.* 1997;112:1656-1663. PMID: 9136845.
44. Ockenga J, Jacobs R, Kemper A, Benschop RJ, Schmidt RE, Manns MP. Lymphocyte subsets and cellular immunity in patients with chronic pancreatitis. *Digestion.* 2000;62:14-21. PMID: 10899720.
45. Ebert MP, Ademmer K, Müller-Ostermeyer F, Friess H, Büchler MW, Schubert W, et al. CD8+CD103+ T cells analogous to intestinal intraepithelial lymphocytes infiltrate the pancreas in chronic pancreatitis. *Am J Gastroenterol.* 1998;93:2141-2147. PMID: 9820387.
46. Schmitz-Winnenthal H, Pietsch DH, Schimmack S, Bonertz A, Udonta F, Ge Y, et al. Chronic pancreatitis is associated with disease-specific regulatory T-cell responses. *Gastroenterology.* 2010;138:1178-1188. PMID: 19931255.
47. Grundsten M, Liu GZ, Permert J, Hjelmstrom P, Tsai JA. Increased central memory T cells in patients with chronic pancreatitis. *Pancreatology.* 2005;5:177-182. PMID: 15849488.
48. Gukovsky I, Li N, Todoric J, Gukovskaya A, Karin M. Inflammation, autophagy, and obesity: common features in the pathogenesis of pancreatitis and pancreatic cancer. *Gastroenterology.* 2013;144:1199-1209. PMID: 23622129.
49. Norman J. The role of cytokines in the pathogenesis of acute pancreatitis. *Am J Surg.* 1998;175:76-83. PMID: 9445247.
50. Szatmary P, Gukovsky I. The role of cytokines and inflammation in the genesis of experimental pancreatitis. *Pancreapedia: Exocrine Pancreas Knowledge Base*, 2016. PMID.
51. Saurer L, Reber P, Schaffner T, Büchler MW, Buri C, Kappeler A, et al. Differential expression of chemokines in normal pancreas and in chronic pancreatitis. *Gastroenterology.* 2000;118:356-367. PMID: 10648464.
52. Gunjaca I, Zunic J, Gunjaca M, Kovac Z. Circulating cytokine levels in acute pancreatitis-model of SIRS/CARS can help in the clinical assessment of disease severity. *Inflammation.* 2012;35:758-763. PMID: 21826480.
53. Shen Y, Cui N, Miao B, Zhao E. Immune dysregulation in patients with severe acute pancreatitis. *Inflammation.* 2011;34:36-42. PMID: 20405190.
54. Bhatia M, Ramnath RD, Chevali L, Guglielmotti A. Treatment with bindarit, a blocker of MCP-1 synthesis, protects mice against acute pancreatitis. *Am J Physiol Gastrointest Liver Physiol.* 2005;288:G1259-G1265. PMID: 15691869.
55. Ishibashi T, Zhao H, Kawabe K, Oono T, Egashira K, Suzuki K, et al. Blocking of monocyte chemoattractant protein-1 (MCP-1) activity attenuates the severity of acute pancreatitis in rats. *J Gastroenterol.* 2008;43:79-85. PMID: 18297440.
56. Zhou GX, Zhu XJ, Ding XL, Zhang H, Chen JP, Qiang H, et al. Protective effects of MCP-1 inhibitor on a rat model of severe acute pancreatitis. *Hepatobiliary Pancreat Dis Int.* 2010;9:201-207. PMID: 20382594.
57. Frossard JL, Lenglet S, Montecucco F, Steffens S, Galan K, Pelli G, et al. Role of CCL-2, CCR-2 and CCR-4 in cerulein-induced acute pancreatitis and pancreatitis-associated lung injury. *J Clin Pathol.* 2011;64:387-393. PMID: 21345872.

58. Nakamura Y, Kanai T, Saeki K, Takabe M, Irie J, Miyoshi J, et al. CCR2 knockout exacerbates cerulein-induced chronic pancreatitis with hyperglycemia via decreased GLP-1 receptor expression and insulin secretion. *Am J Physiol Gastrointest Liver Physiol.* 2013;304:G700-G707. PMID: 23449669.
59. Moreno C, Nicaise C, Gustot T, Quertinmont E, Nagy N, Parmentier M, et al. Chemokine receptor CCR5 deficiency exacerbates cerulein-induced acute pancreatitis in mice. *Am J Physiol Gastrointest Liver Physiol.* 2006;291:G1089-G1099. PMID: 16891300.
60. Bhatia M, Brady M, Zagorski J, Christmas SE, Campbell F, Neoptolemos JP, et al. Treatment with neutralising antibody against cytokine induced neutrophil chemoattractant (CINC) protects rats against acute pancreatitis associated lung injury. *Gut.* 2000;47:838-844. PMID: 11076884.
61. Huang L, Ma J, Tang Y, Chen P, Zhang S, Zhang Y, et al. siRNA-based targeting of fractalkine overexpression suppresses inflammation development in a severe acute pancreatitis rat model. *Int J Mol Med.* 2012;30:514-520. PMID: 22751862.
62. Bhatia M, Hegde A. Treatment with antileukinate, a CXCR2 chemokine receptor antagonist, protects mice against acute pancreatitis and associated lung injury. *Regul Pept.* 2007;138:40-48. PMID: 17014919.
63. Gerard C, Frossard JL, Bhatia M, Saluja A, Gerard NP, Lu B, et al. Targeted disruption of the beta-chemokine receptor CCR1 protects against pancreatitis-associated lung injury. *J Clin Invest.* 1997;100:2022-2027. PMID: 9329966.
64. He M, Horuk R, Bhatia M. Treatment with BX471, a nonpeptide CCR1 antagonist, protects mice against acute pancreatitis-associated lung injury by modulating neutrophil recruitment. *Pancreas.* 2007;34:233-241. PMID: 17312463.
65. Steele CW, Karim SA, Foth M, Rishi L, Leach JD, Porter RJ, et al. CXCR2 inhibition suppresses acute and chronic pancreatic inflammation. *J Pathol.* 2015;237:85-97. PMID: 25950520.
66. Butcher EC, Picker LJ. Lymphocyte homing and homeostasis. *Science.* 1996;272:60-66. PMID: 8600538.
67. Carman CV, Springer TA. Trans-cellular migration: cell-cell contacts get intimate. *Curr Opin Cell Biol.* 2008;20:533-540. PMID: 18595683.
68. Lundberg AH, Fukatsu K, Gaber L, Callicutt S, Kotb M, Wilcox H, et al. Blocking pulmonary ICAM-1 expression ameliorates lung injury in established diet-induced pancreatitis. *Ann Surg.* 2001;233:213-220. PMID: 11176127.
69. Werner J, Z'Graggen K, Fernandez-del Castillo C, Lewandrowski KB, Compton CC, Warshaw AL. Specific therapy for local and systemic complications of acute pancreatitis with monoclonal antibodies against ICAM-1. *Ann Surg.* 1999;229:834-840; discussion 841-842. PMID: 10363897.
70. Rau B, Paszkowski A, Esber S, Gansauge F, Poch B, Beger HG, et al. Anti-ICAM-1 antibody modulates late onset of acinar cell apoptosis and early necrosis in taurocholate-induced experimental acute pancreatitis. *Pancreas.* 2001;23:80-88. PMID: 11451152.
71. Rau B, Bauer A, Wang A, Gansauge F, Weidenbach H, Nevalainen T, et al. Modulation of endogenous nitric oxide synthase in experimental acute pancreatitis: role of anti-ICAM-1 and oxygen free radical scavengers. *Ann Surg.* 2001;233:195-203. PMID: 11176125.
72. Sun W, Watanabe Y, Wang ZQ. Expression and significance of ICAM-1 and its counter receptors LFA-1 and Mac-1 in experimental acute pancreatitis of rats. *World J Gastroenterol.* 2006;12:5005-5009. PMID: 16937496.
73. Goecke H, Forssmann U, Uguccioni M, Friess H, Conejo-Garcia JR, Zimmermann A, et al. Macrophages infiltrating the tissue in chronic pancreatitis express the chemokine receptor CCR5. *Surgery.* 2000;128:806-814. PMID: 11056444.
74. DiDonato JA, Mercurio F, Karin M. NF-kappaB and the link between inflammation and cancer. *Immunol Rev.* 2012;246:379-400. PMID: 22435567.
75. Hayden MS, Ghosh S. NF-kappaB, the first quarter-century: remarkable progress and outstanding questions. *Genes Dev.* 2012;26:203-234. PMID: 22302935.
76. Perkins ND. Integrating cell-signalling pathways with NF-kappaB and IKK function. *Nat Rev Mol Cell Biol.* 2007;8:49-62. PMID: 17183360.
77. Pasparakis M. Role of NF-kappaB in epithelial biology. *Immunol Rev.* 2012;246:346-358. PMID: 22435565.
78. Gukovsky I, Gukovskaya AS, Blinman TA, Zaninovic V, Pandol SJ. Early NF-kappaB activation is associated with hormone-induced pancreatitis. *Am J Physiol Gastrointest Liver Physiol.* 1998;275:G1402-G1414. PMID: 9843778.
79. Steinle AU, Weidenbach H, Wagner M, Adler G, Schmid RM. NF-kappaB/Rel activation in cerulein pancreatitis. *Gastroenterology.* 1999;116:420-430. PMID: 9922324.
80. Pandol SJ, Saluja AK, Imrie CW, Banks PA. Acute pancreatitis: bench to the bedside. *Gastroenterology.* 2007;132:1127-1151. PMID: 17383433.
81. Rakonczay Z Jr, Hegyi P, Takacs T, McCarroll J, Saluja AK. The role of NF-kappaB activation in the pathogenesis of acute pancreatitis. *Gut.* 2008;57:259-267. PMID: 17675325.
82. Gukovsky I, Gukovskaya A. Nuclear factor-kappaB in pancreatitis: Jack-of-all-trades, but which one is more important? *Gastroenterology.* 2013;144:26-29. PMID: 23164573.
83. Algul H, Treiber M, Lesina M, Nakhai H, Saur D, Geisler F, et al. Pancreas-specific RelA/p65 truncation increases susceptibility of acini to inflammation-associated cell death following cerulein pancreatitis. *J Clin Invest.* 2007;117:1490-1501. PMID: 17525802.
84. Neuhöfer P, Liang S, Einwächter H, Schwerdtfeger C, Wartmann T, Treiber M, et al. Deletion of IkappaBalpha activates RelA to reduce acute pancreatitis in mice through up-regulation of Spi2A. *Gastroenterology.* 2013;144:192-201. PMID: 23041330.
85. Chen X, Ji B, Han B, Ernst SA, Simeone D, Logsdon CD. NF-kappaB activation in pancreas induces pancreatic and systemic inflammatory response. *Gastroenterology.* 2002;122:448-457. PMID: 11832459.
86. Baumann B, Wagner M, Aleksic T, von Wichert G, Weber CK, Adler G, et al. Constitutive IKK2 activation in acinar cells is sufficient to induce pancreatitis in vivo. *J Clin Invest.* 2007;117:1502-1513. PMID: 17525799.
87. Altavilla D, Famulari C, Passaniti M, Galeano M, Macri A, Seminara P, et al. Attenuated cerulein-induced pancreatitis in nuclear factor-kappaB-deficient mice. *Lab Invest.* 2003;83:1723-1732. PMID: 14691290.

88. Huang H, Liu Y, Daniluk J, Gaiser S, Chu J, Wang H, et al. Activation of nuclear factor-kappaB in acinar cells increases the severity of pancreatitis in mice. *Gastroenterology*. 2013;144:202-210. PMID: 23041324.
89. Song L, Wormann S, Ai J, Neuhöfer P, Lesina M, Diakopoulos KN, et al. BCL3 Reduces the Sterile Inflammatory Response in Pancreatic and Biliary Tissues. *Gastroenterology*. 2016;150:499-512. PMID: 26526716.
90. Sah RP, Dawra RK, Saluja AK. New insights into the pathogenesis of pancreatitis. *Curr Opin Gastroenterol*. 2013;29:523-530. PMID: 23892538.
91. Ling J, Kang Y, Zhao R, Xia Q, Lee DF, Chang Z, et al. KrasG12D-induced IKK2/beta/NF-kappaB activation by IL-1alpha and p62 feedforward loops is required for development of pancreatic ductal adenocarcinoma. *Cancer Cell*. 2012;21:105-120. PMID: 22264792.
92. Heinrich PC, Behrmann I, Haan S, Hermanns HM, Muller-Newen G, Schaper F. Principles of interleukin (IL)-6-type cytokine signalling and its regulation. *Biochem J*. 2003;374:1-20. PMID: 12773095.
93. Yu H, Lee H, Herrmann A, Buettner R, Jove R. Revisiting STAT3 signalling in cancer: new and unexpected biological functions. *Nat Rev Cancer*. 2014;14:736-746. PMID: 25342631.
94. Shigekawa M, Hikita H, Kodama T, Shimizu S, Li W, Uemura A, et al. Pancreatic STAT3 protects mice against caerulein-induced pancreatitis via PAP1 induction. *Am J Pathol*. 2012;181:2105-2113. PMID: 23064197.
95. Shamoon M, Deng Y, Chen YQ, Bhatia M, Sun J. Therapeutic implications of innate immune system in acute pancreatitis. *Expert Opin Ther Targets*. 2016;20:73-87. PMID: 26565751.
96. Johnson CD. Platelet-activating factor and platelet-activating factor antagonists in acute pancreatitis. *Dig Surg*. 1999;16:93-101. PMID: 10207233.
97. Johnson CD, Kingsnorth AN, Imrie CW, McMahon MJ, Neoptolemos JP, McKay C, et al. Double blind, randomised, placebo controlled study of a platelet activating factor antagonist, lexipafant, in the treatment and prevention of organ failure in predicted severe acute pancreatitis. *Gut*. 2001;48:62-69. PMID: 11115824.
98. Kambhampati S, Park W, Habtezion A. Pharmacologic therapy for acute pancreatitis. *World J Gastroenterol*. 2014;20:16868-16880. PMID: 25493000.
99. Fakhari S, Abdolmohammadi K, Panahi Y, Nikkhoo B, Peirmohammadi H, Rahmani MR, et al. Glycyrrhizin attenuates tissue injury and reduces neutrophil accumulation in experimental acute pancreatitis. *Int J Clin Exp Pathol*. 2014;7:101-109. PMID: 24427330.
100. Cao J, Liu Q. Protective effects of sivelestat in a caerulein-induced rat acute pancreatitis model. *Inflammation*. 2013;36:1348-1356. PMID: 23794035.
101. Polito F, Bitto A, Irrera N, Squadrito F, Fazzari C, Minutoli L, et al. Flavocoxid, a dual inhibitor of cyclooxygenase-2 and 5-lipoxygenase, reduces pancreatic damage in an experimental model of acute pancreatitis. *Br J Pharmacol*. 2010;161:1002-1011. PMID: 20977452.
102. Reding T, Bimmler D, Perren A, Sun LK, Fortunato F, Storni F, et al. A selective COX-2 inhibitor suppresses chronic pancreatitis in an animal model (WBN/Kob rats): significant reduction of macrophage infiltration and fibrosis. *Gut*. 2006;55:1165-1173. PMID: 16322109.
103. Chen KL, Lv ZY, Yang HW, Liu Y, Long FW, Zhou B, et al. Effects of Tocilizumab on Experimental Severe Acute Pancreatitis and Associated Acute Lung Injury. *Crit Care Med*. 2016;44:e664-e677. PMID: 26963319.
104. Ectors N, Maillet B, Aerts R, Geboes K, Donner A, Borchard F, et al. Non-alcoholic duct destructive chronic pancreatitis. *Gut*. 1997;41:263-268. PMID: 9301509.

Chapter 8

Heat shock proteins as modulators of pancreatitis

Rajinder K. Dawra, Vikas Dudeja, and Ashok K. Saluja*

Department of Surgery, University of Miami Miller School of Medicine, Miami, Florida, USA.

Introduction

Heat shock proteins (HSPs) are highly conserved proteins expressed in response to stress in all species. In 1962, Ritossa was the first to observe an altered puffing pattern in giant chromosomes of salivary glands in *Drosophila busckii* after heat shock.[1] On microscopic evaluation, areas of increased transcriptional activity in these giant chromosomes appear swollen and are called puffs. He reported that temperature shock induced well-defined variation in the normal puffing patterns, which is observed during the development of *Drosophila* larvae. After initiation of heat shock, incorporation of ^{3}H-cytidine in puffs started within 3-4 min and peaked after 10 min. In addition to heat shock, this effect could also be reproduced by treatment with 2,4-dinitrophenol (DNP) and sodium salicylate. After the initial report, this important work remained largely ignored until it was rediscovered in 1974. While studying synthesis of proteins by metabolic incorporation of radioactive precursors, Tissieres et al. observed a new pattern of radiolabeled protein synthesis following heat shock.[2] These new proteins were termed HSPs. Interestingly, heat shock activated the synthesis of only a few polypeptides and strongly inhibited the synthesis of most others. Subsequently, it was found that this family of proteins is upregulated in response to a variety of stresses including heat stress, inflammation, ischemia, anoxia, and heavy metals.

HSPs are subdivided according to their molecular weight (MW): HSP110, HSP90 (HSP90a, HSP90b, GRP94), HSP70 (HSP70, HSC70, mHSP70 [GRP75], GRP78),[3-5] HSP60,[6] HSP40,[7,8] HSP27,[9] and HSP10 (GroES)[10,11] and contain both constitutively expressed members and polypeptides whose expression increases many fold in response to stress.

HSP100: This family is comprised of proteins with MW 104-110kDa, and each member has ATPase activity.[12] Members of this family include both constitutively expressed and inducible proteins. There are usually two ATP binding domains; however, a few members have only one ATP binding site. HSP104 is required for inducing thermo tolerance in yeast and appears to disaggregate insoluble proteins. Proteins of this family are localized to different subcellular compartments.[12]

HSP90s: These proteins (MW 82-94kDa) have permanent and abundant expression in eukaryotic cells.[13,14] This family of proteins is involved in regulating cytoskeleton dynamics, cell shape, and motility. Experiments suggest that HSP90 may be involved in cross-linking actin filaments in a calcium (Ca^{2+})-dependent fashion and has critical ATPase activity.

HSP70: The HSP70s are ubiquitous and have both constitutive and inducible members.[15] These are major molecular chaperones of eukaryotes and are present throughout cells. These have highly conserved nucleotide-binding N-termini and relatively variable C-termini domains. Synthesis of inducible members sharply increases in response to stress. The constitutive members are equally important because of their role in protein folding, maturation and proteolysis. HSP72 (HSP70) is the best-known stress inducible cytoplasmic chaperone, while other stress-inducible chaperones are found in other cellular compartments. GRP78 is located in the endoplasmic reticulum while GRP75 is found in mitochondria. HSC71 is present in cytoplasm but is constitutively expressed.

HSP60: This mitochondrial chaperone is coded by a nuclear gene.[6] It is essential for the folding and assembly of newly imported proteins in mitochondria. HSP60 monomers form a complex arrangement as two stacks of seven monomers each. This complex binds to unfolded proteins and catalyze their folding in an ATP-dependent manner.

HSP40: All DnaJ/HSP40 proteins contain a J domain through which they bind to HSP70s and can be categorized into three groups depending upon the presence of other domains.[7] In humans, 41 DnaJ/HSP40 family members have been identified based on genome-wide analysis. HSP40s are considered cochaperones for HSP70s because their binding causes an essential increase in HSP70'sATP

*Corresponding author. Email: asaluja@miami.edu

hydrolysis activity. In the absence of a cochaperone, ATP hydrolysis by HSP70s proceeds slowly, but it is enhanced several fold in the presence of cochaperone (DnaJ/Hsp40s), thereby accelerating the processing of unfolded polypeptides. DnaJ/Hsp40s also help in binding HSP70 to polypeptides, which stabilizes their interaction with the substrates. HSP40 activity is affected by the redox status.[7]

HSP27: These proteins lack ATPase activity but can be phosphorylated.[16-18] They protect other proteins from thermal inactivation and aggregation. The role of phosphorylation has been studied, and the results indicate that transient phosphorylation might play a role in release of unproductively unfolded proteins from HSP27. It is required for suppression of ASK1 cell death signaling and neuroprotection against ischemic injury.[9] Oligomerization of HSP27 is required for chaperone activity, and phosphorylation downregulates its chaperone properties by decreasing oligomerization. HSP27 expression is increased in response to stress, but it follows different kinetics compared to phosphorylation, which is considered its first response to stress.

Ubiquitin: This low MW (~8kDA) heat-inducible protein is constitutively expressed in most mammalian cell types and increases with heat shock. These have a role in protein degradation. Heat shock response stimulates protein degradation, and increased ubiquitin synthesis facilitates the process.[19,20] The ubiquitin genes constitute a multigene family, and three types of mRNA are detectable. The function of ubiquitin is presumed to be labeling polypeptides designated as substrates for intracellular proteases.

Crystallin: The lens structural proteins, crystallin-αA and -αB are also considered to be HSPs.[21] Besides their robust expression in lens, these are also expressed in other tissues. αA-crystallin is expressed in human and mouse pancreas and is involved in modulating activation of AP-1. αA crystallin has also been shown to negatively regulate pancreatic tumorigenesis.[21]

HSP expression in pancreatitis

Cerulein- and L-arginine-induced models of acute pancreatitis (AP) have been used to evaluate heat shock responses during AP development.[22,23] HSP70 mRNA was upregulated when pancreatic lobules were stimulated with supra maximal concentrations of cerulein or heat shocked at 42°C for 60 min.[22] Relative HSP70 expression varied in response to induction of pancreatitis and heat shock.[22] With cerulein-induced pancreatitis, HSP70 levels were increased 6-7 fold, but in response to heat shock the expression levels reached 20-23 fold that of baseline. When ^{35}S-methionine metabolic labeling of rat acinar cells was performed to determine hyperthermia-induced protein expression, the results revealed that overall protein synthesis was reduced by hyperthermia, but proteins with apparent MWs of 90, 72, 59, 58 and 30 kDa were induced. Thermal stress with 42°C led to significantly higher incorporation of radioactivity in at least five acinar proteins with MWs of 90, 72, 59, 58, and 30 kDa apparent molecular weight whereas incubation at 40°C had no such effect.[24] The degree of induction of hyperthermia-induced protein synthesis varied greatly between individual proteins, with and 72-and 90-kDa proteins showing the highest and lowest responses, respectively.[21] Four HSP70 isoforms were expressed in the pancreas in response to thermal stress in vivo.

Heat stress responses were evaluated at 24 h in the pancreases of rats after intraperitoneal injection of L-arginine at 3.0 and 4.5 g/kg.[23] With induction of arginine pancreatitis, there were increases in the expression of HSP27, 70, 60, and 90. A lower L-arginine dose resulted in the highest expression of HSP27 followed by HSP70, 60, and 90.[23] With a higher dose, HSP60 was expressed at a higher level followed by HSP27 and HSP70. HSP27 exists as three isoforms (unphosphorylated, mono-, and diphosphorylated forms) in rat pancreatic acinar cells. HSP27 phosphorylation was stimulated by CCK in vivo and in vitro and by osmotic stress in vitro. HSP27 phosphorylation status was also altered with the monophosphorylated form increasing at 6 h and remaining elevated up to 120 h.[23] The dephosphorylated form was highest at 12 h and decreased there after but was still higher compared to basal level. Injection of a nonpathological dose of L-arginine (3 g/kg) induced a higher ratio of phosphorylated to unphosphorylated HSP27 protein, which indicates that it might be a protective response. HSP27 overexpression is known to confer resistance to heat and other stresses. The mechanism of HSP induction during AP onset has not been the specific subject of any study. Some plausible mechanisms could be (i) decreased ATP levels, (ii) accumulation of unfolded proteins, or (iii) ischemia due to compromised microcirculation.[25] All of these could trigger cellular stress and a heat stress response. In the study by Ritossa, treatment with DNP, also altered the puffing pattern.[1] DNP inhibits oxidative phosphorylation and can decrease intracellular ATP levels, so it could be a strong signal for triggering stress responses. Pancreatitis-causing agents like cerulein, bile acids, palmitoleic acid (POA), and palmitoleic acid ethyl ester (POAEE) decrease ATP levels in the pancreas.[26,27]

HSP-mediated protection from pancreatitis

Based on initial observations that showed that pre-exposure to sublethal stress has a protective effect to subsequent lethal exposure, there are several studies, which have investigated expression of heat stress proteins during AP development.[22-24] In these studies, increased HSP expression was observed during AP. It was hypothesized that this is a protective response of acinar cells, and its preinduction might protect pancreatic acinar cells from subsequent injury. In pancreatitis, injury is initiated in pancreatic acinar cells, which eventually leads to the development of AP. Weber et al. studied autoprotective potential of pancreatic acinar cells by exposing rat pancreatic lobules either to cerulein (100 nM) stimulation or hyperthermia (42°C for 60 min).[22] HSP70 and ubiquitin expression levels in response to cerulein stimulation and hyperthermia were compared to those in unexposed pancreatic lobules. The rationale of using pancreatic lobules rather than pancreatic acinar cells was that cells will undergo minimal processing-related stress. Increased expression of HSP70 mRNA was observed with cerulein hyperstimulation and hyperthermia, but there was no effect on ubiquitin expression. This protective effect was further confirmed by induction of mild edematous pancreatitis in rats using cerulein (10 µg/kg/h, intravenous). Increased HSP70 expression was observed as early as 4 h and peaked by 12 h; however, ubiquitin mRNA levels did not change. It was hypothesized that HSP70 expression during pancreatitis is a self-defense mechanism of pancreatic acinar cells.

The expression of various HSPs and the correlation with reduced AP severity was further investigated by Wagner et al.[24] The authors exposed rat pancreatic acini to heat and analyzed protein expression using ^{35}S-methionine labeling and western blots. They observed that after thermal stress (42°C), pancreatic acini increasingly expressed five proteins of 92, 72, 59, 58, and 30kDa, with HSP70 the most strongly induced 72-kDa protein. After whole-body hyperthermia (42°C for 20 min, using a heat pad and lamp in anesthetized rats), cerulein-induced pancreatic organ damage was greatly reduced.[24] The degree of protection was correlated with the strength of HSP induction. Based on these findings, a causal relationship between hyperthermia-induced HSP expression and protection from subsequent injury to the pancreas was proposed.

Because heat stress induces multiple HSPs, although HSP70 (also known as HSP72) was the major protein, it was not clear that the observed protection against pancreatitis is due to HSP70 overexpression. This issue was investigated by Bhagat et al.,[28] who used in vitro culture of pancreatic lobules to demonstrate that HSP70 overexpression was actually responsible for the observed protective role of heat stress. In this elegant study, selective inhibition of HSP70 overexpression using an antisense approach and pharmacological inhibition (**Figure 1 & 2**) was used to understand the contribution of HSP70 in heat stress-induced protection against AP. In the presence of HSP70 antisense or the pharmacological inhibitor quercetin, protection against cerulein-induced injury was abrogated (**Figure 1 & 2**). These findings indicated that protection against cerulein-induced pancreatitis following heat stress is mediated by HSP70. The role of HSP70 in protection imparted by heat stress against pancreatic injury was further evaluated in vivo by Bhagat et al. (**Figure 3**).[29] When antisense oligonucleotide specific to HSP70 was administered prior to

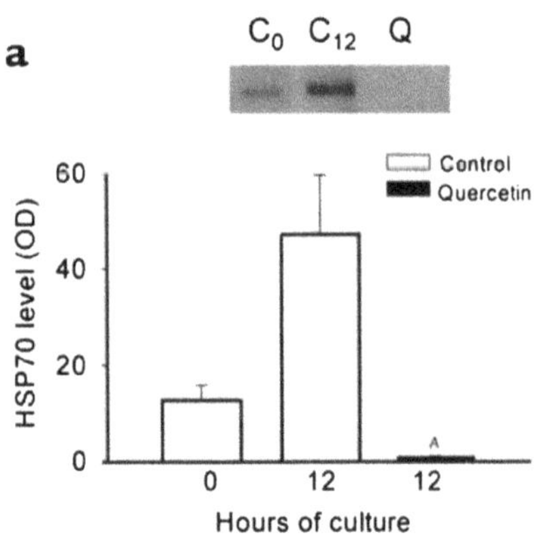

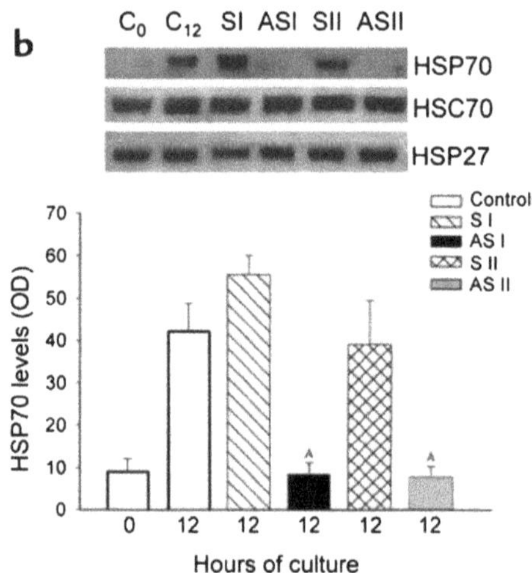

Figure 1. HSP expression following incubation of pancreas fragments with quercetin or antisense/sense HSP70 oligonucleotides. (**a**) C_0, freshly prepared pancreas fragments; C_{12}, pancreas fragments after 12 h of culture; Q, pancreas fragments after 12 h of culture with quercetin (50 µM). HSP70 protein expression was evaluated by western blotting, and relative optical densities are expressed as mean ± SEM for at least three separate experiments in each group. $^{A}P < 0.01$, quercetin-incubated fragments vs. untreated 12 h control fragments. (**b**) C_0, freshly prepared pancreas fragments; C_{12}, pancreas fragments after 12 h of culture; S I, pancreas fragments incubated with sense oligonucleotide S I (1 µM) for 12 h; AS I, pancreas fragments incubated with 14-mer antisense oligonucleotide AS I (1 µM) for 12 h; S II, pancreas fragments incubated with sense oligonucleotide S II (1 µM) for 12 h; AS II, pancreas fragments incubated with 18-mer antisense oligonucleotide AS II (1 µM) for 12 h. Expression of indicated HSPs was assessed by western blotting. Relative optical densities of HSP70 bands are expressed as mean ± SEM for at least three separate experiments in each group. $^{A}P < 0.01$, antisense oligonucleotide-incubated fragments vs. untreated 12 h control fragments. Reproduced with permission from *J Clin Invest.*[28]

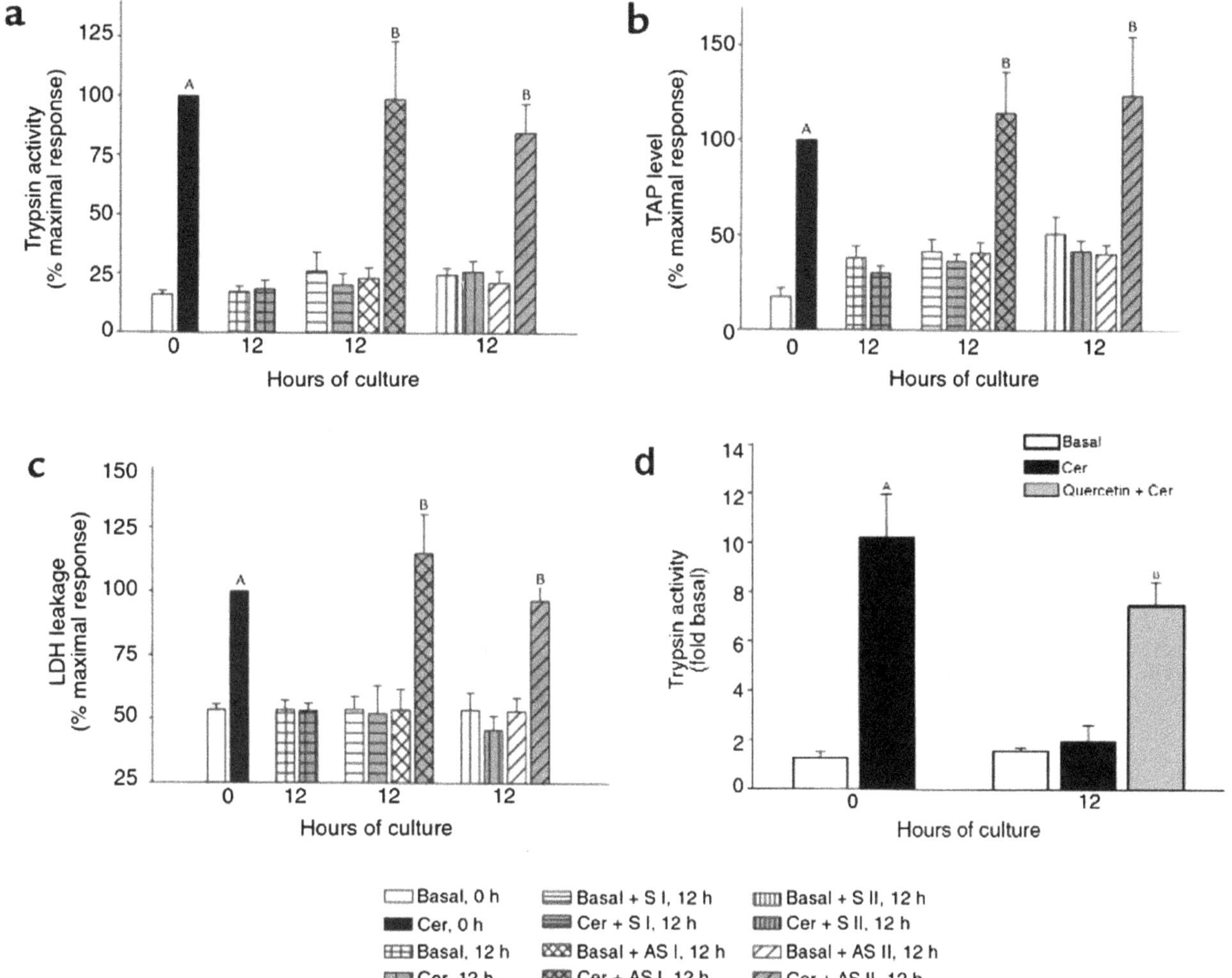

Figure 2. Effect of incubation of pancreas fragments with antisense/sense HSP70 oligonucleotides (1 μM) on trypsinogen activation and cell injury as assessed by LDH release into the medium. Trypsin activity (**a**), TAP levels (**b**), and LDH leakage (**c**) were measured. Values are mean ± SEM from at least three independent experiments and are expressed as the percent of maximal response to cerulein stimulation in freshly prepared pancreas fragments. $^{A}P < 0.05$, cerulein-treated freshly prepared fragment values vs. basal values. $^{B}P < 0.05$, antisense oligonucleotide-incubated cerulein-stimulated fragments vs. cerulein-stimulated 12 h control fragments. (**d**) Quercetin treatment blocked HSP70 induction and restored cerulein-induced trypsinogen activation. Reproduced with permission from *J Clin Invest*.[28]

heat stress, the authors observed expression of other stress proteins except HSP70. The protective effect of preinduced heat stress to cerulein-induced pancreatitis in these animals was lost, indicating that this protective effect is mediated through overexpressed HSP70. But in the group treated with sense-oligonucleotide for HSP70 prior to heat stress, HSP70 overexpression was not affected and the protective effect of heat stress to cerulein-induced pancreatitis was maintained.

HSP70 can also be induced by other means. Bhagat et al. investigated whether sodium arsenite-induced HSP70 overexpression protects against AP, similar to the HSP70 expression by heat stress.[30] It was observed that sodium arsenite-induced HSP70 overexpression provides protection against cerulein- (**Figure 4 & 5**) and L-arginine-induced models of AP. That study demonstrated that the protective effects of heat stress are not due to non-HSP-related heat stress events and are not limited to mild cerulein-induced pancreatitis. Frossard et al. showed that HSP70 induced by β-adrenergic stimulation protected against cerulein-induced pancreatitis, a finding that supports the conclusion that HSP70 has a protective role in pancreatitis irrespective of the mode of induction.[31]

Further evidence of role of HSP70 in modulation of severity of AP came from the clinical studies, where AP severity was related to HSP70 gene polymorphism status. Specifically, HSP 70.2 expression was linked to pancreatitis severity. The HSP70-2G allele has been associated

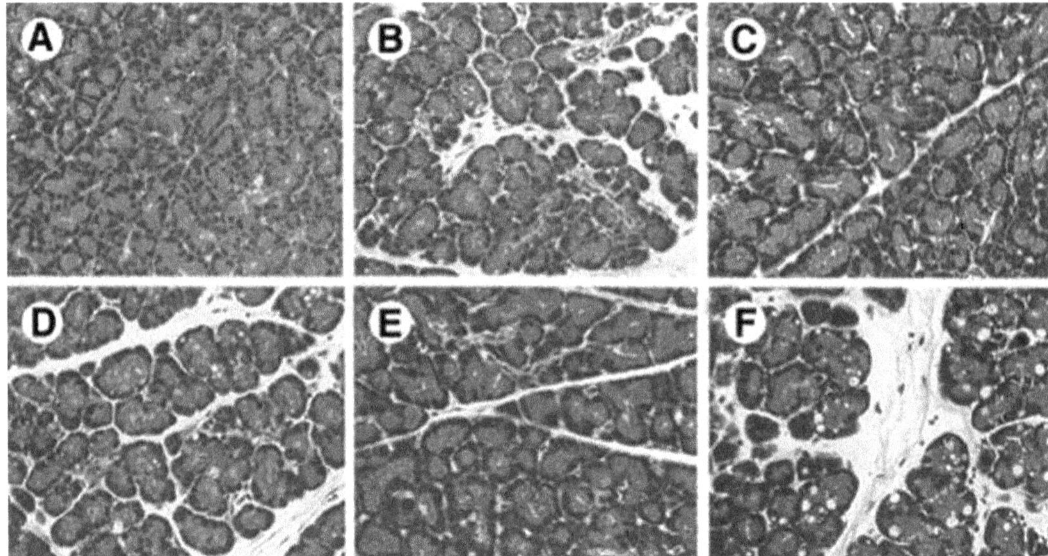

Figure 3. Effects of prior thermal stress and oligonucleotide treatment on morphologic changes induced by supramaximal cerulein in the rat pancreas. Representative light micrographs of H&E-stained pancreas sections from **(A)** control, **(B)** CER-, **(C)** H+CER-, **(D)** H+AS+CER-, **(E)** H+S+CER-, and **(F)** AS+CER-treated rats are shown. Note increased vacuolization/necrosis and leukocyte infiltration in the CER and H+AS+CER groups. Both H+CER- and H+S+CER-treated rats show marked protection, whereas (F) animals given AS-HSP70 before cerulein show more pronounced acinar cell vacuolization/necrosis. Reproduced with permission from *Gastroenterology*.[29]

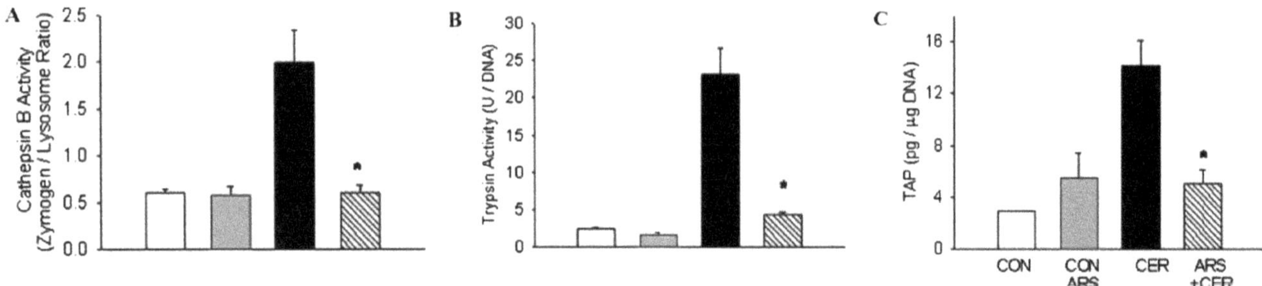

Figure 4. Effect of sodium arsenite pretreatment on cerulein-induced colocalization and trypsinogen activation. (A) Subcellular distribution of cathepsin B. Rats were given a single intraperitoneal injection (10 mg/kg) of sodium arsenite (ARS). After 14 h, pancreatitis was induced in both treated and untreated rats by a single injection of cerulein (CER, 20 µg/kg); rats were sacrificed 2.5 h later. Untreated and ARS alone-treated rats served as controls (CON). Cathepsin B activity in subcellular fractions was measured as described in the text. Values are mean ± SEM for at least three independent experiments, each with at least three or four rats per group. $^*P<0.05$ for ARS + CER rats vs. CER-alone rats. Trypsinogen activation measured as trypsin **(B)** and TAP levels **(C)**. Values are mean ± SEM for three independent experiments. $^*P<0.05$ for ARS + CER rats vs. CER rats. Reproduced with permission from *J Cell Physiol*.[30]

with low HSP70-2 expression and was more prevalent in patients with severe pancreatitis than those with mild disease or a healthy population. Conversely, patients with the "protective" AA genotype are less vulnerable to severe disease and are expected to have better prognoses with far fewer complications. The coexistence of TNF2 and HSP70-2G was detected in 9 of the 49 patients in the severe group, and 6 of these patients experienced infected necrosis with multiple organ failure, and 1 died.[32]

Pancreatic HSP60 is reportedly weakly induced in response to heat stress but has robust expression following water immersion stress.[33] Prior induction of HSP60 was also found to be protective against cerulein-induced pancreatitis as evaluated by different markers of severity. Although HSP60 was the main stress protein overexpressed, water immersion can theoretically induce other proteins and pathways that could be responsible for the observed protection; therefore further confirmation of these findings by targeted changes in HSP60 expression is required.

HSP27 is another inducible stress protein whose protective role has been studied in AP. Kubisch et al. reported that HSP27 overexpression in the pancreas also protects against cerulein-induced pancreatitis.[34] In this study, huHSP27 was

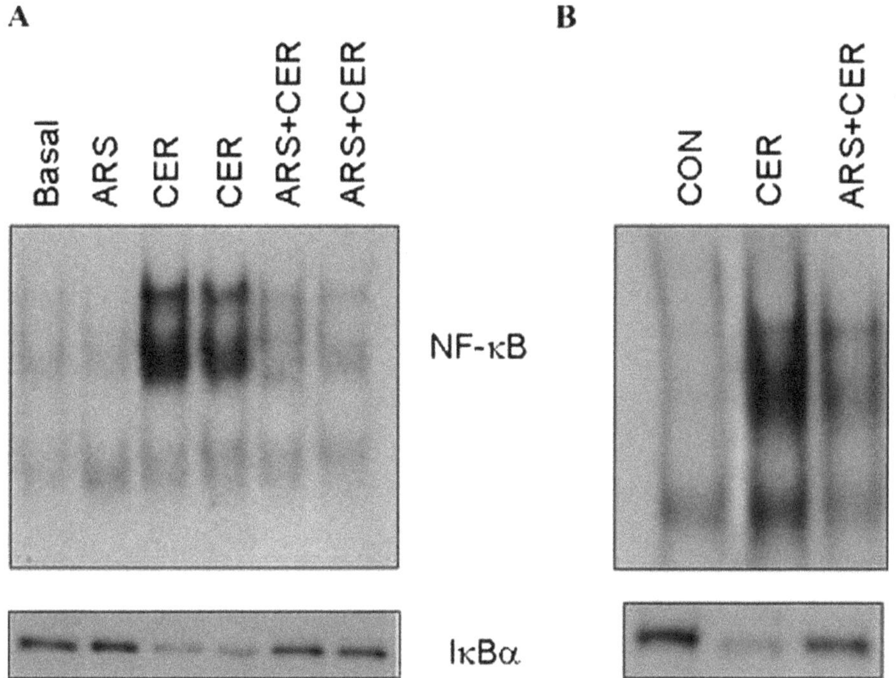

Figure 5. Preinduction of HSP70 expression using sodium arsenite-inhibited, secretagogue-induced NFkB activation in the pancreas. Upper panels show the EMSA of the nuclear fractions, while the lower panels depict IkBa degradation in the cytosolic fraction. Reproduced with permission from *J Cell Physiol.*[30]

overexpressed under the control of a cytomegalovirus promoter. Of all the tissues examined, high huHSP27 expression was found in the pancreas and stomach. The protection was mediated by a phosphorylated form of HSP27 because the effect was not observed when a nonphosphorylatable huHSP27 mutant form was used. HSP27 differs from other HSPs in that it modulates actin dynamics following HSP27 phosphorylation. Microfilament stabilization is thought to be responsible for increased survival of cells recovering from stress.

There is overwhelming evidence to indicate that overexpression of HSP70, -60 or -27 has a protective effect on pancreatitis, and this effect is observed irrespective of the method used for inducing overexpression or the experimental model used for pancreatitis induction. However, in an interesting study by Lunova et al.,[35] acinar cell-specific HSP70 overexpression did not protect against pancreatitis severity but did accelerate recovery.

This some what contradictory finding could be explained by the observation that HSP70 ATPase activity is slow but is accelerated many fold in the presence of its cochaperone HSP40; this protein also helps HSP70 bind to polypeptides. Efficient cleavage of ATP and effective binding to unfolded polypeptides determine HSP70 effectiveness. With targeted HSP70 overexpression, cochaperone availability may become a limitation, which may not be the case with induction of stress proteins by other methods.

Mechanism of HSP overexpression-mediated protection

The mechanism by which HSP overexpression protects against injury in pancreatitis has been investigated in studies where either HSP70, HSP60, or HSP27 was overexpressed. In the studies where HSP70 was overexpressed via heat stress or pharmacological means, activation of trypsinogen to trypsin was significantly inhibited during pancreatitis initiation (**Figures 2 & 4**). Activation of trypsin is observed early and is considered to be the key pathological event in AP.[28,29] Inhibition of trypsin activation by different means is protective[36-38] while disrupting the protective mechanisms by deletion of SPINK1[39,40] or chymotrypsin C[41] accentuate trypsin activation and pancreatitis. The mechanism by which HSP70 prevents trypsin activation has also been investigated. Studies suggest that HSP70 overexpression interferes with colocalization of zymogens and lysosomes, which is a prerequisite for intracellular activation of trypsinogen to trypsin. In nonpancreatic cells, HSP70 has been suggested to influence Ca^{2+} homeostasis.[42] Given the requirement of Ca^{2+} for colocalization of zymogen and lysosomal contents and evidence of HSP70 perturbing Ca^{2+} signaling, HSP70-mediated inhibition of colocalization could be through the attenuation of pathological Ca^{2+} signaling. Another key event in the pathogenesis of AP is activation of nuclear factor kappa B (NFkB), which is independent of trypsin activation and contributes to the development of pancreatitis and associated systemic injury. HSP70 overexpression also provides protection against NFkB activation (**Figure 5**).[30]

Besides the mechanisms described above, other means of HSP-mediated protection in AP have been proposed. All three major components of the cytoskeleton (microfilaments, intermediate filaments, and microtubules) are present in pancreatic acinar cells.[23] Stimulation of acinar cells with supramaximal concentrations of cerulein or induction of AP in vivo leads to a loss of filamentous actin. Arginine administration has also been reported to cause changes in the actin cytoskeleton, including reduced actin staining under the luminal membrane and increased cytoplasmic staining.[23] These early changes are related to acinar cell injury in pancreatitis. HSP27 overexpression is considered to provide protection through regulation of actin.[23] Microfilament stabilization is considered important for the survival of cells recovering from stress. The protective effects of HSP27 overexpression correlate with both overexpression and phosphorylation. HSP70 overexpression has also been shown to protect the cytoskeleton. The stress conditions that induce HSP27 are also known to cause increases in HSP70.[23] The observed protection of HSP27 on the cytoskeleton may also be enhanced in the setting of HSP70 overexpression.

Park et al. reported that HSP27 associates with IkB kinase complex and this interaction is stimulated by treatment with tumor necrosis factor alpha.[43] There are contradictory reports about enhanced association of phosphorylated HSP27 with IkB kinase complex and resulting decreased IkB kinase activity because no increased activity was observed in transgenic mice with overexpression of HSP27.[34]

HSP27 overexpression also did not affect intracellular calcium release in response to cerulein stimulation.Thus, the protective effect of HSP27 overexpression during AP is mainly related to cytoskeleton stabilization. Subcellular redistribution of cathepsin B from the lysosome-enriched fraction to the zymogen granule-enriched fraction was decreased in animals subjected to water immersion; this might indicate that HSP60-mediated protection involves interference with colocalization and a subsequent decrease in trypsin activation.

Conclusion

There is strong experimental evidence to support the hypothesis that HSPs are overexpressed during the development of pancreatitis. Increased HSP expression is a protective response and is observed in multiple models of experimental pancreatitis. Preinduction of HSPs by different means protects from subsequent pancreatitis-induced injury. The mechanism of protection is not fully understood, but prevention of intra-acinar trypsinogen activation, cytoskeleton stabilization, and inhibition of NFkB signaling appear to be the main contributors. Better and safe pharmacological approaches for inducing HSPs could help reduce pancreatitis severity and related complications.

References

1. Ritossa F. A new puffing pattern induced by temperature shock and DNP in drosophila. *Experientia.* 1962; 18: 571-573.
2. Tissieres A, Mitchell HK, Tracy UM. Protein synthesis in salivary glands of Drosophila melanogaster: relation to chromosome puffs. *J Mol Biol.* 1974; 84: 389-398. PMID: 4219221.
3. Lindquist S. The heat-shock response. *Annu Rev Biochem.* 1986; 55: 1151-1191. PMID: 2427013.
4. Lindquist S, Craig EA. The heat-shock proteins. *Annu Rev Genet.* 1988; 22: 631-677. PMID: 2853609.
5. Welch WJ. Mammalian stress response: cell physiology, structure/function of stress proteins, and implications for medicine and disease. *Physiol Rev.* 1992; 72: 1063-1081. PMID: 1438579.
6. Cheng MY, Hartl FU, Horwich AL. The mitochondrial chaperonin hsp60 is required for its own assembly. *Nature.* 1990; 348: 455-458. PMID: 1978929.
7. Qiu XB, Shao YM, Miao S, Wang L. The diversity of the DnaJ/Hsp40 family, the crucial partners for Hsp70 chaperones. *Cell Mol Life Sci.* 2006; 63: 2560-2570. PMID: 16952052.
8. Choi HI, Lee SP, Kim KS, Hwang CY, Lee YR, Chae SK, et al. Redox-regulated cochaperone activity of the human DnaJ homolog Hdj2. *Free Radic Biol Med.* 2006; 40: 651-659. PMID: 16458196.
9. Stetler RA, Gao Y, Zhang L, Weng Z, Zhang F, Hu X, et al. Phosphorylation of HSP27 by protein kinase D is essential for mediating neuroprotection against ischemic neuronal injury. *J Neurosci.* 2012; 32: 2667-2682. PMID: 22357851.
10. Hohfeld J, Hartl FU. Role of the chaperonin cofactor Hsp10 in protein folding and sorting in yeast mitochondria. *J Cell Biol.* 1994; 126: 305-315. PMID: 7913473.
11. Jia H, Halilou AI, Hu L, Cai W, Liu J, Huang B. Heat shock protein 10 (Hsp10) in immune-related diseases: one coin, two sides. *Int J Biochem Mol Biol.* 2011; 2: 47-57. PMID: 21969171.
12. Schirmer EC, Glover JR, Singer MA, Lindquist S. HSP100/Clp proteins: a common mechanism explains diverse functions. *Trends Biochem Sci.* 1996; 21: 289-296. PMID: 8772382.
13. Jackson SE. Hsp90: structure and function. *Top Curr Chem.* 2013; 328: 155-240. PMID: 22955504.
14. Li J, Soroka J, Buchner J. The Hsp90 chaperone machinery: conformational dynamics and regulation by co-chaperones. *Biochim Biophys Acta.* 2012; 1823: 624-635. PMID: 21951723.
15. Mayer MP, Bukau B. Hsp70 chaperones: cellular functions and molecular mechanism. *Cell Mol Life Sci.* 2005; 62: 670-684. PMID: 15770419.
16. Miron T, Vancompernolle K, Vandekerckhove J, Wilchek M, Geiger B. A 25-kD inhibitor of actin polymerization is a low molecular mass heat shock protein. *J Cell Biol.* 1991; 114: 255-261. PMID: 2071672.
17. Benndorf R, Hayess K, Ryazantsev S, Wieske M, Behlke J, Lutsch G. Phosphorylation and supramolecular organization

of murine small heat shock protein HSP25 abolish its actin polymerization-inhibiting activity. *J Biol Chem.* 1994; 269: 20780-20784. PMID: 8051180.

18. Rogalla T, Ehrnsperger M, Preville X, Kotlyarov A, Lutsch G, Ducasse C, et al. Regulation of Hsp27 oligomerization, chaperone function, and protective activity against oxidative stress/tumor necrosis factor alpha by phosphorylation. *J Biol Chem.* 1999; 274: 18947-18956. PMID: 10383393.
19. Friant S, Meier KD, Riezman H. Increased ubiquitin-dependent degradation can replace the essential requirement for heat shock protein induction. *EMBO J.* 2003; 22: 3783-3791. PMID: 12881413.
20. Parag HA, Raboy B, Kulka RG. Effect of heat shock on protein degradation in mammalian cells: involvement of the ubiquitin system. *EMBO J.* 1987; 6: 55-61. PMID: 3034579.
21. Deng M, Chen PC, Xie S, Zhao J, Gong L, Liu J, et al. The small heat shock protein alphaA-crystallin is expressed in pancreas and acts as a negative regulator of carcinogenesis. *Biochim Biophys Acta.* 2010; 1802: 621-631. PMID: 20434541.
22. Weber CK, Gress T, Muller-Pillasch F, Lerch MM, Weidenbach H, Adler G. Supramaximal secretagogue stimulation enhances heat shock protein expression in the rat pancreas. *Pancreas.* 1995; 10: 360-367. PMID: 7792292.
23. Tashiro M, Schafer C, Yao H, Ernst SA, Williams JA. Arginine induced acute pancreatitis alters the actin cytoskeleton and increases heat shock protein expression in rat pancreatic acinar cells. *Gut.* 2001; 49: 241-250. PMID: 11454802.
24. Wagner AC, Weber H, Jonas L, Nizze H, Strowski M, Fiedler F, et al. Hyperthermia induces heat shock protein expression and protection against cerulein-induced pancreatitis in rats. *Gastroenterology.* 1996; 111: 1333-1342. PMID: 8898648.
25. Plusczyk T, Westermann S, Rathgeb D, Feifel G. Acute pancreatitis in rats: effects of sodium taurocholate, CCK-8, and Sec on pancreatic microcirculation. *Am J Physiol Gastrointest Liver Physiol.* 1997; 2722 Pt 1: G310-G320. PMID: 9124355.
26. Voronina SG, Barrow SL, Simpson AW, Gerasimenko OV, da Silva Xavier G, Rutter GA, et al. Dynamic changes in cytosolic and mitochondrial ATP levels in pancreatic acinar cells. *Gastroenterology.* 2010; 138: 1976-1987. PMID: 20102715.
27. Halangk W, Matthias R, Nedelev B, Schild L, Meyer F, Schulz HU, et al. [Modification of energy supply by pancreatic mitochondria in acute experimental pancreatitis]. *Zentralbl Chir.* 1997; 122: 305-308. PMID: 9221643.
28. Bhagat L, Singh VP, Hietaranta AJ, Agrawal S, Steer ML, Saluja AK. Heat shock protein 70 prevents secretagogue-induced cell injury in the pancreas by preventing intracellular trypsinogen activation. *J Clin Invest.* 2000; 106: 81-89. PMID: 10880051.
29. Bhagat L, Singh VP, Song AM, van Acker GJ, Agrawal S, Steer ML, et al. Thermal stress-induced HSP70 mediates protection against intrapancreatic trypsinogen activation and acute pancreatitis in rats. *Gastroenterology.* 2002; 122: 156-165. PMID: 11781290.
30. Bhagat L, Singh VP, Dawra RK, Saluja AK. Sodium arsenite induces heat shock protein 70 expression and protects against secretagogue-induced trypsinogen and NF-kappaB activation. *J Cell Physiol.* 2008; 215: 37-46. PMID: 17941083.
31. Frossard JL, Saluja AK, Mach N, Lee HS, Bhagat L, Hadenque A, et al. In vivo evidence for the role of GM-CSF as a mediator in acute pancreatitis-associated lung injury. *Am J Physiol Lung Cell Mol Physiol.* 2002; 283: L541-L548. PMID: 12169573.
32. Balog A, Gyulai Z, Boros LG, Farkas G, Takacs T, Lonovics J, et al. Polymorphism of the TNF-alpha, HSP70-2, and CD14 genes increases susceptibility to severe acute pancreatitis. *Pancreas.* 2005; 30: e46-e50. PMID: 15714129.
33. Lee HS, Bhagat L, Frossard JL, Hietaranta A, Singh VP, Steer ML, et al. Water immersion stress induces heat shock protein 60 expression and protects against pancreatitis in rats. *Gastroenterology.* 2000; 119: 220-229. PMID: 10889172.
34. Kubisch C, Dimagno MJ, Tietz AB, Welsh MJ, Ernst SA, Brandt-Nedelev B, et al. Overexpression of heat shock protein Hsp27 protects against cerulein-induced pancreatitis. *Gastroenterology.* 2004; 127: 275-286. PMID: 15236192.
35. Lunova M, Zizer E, Kucukoglu O, Schwarz C, Dillmann WH, Wagner M, et al. Hsp72 overexpression accelerates the recovery from caerulein-induced pancreatitis. *PLoS One.* 2012; 7: e39972. PMID: 22792201.
36. Saluja AK, Donovan EA, Yamanaka K, Yamaguchi Y, Hofbauer B,Steer ML. Cerulein-induced in vitro activation of trypsinogen in rat pancreatic acini is mediated by cathepsin B. *Gastroenterology.* 1997; 113: 304-310. PMID: 9207291.
37. Van Acker GJ, Saluja AK, Bhagat L, Singh VP, Song AM, Steer ML. Cathepsin B inhibition prevents trypsinogen activation and reduces pancreatitis severity. *Am J Physiol Gastrointest Liver Physiol.* 2002; 283: G794-G800. PMID: 12181196.
38. Halangk W, Lerch MM, Brandt-Nedelev B, Roth W, Ruthenbuerger M, Reinheckel T, et al. Role of cathepsin B in intracellular trypsinogen activation and the onset of acute pancreatitis. *J Clin Invest.* 2000; 106: 773-781. PMID: 10995788.
39. Nathan JD, Romac J, Peng RY, Peyton M, Macdonald RJ, Liddle RA. Transgenic expression of pancreatic secretory trypsin inhibitor-I ameliorates secretagogue-induced pancreatitis in mice. *Gastroenterology.* 2005; 128: 717-727. PMID: 15765407.
40. Koziel D, Gluszek S, Kowalik A, Chlopek M, Pieciak L. Genetic mutations in SPINK1, CFTR, CTRC genes in acute pancreatitis. *BMC Gastroenterol.* 2015; 15: 70. PMID: 26100556.
41. Szabó A, Ludwig M, Hegyi E, Szepeová R, Witt H, Sahin-Tóth M. Mesotrypsin signature mutation in a chymotrypsin C (CTRC) variant associated with chronic pancreatitis. *J Biol Chem.* 2015; 290: 17282-17292. PMID: 26013824.
42. Kiang JG, Ding XZ, McClain DE. Overexpression of HSP-70 attenuates increases in $[Ca^{2+}]i$ and protects human epidermoid A-431 cells after chemical hypoxia. *Toxicol Appl Pharmacol.* 1998; 149: 185-194. PMID: 9571987.
43. Park KJ, Gaynor RB, Kwak YT. Heat shock protein 27 association with the I kappa B kinase complex regulates tumor necrosis factor alpha-induced NF-kappa B activation. *J Biol Chem.* 2003; 278: 35272-35278. PMID: 12829720.

Chapter 9

Endoplasmic reticulum stress and the unfolded protein response in exocrine pancreas physiology and pancreatitis

Richard T. Waldron[1*], Stephen Pandol[1], Aurelia Lugea[1], and Guy Groblewski[2]

[1]*Cedars Sinai Medical Center, VA Greater Los Angeles Health Care System and University of California, Los Angeles, California;* [2]*Department of Nutritional Sciences, University of Wisconsin, Madison, Wisconsin.*

Endoplasmic Reticulum Stress and the Unfolded Protein Response

The endoplasmic reticulum (ER) plays a pivotal role in cellular homeostasis as it is the site of translation, folding and covalent modification of proteins either destined for secretion or expressed on the surface of other organelles and the plasma membrane. The cytoplasmic surface of the ER membrane is also the primary site of triglyceride, phospholipid, and sterol synthesis and therefore is a hub of membrane synthesis and cellular metabolism. Many studies have established the ER as a major site of intracellular calcium (Ca^{2+}) storage, essential for hormone/neurotransmitter signaling. More recent work has identified unexpected functions of the ER in diverse cellular processes including mitochondrial fission, endosomal dynamics, and autophagy.

Quality control mechanisms for protein folding in the ER were first demonstrated by the identification of glucose-regulated proteins (GRPs) 78 (a.k.a. binding immunoglobulin protein [BiP]) and 94 (a.k.a. heat shock protein [HSP] 90B1/endoplasmin) that reside in the ER lumen.[1] Whereas GRPs have significant homology to heat-shock chaperone proteins, their expression is induced by glucose starvation, sulfhydryl reducing agents, glycosylation inhibitors, and calcium ionophores rather than heat stress. A seminal study demonstrated that enhanced expression of misfolded proteins in the ER induced GRP mRNA expression, thereby establishing the presence of a signaling network from the ER to the nucleus.[2] The concept of an unfolded protein response (UPR) opened the door to a multitude of studies over the last three decades uncovering molecular components and mechanisms of the UPR. These findings have provided important insight into the pathophysiological consequences of ER stress in various disorders from neurodegenerative to metabolic diseases. Perhaps not surprisingly given the high protein secretory capacity and vastly expanded ER in the pancreatic acinar cell, results indicate that the UPR is critical to maintaining acinar cell homeostasis. This review will focus on what is known of the UPR in acinar cell function, as well as recent evidence underscoring its importance in the development and progression of pancreatitis.

The UPR is Comprised of Distinct Functional Components

The UPR is activated when the concentration of unfolded or misfolded proteins present in the ER overwhelms the capacity of resident proteins including molecular chaperones, disulfide isomerases, oxidoreductases, acetylases, and glycosylases to respond to that stress.

Figure 1 illustrates many of the features discussed in this and subsequent sections. Three major pathways of the UPR have been identified; the inositol-requiring enzyme-1 (IRE1), activating transcription factor 6 (ATF6), and protein kinase RNA (PKR)-like ER kinase (PERK) pathways. These transmembrane proteins can sense the level of stress in the ER lumen and transduce signals to the cytoplasm; complex sensing mechanisms involve the binding of either unfolded proteins themselves, or chaperones, (e.g., BiP) that modulate their oligomerization and other individual functional responses.

The level and duration of ER stresses dictate the extent to which each UPR pathway becomes activated. Acutely, new protein synthesis is attenuated to limit the protein load entering the ER. At later times, nuclear signaling induces gene expression to promote protein folding as well as the degradation of misfolded proteins. Under extreme

*Corresponding author. Email: waldronr@cshs.org

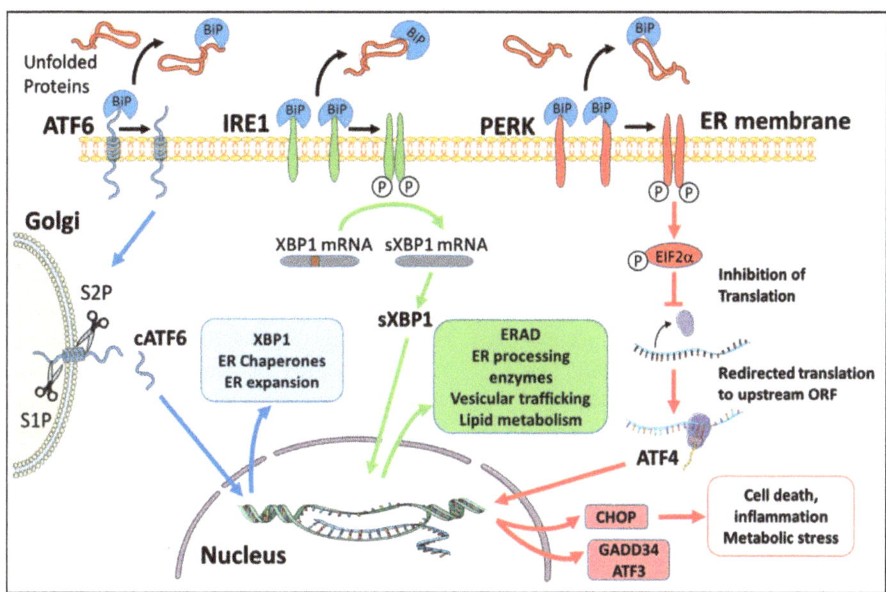

Figure 1. Principal components of the UPR/ER-stress response. ATF6, IRE1, and PERK are ER transmembrane proteins capable of sensing the level of unfolded or misfolded proteins in the ER lumen. The precise mechanism(s) for activating each pathway is unclear and likely involves the displacement of molecular chaperones (e.g., BiP) from the luminal domain of the protein. **ATF6:** Upon activation, ATF6 traffics from the ER to the Golgi via COPII-directed clathrin-coated vesicles. In the Golgi, ATF6 is sequentially cleaved by site-1 and site-2 proteases, freeing the N-terminal transcription factor domain (cATF6) to translocate to the nucleus and promote transcription of UPR target genes. **IRE1:** Activation of IRE1 kinase activity is mediated by *trans*-autophosphorylation causing IRE1 to oligomerize in the ER membrane. Phosphorylated IRE1 exhibits endoribonuclease activity that excises a portion of the XBP1 mRNA, forming a spliced mRNA that generates the transcription factor sXBP1, which translocates to the nucleus and directs the expression of a number of ER-regulators necessary for protein folding, lipid metabolism, vesicular trafficking, and acinar secretory function. **PERK:** Kinase activation and autophosphorylation of PERK phosphorylates the cytosolic eukaryotic translation initiation factor eIF2α, thereby inhibiting global secretory protein translation. As a consequence, translation of select mRNAs including ATF4 is redirected to an upstream open reading frame, giving rise to alternative protein products. ATF4 acts as a transcriptional activator or repressor and directs the synthesis of the transcription factor CHOP, which plays a key role in mediating cell death, inflammation, and metabolic stress.

conditions of ER stress intensity and duration, UPR responses mitigating ER stress are supplanted by those promoting cell death.

The IRE1 and XBP1/spliced XBP1 (sXBP1) pathway

IRE1 was originally identified in yeast as a gene required to enhance the expression of KAR2 (a.k.a. BiP) or 78-kDa glucose-regulated protein (GRP-78) in mammalian cells) during ER stress.[3,4] The name inositol-requiring enzyme-1 was coined based on its role in inositol prototropy in yeast.[5] There are two isoforms, IRE1α and IRE1β, the latter of which is prominent in intestinal epithelia though its function is unclear. This review will focus on IRE1α (i.e., IRE1). IRE1 is a type 1 transmembrane protein with an N-terminal domain in the ER lumen that binds to BiP and a C-terminal serine/threonine protein kinase domain oriented toward the cytoplasm. Displacement of the molecular chaperone BiP from the N-terminus and/or a direct interaction with unfolded proteins has been proposed to activate IRE1 kinase activity. Although kinase activity is required for signaling, the only known substrate characterized is IRE1 itself, which upon trans-autophosphorylation causes IRE1 to oligomerize in the ER membrane.[3,4,6] Phosphorylated IRE1 induces endoribonuclease activity in its C-terminus that excises a portion of the mRNA encoding the transcription factor homologous to ATF/CREB1 (HAC) in yeast[7] or X-box binding protein-1 (XBP1) in mammals.[3,8,9] Spliced XBP1 induces the expression of a number of ER proteins to mitigate ER stress (see below). With high levels of or prolonged ER stress, IRE1 also participates in a process termed “regulated IRE1-dependent decay” (RIDD) of ER membrane-bound and cytosolic mRNAs, as well as IRE1 mRNA to reduce protein synthesis.[10,11] More recently, IRE1 was also reported to cleave microRNAs that control the level of caspase-2, thereby promoting apoptosis.[12] It is proposed that IRE1-mediated XBP1 splicing has a prosurvival output, whereas RIDD has a proapoptotic output.[7] A final consideration is that IRE1 may serve as a link between ER stress and stress kinase activation. IRE1 recruits an adapter protein, TRAF2, to the ER membrane to initiate a signaling cascade that culminates in activation of Jun N-terminal kinase (JNK).[13] Although JNK is a stress kinase that can induce apoptosis, the significance of this activation during physiological ER stress is unclear.

Activated IRE1 mediates the splicing of an intron in XBP1 mRNA that causes a frame-shift during translation, resulting in a new carboxyl terminal domain in the spliced XBP1 (sXBP1) protein. Unspliced XBP1 (MW 29-33 kDa) has a nuclear exclusion signal and rapidly degrades but can act as a negative modulator of the UPR when accumulated in mammalian cells.[14] Conversely, sXBP1 (54-60 kDa) contains a nuclear localization signal and basic leucine-zipper (BZIP) domain that binds to the cis-acting ER stress response element (ERSE) and functions as a potent transcription factor. Genetic profiling and analyses revealed that sXBP1 controls the expression of genes related to the UPR, including chaperone induction, up-regulation of ER-associated degradation (ERAD) machinery, membrane biogenesis, and ER quality control.[15-17] In mammals, sXBP1 also activates the expression of cell type-specific targets linked to cell differentiation, signaling, and DNA damage.[15,18] In pancreatic acinar cells, sXBP1 has been shown to be essential to maintain a differentiated secretory phenotype.[19] This role of sXBP1 was demonstrated using pharmacologic inhibitors of IRE1 endonuclease activity in the acinar cell line, AR42J.[20] Thus, IRE1 inhibition substantially diminished spontaneous amylase secretion by these cells. We also found that inhibition of sXBP1 formation attenuates the synthesis of certain digestive enzymes by acinar cells, as well as secretagogue-induced secretion (unpublished data). That the efficacy of these approaches relies on inhibition of the splicing reaction indicates that the spliced form of XBP1 plays a major role in the biosynthesis and secretion in professional secretory cells. Nevertheless, unspliced XBP1 may yet prove to act in unknown ways to alter acinar cell physiology. Interestingly, the unspliced form was reported to regulate sXBP1 stability, and more recently a role was also proposed for unspliced XBP1 to regulate autophagy via control of the stability of another transcription factor, Foxo1.[21]

The PERK/ATF4 pathway

The protein kinase RNA (PKR)-like ER kinase (PERK) is a type 1 transmembrane protein that, like IRE1, undergoes kinase activation in response to accumulation of misfolded proteins in the ER lumen. Autophosphorylated PERK in turn phosphorylates the cytosolic eukaryotic translation initiation factor eIF2α at Ser51, causing its inactivation. Inactivation of eIF2α, a small G-protein, involves blocking its interaction with a guanine nucleotide exchange factor, thereby locking it in a GDP-bound state. This greatly reduces protein translation and acutely attenuates secretory protein load.[22] Besides PERK, other kinases including general control nonderepressible 2 (GCN2), protein kinase RNA-activated (PKR), and heme-regulated inhibitor (HRI) can promote phosphorylation of eIF2α at Ser51 in response to cellular stresses such as amino acid deprivation, viral infection, and heme deficiency.

In addition to inhibiting general protein translation, PERK activation also increases the translation of mRNAs that contain upstream open reading frames within their 5'-UTR_including the transcription factor ATF4.[23] Under stress conditions and eIF2α inhibition, translation is redirected to the upstream open reading frame, giving rise to an alternative protein product. Only translation from the upstream open reading frame gives rise to a stable form of ATF4, which is a BZIP transcription factor of the cAMP response element-binding protein family that forms homo- and heteromeric dimers with various proteins and can act as a transcriptional activator or repressor. Analysis of transcripts from ATF4 knockout cells support that it regulates a number of genes that are important for secretory cell function.[24] However, the best characterized ATF4 gene targets include CHOP (transcriptional factor C/EBP homologous protein), GADD34 (growth arrest and DNA damage-inducible 34), and activating transcription factor 3 (ATF3). CHOP was reported to play a major role in promoting apoptosis by inducing the expression of pro-apoptotic proteins including Bim, and more recently, DR5 and repressing the expression of anti-apoptotic proteins (e.g., Bcl2).[25-29] An alternate theory put forward by some investigators emphasizes enhanced expression and function of translational machinery to de-energize the cell by consuming excessive amounts of metabolic intermediates, rather than differential induction and suppression of pro- and anti-apoptotic proteins, respectively, as a major role of CHOP.[30,31] Irrespective of the precise pathway, CHOP induction correlates with cell death, and knockout models have established its role as a detrimental signal, including in the exocrine pancreas.

A theme in the regulatory control of UPR is feedback within and/or between the different branches. CHOP (and ATF4) reportedly induces expression of GADD34, a regulatory subunit of protein phosphatase 1. Thus, GADD34 enables a stress-inducible phosphatase that dephosphorylates eIF2α, producing negative feedback to inactivate its own induction (since eif2α Ser51 phosphorylation mediates CHOP expression). Although GADD34 can help restore protein translation, it also promotes the expression of pro-apoptotic proteins, as evidenced by knockout and pharmacologic approaches.[31] ATF3 is also a BZIP transcription factor of the cAMP response element-binding protein family. Its expression can be induced by a number of stresses in addition to the UPR and has been shown to exert both positive and negative effects on cell survival and disease progression.[32] ATF3 was recently shown to interact with an acetyltransferase, Tat-interactive protein

60 (Tip60), that acetylates the major DNA damage kinase Ataxia telangiectasia mutated (ATM) to promote genomic stability during cell stress.[33]

The ATF6 pathway

Two ubiquitously expressed isoforms, ATF6α and ATF6β, are found in mammalian cells. Although they share significant homology, ER localization, and processing, studies in cultured mouse embryonic fibroblasts from double knockout mice indicate that ATF6α and not ATF6β is required for gene transcription induction.[34] Activated ATF6 mediates expansion of the ER and induces the expression of chaperones, foldases, and components of the ERAD pathway.[34,35] ATF6 is a type II ER transmembrane protein, which like IRE1 and PERK, has a C-terminal luminal domain but differs in that it has a BZIP transcription factor domain in the N-terminal cytoplasmic domain. During ER stress, and potentially via the loss of BiP binding, ATF6 emerges from the ER on COPII-coated vesicles and traffics to the Golgi where it is sequentially cleaved by site-1 and site-2 proteases (S1P and S2P).[36] Once released, the N-terminal transcription factor domain (cATF6) translocates to the nucleus and activates UPR target gene transcription.[37,38]

ER Stress, UPR, and Functional Crosstalk in Pancreatitis Models

Synthesis and packaging of proteins for transport is the singular key task of the acinar cell of the exocrine pancreas. Accordingly, the ER of the acinar cell is highly developed, and all of the UPR components described above have been identified in this cell type. The importance of the UPR to exocrine pancreatic function was demonstrated by ablating the *XBP1* gene in mice and expressing an XBP1 transgene in liver to prevent embryonic lethality.[19] These mice have normal morphology of all organs except the exocrine pancreas and salivary glands and die shortly after birth due to poor ER development and digestive enzyme synthesis in the acinar cells, resulting in severe exocrine insufficiency.[19] We have confirmed these results in a mouse with acinar cell-specific conditional knock down of XBP1 (unpublished data). XBP1 deficiency leads to extensive acinar cell loss and severe pathology in the remaining acinar cells, as evidenced by a poorly developed ER network and secretory system, reduced ER chaperone expression, marked reduction in zymogen granules and digestive enzymes, and accumulation of autophagic vacuoles.

The activation of UPR pathways has been demonstrated in several models of experimental pancreatitis.[39-53] In the arginine-induced and high-dose cholecystokinin (CCK) models, there was phosphorylation of PERK and its downstream target eIF2α, ATF4 nuclear translocation, and increased CHOP expression accompanied by BiP and sXBP1 upregulation.[39,41] Under these conditions, there was development of pancreatitis with inflammation and trypsin activation. On the other hand, secretagogues that do not cause pancreatitis, such as bombesin and the CCK analogue JMV-180, caused only increases in BiP and sXBP1.[40,49] The chemical chaperones, tauroursodeoxycholic acid and 4-phenyl butyric acid reduced these markers of ER stress, which was associated with less severe pancreatitis.[47,49] Finally, altering BiP expression has an effect on pancreatitis severity.[45] UPR pathways are involved in both acute and chronic pancreatitis models.[53]

Our understanding of the role of specific UPR system components in physiology and disease remains incomplete. Nevertheless, there are key findings that provide a framework for further investigations. One key finding is that genetic deletion of CHOP results in less severe experimental pancreatitis, suggesting that activation of the PERK-eIF2α pathway leading to increased CHOP expression is important for the development of the pathologic pancreatitis response.[44] Indeed, *Chop-/-* mice exhibited less pancreatic inflammation and histological damage than wild type when challenged with cerulein and lipopolysaccharide.[44]

We showed that sXBP1 expression increases in the pancreas of alcohol-fed animals. Further, we observed that pathologic changes of pancreatitis occur with genetic inhibition of the sXBP1 response to alcohol feeding.[54-56] With inhibition of the sXBP1 response, there was activation of the PERK/eIF2α/ATF4/CHOP pathway associated with the development of pancreatitis. That is, we found that depriving the acinar cell from using the IRE1-sXBP1 to adapt to ER stress was associated with sustained activation of the PERK/eIF2α/ATF4/CHOP pathway and development of pancreatic pathology.[56] From these findings, we postulate that the IRE1/sXBP1 pathway is activated with mild to moderate ER stressors such as alcohol abuse, and pancreas pathology develops when this ER "adaptive" response fails to re-establish ER homeostasis, reinforcing PERK/eIF2α/ATF4/CHOP pathways activation, inflammation, and cell death. These findings also align with our hypotheses that the UPR mediates necessary adaptive responses to stressors to maintain normal exocrine pancreas function (illustrated in the above case with alcohol) and that cellular failure and pancreatitis ensue when the stressors exceed the cell's adaptive capacity or the adaptive response fails to deploy. We anticipate that completion of ongoing proteomic analysis of the ER from XBP1-deficient mice will clarify which key proteins are altered, as well as how the deficiencies are pathologically exacerbated by risk factors such as ethanol consumption.

The findings and hypothesis listed above are consistent with results in other systems showing that CHOP promotes inflammation by regulating cytokine production, inflammatory and cell survival.[57,58] Our studies representing pathologic ER stress mechanisms arising in the exocrine pancreas also complement those attributed to beta cell malfunction in the endocrine pancreas that reportedly contribute to diabetic pathology.[31] Indeed, the links between endocrine and exocrine dysfunction have been insufficiently elucidated despite many years of study, but there is increasing awareness that each of these compartments reciprocally participates in regulating pancreas damage and disease.

ER stress, ERAD, and autophagy

ER stress is also linked with activation of ER-associated degradation (ERAD) and induction of autophagic gene expression, mechanisms to eliminate misfolded proteins and dysfunctional ER.[59,60] These misfolded proteins are proteasomally degraded in conjunction with autophagy to disassemble proteins and recycle their amino acids. Misfolded proteins within the ER are recognized and targeted for ERAD by mechanisms utilizing ER chaperones and quality control systems. Several ERAD regulators are regulated by sXBP1, and both cells and mice deficient in sXBP1 exhibit impairments in ERAD and autophagy activation.[55,56] We reported that *Xbp+/-* mice fed alcohol diets exhibited reduced levels of pancreatic EDEM1, a key ERAD protein. This decrease was associated with marked vacuolization suggesting that a failure of the adaptive IRE1-sXBP1 pathway inhibits ERAD and promotes disordered autophagy.[54-56]

The PERK-eIF2α arm of the UPR induces autophagy through downstream targets including ATF4 and CHOP. Autophagy regulators required for induction and autophagosome formation including REDD1, ATG3, ATG5, ATG7, LC3B, and p62 are transcriptionally upregulated by ATF4 and CHOP.[61,62] These findings highlight the linkage between ER stress and autophagy induction, two important contributors to pancreatitis pathology.

The roles of ER Ca^{2+}, oxidative stress, and other factors in ER stress/UPR

The ER is one of the major storage sites for Ca^{2+} used to generate cytosolic signals to trigger diverse events including secretion and mitosis in all mammalian cells.[63] The role of inositol lipid turnover in Ca^{2+} release from the ER was originally demonstrated in pancreatic acinar cells.[64] Extensive studies established the roles of both intra- and extracellular Ca^{2+} in regulated secretion of zymogens from acinar cells.[65] Localized Ca^{2+} spikes are required for optimal secretagogue-induced amylase release, while global cytosolic Ca^{2+} elevations in acinar cells have been associated with supraphysiological inhibition of secretion and aberrant conversion of trypsinogen to active trypsin. Whereas these events represent widely accepted root causes of initial damage to acinar cells, nuclear factor-kB activation and an inflammatory response are also required for full pancreatitis development.[66] Ca^{2+} stored within the ER has important functions in protein biosynthesis and folding. Membrane-bound (calnexin) or lumenal (calreticulin) lectins are major Ca^{2+}-binding proteins within the ER.[67] These "glycosensor" proteins recycle cargo until its core glycosylation meets a quality standard for packaging and export from the ER en route to the Golgi. Ca^{2+} also regulates the ATPase activity of BiP that in turn regulates its interactions, including those with unfolded proteins.[68]

Whether Ca^{2+} affects the ER stress sensor functions through regulation of specific BiP interaction sites or independently, depletion of Ca^{2+} from the ER is well established as a major inducer of ER stress. Thapsigargin (TG), an irreversible Ca^{2+} pump inhibitor, potently induces cellular XBP1 splicing, as well as the PERK/eif2α/CHOP and ATF6 pathways. TG administration elicits cell type-specific effects ranging from growth arrest to apoptosis. The ER stress associated with TG treatment is caused by perturbation of multiple functions including protein synthesis and folding and formation of cargo-laden transport vesicles. To counterbalance these defects, XBP1s govern several measures that reduce the misfolded protein load, either through chaperone-assisted cycles of redox-dependent refolding, or removal via ERAD.

ER Ca^{2+} depletion and redox alterations are causally linked. Increases in misfolded proteins upregulate the activity and/or gene expression of the folding oxidoreductase, ERO-1L that generates hydrogen peroxide as it restores the balance of oxidized to reduced protein disulfide isomerases. In ongoing studies, we are examining effects of ethanol to perturb the redox status of key proteins of the folding and quality control apparatus, as well as the various cargo molecules (zymogens) in transit to the secretory pathway. The scheme shown in **Figure 2** illustrates aspects of our working hypothesis for these studies.

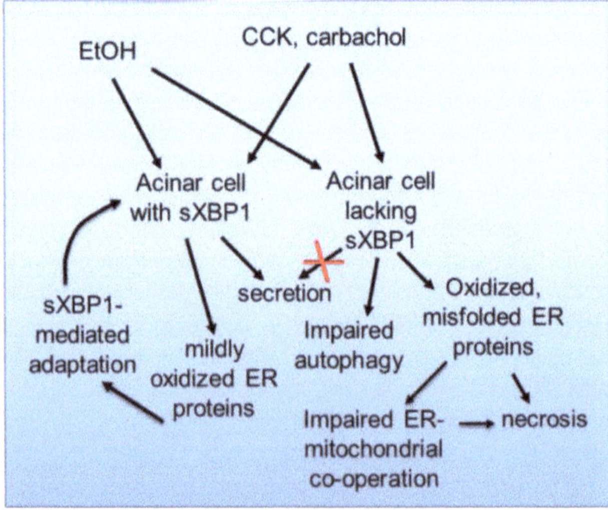

Figure 2. Scheme depicting UPR activation and regulation of ER stress responses. Working hypothesis for adaptation versus pathological outcomes to insults triggering redox perturbations in acinar cells in the presence or absence of the protein unfolded response regulator, spliced XBP1 (sXBP1).

Importantly, the ER stores a major part but not all of the cellular Ca^{2+} used for signaling. Endo-lysosomal "acidic" organelles have also increasingly been implicated in physiological events.[65,69] In particular, specialized Ca^{2+}-ATPases (SERCA3), and release channels (two pore channels and Mcoln1/TRPML1) have been associated with storage and release events, which have been linked to lysosomal functions and autophagy in other cell types.[70,71] Pharmacologic agents that have helped to identify these stores in pancreatic acinar cells include glycyl-L-phenylalanine-beta-naphthylamide (GPN), bafilomycin, and nigericin. Recently it was reported that all these agents release Ca^{2+} from both ER and endolysosomal Ca^{2+} stores. Substantial evidence points to cooperative domains, especially the membranes of distinct organelles such as mitochondrial, lysosomal, or plasma membrane in apposition to the ER. Whereas the most essential among these has not been identified, it seems clear that the multiple Ca^{2+} stores of the ER and other membrane-bound organelles operate interdependently.[72] Recent studies of membrane contact sites uncovered specific complexes (e.g., EGFR-PTP1B, Rab7-VAP via ORP1L or RILP, and STARD3-VAP) that tether segments of ER with endosomes, as well as Nvj1p-Vac8p that mediates nuclear-vacuole tethering.[73-76]

Reversible transcriptional regulation of acinar cell secretory differentiation: compensatory regrowth after damage versus tumorigenesis

A highly specialized transcription factor of the helix-loop-helix (HLH) family termed BHLHA15 or MIST1 was shown to dramatically alter the fate of the ER and secretory pathways. The expression of MIST1 is reportedly regulated by XBP1s.[18] Konieczny and others used a knockout approach to establish that proper pancreatic acinar cell organization and secretory function were MIST1 dependent.[77] Subsequently, *Mist1-/-* mice proved an interesting model to study the role of Ca^{2+} signaling in the acinar cell. The altered balance of ER versus secretory compartments revealed their roles in Ca^{2+} transients and global cytosolic elevations.[78] Research probing the roles of distinct transcriptional pathways in altering the identity of acinar cells continue to reveal the unexpected phenotypic plasticity of this extraordinary cell type.

Mounting evidence indicates that acinar cells can give rise to tumors as well as regenerative self-duplication, both of which occur through an initial loss of acinar cell properties and transition to a dedifferentiated phenotype. In this process, acinar genes such as carboxypeptidase 1 (*CPA1*), pancreatic amylase (*Amy2*), and Ptf-1a are lost, and the expression of some genes important for embryonic development or conferring stem-like properties, including Sox-9, Pdx1, and intermediates of the Wnt/β-catenin signaling pathway, are recapitulated. Dedifferentiation is permissive for proliferation, and in regeneration after damage, it is followed by restoration of the acinar phenotype. In contrast, further phenotypic transition such as acinar-to-ductal metaplasia (ADM) formation may occur in parallel with or leading to pancreatic intraepithelial neoplasia (PanIN) lesions. PanINs represent definitive precursor lesions for pancreatic ductal adenocarcinoma (PDAC), whereas ADMs are only tentatively established as such. Which of these (regrowth or tumorigenic) pathways is followed depends in part on environmental factors including the presence or absence of an inflammatory milieu.

Interestingly, the Map kinases, extracellular signal-regulated kinase 1/2 (ERK1/2), and the BZIP transcription factor c-Jun, are required for dedifferentiation.[79,80] Much evidence also supports a role for ERK-dependent signaling as a critical effector through which KRAS activity promotes PanIN and PDAC formation. MIST1 expression restrains these activities of KRAS and promotes maintenance of the acinar phenotype. Specifically, removing MIST1 was a permissive event for formation of ADM.[81] Mechanisms whereby Ca^{2+}, redox, and UPR pathways impact MIST1 or other transcription factors to modulate phenotypic plasticity remain relatively unexplored. Elucidation of these pathways enable harnessing the replicative potential of dedifferentiated cells and reverse engineering acinar and/or endocrine cells to develop novel stem cell therapies.

Summary

ER stress and oxidative stress are interlocked events regulated by Ca^{2+} and interchanged via intimate membrane contacts in the pancreatic acinar cell. Distinct UPR pathways work to maintain the acinar secretory phenotype and restrain oncogenic signaling (sXBP1, MIST1), while others (CHOP) are proapoptotic. Multiple investigations support the view of sXBP1-mediated signaling as an adaptive branch of UPR that protects/maintains the functional phenotype of the pancreatic acinar cell. Prolonged ER stress impairs homeostatic processes such as endo-/lysosomal function and autophagy (see **Figure 2**). Collectively, such disturbances in acinar cell function lead to pathologic outcomes. In particular, the energetic imbalance and oxidative stress that accompany excessive unfolded ER proteins and impaired ER-mitochondrial cooperation promote necrosis, a form of cell death associated with inflammatory responses. Impaired autophagy may also favor cell death by promoting apoptosis or necrosis. Acinar cell dedifferentiation permits proliferative, stem-like properties with concomitant loss of the acinar phenotype and may give rise to tumorigenic intermediates. However, dedifferentiation must also be contemplated to achieve stem cell therapy since adult tissues are nonproliferative.

References

1. Lee AS, Bell J, Ting J. Biochemical characterization of the 94- and 78-kilodalton glucose-regulated proteins in hamster fibroblasts. *J Biol Chem*. 1984; 259(7): 4616-4621. PMID: 6707023.
2. Kozutsumi Y, Segal M, Normington K, Gething MJ, Sambrook J. The presence of malfolded proteins in the endoplasmic reticulum signals the induction of glucose-regulated proteins. *Nature*. 1988; 332(6163): 462-464. PMID: 3352747.
3. Cox JS, Shamu CE, Walter P. Transcriptional induction of genes encoding endoplasmic reticulum resident proteins requires a transmembrane protein kinase. *Cell*. 1993; 73(6): 1197-1206. PMID: 8513503.
4. Mori K, Ma W, Gething MJ, Sambrook J. A transmembrane protein with a cdc2+/CDC28-related kinase activity is required for signaling from the ER to the nucleus. *Cell*. 1993; 74(4): 743-756. PMID: 8358794.
5. Nikawa J, Yamashita S. IRE1 encodes a putative protein kinase containing a membrane-spanning domain and is required for inositol phototrophy in Saccharomyces cerevisiae. *Mol Microbiol*. 1992; 6(11): 1441-1446. PMID: 1625574.
6. Sidrauski C, Walter P. The transmembrane kinase Ire1p is a site-specific endonuclease that initiates mRNA splicing in the unfolded protein response. *Cell*. 1997; 90(6): 1031-1039. PMID: 9323131.
7. Maurel M, Chevet E, Tavernier J, Gerlo S. Getting RIDD of RNA: IRE1 in cell fate regulation. *Trends Biochem Sci*. 2014; 39(5): 245-254. PMID: 24657016.
8. Calfon M, Zeng H, Urano F, Till JH, Hubbard SR, Harding HP, et al. IRE1 couples endoplasmic reticulum load to secretory capacity by processing the XBP-1 mRNA. *Nature*. 2002; 415(6867): 92-96. PMID: 11780124.
9. Yoshida H, Matsui T, Yamamoto A, Okada T, Mori K. XBP1 mRNA is induced by ATF6 and spliced by IRE1 in response to ER stress to produce a highly active transcription factor. *Cell*. 2001; 107(7): 881-891. PMID: 11779464.
10. Hollien J, Lin JH, Li H, Stevens N, Walter P, Weissman JS. Regulated Ire1-dependent decay of messenger RNAs in mammalian cells. *J Cell Biol*. 2009; 186(3): 323-331. PMID: 19651891.
11. Hollien J, Weissman JS. Decay of endoplasmic reticulum-localized mRNAs during the unfolded protein response. *Science*. 2006; 313(5783): 104-107. PMID: 16825573.
12. Upton JP, Wang L, Han D, Wang ES, Huskey NE, Lim L, et al. IRE1alpha cleaves select microRNAs during ER stress to derepress translation of proapoptotic Caspase-2. *Science*. 2012; 338(6108): 818-822. PMID: 23042294.
13. Urano F, Wang X, Bertolotti A, Zhang Y, Chung P, Harding HP, et al. Coupling of stress in the ER to activation of JNK protein kinases by transmembrane protein kinase IRE1. *Science*. 2000; 287(5453): 664-666. PMID: 10650002.
14. Yoshida H, Oku M, Suzuki M, Mori K. pXBP1(U) encoded in XBP1 pre-mRNA negatively regulates unfolded protein response activator pXBP1(S) in mammalian ER stress response. *J Cell Biol*. 2006; 172(4): 565-575. PMID: 16461360.
15. Lee AH, Iwakoshi NN, Glimcher LH. XBP-1 regulates a subset of endoplasmic reticulum resident chaperone genes in the unfolded protein response. *Mol Cell Biol*. 2003; 23(21): 7448-7459. PMID: 14559994.
16. Shaffer AL, Shapiro-Shelef M, Iwakoshi NN, Lee AH, Qian SB, Zhao H, et al. XBP1, downstream of Blimp-1, expands the secretory apparatus and other organelles, and increases protein synthesis in plasma cell differentiation. *Immunity*. 2004; 21(1): 81-93. PMID: 15345222.
17. Shoulders MD, Ryno LM, Genereux JC, Moresco JJ, Tu PG, Wu C, et al. Stress-independent activation of XBP1s and/or ATF6 reveals three functionally diverse ER proteostasis environments. *Cell Rep*. 2013; 3(4): 1279-1292. PMID: 23583182.
18. Acosta-Alvear D, Zhou Y, Blais A, Tsikitis M, Lents NH, Arias C, et al. XBP1 controls diverse cell type- and condition-specific transcriptional regulatory networks. *Mol Cell*. 2007; 27(1): 53-66. PMID: 17612490.
19. Lee AH, Chu GC, Iwakoshi NN, Glimcher LH. XBP-1 is required for biogenesis of cellular secretory machinery of exocrine glands. *EMBO J*. 2005; 24(24): 4368-4380. PMID: 16362047.
20. Cross BC, Bond PJ, Sadowski PG, Jha BK, Zak J, Goodman JM, et al. The molecular basis for selective inhibition of unconventional mRNA splicing by an IRE1-binding small molecule. *Proc Natl Acad Sci U S A*. 2012; 109(15): E869-E878. PMID: 22315414.
21. Vidal RL, Hetz C. Unspliced XBP1 controls autophagy through FoxO1. *Cell Res*. 2013; 23(4): 463-464. PMID: 23337584.
22. Harding HP, Zhang Y, Ron D. Protein translation and folding are coupled by an endoplasmic-reticulum-resident kinase. *Nature*. 1999; 397(6716): 271-274. PMID: 9930704.
23. Harding HP, Novoa I, Zhang Y, Zeng H, Wek R, Schapira M, et al. Regulated translation initiation controls stress-induced gene expression in mammalian cells. *Mol Cell*. 2000; 6(5): 1099-1108. PMID: 11106749.
24. Fox RM, Andrew DJ. Transcriptional regulation of secretory capacity by bZip transcription factors. *Front Biol (Beijing)*. 2015; 10(1): 28-51. PMID: 25821458.
25. Lu M, Lawrence DA, Marsters S, Acosta-Alvear D, Kimmig P, Mendez AS, et al. Cell death. Opposing unfolded-protein-response signals converge on death receptor 5 to control apoptosis. *Science*. 2014; 345(6192): 98-101. PMID: 24994655.
26. McCullough KD, Martindale JL, Klotz LO, Aw TY, Holbrook NJ. Gadd153 sensitizes cells to endoplasmic reticulum stress by down-regulating Bcl2 and perturbing the cellular redox state. *Mol Cell Biol*. 2001; 21(4): 1249-1259. PMID: 11158311.
27. Puthalakath H, O'Reilly LA, Gunn P, Lee L, Kelly PN, Huntington ND, et al. ER stress triggers apoptosis by activating BH3-only protein Bim. *Cell*. 2007; 129(7): 1337-1349. PMID: 17604722.
28. Oyadomari S, Mori M. Roles of CHOP/GADD153 in endoplasmic reticulum stress. *Cell Death Differ*. 2004; 11(4): 381-389. PMID: 14685163.

29. Tabas I, Ron D. Integrating the mechanisms of apoptosis induced by endoplasmic reticulum stress. *Nat Cell Biol.* 2011; 13(3): 184-190. PMID: 21364565.
30. Marciniak SJ, Yun CY, Oyadomari S, Novoa I, Zhang Y, Jungreis R, et al. CHOP induces death by promoting protein synthesis and oxidation in the stressed endoplasmic reticulum. *Genes Dev.* 2004; 18(24): 3066-3077. PMID: 15601821.
31. Wang S and Kaufman RJ. The impact of the unfolded protein response on human disease. *J Cell Biol* 197(7): 857-867, 2012. PMID: 22733998.
32. Hai T, Jalgaonkar S, Wolford CC, Yin X. Immunohistochemical detection of activating transcription factor 3, a hub of the cellular adaptive-response network. *Methods Enzymol.* 2011; 490: 175-194. PMID: 21266251.
33. Cui H, Guo M, Xu D, Ding ZC, Zhou G, Ding HF, et al. The stress-responsive gene ATF3 regulates the histone acetyltransferase Tip60. *Nat Commun.* 2015; 6: 6752. PMID: 25865756.
34. Adachi Y, Yamamoto K, Okada T, Yoshida H, Harada A, Mori K. ATF6 is a transcription factor specializing in the regulation of quality control proteins in the endoplasmic reticulum. *Cell Struct Funct.* 2008; 33(1): 75-89. PMID: 18360008.
35. Bommiasamy H, Back SH, Fagone P, Lee K, Meshinchi S, Vink E, et al. ATF6alpha induces XBP1-independent expansion of the endoplasmic reticulum. *J Cell Sci.* 2009; 122(Pt 10): 1626-1636. PMID: 19420237.
36. Schindler AJ, Schekman R. In vitro reconstitution of ER-stress induced ATF6 transport in COPII vesicles. *Proc Natl Acad Sci U S A.* 2009; 106(42): 17775-17780. PMID: 19822759.
37. Haze K, Yoshida H, Yanagi H, Yura T, Mori K. Mammalian transcription factor ATF6 is synthesized as a transmembrane protein and activated by proteolysis in response to endoplasmic reticulum stress. *Mol Biol Cell.* 1999; 10(11): 3787-3799. PMID: 10564271.
38. Yoshida H, Haze K, Yanagi H, Yura T, Mori K. Identification of the cis-acting endoplasmic reticulum stress response element responsible for transcriptional induction of mammalian glucose-regulated proteins. Involvement of basic leucine zipper transcription factors. *J Biol Chem.* 1998; 273(50): 33741-33749. PMID: 9837962.
39. Kubisch CH, Sans MD, Arumugam T, Ernst SA, Williams JA, Logsdon CD. Early activation of endoplasmic reticulum stress is associated with arginine-induced acute pancreatitis. *Am J Physiol Gastrointest Liver Physiol.* 2006; 291(2): G238-G245. PMID: 16574987.
40. Kubisch CH, Logsdon CD. Secretagogues differentially activate endoplasmic reticulum stress responses in pancreatic acinar cells. *Am J Physiol Gastrointest Liver Physiol.* 2007; 292(6): G1804-G1812. PMID: 17431218.
41. Kubisch CH, Logsdon CD. Endoplasmic reticulum stress and the pancreatic acinar cell. *Expert Rev Gastroenterol Hepatol.* 2008; 2(2): 249-260. PMID: 19072360.
42. Malo A, Krüger B, Seyhun E, Schäfer C, Hoffmann RT, Göke B, et al. Tauroursodeoxycholic acid reduces endoplasmic reticulum stress, trypsin activation, and acinar cell apoptosis while increasing secretion in rat pancreatic acini. *Am J Physiol Gastrointest Liver Physiol.* 2010; 299(4): G877-G886. PMID: 20671193.
43. Kowalik AS, Johnson CL, Chadi SA, Weston JY, Fazio EN, Pin CL. Mice lacking the transcription factor Mist1 exhibit an altered stress response and increased sensitivity to caerulein-induced pancreatitis. *Am J Physiol Gastrointest Liver Physiol.* 2007; 292(4): G1123-G1132. PMID: 17170023.
44. Suyama K, Ohmuraya M, Hirota M, Ozaki N, Ida S, Endo M, et al. C/EBP homologous protein is crucial for the acceleration of experimental pancreatitis. *Biochem Biophys Res Commun.* 2008; 367(1): 176-182. PMID: 18166146.
45. Ye R, Mareninova OA, Barron E, Wang M, Hinton DR, Pandol SJ, et al. Grp78 heterozygosity regulates chaperone balance in exocrine pancreas with differential response to cerulein-induced acute pancreatitis. *Am J Pathol.* 2010; 177(6): 2827-2836. PMID: 20971738.
46. Fazio EN, Dimattia GE, Chadi SA, Kernohan KD, Pin CL. Stanniocalcin 2 alters PERK signalling and reduces cellular injury during cerulein induced pancreatitis in mice. *BMC Cell Biol.* 2011; 12: 17. PMID: 21545732.
47. Seyhun E, Malo A, Schäfer C, Moskaluk CA, Hoffmann RT, Göke B, et al. Tauroursodeoxycholic acid reduces endoplasmic reticulum stress, acinar cell damage, and systemic inflammation in acute pancreatitis. *Am J Physiol Gastrointest Liver Physiol.* 2011; 301(5): G773-G782. PMID: 21778463.
48. Zeng Y, Wang X, Zhang W, Wu K, Ma J. Hypertriglyceridemia aggravates ER stress and pathogenesis of acute pancreatitis. *Hepatogastroenterology.* 2012; 59(119): 2318-2326. PMID: 22389298.
49. Malo A, Krüger B, Göke B, Kubisch CH. 4-Phenylbutyric acid reduces endoplasmic reticulum stress, trypsin activation, and acinar cell apoptosis while increasing secretion in rat pancreatic acini. *Pancreas.* 2013; 42(1): 92-101. PMID: 22889983.
50. Beer S, Zhou J, Szabó A, Keiles S, Chandak GR, Witt H, et al. Comprehensive functional analysis of chymotrypsin C (CTRC) variants reveals distinct loss-of-function mechanisms associated with pancreatitis risk. *Gut.* 2013; 62(11): 1616-1624. PMID: 22942235.
51. Li N, Wu X, Holzer RG, Lee JH, Todoric J, Park EJ, et al. Loss of acinar cell IKKα triggers spontaneous pancreatitis in mice. *J Clin Invest.* 2013; 123(5): 2231-2243. PMID: 23563314.
52. Wu L, Cai B, Zheng S, Liu X, Cai H, Li H. effect of emodin on endoplasmic reticulum stress in rats with severe acute pancreatitis. *Inflammation.* 2013; 36(5): 1020-1029. PMID: 23605470.
53. Sah RP, Garg SK, Dixit AK, Dudeja V, Dawra RK, Saluja AK. Endoplasmic reticulum stress is chronically activated in chronic pancreatitis. *J Biol Chem.* 2014; 289(40): 27551-27561. PMID: 25077966.
54. Pandol SJ, Gorelick FS, Lugea A. Environmental and genetic stressors and the unfolded protein response in exocrine pancreatic function - a hypothesis. *Front Physiol.* 2011; 2: 8. PMID: 21483727.
55. Lugea A, Waldron RT, French SW, Pandol SJ. Drinking and driving pancreatitis: links between endoplasmic reticulum stress and autophagy. *Autophagy.* 2011; 7(7): 783-785. PMID: 21460613.
56. Lugea A, Tischler D, Nguyen J, Gong J, Gukovsky I, French SW, et al. Adaptive unfolded protein response attenuates

alcohol-induced pancreatic damage. *Gastroenterology*. 2011; 140(3): 987-997. PMID: 21111739.

57. Goodall JC, Wu C, Zhang Y, McNeill L, Ellis L, Saudek V, et al. Endoplasmic reticulum stress-induced transcription factor, CHOP, is crucial for dendritic cell IL-23 expression. *Proc Natl Acad Sci U S A*. 2010; 107(41): 17698-17703. PMID: 20876114.
58. Malhi H, Kropp EM, Clavo VF, Kobrossi CR, Han J, Mauer AS, et al. C/EBP Homologous Protein-induced Macrophage Apoptosis Protects Mice from Steatohepatitis. *J Biol Chem*. 2013; 288(26): 18624-18642. PMID: 23720735.
59. Brodsky JL, Wojcikiewicz RJ. Substrate-specific mediators of ER associated degradation (ERAD). *Curr Opin Cell Biol*. 2009; 21(4): 516-521. PMID: 19443192.
60. Yoshida Y, Tanaka K..Lectin-like ERAD players in ER and cytosol. *Biochim Biophys Acta*. 2010; 1800(2): 172-180. PMID: 19665047.
61. B'chir W, Maurin AC, Carraro V, Averous J, Jousse C, Muranishi Y, et al. The eIF2α/ATF4 pathway is essential for stress-induced autophagy gene expression. *Nucleic Acids Res*. 2013; 41(16): 7683-7699. PMID: 23804767.
62. Rouschop KM, van den Beucken T, Dubois L, Niessen H, Bussink J, Savelkouls K, et al. The unfolded protein response protects human tumor cells during hypoxia through regulation of the autophagy genes MAP1LC3B and ATG5. *J Clin Invest*. 2010; 120(1): 127-141. PMID: 20038797.
63. Berridge MJ. Inositol trisphosphate and calcium signalling. *Nature*. 1993; 361(6410): 315-325. PMID: 8381210.
64. Streb H, Irvine RF, Berridge MJ, Schulz I. Release of Ca^{2+} from a nonmitochondrial intracellular store in pancreatic acinar cells by inositol-1,4,5-trisphosphate. *Nature*. 1983; 306(5938): 67-69. PMID: 6605482.
65. Gerasimenko JV, Gerasimenko OV, Petersen OH. The role of Ca^{2+} in the pathophysiology of pancreatitis. *J Physiol*. 2014; 592(Pt 2): 269-280. PMID: 23897234.
66. Sah RP, Dawra RK, Saluja AK. New insights into the pathogenesis of pancreatitis. *Curr Opin Gastroenterol*. 2013; 29(5): 523-530. PMID: 23892538.
67. Wang WA, Groenendyk J, Michalak M. Calreticulin signaling in health and disease. *Int J Biochem Cell Biol*. 2012; 44(6): 842-846. PMID: 22373697.
68. Behnke J, Feige MJ, Hendershot LM. BiP and its nucleotide exchange factors Grp170 and Sil1: mechanisms of action and biological functions. *J Mol Biol*. 2015; 427(7): 1589-1608. PMID: 25698114.
69. Patel S, Muallem S. Acidic Ca^{2+} stores come to the fore. *Cell Calcium*. 2011; 50(2): 109-112. PMID: 21497395.
70. Medina DL, Di Paola S, Peluso I, Armani A, De Stefani D, Venditti R, et al. Lysosomal calcium signalling regulates autophagy through calcineurin and TFEB. *Nat Cell Biol*. 2015; 17(3): 288-299. PMID: 25720963.
71. Venkatachalam K, Wong CO, Montell C. Feast or famine: role of TRPML in preventing cellular amino acid starvation. *Autophagy*. 2013; 9(1): 98-100. PMID: 23047439.
72. Ronco V, Potenza DM, Denti F, Vullo S, Gagliano G, Tognolina M, et al. A novel Ca^{2+}-mediated cross-talk between endoplasmic reticulum and acidic organelles: implications for NAADP-dependent Ca^{2+} signalling. *Cell Calcium*. 2015; 57(2): 89-100. PMID: 25655285.
73. Alpy F, Rousseau A, Schwab Y, Legueux F, Stoll I, Wendling C, et al. STARD3 or STARD3NL and VAP form a novel molecular tether between late endosomes and the ER. *J Cell Sci*. 2013; 126(Pt 23): 5500-5512. PMID: 24105263.
74. Eden ER, White IJ, Tsapara A, Futter CE. Membrane contacts between endosomes and ER provide sites for PTP1B-epidermal growth factor receptor interaction. *Nat Cell Biol*. 2010; 12(3): 267-272. PMID: 20118922.
75. Rocha N, Kuijl C, van der Kant R, Janssen L, Houben D, Janssen H, et al. Cholesterol sensor ORP1L contacts the ER protein VAP to control Rab7-RILP-p150 Glued and late endosome positioning. *J Cell Biol*. 2009; 185(7): 1209-1225. PMID: 19564404.
76. Penny CJ, Kilpatrick BS, Eden ER, Patel S. Coupling acidic organelles with the ER through Ca^{2+} microdomains at membrane contact sites. *Cell Calcium*. 2015; 58(4): 387-396. PMID: 25866010.
77. Pin CL, Rukstalis JM, Johnson C, Konieczny SF. The bHLH transcription factor Mist1 is required to maintain exocrine pancreas cell organization and acinar cell identity. *J Cell Biol*. 2001; 155(4): 519-530. PMID: 11696558.
78. Luo X, Shin DM, Wang X, Konieczny SF, Muallem S. Aberrant localization of intracellular organelles, Ca^{2+} signaling, and exocytosis in Mist1 null mice. *J Biol Chem*. 2005; 280(13): 12668-12675. PMID: 15665001.
79. Collins MA, Yan W, Sebolt-Leopold JS, Pasca di Magliano M. MAPK signaling is required for dedifferentiation of acinar cells and development of pancreatic intraepithelial neoplasia in mice. *Gastroenterology*. 2014; 146(3): 822-834 e827. PMID: 24315826.
80. Guo L, Sans MD, Hou Y, Ernst SA, Williams JA. c-Jun/AP-1 is required for CCK-induced pancreatic acinar cell dedifferentiation and DNA synthesis in vitro. *Am J Physiol Gastrointest Liver Physiol*. 2012; 302(12): G1381-G1396. PMID: 22461029.
81. Shi G, DiRenzo D, Qu C, Barney D, Miley D, Konieczny SF. Maintenance of acinar cell organization is critical to preventing Kras-induced acinar-ductal metaplasia. *Oncogene*. 2013; 32(15): 1950-1958. PMID: 22665051.

Chapter 10

Spontaneous pancreatitis in genetically modified animal strains

Yan Bi[1] and Baoan Ji[2*]

[1]*Department of Gastroenterology and Hepatology, Mayo Clinic, Jacksonville, FL;*
[2]*Department of Cancer Biology, Mayo Clinic, Jacksonville, FL.*

Introduction

Dysregulation of multiple signaling pathways in the pancreas is proposed to be involved the initiation of pancreatitis. Genetic manipulation in experimental animals has been used to understand the critical roles of these pathways during the pathogenesis of pancreatitis. In general, the genetic approaches that specifically target these specific molecules are superior to pharmacological methods. Additionally, genetic modification of the initiator genes observed in human pancreatitis can help create clinically relevant animal models. These models will be valuable for studying the mechanisms of pancreatitis and testing preclinical therapeutic and preventive interventions. In this review, we will focus on the impact of trypsin, nuclear factor kappa B (NF-κB), endoplasmic reticulum (ER) stress, Ras, autophagy, cyclooxygenase (Cox)-2 and several others on pancreatitis. We will also discuss efforts to create animal models for human hereditary pancreatitis, cystic fibrosis, and autoimmune pancreatitis.

Animal Models Targeting Trypsinogen Activation

Trypsin and pancreatitis

The exocrine pancreas synthesizes digestive enzymes to facilitate digestion. More than a century ago, Chiari proposed that acute pancreatitis (AP) was an autodigestive disease.[1] During the past two decades, researchers discovered that trypsinogen is prematurely activated in various animal models of pancreatitis and human pancreatitis.[2-6] Because trypsin is capable of degrading proteins and initiating other zymogen activation cascades, premature activation of trypsinogen in pancreatic acinar cells is considered a key initiator of this disease. This notion is strongly supported by the observation that gain-of-function cationic trypsinogen (PRSS1) mutations and loss-of-function mutations of the potent pancreatic protease inhibitor Kazal type 1 (SPINK1) are associated with hereditary pancreatitis (HP).[7-14] The mechanisms of trypsinogen activation have been extensively studied.[15-18] However, the roles of intracellular trypsin have only recently been directly investigated. In transgenic mouse models, expression of active trypsin or mutant PRSS1 caused pancreatitis, and the expression of the trypsin inhibitor SPINK1 ameliorated experimental pancreatitis.[13,19-21] Genetic deletion of trypsinogen 7, the most prominent trypsinogen in mice, blunted trypsinogen activation and caused a 50% reduction in acinar necrosis following caerulein challenge.[22]

Models with direct trypsinogen activation

Because pharmacological inhibitors have nonspecific effects, and the stimuli used to induce pancreatitis activate multiple signaling pathways in addition to activating trypsinogen,[23] the direct effects of intracellular trypsin activity cannot be examined using these approaches. However, a recent study reported the development of a mutant trypsinogen that could be activated intracellularly by PACE, an endogenous protease named paired basic amino acid cleaving enzyme.[24] This new construct (PACE-trypsinogen) allowed direct examination of the effects of intracellular trypsin on pancreatic acinar cells for the first time. In *in vitro* studies, PACE-trypsinogen was expressed by means of adenoviral vector in the secretory pathway and was activated within acinar cells. Expression of PACE-trypsinogen induced the apoptosis of pancreatic acinar cells. Cell death was blocked by the trypsin inhibitor pefabloc, but it was not completely blocked by the pancaspase inhibitor benzyloxycarbonyl-VAD, indicating that caspase-independent pathways were also involved. However, intracellular trypsin had no significant effect on the activity of the proinflammatory transcription factor NF-κB. In contrast, extracellular trypsin caused cell damage and dramatically increased NF-κB activity. These data indicate that

*Corresponding author. Email: ji.baoan@mayo.edu

the effects of active trypsin on pancreatic acinar cells are determined by its localization.[24] For *in vivo* studies, a new mouse model of this construct was developed. These mice were engineered to conditionally express an endogenously activated trypsinogen within pancreatic acinar cells after Cre-mediated recombination (**Figure 1B**)[19]. The acinar specificity was achieved by crossing these mice with mice harboring pancreatic elastase I promoter-driven CreERT, a tamoxifen-inducible Cre (**Figure 2A**).[25] These frequently used pancreatic-specific Cre mice are described in **Figure 2B**. Interestingly, initiation of AP was observed at high (homozygous) but not low (heterozygous) expression levels of PACE-trypsinogen. Rapid caspase-3 activation and apoptosis with delayed necrosis was observed, and lost acinar cells were replaced with abundant fatty tissue and limited fibrosis. These findings indicated that intra-acinar activation of trypsinogen is sufficient to initiate AP. This novel model will provide a powerful tool for improving our understanding of the basic mechanisms that occur during the initiation of pancreatitis.[19]

A model with SPINK inactivation

SPINK1 (Serine Protease Inhibitor Kazal-type 1), also known as pancreatic secretory trypsin inhibitor (PSTI), was originally identified as a trypsin inhibitor in 1948 by Kazal et al.[26] SPINK1 is synthesized by the acinar cells of the pancreas and binds to trypsin to prevent further activation of pancreatic enzymes. Thus, a lack of SPINK1 may result in the premature conversion of trypsinogen into active trypsin in acinar cells, leading to autodigestion of the exocrine pancreas by activated proteases. The detailed functions and roles of SPINK1in pancreatic diseases have been previously reviewed.[27,28] In 2000, Witt et al. showed that mutations in the SPINK1 gene were associated with chronic pancreatitis,[14] and since then there have been many reports on the association between mutations in SPINK1 genes and patients with pancreatitis.[29-31]

In mice, SPINK3 is the homolog of human SPINK1. Upregulation of SPINK 3 provides a protective mechanism in caerulein-induced pancreatitis,[32] and knockdown of SPINK3 (Spink3$^{-/-}$ mice) enhances trypsin activity in pancreatic acinar cells.[33] The pancreas of Spink3$^{-/-}$ mice usually develops for up to 15.5 days after fertilization; however, autophagic degeneration of acinar cells, but not ductal or islet cells, begins after 16.5 days. Rapid onset of cell death occurs in the pancreas and duodenum within a few days after birth and results in death by 14.5 days after birth. There is limited inflammatory cell infiltration and no signs of apoptosis. At 7.5 days after birth, residual ductlike

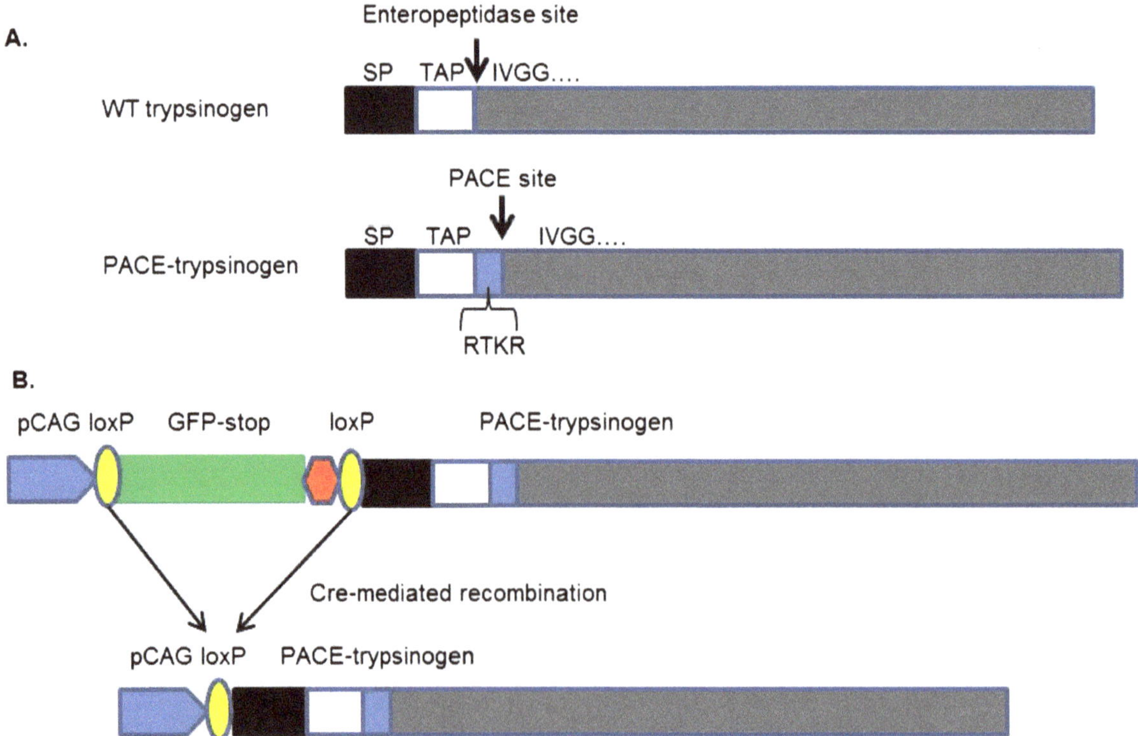

Figure 1. Expression of a trypsinogen that can be activated intracellularly. A. Wild-type trypsinogen is normally activated in the duodenum by enteropeptidase (top). A mutant trypsinogen was developed by the insertion of an amino acid sequence motif RTKR immediate before the active trypsin. The RTKR sequence can be recognized and cleaved by PACE. B. In a conditional transgenic mouse line, PACE-trypsinogen expression was blocked by a loxp-GFP-stop-loxP cassette until Cre medicated recombination.[19,24]

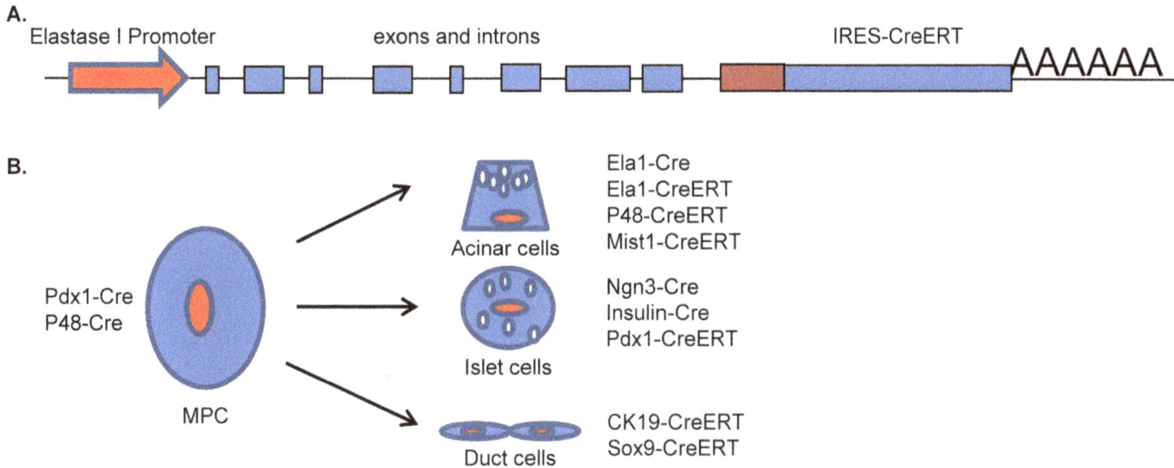

Figure 2. Commonly used cell-specific Cre mouse lines for pancreatic research. A. For inducible pancreatic acinar specific gene targeting, a tamoxifen-inducible Cre (CreERT) was introduced in a bacterial artificial chromosome containing the pancreatic elastase I gene. The full length promoter of elastase I gave highly efficient and specific CreERT expression in acinar cells. B. pdx1 and p48 (Ptf1a) are transcription factors expressed early in pancreatic multipotent progenitor cells (MPC). Cre driven by these promoters will be active in acinar, ductal, and endocrine cells. Pancreatic elastase I promoter is pancreatic acinar-cell specific. Although P48 and Mist1 are activated early in MPC, in adults they are expressed only in acinar cells. Therefore, using the tamoxifen-inducible CreERT system in adults, these gene promoters will only induce recombination in pancreatic acinar cells. Similarly, Pdx1 promoter is active only in endocrine cells of the adult pancreas. Ngn3 drives differentiation of endocrine islets. Cre expression driven by this gene promoter will occur in all pancreatic endocrine lineages. Insulin promoter is specific to beta cells. For pancreatic duct cells, CK19 and Sox9 promoters can be used. However, these genes are also expressed in many other organs.

cells in the tubular complexes strongly express pancreatic duodenal homeodomain-containing protein 1, a marker of pancreatic stem cells, without any sign of acinar cell regeneration. These findings indicate that the progressive disappearance of acinar cells in Spink3$^{-/-}$ mice was due to autophagic cell death and impaired regeneration, suggesting that SPINK3 maintains the integrity and regeneration of acinar cells.[34] Although SPINK3 is also expressed in the kidney, lung, and a small proportion of cells in the gastrointestinal tract and liver,[35] pancreas-specific transgenic expression of SPINK rescues SPINK3$^{-/-}$ mice and restores a normal pancreatic phenotype, supporting the critical role of SPINK3 in pancreatic homeostasis.[20,36]

Hereditary pancreatitis-related models

Hereditary pancreatitis (HP) is a rare form of pancreatitis.[37] The first family with HP was described by Comfort and Steinberg in 1952.[38] Using genetic linkage studies, the HP locus was independently narrowed to the long arm of chromosome 7 by Le Bodic, Whitcomb, and Pandya in 1996.[39-41] Shortly afterward, Whitcomb et al.[7] identified an Arg-His substitution at residue 122 of the cationic trypsinogen gene (PRSS1) in HP through mutational analysis. It was originally named R117H based on the chymotrypsin numbering system, and was renamed R122H following the recommendations for gene mutation nomenclature.[42,43] Subsequently, a number of gain-of-function PRSS1 mutations were identified. The most common ones were R122H, A16V, and N29I.[44] Clinically, HP is characterized by recurrent AP with an unusual early onset of the disease (5-23 years of age) and the development of chronic pancreatitis. Importantly, the cumulative risk of pancreatic cancer after the onset of symptoms is 44% at 70 years after the onset of the disease in HP patients. The calculated standardized incidence ratio of pancreatic cancer from the European registry of hereditary pancreatitis and pancreatic cancer cohort after correction for age, history of smoking, nationality, and surgical intervention was 67.[45]

Several groups have tried to generate an animal model mimicking the mutations harbored in HP patients, but with limited success. In one model, human PRSS1 mutant R122H transgenic mice were generated under using a 213-bp fragment of the rat elastase promoter/enhancer.[46] PRSS1 was expressed in small amounts in zymogen granules. No spontaneous development of pancreatitis was observed. However, serum pancreatic lipase levels or activity was higher in these animals after induction of pancreatitis compared with controls. Repeated caerulein insults resulted in a slightly more severe pancreatitis. This rather small difference compared with controls could have been caused by the low expression of the transgene in the mouse pancreas.[46]

Another transgenic mouse was generated in which the expression of the mouse PRSS1 mutant R122H (R122H_mPRSS1) was expressed using a rat elastase promoter.[13] Acinar cell damage was detectable by 7 weeks of age with increasing inflammatory infiltrates at 12 weeks. Fibrosis was evident in 24-week-old animals. The highest penetrance of this phenotype reached 40% after 1 year of age. The inflammatory phenotype varied in both extent and severity among the animals. It is surprising that the rapid response of the transgenic animals to caerulein injection was indistinguishable from that of the wild-type (WT). In contrast, 1 week after injection the inflammatory phenotype in the WT animals largely resolved, while the R122H_mPRSS1 transgenic animals displayed extensive collagen deposition in the periacinar and interlobular areas, indicating a chronic inflammatory response. This was the first genetic model of chronic pancreatitis in which a genetic alteration resulted in a predicted phenotype. Unfortunately, there have been no follow-up studies published since 2006. Therefore, this model might be "lost" during breeding, probably because of unstable gene expression from the small elastase promoter.

In another recent study, Athwal et al. developed a transgenic mouse model system using WT human PRSS1 and two HP-associated mutants (R122H and N29I) using a rat elastase promoter.[47] The transgenic animals revealed pathological changes similar to those of chronic pancreatitis, particularly in aging (> 9 months of age) animals. These changes occurred spontaneously in up to 10% of the animals that expressed the transgenes. When a supra-physiological dose (50 µg/kg) of caerulein was administered to the WT and PRSS1 transgenic strains, no differences in pancreatic response were observed. However, when these animals were treated with a lower dose of caerulein (20 µg/kg), the transgenic animals from each of the three transgenic strains displayed more severe pancreatitis than WT animals. The transgenic expression of PRSS1 promoted apoptotic rather than necrotic cell death. It is intriguing that no differences in phenotype were observed among these transgenic strains, and that the supra-physiological dose of caerulein did not cause more severe pancreatitis in the transgenic mice compared with the WT mice.

Animal Models Induced by Modulating NF-κB Activity

Introduction of NF-κB

The NF-κB transcription factor family is expressed in almost all cell types and tissues, and specific NF-κB binding sites are present in the promoters/enhancers of a large number of genes. These genes regulate inflammation, immunity, cell proliferation, differentiation, and survival.[48] NF-κB consists of five proteins, p65 (RelA), RelB, c-Rel, p105/p50 (NF-κB1), and p100/52 (NF-κB2) that associate with each other to form distinct transcriptionally active homo- and heterodimeric complexes. Among these, p65, RelB, and c-Rel contain c-terminal transactivation domains. p50 and p52 are generated by processing of the precursor molecules p105 and p100, respectively. The p50/65 heterodimer represents the most abundant form of Rel dimers and is expressed in almost all cell types. However, not all combinations of Rel dimers are transcriptionally active. DNA-bound p50 and p52 homo- and heterodimers have been found to repress κB-dependent transcription. In most unstimulated cells, NF-κB dimers are retained in an inactive form in the cytosol through their interaction with IκB proteins. Degradation of these inhibitors upon phosphorylation by the IκB kinase (IKK) complex leads to nuclear translocation of NF-κB and induction of the transcription of target genes.[49-52]

The canonical IKKs, IKKα, and IKKβ, form a complex with the regulatory adaptor protein NF-κB essential modulator (NEMO), which is also known as IKKγ. IKKα and IKKβ are Ser/Thr kinases that phosphorylate the NF-κB inhibitor IκB proteins, resulting in their poly-ubiquitination and subsequent proteasomal degradation. This allows NF-κB to translocate to the nucleus and bind to specific DNA elements. Despite extensive sequence similarity, IKKα and IKKβ have largely distinct functions because they have different substrate specificities and modes of regulation. IKKβ (and IKKγ) are essential for rapid NF-κB activation by proinflammatory signaling cascades, such as those triggered by tumor necrosis factor alpha (TNFα) or lipopolysaccharide (LPS). In contrast, IKKα participates in the activation of a specific form of NF-κB in response to a subset of TNF family members and may also serve to attenuate IKKβ-driven NF-κB activation.[53] Based on sequence similarities with IKKα and IKKβ, two IKK-related kinases, TANK binding kinase 1 (TBK1) and IKKε (also known as IKK-inducible or IKK-i), were discovered. IKKε and TBK1 are known as noncanonical IKKs. These protein kinases are important for the activation of interferon response factors 3 and 7. NF-κB is activated in most inflammatory diseases including animal models of AP.[54,55] Moreover, IKKs are also involved in kinase- and NF-κB-independent activities.[53,56-58]

Activation of IKK2 (IKKB)-induced pancreatitis

To specifically address the roles of NF-κB in pancreatitis, the active form of NF-κB subunit can be expressed in the pancreas. IKK contains a canonical MAP kinase activation loop motif in which phosphorylation of both serine residues is necessary for activation. Mutation of both serine residues to glutamate residues mimics the effect of p-serine and generates high kinase activity.[59,60] An early attempt to conditionally overexpress the constitutively active mutant of IKK2 in the pancreas used a tetracycline-inducible system. To achieve transgene expression in the pancreas, tetO-IKK2-EE (EE denotes serine to glutamate mutations) animals were crossed with CMV-reverse tetracycline-responsive transactivator (rtTA) mice.[61] In these double transgenic animals, doxycycline treatment induced expression of IKK2-EE in pancreatic acinar cells, resulting in moderate activation of the IKK complex. IKK2 expression in the pancreas had a mosaic pattern, and the activation level of the NF-κB cascade induced by IKK2 was considerably lower compared with that observed after supramaximal caerulein stimulation, but it still led to the formation of the leucocyte infiltrates observed after 4 weeks of doxycycline stimulation. The infiltrates were mainly composed of B lymphocytes and macrophages. However, only minor damage to pancreatic tissue was observed, indicating that a moderate level of activation is not sufficient to induce pancreatic damage in mice.[62]

The influence of expression and thus activation level of NF-κB on the development of AP was confirmed by a second study from the same group of investigators published a few months later. In the new transgene system, transgenic mice expressing the rtTA gene under the control of a rat elastase promoter were generated to mediate acinar cell-specific expression of IKK2 alleles. Expression of dominant-negative IKK2 ameliorated caerulein-induced pancreatitis but did not affect trypsinogen activation. Expression of constitutively active IKK2 was sufficient to induce AP, including increased edema, cellular infiltrates, necrosis, serum lipase levels, and pancreatic fibrosis.[63] These phenotypes were likely caused by increased expression levels from the tandem $(tetO)_7$ Promoter (64).

Activation of the IKK2/NF-κB signaling pathway causing AP was further confirmed by transgenic mice that encode the NF-κB p65 subunit or constitutively active IKK2 in pancreatic acinar cells.[65] Transgenic expression of p65 led to compensatory expression of the inhibitory subunit IKB-α. Therefore, there was no increased NF-κB activity or clear phenotype. However, p65 transgenic mice had higher levels of NF-κB activity in acinar cells and increased levels of inflammation in pancreatic tissue upon caerulein challenge. In contrast, pancreas-specific expression of active IKK2 directly increased the activity of NF-κB in acinar cells and induced pancreatitis. Prolonged activity of IKK2 resulted in the activation of stellate cells, loss of acinar cells, and initiation of fibrosis, which are the characteristics of chronic pancreatitis. Co-expression of IKK2 and p65 further increased the expression levels of inflammatory mediators and the severity of pancreatitis.[65] In addition, this pathway also orchestrated oncogenic Ras-induced inflammation and tumorigenesis, which are further discussed below.[66]

Overall, these findings indicate that NF-κB activity increased the severity of pancreatic inflammation, and strategies to inactivate NF-κB may be used to treat patients with acute or chronic pancreatitis. However, selective truncation of the p65 gene (**Figure 3**), which leads to the reduction the NF-κB activity in pancreatic exocrine cells, surprisingly led to both severe injury of the acinar cells and systemic adverse events.[67] This is because the expression and induction of the protective pancreas-specific acute phase protein pancreatitis-associated protein 1 (PAP1) depends on RelA/p65. Lentiviral gene transfer of PAP1 cDNA reduced the severity of pancreatitis in mice with selective truncation of RelA/p65. Opposing functions of RelA/p65 on AP in different cell types have been reported. For example, RelA/p65 activation in myeloid cells promotes the pathogenesis of CP but protects against chronic inflammation in acinar cells.[68]

The assembled data argue that NF-κB functions more generally as a central regulator of stress responses and regulates both inflammation and cell survival. Coupling stress responsiveness and antiapoptotic pathways through the use

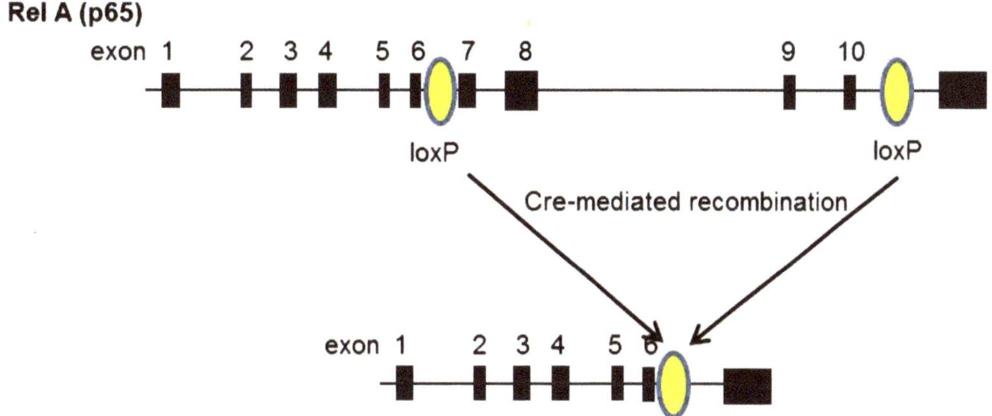

Figure 3. An example of tissue specific gene deletion. Two identical loxp sites flank several exons of the p65 gene. Cre mediated recombination removes the sequences between these two sites, causing gene truncation or deletion.

of a common transcription factor may result in increased cell survival following stress insults.[56]

Functional roles of IKK1 (IKKα)

IκB kinase α (IKKα) is a subunit of the IKK complex, which functions together with IKKβ and IKKγ/NEMO. Although it is involved in the regulation of NK-κB activity by phosphorylation of IκB proteins, which triggers their degradation, IKKα is not required for degradation of IκB by proinflammatory stimuli. IKKα is more important in alternative NF-κB signaling in which RelB:p52 dimers are activated.[53] Global loss of IKKα perturbs multiple morphogenetic events, including limb and skeletal patterning and the proliferation and differentiation of epidermal keratinocytes.[53,69,70] Pancreatic-specific IKKα ablation using PDX-CRE results in acinar cell vacuolization and death, fibrosis, and inflammation, resembling chronic pancreatitis in humans. These studies indicate that IKKα plays a central role in maintaining pancreatic acinar cell homeostasis.[71,72] The role of IKKα in maintaining pancreatic homeostasis is independent of NF-κB or its protein kinase activity reflected in inactive IKK1 knock-in mutant mice, which exhibit no pancreatic abnormalities. In contrast, the loss of IKKα in acinar cells diminished autophagic protein degradation and caused the accumulation of p62 aggregates and ER stress. Pancreatic-specific p62 ablation ameliorated pancreatitis in IKKα deficient mice.[71]

IκB-α mutation/deletion and pancreatitis

One of the key target genes induced by NF κB is its inhibitor IκBα, which in turn inhibits NF-κB activity and thus establishes a feedback regulation mechanism for controlling NF-κB activity.[73] Therefore, IκB-α deficiency results in a sustained NF-κB response and severe widespread dermatitis in mice.[74] Although they appear normal at birth, IκB-α-/- mice exhibit severe runting, skin defects, and extensive granulopoiesis postnatally and typically die after 8 days.[75]

In a mouse model where the 2 well-defined κB enhancer elements and 4 additional κB-like sites in the IκBα promoter were altered and therefore defective in response to NF-κB activation-induced negative feedback, the mice became sick, had elevated serum cytokine levels, and died at 13 to 15 months of age. These mice were found to be hypersensitive to LPS-induced proinflammatory cytokine production and lethality. Pancreas, liver, and lung tissues derived from these mice at 3 months of age showed extensive perivascular lymphocytic infiltration. Immunohistochemical analysis revealed a phenotype resembling Sjögren's syndrome, an autoimmune disorder.[76]

Pancreas-specific ablation of IκB-α also led to increased basal NF-κB activity with small increases in cytokine and chemokine levels. In stark contrast, the basal increase of NF-κB did not cause any overt phenotype in the pancreas, but caerulein- and L-arginine-induced pancreatitis was ameliorated in IKB-$\alpha^{-/-}$ mice.[77] The amelioration of pancreatitis was lost in the mice when p65 was also ablated, indicating that the protective effects of IκB deletion were mediated by p65. These results were consistent with a previous study by this group reporting that pancreas-specific RelA/p65 truncation increased the susceptibility of acini to inflammation-associated cell death following caerulein-induced pancreatitis.[67] They concluded that acinar-cell NF-κB activation exerts a protective role in AP.

In summary, NF-κB regulates both cell survival and inflammation. The extent and mode of NF-κB manipulation, and the cellular context can have profoundly different consequences. The paradox that activation of IKK2 or p65 leads to both aggravation and amelioration of pancreatitis reflects the complicated roles of NF-κB signaling. The complexities of the NF-κB system, with both pro- and anti-inflammatory effects, have been discussed in an editorial.[78]

Ras signaling and pancreatitis

Ras proteins function as binary molecular switches that, when turned on in the GTP-bound state, interact with downstream signaling molecules to activate a wide variety of intracellular signaling networks regulating proliferation, differentiation, apoptosis, and cell migration.[79] Ras mutations lead to increased Ras activity and are observed in ~30% of all cancers. In particular, K-Ras mutations are found in nearly every pancreatic cancer, which is the fourth leading cause of cancer-related death in USA.[80] That mutant Ras is oncogenic has been shown in many *in vivo* and *in vitro* studies.[81] However, its role in the development of inflammation and fibrosis was not appreciated until recently.[66,82,83]

It is well known that activation of Ras mutations can induce either proliferation at low levels or senescence at high levels. In mice bearing targeted pancreas-specific activating mutations at the native K-Ras locus that promote low levels of Ras activity, pancreatic histology was normal at the early stages. Only a small subset of cells displayed hyperproliferation and tumorigenesis when the levels of Ras activity were significantly elevated.[84] Evidence for the existence of a threshold of Ras pathway activity in pancreatic pathology comes from studies of high levels of mutant K-Ras expression using a transgenic approach (**Figure 4A**).[82] Although the expression of endogenous levels of mutant K-Ras results in minimal change in the pancreas, higher levels of expression generate Ras pathway activity that mimics what is observed in pancreatic cancer cells. In this model, increased Ras activity in pancreatic

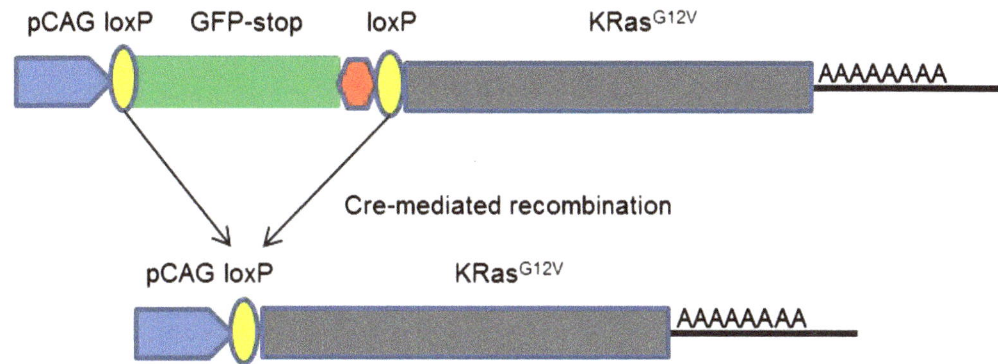

B.

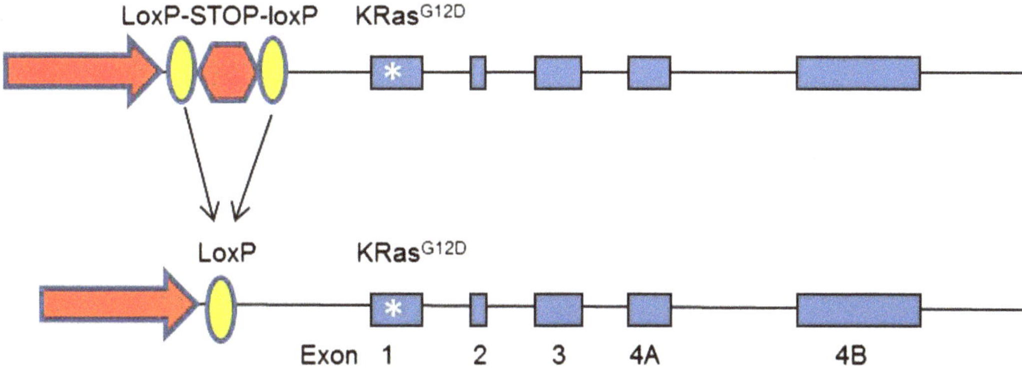

Figure 4. Different expression levels in transgene and knock-in models. (A) Mutant KRas was expressed at high level from a strong CMV chimeric promoter (pCAG) after Cre recombination. (B) A mutation was knocked into the endogenous KRas exon (*). Upon Cre recombination, the mutant KRas was expressed from its native promoter at physiological levels.

acinar cells caused rapid and abundant development of inflammatory cell infiltration, fibrosis, acinar cell loss, and atrophy. This model confirms that elevation of Ras activity is sufficient to cause chronic pancreatitis-like changes. These data suggest that the level of Ras pathway activity, rather than the presence of mutations, is biologically important.

Transgenic overexpression of mutant K-Ras provides proof-of-concept that high Ras activity will cause an inflammatory response with drastic fibrosis. However, under physiological conditions, humans or mice with knock-in mutant Ras express only endogenous levels of mutant K-Ras. While expression of oncogenic Ras at physiological levels in a K-Ras knock-in model generally does not directly cause pathological outcomes (**Figure 4B**),[85] the presence of mutations predispose to significant elevation of Ras activity by various etiologic stimuli.[66]

Stimuli that cause only transient up-regulation of Ras activity in WT animals induced enhanced and prolonged stimulation in animals bearing oncogenic K-Ras. Importantly, this increased Ras signaling led to the development of chronic inflammatory changes similar to those observed in transgenic K-Ras mice with high Ras activity. Further study demonstrated that inflammatory or physiologic stimuli triggered an NF-κB-mediated positive feedback mechanism involving Cox-2 that amplified Ras activity to pathological levels. Because a large proportion of the adult human population possess Ras mutations, disruption of this positive feedback loop may be an important strategy for cancer prevention.[66] It may be puzzling why stimulation is needed for "constitutively active" mutant

Ras to increase in activity and cause pathology. However, it has been demonstrated that oncogenic K-Ras is not constitutively active, as has been believed, but can be readily activated by upstream stimuli leading to prolonged strong Ras activity.[79] These data indicate that in addition to targeting K-Ras downstream effectors, interventions to reduce K-Ras activation may have important cancer-preventive value, especially in patients with oncogenic Ras mutations.

ER Stress and Pancreatitis

Pancreatic acinar cells are specialized for the production of many digestive enzymes. The enzyme proteins are produced in the ER, a multifunctional organelle responsible for the synthesis and folding of proteins in the secretory pathway. When misfolded proteins in the ER exceed the capacity of ER chaperones (e.g., GRP78), the unfolded protein response (UPR) will be activated. In mammalian cells, the UPR is transduced by 3 ER-localized transmembrane protein sensors, activating transcription factor 6α (ATF6α), inositol-requiring kinase 1α (IRE1α), and PKR-like ER kinase (PERK). ATF6α leads to increased transcription of ER chaperones, including GRP78 (BiP) and protein foldases. Activation of IRE1 induces the splicing and activation of XBP1 to its active transcription factor form (sXBP1), which also regulates the expression of various chaperones, foldases, and other protective molecules. PERK activation leads to phosphorylation of eukaryotic initiation factor (eIF)-2α and results in decreased protein translation. At a certain level, the UPR mechanisms decrease protein misfolding and alleviate stress by shutting down translation and upregulating protective molecules. However, prolonged and severe UPRs can lead to apoptosis by upregulating the transcription factor C/EBP-homologous protein (CHOP) and the IRE1-activated JNK pathway. Severe ER stress also impairs cellular homeostasis through ER calcium leakage, mitochondrial damage, oxidative stress, energy depletion, and activation of caspases. ER stress triggered by protein misfolding represents a potential disease mechanism for pancreatitis.[16,86-90] Genetic deletion of GRP78 leads to peri-implantation lethality.[91] Grp78 heterozygosity regulates ER chaperone balance against a dietary- and genetic background, and improved ER protein folding may be protective against pancreatitis.[92] Pancreata that have a genetic deletion of CHOP are histologically normal, and the role of CHOP in pancreatitis remains controversial.[93,94]

XBP1 and pancreatitis

Pancreatic acinar-specific disruption of Xbp1 in adult pancreatic acinar cells with Mist1-CreERT led to the activation of the UPR, extensive apoptosis followed by a rapid recovery phase that included expansion of the centroacinar cell compartment, formation of tubular complexes that contained Hes1- and Sox9-expressing cells, and regeneration of acinar cells that expressed Mist1 from the residual, surviving Xbp1+ cell population. This study suggests that XBP1 is required for the homeostasis of adult acinar cells in mice.[95] In ethanol-fed Xbp1$^{+/-}$ mice, ER stress was associated with disorganized and dilated ER, loss of zymogen granules, accumulation of autophagic vacuoles, and increased acinar cell death.[96]

PERK and pancreatitis

The exocrine and endocrine pancreas developed normally in Perk$^{-/-}$ mice. Postnatally, ER distention and activation of the ER stress transducer IRE1α accompanied increased cell death and led to progressive diabetes mellitus and exocrine pancreatic insufficiency.[97] In another study with pancreatic specific PERK ablation (Ela-CRE), there was no evidence of perturbations in ER-stress, but acinar cells succumbed to a nonapoptotic form of cell death, oncosis, which is associated with a pronounced inflammatory response and induction of pancreatitis stress response genes.[98] In the same study, the effects of activating transcription factor 4 (ATF4) on the pancreas were evaluated in ATF4-deficient mice because translation of the ATF4 transcription factor is positively regulated by PERK activation. In these mice, the exocrine pancreata of neonatal (P4) mice were severely underdeveloped, and the number of acini and the acinar cell size were greatly reduced. The pancreatic acini were dispersed and often were not in close proximity to neighboring acini, resulting in an expanded extracellular space. Moreover, ATF4-deficient acinar cells appeared smaller with substantially less zymogen granule content, which correlated with an increase in the diameter of the centroacinar duct. In adults the centroacinar duct was greatly expanded resulting in a tubular appearance of the exocrine pancreas with numerous adipocytes.[98]

Cystic Fibrosis (CF)

CF is caused by mutations in the gene encoding the cystic fibrosis transmembrane conductance regulator (*CFTR*). The CFTR protein is highly expressed in pancreatic duct epithelia. CFTR is an ion channel that conducts chloride and thiocyanate ions across epithelial cell membranes. Mutations in the *CFTR* gene lead to dysregulation of epithelial fluid transport in the lung, pancreas, and other organs. In the CF pancreas, a high protein concentration resulting from a low flow of secretions causes precipitation in the duct, leading to obstruction and damage. These changes in the CF pancreas begin *in utero*. Eventually, this process results in the obstruction of ducts by mucus, the destruction of acini, severe inflammation, generalized fibrosis, and fat replacement.[99]

Mouse models of CF

Since the discovery of *CFTR* gene in 1989,[100] many genetic mouse models have been developed to study the pathophysiology of CF and to test experimental therapies prior to clinical trials.[101,102] All *CFTR*-mutant mice develop prominent intestinal disease similar to that seen in human CF, and die from intestinal obstruction during the first month of life. Although the lung and pancreas are the organs severely affected in human CF, mouse models with *CFTR* mutations lack obvious lung and pancreas histology except in one study.[101] In that study, $Cftr^{-/-}$ mice were weaned to a liquid diet to minimize bowel obstruction and optimize long-term viability. Under these conditions, the intercalated, intralobular and interlobular ducts, and acinar lumina of the exocrine pancreas of the $Cftr^{-/-}$ animals were dilated and filled with inspissated material. There was also mild inflammation and acinar cell drop out. Quantitative measurements of the pancreas showed significant acinar atrophy and increased acinar volume compared with age-matched WT littermates.[103] $Cftr^{-/-}$ mice were also more sensitive to caerulein-induced severe pancreatitis than WT mice.[104,105]

When human *CFTR* (*hCFTR*) was expressed in $Cftr^{-/-}$ mice under the control of the rat intestinal fatty acid-binding protein gene promoter, the mice survived and showed functional correction of ileal goblet cell and crypt cell hyperplasia and cyclic adenosine monophosphate-stimulated chloride secretion. These results support the concept that transfer of the *hCFTR* gene may be a useful strategy for correcting physiologic defects in patients with CF.[106]

Pig models of CF

Because pigs share many anatomical and physiological features with humans, pigs with *CFTR* gene disruptions or mutations (DeltaF508) were generated by adeno-associated virus (rAAV)-mediated gene targeting.[107] Newborn pigs lacking CFTR exhibited defective chloride transport and developed meconium ileus, exocrine pancreatic destruction, and focal biliary cirrhosis, replicating the abnormalities seen in newborn humans with CF. The $Cftr^{-/-}$ porcine pancreas was smaller than that in WT controls. Microscopic examination revealed small, degenerative lobules with increased loose adipose and myxomatous tissue, as well as scattered-to-moderate cellular inflammation. Residual acini had diminished amounts of eosinophilic zymogen granules. Ducts were variably dilated and obstructed by eosinophilic material plus neutrophils and macrophages mixed with cellular debris. Pancreatic endocrine tissue was spared. These changes are similar to those seen in human CF.[108,109] $Cftr^{DF508/DF508}$ pancreata had reduced parenchyma compared with those in $Cftr^{+/+}$ mice, but the destruction was slightly less severe than in $Cftr^{-/-}$ because this mutant has residual CFTR activity.[110] The pig model may provide opportunities to address persistent questions about CF pathogenesis and accelerate the discovery of strategies for prevention and treatment.

Ferret model of CF

The domestic ferret is also an alternative species to be used for modeling human CF because ferrets and humans share similar airway cytoarchitecture and *CFTR* gene expression patterns. A *CFTR* gene-deficient domestic ferret model has been developed using rAAV-mediated gene targeting of exon 10 in fibroblasts and nuclear transfer cloning.[111] Neonatal CFTR-knockout ferrets demonstrated many of the characteristics of human CF disease. The pancreata of newborn $Cftr^{-/-}$ ferrets were normal at the gross level, but histologic lesions were evident, with acinar lumen and duct dilation in all animals. Overall, the level of histopathology in the newborn $Cftr^{-/-}$ ferret pancreas appears quite similar to that seen in CF infants and significantly less severe than the extensive destruction observed in the exocrine pancreas of newborn CF pigs.[112] Further evaluation of older CF animals indicated that 85% of these CF animals had significant loss of the exocrine pancreas with associated fibrosis, ductal proliferation, and plugging of intralobular ducts. Interestingly, some of the CF animals had fewer histological changes, with only focal loss of exocrine parenchyma and cystic dilation of ducts. These findings demonstrate that the ferret model retains the variability in pancreatic phenotypes also seen in CF patients, where 10% to 15% of CF patients retain partial or complete exocrine pancreas function. Modifier genes are the most likely explanation for the pancreatic sufficiency.[113]

Inflammatory Factors/Growth Factors/Cytokines and Pancreatitis

Transforming growth factor-beta (TGF-β)

TGF-β 1 proteins are central regulators of pancreatic cell function and play key roles in pancreatic development and disease.[114] In transgenic mice that express TGF-β1 in the pancreatic islet cells directed by a human insulin promoter, fibroblast proliferation and abnormal deposition of macrophages and neutrophils in the extracellular matrix were observed from birth onward, and replaced almost the entire exocrine pancreas. TGF-β1 inhibited proliferation of acinar cells and resulted in small islet-cell clusters. These findings suggest that TGF-β1 might mediate diseases associated with extracellular matrix deposition, such as chronic pancreatitis.[115]

In a mouse model in which TGF-β signaling was inactivated in pancreas by overexpressing a dominant-negative mutant form of the TGF-β type II receptor under the control of the pS2/TFF1 promoter, the mice showed marked increases in MHC class II molecules and matrix metalloproteinase expression in pancreatic acinar cells. These mice also showed increased susceptibility to caerulein-induced pancreatitis. Therefore, TGF-β signaling seems to be essential either for maintaining normal immune homeostasis and suppressing autoimmunity or for preserving the integrity of pancreatic acinar cells.[116] Remarkably, in another study from the same group, attenuated caerulein-induced pancreatic fibrosis was reported in these mice.[117]

The dominant-negative mutant type II TGF-β receptor (DNR), the extracellular and transmembrane domains of TβRII, blocks signaling of all three TGF-β isoforms. In transgenic mice expressing DNR with a mouse MT1 promoter, the pancreas showed severe abnormalities, including ductular transformation, neo-angiogenesis, inter- and intralobular fibrosis, and adipose replacement of acini in the exocrine pancreas.[118] These mice exhibited reduced pancreatitis in response to caerulein compared with WT control mice, indicating that a functional TGF-β signaling pathway may be required for caerulein to induce AP.[119]

In mice with conditional knockout of the TGFβ type II receptor by an S100A4/fibroblast-specific protein 1 (FSP1) Cre, which is expressed in dendritic cells (DCs) and fibroblasts, autoimmune pancreatitis (AIP) spontaneously developed by 6 weeks of age. Adoptive transfer of bone marrow-derived DC from Tgfbr2 KO mice into 2-week-old syngeneic WT mice resulted in reproduction of pancreatitis within 6 weeks. In contrast, adoptive transfer of Tgfbr2 KO DC to adult mice failed to induce pancreatitis, suggesting a developmental event in AIP pathogenesis. This model illustrates the role of TGFβ for maintaining myeloid DC immune tolerance.[120]

COX-2

Cyclooxygenases (COX-1 and -2) are rate-limiting enzymes in the production of prostaglandins. COX-1 expression is generally constitutive, whereas COX-2 is usually induced by stimuli involved in inflammatory responses.[121] Overexpression of COX-2 in transgenic mice using a bovine keratin-5 promoter caused a chronic pancreatitis-like state by 3 months of age. By 6 to 8 months, strongly dysplastic features suggestive of pancreatic ductal adenocarcinoma emerged in the metaplastic ducts. The abnormal pancreatic phenotype can be completely prevented by maintaining mice on a diet containing celecoxib, a well-characterized COX-2 inhibitor.[122] In contrast, COX-2 over expression in pancreatic acinar cells increased pancreas size but did not affect histology within 5-6 months. After 8 months, COX-2-expressing mice developed chronic inflammation and numerous pancreatic cysts (ductal ectasia). None of the COX-2-expressing mice developed PanINs or tumors within 1 year. However, co-expression of Cox-2 and mutant KRas caused dramatic inflammation resembling severe chronic pancreatitis and abundant PanINs.[66] In line with this study, COX-2 but not COX-1 deficiency attenuated the severity of AP.[123]

Interleukin-1 beta (IL-1β)

Pancreatitis is associated with the increase of numerous cytokine/chemokines.[124] A transgenic approach can be used to study the function of these factors. For example, IL-1β is a proinflammatory cytokine involved in many inflammation pathways. In a transgenic mouse model in which a rat elastase promoter drives the expression of human IL-1β, the pancreas was atrophied, and there was increased acinar proliferation and apoptosis, which is typical of chronic pancreatitis. Older mice displayed acinar-ductal metaplasia but did not develop neoplasia.[125]

Lymphotoxin (LT) α and β

LTα and LTβ are cytokines of the TNF superfamily and are involved in the regulation of immunity. LTα and β mRNA levels were increased in pancreatic tissues from patients with AIP. Acinar-specific overexpression of LTαβ (Ela1-LTαβ) in mice led to an autoimmune disorder with various features similar to AIP. Chronic inflammation developed only in the pancreas but was sufficient to cause systemic autoimmunity. Acinar-specific overexpression of LTαβ did not cause autoimmunity in lymphocyte-deficient mice.[126] This transgenic mouse model has the critical features of human AIP, including progressive pancreatitis and the formation of B- and T-cell zones that are reminiscent of tertiary lymphoid tissues. Most surprisingly, the overexpression of LT in the pancreas was sufficient to trigger a systemic autoimmune response that involved distant organs.[127]

Other Models

Autophagy

Autophagy degrades intracellular protein aggregates and damaged or unneeded organelles through a lysosome-driven process and recycles components vital for cell survival. There are 3 major autophagic pathways, chaperone-mediated autophagy, microautophagy, and macroautophagy.[128] The major form of autophagy is macroautophagy.

Impaired autophagic flux can lead to the formation of large vacuoles resulting fom the fusion of autophagic vacuoles. Accumulation of large vacuoles in acinar cells is a prominent feature of pancreatitis, and most of these vacuoles are predominantly autolysosomes accompanied by increased LC3-II and p62, which are signs of increased and defective autophagy.[129] Impaired autophagy can cause accumulation of damaged mitochondria, resulting in decreased ATP production, reactive oxygen species (ROS) overproduction, inflammasome activation, and ultimately cell death.[130] Impaired autophagy also induces the accumulation of aggregates that contain p62, a signaling hub for oxidative stress and NF-κB pathways.[131] In addition, autophagic dysfunction mediates the accumulation of active trypsin in acinar cells, another key mechanism of pancreatitis.[129]

The assembly of Atg5-Atg12-Atg16 and the Atg5-Atg12-Atg16-mediated conjugation of LC3-I with phosphatidylethanolamine is key to the formation of autophagosomes. Therefore, the absence of Atg5 blocks autophagic processing, leading to the accumulation of protein aggregates and damaged organelles.[132]. The role of Atg5 was recently studied in pancreas-specific Atg5-deficient mice by crossing $Atg5^{flox/flox}$ with Ptf1aCre mice.[133] Pancreata were normal in 1-week-old Atg5 deficient mice. However, the loss of Atg5 resulted in edematous and enlarged pancreata by 4 weeks of age. With increasing age, the pancreata became atrophic, and the mice lost a significant amount of body weight. Histologically, acinar cells exhibited early cytoplasmic vacuolization and acquired a hypertrophic phenotype. Evidence of incremental fibrosis, pancreatic stellate cell activation, duct-like structures, inflammation, proliferation, apoptosis, and necrosis were evident. Blocked autophagic degradation was also evidenced by the accumulation of improperly formed autophagosomes containing various cellular constituents. Increased serum lipase activity, increased trypsin, and cathepsin B activity were found in pancreatic tissue. Defective pancreatic autophagy leads to the accumulation of p62, damaged mitochondria, increased ROS, and terminal ER stress. ROS and p62 activate Nrf2/Nqo1/p53 signaling, thereby exacerbating cellular stress, necrosis/apoptosis, inflammation, and fibrosis. Surprisingly, the development of CP was much less pronounced in female mice than in male mice. Antioxidative treatment prevents the progression of CP in male mice.[133] This study represents the first detailed analysis of the effects of genetic ablation of a key autophagy mediator in the pancreas.[134]

Keratin K8 and K18

K8 and K18 are the major components of the intermediate-filament cytoskeleton of simple epithelia. Transgenic mice expressing the human K8 (KRT8) gene exhibited a moderate increase in keratin-content of the epithelia.[135] These mice displayed progressive exocrine pancreas alterations, including dysplasia, loss of acinar architecture, redifferentiation of acinar cells to ductal cells, inflammation, fibrosis, substitution of exocrine tissue by adipose tissue, increased cell proliferation, and apoptosis. These results indicate that simple epithelial keratins play a relevant role in the regulation of exocrine pancreas homeostasis.[136] In contrast, another study showed that K8- and K18-overexpressing pancreata were histologically similar to those of WT mice, whereas K8/K18 pancreata displayed age-enhanced vacuolization and atrophy of the exocrine pancreas. Zymogen granules in K8/K18 pancreata were 50% smaller and more dispersed than when in the normal apical concentration.[137]

Liver X receptors (LXR)

LXRα and LXRβ are nuclear receptors belonging to the ligand-activated transcription factor superfamily and play a key role in controlling lipid and glucose metabolism. The ligands for LXRs are 22-hydroxycholesterol, 24(S)-hydroxycholesterol, 25-epoxycholesterol, and 27-hydroxycholesterol, which at physiological concentrations, bind to and activate these receptors. $LXR\beta^{-/-}$ mice showed pancreatic exocrine insufficiency with reduced serum levels of amylase and lipase, and the pancreas pathology indicated chronic inflammatory infiltration and increased apoptosis without compensatory proliferation in the ductal epithelium.[138,139]

The serum response factor (SRF)

SRF is a transcription factor regulating many immediate early genes and has been implicated in the control of differentiation, growth, and cell death. Using pancreatic-specific disruption of this gene, it was shown that SRF is indispensable for pancreatic ontogenesis; and after weaning, these mice developed profound pancreatitis. At 4 months of age, the exocrine pancreas had completely disappeared in most animals and was replaced by adipose tissue. Interestingly, the organization and function of the endocrine islets of Langerhans remained well preserved even though PDX-Cre also targets the deletion of SRF in those cells.[140]

Cilia

Defects in cilia formation or function have been implicated in several human genetic diseases, including polycystic kidney disease (PKD). Pancreatic lesions are found in approximately 10% of PKD patients, suggesting a connection between cilia defects and pancreatic pathologies. *Kif3a*, the gene encoding for a subunit of the kinesin-2 complex that is essential for cilia formation, was conditionally inactivated in pancreatic epithelia using PDX-Cre. The pancreata of these mutant mice displayed a loss of acinar cells shortly after birth and an acinar-to-ductal metaplasia and periductal fibrosis by 2 weeks after birth. At 12 weeks, the acinar cells were replaced by adipose tissue.

At 6 months, the pancreata in these mice were composed of cysts that enlarged over time.[141,142]

Summary

The recent use of genetically engineered mice in pancreatic research has greatly improved our understanding of the molecular mechanisms of pancreatitis. Genetic approaches have also assisted the development of clinically relevant models of pancreatitis. In general, the genetic approaches are believed to be more specific than pharmacological compounds for targeting a particular pathway. However, caution should be used when interpreting the results of genetic studies. Expression of a transgene at an irrelevant level may give rise to artificial effects or no phenotype. Expression of an irrelevant gene (e.g., toxin) may not reflect pathogenesis in humans. Genetic deletion of a gene may cause paradoxical effects because many genes (e.g., ER stress related genes, NF-κB) are important in the pathogenesis of inflammation but are also critical for homeostasis. Because of species-specific gene functions, different phenotypic patterns, or no phenotypes, may develop when mouse counterparts are targeted. "Off target" effects should also be considered because a single gene may regulate many pathways. In addition, pancreatitis is caused by multifaceted mechanisms.[143] Thus most of the genetically engineered pancreatitis models, which are created by targeting 1 gene may not be appropriate for testing general preventive and therapeutic interventions. It should also be noted that pancreatitis initiation, progression, and regression involve interactions between pancreatic parenchymal cells and inflammatory cells (CD11c-Cre, LysM-Cre, F4/80-Cre, etc), stellate cells (SMA-Cre), and endothelial cells (VECadherin-CreERT) that can also be targeted. Using these cell-specific Cre to target gene expression in the specific cell population is also of great interest in pancreatitis research.

Acknowledgements

The project described was supported by P50 CA102701 and K12 CA90628 from the National Cancer Institute and W81XWH-15-1-0257 from the Department of Defense. This publication was also supported by the CTSA Grant UL1 TR000135 from the National Center for Advancing Translational Sciences (NCATS), a component of the National Institutes of Health. The content is solely the responsibility of the authors and does not necessarily represent the official views of the National Institutes of Health or the Department of Defense. We also thank Ms. Kelly E. Viola, ELS, for critical editing.

References

1. Chiari H. Über die Selbstverdauung des menschlichen Pankreas. *Zeitschrift für Heilkunde* 1896; 17: 69-96.
2. Gilliland L and Steer ML. Effects of ethionine on digestive enzyme synthesis and discharge by mouse pancreas. *Am J Physiol Gastrointest Liver Physiol.* 1980; 239: G418-426. PMID: 6159794.
3. Koike H, Steer ML, and Meldolesi J. Pancreatic effects of ethionine: blockade of exocytosis and appearance of crinophagy and autophagy precede cellular necrosis. *Am J Physiol Gastrointest Liver Physiol.* 1982; 242: G297-307. PMID: 7065251.
4. Bialek R, Willemer S, Arnold R, and Adler G. Evidence of intracellular activation of serine proteases in acute cerulein-induced pancreatitis in rats. *Scand J Gastroenterol.* 1991; 26: 190-196. PMID: 1707179.
5. Willemer S,Bialek R, and Adler G. Localization of lysosomal and digestive enzymes in cytoplasmic vacuoles in caerulein-pancreatitis. *Histochemistry.* 1990; 94: 161-170. PMID: 2358374.
6. Leach SD, Modlin IM, Scheele GA, and Gorelick FS. Intracellular activation of digestive zymogens in rat pancreatic acini. Stimulation by high doses of cholecystokinin. *J Clin Invest.* 1991; 87: 362-366. PMID: 1985109.
7. Whitcomb DC, Gorry MC, Preston RA, Furey W, Sossenheimer MJ, Ulrich CD, et al. Hereditary pancreatitis is caused by a mutation in the cationic trypsinogen gene. *Nat Genet.* 1996; 14: 141-145. PMID: 8841182.
8. Whitcomb DC. Hereditary pancreatitis: new insights into acute and chronic pancreatitis. *Gut.* 1999; 45: 317-322. PMID: 10446089.
9. Weber P, Keim V, and Zimmer KP. Hereditary pancreatitis and mutation of the trypsinogen gene. *Arch Dis Child.* 1999; 80: 473-474. PMID: 10208958.
10. Blackstone M. Premature trypsin activation in hereditary pancreatitis. *Gastroenterology.* 1998; 115: 796-799. PMID: 9742004.
11. Wyllie R. Hereditary pancreatitis. *Am J Gastroenterol.* 1997; 92: 1079-1080. PMID: 9219774.
12. Sahin-Toth M and Toth M. Gain-of-function mutations associated with hereditary pancreatitis enhance autoactivation of human cationic trypsinogen. *Biochem Biophys Res Commun.* 2000; 278: 286-289. PMID: 11097832.
13. Archer H, Jura N, Keller J, Jacobson M, and Bar-Sagi D. A mouse model of hereditary pancreatitis generated by transgenic expression of R122H trypsinogen. *Gastroenterology.* 2006; 131: 1844-1855. PMID: 17087933.
14. Witt H, Luck W, Hennies HC, Classen M, Kage A, Lass U, et al. Mutations in the gene encoding the serine protease inhibitor, Kazal type 1 are associated with chronic pancreatitis. *Nat Genet* 2000; 25: 213-216. PMID: 10835640.
15. van Acker GJ, Perides G, and Steer ML. Co-localization hypothesis: a mechanism for the intrapancreatic activation of digestive enzymes during the early phases of acute pancreatitis. *World J Gastroenterol.* 2006; 12: 1985-1990. PMID: 16610045.
16. Sah RP, Garg P, and Saluja AK. Pathogenic mechanisms of acute pancreatitis. *Curr Opinion Gastroenterol.* 2012; 28: 507-515. PMID: 22885948.
17. Gukovsky I, Pandol SJ, and Gukovskaya AS. Organellar dysfunction in the pathogenesis of pancreatitis. *Antioxid Redox Signal.* 2011; 15: 2699-2710. PMID: 21834686.
18. Petersen OH, Gerasimenko OV, Tepikin AV, and Gerasimenko JV. Aberrant Ca(2+) signalling through acidic calcium stores in pancreatic acinar cells. *Cell Calcium.* 2011; 50: 193-199. PMID: 21435718.

19. Gaiser S, Daniluk J, Liu Y, Tsou L, Chu J, Lee W, et al. Intracellular activation of trypsinogen in transgenic mice induces acute but not chronic pancreatitis. *Gut*. 2011; 60: 1379-1388. PMID: 21471572.
20. Nathan JD, Romac J, Peng RY, Peyton M, Macdonald RJ, and Liddle RA. Transgenic expression of pancreatic secretory trypsin inhibitor-I ameliorates secretagogue-induced pancreatitis in mice. *Gastroenterology*. 2005; 128: 717-727. PMID: 15765407.
21. Romac JM, Shahid RA, Choi SS, Karaca GF, Westphalen CB, Wang TC, et al. Pancreatic Secretory Trypsin Inhibitor 1 Reduces the Severity of Chronic Pancreatitis in Mice Overexpressing Interleukin-1beta in the Pancreas. *Am J Physiol Gastrointest Liver Physiol*. 2011; 302: G535-G541. PMID: 22173919.
22. Dawra R, Sah RP, Dudeja V, Rishi L, Talukdar R, Garg P, et al. Intra-acinar trypsinogen activation mediates early stages of pancreatic injury but not inflammation in mice with acute pancreatitis. *Gastroenterology*. 2011; 141: 2210-2217 e2212. PMID: 21875495.
23. Han B, Ji B, and Logsdon CD. CCK independently activates intracellular trypsinogen and NF-kappaB in rat pancreatic acinar cells. *Am J Physiol Cell Physiol*. 2001; 280: C465-C472. PMID: 11171565.
24. Ji B, Gaiser S, Chen X, Ernst SA, and Logsdon CD. Intracellular trypsin induces pancreatic acinar cell death but not NF-kappaB activation. *J Biol Chem*. 2009; 284: 17488-17498. PMID: 19383608.
25. Ji B, Song J, Tsou L, Bi Y, Gaiser S, Mortensen R, et al. Robust acinar cell transgene expression of CreErT via BAC recombineering. *Genesis*. 2008; 46: 390-395. PMID: 18693271.
26. Kazal LA, Spicer DS, and Brahinsky RA. Isolation of a crystalline trypsin inhibitor-anticoagulant protein from pancreas. *J Am Chem Soc*. 1948; 70: 3034-3040. PMID: 18882536.
27. Marchbank T, Freeman TC, and Playford RJ. Human pancreatic secretory trypsin inhibitor. Distribution, actions and possible role in mucosal integrity and repair. *Digestion*. 59: 167-174,1998. PMID: 9643675.
28. Ohmuraya M and Yamamura K. Roles of serine protease inhibitor Kazal type 1 (SPINK1) in pancreatic diseases. *Exp Anim*. 2011; 60: 433-444. PMID: 22041280.
29. LaRusch J, Solomon S, and Whitcomb DC. Pancreatitis Overview. *GeneReviews*. 2014. Available at http://www.ncbi.nlm.nih.gov/books/NBK190101/.
30. Paju A and Stenman UH. Biochemistry and clinical role of trypsinogens and pancreatic secretory trypsin inhibitor. *Critical reviews in clinical laboratory sciences*. 2006; 43: 103-142. PMID: 16517420.
31. Awano H, Lee T, Yagi M, Masamune A, Kume K, Takeshima Y, et al. Childhood-onset hereditary pancreatitis with mutations in the CT gene and SPINK1 gene. *Pediatrics international*. 2013; 55: 646-649. PMID: 24134754.
32. Neuschwander-Tetri BA, Fimmel CJ, Kladney RD, Wells LD, and Talkad V. Differential expression of the trypsin inhibitor SPINK3 mRNA and the mouse ortholog of secretory granule protein ZG-16p mRNA in the mouse pancreas after repetitive injury. *Pancreas*. 2004; 28: e104-e111. PMID: 15097871.
33. Ohmuraya M, Hirota M, Araki K, Baba H, and Yamamura K. Enhanced trypsin activity in pancreatic acinar cells deficient for serine protease inhibitor kazal type 3. *Pancreas*. 2006; 33: 104-106. PMID: 16804421.
34. Ohmuraya M, Hirota M, Araki M, Mizushima N, Matsui M, Mizumoto T, et al. Autophagic cell death of pancreatic acinar cells in serine protease inhibitor Kazal type 3-deficient mice. *Gastroenterology*. 2005; 129: 696-705. PMID: 16083722.
35. Sakata K, Ohmuraya M, Araki K, Suzuki C, Ida S, Hashimoto D, et al. Generation and analysis of serine protease inhibitor kazal type 3-cre driver mice. *Exp Anim*. 2014; 63: 45-53. PMID: 24521862.
36. Romac JM, Ohmuraya M, Bittner C, Majeed MF, Vigna SR, Que J, et al. Transgenic expression of pancreatic secretory trypsin inhibitor-1 rescues SPINK3-deficient mice and restores a normal pancreatic phenotype. *Am J Physiol Gastrointest Liver Physiol*. 2010; 298: G518-G524. PMID: 20110462.
37. Solomon S and Whitcomb DC. Genetics of pancreatitis: an update for clinicians and genetic counselors. *Curr Gastroenterol Rep*. 2012; 14: 112-117. PMID: 22314809.
38. Comfort MW and Steinberg AG. Pedigree of a family with hereditary chronic relapsing pancreatitis. *Gastroenterology*. 1952; 21: 54-63. PMID: 14926813.
39. Le Bodic L, Bignon JD, Raguenes O, Mercier B, Georgelin T, Schnee M, et al. The hereditary pancreatitis gene maps to long arm of chromosome 7. *Hum Mol Genet*. 1996; 5: 549-554. PMID: 8845851.
40. Whitcomb DC, Preston RA, Aston CE, Sossenheimer MJ, Barua PS, Zhang Y, et al. A gene for hereditary pancreatitis maps to chromosome 7q35. *Gastroenterology*. 1996; 110: 1975-1980. PMID: 8964426.
41. Pandya A, Blanton SH, Landa B, Javaheri R, Melvin E, Nance WE, et al. Linkage studies in a large kindred with hereditary pancreatitis confirms mapping of the gene to a 16-cM region on 7q. *Genomics*. 1996; 38: 227-230. PMID: 8954806.
42. Chen JM and Ferec C. Genes, cloned cDNAs, and proteins of human trypsinogens and pancreatitis-associated cationic trypsinogen mutations. *Pancreas*. 2000; 21: 57-62. PMID: 10881933.
43. Antonarakis SE. Recommendations for a nomenclature system for human gene mutations. Nomenclature Working Group. *Human mutation*. 1998; 11: 1-3. PMID: 9450896.
44. Nemeth BC and Sahin-Toth M. Human cationic trypsinogen (PRSS1) variants and chronic pancreatitis. *Am J Physiol Gastrointest Liver Physiol*. 2014; 306: G466-G473. PMID: 24458023.
45. Weiss FU. Pancreatic cancer risk in hereditary pancreatitis. *Front Physiol*. 5: 70,2014. PMID: 24600409.
46. Selig L, Sack U, Gaiser S, Kloppel G, Savkovic V, Mossner J, et al. Characterisation of a transgenic mouse expressing R122H human cationic trypsinogen. *BMC Gastroenterol*. 2006; 6: 30. PMID: 17069643.
47. Athwal T, Huang W, Mukherjee R, Latawiec D, Chvanov M, Clarke R, et al. Expression of human cationic trypsinogen

(PRSS1) in murine acinar cells promotes pancreatitis and apoptotic cell death. *Cell Death Dis*. 2014; 5: e1165. PMID: 24722290.

48. DiDonato JA, Mercurio F, and Karin M. NF-kappaB and the link between inflammation and cancer. *Immunological Rev*. 2012; 246: 379-400. PMID: 22435567.
49. Sen R and Baltimore D. Inducibility of kappa immunoglobulin enhancer-binding protein Nf-kappa B by a posttranslational mechanism. *Cell*. 1986; 47: 921-928. PMID: 3096580.
50. Hinz M and Scheidereit C. The IkappaB kinase complex in NF-kappaB regulation and beyond. *EMBO Reports*. 2014; 15: 46-61. PMID: 24375677.
51. Napetschnig J and Wu H. Molecular basis of NF-kappaB signaling. *Ann Rev Biophys*. 42: 443-468,2013. PMID: 23495970.
52. Hoffmann A and Baltimore D. Circuitry of nuclear factor kappaB signaling. *Immunol Rev*. 2006; 210: 171-186. PMID: 16623771.
53. Hacker H and Karin M. Regulation and function of IKK and IKK-related kinases. 2006; *Sci STKE*. 2006: re13. PMID: 17047224.
54. Grady T, Liang P, Ernst SA, and Logsdon CD. Chemokine gene expression in rat pancreatic acinar cells is an early event associated with acute pancreatitis. *Gastroenterology*. 1997; 113: 1966-1975. PMID: 9394737.
55. Sah RP, Dawra RK, and Saluja AK. New insights into the pathogenesis of pancreatitis. *Curr Opinion Gastroenterol*. 2013; 29: 523-530. PMID: 23892538.
56. Oeckinghaus A and Ghosh S. The NF-kappaB family of transcription factors and its regulation. *Cold Spring Harb Perspect Biol*. 2009; 1: a000034. PMID: 20066092.
57. Verhelst K, Verstrepen L, Carpentier I, and Beyaert R. IkappaB kinase epsilon (IKKepsilon): a therapeutic target in inflammation and cancer. *Biochem Pharmacol*. 2013; 85: 873-880. PMID: 23333767.
58. Shen RR and Hahn WC. Emerging roles for the non-canonical IKKs in cancer. *Oncogene*. 2011; 30: 631-641. PMID: 21042276.
59. Delhase M, Hayakawa M, Chen Y, and Karin M. Positive and negative regulation of IkappaB kinase activity through IKKbeta subunit phosphorylation. *Science*. 1999; 284: 309-313. PMID: 10195894.
60. Mercurio F, Zhu H, Murray BW, Shevchenko A, Bennett BL, Li J, et al. IKK-1 and IKK-2: cytokine-activated IkappaB kinases essential for NF-kappaB activation. *Science*. 1997; 278: 860-866. PMID: 9346484.
61. Kistner A, Gossen M, Zimmermann F, Jerecic J, Ullmer C, Lubbert H, et al. Doxycycline-mediated quantitative and tissue-specific control of gene expression in transgenic mice. *Proc Natl Acad Sci U S A*. 1996; 93: 10933-10938. PMID: 8855286.
62. Aleksic T, Baumann B, Wagner M, Adler G, Wirth T, and Weber CK. Cellular immune reaction in the pancreas is induced by constitutively active IkappaB kinase-2. *Gut*. 2007; 56: 227-236. PMID: 16870717.
63. Baumann B, Wagner M, Aleksic T, von Wichert G, Weber CK, Adler G, et al. Constitutive IKK2 activation in acinar cells is sufficient to induce pancreatitis in vivo. *J Clin Invest*. 2007; 117: 1502-1513. PMID: 17525799.
64. Herrmann O, Baumann B, de Lorenzi R, Muhammad S, Zhang W, Kleesiek J, et al. IKK mediates ischemia-induced neuronal death. *Nature Med*. 2005; 11: 1322-1329,. PMID: 16286924.
65. Huang H, Liu Y, Daniluk J, Gaiser S, Chu J, Wang H, et al. Activation of nuclear factor-kappaB in acinar cells increases the severity of pancreatitis in mice. *Gastroenterology*. 2013; 144: 202-210,. PMID: 23041324.
66. Daniluk J, Liu Y, Deng D, Chu J, Huang H, Gaiser S, et al. An NF-kappaB pathway-mediated positive feedback loop amplifies Ras activity to pathological levels in mice. *J Clin Invest*. 2012; 122: 1519-1528. PMID: 22406536.
67. Algul H, Treiber M, Lesina M, Nakhai H, Saur D, Geisler F, et al. Pancreas-specific RelA/p65 truncation increases susceptibility of acini to inflammation-associated cell death following cerulein pancreatitis. *J Clin Invest*. 2007; 117: 1490-1501. PMID: 17525802.
68. Treiber M, Neuhofer P, Anetsberger E, Einwachter H, Lesina M, Rickmann M, et al. Myeloid, but not pancreatic, RelA/p65 is required for fibrosis in a mouse model of chronic pancreatitis. *Gastroenterology*. 2011; 141: 1473-1485. PMID: 21763242.
69. Rothwarf DM and Karin M. The NF-kappa B activation pathway: a paradigm in information transfer from membrane to nucleus. *Sci STKE*. 1999; 1999: RE1. PMID: 11865184.
70. Hu Y, Baud V, Delhase M, Zhang P, Deerinck T, Ellisman M, et al. Abnormal morphogenesis but intact IKK activation in mice lacking the IKKalpha subunit of IkappaB kinase. *Science*. 1999; 284: 316-320. PMID: 10195896.
71. Li N, Wu X, Holzer RG, Lee JH, Todoric J, Park EJ, et al. Loss of acinar cell IKKalpha triggers spontaneous pancreatitis in mice. *J Clin Invest*. 2013; 123: 2231-2243. PMID: 23563314.
72. Liu B, Xia X, Zhu F, Park E, Carbajal S, Kiguchi K, et al. IKKalpha is required to maintain skin homeostasis and prevent skin cancer. *Cancer Cell*. 2008; 14: 212-225. PMID: 18772111.
73. Sun SC, Ganchi PA, Ballard DW, and Greene WC. NF-kappa B controls expression of inhibitor I kappa B alpha: evidence for an inducible autoregulatory pathway. *Science*. 1993; 259: 1912-1915. PMID: 8096091.
74. Klement JF, Rice NR, Car BD, Abbondanzo SJ, Powers GD, Bhatt PH, et al. IkappaBalpha deficiency results in a sustained NF-kappaB response and severe widespread dermatitis in mice. *Mol Cell Biol*. 1996; 16: 2341-2349. PMID: 8628301.
75. Beg AA,Sha WC,Bronson RT and Baltimore D. Constitutive NF-kappa B activation, enhanced granulopoiesis, and neonatal lethality in I kappa B alpha-deficient mice. *Genes Dev*. 1995; 9: 2736-2746. PMID: 7590249.
76. Peng B, Ling J, Lee AJ, Wang Z, Chang Z, Jin W, et al. Defective feedback regulation of NF-kappaB underlies Sjogren's syndrome in mice with mutated kappaB enhancers of the IkappaB alpha promoter. *Proc Natl Acad Sci U S A*. 2010; 107: 15193-15198. PMID: 20696914.
77. Neuhofer P, Liang S, Einwachter H, Schwerdtfeger C, Wartmann T, Treiber M, et al. Deletion of IkappaBalpha activates RelA to reduce acute pancreatitis in mice through

up-regulation of Spi2A. *Gastroenterology*. 2013; 144: 192-201. PMID: 23041330.
78. Gukovsky I and Gukovskaya A. Nuclear factor-kappaB in pancreatitis: Jack-of-all-trades, but which one is more important? *Gastroenterology*. 2013; 144: 26-29. PMID: 23164573.
79. Huang H, Daniluk J, Liu Y, Chu J, Li Z, Ji B, et al. Oncogenic K-Ras requires activation for enhanced activity. *Oncogene*. 2013; 33: 532-535. PMID: 23334325.
80. Siegel RL, Miller KD, and Jemal A. Cancer statistics, *CA Cancer J Clin*. 2016; 66: 7-30. PMID: 26742998.
81. Stephen AG, Esposito D, Bagni RK, and McCormick F. Dragging ras back in the ring. *Cancer Cell*. 2014; 25: 272-281. PMID: 24651010.
82. Ji B, Tsou L, Wang H, Gaiser S, Chang DZ, Daniluk J, et al. Ras activity levels control the development of pancreatic diseases. *Gastroenterology*. 2009; 137: 1072-1082, 1082 e1071-1076. PMID: 19501586.
83. Logsdon CD and Ji B. Ras activity in acinar cells links chronic pancreatitis and pancreatic cancer. *Clin Gastroenterol Hepatol*. 2009; 7(11 Suppl): S40-S43. PMID: 19896097.
84. Aguirre AJ, Bardeesy N, Sinha M, Lopez L, Tuveson DA, Horner J, et al. Activated Kras and Ink4a/Arf deficiency cooperate to produce metastatic pancreatic ductal adenocarcinoma. *Genes Dev*. 2003; 17: 3112-3126. PMID: 14681207.
85. Hingorani SR, Petricoin EF, Maitra A, Rajapakse V, King C, Jacobetz MA, et al. Preinvasive and invasive ductal pancreatic cancer and its early detection in the mouse. *Cancer Cell*. 2003; 4: 437-450. PMID: 14706336.
86. Kubisch CH and Logsdon CD. Endoplasmic reticulum stress and the pancreatic acinar cell. *Expert Rev Gastroenterol Hepatol*. 2008; 2: 249-260. PMID: 19072360.
87. Garg AD, Kaczmarek A, Krysko O, Vandenabeele P, Krysko DV, and Agostinis P. ER stress-induced inflammation: does it aid or impede disease progression? *Trends Mol Med*. 2012; 18: 589-598. PMID: 22883813.
88. Adolph TE, Niederreiter L, Blumberg RS, and Kaser A. Endoplasmic reticulum stress and inflammation. *Digestive Dis*. 2012; 30: 341-346. PMID: 22796794.
89. Dufey E, Sepulveda D, Rojas-Rivera D, and Hetz C. Cellular mechanisms of endoplasmic reticulum stress signaling in health and disease. 1. An overview. *Am J Physiol Cell Physiol*. 2014; 307: C582-C594. PMID: 25143348.
90. Lugea A, Waldron RT, and Pandol SJ. Pancreatic adaptive responses in alcohol abuse: Role of the unfolded protein response. *Pancreatology*. 2015;(4 Suppl): S1-S5. PMID: 25736240.
91. Luo S, Mao C, Lee B, and Lee AS. GRP78/BiP is required for cell proliferation and protecting the inner cell mass from apoptosis during early mouse embryonic development. *Mol Cell Biol*. 2006; 26: 5688-5697. PMID: 16847323.
92. Ye R, Mareninova OA, Barron E, Wang M, Hinton DR, Pandol SJ, et al. Grp78 heterozygosity regulates chaperone balance in exocrine pancreas with differential response to cerulein-induced acute pancreatitis. *Am J Pathol*. 2010; 177: 2827-2836. PMID: 20971738.
93. Weng TI, Wu HY, Chen BL, Jhuang JY, Huang KH, Chiang CK, et al. C/EBP homologous protein deficiency aggravates acute pancreatitis and associated lung injury. *World J Gastroenterol*. 2013; 19: 7097-7105. PMID: 24222953.
94. Suyama K, Ohmuraya M, Hirota M, Ozaki N, Ida S, Endo M, et al. C/EBP homologous protein is crucial for the acceleration of experimental pancreatitis. *Biochem Biophys Res Commun*. 2008; 367: 176-182. PMID: 18166146.
95. Hess DA, Humphrey SE, Ishibashi J, Damsz B, Lee AH, Glimcher LH, et al. Extensive pancreas regeneration following acinar-specific disruption of Xbp1 in mice. *Gastroenterology*. 2011; 141: 1463-1472. PMID: 21704586.
96. Lugea A, Tischler D, Nguyen J, Gong J, Gukovsky I, French SW, et al. Adaptive unfolded protein response attenuates alcohol-induced pancreatic damage. *Gastroenterology*. 2011; 140: 987-997. PMID: 21111739.
97. Harding HP, Zeng H, Zhang Y, Jungries R, Chung P, Plesken H, et al. Diabetes mellitus and exocrine pancreatic dysfunction in perk-/- mice reveals a role for translational control in secretory cell survival. *Mol Cell*. 2001; 7: 1153-1163. PMID: 11430819.
98. Iida K, Li Y, McGrath BC, Frank A, and Cavener DR. PERK eIF2 alpha kinase is required to regulate the viability of the exocrine pancreas in mice. *BMC Cell Biol*. 2007; 8: 38. PMID: 17727724.
99. Wilschanski M and Novak I. The cystic fibrosis of exocrine pancreas. *Cold Spring Harb Perspect Med*. 2013; 3: a009746. PMID: 23637307.
100. Riordan JR, Rommens JM, Kerem B, Alon N, Rozmahel R, Grzelczak Z, et al. Identification of the cystic fibrosis gene: cloning and characterization of complementary DNA. *Science*. 1989; 245: 1066-1073. PMID: 2475911.
101. Wilke M, Buijs-Offerman RM, Aarbiou J, Colledge WH, Sheppard DN, Touqui L, et al. Mouse models of cystic fibrosis: phenotypic analysis and research applications. *J Cyst Fibrosis*. 2011; 10(Suppl2): S152-S171. PMID: 21658634.
102. Dorin JR, Farley R, Webb S, Smith SN, Farini E, Delaney SJ, et al. A demonstration using mouse models that successful gene therapy for cystic fibrosis requires only partial gene correction. *Gene Therapy*. 1996; 3: 797-801. PMID: 8875228.
103. Durie PR, Kent G, Phillips MJ, and Ackerley CA. Characteristic multiorgan pathology of cystic fibrosis in a long-living cystic fibrosis transmembrane regulator knockout murine model. *Am J Pathol*. 2004; 164: 1481-1493. PMID: 15039235.
104. Dimagno MJ, Lee SH, Hao Y, Zhou SY, McKenna BJ, and Owyang C. A proinflammatory, antiapoptotic phenotype underlies the susceptibility to acute pancreatitis in cystic fibrosis transmembrane regulator (-/-) mice. *Gastroenterology*. 2005; 129: 665-681. PMID: 16083720.
105. DiMagno MJ, Lee SH, Owyang C, and Zhou SY. Inhibition of acinar apoptosis occurs during acute pancreatitis in the human homologue DeltaF508 cystic fibrosis mouse. *Am J Physiol Gastrointest Liver Physiol*. 2010; 299: G400-G412. PMID: 20522641.

106. Zhou L, Dey CR, Wert SE, DuVall MD, Frizzell RA, and Whitsett JA. Correction of lethal intestinal defect in a mouse model of cystic fibrosis by human CFTR. *Science*. 1994; 266: 1705-1708. PMID: 7527588.
107. Rogers CS, Hao Y, Rokhlina T, Samuel M, Stoltz DA, Li Y, et al. Production of CFTR-null and CFTR-DeltaF508 heterozygous pigs by adeno-associated virus-mediated gene targeting and somatic cell nuclear transfer. *J Clin Invest*. 2008; 118: 1571-1577. PMID: 18324337.
108. Rogers CS, Stoltz DA, Meyerholz DK, Ostedgaard LS, Rokhlina T, Taft PJ, et al. Disruption of the CFTR gene produces a model of cystic fibrosis in newborn pigs. *Science*. 2008; 321: 1837-1841. PMID: 18818360.
109. Imrie JR, Fagan DG, and Sturgess JM. Quantitative evaluation of the development of the exocrine pancreas in cystic fibrosis and control infants. *Am J Pathol*. 1979; 95: 697-708. PMID: 453330.
110. Ostedgaard LS, Meyerholz DK, Chen JH, Pezzulo AA, Karp PH, Rokhlina T, et al. The DeltaF508 mutation causes CFTR misprocessing and cystic fibrosis-like disease in pigs. *Science Transl Med*. 2011; 3: 74ra24. PMID: 21411740.
111. Sun X, Yan Z, Yi Y, Li Z, Lei D, Rogers CS, et al. Adeno-associated virus-targeted disruption of the CFTR gene in cloned ferrets. *J Clin Invest*. 2008; 118: 1578-1583. PMID: 18324338.
112. Sun X, Sui H, Fisher JT, Yan Z, Liu X, Cho HJ, et al. Disease phenotype of a ferret CFTR-knockout model of cystic fibrosis. *J Clin Invest*. 2010; 120: 3149-3160. PMID: 20739752.
113. Sun X, Olivier AK, Yi Y, Pope CE, Hayden HS, Liang B, et al. Gastrointestinal pathology in juvenile and adult CFTR-knockout ferrets. *Am J Pathol*. 2014; 184: 1309-1322. PMID: 24637292.
114. Rane SG, Lee JH, and Lin HM. Transforming growth factor-beta pathway: role in pancreas development and pancreatic disease. *Cytokine Growth Factor Rev*. 2006; 17: 107-119. PMID: 16257256.
115. Lee MS, Gu D, Feng L, Curriden S, Arnush M, Krahl T, et al. Accumulation of extracellular matrix and developmental dysregulation in the pancreas by transgenic production of transforming growth factor-beta 1. *Am J Pathol*. 1995; 147: 42-52. PMID: 7604884.
116. Hahm KB, Im YH, Lee C, Parks WT, Bang YJ, Green JE, et al. Loss of TGF-beta signaling contributes to autoimmune pancreatitis. *J Clin Invest*. 105: 1057-1065,2000. PMID: 10772650.
117. Yoo BM, Yeo M, Oh TY, Choi JH, Kim WW, Kim JH, et al. Amelioration of pancreatic fibrosis in mice with defective TGF-beta signaling.. *Pancreas*. 2005; 30: e71-79. PMID: 15782092.
118. Bottinger EP, Jakubczak JL, Roberts IS, Mumy M, Hemmati P, Bagnall K, et al. Expression of a dominant-negative mutant TGF-beta type II receptor in transgenic mice reveals essential roles for TGF-beta in regulation of growth and differentiation in the exocrine pancreas. *EMBO J*. 199716: 2621-2633. PMID: 9184209.
119. Wildi S, Kleeff J, Mayerle J, Zimmermann A, Bottinger EP, Wakefield L, et al. Suppression of transforming growth factor beta signalling aborts caerulein induced pancreatitis and eliminates restricted stimulation at high caerulein concentrations. *Gut*. 2007; 56: 685-692. PMID: 17135311.
120. Boomershine CS, Chamberlain A, Kendall P, Afshar-Sharif AR, Huang H, Washington MK, et al. Autoimmune pancreatitis results from loss of TGFbeta signalling in S100A4-positive dendritic cells. *Gut*. 58: 1267-1274. PMID: 19625278.
121. FitzGerald GA. COX-2 and beyond: Approaches to prostaglandin inhibition in human disease. *Nat Rev Drug Discov*. 2003; 2: 879-890. PMID: 14668809.
122. Colby JK, Klein RD, McArthur MJ, Conti CJ, Kiguchi K, Kawamoto T, et al. Progressive metaplastic and dysplastic changes in mouse pancreas induced by cyclooxygenase-2 overexpression. *Neoplasia*. 2008; 10: 782-796. PMID: 18670639.
123. Ethridge RT, Chung DH, Slogoff M, Ehlers RA, Hellmich MR, Rajaraman S, et al. Cyclooxygenase-2 gene disruption attenuates the severity of acute pancreatitis and pancreatitis-associated lung injury. *Gastroenterology*. 2002; 123: 1311-1322. PMID: 12360491.
124. Ji B,Chen XQ, Misek DE, Kuick R, Hanash S, Ernst S, et al. Pancreatic gene expression during the initiation of acute pancreatitis: identification of EGR-1 as a key regulator. *Physiol Genomics*. 2003; 14: 59-72. PMID: 12709512.
125. Marrache F, Tu SP, Bhagat G, Pendyala S, Osterreicher CH, Gordon S, et al. Overexpression of interleukin-1beta in the murine pancreas results in chronic pancreatitis. *Gastroenterology*. 2008; 135: 1277-1287. PMID: 18789941.
126. Seleznik GM, Reding T, Romrig F, Saito Y, Mildner A, Segerer S, et al. Lymphotoxin beta receptor signaling promotes development of autoimmune pancreatitis. *Gastroenterology*. 2012; 143: 1361-1374. PMID: 22863765.
127. Algul H and Chari ST. Lymphotoxin in the pathogenesis of autoimmune pancreatitis: a new player in the field. *Gastroenterology*. 2012; 143: 1147-1150. PMID: 23000229.
128. Glick D, Barth S, and Macleod KF. Autophagy: cellular and molecular mechanisms. *J Pathol*. 2010; 221: 3-12. PMID: 20225336.
129. Mareninova OA, Hermann K, French SW, O'Konski MS, Pandol SJ, Webster P, et al. Impaired autophagic flux mediates acinar cell vacuole formation and trypsinogen activation in rodent models of acute pancreatitis. *J Clin Invest*. 2009; 119: 3340-3355. PMID: 19805911.
130. Green DR, Galluzzi L, and Kroemer G. Mitochondria and the autophagy-inflammation-cell death axis in organismal aging. *Science*. 2011; 333: 1109-1112. PMID: 21868666.
131. Nezis IP and Stenmark H. p62 at the interface of autophagy, oxidative stress signaling, and cancer. *Antioxid Redox Signal*. 2012; 17: 786-793. PMID: 22074114.
132. Mizushima N and Komatsu M. Autophagy: renovation of cells and tissues. *Cell*. 2011; 147: 728-741. PMID: 22078875.
133. Diakopoulos KN, Lesina M, Wormann S, Song L, Aichler M, Schild L, et al. Impaired autophagy induces chronic atrophic pancreatitis in mice via sex- and nutrition-dependent processes. *Gastroenterology*. 2015; 148: 626-638 e617. PMID: 25497209.

134. Gukovsky I and Gukovskaya AS. Impaired autophagy triggers chronic pancreatitis: lessons from pancreas-specific atg5 knockout mice. *Gastroenterology*. 2015; 148: 501-505. PMID: 25613315.
135. Casanova L, Bravo A, Were F, Ramirez A, Jorcano JJ, and Vidal M. Tissue-specific and efficient expression of the human simple epithelial keratin 8 gene in transgenic mice. *J Cell Sci*. 1995; 108: 811-820. PMID: 7539440.
136. Casanova ML, Bravo A, Ramirez A, Morreale de Escobar G, Were F, Merlino G, et al. Exocrine pancreatic disorders in transgenic mice expressing human keratin 8. *J Clin Invest*. 1999; 103: 1587-1595. PMID: 10359568.
137. Toivola DM, Nakamichi I, Strnad P, Michie SA, Ghori N, Harada M, et al. Keratin overexpression levels correlate with the extent of spontaneous pancreatic injury. *Am J Pathol*. 2008; 172: 882-892. PMID: 18349119.
138. Alberti S, Schuster G, Parini P, Feltkamp D, Diczfalusy U, Rudling M, et al. Hepatic cholesterol metabolism and resistance to dietary cholesterol in LXRbeta-deficient mice. *J Clin Invest*. 2001; 107(5): 565-573. PMID: 11238557.
139. Gabbi C, Kim HJ, Hultenby K, Bouton D, Toresson G, Warner M, et al. Pancreatic exocrine insufficiency in LXRbeta-/- mice is associated with a reduction in aquaporin-1 expression. *Proc Natl Acad Sci U S A*. 2008; 105: 15052-15057. PMID: 18806227.
140. Miralles F, Hebrard S, Lamotte L, Durel B, Gilgenkrantz H, Li Z, et al. Conditional inactivation of the murine serum response factor in the pancreas leads to severe pancreatitis. *Lab Invest*. 2006; 86: 1020-1036. PMID: 16894357.
141. Cano DA, Sekine S, and Hebrok M. Primary cilia deletion in pancreatic epithelial cells results in cyst formation and pancreatitis. *Gastroenterology*. 2006; 131: 1856-1869. PMID: 17123526.
142. Schmid RM and Whitcomb DC. Genetically defined models of chronic pancreatitis. *Gastroenterology*. 2006; 131: 2012-2015. PMID: 17123529.
143. Ji B and Logsdon CD. Digesting new information about the role of trypsin in pancreatitis. *Gastroenterology*. 2011; 141: 1972-1975. PMID: 22033179.

Chapter 11

Pathogenesis of pain in chronic pancreatitis

Dana Dominguez* and Kimberly Kirkwood

University of California, San Francisco School of Medicine, San Francisco, California, USA.

Introduction

Severe, disabling abdominal pain is the hallmark of chronic pancreatitis. Currently available treatments for pancreatitis pain are inadequate and expensive, both in healthcare dollars and lost productivity. Pain is the most common reason for hospitalization among chronic pancreatitis patients, and as many as 40% require three or more admissions for pain management during their lifetime.[1] Developing improved treatments will require a better understanding of the mechanisms of chronic visceral pain, a subject that has recently gained attention with the development of suitable animal models and reproducible experimental measures of sustained pancreatic pain.

Manifestations and Treatment of Pancreatic Pain

Pain theories

Traditional theories of the origin of pancreatic pain in chronic pancreatitis focused on structural abnormalities causing ductal hypertension.[2] Such abnormalities ranged from stones and strictures, to fibrosis due to toxic effects, and ischemia.[3] While this ductal obstruction theory is logical, studies of patients with chronic pancreatitis have failed to show a correlation between ductal pressure and pain levels; moreover, ductal pressures do not accurately predict the success of ductal decompression procedures.[4-7] In fact, Bornman et al. demonstrated that there was no significant difference in either the anatomy or the morphological changes between groups of patients with either painful or painless pancreatitis.[8] Rather than a single mechanism of pain, recent research has favored a more complex relationship between these structural and morphological components and their interaction with neurobiological mechanisms.[9] Nociceptive pathways, inflammatory mediators, and sensitization of both central and peripheral pathways have been shown to play important roles in pancreatic pain.[10]

Chronic pain syndrome: A downward spiral

Among the many clinical sequelae of chronic pancreatitis, pain has been shown to be the most important factor affecting quality of life.[11] The pain often becomes the focal point around which work, leisure activities, and relationships must revolve. Two types of pain patterns have been identified among these patients: type A, characterized by intermittent flares of pain, and type B, consisting of prolonged periods of persistent pain of varying severity.[12] In the largest study of pain in chronic pancreatitis, Mullady et al. showed that those who exhibit more type B pain of a more constant nature have lower quality of life measures.[1] In a study of 265 patients, Wehler et al. demonstrated that as abdominal pain index scores increased across subgroups, there was a significant and profound decrease in all quality of life indices. Because eating can trigger pain exacerbations, patients typically respond by decreasing food intake. Many patients also suffer nutrient malabsorption due to pancreatic exocrine insufficiency, and this combination leads to progressive weight loss and malnutrition. Decreased body mass index has been correlated with impairment in quality of life measurements.[13]

Medical treatment

The mainstay therapy for chronic pancreatitis is the symptomatic treatment of pain. Since we have a limited understanding of chronic pancreatic pain pathogenesis, treatment is limited to a supportive care regimen targeting symptoms rather than etiologies of the pain.[14] Therapeutic regimens rely heavily on opioid analgesics, which lead to

*Corresponding author. Email: d.dominguez@alamedahealthsystem.org

both physiological and psychological dependence, as well as tolerance requiring escalating doses. The undesirable side effects of these drugs reduce patient well-being through physical symptoms such as somnolence, impaired cognitive function, and constipation. The side effects of existing therapeutics combine with inadequately treated pain to produce the detrimental socioeconomic effects of inability to work or, in some cases, even to leave the house.[15] The results of some studies even support the possible role of long-term opioid treatment in the development of hyperalgesia and allodynia, which further exacerbate pain syndromes.[16] Newer approaches typically use multimodal combinations of agents that target inflammation, nerve injury, and descending pathways, with the goal of reducing narcotic dosages and achieving synergistic effects. Examples of this include the addition of the gabapentoid pregabalin, as well as the antioxidant methionine, both of which have been shown to improve pain in chronic pancreatitis.[17,18] Despite these advances, ideal medical treatments remain elusive due to the lack of reliable trials comparing various treatment regimens, as well as heterogeneity in pain patterns.[14,19]

Interventional treatment

For pain that is refractory to medical management, an array of procedures have been used with risk and side effect profiles that roughly parallel their efficacies and durabilities in improving pain.

Peripheral nerve ablation

One of the original approaches was endoscopic injection of anti-inflammatory, analgesic, or ablative agents into the celiac ganglia through which most of the pancreatic afferents pass.[20] In a prospective study by Gress and colleagues, of 90 patients with chronic pancreatitis, only 55% of patients reported significant improvement in pain scores following endoscopic ultrasound-guided celiac plexus block, and only 10% had lasting benefit from the procedure at 24 weeks.[21] Rare but serious side effects included motor nerve impairment and exacerbation of pain. Therefore, it is no longer recommended as a routine therapy for patients with intractable benign pancreatic pain, but it is still used to improve quality of remaining life for some patients with severe pain from pancreatic cancer.[22] Newer therapies have been developed utilizing percutaneous radiofrequency ablation to achieve site-directed ablation of splanchnic nerves. Demonstrated first in a small cohort of patients with chronic nonmalignant abdominal pain by Garcea et al. in 2005,[23] this approach was used by Verhaegh et al. in 2013 on a cohort of 11 chronic pancreatitis patients. They found a 50%-75% reduction in pain scores in more than half of patients, and a median pain free period of 45 weeks.[24] While these early results are promising, the durability of the effect remains a limitation, and evidence for success of repeat interventions is lacking. Surgical resection of segments of these peripheral splanchnic nerves via a minimally invasive approach, so-called thoracoscopic splanchnicectomy, has also been shown to be effective for short-term pain relief, but durable improvement remains elusive for 50% of patients after 15 months.[25] For these reasons, peripheral nerve interventions play a limited role in the clinical management of patients with severe chronic pancreatitis pain. They may, for example, be useful as a bridge therapy to reduce narcotic dependence, and, in suitable cases, may allow a patient to gain weight in preparation for a more durable, and higher risk, surgical procedure.

Pancreatic drainage

For a select minority of patients with diffuse dilation of the main pancreatic duct, typically due to anatomic, fibrotic, or calculus obstruction at or near the insertion of the pancreatic duct into the common channel, endoscopic or surgical drainage into the small intestine may be beneficial. Endoscopically, this is typically achieved via a transampullary approach during endoscopic retrograde cholangiopancreatography (ERCP) with sphincterotomy, dilation, and possibly stenting.[28] For patients with large duct disease, decompression can improve pain; however, repeat endoscopic therapy is often needed as more than half of patients will have recurrence of pain.[26] Extracorporeal shockwave lithotripsy (ESWL) can also be used as an adjunct with ERCP in patients with large duct stones.[27] Surgical drainage procedures have evolved over time, and the modern lateral pancreaticojejunostomy now typically includes resection of a portion of the pancreatic head (Frey procedure) to provide wide open drainage of pancreatic juice into the limb of the jejunum. One study of 29 chronic pancreatitis patients treated with the Frey procedure reported long-term pain relief in 90% at 1 year.[28] To date, only two large randomized control trials have compared surgical drainage with endoscopic drainage modalities. Both studies demonstrated significantly better long-term pain relief in surgically treated patients. Dite et al. demonstrated that 37% of patients in the surgical group remained pain-free at their 5-year follow-up.[29] There were no significant differences in the number of adverse events between the two cohorts.[29,30]

Pancreatic resection

For the majority of patients with debilitating chronic pancreatitis pain, the main pancreatic duct is not diffusely dilated, and drainage is not feasible. These patients with so-called "small duct" disease who fail non-surgical management due to uncontrolled pain and its sequelae, and/or intolerance of the side effects of high-dose narcotics, are relegated to the last ditch surgical alternative of resection. In general, the likelihood of pain relief and surgical diabetes both scale with the percentage of pancreas removed, with more recent long-term follow-up data diminishing enthusiasm for resection. In a study of 224 patients, Riediger et al. evaluated surgical partial resections for chronic pancreatitis including pylorus-preserving pancreaticoduodenectomy (PPPD), duodenum-preserving pancreatic head resection (DPPHR), classic Whipple, distal pancreatectomy, and central pancreatic resection. With a median follow-up of 56.3 months, 60% of patients remained pain free at last follow-up. Although subgroup analysis by resection type did not demonstrate a significant correlation with pain outcomes, patient selection likely plays an important role.[31] An advantage of more aggressive resections such as total pancreatectomy may be the added resection of pancreatic nerve ganglia.[20] With more generalizable results showing improved glycemic control among patients who undergo total pancreatectomy with islet cell harvest and auto transplantation.[32,33] This procedure has recently gained some favor; however, the refractory nature of pain in a substantial fraction of these patients, even following the resource-intensive removal of the entire gland, remains both confusing and frustrating.[34] This group of patients provides us with an interesting glimpse into the complexity of the extrapancreatic pathways that contribute to sustained pancreatic pain.

Models

Whereas pancreatic atrophy and fibrosis can be induced experimentally in a variety of ways, measures of visceral pain have proven more difficult. Studies in rats qualitatively evaluated spontaneous activity using video tracking and abdomen sensitivity to mechanical and electrical stimulation.[35] The most widely used of these rat models was developed in 1996 by Puig et al. who injected trinitrobenzene sulfonic acid (TNBS) directly into the pancreatic duct of rats to induce early severe acute pancreatitis that evolved over weeks into painful chronic pancreatitis.[36] In 2005, Winston et al. further characterized and modified this model to provide better face validity and generalization to human disease.[35] This model has proved invaluable in providing insight into the complex nature of pain from chronic pancreatitis. Further progress in identifying specific pathways that might be therapeutic targets, however, was hampered by the lack of a murine model in which putative mediators could be genetically deleted.

Adaptation of the TNBS model to mice was fraught with early experimental failure related to the high mortality of severe acute pancreatitis in physiologically fragile mice. Our laboratory adapted the model to mice by dramatically reducing the TNBS dose and providing perioperative fluid resuscitation during the first 24 hours.[37] The resultant chronic pancreatitis is apparent after 1-2 weeks with severe fibrosis, monocyte infiltration, atrophy, and fatty replacement of the gland. We use Von Frey filament probing of the abdomen to demonstrate referred mechanical hyperalgesia, in which heightened withdrawal responses are measured to a mildly painful stimulus, as well as allodynia, in which probes that do not cause pain in control mice evoke withdrawal responses. TNBS-injected mice also show reduced spontaneous activity (distance and time) on a running wheel and longer periods of immobility during open field testing. This model can be used to examine both peripheral and central mechanisms of sustained pain and for comparison with models of somatic pain such as peripheral or spinal nerve ligation, so that both shared and unique pathways can be identified.

Components of Pancreatic Pain

Nociceptive neurons

In addition to parasympathetic cholinergic innervation from the vagus nerve and sympathetic innervation mainly derived from the celiac ganglia, the pancreas is also innervated by nociceptive sensory neurons. These afferent neurons have their cell bodies in the dorsal root ganglia (DRG), and they give off projections that map to the dorsal horn of the spinal cord (**Figure 1**).[10] They are responsible for transmitting noxious visceral stimuli from the pancreas and the relay of this information to the central nervous system (CNS).

Uncontrolled proteolysis

The pancreas is rich in cysteine and serine proteases that can be released following a variety of insults and are known to directly or indirectly activate nociceptive neurons. Using a near infrared-labeled activity-based probe that covalently modifies active cathepsins, our laboratory found significant accumulation of cathepsins B, L, and S in both the inflamed rodent pancreas and juice from patients with painful chronic pancreatitis.[38] Cathepsins, in turn, cleave and activate trypsinogens, yielding active trypsins, some of which are resistant to endogenous degradation by ubiquitous inhibitors, and are thereby free to bind and activate receptors on peptidergic neurons.[39] Following activation, these neurons release neuropeptides and inflammatory mediators including calcitonin gene related peptide (CGRP), substance P (SP), vasoactive intestinal polypeptide (VIP), and bradykinin that act both peripherally where they promote vasodilation, plasma extravasation, and neutrophil infiltration (so called neurogenic inflammation) and centrally where they activate central pain pathways.[40]

Sensory neuron receptors

Vanilloid receptors

One of the best characterized pain receptors is transient receptor potential vanilloid 1 (TRPV1). A member of the family of vanilloid nociceptive receptors found on sensory neurons, it functions as a nonselective cation channel, permitting sodium and calcium flow into cells, leading to depolarization of the cell membrane and release of neurotransmitters such as SP and CGRP.[10] Originally known as the capsaicin receptor, it is activated by heat and local acidification, as well as multiple endogenous chemical mediators including leukotrienes and arachadonic acid metabolites.[41] Caterina et al. used TRPV1 knockout mice to clearly demonstrate the role of TRPV1 in nociception and tissue-injury induced hyperalgesia.[42] We showed that TRPV1 plays an important role in nociceptive mediation in acute pancreatitis through inducing SP and CGRP release by pancreatic sensory nerves, thereby increasing *c-fos* expression in the rat spinal cord. Administration of a TRPV1 antagonist attenuated this effect.[43] TRPV1 is upregulated in chronic pancreatitis and is a mediator of hyperalgesia and inflammation in this condition.[44] Additionally, it has been implicated to have interactions with other TRP receptors, as well as protease-activated receptor 2 (PAR2), a G-protein coupled receptor with unique roles in inflammation and pain sensitization,[10] described below.

TRPV1 can work alone or in concert with other TRP receptors such as TRP ankyrin 1 (TRPA1), to amplify nociceptive signaling. Required for sensory neuron excitation, TRPA1 functions as a "gatekeeper" of chronic inflammation by serving two major roles: controlling the peripheral release of inflammatory neuropeptides and facilitating neuronal activation by inflammatory mediators released through local tissue injury.[45] Though it had been previously shown to mediate inflammation and visceral pain in acute pancreatitis,[46] the first evidence of TRPA1's direct role in pain from chronic pancreatitis came in 2013 with the establishment of a TNBS murine model of chronic pancreatitis. In this model of painful chronic pancreatitis following severe acute pancreatitis, we found that compared with wild-type controls, TRPA1 knockout mice had less inflammation and fibrosis and markedly reduced pain indices including referred mechanical hyperalgesia, spontaneous running activity, and mobility in open field testing.[37]

Studies in the past decade using knockout mice,[42,47,48] TRPA1 knockdowns,[49] and antagonists,[50] have shown that TRPA1 works in concert with TRPV1 to mediate inflammation-induced stimulus transmission in sensory neurons. Evidence for direct interaction between the two channels was shown by Staruschenko et al. using Förster resonance energy transfer (FRET) constructs of the respective channels.[51] TRPA1 and TRPV1 were recently implicated in the transition from acute to chronic inflammation in the pancreas. Schwartz et al. used a cerulein model of acute pancreatitis to demonstrate that morphologic acute to chronic changes are mitigated by TRP antagonists.[52]

Increasing evidence also supports a role for TRPV4 in pancreatic pain. TRPV4 is directly activated by shear stress, osmotic stimuli, and lipid mediators, as well as indirectly via G-protein coupled receptors that regulate TRP channels.[53,54] TRPV4 knockout mice[55] and TRPV4 knockdowns[56] have demonstrated abnormal osmotic regulation and decreased responses to changes in pressure and tonicity. Alessandri et al. proposed the attractive notion that the "soup" of inflammatory mediators that surround local tissue injury, including bradykinin, SP, prostaglandin E2 (PGE_2), serotonin, and histamine, among others, may induce mechanical hyperalgesia through activation of TRPV4, sensitizing it for a triggering event. They demonstrated that activation of TRPV4 by hypotonic saline is enhanced in the presence of PGE2 and increases nociceptive behavior in rats. These effects are absent in TRPV4 knockout rats.[56] They also showed the involvement of protein kinase A and C intracellular second messenger pathways in TRPV4 activation.[57] This activation in turn mediates pain transmission through subsequent activation of nociceptive spinal neurons in the superficial laminae of the spinal cord. In the pancreas, we showed that injection of a TRPV4 agonist into the pancreatic duct increases c-Fos-like immunoreactivity expression in the spinal cord in the input regions of pancreatic sensory neurons located by retrograde tracing, suggesting that TRPV4 could play a role in pain signaling in the inflamed pancreas.[46] Further experiments are needed to clarify the importance of TRPV4 in acute and chronic pancreatic inflammatory pain.

Protease-activated receptor 2

Protease-activated receptor 2 (PAR2) is one of four GPCRs activated by serine proteases such as trypsin and thrombin. These proteases cleave an N-terminal fragment, revealing a tethered receptor agonist (ligand), which can then bind and activate signaling pathways.[58] Steinhoff et al. provided the initial evidence of a neurogenic inflammatory role for PAR2 by demonstrating its co-expression with neuropeptides CGRP and SP in DRG neurons. PAR2 activation leads to neuropeptide release in peripheral tissues, as well as the spinal cord, increasing local inflammation and edema.[59]

In addition to causing the direct release of inflammatory neuropeptides from sensory neurons, activated PAR2 leads to increased intracellular calcium, which lowers the threshold for TRP channel activation by other inflammatory mediators and products of tissue injury, so-called "sensitization." Thus, the addition of trypsin or PAR2-activating peptide (AcPep) in dorsal root ganglion cell culture leads to significantly increased capsaicin-evoked CGRP release, an indication of PAR2 sensitization of TRPV1. *In vivo*, pre-injection of AcPep into the pancreatic duct increases capsaicin-induced FOS expression in pancreatic spinal cord segments compared with the control peptide, suggesting that PAR2 sensitizes TRPV1 in the pancreas.[60] Under normal physiologic conditions, concentrations of active trypsin in the pancreas are low due to its release in a zymogen form as trypsinogen. However, following pancreatic inflammation, early activation of trypsins by cysteine proteases, as well as the recruitment of mast cells that release tryptase, can, in turn, activate PAR2.[61] Indirect evidence of the importance of mast cell products in chronic pancreatitis pain derives from the observation that mast cells are present in significantly higher numbers in patients with painful chronic pancreatitis than in patients with nonpainful pancreatitis (33.8 vs. 9.4 average mast cells/10 high-power fields; $P < 0.01$) or with healthy controls (33.8 vs. 6.1 average mast cells/10 high-power fields, $P < 0.01$).[62] Intraductal injection of trypsin into the pancreatic duct of mice in sub-inflammatory concentrations increases FOS expression in pancreatic-specific spinal cord DRG. This effect is mitigated by pretreatment with AcPep, indicating that PAR2 and trypsin may share this pain pathway.[63] PAR2 activation in these neurons leads to sustained hyperalgesia.[64] Thus, serine proteases contribute to pancreatic pain via multiple pathways mediated by PAR2 activation.[39]

PAR2 has also been shown to sensitize both TRPV4 and TRPA1 and thereby lower the threshold for activation of pancreatic sensory neurons.[65,66] PAR2-mediated sensitization of these TRP channels has been associated with neuropathic pain induced by the chemotherapy agent paclitaxel, which indicates that these pathways have clinical importance.[67] Peripheral sensitization represents an important pathway by which the painful effects of inflammatory mediators that result from tissue injury are amplified and sustained.

Nerve growth factor and receptor tyrosine kinase A

Nerve growth factor (NGF), a protein that contributes to the development and survival of neurons, also plays an important role in the peripheral sensitization of sensory neurons.[68] It acts mainly through its high affinity tyrosine kinase receptor TrkA, which is found in highest concentration within the pancreas in the perineurium. Co-expression of TrkA with NGF is increased in the pancreas from patients with chronic pancreatitis.[69] NGF exerts its effects through multiple mechanisms including a direct effect on ion channels, posttranslational modifications by second messengers, and translocation of the NGF/trkA complex to the nucleus where it regulates transcriptional modifications to certain genes.[70] Early evidence for its role in mediating visceral pain came from expression studies by McMahon et al. in 1994, demonstrating that almost all afferent neurons innervating visceral targets express trkA, while its expression in those innervating skeletal muscle is very low.[71] Immunodepletion studies using trkA-IgG on cultured neurons showed sustained hypoalgesia and CGRP downregulation.[72] This is further supported by studies that used animals lacking the trkA gene, which also experienced a significant hypoalgesic state.[73] This same hypoalgesic effect was noted after rats with chronic pancreatitis were treated with an NGF blocking antibody, which significantly increased A-type potassium currents, thereby decreasing the likelihood of depolarization.[74] Conversely, both neonatal and adult rats injected with excess exogenous NGF show profound behavioral hyperalgesia.[75] Recent reports suggest that NGF/trkA can sensitize neurons via interaction with the vanilloid receptor TRPV1, and NGF can regulate TRPV1 expression through both transcriptional and posttranslational mechanisms (**Figure 1**).[70]

Neurokinin receptor 1

SP and neurokinins A (NKA) and B (NKB) are the main tachykinins involved in sensory neural transmission and nociception. SP and NKA share a receptor, neurokinin receptor 1 (NK-1R), and NKB binds preferentially to neurokinin receptor 2 (NK-2R).[76] By studying human pancreatic tissue, Di Sabastiano et al. found that although there is an increase in SP surrounding pancreatic nerve fibers, there is no concomitant increase in the gene encoding SP. This observation led to the early understanding that SP is synthesized in extrapancreatic ganglia and transported to the pancreas.[77] Thus, activation of peripheral sensory nerve endings leads to the release of SP and CGRP peripherally within the pancreas, where they promote neurogenic inflammation in a positive feedback loop that leads to amplification of inflammatory pain, and centrally, where SP binds to NK-1R in the dorsal horn of the spinal cord and activates central pain pathways.[78,79] Shrikhande et al. was the first to examine NK-1R expression in pancreata from patients with painful chronic pancreatitis. They established a definitive relationship between mRNA levels and pain intensity, frequency, and duration in these patients.[80]

Central Sensitization

Nervous system support cells

Microglia

Microglia are CNS immune cells that respond to tissue injury by switching from a quiescent to an active state, in which they secrete inflammatory mediators to recruit other immune cells and promote cellular hypertrophy and proliferation.[81,82] Their function in the CNS is similar to that of macrophages in peripheral tissues.

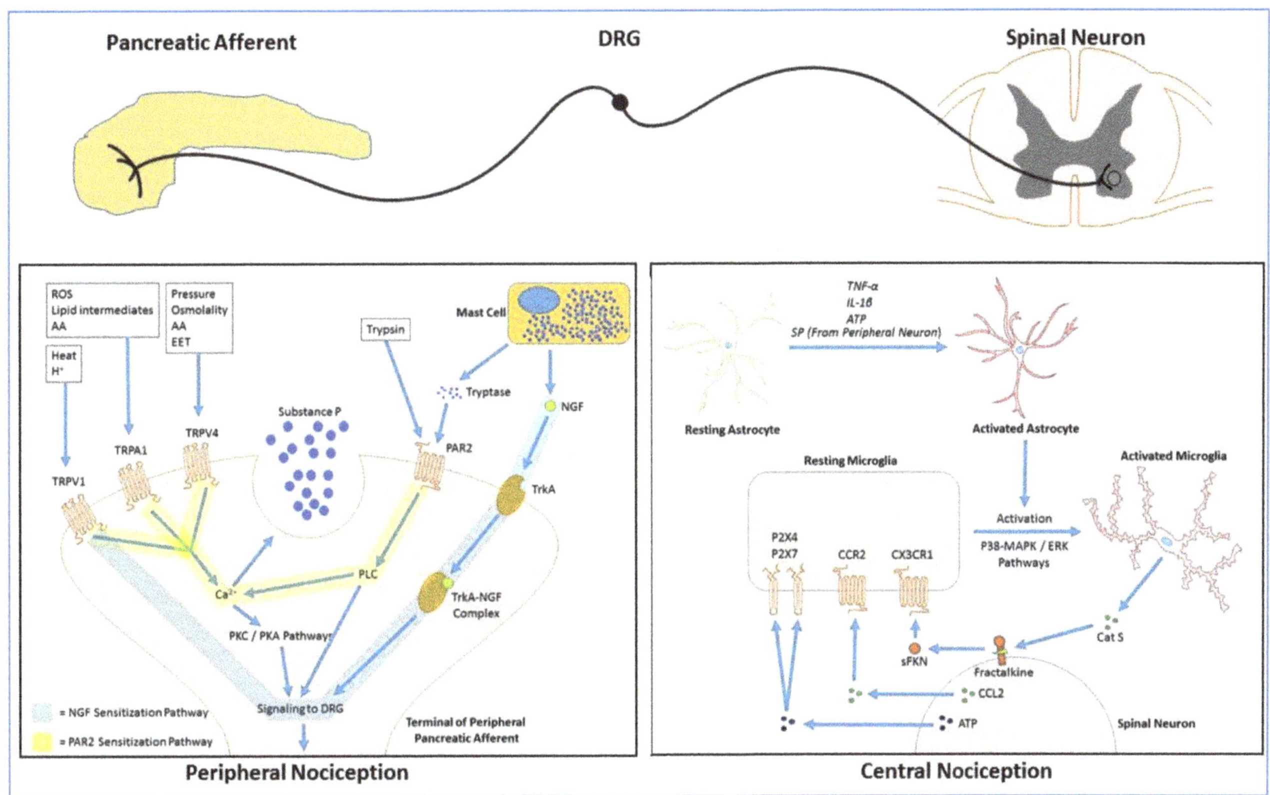

Figure 1. Pathways of pancreatic pain signal transmission in chronic pancreatitis with an emphasis on sensitization mechanisms.

How are microglia activated?

The initial activation likely occurs through multiple pathways. Excitation of nociceptive neurons leads to release of the chemokine CCL2 that binds to its receptor CCR2 on microglia, a critical signaling event in microglial activation[83] that promotes pain signal amplification (**Figure 1**). Another potential pathway is through the receptors P2X4 and P2X7, which are upregulated in microglia after nerve injury and activated in response to injury by ATP released by primary sensory and dorsal horn neurons, as well as dorsal horn astrocytes.[84] P38, a mitogen-activated protein kinase (MAPK) has been implicated as a major participant in the activation of spinal microglia (**Figure 1**). Originally demonstrated in a neuropathic pain model using sciatic nerve ligation, Jin et al. showed early p38 activation in spinal microglia (12-24 h after injury), with subsequent activation in DRG neurons.[85] A p38-inhibitor prevents the development of pain hypersensitivity.[81] P38 activation was also reported in a rat model of chronic pancreatitis pain by Liu et al., suggesting that this pathway is important in sustained visceral pain.[86] Once activated, these loops can function without further external stimulus. Thus, excitation of nociceptive spinal neurons leads to spinal microglia activation via multiple parallel pathways that provide an efficient means to amplify inflammatory nociceptive signals.

How does microglial activation cause sustained pain?

It is well established that nervous system support cells participate in maintaining neuropathic pain pathways in somatic pain models.[81,87,88] Activation of spinal microglia leads to the release of the soluble chemokine fractalkine (FKN), which is expressed in CNS sensory neurons as a transmembrane protein that can be cleaved to a soluble form (**Figure 1**). This was originally shown to occur after excitotoxic stimuli, suggesting that FKN cleavage represented an early event in the neurogenic inflammatory process.[89] It is now known that membrane-bound FKN is cleaved by the cysteine protease cathepsin S (Cat S), which is secreted peripherally by macrophages and centrally by activated microglia.[90] Cat S cleaves FKN on dorsal horn neurons, releasing its soluble form, which then binds its own receptor CX3CR1.[91] This receptor is only expressed in activated microglia,[92] and binding further activates the p38 pathway in a positive feedback loop. Using the rat model of peripheral nerve ligation, Clark et al. showed that a Cat S inhibitor reduced pain behavior 7 and 14 days after sciatic nerve ligation in rats, whereas it did not prevent the initial development of pain. This suggests that Cat S is important in the maintenance of neuropathic pain, rather than the development of hyperalgesia.[91] The release of Cat S and subsequent binding and activation of the p38 pathway is dependent on microglial activation.

Peripherally, extracellular inflammatory agents including NGF, trypsin, and tryptase sensitize and activate pancreatic afferent nociceptive neurons through integrative calcium signaling pathways. Centrally, sensitization is mediated through positive feedback loops among dorsal horn neurons and the activated neuronal supporting cells microglia and astrocytes, via Cat S-mediated cleavage and release of soluble FKN. Abbreviations: AA, arachadonic acid metabolites; Cat S, cathepsin S; CCL2, chemokine ligand 2; CCR2, chemokine receptor 2; DRG, dorsal root ganglia; EET, epoxyeicosatrienoic acids; ERK, extracellular signal-related kinase pathway; FKN, fractalkine; MAPK, mitogen-activated protein kinase pathway; NGF, nerve growth factor; PAR2, protease-activated receptor 2; PKA, protein kinase A; PKC, protein kinase C; PLC, phospholipase C; ROS, reactive oxygen species; sFKN, soluble fractalkine; SP, substance P; TrkA, trypomyosin-related kinase A; TRPV, transient receptor potential vanilloids.

Recent evidence supports the importance of activated microglia in the development and maintenance of sustained visceral pain. In a rat model of TNBS-induced chronic pancreatitis, Liu et al. found that the microglial activation inhibitor minocycline significantly decreased nociceptive behavior, and that withdrawal of minocycline caused a return to baseline. Also, pretreatment with minocycline prior to TNBS injection prevented chronic visceral hyperalgesia for as long as 3 weeks.[86] We found similar results in the TNBS-induced chronic pancreatitis mice treated with minocycline, with normalization of the expected heightened responses to Von Frey filament probing (unpublished results). These data suggest that microglial activation may play an important role in sustained pancreatic pain.

Astrocytes

Astrocytes demonstrate activated morphology in neuropathic pain models,[93] and drugs used to treat pain in these experimental conditions attenuate activation.[88,94] Activation of astrocytes by mediators such as ATP, SP, prostaglandins, and glutamate released by sensory nerves in response to injury, stimulates release of pro-inflammatory mediators. These mediators include cytokines such as interleukin (IL)-1β, IL-6 and tumor necrosis factor-α, as well as the molecules that activate them, including ATP and prostaglandins.[88] Multiple intracellular signaling pathways have been implicated in the regulation of astrocyte activation, including p38, c-Jun-N-terminal kinase (JNK) and, perhaps most importantly, the extracellular signal-regulated kinase (ERK) pathway.[54] Zhuang et al. demonstrated increased expression of phosphorylated ERK in both microglia and dorsal horn astrocytes 10 days after spinal nerve ligation.

In this study, intrathecal injection of an ERK inhibitor significantly reduced mechanical allodynia.[96] In the rat TNBS chronic pancreatitis pain model, Feng et al. reported an increase in glial fibrillary acidic protein (GFAP), an astrocyte marker upregulated in somatic models of neuropathic pain. This study also importantly demonstrated that attenuation of neuropathic pain in this model was possible using L-α-aminoadipate (LAA), a specific inhibitor of astrocyte activation,[97] suggesting a potential therapeutic target.

Reorganization

Observational studies in humans with chronic visceral pain have led to the notion that changes in inhibitory and amplification processes in the CNS contribute to reorganization of referred pain signal mapping. Mertz et al. meticulously mapped pain patterns in patients with inflammatory bowel syndrome (IBS). In response to rectal distension, IBS patients have increased hypersensitivity in areas remote from the stimulus, as well as larger overall pain areas compared with healthy controls. These changes are associated with increased thalamic activation, suggesting that increased afferent signaling from the gut may lead to perceptual reorganization of pain signals.[98] Interestingly, in contrast to these results, Dimcevski and colleagues reported that chronic pancreatitis patients have hypoalgesia in response to balloon distension of viscera surrounding the pancreas compared with healthy controls.[99] It is worth noting that duodenal distension is less well established as a marker of referred visceral hyperalgesia than rectal distension, which could contribute to these results. In other studies by this group, electrical visceral pain stimulation in chronic pancreatitis patients was associated with reduced evoked potential latency in the brain, thereby suggesting that central modulation of pain pathways contributes to visceral hypersensitivity. Similar to prior findings in IBS patients, chronic pancreatitis patients also show an increase in the mean areas of referred pain following electrical visceral stimulation, suggesting reorganization of pain perception.[100]

Opioid-induced hyperalgesia

Opioids are the mainstay of treatment for patients with severe chronic pancreatitis pain. As early as the 19th century, it was recognized that chronic opioid use leads not only to tolerance and physical and psychological dependence, but ironically, to increased sensitivity to painful stimuli or opioid-induced hyperalgesia (OIH). Unlike opioid tolerance, OIH cannot be mitigated by increased dosage regimens.[101] Multiple studies in animal models have shown reductions in mechanical and thermal thresholds to nociceptive stimuli with opioid treatment.[102-104] Similarly, multiple clinical studies in humans describe varying levels of hyperalgesic states among both patients and healthy controls treated with chronic opioids.[105-108]

Much remains to be defined regarding these hyperalgesic mechanisms, but they are thought to be closely intertwined with the pathways of opioid tolerance. Pathways involving the N-methyl-D-aspartate receptor (NMDAR), spinal glutamate activity, protein kinase C activity, and spinal dynorphin have all been implicated as vital to both tolerance and hyperalgesia.[109] It is likely that this phenomenon contributes, in part, to the exasperation experienced by both patients and physicians at the progressive worsening of chronic pancreatitis pain experienced by some patients on escalating opioid dosages.

Conclusion

Research into the mechanisms of chronic pancreatitis pain has been accelerated by the recent availability of validated rat and mouse models. These have provided interested investigators with a wider array of reproducible measures of experimental visceral pain. Emerging models illustrate the complexity, redundancy, interconnectedness, and plasticity of chronic visceral pain pathways. Current treatments do not address the underlying mechanisms of sensitization and amplification of either peripheral or central pain signals, which may partially explain the high level of medical and surgical treatment failure. Integrative channels in the periphery offer potentially high-leverage targets, as do positive feedback loops in the spinal cord, where selective inhibition could have profound beneficial results. The development of clinically useful inhibitors of these potential targets is expected to improve both treatment efficacy and quality of life for patients with debilitating chronic pancreatitis pain.

References

1. Mullady DK, Yadav D, Amann ST, O'Connell MR, Barmada MM, Elta GH, et al. Type of pain, pain-associated complications, quality of life, disability and resource utilisation in chronic pancreatitis: a prospective cohort study. *Gut*. 2011; 60(1): 77-84. PMID: 21148579.
2. Bradley EL 3rd. Pancreatic duct pressure in chronic pancreatitis. *Am J Surg*. 1982; 144(3): 313-316. PMID: 7114368.
3. Demir IE, Tieftrunk E, Maak M, Friess H, Ceyhan GO. Pain mechanisms in chronic pancreatitis: of a master and his fire. *Langenbecks Arch Surg*. 2011; 396(2): 151-160. PMID: 21153480.
4. Ebbehoj N. Pancreatic tissue fluid pressure and pain in chronic pancreatitis. *Dan Med Bull*. 1992; 39(2): 128-133. PMID: 1611919.
5. Ebbehøj N, Borly L, Bülow J, Henriksen JH, Heyeraas KJ, Rasmussen SG. Evaluation of pancreatic tissue fluid pressure measurements intraoperatively and by sonographically guided fine-needle puncture. *Scand J Gastroenterol*. 1990; 25(11): 1097-1102. PMID: 2274734.
6. Ebbehøj N, Borly L, Madsen P, Matzen P. Pancreatic tissue fluid pressure during drainage operations for chronic pancreatitis. *Scand J Gastroenterol*. 1990; 25(10): 1041-1045. PMID: 2263876.
7. Ebbehøj N, Borly L, Madsen P, Matzen P. Comparison of regional pancreatic tissue fluid pressure and endoscopic retrograde pancreatographic morphology in chronic pancreatitis. *Scand J Gastroenterol*. 1990; 25(7): 756-760. PMID: 2396092.
8. Bornman PC, Marks IN, Girdwood AW, Berberat PO, Gulbinas A, Büchler MW. Pathogenesis of pain in chronic pancreatitis: ongoing enigma. *World J Surg*. 2003; 27(11): 1175-1182. PMID: 14574490.
9. Drewes AM, Krarup AL, Detlefsen S, Malmstrøm ML, Dimcevski G, Funch-Jensen P, et al. Pain in chronic pancreatitis: the role of neuropathic pain mechanisms. *Gut*. 2008; 57(11): 1616-1627. PMID: 18566105.
10. Pasricha PJ. Unraveling the mystery of pain in chronic pancreatitis. *Nat Rev Gastroenterol Hepatol*. 2012; 9(3): 140-151. PMID: 22269952.
11. Pezzilli R, Morselli Labate AM, Ceciliato R, Frulloni L, Cavestro GM, Comparato G, et al. Quality of life in patients with chronic pancreatitis. *Dig Liver Dis*. 2005; 37(3): 181-189. PMID: 15888283.
12. Ammann RW, Muellhaupt B. The natural history of pain in alcoholic chronic pancreatitis. *Gastroenterology*. 1999; 116(5): 1132-1140. PMID: 10220505.
13. Wehler M, Nichterlein R, Fischer B, Farnbacher M, Reulbach U, Hahn EG, et al. Factors associated with health-related quality of life in chronic pancreatitis. *Am J Gastroenterol*. 2004; 99(1): 138-146. PMID: 14687155.
14. Gachago C, Draganov PV. Pain management in chronic pancreatitis. *World J Gastroenterol*. 2008; 14(20): 3137-3148. PMID: 18506917.
15. Savage SR. Long-term opioid therapy: assessment of consequences and risks. *J Pain Symptom Manage*. 1996; 11(5): 274-286. PMID: 8636626.
16. Mao J, Price DD, Mayer DJ. Mechanisms of hyperalgesia and morphine tolerance: a current view of their possible interactions. *Pain*. 1995; 62(3): 259-274. PMID: 8657426.
17. Olesen SS, Bouwense SA, Wilder-Smith OH, van Goor H, Drewes AM. Pregabalin reduces pain in patients with chronic pancreatitis in a randomized, controlled trial. *Gastroenterology*. 2011; 141(2): 536-543. PMID: 21683078.
18. Talukdar R, Murthy HV, Reddy DN. Role of methionine containing antioxidant combination in the management of pain in chronic pancreatitis: A systematic review and meta-analysis. *Pancreatology*. 2015; 15(2): 136-144. PMID: 25648074.
19. Ballantyne JC, Mao J. Opioid therapy for chronic pain. *N Engl J Med*. 2003; 349(20): 1943-1953. PMID: 14614170.
20. D'Haese JG, Ceyhan GO, Demir IE, Tieftrunk E, Friess H. Treatment options in painful chronic pancreatitis: a systematic review. *HPB (Oxford)*. 2014; 16(6): 512-521. PMID: 24033614.
21. Gress F, Schmitt C, Sherman S, Ciaccia D, Ikenberry S, Lehman G. Endoscopic ultrasound-guided celiac plexus block for managing abdominal pain associated with chronic pancreatitis: a prospective single center experience. *Am J Gastroenterol*. 2001; 96(2): 409-416. PMID: 11232683.

22. Michaels AJ, Draganov PV. Endoscopic ultrasonography guided celiac plexus neurolysis and celiac plexus block in the management of pain due to pancreatic cancer and chronic pancreatitis. *World J Gastroenterol.* 2007; 13(26): 3575-3580. PMID: 17659707.
23. Garcea G, Thomasset S, Berry DP, Tordoff S. Percutaneous splanchnic nerve radiofrequency ablation for chronic abdominal pain. *ANZ J Surg.* 2005; 75(8): 640-644. PMID: 16076323.
24. Verhaegh BP, van Kleef M, Geurts JW, Puylaert M, van Zundert J, Kessels AG, et al. Percutaneous radiofrequency ablation of the splanchnic nerves in patients with chronic pancreatitis: results of single and repeated procedures in 11 patients. *Pain Pract.* 2013; 13(8): 621-626. PMID: 23301539.
25. Baghdadi S, Abbas MH, Albouz F, Ammori BJ. Systematic review of the role of thoracoscopic splanchnicectomy in palliating the pain of patients with chronic pancreatitis. *Surg Endosc.* 2008; 22(3): 580-588. PMID: 18163168.
26. Costamagna G, Bulajic M, Tringali A, Pandolfi M, Gabbrielli A, Spada C, et al. Multiple stenting of refractory pancreatic duct strictures in severe chronic pancreatitis: long-term results. *Endoscopy.* 2006; 38(3): 254-259. PMID: 16528652.
27. Tandan M1, Reddy DN, Talukdar R, Vinod K, Santosh D, Lakhtakia S, et al. Long-term clinical outcomes of extracorporeal shockwave lithotripsy in painful chronic calcific pancreatitis. *Gastrointest Endosc.* 2013; 78(5): 726-733. PMID: 23891416.
28. Ueda J, Miyasaka Y, Ohtsuka T, Takahata S, Tanaka M. Short- and long-term results of the Frey procedure for chronic pancreatitis. *J Hepatobiliary Pancreat Sci.* 2015; 22(3): 211-216. PMID: 25339262.
29. Díte P, Ruzicka M, Zboril V, Novotný I. A prospective, randomized trial comparing endoscopic and surgical therapy for chronic pancreatitis. *Endoscopy.* 2003; 35(7): 553-558. PMID: 12822088.
30. Cahen DL, Gouma DJ, Nio Y, Rauws EA, Boermeester MA, Busch OR, et al. Endoscopic versus surgical drainage of the pancreatic duct in chronic pancreatitis. *N Engl J Med.* 2007; 356(7): 676-684. PMID: 17301298.
31. Riediger H1, Adam U, Fischer E, Keck T, Pfeffer F, Hopt UT, et al. Long-term outcome after resection for chronic pancreatitis in 224 patients. *J Gastrointest Surg.* 2007; 11(8): 949-959; discussion 959-960. PMID: 17534689.
32. Georgiev G, Beltran del Rio M, Gruessner A, Tiwari M, Cercone R, Delbridge M, et al. Patient quality of life and pain improve after autologous islet transplantation (AIT) for treatment of chronic pancreatitis: 53 patient series at the University of Arizona. *Pancreatology.* 2015; 15(1): 40-45. PMID: 25455347.
33. Walsh RM, Saavedra JR, Lentz G, Guerron AD, Scheman J, Stevens T, et al. Improved quality of life following total pancreatectomy and auto-islet transplantation for chronic pancreatitis. *J Gastrointest Surg.* 2012; 16(8): 1469-1477. PMID: 22673773.
34. Sutherland DE, Radosevich DM, Bellin MD, Hering BJ, Beilman GJ, Dunn TB, et al. Total pancreatectomy and islet autotransplantation for chronic pancreatitis. *J Am Coll Surg.* 2012; 214(4): 409-424; discussion 424-426. PMID: 22397977.
35. Winston JH, He ZJ, Shenoy M, Xiao SY, Pasricha PJ. Molecular and behavioral changes in nociception in a novel rat model of chronic pancreatitis for the study of pain. *Pain.* 2005; 117(1-2): 214-222. PMID: 16098667.
36. Puig-Diví V, Molero X, Salas A, Guarner F, Guarner L, Malagelada JR. Induction of chronic pancreatic disease by trinitrobenzene sulfonic acid infusion into rat pancreatic ducts. *Pancreas.* 1996; 13(4): 417-424. PMID: 8899803.
37. Cattaruzza F, Johnson C, Leggit A, Grady E, Schenk AK, Cevikbas F, et al. Transient receptor potential ankyrin 1 mediates chronic pancreatitis pain in mice. *Am J Physiol Gastrointest Liver Physiol.* 2013; 304(11): G1002-G1012. PMID: 23558009.
38. Lyo V, Cattaruzza F, Kim TN, Walker AW, Paulick M, Cox D, et al. Active cathepsins B, L, and S in murine and human pancreatitis. *Am J Physiol Gastrointest Liver Physiol.* 2012; 303(8): G894-G903. PMID: 22899821.
39. Cattaruzza F, Amadesi S, Carlsson JF, Murphy JE, Lyo V, Kirkwood K, et al. Serine Proteases and Protease-activated Receptor 2 Mediate the Proinflammatory and Algesic Actions of Diverse Stimulants. *Br J Pharmacol.* 2014; 171(16): 3814-3826. PMID: 24749982.
40. Larsson LI. Innervation of the pancreas by substance P, enkephalin, vasoactive intestinal polypeptide and gastrin/CCK immunoractive nerves. *J Histochem Cytochem.* 1979; 27(9): 1283-1284. PMID: 479572.
41. Hwang SW, Cho H, Kwak J, Lee SY, Kang CJ, Jung J, et al. Direct activation of capsaicin receptors by products of lipoxygenases: endogenous capsaicin-like substances. *Proc Natl Acad Sci U S A.* 2000; 97(11): 6155-6160. PMID: 10823958.
42. Caterina MJ, Leffler A, Malmberg AB, Martin WJ, Trafton J, Petersen-Zeitz KR, et al. Impaired nociception and pain sensation in mice lacking the capsaicin receptor. *Science.* 2000; 288(5464): 306-313. PMID: 10764638.
43. Wick EC, Hoge SG, Grahn SW, Kim E, Divino LA, Grady EF, et al. Transient receptor potential vanilloid 1, calcitonin gene-related peptide, and substance P mediate nociception in acute pancreatitis. *Am J Physiol Gastrointest Liver Physiol.* 2006; 290(5): G959-G969. PMID: 16399878.
44. Liddle RA. The role of Transient Receptor Potential Vanilloid 1 (TRPV1) channels in pancreatitis. *Biochim Biophys Acta.* 2007; 1772(8): 869-878. PMID: 17428642.
45. Bautista DM, Pellegrino M, Tsunozaki M. TRPA1: A gatekeeper for inflammation. *Annu Rev Physiol.* 2013; 75: 181-200. PMID: 23020579.
46. Ceppa E, Cattaruzza F, Lyo V, Amadesi S, Pelayo JC, Poole DP, et al. Transient receptor potential ion channels V4 and A1 contribute to pancreatitis pain in mice. American journal of physiology. *Am J Physiol Gastrointest Liver Physiol.* 2010; 299(3): G556-G571. PMID: 20539005.
47. Bautista DM, Jordt SE, Nikai T, Tsuruda PR, Read AJ, Poblete J, et al. TRPA1 mediates the inflammatory actions of environmental irritants and proalgesic agents. *Cell.* 2006; 124(6): 1269-1282. PMID: 16564016.
48. Kwan KY, Allchorne AJ, Vollrath MA, Christensen AP, Zhang DS, Woolf CJ, et al. TRPA1 contributes to cold, mechanical, and chemical nociception but is not essential for hair-cell transduction. *Neuron.* 2006; 50(2): 277-289. PMID: 16630838.

49. Obata K, Katsura H, Mizushima T, Yamanaka H, Kobayashi K, Dai Y, et al. TRPA1 induced in sensory neurons contributes to cold hyperalgesia after inflammation and nerve injury. *J Clin Invest*. 2005; 115(9): 2393-2401. PMID: 16110328.
50. Petrus M, Peier AM, Bandell M, Hwang SW, Huynh T, Olney N, et al. A role of TRPA1 in mechanical hyperalgesia is revealed by pharmacological inhibition. *Mol Pain*. 2007; 3: 40. PMID: 18086313.
51. Staruschenko A, Jeske NA, Akopian AN. Contribution of TRPV1-TRPA1 interaction to the single channel properties of the TRPA1 channel. *J Biol Chem*. 2010; 285(20): 15167-15177. PMID: 20231274.
52. Schwartz ES, La JH, Scheff NN, Davis BM, Albers KM, Gebhart GF. TRPV1 and TRPA1 antagonists prevent the transition of acute to chronic inflammation and pain in chronic pancreatitis. *J Neurosci*. 2013; 33(13): 5603-5611. PMID: 23536075.
53. Nilius B. TRP channels in disease. *Biochim Biophys Acta*. 2007; 1772(8): 805-812. PMID: 17368864.
54. Poole DP, Amadesi S, Veldhuis NA, Abogadie FC, Lieu T, Darby W, et al. Protease-activated receptor 2 (PAR2) protein and transient receptor potential vanilloid 4 (TRPV4) protein coupling is required for sustained inflammatory signaling. *J Biol Chem*. 2013; 288(8): 5790-5802. PMID: 23288842.
55. Liedtke W, Friedman JM. Abnormal osmotic regulation in trpv4-/- mice. *Proc Natl Acad Sci U S A*. 2003; 100(23): 13698-13703. PMID: 14581612.
56. Alessandri-Haber N, Joseph E, Dina OA, Liedtke W, Levine JD. TRPV4 mediates pain-related behavior induced by mild hypertonic stimuli in the presence of inflammatory mediator. *Pain*. 2005; 118(1-2): 70-79. PMID: 16213085.
57. Alessandri-Haber N, Dina OA, Joseph EK, Reichling D, Levine JD. A transient receptor potential vanilloid 4-dependent mechanism of hyperalgesia is engaged by concerted action of inflammatory mediators. *J Neurosci*. 2006; 26(14): 3864-3874. PMID: 16597741.
58. Vu TK, Hung DT, Wheaton VI, Coughlin SR. Molecular cloning of a functional thrombin receptor reveals a novel proteolytic mechanism of receptor activation. *Cell*. 1991; 64(6): 1057-1068. PMID: 1672265.
59. Steinhoff M, Vergnolle N, Young SH, Tognetto M, Amadesi S, Ennes HS, et al. Agonists of proteinase-activated receptor 2 induce inflammation by a neurogenic mechanism. *Nat Med*. 2000; 6(2): 151-158. PMID: 10655102.
60. Hoogerwerf WA, Zou L, Shenoy M, Sun D, Micci MA, Lee-Hellmich H, et al. The proteinase-activated receptor 2 is involved in nociception. *J Neurosci*. 2001; 21(22): 9036-9042. PMID: 11698614.
61. Déry O, Corvera CU, Steinhoff M, Bunnett NW. Proteinase-activated receptors: novel mechanisms of signaling by serine proteases. *Am J Physiol Cell Physiol*. 1998; 274: C1429-C1452. PMID: 9696685.
62. Hoogerwerf WA, Gondesen K, Xiao SY, Winston JH, Willis WD, Pasricha PJ. The role of mast cells in the pathogenesis of pain in chronic pancreatitis. *BMC Gastroenterol*. 2005; 5: 8. PMID: 15745445.
63. Hoogerwerf WA, Shenoy M, Winston JH, Xiao SY, He Z, Pasricha PJ. Trypsin mediates nociception via the proteinase-activated receptor 2: a potentially novel role in pancreatic pain. *Gastroenterology*. 2004; 127(3): 883-891. PMID: 15362043.
64. Vergnolle N, Bunnett NW, Sharkey KA, Brussee V, Compton SJ, Grady EF, et al. Proteinase-activated receptor-2 and hyperalgesia: A novel pain pathway. *Nat Med*. 2001; 7(7): 821-816. PMID: 11433347.
65. Dai Y, Wang S, Tominaga M, Yamamoto S, Fukuoka T, Higashi T, et al. Sensitization of TRPA1 by PAR2 contributes to the sensation of inflammatory pain. *J Clin Invest*. 2007; 117(7): 1979-1987. PMID: 17571167.
66. Grant AD, Cottrell GS, Amadesi S, Trevisani M, Nicoletti P, Materazzi S, et al. Protease-activated receptor 2 sensitizes the transient receptor potential vanilloid 4 ion channel to cause mechanical hyperalgesia in mice. *J Physiol*. 2007; 578: 715-733. PMID: 17124270.
67. Chen Y, Yang C, Wang ZJ. Proteinase-activated receptor 2 sensitizes transient receptor potential vanilloid 1, transient receptor potential vanilloid 4, and transient receptor potential ankyrin 1 in paclitaxel-induced neuropathic pain. *Neuroscience*. 2011; 193: 440-451. PMID: 21763756.
68. Woolf CJ, Safieh-Garabedian B, Ma QP, Crilly P, Winter J. Nerve growth factor contributes to the generation of inflammatory sensory hypersensitivity. *Neuroscience*. 1994; 62: 327-331. PMID: 7530342.
69. Friess H, Zhu ZW, di Mola FF, Kulli C, Graber HU, Andren-Sandberg A, et al. Nerve growth factor and its high-affinity receptor in chronic pancreatitis. *Ann Surg*. 1999; 230(5): 615-624. PMID: 10561084.
70. Zhu Y, Colak T, Shenoy M, Liu L, Pai R, Li C, et al. Nerve growth factor modulates TRPV1 expression and function and mediates pain in chronic pancreatitis. *Gastroenterology*. 2011; 141(1): 370-377. PMID: 21473865.
71. McMahon SB, Armanini MP, Ling LH, Phillips HS. Expression and coexpression of Trk receptors in subpopulations of adult primary sensory neurons projecting to identified peripheral targets. *Neuron*. 1994; 12(5): 1161-1171. PMID: 7514427.
72. McMahon SB, Bennett DL, Priestley JV, Shelton DL. The biological effects of endogenous nerve growth factor on adult sensory neurons revealed by a trkA-IgG fusion molecule. *Nat Med*. 1995; 1(8): 774-780. PMID: 7585179.
73. Barbacid M. The Trk family of neurotrophin receptors. *J Neurobiol*. 1994; 25(11): 1386-1403. PMID: 7852993.
74. Zhu Y, Mehta K, Li C, Xu GY, Liu L, Colak T, et al. Systemic administration of anti-NGF increases A-type potassium currents and decreases pancreatic nociceptor excitability in a rat model of chronic pancreatitis. *Am J Physiol Gastrointest Liver Physiol*. 2012; 302(1): G176-G181. PMID: 22038828.
75. Lewin GR, Ritter AM, Mendell LM. Nerve growth factor-induced hyperalgesia in the neonatal and adult rat. *J Neurosci*. 1993; 13(5): 2136-2148. PMID: 8478693.
76. Mantyh PW, Mantyh CR, Gates T, Vigna SR, Maggio JE. Receptor binding sites for substance P and substance K in the canine gastrointestinal tract and their possible role in inflammatory bowel disease. *Neuroscience*. 1988;(3): 817-837. PMID: 2457186.
77. Di Sebastiano P, di Mola FF, Di Febbo C, Baccante G, Porreca E, Innocenti P, et al. Expression of interleukin 8

(IL-8) and substance P in human chronic pancreatitis. *Gut.* 2000; 47(3): 423-428. PMID: 10940282.
78. Grady EF, Yoshimi SK, Maa J, Valeroso D, Vartanian RK, Rahim S, et al. Substance P mediates inflammatory oedema in acute pancreatitis via activation of the neurokinin-1 receptor in rats and mice. *Br J Pharmacol.* 2000; 130(3): 505-512. PMID: 10821777.
79. Hutter MM, Wick EC, Day AL, Maa J, Zerega EC, Richmond AC, et al. Transient receptor potential vanilloid (TRPV-1) promotes neurogenic inflammation in the pancreas via activation of the neurokinin-1 receptor (NK-1R). *Pancreas.* 2005; 30(3): 260-265. PMID: 15782105.
80. Shrikhande SV, Friess H, di Mola FF, Tempia-Caliera A, Conejo Garcia JR, Zhu Z, et al. NK-1 receptor gene expression is related to pain in chronic pancreatitis. *Pain.* 2011; 91(3): 209-217. PMID: 11275376.
81. Tsuda M, Inoue K, Salter MW. Neuropathic pain and spinal microglia: a big problem from molecules in "small" glia. *Trends Neurosci.* 2005; 28(2): 101-107. PMID: 15667933.
82. Wen YR, Tan PH, Cheng JK, Liu YC, Ji RR. Microglia: a promising target for treating neuropathic and postoperative pain, and morphine tolerance. *J Formos Med Assoc.* 2011; 110(8): 487-494. PMID: 21783017.
83. Thacker MA, Clark AK, Bishop T, Grist J, Yip PK, Moon LD, et al. CCL2 is a key mediator of microglia activation in neuropathic pain states. *Eur J Pain.* 2009; 13(3): 263-272. PMID: 18554968.
84. Tsuda M, Shigemoto-Mogami Y, Koizumi S, Mizokoshi A, Kohsaka S, Salter MW, et al. P2X4 receptors induced in spinal microglia gate tactile allodynia after nerve injury. *Nature.* 2003; 424(6950): 778-783. PMID: 12917686.
85. Jin SX, Zhuang ZY, Woolf CJ, Ji RR. p38 mitogen-activated protein kinase is activated after a spinal nerve ligation in spinal cord microglia and dorsal root ganglion neurons and contributes to the generation of neuropathic pain. *J Neurosci.* 2003; 23(10): 4017-4022. PMID: 12764087.
86. Liu PY, Lu CL, Wang CC, Lee IH, Hsieh JC, Chen CC, et al. Spinal microglia initiate and maintain hyperalgesia in a rat model of chronic pancreatitis. *Gastroenterology.* 2012; 142(1): 165-173. PMID: 21963786.
87. Smith HS. Activated microglia in nociception. *Pain Physician.* 2010; 13(3): 295-304. PMID: 20495595.
88. Watkins LR, Milligan ED, Maier SF. Glial activation: a driving force for pathological pain. *Trends Neurosci.* 2001; 24(8): 450-455. PMID: 11476884.
89. Chapman GA, Moores K, Harrison D, Campbell CA, Stewart BR, Strijbos PJ. Fractalkine cleavage from neuronal membranes represents an acute event in the inflammatory response to excitotoxic brain damage. *J Neurosci.* 2000; 20(15): RC87. PMID: 10899174.
90. Barclay J, Clark AK, Ganju P, Gentry C, Patel S, Wotherspoon G, et al. Role of the cysteine protease cathepsin S in neuropathic hyperalgesia. *Pain.* 2007; 130(3): 225-234. PMID: 17250968.
91. Clark AK, Yip PK, Grist J, Gentry C, Staniland AA, Marchand F, et al. Inhibition of spinal microglial cathepsin S for the reversal of neuropathic pain. *Proc Natl Acad Sci U S A.* 2007; 104(25): 10655-10660. PMID: 17551020.
92. Clark AK, Yip PK, Malcangio M. The liberation of fractalkine in the dorsal horn requires microglial cathepsin S. *J Neurosci.* 2009; 29(21): 6945-6954. PMID: 19474321.
93. Garrison CJ, Dougherty PM, Kajander KC, Carlton SM. Staining of glial fibrillary acidic protein (GFAP) in lumbar spinal cord increases following a sciatic nerve constriction injury. *Brain Res.* 1991; 565(1): 1-7. PMID: 1723019.
94. Garrison CJ, Dougherty PM, Carlton SM. GFAP expression in lumbar spinal cord of naive and neuropathic rats treated with MK-801. *Exp Neurol.* 1994; 129(2): 237-243. PMID: 7957738.
95. Ji RR, Kawasaki Y, Zhuang ZY, Wen YR, Decosterd I. Possible role of spinal astrocytes in maintaining chronic pain sensitization: review of current evidence with focus on bFGF/JNK pathway. *Neuron Glia Biol.* 2006; 2(4): 259-269. PMID: 17710215.
96. Zhuang ZY, Gerner P, Woolf CJ, Ji RR. ERK is sequentially activated in neurons, microglia, and astrocytes by spinal nerve ligation and contributes to mechanical allodynia in this neuropathic pain model. *Pain.* 2005; 114(1-2): 149-159. PMID: 15733640.
97. Feng QX, Wang W, Feng XY, Mei XP, Zhu C, Liu ZC, et al. Astrocytic activation in thoracic spinal cord contributes to persistent pain in rat model of chronic pancreatitis. *Neuroscience.* 2010; 167(2): 501-509. PMID: 20149842.
98. Mertz H. Role of the brain and sensory pathways in gastrointestinal sensory disorders in humans. *Gut.* 2002; 51 Suppl 1: i29-33. PMID: 12077061.
99. Dimcevski G, Schipper KP, Tage-Jensen U, Funch-Jensen P, Krarup AL, Toft E, et al. Hypoalgesia to experimental visceral and somatic stimulation in painful chronic pancreatitis. *Eur J Gastroenterol Hepatol.* 2006; 18(7): 755-764. PMID: 16772833.
100. Dimcevski G, Sami SA, Funch-Jensen P, Le Pera D, Valeriani M, Arendt-Nielsen L, et al. Pain in chronic pancreatitis: the role of reorganization in the central nervous system. *Gastroenterology.* 2007; 132(4): 1546-1556. PMID: 17408654.
101. Lee M, Silverman SM, Hansen H, Patel VB, Manchikanti L. A comprehensive review of opioid-induced hyperalgesia. *Pain Physician.* 2011; 14(2): 145-161. PMID: 21412369.
102. Célèrier E, Laulin J, Larcher A, Le Moal M, Simonnet G. Evidence for opiate-activated NMDA processes masking opiate analgesia in rats. *Brain Res.* 1999; 847(1): 18-25. PMID: 10564731.
103. Mao J, Sung B, Ji RR, Lim G. Chronic morphine induces downregulation of spinal glutamate transporters: implications in morphine tolerance and abnormal pain sensitivity. *J Neurosci.* 2002; 22(18): 8312-8323. PMID: 12223586.
104. Vanderah TW, Ossipov MH, Lai J, Malan TP Jr, Porreca F. Mechanisms of opioid-induced pain and antinociceptive tolerance: descending facilitation and spinal dynorphin. *Pain.* 2001; 92(1-2): 5-9. PMID: 11323121.
105. Chu LF, Clark DJ, Angst MS. Opioid tolerance and hyperalgesia in chronic pain patients after one month of oral morphine therapy: a preliminary prospective study. *J Pain.* 2006; 7(1): 43-48. PMID: 16414554.
106. Compton P, Charuvastra VC, Ling W. Pain intolerance in opioid-maintained former opiate addicts: effect of long-acting maintenance agent. *Drug Alcohol Depend.* 2001; 63(2): 139-146. PMID: 11376918.

107. Hay JL, White JM, Bochner F, Somogyi AA, Semple TJ, Rounsefell B. Hyperalgesia in opioid-managed chronic pain and opioid-dependent patients. *J Pain*. 2009; 10(3): 316-322. PMID: 19101210.
108. Reznikov I, Pud D, Eisenberg E. Oral opioid administration and hyperalgesia in patients with cancer or chronic nonmalignant pain. *Br J Clin Pharmacol*. 2005; 60(3): 311-318. PMID: 16120071.
109. Mao J. Opioid-induced abnormal pain sensitivity: implications in clinical opioid therapy. *Pain*. 2002; 100(3): 213-217. PMID: 12467992.

Chapter 12

The effects of bile acids on pancreatic ductal cells

Viktória Venglovecz[1*], Zoltán Rakonczay Jr.[2,3], and Péter Hegyi[2,4]

[1]Department of Pharmacology and Pharmacotherapy; [2]First Department of Medicine, University of Szeged, Szeged, Hungary;
[3]Department of Pathophysiology, University of Szeged, Szeged, Hungary;
[4]MTA-SZTE Translational Gastroenterology, Research Group, Szeged, Hungary.

Introduction

Bile acids (BAs) are natural end products of cholesterol metabolism.[1] The physiological functions of BAs are the emulsification of lipid aggregates and solubilization of lipids in an aqueous environment. The major BAs in humans are chenodeoxycholic acid (CDCA) and cholic acid (CA), which are known as primary BAs since they are synthesized in the liver.[2] Before secretion by hepatocytes, primary BAs are conjugated with either taurine or glycine, which increases their polarity and water solubility. Secondary bile acids such as deoxycholic acid (DCA) and lithocholic acid (LCA) are produced in the colon by bacterial dehydroxylation of the primary BAs. Under physiological conditions, BAs are temporarily stored in the gallbladder and released to the intestine. Most BAs are then efficiently reabsorbed from the ileum and transported back to the liver via the portal vein (enterohepatic circulation). Under normal, physiological conditions, BAs cannot access the pancreas. However, under pathophysiological conditions such as obstruction of the ampulla of Vater by an impacted gallstone, bile can enter into the pancreatic ducts and trigger pancreatitis.[3] Unfortunately, we do not know the concentration of BAs that can reach the pancreatic ductal cells under pathological conditions. It probably varies among patients and mainly depends on the duration of ampullary gallstone obstruction. However, previous studies have shown that relatively low concentrations of BAs (25-200 μM) can alter intracellular calcium (Ca^{2+}) signaling and cause acinar cell death.[4,5] The close relationship between gallstone passage and the development of acute pancreatitis (AP) has been known for more than 100 years[3] and has been confirmed in a number of studies.[6-8] However, the pathogenesis underlying the development of biliary AP is not well understood.

Most of the research investigating the pathomechanism of AP has been done on pancreatic acinar cells. These studies have demonstrated that the central intra-acinar events in pancreatitis are increased intra-acinar Ca^{2+} concentration, premature activation of trypsinogen, and activation of the proinflammatory transcription factor nuclear factor-κB (NF-κB), which leads to pancreatic injury.[9-14] One of the most toxic BAs to acinar cells is the secondary BA taurolithocholic acid (TLC) that forms from LCA after reabsorption from the intestine. The sulfated form of TLC (TLCS) induces Ca^{2+} signaling in pancreatic acinar cells via an inositol 1,4,5-trisphosphate (IP_3)-dependent mobilization of sequestered intracellular Ca^{2+}.[5] Elevated interacellur free Ca^{2+} concentration $[(Ca^{2+})_i]$ can lead to enzyme activation[13] and/or cell death[4] and leads to severe acute necrotizing pancreatitis. Since increased $[Ca^{2+}]$ is a critical step in the initiation of acinar cell injury, several studies have focused on the prevention of cytosolic Ca^{2+} overload. The Ca^{2+} chelator, caffeine and its dimethylxanthine metabolites efficiently decreased TLCS-induced Ca^{2+} elevation and cell death on isolated pancreatic acinar cells. Caffeine also reduced the severity of TLCS-induced AP, most likely by inhibiting IP_3R-mediated Ca^{2+} signaling.[15] In another aspect, blocking Ca^{2+} entry by pharmacological inhibition of the store-operated Ca^{2+} channel Orai-1 has also proven effective against TLCS-induced acinar cell necrosis.[16] The target of the sustained Ca^{2+} signal is the Ca^{2+}-activated phosphatase calcineurin, which plays a central role in intra-acinar activation of zymogens and NF-κB.[17] In addition to Ca^{2+}, other cellular mechanisms are also involved in BA-induced acinar injury, such as mitochondrial dysfunction,[18,19] depletion of cytosolic ATP,[20] and increased reactive oxygen species (ROS) production.[21]

In contrast to acinar cells, the role of pancreatic ductal epithelial cells (PDECs) in biliary AP pathogenesis has received much less attention, despite being the first pancreatic cell type exposed to the refluxed bile. Pancreatic ducts can be divided into three main types on the basis of their size and location: main, interlobular, and intralobular ducts. The main duct mostly collects and drains the juice secreted by

*Corresponding author. Email: venglovecz.viktoria@med.u-szeged.hu

other branches of the ductal tree, whereas intra-/interlobular ducts are the main sites of HCO_3^- secretion. Although, several studies have shown that ductal fluid and HCO_3^- secretion are crucially important to maintain pancreas integrity,[22-25] the role of PDECs in AP development has only been highlighted recently. *In vivo* studies have shown that pancreatic hypersecretion (with hypoproteinemia) occurs in the early phase of AP, which develops into hyposecretion during pancreatitis onset.[23-25] This hypersecretion may represent a defense mechanism by washing out toxic factors from the pancreas. The beneficial effect of fluid hypersecretion is further supported by studies in which secretin, one of the major secretagogues of ductal fluid secretion, was shown to reduce the severity of cerulein-induced AP.[26,27] In addition, impaired or insufficient ductal fluid secretion, such as observed in cystic fibrosis, increases the risk of AP.[28,29] Taken together, these data strongly suggest that PDECs represent an important and essential protective mechanism in the exocrine pancreas.

Effect of BAs on the Main Pancreatic Duct

In the 1980s, it was postulated that breakdown of the pancreatic duct permeability barrier is a risk factor for AP development. Researchers then extensively investigated the effect of BAs on main pancreatic duct morphology and permeability. In these *in vivo* studies, various BAs were perfused through the cannulated main duct, and the permeability of the pancreatic duct mucosal barrier was measured using different techniques.[30-34] The results revealed that high concentrations (2-15 mM) of BAs rendered the ducts permeable to molecules as large as 20,000-Daltons, whereas they are normally impermeable to molecules over 3,000 Daltons.[30,31] BAs in millimolar concentrations also increase the permeability of the main duct to Cl^- and HCO_3^-.[32-34] The effect of dihydroxy BAs was significantly greater than the effect of trihydroxy BAs on the permeability of these anions, probably because trihydroxy BAs are less lipid soluble and therefore less cytotoxic. The changes in ductal permeability were in accordance with changes in ductal epithelia morphology. Perfusion with higher concentrations (15 mM) disrupted cell integrity, leading to ductal epithelium flattening and cell loss.[30] This harmful effect of BAs is not surprising given their detergent properties.

It was also highlighted that infected bile is more harmful to the duct cells than sterile bile.[30,33,34] Its higher toxicity is likely due to bacterial deconjugation, which produces more toxic unconjugated BAs. The toxicity of BAs mainly depends on their solubility and the degree of ionization. At neutral pH, unconjugated bile acids exist in an unionized,[35] electrically neutral form and therefore can pass easily through the cell membrane. In contrast, glycine- and taurine-conjugated BAs have a lower pK_a (around 4 and 2 respectively), are ionized at neutral pH,[35] and are therefore less lipid soluble.

Although, *in vivo* animal studies are important, their relevance to human disease is doubtful. One of the major problems with these studies is that BAs were used in relatively high concentrations; probably higher than would be present in the pancreatic duct following reflux. Moreover, at these extremely high concentrations, BAs caused excessive and uncontrolled destruction of both acini and ducts.

In vitro studies have allowed the investigation of more pathophysiologically relevant effects of BAs on the ductal epithelium. Okolo et al. studied the effects of BAs (100 μM to 2 mM) on the ion conductances and monolayer resistance of cultured PDECs isolated from dog accessory pancreatic duct.[36] They found that taurodeoxycholic acid (TDCA) and taurochenodeoxycholic acid caused concentration-dependent increases in both chloride (Cl^-) and potassium (K^+) conductances, whereas the trihydroxy BA taurocholic acid was completely ineffective. The increases in Cl^- and K^+ conductances were mediated via $[Ca^{2+}]_i$ elevation and blocked by 4,4′-diisothiocyanostilbene-2,2′-disulfonic acid (DIDS) and charybdotoxin, respectively. Using Ussing chambers, they could localize the Cl^- and K^+ conductances to the apical and basolateral membranes of PDECs, respectively. In addition, they showed that only higher BA concentrations decreased the monolayer transepithelial resistance. Similar results have been found in bovine PDECs, in which TDCA markedly increased transepithelial ion transport and decreased tissue electrical resistance.[37] On the other hand, TDCA caused dose-dependent mucosal damage,[38] and at higher concentrations, extensive loss of the epithelial cell lining.[37]

Effect of BAs on the Intra-/Interlobular Pancreatic Ducts

The earlier studies described above characterized the effects of BAs on main pancreatic duct permeability and morphology; no information was available about their effects on the smaller ducts. However, the development of microdissection techniques for isolating the small intra-/interlobular ducts led to a breakthrough in our understanding of ductal cell physiology.[39]

The main physiological function of the intra-/interlobular pancreatic ductal cells is to secrete a HCO_3^--rich alkaline fluid that washes digestive enzymes out of the gland and neutralizes acid chyme in the duodenum.[39] The effects of BAs on HCO_3^- secretion have been intensively investigated in the last few years,[40-42] and the results of these studies suggest a complex role of ductal cells in the pathomechanism of biliary AP.

Our research group has shown that both basolateral and luminal administration of either nonconjugated or glycine-conjugated forms of CDCA causes a dose-dependent intracellular acidification in guinea pig PDECs.[42] Interestingly, basolateral administration of 1 mM CDCA for

6–8 min damaged membrane integrity, and the cells rapidly lost the fluorescent dye. The same concentration of CDCA on the luminal membrane had no toxic effects. Okolo et al. also found differences between the effects of BAs on the luminal and basolateral membranes.[36] In addition, both CDCA and glycochenodeoxycholate (GCDCA) induced a dose-dependent increase in $[Ca^{2+}]_i$ via phospholipase C- and IP_3 receptor-mediated mechanisms. GCDCA had a smaller effect on intracellular pH (pH_i) and $[Ca^{2+}]_i$ than CDCA, most likely because conjugated BAs are ionized at neutral pH and therefore require active transport mechanisms for cellular uptake.

We also found that the effect of CDCA on ductal HCO_3^- efflux is concentration dependent.[42] At a low concentration (0.1 mM), CDCA significantly stimulated HCO_3^- efflux by a DIDS-sensitive Cl^-/HCO_3^- exchange mechanism. The stimulatory effect of CDCA was only observed when CDCA was added to the lumen of the ducts and was dependent on Ca^{2+} mobilization. In contrast, a high concentration of CDCA (1 mM) induced pathologic Ca^{2+} signaling and strongly inhibited HCO_3^- efflux. This inhibitory effect of high-concentration CDCA was independent of $[Ca^{2+}]_i$ changes and was observed when CDCA was applied to either the luminal or basolateral membrane of the ducts.[42] The effect of the conjugated GCDCA on pH_i and $[Ca^{2+}]_i$ suggest that although GCDCA can enter the cells, likely by a transporter-mediated mechanism, it had no effect on HCO_3^- efflux at either high or low concentrations.

The concentration-dependent differences in the effects of CDCA suggest that nonconjugated BAs have a specific mode of action on PDECs that strongly depends on their concentration. The key is to identify the cellular mechanisms by which BAs exert these opposite effects. Perides et al. recently described the presence of a G-protein-coupled bile acid receptor-1 (GPBAR1 also known as TGR5) on the apical membrane of acinar cells.[43] They showed that GPBAR1 knockout mice were completely protected against TLCS-induced pancreatitis and suggested that this receptor has a central role in the BA-induced acinar cell injury in mice. In contrast, guinea pig pancreatic ductal cells do not express GPBAR1,[41] suggesting that this receptor is not involved in the effect of CDCA on PDECs.

Stimulatory effect of low concentrations of BAs

Since CDCA only increases HCO_3^- efflux when applied to the luminal membrane, it is likely that the stimulatory effect of CDCA is due to activation of one or more Ca^{2+}-dependent apical transporters. The SLC26 anion transporters[44,45] and the Ca^{2+}-activated Cl^- channel (CaCC) are known to be activated by increased $[Ca^{2+}]_i$ suggesting that these transporters could be the target for the CDCA-induced Ca^{2+} increase.

Using the whole cell configuration of the patch clamp technique, CDCA failed to activate CaCC but induced a robust and reversible increase in K^+ currents.[41] The activated currents could be blocked by the specific large-conductance Ca^{2+}-activated K^+ channel (BK) inhibitor, iberiotoxin. In contrast, the small- and intermediate Ca^{2+}-activated K^+ channel inhibitors, UCL1684 and TRAM34 had no effect on the CDCA-activated currents. Luminal administration of iberiotoxin completely blocked the stimulatory effect of CDCA on HCO_3^- efflux in microperfused ducts. In contrast, basolaterally applied iberiotoxin had no effect on luminal CDCA-stimulated HCO_3^- efflux. These data strongly indicate that BK channels play a central role in the stimulatory effect of CDCA on HCO_3^- efflux and that they are localized to the luminal membrane of ductal cells. This latter hypothesis has been confirmed by immunohistochemistry showing strong BK channel expression at the apical membrane of guinea pig intra/interlobular ducts.[41] Moreover, activation of BK channels by luminal administration of the pharmacological compound NS11021 increased HCO_3^- efflux in a manner similar to CDCA. Our hypothesis is that apical BK channel activation leads to hyperpolarization of the apical plasma membrane, which in turn increases the electrochemical driving force for anion efflux through SLC26 anion exchangers (**Figure 1**). The cystic fibrosis transmembrane conductance regulator (CFTR) Cl^- channel is one of the major ion channels on the apical membrane of PDECs which interacts with the Cl^-/HCO_3^- exchanger and thereby plays an essential role in HCO_3^- efflux. The possible role of this ion channel has also been raised in the stimulatory effect of CDCA.[46] CFPAC-1 is a human, pancreatic ductal cell line that is deficient for CFTR but expresses the SLC26A6 anion exchanger. Administration of 0.1 mM CDCA had no effect on HCO_3^- efflux in these cells. However, after the transduction of CFPAC-1 cells with wild-type CFTR, CDCA significantly stimulated HCO_3^- efflux. Patch clamp experiments showed that CDCA had no effect on the activity of this channel, although it requires CFTR expression to exert its stimulatory effect.[46]

Recent studies by Kowal et al. indicated that ATP release and purinergic receptor activation are also involved in the stimulatory effect of CDCA.[47,48] Using a pancreatic ductal cell line (Capan-1) they showed that CDCA induces dose-dependent ATP release via both vesicular and nonvesicular mechanisms; this is more pronounced when CDCA is applied to the luminal membrane. Extracellular ATP then binds to P2 receptors leading to increased $[Ca^{2+}]_i$ which may be involved in the activation of Ca^{2+}-activated ion channels such as BK channels (**Figure 1**). Capan-1 cells express the GPBAR1 receptor that is activated by CDCA; although activation of this receptor is not involved in CDCA-induced ATP release.

The stimulatory effect of low CDCA concentrations highlights the importance of ductal fluid secretion in the

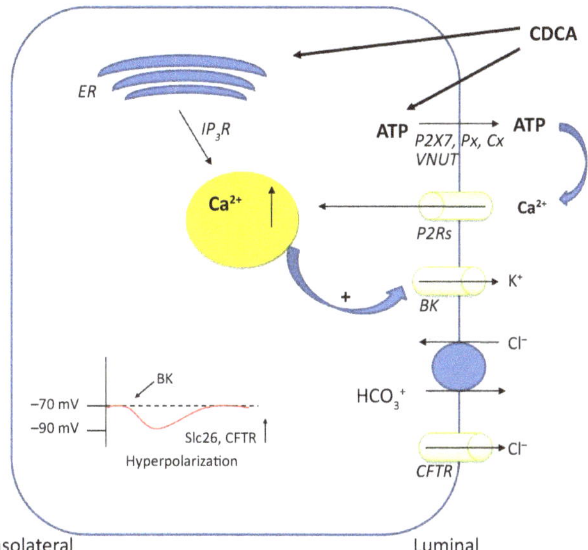

Figure 1. Cellular mechanism of the stimulatory effect of CDCA. A low CDCA concentration (0.1 mM) elevates $[Ca^{2+}]_i$ by two distinct mechanisms: (1) release of Ca^{2+} from the ER lumen by an IP_3R- and PLC-mediated pathway and (2) extracellular ATP-induced Ca^{2+} influx directly and indirectly through P2X and P2Y receptors, respectively. The increase in $[Ca^{2+}]_i$ activates BK channels that leads to the hyperpolarization of the plasma membrane that subsequently increases the electrochemical driving force for anion secretion through CFTR and SLC26 anion exchangers. BK: large conductance Ca^{2+}-activated K^+ channel, Ca^{2+}: calcium, CDCA: chenodeoxycholic acid, CFTR: cystic fibrosis transmembrane conductance regulator Cl^- channel, Cx: connexin, ER: endoplasmic reticulum, IP_3R: inositol 1,4,5-trisphosphate receptor, PLC: phospholipase C, Px: pannexin, VNUT: vesicular nucleotide, +: stimulation.

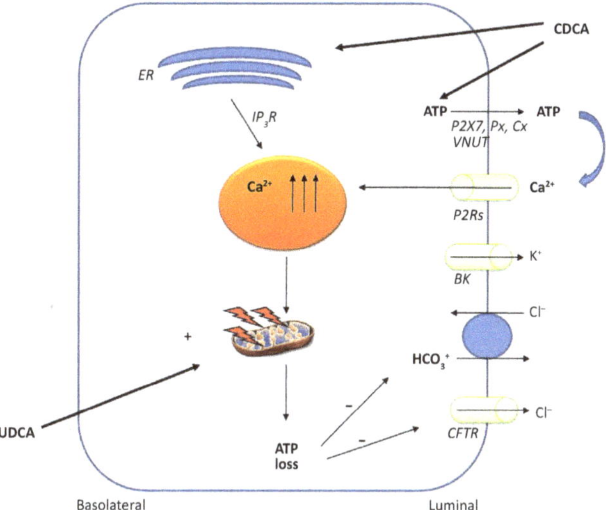

Figure 2. Cellular mechanism of the inhibitory effect of CDCA. A high concentration of CDCA (1 mM) induces toxic $Ca^{2+}{}_i$ signaling, mitochondrial damage, and ATP_i depletion that leads to the inhibition of acid-base transporters of PDECs. A 24-h pretreatment of the ducts with UDCA (0.5 mM) can prevent the toxic effect of CDCA by stabilizing the mitochondrial membrane. BK: large conductance Ca^{2+}-activated K^+ channel, Ca^{2+}: calcium, CDCA: chenodeoxycholic acid, CFTR: cystic fibrosis transmembrane conductance regulator Cl^- channel, Cx: connexin, ER: endoplasmic reticulum, IP_3R: inositol 1,4,5-trisphosphate receptor, Px: pannexin, UDCA: ursodeoxycholic acid, VNUT: vesicular nucleotide, -: inhibition, +: protective effect.

protection of the pancreas. The increased fluid volume can be beneficial in several ways:

(i) High HCO_3^- concentrations in the secreted fluid promote the deprotonation of BAs to less toxic bile salts.
(ii) The increased volume of fluid decreases ductal BA concentration.
(iii) The greater ductal flow may push stones through the papilla of Vater to clear the obstruction.
(iv) Increased fluid secretion may wash out the toxic BAs from the ductal tree to avoid pancreatic injury.

Inhibitory effect of high concentrations of bile acids

If the stimulated secretion is not able to wash out BAs from the ductal tree, the luminal concentrations of BAs will increase further. In this situation, high CDCA concentrations cause pathologic Ca^{2+} signaling and inhibition of the acid/base transporters of PDECs.[42] We have provided evidence that mitochondrial damage and depletion of intracellular ATP (ATP_i) are the most crucial factors in the toxic effect of CDCA on pancreatic ductal secretion.[40] Administration of 1 mM CDCA to PDECs for 10 minutes causes swelling of the mitochondria and disruption of their inner membranes. Damage of the mitochondria markedly and irreversibly reduce ATP_i. Exposure of pancreatic ducts to carbonyl cyanide m-chlorophenyl hydrazone and deoxyglucose/iodoacetamide (inhibitors of oxidative phosphorylation and the glycolytic pathway respectively) fully mimic the effect of 1 mM CDCA. These data indicate that CDCA inhibits both the oxidative and glycolytic pathways in PDECs. In addition, ATP_i depletion is crucial in the inhibitory effect of CDCA on ductal ion transport mechanisms. In the absence of ATP_i the acid/base transporters do not work properly, which leads to impaired fluid secretion and finally cell death (**Figure 2**). In this case, BAs could reach the acinar cells, either by diffusion up the ductal tree or leakage into the gland interstitium, where they will switch on pathologic Ca^{2+} signaling and trigger AP. We have also shown that the CDCA-induced mitochondrial injury is due to the opening of mitochondrial permeability transition pore (mPTP), which leads to mitochondrial swelling/dysfunction and consequently inhibition of ATP synthesis.[49] Studies of hepatocytes have demonstrated that the toxic effect of hydrophobic BAs can be attenuated by the hydrophilic BA ursodeoxycholic acid (UDCA).[50–53] These studies have shown that the cytoprotective effect of UDCA is largely based on its ability to stabilize the mitochondrial membrane by inhibiting BA-induced mPTP opening. A 24-h

Table 1. Summary of the effect of bile acids on pancreatic ductal epithelial cells.

	Species	Duct type	Bile acid	mM	Effect	Ref.
In vivo studies	Rat	Main duct	Human bile		Sterile bile: Increased ionic flux, cell oedema Infected bile: loss of integrity	30
	Cat	Main duct	CA, GDCA, GCA, TCA, CDCA, GCDCA, DCA	1.5, 2, 15–42	Increased permeability	2, 3, 26, 31
In vitro studies	Dog	Accessory duct	TDCA, TCDCA	0.1–2	Increased Cl^- and K^+ conductances	36
	Bovine	Main duct	TDCA	0.05–5	Increased transepithelial ion transport, decreased electrical resistance and loss of epithelial cell lining	37, 38
	Guinea pig	Intra-interlobular ducts	CDCA	0.1–1	Low dose: Increased HCO_3^- efflux High dose: Inhibited HCO_3^- efflux	40–42
Studies on cell lines	Capan-1		CDCA	0.3–1	ATP release	47
	CFPAC-1		CDCA	0.1	Increased HCO_3^- efflux in the presence of CFTR	46

CA: cholic acid, CDCA: chenodeoxycholic acid, DCA: deoxycholic acid, GCA: glycocholic acid, GCDCA: glycochenodeoxycholic acid, GDCA: glycodeoxycholic acid, TCA: taurocholic acid, TCDCA: taurochenodeoxycholic acid, TDCA: taurodeoxycholic acid.

pretreatment of the pancreatic ducts with 0.5 mM UDCA significantly decreased CDCA-induced mitochondrial injury by inhibiting CDCA-induced mPTP and ATP_i loss and reduced the inhibitory effect of CDCA on the acid/base transporters.[49] Moreover, the protective effect of UDCA on the mitochondria is associated with an anti-apoptotic effect, which raises the possibility of therapeutic UDCA use for bile-induced AP.

Conclusion

Taken together, both *in vivo* and *in vitro* studies indicate that once BAs reach the ductal epithelium, they exert a harmful or beneficial effect on PDECs depending on their concentration (**Table 1**). This biphasic effect of BAs on ductal secretion may be a significant factor in the pathomechanism of biliary AP.

Acknowledgement

This work was supported by Hungarian Scientific Research Fund (K116634 to P.H. and the Momentum Grant of the Hungarian Academy of Sciences LP201X-10/2014 to P.H.).

References

1. Danielsson H, Sjövall J. Bile acid metabolism. *Annu Rev Biochem.* 1975; 44: 233-253. PMID 1094911.
2. Swell L, Gustafsson J, Danielsson H, Schwartz CC, Halloran LG, Vlahcevic ZR. Bile acid synthesis in humans. *Cancer Res.* 1981; 41: 3757-3758. PMID 7260942.
3. Opie E. The etiology of acute haemorrhagic pancreatitis. *Bull Johns Hopkins Hosp.* 1901; 12: 182-188.
4. Kim JY, Kim KH, Lee JA, Namkung W, Sun AQ, Ananthanarayanan M, et al. Transporter-mediated bile acid uptake causes Ca^{2+}-dependent cell death in rat pancreatic acinar cells. *Gastroenterology.* 2002; 122: 1941-1953. PMID 12055600.
5. Voronina S, Longbottom R, Sutton R, Petersen OH, Tepikin A. Bile acids induce calcium signals in mouse pancreatic acinar cells: implications for bile-induced pancreatic pathology. *J Physiol.* 2002; 540: 49-55. PMID 11927668.
6. Niederau C, Niederau M, Lüthen R, Strohmeyer G, Ferrell LD, Grendell JH. Pancreatic exocrine secretion in acute experimental pancreatitis. *Gastroenterology.* 1990; 99: 1120-1127. PMID 2394333.
7. Pandol SJ, Saluja AK, Imrie CW, Banks PA. Acute pancreatitis: bench to the bedside. *Gastroenterology.* 2007; 132: 1127-1151. PMID 17383433.
8. Senninger N. Bile-induced pancreatitis. *Eur Surg Res.* 1992; 24 Suppl 1: 68-73. PMID 1601026.
9. Bialek R, Willemer S, Arnold R, Adler G. Evidence of intracellular activation of serine proteases in acute cerulein-induced pancreatitis in rats. *Scand J Gastroenterol.* 1991; 26: 190-196. PMID 1707179.
10. Grady T, Mah'Moud M, Otani T, Rhee S, Lerch MM, Gorelick FS. Zymogen proteolysis within the pancreatic acinar cell is associated with cellular injury. *Am J Physiol Gastrointest Liver Physiol.* 1998; 275: G1010-G1017. PMID 9815031.
11. Grady T, Saluja A, Kaiser A, Steer M. Edema and intrapancreatic trypsinogen activation precede glutathione depletion during caerulein pancreatitis. *Am J Physiol Gastrointest Liver Physiol.* 1996; 271: G20-G26. PMID 8760102.
12. Gukovsky I, Gukovskaya AS, Blinman TA, Zaninovic V, Pandol SJ. Early NF-kappaB activation is associated with hormone-induced pancreatitis. *Am J Physiol Gastrointest Liver Physiol.* 1998; 275: G1402-G1414. PMID 9843778.

13. Raraty M, Ward J, Erdemli G, Vaillant C, Neoptolemos JP, Sutton R, et al. Calcium-dependent enzyme activation and vacuole formation in the apical granular region of pancreatic acinar cells. *Proc Natl Acad Sci U S A.* 2000; 97: 13126-13131. PMID 11087863.
14. Saluja AK, Lerch MM, Phillips PA, Dudeja V. Why does pancreatic overstimulation cause pancreatitis? *Annu Rev Physiol.* 2007; 69: 249-269. PMID 17059357.
15. Huang W, Cane MC, Mukherjee R, Szatmary P, Zhang X, Elliott V, et al. Caffeine protects against experimental acute pancreatitis by inhibition of inositol 1,4,5-trisphosphate receptor-mediated Ca^{2+} release. *Gut.* 2015 Dec 7 [Epub ahead of print]. PMID: 26642860.
16. Wen L, Voronina S, Javed MA, Awais M, Szatmary P, Latawiec D, et al. Inhibitors of ORAI1 Prevent Cytosolic Calcium-Associated Injury of Human Pancreatic Acinar Cells and Acute Pancreatitis in 3 Mouse Models. *Gastroenterology.* 2015; 149(2): 481-492.e7. PMID: 25917787.
17. Muili KA, Jin S, Orabi AI, Eisses JF, Javed TA, Le T, et al. Pancreatic acinar cell nuclear factor kappaB activation because of bile acid exposure is dependent on calcineurin. *J Biol Chem.* 2013; 288(29): 21065-21073. PMID: 23744075.
18. Mukherjee R, Mareninova OA, Odinokova IV, Huang W, Murphy J, Chvanov M, et al. Mechanism of mitochondrial permeability transition pore induction and damage in the pancreas: inhibition prevents acute pancreatitis by protecting production of ATP. *Gut.* 2016; 65(8): 1333-1346. PMID: 26071131.
19. Voronina SG, Barrow SL, Gerasimenko OV, Petersen OH, Tepikin AV. Effects of secretagogues and bile acids on mitochondrial membrane potential of pancreatic acinar cells: comparison of different modes of evaluating DeltaPsim. *J Biol Chem.* 2004; 279(26): 27327-27338. PMID: 15084611.
20. Voronina SG, Barrow SL, Simpson AW, Gerasimenko OV, da Silva Xavier G, Rutter GA, et al. Dynamic changes in cytosolic and mitochondrial ATP levels in pancreatic acinar cells. *Gastroenterology.* 2010; 138(5): 1976-1987. PMID: 20102715.
21. Booth DM, Murphy JA, Mukherjee R, Awais M, Neoptolemos JP, Gerasimenko OV, et al. Reactive oxygen species induced by bile acid induce apoptosis and protect against necrosis in pancreatic acinar cells. *Gastroenterology.* 2011; 140(7): 2116-2125. PMID: 21354148.
22. Argent BE, Gray MA, Steward MC, Case RM. Cell physiology of pancreatic ducts. In: Johnson LR, ed. *Physiology of the Gastrointestinal Tract.* Oxford, Academic Press; 2012: 1399-1424.
23. Czakó L, Yamamoto M, Otsuki M. Exocrine pancreatic function in rats after acute pancreatitis. *Pancreas.* 1997; 15: 83-90. PMID 9211497.
24. Czakó L, Yamamoto M, Otsuki M. Pancreatic fluid hypersecretion in rats after acute pancreatitis. *Dig Dis Sci.* 1997; 42: 265-272. PMID 9052504.
25. Hegyi P, Czako L, Takacs T, Szilvassy Z, Lonovics J. Pancreatic secretory responses in L-arginine-induced pancreatitis: comparison of diabetic and nondiabetic rats. *Pancreas.* 1999; 19: 167-174. PMID 10438164.
26. Renner IG, Wisner JR Jr. Ceruletide-induced acute pancreatitis in the dog and its amelioration by exogenous secretin. *Int J Pancreatol.* 1986; 1: 39-49. PMID 3693975.
27. Renner IG, Wisner JR Jr, Rinderknecht H. Protective effects of exogenous secretin on ceruletide-induced acute pancreatitis in the rat. *J Clin Invest.* 1983; 72: 1081-1092. PMID 6193140.
28. Durie PR. The pathophysiology of the pancreatic defect in cystic fibrosis. *Acta Paediatr Scand Suppl.* 1989; 363: 41-44. PMID 2701923.
29. Durie PR. Pancreatitis and mutations of the cystic fibrosis gene. *N Engl J Med.* 1998; 339: 687-688. PMID 9725928.
30. Armstrong CP, Taylor TV, Torrance HB. Effects of bile, infection and pressure on pancreatic duct integrity. *Br J Surg.* 1985; 72: 792-795. PMID 3899241.
31. Farmer RC, Tweedie J, Maslin S, Reber HA, Adler G, Kern H. Effects of bile salts on permeability and morphology of main pancreatic duct in cats. *Dig Dis Sci.* 1984; 29: 740-751. PMID 6745035.
32. Reber HA, Tweedie JH. Effects of a bile salt on the permeability of the pancreatic duct to macromolecules. *Surg Forum.* 1981; 32: 219-221.
33. Reber HA, Mosley JG. The effect of bile salts on the pancreatic duct mucosal barrier. *Br J Surg.* 1980; 67: 59-62. PMID 7357247.
34. Reber HA, Roberts C, Way LW. The pancreatic duct mucosal barrier. *Am J Surg.* 1979; 137: 128-134. PMID 31807.
35. Carey J. Bile salt metabolism in man. In: Nair P, Kritchevsky D, eds. *The Bile Acids Chemistry, Physiology, and Metabolism.* New York: Plenum Pub Corp.; 1973: 55.
36. Okolo C, Wong T, Moody MW, Nguyen TD. Effects of bile acids on dog pancreatic duct epithelial cell secretion and monolayer resistance. *Am J Physiol Gastrointest Liver Physiol.* 2002; 283: G1042-G1050. PMID 12381517.
37. Alvarez C, Fasano A, Bass BL. Acute effects of bile acids on the pancreatic duct epithelium in vitro. *J Surg Res.* 1998; 74: 43-46. PMID 9536972.
38. Alvarez C, Nelms C, D'Addio V, Bass BL. The pancreatic duct epithelium in vitro: bile acid injury and the effect of epidermal growth factor. *Surgery.* 1997; 122: 476-483; discussion 483-484. PMID 9288155.
39. Argent BE, Arkle S, Cullen MJ, Green R. Morphological, biochemical and secretory studies on rat pancreatic ducts maintained in tissue culture. *Q J Exp Physiol.* 1986; 71: 633-648. PMID 3024200.
40. Maléth J, Venglovecz V, Rázga Z, Tiszlavicz L, Rakonczay Z Jr, Hegyi P. Non-conjugated chenodeoxycholate induces severe mitochondrial damage and inhibits bicarbonate transport in pancreatic duct cells. *Gut.* 2011; 60: 136-138. PMID 20732916.
41. Venglovecz V, Hegyi P, Rakonczay Z Jr, Tiszlavicz L, Nardi A, Grunnet M, et al. Pathophysiological relevance of apical large-conductance Ca^{2+}-activated potassium channels in pancreatic duct epithelial cells. *Gut.* 2011; 60: 361-369. PMID 20940280.
42. Venglovecz V, Rakonczay Z Jr, Ozsvári B, Takács T, Lonovics J, Varró A, et al. Effects of bile acids on pancreatic ductal bicarbonate secretion in guinea pig. *Gut.* 2008; 57: 1102-1112. PMID 18303091.

43. Perides G, Laukkarinen JM, Vassileva G, Steer ML. Biliary acute pancreatitis in mice is mediated by the G-protein-coupled cell surface bile acid receptor Gpbar1. *Gastroenterology*. 2010; 138: 715-725. PMID 19900448.
44. Namkung W, Lee JA, Ahn W, Han W, Kwon SW, Ahn DS, et al. Ca^{2+} activates cystic fibrosis transmembrane conductance regulator- and Cl^--dependent HCO3 transport in pancreatic duct cells. *J Biol Chem*. 2003; 278: 200-207. PMID 12409301.
45. Zsembery A, Strazzabosco M, Graf J. Ca^{2+}-activated Cl^- channels can substitute for CFTR in stimulation of pancreatic duct bicarbonate secretion. *FASEB J*. 2000; 14: 2345-2356. PMID 11053257.
46. Ignáth I, Hegyi P, Venglovecz V, Székely CA, Carr G, Hasegawa M, et al. CFTR expression but not Cl^- transport is involved in the stimulatory effect of bile acids on apical $Cl^-/HCO3^-$ exchange activity in human pancreatic duct cells. *Pancreas*. 2009; 38: 921-929. PMID 19752774.
47. Kowal JM, Haanes KA, Christensen NM, Novak I. Bile acid effects are mediated by ATP release and purinergic signalling in exocrine pancreatic cells. *Cell Commun Signal*. 2015; 13: 28. PMID: 26050734.
48. Kowal JM, Yegutkin GG, Novak I. ATP release, generation and hydrolysis in exocrine pancreatic duct cells. *Purinergic Signal*. 2015; 11(4): 533-550. PMID: 26431833.
49. Katona M, Hegyi P, Kui B, Balla Z, Rakonczay Z Jr., Razga Z, et al. A novel, protective role of ursodeoxycholate in bile-induced pancreatic ductal injury. *Am J Physiol Gastrointest Liver Physiol*. 2016; 310(3): G193-G204. PMID: 26608189.
50. Botla R, Spivey JR, Aguilar H, Bronk SF, Gores GJ. Ursodeoxycholate (UDCA) inhibits the mitochondrial membrane permeability transition induced by glycochenodeoxycholate: a mechanism of UDCA cytoprotection. *J Pharmacol Exp Ther*. 1995; 272(2): 930-938. PMID: 7853211.
51. Pusl T, Vennegeerts T, Wimmer R, Denk GU, Beuers U, Rust C. Tauroursodeoxycholic acid reduces bile acid-induced apoptosis by modulation of AP-1. *Biochem Biophys Res Commun*. 2008; 367(1): 208-212. PMID: 18164257.
52. Rodrigues CM, Fan G, Ma X, Kren BT, Steer CJ. A novel role for ursodeoxycholic acid in inhibiting apoptosis by modulating mitochondrial membrane perturbation. *J Clin Invest*. 1998; 101(12): 2790-2799. PMID: 9637713.
53. Rodrigues CM, Fan G, Wong PY, Kren BT, Steer CJ. Ursodeoxycholic acid may inhibit deoxycholic acid-induced apoptosis by modulating mitochondrial transmembrane potential and reactive oxygen species production. *Mol Med*. 1998; 4(3): 165-178. PMID: 9562975.

Chapter 13

Alcohol and the pancreas

Minoti V. Apte, Romano C. Pirola, and Jeremy S. Wilson*

Pancreatic Research Group, South Western Sydney Clinical School, University of New South Wales, Sydney, and Ingham Institute for Applied Medical Research, Liverpool, New South Wales, Australia.

Introduction

Damage to the pancreas as a result of alcohol[†] abuse was first recognized as early as 200 years ago, with reports published in 1815 describing an association between heavy drinking and the development of pancreatitis.[1,2] This was subsequently confirmed by Freidrich[3] in 1878 and Fitz[4] in 1889, using a more detailed analytical approach.

Alcoholic pancreatitis is now generally recognized to have both acute and chronic manifestations. An acute episode of pancreatic necroinflammation (acute pancreatitis [AP]) is characterized by acute abdominal pain and raised serum amylase and lipase levels. Repeated attacks of necroinflammation can then lead to chronic changes in the pancreas including acinar atrophy and fibrosis (chronic pancreatitis), with patients suffering from chronic pain, symptoms of pancreatic insufficiency (i.e., maldigestion), and in advanced cases, diabetes.

Despite the well-established association between alcohol abuse and pancreatitis, there is an acknowledged clinical paradox in the field. On one hand, the risk of developing the disease increases with increasing alcohol consumption, but only a minority of heavy drinkers (<5%) develop clinically evident pancreatic disease.[6,7] This implies that additional factors may confer susceptibility to alcoholic pancreatitis in some drinkers.

Epidemiology of alcoholic pancreatitis

Alcohol abuse is ranked as the second most common cause of AP (after gallstone disease),[8] but is well established as the single most common cause of *chronic* pancreatitis, with an attributable risk of 40%.[9,10] A population-based cohort study reported that alcohol increases the risk of pancreatitis in a dose-dependent manner,[5] while a large case-control study proposed a threshold of five drinks per day as the baseline for the risk of developing alcoholic chronic pancreatitis.[7] A meta-analysis of several relevant studies has calculated the threshold to be four drinks per day for chronic pancreatitis.[11] If patients continue to drink at the same level as that prior to the first attack of pancreatitis, their risk of repeated acute attacks leading to chronic pancreatic injury is around 41%, with reduced drinking the risk falls to 23%, and it decreases to 14% with abstinence or occasional alcohol intake.[12]

Although the increased risk of pancreatitis with alcohol abuse is unquestioned, it is well acknowledged that the overall frequency of the disease (at least in terms of overt clinical illness) is low, with clinically evident AP seen in only up to 3%-5% of heavy drinkers.[5,13,14] Dreiling and Koller reported that among 100 alcoholics, 5 will develop clinical AP, 15 will develop alcoholic cirrhosis, while only 1 will develop clinical evidence of both diseases.[15] Thus in the clinical setting, a diagnosis of alcoholic pancreatitis will be less frequent than that of alcoholic liver disease. Interestingly, autopsy studies have revealed that the frequency of both disorders in alcoholics is much higher; approximately 40%-50% of patients diagnosed with alcoholic pancreatitis during their lifetime manifest signs of liver injury at autopsy.[16]

Natural history and clinical features

The onset of alcoholic pancreatitis usually occurs in the fourth decade, and the majority of patients are male with a history of heavy drinking (80-100 g of alcohol per day) for at least 5 years.[8] Alcoholic AP rarely occurs after a single binge.[17,18] Patients usually present with acute abdominal pain, raised serum levels of pancreatic enzymes (particularly serum amylase and lipase over 3 times the upper limit of normal), and evidence of pancreatic injury in imaging studies. Severe AP occurs in a minority of cases and can be fatal. As noted earlier, if the patient recovers but continues to drink, the disease progresses to a chronic stage

[†] *Note: The terms "alcohol" and "ethanol" are used interchangeably in this Chapter.*

*Corresponding author. Email: js.wilson@unsw.edu.au

characterized by atrophy and fibrosis of the pancreas, with patients developing chronic, often intractable, abdominal pain and signs of exocrine and endocrine insufficiency such as maldigestion and diabetes.

Disease progression from the initial attack of acute pancreatic necroinflammation to chronic, irreversible injury is now accepted to occur via repeated attacks of AP, each resulting in increasing residual damage to the gland and eventually leading to chronic pancreatic damage. Evidence in support of this necrosis-fibrosis sequence, a concept first postulated by Comfort in 1946,[19] comes from both clinical and experimental studies. A large prospective study demonstrated that clinical manifestations of chronic pancreatitis (exocrine and endocrine dysfunction) were more likely to occur in alcoholics with recurrent acute inflammation of the gland, suggesting that these acute episodes may eventually lead to chronic damage.[20] Recently, smoking, a lifestyle factor commonly associated with heavy drinking, has been reported to accelerate the progression of alcoholic chronic pancreatitis, as evidenced by earlier development of calcification and diabetes in patients who drink and smoke.[21] Experimental evidence in support of the necrosis-fibrosis sequence is provided by the finding that repeated episodes of acute experimental pancreatitis produce changes (albeit transient) resembling chronic pancreatitis, including fatty infiltration, acinar atrophy, and fibrosis.[22,23] Particularly relevant to alcoholic chronic pancreatitis are two recent experimental studies reporting the development of low-grade pancreatic fibrosis in alcohol-fed rats[24] and mice[25] subjected to repeated episodes of cerulein-induced pancreatic necroinflammation and in alcohol-fed rats subjected to repeated endotoxin challenge.[26]

Pathogenesis of Alcoholic Pancreatitis

Researchers examining the pathogenesis of alcoholic pancreatitis have usually adopted two approaches: (i) to study direct toxic effects of alcohol on the pancreas (**Figure 1**), given the fact that the risk of developing pancreatitis increases with increasing alcohol intake, and (ii) to identify individual susceptibility factors based on the knowledge that only a minority of heavy drinkers develop clinically evident pancreatitis.

Direct effects of alcohol on the pancreas

Effects of alcohol on pancreatic ducts

The earliest studies on the effects of alcohol on the pancreas were focused on the sphincter of Oddi (SO), with researchers taking their cues from Opie's original observations of SO dysfunction as a potential mechanism for gallstone pancreatitis.[27] The "large duct/sphincteric" theories of pancreatitis comprised the biliary-pancreatic reflux theory, duodeno-pancreatic reflux theory, and stimulation-obstruction theory. The central hypothesis for each of these was that alterations in SO motility secondary to alcohol exposure, play a major role in pancreatitis development. A spasmogenic effect (increased SO tone) of alcohol on the sphincter has been reported in an experimental model involving possums,[28] and it was postulated that the resultant reduction in trans-sphincteric flow may partially explain the decrease in pancreatic secretion observed after acute alcohol intake in humans.[29] However, studies on the effects of alcohol on SO tone and exocrine secretion in humans have reported contradictory findings, resulting in a gradual loss of interest in the large duct theories of alcoholic pancreatitis (a detailed discussion of these theories can be found in previously published reviews[30-32]).

In the 1970s, research focus shifted to the small pancreatic ducts, largely inspired by the work of Henri Sarles and his coworkers who postulated that a blockage of small pancreatic ductules by protein plugs (precipitated and calcified protein deposits) led to increased local duct damage as well as upstream pressure, acinar atrophy, and fibrosis.[33] They also proposed that contact of the calculi with the duct mucosa and duct wall resulted in ulceration and scarring, with further obstruction of the ducts eventually causing acinar cell atrophy.[33] Pertinent to this theory are reports that alcoholics have an increased tendency for protein precipitation in pancreatic juice.[34] Support for the concept is also provided by experimental studies using a rat model of alcohol administration, which demonstrated that alcohol alters the levels of two lithogenic proteins in pancreatic secretions. The first is lithostathine (also called pancreatic stone protein), a 144-amino acid protein secreted by acinar cells that when hydrolyzed by enzymes such as trypsin is converted to a highly precipitable 133-amino acid peptide called lithostathine S1. Messenger RNA levels of pancreatic lithostathine have been shown to be significantly increased in alcohol-fed rats.[35] The second is GP2, a glycoprotein that is the most abundant protein component of zymogen granule membranes.[36] GP2 is secreted into pancreatic ducts via exocytosis from acinar cells along with digestive enzymes or directly released from apical plasma membranes via an enzymatic process. This glycoprotein has unique properties for self aggregation in pancreatic juice. Chronic alcohol administration to rats decreases pancreatic GP2 content,[37] possibly due to increased secretion of GP2 into the pancreatic juice, where it may form fibrillar aggregates that act as a nidus for protein and Ca^{2+} precipitation.

Another determinant of lithogenicity of pancreatic juice is pancreatic secretion viscosity. Sarles and colleagues were the first to show that patients with alcoholic pancreatitis have increased sweat electrolyte levels, suggestive of cystic fibrosis transmembrane regulator (CFTR) dysfunction.[38] The resultant increase in pancreatic secretion viscosity could predispose to protein plug

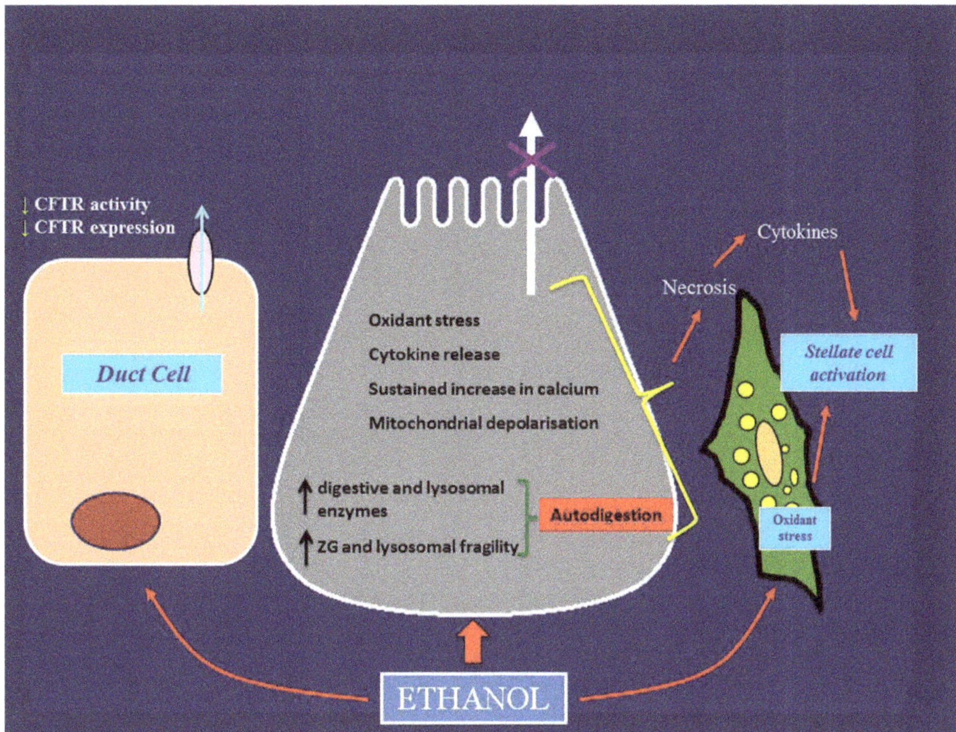

Figure 1. Alcohol and its metabolites exert detrimental effects on acinar, stellate, and duct cells in the exocrine pancreas.
Effects on acinar cells:

- Increased synthesis of digestive and lysosomal enzymes, associated with decreased exocytosis and increased fragility of lysosomal and zymogen granule membranes, thus predisposing the cell to premature intracellular enzyme activation and autodigestion
- Damage to subcellular membranes, proteins, and nucleic acids by reactive oxygen species (ROS) formed during ethanol metabolism
- Sustained increase in intracellular calcium (Ca^{2+}) leading to mitochondrial depolarization and cell death
- Release of cytokines by injured acinar cells, which can damage neighboring cells

Effects on pancreatic stellate cells (PSCs):

- Activation of PSCs by ethanol and its metabolites and by cytokines from acinar cells and inflammatory cells, leading to production of excessive extracellular matrix proteins (fibrosis) and synthesis of endogenous cytokines that can further activate the cells in an autocrine manner, leading to progressive fibrosis, even in the absence of the initial trigger

Effects on ductal cells:

- Decreased CFTR expression and activity, leading to impaired duct cell function

formation, and consequently, chronic changes in the pancreas. Interestingly, CFTR gene mutations that affect duct cell function are strongly associated with idiopathic chronic pancreatitis,[39,40] suggesting that ductular dysfunction contributes to pancreatic injury. In this regard, Hegyi and colleagues recently published evidence of detrimental effects of alcohol on CFTR expression and function in pancreatic ductal cells.[41] These will be discussed in more detail below in the section on effects of alcohol at a cellular level in the pancreas.

Cellular effects of alcohol

The large and small duct theories noted above were insufficient in terms of fully explaining alcoholic pancreatitis pathogenesis. Consequently, researchers' attention over the past four decades has been focused on the acinar cell (the major functional unit of the exocrine pancreas), PSC (the key player in pancreatic fibrosis), and most recently, the ductal cell (**Figure 1**).

The acinar cell is an enzyme factory that synthesizes and secretes significant quantities of digestive enzymes in response to a meal. It is well established that this enzyme synthetic capacity places the cell at a unique risk of injury via a process called autodigestion if the digestive enzymes are prematurely activated within the cells. As detailed below, in vitro and in vivo experiments have provided strong evidence that alcohol exposure predisposes the acinar cell to autodigestive injury.

Most of the detrimental effects of alcohol on the pancreas are likely mediated by the metabolism of alcohol to toxic metabolites within the gland, via both oxidative and nonoxidative pathways. Oxidation of alcohol to acetaldehyde is mainly catalyzed by the enzyme alcohol dehydrogenase (ADH) with some contribution from cytochrome P4502E1 (CYP2E1) and, to a lesser extent, from catalase. Studies with rat pancreatic acinar cells have shown the presence of ADH activity in the pancreas, with kinetics suggestive of ADH III (an isoform of ADH with low affinity and high Km for alcohol).[42,43] This ADH activity was found to be resistant to inhibition by 4-methylpyrazole (4-MP), which is a specific inhibitor of the ADH I isoform. However, a study using human pancreatic tissue has reported that the predominant class of ADH in human pancreatic acini is ADH I, with ADH III contributing little to pancreatic alcohol oxidation.[44] The differences in ADH isozymes and their resulting kinetic properties may reflect species differences between the rodent and human pancreas. CYP2E1 is also known to be present in the pancreas, and its activity is induced by alcohol administration in a manner similar to hepatic CYP2E1.[45] A byproduct of the oxidative pathway of alcohol metabolism is the generation of ROS that can damage lipid membranes, proteins, and cellular DNA. Increased ROS levels associated with a concurrent depletion of antioxidant factors (e.g., the ROS scavenger glutathione) leads to oxidant stress within the cell. Alcohol-induced pancreatic oxidant stress has been demonstrated in alcohol-fed experimental animals and humans with alcoholic pancreatitis.[46,47]

The nonoxidative pathway of alcohol metabolism involves the esterification of alcohol with fatty acids to form fatty acid ethyl esters (FAEEs). This reaction is catalyzed by FAEE synthases that remain to be fully characterized, but two enzymes implicated to date include carboxylester lipase and triglyceride lipase. Notably, FAEE synthase activity in the pancreas was calculated to be several fold higher than that observed in the liver.[48] Indeed, a number of studies have reported FAEE accumulation in the human and rat pancreas after alcohol intake.[42,49-51] It is also important to note that FAEE concentrations found in the pancreas of alcohol-fed rats are sufficient to induce damage to the subcellular organelles of pancreatic acinar cells.[49,52] The mechanisms by which FAEEs exert their toxic effects include : (i) direct interaction of the compounds with cellular membranes,[53] (ii) stimulation of cholesteryl ester synthesis by transesterification,[54] and (iii) release of free fatty acids by hydrolysis of FAEEs, a process thought to contribute to FAEE-induced mitochondrial damage.[54]

Experimental studies have demonstrated that the oxidative pathway is the predominant route for alcohol metabolism in the pancreas.[42,43] However, this does not diminish the potential importance of the nonoxidative pathway, since as noted above, products from this pathway are generated in amounts sufficient to cause subcellular injury. Whether there is a direct link between the two pathways is not yet clear. In isolated pancreatic acini, FAEE synthesis was reportedly increased in the presence of inhibitors of the oxidative pathway, while in vivo infusion of alcohol with ADH inhibitors resulted in increased FAEE accumulation in the pancreas.[55] Although these studies did not clearly demonstrate actual inhibition of alcohol oxidation in the pancreas, the findings suggest that the pancreas may be able to modulate alcohol metabolism based on the substrate and enzyme availabilities for the two different pathways.

The other cell type in the pancreas with a capacity for alcohol metabolism is the PSC (now established as the key cell responsible for producing fibrosis in the pancreas.[56,57] PSCs exhibit 4-methylpyrazole-sensitive ADH activity, with kinetics of alcohol oxidation consistent with ADH I.[57] In support of these findings, is a recent study demonstrating the presence of an ADH I isozyme (ADH1C) in quiescent human PSCs, and it was inhibited by pyrazole.[44] Notably, the researchers also showed that ADH1C expression was increased in activated human PSCs in chronic pancreatitis. Whether PSCs have a capacity for nonoxidative ethanol metabolism is not known.

Effects of alcohol on acinar cells

Chronic alcohol administration to rats has been shown to increase synthesis of the digestive enzymes trypsinogen, chymotrypsinogen, and lipase and the lysosomal enzyme cathepsin B within acinar cells[58,59] and reduce enzyme secretion by acinar cells, possibly secondary to acetaldehyde-induced microtubular dysfunction.[60] Alcohol-induced reorganization of the apical cytoskeleton, as reported by Siegmund et al. using isolated acinar cells,[61] may also play a role in impairing enzyme secretion. These effects perturb exocytosis and cause intracellular enzyme accumulation. At the same time, alcohol decreases the stability of the membranes of zymogen granules and lysosomes, which contain digestive and lysosomal enzymes, respectively.[62,63] Lysosomal membrane instability may be mediated by cholesteryl esters[64] and FAEEs,[52] substances known to accumulate in the pancreas after chronic alcohol consumption,[50,65] while zymogen granules instability is postulated to be the result of loss of a glycoprotein GP2, which is important for granule shape and stability.[37] The alcohol-induced increase in digestive and lysosomal enzyme contents accompanied by decreased stability of the organelles that contain these enzymes increases the potential for contact between digestive and lysosomal enzymes. In the presence of an appropriate trigger factor, premature intracellular activation of digestive enzymes can occur, leading to autodigestive injury of the gland.

Effects of alcohol on two major homeostatic mechanisms that maintain cellular integrity, namely, the unfolded protein response (UPR)/endoplasmic reticulum (ER) stress and autophagy, have attracted some attention in recent years. In vivo and in vitro studies demonstrated that exposure to alcohol causes an adaptive increase in the UPR (as evidenced by increased spliced XBP1 expression) in acinar cells, possibly to deal with the alcohol-induced increased production of enzymes within the cells.[66] This may be a protective response, since exposure to alcohol alone does not cause overt acinar damage. However, in the presence of an additional injurious agent (e.g., high-dose cerulein and possibly endotoxins or smoking), this adaptive response may be overwhelmed, leading to frank ER stress and cellular damage.[67,68] With regard to autophagy, in vivo studies using alcohol-fed rodents have demonstrated a significant decrease in LAMP2, a protein essential for autolysosome formation.[69] The resultant impairment of autophagic flux could lead to accumulation of misfolded proteins and damaged organelles within the acinar cell, eventually causing acinar death.

In recent years, downstream signaling pathways involved in the effects of alcohol and its metabolites on acinar cells have also been examined. Alcohol, acetaldehyde, and FAEEs induce the expression of nuclear factor (NF)-κB and AP-1, transcription factors that regulate cytokine expression.[42] FAEEs have also been shown to cause perturbations of intracellular Ca^{2+}. Criddle et al. reported that exposure of pancreatic acinar cells in vitro to the FAEE palmitoleic acid ethyl ester (PAEE) caused a sustained rise in cytosolic Ca^{2+} as a consequence of increased Ca^{2+} release from intracellular sources such as the ER (via stimulation of inositol triphosphate receptors) and decreased clearance of Ca^{2+} due to dysfunction of the Ca^{2+} ATPase pumps in the ER and plasma membrane.[70] The ATPase pump dysfunction is dependent on the hydrolysis of PAEE to its free fatty acid palmitoleic acid, which leads to uncoupled mitochondrial oxidative phosphorylation and deficient ATP production.

An additional source for increased intracellular Ca^{2+} in alcohol-exposed acinar cells is via increased influx of extracellular Ca^{2+}, as has been reported in mouse acinar cells incubated with physiological concentrations of cholecystokinin (CCK) and intoxicating concentrations of alcohol (50mM).[70] Inhibition of alcohol oxidation by 4-methylpyrazole or preincubation with the antioxidant cinnamtannin-B prevented the alcohol-induced Ca^{2+} influx.[71] These findings indicate that alcohol oxidation and subsequent ROS generation may play an important role in this process. It is thought that the sustained rise in intracellular Ca^{2+} leads to mitochondrial Ca^{2+} overload and mitochondrial depolarization, eventually causing acinar cell death.

Effects of alcohol on PSCs

A characteristic histologic feature of alcoholic chronic pancreatitis is abundant pancreatic fibrosis. Activated PSCs are now known to play a central role in pancreatic fibrogenesis.[56] With regard to alcoholic pancreatitis, both human and rat PSCs are directly activated by alcohol at clinically relevant concentrations ranging from 10 mM (encountered during social drinking) to 50 mM (seen with heavy alcohol consumption).[57,72] Inhibitor studies have determined that this alcohol-induced PSC activation is mediated by oxidation of alcohol to acetaldehyde and the subsequent generation of oxidant stress.[57,72] Alcohol and acetaldehyde increase the secretion of MMP2 by PSCs. MMP2 digests basement membrane collagen (collagen IV) and facilitates deposition of fibrillary collagen (collagen I).[73] Interestingly, alcohol has also been reported to stimulate the synthesis of endogenous cytokines such as interleukin (IL)-8 and connective tissue growth factor by PSCs.[72] These endogenous cytokines could act on PSC membranes via autocrine pathways to further perpetuate PSC activation. In addition, alcohol has been shown to inhibit PSC apoptosis, thereby prolonging survival of activated cells in the pancreas.[74]

Of relevance to alcoholic pancreatitis is another potential activating factor for PSCs, namely, bacterial endotoxins. Increased gut permeability is a known consequence of alcohol consumption that can facilitate translocation of gut bacteria into the circulation and result in increased circulating endotoxin levels.[75,76] In vivo studies have demonstrated a key role for lipopolysaccharide (LPS), an endotoxin found in the cell wall of Gram-negative bacteria such as *Escherichia coli*, in the initiation and progression of alcoholic pancreatitis.[26,77] Similar to alcohol, LPS has been shown to activate PSCs (as assessed by αSMA expression) and inhibit PSC apoptosis.[26,74] Importantly, alcohol and LPS together exert synergistic effects on PSC activation and apoptosis.[26,74]

Signaling pathways implicated in the effects of alcohol and its metabolites on PSCs include the three major components– ERK1/2, p38 kinase (p38K) and c-jun amino terminal kinase (JNK) – of the mitogen-activated protein kinase (MAPK) pathway.[42,78] Alcohol and acetaldehyde also activate protein kinase C (PKC) and PI3K, two pathways upstream of the MAPK cascade.[78] The synergistic effects of alcohol and endotoxin noted earlier are likely mediated via LPS-induced upregulation of the LPS receptor Toll-like receptor 4 (TLR4) on PSCs[26] and downstream activation of NFκB.[79] These findings are relevant to the observed LPS-induced decrease in apoptosis of PSCs because NFκB can induce anti-apoptotic proteins such as IAPs (inhibitors of apoptosis proteins)[80] and may explain the LPS-induced inhibition of PSC apoptosis. For a majority of the pathways noted above that are stimulated by the binding of relevant ligands to their receptors, the common downstream event is most likely intracellular Ca^{2+} modulation. A recent study showed that activation of the bradykinin 2 receptor on PSCs by bradykinin (formed in the extracellular matrix due to cleavage of its precursor kininogen by kallikreinin released from FAEE-injured acinar cells), leads to a sustained increase in Ca^{2+} within PSCs, resulting in their proliferation and activation, which would further perpetuate fibrosis.[81]

Effects of alcohol on ductal cells

Although Sarles and colleagues[38] drew attention to CFTR abnormalities and pancreatic duct changes several decades ago, there was little research into the effects of alcohol on ductal cells until recent work by Maleth et al.[41] The authors report increased sweat chloride levels (suggesting impaired CFTR function) in patients who acutely abused alcohol and long-term alcohol dependent patients, while healthy volunteers had normal sweat chloride levels. Pancreatic CFTR expression (at both mRNA and protein levels) was reduced in patients with alcoholic AP. In alcoholic chronic pancreatitis, decreased membrane expression of CFTR was associated with increased CFTR mRNA and protein expression in the cytoplasm, suggesting translocation of CFTR from the membrane to the cytosol and/or misfolding of proteins in the ER leading to their cytoplasmic accumulation. In human pancreatic ductal epithelial cells exposed to alcohol and fatty acids, fluid and bicarbonate secretion and CFTR activity were significantly reduced.[41] These changes were associated with increased cellular Ca^{2+} concentrations, decreased ATP levels, and mitochondrial depolarization. Using mouse and guinea pig pancreatic ducts and human pancreatic duct cell lines, the authors also showed that incubation with high-dose alcohol plus the FAEE metabolite palmitoleic acid, decreased CFTR mRNA levels and CFTR stability. Notably, CFTR knockout mice administered ethanol and fatty acids developed a more severe form of pancreatitis than wild-type mice. Thus, this study implicates CFTR dysfunction in ductal cells as a major factor in alcohol-induced pancreatic injury and postulates that the effects of alcohol on pancreatic ducts are mediated by the nonoxidative metabolites of alcohol.[41]

Individual susceptibility to alcoholic pancreatitis

Based on the studies described above, direct toxic effects of alcohol and its metabolites on pancreatic cells likely occur in all heavy drinkers, at least at subclinical levels. However, clinically overt pancreatitis only occurs in a minority of alcoholics, indicating that an additional hit/insult or a factor that confers specific susceptibility is essential to trigger clinical disease. Concerted efforts are underway to identify this trigger factor/susceptibility factor (summarized in **Table 1**), but no particular factor has been unequivocally demonstrated to play this role.

The key comparison when assessing susceptibility factors should be between alcoholics *with* alcoholic pancreatitis and alcoholics *without* pancreatitis so that the index and the control groups differ in only one variable: the presence or absence of pancreatitis. This comparison has not always been made, with many studies limited to the use of a healthy population as a control group. Nonetheless, numerous potential factors have been examined in the past three decades, each of which usually falls into one of two groups: hereditary factors and lifestyle/environmental factors.

Hereditary factors

The hereditary factors assessed to date can be grouped into genes relevant to the alcohol metabolizing pathway, digestive enzymes and their inhibitors, CFTR, growth factors and cytokines, blood group antigens, and genes relevant to tight junction proteins that regulate mucosal permeability.

Alcohol metabolizing enzymes

As noted earlier, the deleterious effects of alcohol on the pancreas are most likely related to the direct toxic effects of its metabolites (acetaldehyde, FAEEs, and ROS) on the gland. Altered activities of alcohol metabolizing enzymes, particularly ADH, ALDH, CYP2E1, and FAEE synthases, may lead to harmful metabolite accumulation and tissue injury.

Oxidative pathway of alcohol metabolism

The major enzymes involved in alcohol oxidation are ADH and acetaldehyde dehydrogenase (ALDH).[82] These enzymes have several isoforms and are encoded by different genes that can have several allelic variants that influence the ethanol metabolism rate.[83] Differences in distributions of the allelic variants can also occur between different tissues in the body or different ethnic groups. Human ADH enzymes are classified into five classes based on amino acid sequence and structural similarities. The Class I ADH enzymes (ADH1A, ADH1B, and ADH1C) are the major enzymes involved in ethanol clearance in the liver. ALDH enzymes are classified into two groups: cytosolic ALDH 1 and mitochondrial ALDH2. Oxidation of acetaldehyde to acetate is mainly carried out by ALDH2.

The best-studied ADH gene with regard to alcoholic pancreatitis susceptibility is the ADH1B gene. Studies in Asian populations have reported that the ADH1B*2 allele is predominant. This encodes for the highly active B2-ADH subunit which oxidizes alcohol to acetaldehyde at a faster rate than the subunit encoded by the ADH1*B1 allele.[84,85] Three studies from Japan have shown that ADH1B*2 allele frequency is increased in patients with alcoholic pancreatitis compared to alcoholics without pancreatitis.[85-87] A decreased frequency of the ADH1*B1 allele has also

Table 1. Individual Susceptibility Factors

Factor	Association	Reference
Inherited factors		
Human leukocyte antigen	No	Wilson et al., 1984[113]
α1-antitrypsin deficiency	No	Haber et al., 1991[114]
Cystic fibrosis genotype	No	Norton et al., 1998[115]
Cytochrome P4502E1 polymorphism	No	Frenzer et al., 2002[116]
ADH genotype	Yes	Matsumoto et al., 1996[87]
	Yes	Maruyama et al., 1999[86]
	No	Frenzer et al., 2002[116]
	Yes	Shimosegawa et al., 2008[85]
	Yes	Maruyama et al., 2008[88]
	Yes	*Zhong et al., 2015[89]
Anionic trypsinogen gene mutation	Yes	*Witt et al., 2006[96]
	Yes	*Whitcomb et al., 2012[94]
	Yes	*Derikx et al., 2015[95]
PSTI/SPINK1 mutations	Yes	Witt et al., 2001[97]
TNFα, TGFα, IL10, IFNγ polymorphisms	No	*Schneider et al., 2004[117]
Detoxifying enzymes		
- Glutathione S-transferase	No	Frenzer et al., 2002[116]
- UDP-glucuronosyl transferase	Yes	*Ockenga et al., 2003[118]
Carboxylester lipase (CEL) polymorphism	Yes	Miyasaka et al., 2005[91]
	No	*Ragvin et al., 2013[119]
Hybrid allele of CEL (CEL-HYB)	Yes	*Fjeld et al., 2015[92]
Lifestyle factors		
Drinking pattern	No	Wilson et al., 1985[18]
Beverage type	No	Wilson et al., 1985[18]
	Yes	*Nakamura et al., 2003[120]
Diet	No	Wilson et al., 1985[18]
Smoking	Yes	Lowenfels et al., 1987[121]
	No	Haber et al., 1993[122]
Obesity	Yes	*Ammann et al., 2010[109]

* These studies did not include alcoholics without pancreatitis as controls.

been reported in the Japanese population and is thought to reduce vulnerability to alcoholic pancreatitis.[87,88] Zhong et al. recently published a meta-analysis of eight case-control studies examining the association of ADH1B, ADH1C, and ALDH2 variants in alcoholic pancreatitis.[89] In Asian patients, a higher risk of alcoholic pancreatitis was found for carriers of the ADH1B*2 allele, but there was a lower risk for those with the ALDH2*2 allele that encodes a metabolically inactive protein. In the non-Asian population, the ADH1C*2 allele was associated with a decreased risk of alcoholic pancreatitis.

The gene for CYP2E1 (which also plays a role in alcohol oxidation as noted earlier) has been shown to have polymorphisms in both the promoter region as well as in intron 6.[90] Some of these polymorphisms are associated with altered CYP2E1 function, but none have been found to be associated with increased risk of alcoholic pancreatitis when compared to alcoholics without pancreatitis.

Nonoxidative pathway of alcohol metabolism

This pathway is catalyzed by FAEE synthases. A Japanese study compared alcoholics with and without pancreatitis and reported a positive association between the risk of developing alcoholic pancreatitis and a gene polymorphism for the FAEE synthase enzyme, carboxyl ester lipase (CEL).[91] However, the functional significance of this polymorphism has not been elucidated, and the study findings were not corroborated in a study of European subjects.

More recently, Fjeld and colleagues reported an association between a hybrid allele of the CEL gene (CEL-HYB) and alcoholic chronic pancreatitis.[92] However, the controls were healthy volunteers and not alcoholics without pancreatitis. The authors also assessed the functional consequences of the CEL-HYB gene in vitro using HEK293 cells. They found that the resulting CEL-HYB protein might impair autophagy within the cells, leading to their death.

Digestive enzyme gene mutations

Several studies have examined the possible association between mutations of genes related to digestive enzymes, their inhibitors, and alcoholic pancreatitis. The genes assessed include cationic trypsinogen (PRSS1), anionic trypsinogen (PRSS2), chymotrypsinogen, secretory trypsin inhibitor (PSTI) also known as serine protease inhibitor Kazal type 1 (SPINK-1), mesotrypsin, and chymotrypsin C (CTRC)(see review[93]).

Two recent genome-wide association studies (GWASs) from North America[94,95] and from Europe[95] (95) have reported that a single nucleotide polymorphism rs10273639 located in the 5'-promoter region of the cationic trypsinogen gene PRSS1 was associated with a decrease in alcoholic pancreatitis risk. This polymorphism was not associated with nonalcoholic chronic pancreatitis or with alcoholic liver disease; however, the studies did not include alcoholics without pancreatitis or liver disease as controls. The authors postulated that rs10273639 may affect expression of trypsinogen, but the functional significance of the polymorphism remains to be clarified. With regard to the anionic trypsinogen gene *PRSS2*, it has been reported that a protective variant (G191R) that produces a form of trypsin that is easily degraded is significantly less common in patients with alcoholic chronic pancreatitis compared to healthy controls.[96] Again, the prevalence of this variant in alcoholics without pancreatitis was not tested.

An association between mutated SPINK1 and alcoholic pancreatitis has also been described. The N34S mutation, a c.101A>G transition leading to substitution of asparagine by serine at codon 34, was found in 5.8% patients with alcoholic pancreatitis compared to 1.0% alcoholic controls without pancreatitis.[97] A study of Romanian patients reported that 5% of patients with ACP had the N34S mutation compared to 1% of healthy controls.[98] A recent meta-analysis found a significant association of the N34S mutation with alcoholic pancreatitis with an odds ratio of 4.98 (95% confidence interval: 3.16-7.85), but the association was weakest among categories analyzed including tropical pancreatitis, idiopathic chronic pancreatitis, and hereditary pancreatitis.[99] Despite the reported association with alcoholic pancreatitis, since the N34S mutated human SPINK1 does not show any altered trypsin inhibitor capacity,[100] the functional consequences of this mutation are unclear.

Two variants of chymotrypsin C (CTRC, a minor isoform of chymotrypsin) have been reported more often in German patients with alcoholic pancreatitis (2.9%) than in patients with alcoholic liver disease (0.7%).[101] In a Chinese population, more CTRC variants were detected in chronic pancreatitis patients, but the overall frequency of mutations was 2.3% and thus lower than in the German study.[102]

Claudin 2 mutations

Claudin-2 is a tight junction protein encoded by the gene CLDN2. In tissue sections of chronic pancreatitis, claudin-2 was expressed in acinar and ductal cells.[94] The two GWASs noted earlier identified two single nucleotide polymorphisms of the CLDN2 gene involving the CLDN2-RIPPLY1-MORC4 locus (Xp23.3, SNPs rs7057398 and rs12688220). A decreased risk of alcoholic pancreatitis was found in association with rs12688220; however, the functional significance of this SNP is not clear. Interestingly, aberrant expression of the claudin-2 protein along basolateral membranes of acinar cells was found in pancreatic sections from chronic pancreatitis patients with the high-risk SNP rs7057398. Again, the functional significance of this aberrant expression is unclear, but it is possible that the SNP alters the function of claudin-2 in the intestine, thereby influencing intestinal mucosal permeability and facilitating the translocation of gut bacteria with consequent endotoxinemia. As discussed later, endotoxinemia (a well reported feature in alcoholics) may be a susceptibility factor for alcoholic pancreatitis. Interestingly, upregulation of claudin-2 has been implicated in increased intestinal permeability in Crohn's disease.[103]

CFTR mutations

As noted earlier, both animal and human studies have revealed that CFTR function and expression are impaired by alcohol. However, there is little evidence to implicate CFTR mutations in the pathogenesis of alcoholic pancreatitis. A small study from Brazil showed that patients with alcoholic pancreatitis had a higher frequency of the T5/T7 genotype in the noncoding region of thymidines in intron 8, suggesting reduced transcription of the CFTR gene.[104] However, additional, larger studies are needed to fully elucidate the role of CFTR mutations in alcoholic pancreatitis.

Other hereditary factors

Numerous other hereditary factors have been examined in alcoholic pancreatitis including blood group antigens, human leukocyte antigen (HLA) serotypes, α-1-antitrypsin phenotypes, the cytokines transforming growth factor β (TGFβ), tumor necrosis factor α (TNFα), IL-10, interferon gamma, and detoxifying enzymes such as UDP glucuronosyltransferase (UGT1A7) and glutathione S-transferase (see review[93]). Most of these studies have failed to show any associations of these genes with alcoholic pancreatitis, although a recent report described a positive association between the risk of developing alcoholic pancreatitis and fucosyl transferase (FUT2) nonsecretor status, as well as with ABO blood group B status.[105]

Lifestyle/environmental factors

Dietary intake, amount and type of alcohol consumed, drinking pattern, lipid intolerance, and smoking (see reviews[93,106]) have all been examined for their possible role in alcoholic pancreatitis. Appropriately controlled studies have ruled out any role for dietary factors, particularly macronutrients, in alcoholic pancreatitis. However, similar studies of dietary antioxidants and other micronutrients remain to be performed. Alcoholic beverage type and drinking pattern have also not been clearly shown to influence the risk of alcoholic pancreatitis.

The role of smoking as a trigger factor for alcoholic pancreatitis has been a particularly fraught subject (see reviews[93,106]). Since a large proportion of heavy drinkers are also smokers, it is difficult to unequivocally demonstrate an independent role of smoking in the initiation of pancreatitis. Law et al. performed a retrospective study adjusting for alcohol and other risk factors and concluded that smoking is independently associated with chronic pancreatitis.[107] However, the authors acknowledged that factors such as recall bias impeded their ability to accurately stratify the extent of smoking and alcohol use. In a recent review on the subject, Yadav and Lowenfels noted that "although smoking increases the risk of chronic pancreatitis independently, the effects of smoking are stronger for alcohol-related chronic pancreatitis."[108] In this regard, there is some evidence to suggest that smoking accelerates the progression of alcoholic chronic pancreatitis by promoting the development of pancreatic calcifications and endocrine dysfunction.[21]

Obesity is another possible risk factor for alcoholic pancreatitis. Ammann et al. prospectively recruited 227 patients with alcoholic chronic pancreatitis and age- and sex-matched healthy subjects as controls.[109] In patients with alcoholic chronic pancreatitis, obesity (body mass index >30) prior to disease onset was 5-fold more frequent than in healthy controls. However, obesity did not influence disease progression. Notably, an earlier study reported that obesity was highly prevalent in asymptomatic alcoholics compared to the general population.[110] In view of this observation and the fact that the study by Ammann and colleagues did not include alcoholics without pancreatitis as controls, it is difficult to clearly attribute a role to obesity as a susceptibility factor for alcoholic pancreatitis.[109] Thus, in terms of "environmental" factors, a clear susceptibility factor for alcoholic pancreatitis remains to be identified.

A potential cofactor that should be explored for its role in clinical alcoholic pancreatitis is endotoxinemia. Serum endotoxin levels are known to be increased in alcoholics, even after a single binge.[111] This is likely due to the alcohol-induced increase in gut permeability permitting translocation of gram-negative bacteria (such as *E. coli*) across the mucosal barrier, and impaired clearance of endotoxin by Kupffer cells in the liver.[75,76] In this regard, alcohol has been shown to increase the permeability of Caco-2 intestinal epithelial cell monolayers via CYP2E1-induced oxidant stress, which in turn induces the circadian clock proteins CLOCK and PER2.[112] Experimental evidence supporting a role for endotoxins as a susceptibility factor in alcoholic pancreatitis, comes from a study by Vonlaufen et al.[26] The authors convincingly demonstrated that endotoxin (LPS) challenge in alcohol-fed rats initiated overt pancreatic injury and stimulated progression to chronic disease manifesting as acinar atrophy and fibrosis.

Taken together, existing clinical studies have not unequivocally identified a hereditary or environmental susceptibility factor for alcoholic pancreatitis. However, studies with experimental models suggest that bacterial endotoxins are a promising candidate worthy of further study. Future work could include assessments of genetic polymorphisms of factors related to endotoxin-related molecules such as the LPS receptor TLR4 and its adapter proteins CD14 and MD2. Other susceptibility factors that remain to be fully examined include proteins relevant to cellular antioxidant defenses and minor CFTR mutations.

Conclusion

The association of alcohol abuse and pancreatitis has been recognized for over two centuries. In the past four decades, considerable advances have been made in our understanding of the pathogenesis of this disease, with elucidation of the detrimental effects of alcohol on the functions of three major pancreas cell types: acinar, ductal, and PSCs. The baseline damage caused by alcohol on the pancreas is now better understood; however, the major challenge in the field remains, that is, to unravel the reasons why only certain heavy drinkers develop the disease. Despite concerted research efforts specific susceptibility/trigger factors that could cause overt pancreatitis in alcoholics remain to be determined. Alcoholic pancreatitis is likely a multifactorial and polygenic condition, and further work is needed to fully characterize the putative pathogenic pathways responsible for the clinical disease.

References

1. Claessen H. *Die Krankheiten des Pankreas [The Diseases of the Pancreas]*. Cologne, Germany: Dumont-Schaumburg; 1884.
2. Fleischmann G. *Leichenöffnungen [Autopsies]*. Erlangen, Germany: Johann Jakob Palm; 1815.
3. Freidreich N. *Disease of the pancreas*. New York, NY: William Wood; 1878.
4. Fitz RH. Acute pancreatitis: a consideration of pancreatic hemorrhage, hemorrhagic, suppurative, and gangrenous pancreatitis, and of disseminated fat-necrosis. *Boston Med Surg J*. 1889; 120: 181-187.
5. Kristiansen L, Gronbaek M, Becker U, Tolstrup JS. Risk of pancreatitis according to alcohol drinking habits: a population-based cohort study. *Am J Epidemiol*. 2008; 168: 932-937. PMID: 18779386.
6. Durbec JP, Sarles H. Multicenter survey of the etiology of pancreatic diseases. Relationship between the relative risk of developing chronic pancreaitis and alcohol, protein and lipid consumption. *Digestion*. 1978; 18: 337-350. PMID: 750261.
7. Yadav D, Hawes RH, Brand RE, Anderson MA, Money ME, Banks PA, et al. Alcohol consumption, cigarette smoking, and the risk of recurrent acute and chronic pancreatitis. *Arch Intern Med*. 2009; 169: 1035-1045. PMID: 19506173.
8. Yadav D, Lowenfels AB. Trends in the epidemiology of the first attack of acute pancreatitis: a systematic review. *Pancreas*. 2006; 33: 323-330. PMID: 17079934.
9. Cote GA, Yadav D, Slivka A, Hawes RH, Anderson MA, Burton FR, et al. Alcohol and smoking as risk factors in an epidemiology study of patients with chronic pancreatitis. *Clin Gastroenterol Hepatol*. 2011; 9: 266-273, PMID: 21029787.
10. Frulloni L, Gabbrielli A, Pezzilli R, Zerbi A, Cavestro GM, Marotta F, et al. Chronic pancreatitis: report from a multicenter Italian survey (PanCroInfAISP) on 893 patients. *Dig Liver Dis*. 2009; 41: 311-317. PMID: 19097829.
11. Irving HM, Samokhvalov AV, Rehm J. Alcohol as a risk factor for pancreatitis. A systematic review and meta-analysis. *JOP*. 2009; 10: 387-392. PMID: 19581740.
12. Takeyama Y. Long-term prognosis of acute pancreatitis in Japan. *Clin Gastroenterol Hepatol*. 2009; 711 Suppl: S15-S17. PMID: 19896091.
13. Lankisch PG, Lowenfels AB, Maisonneuve P. What is the risk of alcoholic pancreatitis in heavy drinkers? *Pancreas*. 2002; 25: 411-412. PMID: 12409838.
14. Yadav D. Recent advances in the epidemiology of alcoholic pancreatitis. *Curr Gastroenterol Rep*. 2011; 13: 157-165. PMID: 21243451.
15. Dreiling DA, Koller M. The natural history of alcoholic pancreatitis: update 1985. *Mt Sinai J Med*. 1985; 52: 340-342. PMID: 3874352.
16. Sarles H. *Alcoholic pancreatitis*. New York, NY, McGraw Hill; 1992.
17. Phillip V, Huber W, Hagemes F, Lorenz S, Matheis U, Preinfalk S, et al. Incidence of acute pancreatitis does not increase during Oktoberfest, but is higher than previously described in Germany. *Clin Gastroenterol Hepatol*. 2011; 9: 995-1000. PMID: 21723238.
18. Wilson JS, Bernstein L, McDonald C, Tait A, McNeil D, Pirola RC. Diet and drinking habits in relation to the development of alcoholic pancreatitis. *Gut*. 1985; 26: 882-887. PMID: 4029715.
19. Comfort HW, Gambill EE, Baggenstoss AH. Chronic relapsing pancreatitis: a study of 29 cases without associated disease of the biliary or gastrointestinal tract. *Gastroenterology*. 1946; 6: 239-285. PMID: 20985712.
20. Ammann RW, Muellhaupt B. Progression of alcoholic acute to chronic pancreatitis. *Gut*. 1994; 35: 552-556. PMID: 8174996.
21. Maisonneuve P, Lowenfels AB, Mullhaupt B, Cavallini G, Lankisch PG, Andersen JR, et al. Cigarette smoking accelerates progression of alcoholic chronic pancreatitis. *Gut*. 2005; 54: 510-514. PMID: 15753536.
22. Elsasser HP, Haake T, Grimmig M, Adler G, Kern HF. Repetitive cerulein-induced pancreatitis and pancreatic fibrosis in the rat. *Pancreas*. 1992; 7: 385-390. PMID: 1594561.
23. Neuschwander-Tetri BA, Burton FR, Presti ME, Britton RS, Janney CG, Garvin PR, et al. Repetitive self-limited acute pancreatitis induces pancreatic fibrogenesis in the mouse. *Dig Dis Sci*. 2000; 45: 665-674. PMID: 10759232.
24. Deng X, Wang L, Elm MS, Gabazadeh D, Diorio GJ, Eagon PK, et al. Chronic alcohol consumption accelerates fibrosis in response to cerulein-induced pancreatitis in rats. *Am J Pathol*. 2005; 166: 93-106. PMID: 15632003.
25. Perides G, Tao X, West N, Sharma A, Steer ML. A mouse model of ethanol dependent pancreatic fibrosis. *Gut*. 2005; 54: 1461-1467. PMID: 15870229.
26. Vonlaufen A, Xu Z, Daniel B, Kumar RK, Pirola R, Wilson J, et al. Bacterial endotoxin: a trigger factor for alcoholic pancreatitis? Evidence from a novel, physiologically relevant animal model. *Gastroenterology*. 2007; 133: 1293-1303. PMID: 17919500.
27. Opie EL. The etiology of acute haemorrhagic pancreatitis. *Bull John Hopkins Hosp*. 1901; 12: 182-188.
28. Sonoda Y, Woods CM, Toouli J, Saccone GTP. Intragastric ethanol reduces sphincter of Oddi function in the anaesthetised Australian possum. *Pancreas*. 2005; 31: 469.
29. Hajnal F, Flores MC, Radley S, Valenzuela JE. Effect of alcohol and alcoholic beverages on meal-stimulated pancreatic secretion in humans. *Gastroenterology*. 1990; 98: 191-196. PMID: 2293577.
30. Apte MV, Haber PS, Norton ID, Wilson JS. Alcohol and the pancreas. *Addict Biol*. 1998; 3: 137-150. PMID: 26734819.
31. Apte MV, Pirola RC, Wilson JS. Molecular mechanisms of alcoholic pancreatitis. *Dig Dis*. 2005; 23: 232-240. PMID: 16508287.
32. Apte MV, Pirola RC, Wilson JS. Mechanisms of alcoholic pancreatitis. *J Gastroenterol Hepatol*. 2010; 25: 1816-1826. PMID: 21091991.
33. Sarles H. Chronic calcifying pancreatitis - chronic alcoholic pancreatitis. *Gastroenterology*. 1974; 66: 604-616. PMID: 4595185.
34. Renner IG, Rinderknecht H, Valenzuela JE, Douglas AP. Studies of pure pancreatic secretions in chronic alcoholic

subjects without pancreatic insufficiency. *Scand J Gastroenterol.* 1980; 15: 241-244. PMID: 7384747.

35. Apte MV, Norton ID, Haber PS, McCaughan GW, Korsten MA, Pirola RC, et al. Both ethanol and protein deficiency increase messenger RNA levels for pancreatic lithostathine. *Life Sci.* 1996; 58: 485-492. PMID: 8569421.
36. Rindler MJ, Hoops TC. The pancreatic membrane protein GP2 localises specifically to secretory granules and is shed into the pancreatic juice as a protein aggregate. *Eur J Cell Biol.* 1990; 53: 154-163.
37. Apte MV, Norton ID, Haber PS, Korsten MA, McCaughan GW, Pirola RC, et al. Chronic ethanol administration decreases rat pancreatic GP2 content. *Biochim Biophys Acta.* 1997; 1336: 89-98. PMID: 9271254.
38. Sarles H, Sarles JC, Camatte R, Muratore R, Gaini M, Guien C, et al. Observations on 205 confirmed cases of acute pancreatitis, recurring pancreatitis, and chronic pancreatitis. *Gut.* 1965; 6: 545-559. PMID: 5857891.
39. Cohn JA, Neoptolemos JP, Feng J, Yan J, Jiang Z, Greenhalf W, et al. Increased risk of idiopathic chronic pancreatitis in cystic fibrosis carriers. *Hum Mutat.* 2005; 26: 303-307. PMID: 16134171.
40. Sharer N, Schwarz M, Malone G, Howarth A, Painter J, Super M, et al. Mutations of the cystic fibrosis gene in patients with chronic pancreatitis. *N Engl J Med.* 1998; 339: 645-652. PMID: 9725921.
41. Maleth J, Balazs A, Pallagi P, Balla Z, Kui B, Katona M, et al. Alcohol disrupts levels and function of the cystic fibrosis transmembrane conductance regulator to promote development of pancreatitis. *Gastroenterology.* 2015; 148: 427-439. PMID: 25447846.
42. Gukovskaya AS, Mouria M, Gukovsky I, Reyes CN, Kasho VN, Faller LD, et al. Ethanol metabolism and transcription factor activation in pancreatic acinar cells in rats. *Gastroenterology.* 2002; 122: 106-118. PMID: 11781286.
43. Haber PS, Apte MV, L. AT, Norton ID, Korsten MA, Pirola RC, et al. Metabolism of ethanol by rat pancreatic acinar cells. *J Lab Clin Med.* 1998; 132: 294-302. PMID: 9794700.
44. Chiang CP, Wu CW, Lee SP, Chung CC, Wang CW, Lee SL, et al. Expression pattern, ethanol-metabolizing activities, and cellular localization of alcohol and aldehyde dehydrogenases in human pancreas: implications for pathogenesis of alcohol-induced pancreatic injury. *Alcohol Clin Exp Res.* 2009; 33: 1059-1068. PMID: 19382905.
45. Norton I, Apte M, Haber P, McCaughan G, Korsten M, Pirola R, et al. P4502E1 is present in rat pancreas and is induced by chronic ethanol administration. *Gastroenterology.* 1996; 110: A1280.
46. Casini A, Galli A, Pignalosa P, Frulloni L, Grappone C, Milani S, et al. Collagen type I synthesized by pancreatic periacinar stellate cells (PSC) co-localizes with lipid peroxidation-derived aldehydes in chronic alcoholic pancreatitis. *J Pathol.* 2000; 192: 81-89. PMID: 10951404.
47. Norton ID, Apte MV, Lux O, Haber PS, Pirola RC, Wilson JS. Chronic ethanol administration causes oxidative stress in the rat pancreas. *J Lab Clin Med.* 1998; 131: 442-446. PMID: 9605109.
48. Laposata EA, Lange LG. Presence of nonoxidative ethanol metabolism in human organs commonly damaged by ethanol abuse. *Science.* 1986; 231: 497-499. PMID: 3941913.
49. Haber PS, Apte MV, Moran C, Applegate TL, Pirola RC, Korsten MA, et al. Non-oxidative metabolism of ethanol by rat pancreatic acini. *Pancreatology.* 2004; 4(2): 82-89. PMID: 15056978.
50. Lange LG. Nonoxidative ethanol metabolism: formation of fatty acid ethyl esters by cholesterol esterase. *Proc Natl Acad Sci U S A.* 1982; 79: 3954-3957. PMID: 6955782.
51. Werner J, Laposata M, Fernández-del Castillo C, Saghir M, Iozzo RV, Lewandrowski KB, et al. Pancreatic injury in rats induced by fatty acid ethyl ester, a nonoxidative metabolite of alcohol. *Gastroenterology.* 1997; 113: 286-294. PMID: 9207289.
52. Haber PS, Wilson JS, Apte MV, Pirola RC. Fatty acid ethyl esters increase rat pancreatic lysosomal fragility. *J Lab Clin Med.* 1993; 121: 759-764. PMID: 8505587.
53. Hungund BL, Goldstein DB, Villegas F, Cooper TB. Formation of fatty acid ethyl esters during chronic ethanol treatment in mice. *Biochem Pharmacol.* 1988; 37: 3001-3004. PMID: 3395375.
54. Lange LG, Sobel BE. Mitochondrial dysfunction induced by fatty acid ethyl esters, myocardial metabolites of ethanol. *J Clin Invest.* 1983; 72: 724-731. PMID: 6308061.
55. Werner J, Saghir M, Fernandez-del Castillo C, Warshaw AL, Laposata M. Linkage of oxidative and nonoxidative ethanol metabolism in the pancreas and toxicity of nonoxidative ethanol metabolites for pancreatic acinar cells. *Surgery.* 2001; 129: 736-744. PMID: 11391373.
56. Apte M, Pirola RC, Wilson JS. Pancreatic stellate cell: physiologic role, role in fibrosis and cancer. *Curr Opin Gastroenterol.* 2015; 31: 416-423. PMID: 26125317.
57. Apte MV, Phillips PA, Fahmy RG, Darby SJ, Rodgers SC, McCaughan GW, et al. Does alcohol directly stimulate pancreatic fibrogenesis? Studies with rat pancreatic stellate cells. *Gastroenterology.* 2000; 118: 780-794. PMID: 10734030.
58. Apte MV, Wilson JS, Korsten MA, McCaughan GW, Haber PS, Pirola RC. Effects of ethanol and protein deficiency on pancreatic digestive and lysosomal enzymes. *Gut.* 1995; 36: 287-293. PMID: 7533742.
59. Apte MV, Wilson JS, McCaughan GW, Korsten MA, Haber PS, Norton ID, et al. Ethanol-induced alterations in messenger RNA levels correlate with glandular content of pancreatic enzymes. *J Lab Clin Med.* 1995; 125: 634-640. PMID: 7738427.
60. Ponnappa BC, Hoek JB, Waring AJ, Rubin E. Effect of ethanol on amylase secretion and cellular calcium homeostasis in pancreatic acini from normal and ethanol-fed rats. *Biochem Pharmacol.* 1987; 36: 69-79. PMID: 2432902.
61. Siegmund E, Luthen F, Kunert J, Weber H. Ethanol modifies the actin cytoskeleton in rat pancreatic acinar cells--comparison with effects of CCK. *Pancreatology.* 2004; 4: 12-21. PMID: 14988654.
62. Haber PS, Wilson JS, Apte MV, Korsten MA, Pirola RC. Chronic ethanol consumption increases the fragility of rat pancreatic zymogen granules. *Gut.* 1994; 35: 1474-1478. PMID: 7525419.
63. Wilson JS, Korsten MA, Apte MV, Thomas MC, Haber PS, Pirola RC. Both ethanol consumption and protein deficiency increase the fragility of pancreatic lysosomes. *J Lab Clin Med.* 1990; 115: 749-755. PMID: 2366035.

64. Wilson JS, Apte MV, Thomas MC, Haber PS, Pirola RC. Effects of ethanol, acetaldehyde and cholesteryl esters on pancreatic lysosomes. *Gut*. 1992; 33: 1099-1104. PMID: 1398235.
65. Wilson JS, Colley PW, Sosula L, Pirola RC. Alcohol causes a fatty pancreas. A rat model of ethanol-induced pancreatic steatosis. *Alcohol Clin Exp Res*. 1982; 6: 117-121. PMID: 7041679.
66. Lugea A, Tischler D, Nguyen J, Gong J, Gukovsky I, French SW, et al. Adaptive unfolded protein response attenuates alcohol-induced pancreatic damage. *Gastroenterology*. 2011; 140: 987-997. PMID: 21111739.
67. Lugea A, Waldron RT, Pandol SJ. Pancreatic adaptive responses in alcohol abuse: Role of the unfolded protein response. *Pancreatology*. 2015; 154 Suppl: S1-S5. PMID: 25736240.
68. Xu Z, Pothula S, Pandol S, Pirola R, Wilson J, Apte M. Smoking worsens the fibrosis of alcoholic chronic pancreatitis via activation of pancreatic stellate cells. *Pancreas*. 2015; 44: 1426.
69. Fortunato F, Burgers H, Bergmann F, Rieger P, Buchler MW, Kroemer G, et al. Impaired autolysosome formation correlates with LAMP-2 depletion: role of apoptosis, autophagy, and necrosis in pancreatitis. *Gastroenterology*. 2009; 137: 350-360. PMID: 19362087.
70. Criddle DN, Murphy J, Fistetto G, Barrow S, Tepikin AV, Neoptolemos JP, et al. Fatty acid ethyl esters cause pancreatic calcium toxicity via inositol trisphosphate receptors and loss of ATP synthesis. *Gastroenterology*. 2006; 130: 781-793. PMID: 16530519.
71. Fernández-Sánchez M, del Castillo-Vaquero A, Salido GM, González A. Ethanol exerts dual effects on calcium homeostasis in CCK-8-stimulated mouse pancreatic acinar cells. *BMC Cell Biol*. 2009; 10: 77. PMID: 19878551.
72. Masamune A, Satoh A, Watanabe T, Kikuta K, Satoh M, Suzuki N, et al. Effects of ethanol and its metabolites on human pancreatic stellate cells. *Dig Dis Sci*. 2010; 55: 204-211. PMID: 19165599.
73. Phillips PA, McCarroll JA, Park S, Wu M-J, Korsten MA, Pirola RC, et al. Pancreatic stellate cells secrete matrix metalloproteinases - implications for extracellular matrix turnover. *Gut*. 2003; 52: 275-282. PMID: 12524413.
74. Vonlaufen A, Phillips PA, Xu Z, Zhang X, Yang L, Pirola RC, et al. Withdrawal of alcohol promotes regression while continued alcohol intake promotes persistence of LPS-induced pancreatic injury in alcohol-fed rats. *Gut*. 2011; 60: 238-246. PMID: 20870739.
75. Bode C, Kugler V, Bode JC. Endotoxemia in patients with alcoholic and non-alcoholic cirrhosis and in subjects with no evidence of chronic liver disease following acute alcohol excess. *J Hepatol*. 1987; 4: 8-14. PMID: 3571935.
76. Bode JC, Parlesak A, Bode C. Gut derived bacterial toxins (endotoxin) and alcohol liver disease. In: Argawal DP, Seitz HK, eds. *Alcohol in Health and Disease*. New York, NY: Marcel Dekker; 2001: 369-386.
77. Fortunato F, Deng X, Gates LK, McClain CJ, Bimmler D, Graf R, et al. Pancreatic response to endotoxin after chronic alcohol exposure: switch from apoptosis to necrosis? *Am J Physiol Gastrointest Liver Physiol*. 2006; 290: G232-G241. PMID: 15976389.
78. McCarroll JA, Phillips PA, Park S, Doherty E, Pirola RC, Wilson JS, et al. Pancreatic stellate cell activation by ethanol and acetaldehyde: is it mediated by the mitogen-activated protein kinase signaling pathway? *Pancreas*. 2003; 27: 150-160. PMID: 12883264.
79. Masamune A, Kikuta K, Watanabe T, Satoh K, Satoh A, Shimosegawa T. Pancreatic stellate cells express Toll-like receptors. *J Gastroenterol*. 2008; 43: 352-362. PMID: 18592153.
80. Bhanot UK, Möller P. Mechanisms of parenchymal injury and signaling pathways in ectatic ducts of chronic pancreatitis: implications for pancreatic carcinogenesis. *Lab Invest*. 2009; 89: 489-497. PMID: 19308045.
81. Gryshchenko O, Gerasimenko JV, Gerasimenko OV, Petersen OH. Ca^{2+} signals mediated by bradykinin type 2 receptors in normal pancreatic stellate cells can be inhibited by specific Ca^{2+} channel blockade. *J Physiol*. 2016; 594: 281-293. PMID: 26442817.
82. Lieber CS. Metabolism of ethanol. In Lieber CS, ed. *Medical and Nutritional Complications of Alcoholism*. Lieber CS. New York, NY: Plenum Publishing Corporation; 1992: 1-35.
83. Zakhari S. Overview: how is alcohol metabolized by the body? *Alcohol Res Health*. 2006; 29: 245-254. PMID: 17718403.
84. Bosron WF, Li TK. Genetic polymorphism of human liver alcohol and aldehyde dehydrogenases, and their relationship to alcohol metabolism and alcoholism. *Hepatology*. 1986; 6: 502-510. PMID: 3519419.
85. Shimosegawa T, Kume K, Masamune A. SPINK1, ADH2, and ALDH2 gene variants and alcoholic chronic pancreatitis in Japan. *J Gastroenterol Hepatol*. 2008; 23 Suppl 1: S82-S86. PMID: 18336671.
86. Maruyama K, Takahashi H, Matsushita S, Nakano M, Harada H, Otsuki M, et al. Genotypes of alcohol-metabolizing enzymes in relation to alcoholic chronic pancreatitis in Japan. *Alcohol Clin Exp Res*. 1999; 234 Suppl: 85s-91s. PMID: 10235286.
87. Matsumoto M, Takahashi H, Maruyama K, Higuchi S, Matsushita S, Muramatsu T, et al. Genotypes of alcohol-metabolizing enzymes and the risk for alcoholic chronic pancreatitis in Japanese alcoholics. *Alcohol Clin Exp Res*. 1996; 209 Suppl: 289a-292a. PMID: 8986224.
88. Maruyama K, Harada S, Yokoyama A, Naruse S, Hirota M, Nishimori I, et al. Association analysis among polymorphisms of the various genes and chronic alcoholic pancreatitis. *J Gastroenterol Hepatol*. 2008; 23 Suppl 1: S69-S72. PMID: 18336668.
89. Zhong Y, Cao J, Zou R, Peng M. Genetic polymorphisms in alcohol dehydrogenase, aldehyde dehydrogenase and alcoholic chronic pancreatitis susceptibility: a meta-analysis. *Gastroenterol Hepatol*. 2015; 38: 417-425. PMID: 25541509.
90. Verlaan M, te Morsche RH, Roelofs HM, Laheij RJ, Jansen JB, Peters WH, et al. Genetic polymorphisms in alcohol-metabolizing enzymes and chronic pancreatitis. *Alcohol Alcoholism*. 2004; 39: 20-24. PMID: 14691069.
91. Miyasaka K, Ohta M, Takano S, Hayashi H, Higuchi S, Maruyama K, et al. Carboxylester lipase gene polymorphism as a risk of alcohol-induced pancreatitis. *Pancreas*. 2005; 30: e87-e91. PMID: 15841033.

92. Fjeld K, Weiss FU, Lasher D, Rosendahl J, Chen JM, Johansson BB, et al. A recombined allele of the lipase gene CEL and its pseudogene CELP confers susceptibility to chronic pancreatitis. *Nat Genet*. 2015; 47: 518-522. PMID: 25774637.
93. Apte MV, Pirola RC, Wilson JS. Individual susceptibility to alcoholic pancreatitis. *J Gastroenterol Hepatol*. 2008; 23 Suppl 1: S63-S68. PMID: 18336667.
94. Whitcomb DC, LaRusch J, Krasinskas AM, Klei L, Smith JP, Brand RE, et al. Common genetic variants in the CLDN2 and PRSS1-PRSS2 loci alter risk for alcohol-related and sporadic pancreatitis. *Nat Genet*. 2012; 44: 1349-1354. PMID: 23143602.
95. Derikx MH, Kovacs P, Scholz M, Masson E, Chen JM, Ruffert C, et al. Polymorphisms at PRSS1-PRSS2 and CLDN2-MORC4 loci associate with alcoholic and non-alcoholic chronic pancreatitis in a European replication study. *Gut*. 2015; 64: 1426-1433. PMID: 25253127.
96. Witt H, Sahin-Toth M, Landt O, Chen JM, Kahne T, Drenth JP, et al. A degradation-sensitive anionic trypsinogen (PRSS2) variant protects against chronic pancreatitis. *Nat Genet*. 2006; 38: 668-673. PMID: 16699518.
97. Witt H, Luck W, Becker M, Bohmig M, Kage A, Truninger K, et al. Mutation in the SPINK1 trypsin inhibitor gene, alcohol use, and chronic pancreatitis. *JAMA*. 2001; 285: 2716-2717. PMID: 11386926.
98. Diaconu BL, Ciobanu L, Mocan T, Pfutzer RH, Scafaru MP, Acalovschi M, et al. Investigation of the SPINK1 N34S mutation in Romanian patients with alcoholic chronic pancreatitis. A clinical analysis based on the criteria of the M-ANNHEIM classification. *J Gastrointestin Liver Dis*. 2009; 18: 143-150. PMID: 19565042.
99. Aoun E, Chang CC, Greer JB, Papachristou GI, Barmada MM, Whitcomb DC. Pathways to injury in chronic pancreatitis: decoding the role of the high-risk SPINK1 N34S haplotype using meta-analysis. *PLoS One*. 2008; 3: e2003. PMID: 18414673.
100. Kuwata K, Hirota M, Shimizu H, Nakae M, Nishihara S, Takimoto A, et al. Functional analysis of recombinant pancreatic secretory trypsin inhibitor protein with amino-acid substitution. *J Gastroenterol*. 2002; 37: 928-934. PMID: 12483248.
101. Rosendahl J, Witt H, Szmola R, Bhatia E, Ozsvari B, Landt O, et al. Chymotrypsin C (CTRC) variants that diminish activity or secretion are associated with chronic pancreatitis. *Nat Genet*. 2008; 40: 78-82. PMID: 18059268.
102. Chang MC, Chang YT, Wei SC, Liang PC, Jan IS, Su YN, et al. Association of novel chymotrypsin C gene variations and haplotypes in patients with chronic pancreatitis in Chinese in Taiwan. *Pancreatology*. 2009; 9: 287-292. PMID: 19407484.
103. Zeissig S, Burgel N, Gunzel D, Richter J, Mankertz J, Wahnschaffe U, et al. Changes in expression and distribution of claudin 2, 5 and 8 lead to discontinuous tight junctions and barrier dysfunction in active Crohn's disease. *Gut*. 2007; 56: 61-72. PMID: 16822808.
104. da Costa MZ, Guarita DR, Ono-Nita SK, Nogueira Jde A, Nita ME, Paranagua-Vezozzo DC, et al. CFTR polymorphisms in patients with alcoholic chronic pancreatitis. *Pancreatology*. 2009; 9: 173-181. PMID: 19077469.
105. Weiss FU, Schurmann C, Guenther A, Ernst F, Teumer A, Mayerle J, et al. Fucosyltransferase 2 (FUT2) non-secretor status and blood group B are associated with elevated serum lipase activity in asymptomatic subjects, and an increased risk for chronic pancreatitis: a genetic association study. *Gut*. 2015; 64: 646-656. PMID: 25028398.
106. Witt H, Apte MV, Keim V, Wilson JS. Chronic pancreatitis: challenges and advances in pathogenesis, genetics, diagnosis, and therapy. *Gastroenterology*. 2007; 132: 1557-1573. PMID: 17466744.
107. Law R, Parsi M, Lopez R, Zuccaro G, Stevens T. Cigarette smoking is independently associated with chronic pancreatitis. *Pancreatology*. 2010; 10: 54-59. PMID: 20332662.
108. Yadav D, Lowenfels AB. The epidemiology of pancreatitis and pancreatic cancer. *Gastroenterology*. 2013; 144: 1252-1261. PMID: 23622135.
109. Ammann RW, Raimondi S, Maisonneuve P, Mullhaupt B. Is obesity an additional risk factor for alcoholic chronic pancreatitis? *Pancreatology*. 2010; 10: 47-53. PMID: 20332661.
110. Wannamethee SG, Shaper AG. Alcohol, body weight, and weight gain in middle-aged men. *Am J Clin Nutr*. 2003; 77: 1312-1317. PMID: 12716687.
111. Bala S, Marcos M, Gattu A, Catalano D, Szabo G. Acute binge drinking increases serum endotoxin and bacterial DNA levels in healthy individuals. *PLoS One*. 2014; 9: e96864. PMID: 24828436.
112. Forsyth CB, Voigt RM, Shaikh M, Tang Y, Cederbaum AI, Turek FW, et al. Role for intestinal CYP2E1 in alcohol-induced circadian gene-mediated intestinal hyperpermeability. *Am J Physiol Gastrointest Liver Physiol*. 2013; 305: G185-G195. PMID: 23660503.
113. Wilson JS, Gossat D, Tait A, Rouse S, Juan XJ, Pirola RC. Evidence for an inherited predisposition to alcoholic pancreatitis. A controlled HLA typing study. *Dig Dis Sci*. 1984; 29: 727-730. PMID: 6589150.
114. Haber PS, Wilson JS, McGarity BH, Hall W, Thomas MC, Pirola RC. Alpha 1 antitrypsin phenotypes and alcoholic pancreatitis. *Gut*. 1991; 32: 945-948. PMID: 1885078.
115. Norton ID, Apte MV, Dixson H, Trent RJ, Pirola RC, Wilson JS. Cystic fibrosis genotypes and alcoholic pancreatitis. *J Gastroenterol Hepatol*. 1998; 13: 496-500. PMID: 9641647.
116. Frenzer A, Butler WJ, Norton ID, Wilson JS, Apte MV, Pirola RC, et al. Polymorphism in alcohol-metabolizing enzymes, glutathione S-transferases and apolipoprotein E and susceptibility to alcohol-induced cirrhosis and chronic pancreatitis. *J Gastroenterol Hepatol*. 2002; 17: 177-182. PMID: 11966948.
117. Schneider A, Barmada MM, Slivka A, Martin JA, Whitcomb DC. Transforming growth factor-beta1, interleukin-10 and interferon-gamma cytokine polymorphisms in patients with hereditary, familial and sporadic chronic pancreatitis. *Pancreatology*. 2004; 4: 490-494. PMID: 15316224.
118. Ockenga J, Vogel A, Teich N, Keim V, Manns MP, Strassburg CP. UDP glucuronosyltransferase (UGT1A7) gene polymorphisms increase the risk of chronic pancreatitis and pancreatic cancer. *Gastroenterology*. 2003; 124: 1802-1808. PMID: 12806614.

119. Ragvin A, Fjeld K, Weiss FU, Torsvik J, Aghdassi A, Mayerle J, et al. The number of tandem repeats in the carboxyl-ester lipase (CEL) gene as a risk factor in alcoholic and idiopathic chronic pancreatitis. *Pancreatology*. 2013; 13: 29-32. PMID: 23395566.
120. Nakamura Y, Ishikawa A, Sekiguchi S, Kuroda M, Imazeki H, Higuchi S. Spirits and gastrectomy increase risk for chronic pancreatitis in Japanese male alcoholics. *Pancreas*. 2003; 26: e27-e31. PMID: 12604924.
121. Lowenfels AB, Zwemer FL, Jhangiani S, Pitchumoni CS. Pancreatitis in a native American Indian population. *Pancreas*. 1987; 2: 694-697. PMID: 3438307.
122. Haber PS, Wilson JS, Pirola RC. Smoking and alcoholic pancreatitis. *Pancreas*. 1993; 8: 568-572. PMID: 8302794.

Chapter 14

Effects of alcohol on pancreatic ductal function

József Maléth[1,2], Zoltán Rakonczay[1,3], Viktória Venglovecz[4], and Péter Hegyi[1,2,5*]

[1]*First Department of Medicine, University of Szeged, Szeged, Hungary;*
[2]*MTA-SZTE Translational Gastroenterology Research Group, Szeged, Hungary;*
[3]*Department of Pathophysiology, University of Szeged, Szeged, Hungary;*
[4]*Department of Pharmacology and Pharmacotherapy, University of Szeged, Szeged, Hungary;*
[5]*Centre for Translational Medicine, Institute for Translational Medicine & 1st Department of Medicine, Department of Translational Medicine, University of Pécs.*

Importance of the pancreatic ductal HCO_3^- secretion

The exocrine pancreas secretes ~1.5 L of alkaline, isotonic fluid that washes digestive enzymes from the lumens of the pancreatic ducts and neutralizes the acidic gastric content entering the duodenum.[1,2] This alkaline pancreatic secretion plays an important role in gland physiology and pathophysiology, protecting the pancreatic tissue from damage. Findings from the last two decades support this hypothesis and demonstrate that pancreatic acinar cells will suffer severe damage if pancreatic ductal secretion is impaired. Freedman et al. observed that pancreatic ductal secretion is impaired in cystic fibrosis transmembrane conductance regulator (*cftr*) knockout mice, resulting in a more acidic (pH 6.6 ± 0.04) pancreatic juice compared to wild-type animals (pH 8.12 ± 0.06).[3] In addition, the lack of CFTR chloride (Cl^-) channel activity caused a defect in the apical membrane transport of the acinar cells. The findings of Reber et al. showed that in cat pancreas, the basal parenchymal pH was ~7.35, which decreased to ~7.25 after the induction of chronic pancreatitis (CP).[4] Moreover, ethanol administration decreased the extracellular pH of the pancreatic tissue to ~7.1 and reduced pancreatic blood flow to 40%. In a rat model, acute pancreatitis (AP) development was affected by contrast solution pH during endoscopic retrograde cholangiopancreatography.[5] Contrast solution at pH 6.0-6.9 injected into the main pancreatic ducts induced pancreatic edema, increased serum amylase activity, neutrophil infiltration, and histological damage. Pancreatic injury correlated with the lower pH. Conversely, pH 7.3 solution caused only mild pancreatic injury. Bhoomagoud et al. showed that the decrease of extracellular pH from 7.6 to 6.8 augmented secretagogue-induced zymogen activation and acinar cell injury *in vitro* and enhanced cerulein-induced trypsinogen activation and pancreatic edema *in vivo*.[6] Our group further proved the importance of the pancreatic ductal secretion; we demonstrated that the autoactivation of trypsinogen is a pH-dependent process, with accelerated autoactivation on acidic pH meaning that HCO_3^- secretion protects the pancreas from untimely trypsinogen autoactivation.[7] Evidence suggests that decreased pancreatic ductal bicarbonate secretion can affect AP severity.

Mechanism of bicarbonate secretion in pancreatic ductal cells

The major site of fluid and bicarbonate (HCO_3) secretion are the pancreatic ductal epithelial cells (PDECs) of the small intercalated and intralobular ducts.[8] The maximal HCO_3^- concentration in the ductal lumen can vary among species; importantly, human PDECs can produce 140 mM maximal intraluminal HCO_3^- concentration, as can guinea pigs.[2]

The complex process of pancreatic ductal HCO_3^- secretion can be divided to two steps: HCO_3^- accumulation across the basolateral membrane followed by the secretion via the apical membrane into the lumen. Basolateral accumulation is mediated by the sodium (Na^+)/HCO_3^- cotransporter (NBCe1-B), which operates with 1 Na^+: 2 HCO_3^- stoichiometry.[9] The passive diffusion of CO_2 through the basolateral membrane may also contribute to the HCO_3^- accumulation, which is followed by the carbonic anhydrase-mediated conversion of CO_2 to HCO_3^-.[10] On the luminal PDEC membrane, the molecules central to HCO_3^- secretion are the electrogenic Cl^-/HCO_3^- exchangers (SLC26A6 and possibly A3, which operates with a 1 Cl^-: 2 HCO_3^- stoichiometry).[11] Another important protein is the CFTR Cl^- channel, which plays an important role in the

*Corresponding author. Email: hegyi.peter@med.u-szeged.hu

ductal HCO_3^- secretion in humans and animals to produce a high intraluminal HCO_3^- concentration.[12] This electrogenic apical Cl^-/HCO_3^- exchange allows PDECs to transport HCO_3^- into the ductal lumen and establish 140 mM intraluminal HCO_3^- concentration during stimulated secretion.[1,2] The details and molecular background of the pancreatic ductal HCO_3^- secretion were recently reviewed elsewhere.[1,13,14]

Effects of ethanol and ethanol metabolites on the pancreatic ductal bicarbonate secretion

One of the most common causes of AP is heavy alcohol abuse. The inhibitory effect of alcohol on pancreatic secretion was first suggested decades ago.[15] Yamamoto et al. found that in the guinea pig, 0.3-30 mM and 100 mM ethanol augmented and inhibited secretin-stimulated pancreatic ductal fluid secretion, respectively.[16] The authors focused on the effects of ethanol in that study; but others have highlighted the harmful effects of various ethanol metabolites in different organs. *In vivo* ethanol metabolism is carried out by two independent pathways.[17,18] The oxidative pathway occurs dominantly in the liver and generates acetaldehyde, whereas, the nonoxidative pathway combines ethanol and fatty acids (FAs) and produces fatty acid ethyl esters (FAEEs) in the pancreas, brain, and heart, tissues typically damaged by excessive ethanol consumption.[17] Compared with the liver, FAEE synthase activity in the pancreas is more likely to cause local accumulation of nonoxidative ethanol metabolites.[19] FAEE can also be hydrolyzed, leading to the intracellular accumulation of FAs that can strongly bind to mitochondrial membrane proteins and thus uncouple oxidative phosphorylation.[20] Clinical studies[21] and experimental animal models suggest that *in vivo* ethanol administration does not induce pancreatitis by itself but sensitizes the pancreas to other triggers.[22] Ethanol was shown to destabilize lysosomes and zymogen granules,[23] sensitize pancreatic mitochondria to activate mitochondrial permeability transition pore (MPTP) leading to mitochondrial failure,[24] modulate the immune response via sensitizing nuclear factor-κB activation in pancreatic acinar cells[25] and cause oxidative ER stress, which activates an unfolded protein response and increases XBP1 levels and activity.[26] Criddle et al. found that FAEEs and FAs but not ethanol cause pancreatic acinar cell damage via sustained intracellular calcium (Ca^{2+}) elevation, mitochondrial dysfunction, ATP depletion and intra-acinar trypsinogen activation leading to cell necrosis.[27-30] Ethanol metabolites were also shown to perturb exocytosis processes in cultured rat pancreatic acini causing apical blockade and basolateral exocytosis.[31] Moreover, Werner et al. showed that FAEE infusion induced pancreatic edema, pancreatic trypsinogen activation, and vacuolization of acinar cells.[32] The role of stellate cell activation was also recently highlighted in the ethanol-induced pancreatic injury;[33] however, there is no direct evidence concerning the involvement of ductal epithelial cells in the pathogenesis of alcohol-induced pancreatitis.

Importantly, Sarles et al. described that the initial pancreatic damage during alcohol-induced chronic calcifying pancreatitis is the formation of mucoprotein plugs in the small pancreatic ducts.[34] In addition, the sweat Cl^- and Na^+ concentrations of these patients were also significantly elevated compared to the control group.[34] These changes are very similar to the alterations of the exocrine pancreas in cystic fibrosis, the most common genetic mutation in the Caucasian population, which is associated with exocrine pancreatic insufficiency[35] and an increased risk of pancreatitis.[36] Although the observations of Sarles are more than 50 years old, the connection between ethanol-induced pancreatic damage and ductal secretory dysfunction has not yet been investigated in detail.

Recently, we employed several overlapping *in vivo* and *in vitro* experimental models to demonstrate that ethanol and FA dose-dependently reduce CFTR expression and activity in PDECs and inhibit fluid and HCO_3^- secretion in the pancreas.[37,38] We observed that the sweat Cl^- concentration (Cl^-_{sw}) was significantly elevated after heavy alcohol intake by human subjects; however, Cl^-_{sw} normalized when the patients were sober.[38] In human tissue samples from patients suffering from alcohol-induced AP or CP, we detected a significant decrease in the CFTR expression at the apical membranes of the pancreatic ducts. Interestingly, in experimental models we found that a low concentration (10 mM) of ethanol stimulated both the apical Cl^-/HCO_3^- exchange and CFTR channel activity. However, at a high concentration (100 mM), a strong inhibitory effect was detected for HCO_3^- secretion, CFTR activity, and pancreatic fluid secretion *in vivo* and *in vitro*. This biphasic effect of ethanol is very similar to the dose-dependent effects of nonconjugated bile acids on pancreatic ductal functions.[39] Similarly to 100 mM ethanol, FAs augmented pancreatic fluid and HCO_3^- secretion. The oxidative ethanol metabolite acetaldehyde and FAEEs have no such effects. Inhibition of CFTR by ethanol and FAs was associated with a sustained increase in concentrations of intracellular Ca^{2+} and decreased 3',5'-cyclic adenosine monophosphate (cAMP) levels, mitochondrial membrane depolarization, and a consequent drop of intracellular ATP. Intracellular ATP supplementation via a patch pipette almost completely prevented inhibition of CFTR activity by ethanol and FA.[37] We also showed that the decrease in CFTR expression and plasma membrane density in response to administration of ethanol, palmitoleic acid, or palmitoleic acid ethyl ester was caused by the combination of accelerated plasma membrane turnover at the apical membrane and impaired protein folding in the endoplasmic reticulum.[38]

Alcohol-induced CFTR dysfunction in the pathogenesis of pancreatic damage

As demonstrated above, ethanol and its metabolites have a strong inhibitory effect on pancreatic HCO_3^- and fluid secretion by reducing CFTR function and expression (**Figure 1**). In addition to these experimental observations, other data suggest that CFTR function can affect AP pathogenesis and severity.

DiMagno et al. showed that CFTR deletion results in continuous overexpression of proinflammatory cytokine genes; moreover, these mice develop more severe AP upon cerulein hyperstimulation compared to wild-type animals.[40] The authors observed increased pancreatic edema, neutrophil infiltration, and mRNA expression of multiple inflammatory mediators. While acinar cell injury was not different, acinar cell apoptosis was decreased in CFTR knockout mice, which also had mild exocrine pancreatic insufficiency as indicated by impaired *in vivo* pancreatic secretion in response to cholecystokinin and reduced pancreatic digestive enzyme mRNA and protein levels. These results were reproduced in ΔF508 mutant mice.[41] These observations are important, although the authors focused on the alterations of acinar cells, whereas CFTR is expressed on the apical membrane of pancreatic ductal cells. The lack of pancreatic CFTR expression impairs ductal fluid and bicarbonate secretion, and any alterations of the acinar cells might be presumably indirect. Our group recently demonstrated that CFTR knockout mice display more severe AP induced by intraperitoneal injection of ethanol and palmitic acid.[38] All laboratory and histological parameters were significantly elevated in CFTR knockout mice compared to wild-type controls, including the extension of necrosis. These data have potential clinical relevance since we detected markedly decreased CFTR mRNA and protein expression in small pancreatic ducts using pancreatic tissue samples from patients diagnosed with alcohol-induced AP.[38] A study by Pallagi et al. confirmed the potential role of CFTR and pancreatic ductal secretion in the pathogenesis of AP.[42] Their study used Na^+/H^+ exchanger regulatory factor-1 (NHERF-1) knockout mice that lack a cytosolic scaffolding protein involved in the apical targeting and retention of membrane proteins. They observed lower CFTR expression in the apical membrane of pancreatic ducts and decreased pancreatic bicarbonate and fluid secretion. Cerulein hyperstimulation and sodium taurocholate infusion into the pancreas induced more severe pancreatitis, further confirming the importance of CFTR-mediated pancreatic secretion.

Alcohol-induced CFTR dysfunction and therefore impaired HCO_3^- secretion also seem to be involved in the

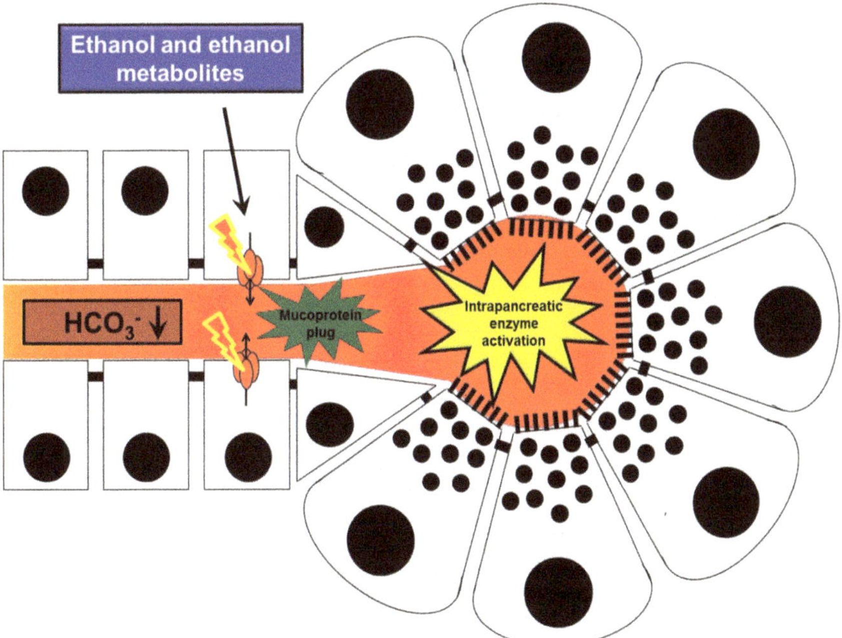

Figure 1. The effects of ethanol and ethanol metabolites on pancreatic ductal function. Under physiological conditions,the CFTR Cl^- channel (red) is expressed on the luminal membrane of small inter/intralobular pancreatic ducts and significantly contributes to pancreatic HCO_3^- secretion to maintain the alkaline intraluminal pH. During alcohol-induced AP or CP, CFTR function and expression are markedly reduced by ethanol and its metabolites, which leads to impaired HCO_3^- and fluid secretion and consequently decreased intraluminal pH. Under these conditions, the wash out of the luminal content is insufficient to prevent the formation of intraluminal protein plugs. The intraductal obstruction will lead to intrapancreatic enzyme activation in AP and to pancreatic atrophy and exocrine pancreatic insufficiency in CP.

pathogeneses of AP and CP. In CP, pancreas destruction can be observed due to chronic inflammation, exocrine pancreatic insufficiency, decreased pancreatic fluid and bicarbonate secretion, fibrosis, and tissue calcification. As an underlying mechanism for this decreased secretion, CFTR dysfunction due to mislocalized protein expression in pancreatic ductal cells has been observed in different forms of CP. Using human pancreatic tissue samples, Ko et al. found that CFTR is mislocalized in alcoholic, obstructive, and idiopathic CP.[43] The decreased expression of CFTR observed in different forms of CP could explain impaired PDEC function.[43] Impaired fluid and HCO_3^- secretion lead to lower intraluminal pH, decreased wash out of the digestive enzymes, and more viscous, protein-rich ductal fluid (**Figure 1**).[44] These changes promote the formation of intraluminal protein gel or plugs that are among the earliest histological features of CP.[34] Intraductal obstruction can lead to pancreatic atrophy, ductal mucinous hyperplasia,[45] goblet cell metaplasia, and protein plugs might also underlie pancreatic stone formation.[44]

Acknowledgement

This work was supported by the Hungarian Scientific Research Fund (K116634 to P.H., K109756 to V.V., and PD115974 to M.J.) and the Momentum Grant of the Hungarian Academy of Sciences (LP2014-10/2014 to P.H.).

References

1. Lee MG, Ohana E, Park HW, Yang D, Muallem S. Molecular mechanism of pancreatic and salivary gland fluid and HCO_3 secretion. *Physiol Rev*. 2012; 92: 39-74. PMID: 22298651.
2. Argent BE, Gray MA, Steward MC, Case RM. Cell physiology of pancreatic Ducts. In: Johnson LR, Barrett KE, Ghisan FK, Merchant JL, Said HM, Wood JD, eds. *Physiology of the Gastrointestinal Tract*. 5th ed. Oxford, Academic Press; 2012: 1399-1424.
3. Freedman SD, Kern HF, Scheele GA. Pancreatic acinar cell dysfunction in CFTR(-/-) mice is associated with impairments in luminal pH and endocytosis. *Gastroenterology*. 2001; 121: 950-957. PMID: 11606508.
4. Reber HA, Karanjia ND, Alvarez C, Widdison AL, Leung FW, Ashley SW, et al. Pancreatic blood flow in cats with chronic pancreatitis. *Gastroenterology*. 1992; 103: 652-659. PMID: 1634080.
5. Noble MD, Romac J, Vigna SR, Liddle RA. A pH-sensitive, neurogenic pathway mediates disease severity in a model of post-ERCP pancreatitis. *Gut*. 2008; 57: 1566-1571. PMID: 18625695.
6. Bhoomagoud M, Jung T, Atladottir J, Kolodecik TR, Shugrue C, Chaudhuri A, et al. Reducing extracellular pH sensitizes the acinar cell to secretagogue-induced pancreatitis responses in rats. *Gastroenterology* 2009; 137: 1083-1092. PMID: 19454288.
7. Pallagi P, Venglovecz V, Rakonczay Z Jr, Borka K, Korompay A, Ozsvari B, et al. Trypsin reduces pancreatic ductal bicarbonate secretion by inhibiting CFTR Cl^- channels and luminal anion exchangers. *Gastroenterology*. 2011; 141: 2228-2239, e2226. PMID: 21893120.
8. Bolender RP. Stereological analysis of the guinea pig pancreas. I. Analytical model and quantitative description of nonstimulated pancreatic exocrine cells. *J Cell Biol*. 1974; 61: 269-287. PMID: 4363955.
9. Ishiguro H, Steward MC, Lindsay AR, Case RM. Accumulation of intracellular $HCO3^-$ by Na^+-$HCO3^-$ cotransport in interlobular ducts from guinea-pig pancreas. *J Physiol*. 1996; 495: 169-178. PMID: 8866360.
10. Dyck WP, Hightower NC, Janowitz HD. Effect of acetazolamide on human pancreatic secretion. *Gastroenterology*. 1972; 62: 547-552. PMID: 5020866.
11. Shcheynikov N, Wang Y, Park M, Ko SB, Dorwart M, Naruse S, et al. Coupling modes and stoichiometry of Cl^-/HCO_3^- exchange by slc26a3 and slc26a6. *J Gen Physiol*. 2006; 127: 511-524. PMID: 16606687.
12. Zeng W, Lee MG, Yan M, Diaz J, Benjamin I, Marino CR, et al. Immuno and functional characterization of CFTR in submandibular and pancreatic acinar and duct cells. *Am J Physiol Cell Physiol*. 1997; 273: C442-C455. PMID: 9277342.
13. Maleth J, Hegyi P. Calcium signaling in pancreatic ductal epithelial cells: an old friend and a nasty enemy. *Cell Calcium*. 2014; 55: 337-345. PMID: 24602604.
14. Ahuja M, Jha A, Maleth J, Park S, Muallem S. cAMP and Ca^{2+} signaling in secretory epithelia: crosstalk and synergism. *Cell Calcium*. 2014; 55: 385-393. PMID: 24613710.
15. Hajnal F, Flores MC, Valenzuela JE. Pancreatic secretion in chronic alcoholics. Effects of acute alcohol or wine on response to a meal. *Dig Dis Sci*. 1993; 38: 12-17. PMID: 8420743.
16. Yamamoto A, Ishiguro H, Ko SB, Suzuki A, Wang Y, Hamada H, et al. Ethanol induces fluid hypersecretion from guinea-pig pancreatic duct cells. *J Physiol*. 2003; 551: 917-926. PMID: 12847207.
17. Laposata EA, Lange LG. Presence of nonoxidative ethanol metabolism in human organs commonly damaged by ethanol abuse. *Science*. 1986; 231: 497-499. PMID: 3941913.
18. Patton S, McCarthy RD. Conversion of alcohol to ethyl esters of fatty acids by the lactating goat. *Nature*. 1966; 209: 616-617. PMID: 5950784.
19. Gukovskaya AS, Mouria M, Gukovsky I, Reyes CN, Kasho VN, Faller LD, et al. Ethanol metabolism and transcription factor activation in pancreatic acinar cells in rats. *Gastroenterology*. 2002; 122: 106-118. PMID: 11781286.
20. Lange LG, Sobel BE. Mitochondrial dysfunction induced by fatty acid ethyl esters, myocardial metabolites of ethanol. *J Clin Invest*. 1983; 72: 724-731. PMID: 6308061.
21. Yadav D, Lowenfels AB. The epidemiology of pancreatitis and pancreatic cancer. *Gastroenterology*. 2013; 144: 1252-1261. PMID: 23622135.
22. Pandol SJ, Periskic S, Gukovsky I, Zaninovic V, Jung Y, Zong Y, et al. Ethanol diet increases the sensitivity of rats to pancreatitis induced by cholecystokinin octapeptide. *Gastroenterology*. 1999; 117: 706-716. PMID: 10464148.
23. Wilson JS, Apte MV, Thomas MC, Haber PS, Pirola RC. Effects of ethanol, acetaldehyde and cholesteryl esters on

pancreatic lysosomes. *Gut*. 1992; 33: 1099-1104. PMID: 1398235.

24. Shalbueva N, Mareninova OA, Gerloff A, Yuan J, Waldron RT, Pandol SJ, et al. Effects of oxidative alcohol metabolism on the mitochondrial permeability transition pore and necrosis in a mouse model of alcoholic pancreatitis. *Gastroenterology*. 2013; 144: 437-446, e436. PMID: 23103769.
25. Satoh A, Gukovskaya AS, Reeve JR Jr, Shimosegawa T, Pandol SJ. Ethanol sensitizes NF-kappaB activation in pancreatic acinar cells through effects on protein kinase C-epsilon. *Am J Physiol Gastrointest Liver Physiol*. 2006; 291: G432-G438. PMID: 16574982.
26. Lugea A, Tischler D, Nguyen J, Gong J, Gukovsky I, French SW, et al. Adaptive unfolded protein response attenuates alcohol-induced pancreatic damage. *Gastroenterology*. 2011; 140: 987-997. PMID: 21111739.
27. Petersen OH, Tepikin AV, Gerasimenko JV, Gerasimenko OV, Sutton R, Criddle DN. Fatty acids, alcohol and fatty acid ethyl esters: toxic Ca^{2+} signal generation and pancreatitis. *Cell Calcium*. 2009; 45: 634-642. PMID: 19327825.
28. Gerasimenko JV, Lur G, Ferdek P, Sherwood MW, Ebisui E, Tepikin AV, et al. Calmodulin protects against alcohol-induced pancreatic trypsinogen activation elicited via Ca^{2+} release through IP_3 receptors. *Proc Natl Acad Sci U S A*. 2011; 108: 5873-5878. PMID: 21436055.
29. Criddle DN, Raraty MG, Neoptolemos JP, Tepikin AV, Petersen OH, Sutton R. Ethanol toxicity in pancreatic acinar cells: mediation by nonoxidative fatty acid metabolites. *Proc Natl Acad Sci U S A*. 2004; 101: 10738-10743. PMID: 15247419.
30. Criddle DN, Murphy J, Fistetto G, Barrow S, Tepikin AV, Neoptolemos JP, et al. Fatty acid ethyl esters cause pancreatic calcium toxicity via inositol trisphosphate receptors and loss of ATP synthesis. *Gastroenterology*. 2006; 130: 781-793. PMID: 16530519.
31. Dolai S, Liang T, Lam PP, Fernandez NA, Chidambaram S, Gaisano HY. Effects of ethanol metabolites on exocytosis of pancreatic acinar cells in rats. *Gastroenterology*. 2012; 143: 832-843, e831-e837. PMID: 22710192.
32. Werner J, Laposata M, Fernández-del Castillo C, Saghir M, Iozzo RV, Lewandrowski KB, et al. Pancreatic injury in rats induced by fatty acid ethyl ester, a nonoxidative metabolite of alcohol. *Gastroenterology*. 1997; 113: 286-294. PMID: 9207289.
33. Apte MV, Pirola RC, Wilson JS. Mechanisms of alcoholic pancreatitis. *J Gastroenterol Hepatol*. 2010; 25: 1816-1826. PMID: 21091991.
34. Sarles H, Sarles JC, Camatte R, Muratore R, Gaini M, Guien C, et al. Observations on 205 confirmed cases of acute pancreatitis, recurring pancreatitis, and chronic pancreatitis. *Gut*. 1965; 6: 545-559. PMID: 5857891.
35. Kristidis P, Bozon D, Corey M, Markiewicz D, Rommens J, Tsui LC, et al. Genetic determination of exocrine pancreatic function in cystic fibrosis. *Am J Hum Genet*. 1992; 50: 1178-1184. PMID: 1376016.
36. Ooi CY, Dorfman R, Cipolli M, Gonska T, Castellani C, Keenan K, et al. Type of CFTR mutation determines risk of pancreatitis in patients with cystic fibrosis. *Gastroenterology*. 2011; 140: 153-161. PMID: 20923678.
37. Judak L, Hegyi P, Rakonczay Z Jr, Maleth J, Gray MA, Venglovecz V. Ethanol and its non-oxidative metabolites profoundly inhibit CFTR function in pancreatic epithelial cells which is prevented by ATP supplementation. *Pflugers Arch*. 2014; 466: 549-562. PMID: 23948742.
38. Maleth J, Balazs A, Pallagi P, Balla Z, Kui B, Katona M, et al. Alcohol disrupts levels and function of the cystic fibrosis transmembrane conductance regulator to promote development of pancreatitis. *Gastroenterology*. 2015; 148: 427-439, e416. PMID: 25447846.
39. Venglovecz V, Rakonczay Z Jr, Ozsvari B, Takacs T, Lonovics J, Varro A, et al. Effects of bile acids on pancreatic ductal bicarbonate secretion in guinea pig. *Gut*. 2008; 57: 1102-1112. PMID: 18303091.
40. Dimagno MJ, Lee SH, Hao Y, Zhou SY, McKenna BJ, Owyang C. A proinflammatory, antiapoptotic phenotype underlies the susceptibility to acute pancreatitis in cystic fibrosis transmembrane regulator (-/-) mice. *Gastroenterology*. 2005; 129: 665-681. PMID: 16083720.
41. DiMagno MJ, Lee SH, Owyang C, Zhou SY. Inhibition of acinar apoptosis occurs during acute pancreatitis in the human homologue DeltaF508 cystic fibrosis mouse. *Am J Physiol Gastrointest Liver Physiol*. 2010; 299: G400-G412. PMID: 20522641.
42. Pallagi P, Balla Z, Singh AK, Dosa S, Ivanyi B, Kukor Z, et al. The role of pancreatic ductal secretion in protection against acute pancreatitis in mice. *Crit Care Med*. 2014; 42: e177-e188. PMID: 24368347.
43. Ko SB, Mizuno N, Yatabe Y, Yoshikawa T, Ishiguro H, Yamamoto A, et al. Corticosteroids correct aberrant CFTR localization in the duct and regenerate acinar cells in autoimmune pancreatitis. *Gastroenterology*. 2010; 138: 1988-1996. PMID: 20080093.
44. Ko SB, Azuma S, Yoshikawa T, Yamamoto A, Kyokane K, Ko MS, et al. Molecular mechanisms of pancreatic stone formation in chronic pancreatitis. *Front Physiol*. 2012; 3: 415. PMID: 23133422.
45. Allen-Mersh TG. What is the significance of pancreatic ductal mucinous hyperplasia? *Gut*. 1985; 26: 825-833. PMID: 4018649.

Chapter 15

Smoking-induced pancreatitis and pancreatic cancer

Mouad Edderkaoui[1*] and Edwin Thrower[2*]

[1]*Cedars-Sinai Medical Center, VA-West Los Angeles & University of California, Los Angeles, California, USA;*
[2]*Yale University & VA CT Healthcare, New Haven, Connecticut, USA.*

Introduction

Multiple clinical studies have shown that smoking tobacco, particularly cigarettes, elevates the risk for developing pancreatic diseases such as pancreatitis and cancer.[1,2] Furthermore, risk increases as a function of the amount of tobacco consumed. Smoking tobacco has often been linked as a cofactor with alcohol abuse in predisposition to pancreatic disorders. However, the inclusion of smokers that do not drink alcohol in some of these studies has highlighted that cigarette smoking can be considered an independent risk factor. Despite significant clinical advancements in this field, scientific data exploring how tobacco toxins affect the pancreas at the cellular level are scarce.[2] In this review, we summarize clinical and scientific knowledge regarding the effects of tobacco on the pancreas and how they may contribute to disease development and progression.

Role of Tobacco in Development of Pancreatic Disease: Pancreatitis

Clinical evidence

An exact role for tobacco intake as a risk factor in pancreatitis has been difficult to determine as chronic tobacco consumption is frequently associated with chronic alcohol abuse. More than 80% of patients with alcoholic chronic pancreatitis (ACP) are smokers, and tobacco has largely been considered to potentiate alcohol toxicity.[3-5] A retrospective cohort study of ACP showed that cigarette smoking altered the average age at diagnosis; it was an average of 5 years earlier in smokers, who were also at an increased risk of pancreatic calcification.[4] These findings were validated in a recent study that also found a concentration-dependent relationship between ACP course and tobacco consumption.[5] Tobacco intake was measured in "pack years," defined as the number of cigarettes per day multiplied by the number of years of smoking divided by 20 (20 cigarettes/pack). At a 10-pack year threshold, no differences in ACP outcome were observed.

At a 20-pack year threshold, the diagnosis of ACP was made earlier, and patients had more frequent calcifications. Similar results were observed for a 30-pack year threshold, along with increased pancreatic exocrine insufficiency.

Although these studies imply that tobacco use potentiates alcohol's effects in pancreatitis, convincing data has emerged from several case-control and cohort studies that strongly support an *independent* association between smoking and pancreatitis.[4,6-14] The major findings from these studies are detailed in **Table 1**. All of these investigations conclude that smoking tobacco increases the risk for developing chronic pancreatitis (CP) independently of alcohol. For example, one U.S. study showed that compared with never-smokers, the odds ratio (OR) for developing CP in smokers with <12 pack years was 1.34 (95% confidence interval [CI] 0.90-2.01), with 12-35 pack years it increased to 2.15 (95% CI 1.46-3.17), and with >35 pack years, the OR was 4.59 (95% CI 2.91-7.25). Furthermore, a stratified analysis revealed a direct correlation between the level of smoking and CP for both sexes of Caucasians and "ever drinkers" (lifetime consumption of >20 alcoholic drinks) but not in the Black/African American population. While there was a trend toward increased risk in the African American community, the CIs also increased, perhaps owing to the small number of subjects.[15] Data from the Iowa Women's Health Study also support a link between smoking levels and an increased OR for CP; heavy smoking (40+ vs. 0 pack years) was associated with a twofold increase in OR for CP, regardless of alcohol use.[16] The fact that the study targeted females ≥65 years old also suggests that smoking may be a specific factor for developing CP in older women.

In Japan, a nationwide survey was conducted to clarify the epidemiological features of patients with CP.[7] As it was a cross-sectional nationwide survey without healthy controls, the researchers did not estimate whether

*Corresponding authors. Email: mouad.edderkaoui@cshs.org, edwin.thrower@yale.edu

Table 1. Summary of recent clinical studies on smoking as a risk factor in pancreatitis.

Study	Study type	No. of subjects	Sex	Alcohol intake	Smoking status	Key observations
Talamini et al. (1999)[11]	Case-control	Total (n) = 1,330 CP = 571 Con = 700	M	0 to 80 g/day	0 to >10 cigarettes/day	• CP patients drank and smoked more than controls • Smoking (1-10 cigarettes/day) greater risk factor for CP than drinking 41-80 g alcohol/day
Lin et al. (2000)[17]	Case-control	Total (n) = 266 CP = 91 Con = 175	M	0 to ≥100g/day	Non-smokers[a] Ex-smokers Current-smokers Mild Moderate Heavy	• Smoking associated with an independent and dose-dependent increase in CP risk • Cigarette smoking associated with higher risk at two alcohol consumption levels (0-28, ≥29 g alcohol/day)
Tolstrup et al. (2009)[1,12]	Cohort	Total (n) = 17,905 P = 235	M, F	Abstainer <7 to >20 drinks/wk	Never[b] Ex (former) Current Mild Moderate Heavy	• 2-3-Fold increased risk of pancreatitis associated with moderate and heavy smoking • Dose-dependent association between smoking and P • Former smokers showed elevated risk (~2-fold) for AP but not CP • Alcohol intake associated with increased risk of pancreatitis • P cases (46%) attributed to smoking
Yadav et al. (2009)[15]	Cohort (NAPS2)	Total (n) = 1,695 CP = 540 RAP = 460 Con = 695	M, F	Abstainer <0.5 to ≥5 drinks/day	Never[c] Ever Mild Moderate Heavy	• Heavy smoking and alcohol intake are independent risk factors for CP • Cigarette smoking was an independent, dose-dependent risk factor for CP and RAP
Law et al. (2010)[8]	Cross-sectional	Total (n) = 235 CP = 79	M, F	Abstainer 0 to ≥10 drinks/wk	Never Ex-smoker Current	• Current but not former smoking significantly associated with CP • Approximately 2-fold increased risk associated with current smoking
Cote et al. (2011)[6]	Epidemiological (NAPS2)	Total (n) =1,234 CP = 539 Con = 695	M, F	Abstainer <0.5 to ≥5 drinks/day	Never[c] Ever Mild Moderate Heavy	• Independent association between smoking and idiopathic CP
Sadr-Azodi et al. (2011)[10]	Cohort	Total (n) = 84,667 AP = 307	M,F	0 to ≥400 g/month	Never[d] Former Current	• Duration of smoking increases risk for non-gallstone related AP • Two decades of smoking cessation decreases risk for AP
Rebours et al. (2012)[5]	Cohort	Total (n) = 108 CP = 79	M,F	Median, 145 g/day; range 40-500 g/day	Current[e] Ex-daily	• 10 pack-year threshold, no differences in ACP outcome • 15 pack-year threshold, ACP diagnosis made earlier (36 vs. 46 years) • 20 pack-year threshold, ACP occurs earlier with more calcifications (seen at 30 pack-year also) • Tobacco accelerates ACP course in a dose-dependent fashion

(Continued)

Table 1. Continued

Study	Study type	No. of subjects	Sex	Alcohol intake	Smoking status	Key observations
DiMagno et al. (2013)[18]	Case-control	Total (n) = 6,505 PEP = 211 Severe PEP = 22 Control = 348	M,F	Current Former Never	Current[f] Former Never	• 6,505 patients had 8,264 ERCPs • 211 had PEP and 22 had severe PEP • Smoking identified as *protective* variable for PEP
Maire et al. (2014)[19]	Cohort	Total (n) = 96 Type 1 AIP = 28 Type 2 AIP = 9	M,F	Abstainer	Non-smokers[g] Current Ex-smokers	• 76% patients were high smokers and 24% low smokers • High smokers presented more frequently with DM (50% vs. 27%, $P = 0.04$) and imaging of pancreatic damage (59% vs. 34%, $P = 0.02$) than low smokers • No protective effect of smoking in the patient subgroup with type 2 AIP and ulcerative colitis • In patients with AIP, high tobacco intake associated with risks of pancreatic damage and DM
Yang et al. (2014)[13]	Population-based, cross-sectional study	Total (n) = 23,294 AP= 45	M, F	Abstainer <56.2 drink-year ≥56.2 drink-year Drink year = (vol. of alcohol/day) × (length of drinking in years)	Non-smokers[h] Current: Mild Heavy	• Smoking was associated with an increased risk of developing AP • Dose-dependent association seen with tobacco, particularly in those who smoked at least 15 pack years
Hirota et al. (2014)[7]	Cross-sectional nationwide survey	Total (n) P = 1,734 ACP = 1,171 AP = 37 AIP = 12	M, F	Abstainer Ethanol <80 or ≥80 g/day	Never[i] Current Former (past) Ever	• Alcoholic (67.5%) most common and idiopathic (20%) second most common cause of CP • Comorbid DM and PC occurred more frequently in ever-smokers, independent of drinking status • In non-drinkers, incidences of DM and PC were higher in ever-smokers than never-smokers • Smoking was an independent factor of DM and PC in CP patients
Lin et al. (2014)[9]	Population-based cohort study	Total (n) = 35,642 AP = 54 CP = 12	M, F	Never Social (<once/wk) Regular (≥once/week, not intoxicated) Heavy (>once per week, intoxicated)	Never[j] Current Former	• Neither current nor ever-smoking was associated with the incidence of pancreatitis • Dose-response analysis also showed no association between smoking and pancreatitis • Regular and heavy alcohol drinking were associated with an increased incidence of pancreatitis
Yuhara et al. (2014)[14]	Systemic review and meta-analysis	Variable criteria (values taken from multiple studies)	M, F	Variable criteria (definitions vary between multiple studies)	Variable criteria (definitions vary between multiple studies)	• Thorough review of literature for studies that have smoking exposure and AP, as well as relative risk/odds ratio calculations • A total of 5 case-control or cohort studies were considered for meta-analysis after screening 451 records using rigorous selection criteria • Both current and former smoking were associated with AP independently of alcohol abuse

(Continued)

Table 1. Continued

Study	Study type	No. of subjects	Sex	Alcohol intake	Smoking status	Key observations
Alsamarrai et al. (2014)[20]	Systemic review and meta-analysis	Variable criteria (values taken from multiple studies)	M, F	Variable criteria (definitions vary between multiple studies)	Variable criteria (definitions vary between multiple studies)	• Searched three databases for prospective cohort studies of modifiable risk for AP, CP, and pancreatic cancer • A total of 51 population-based studies with 3 million individuals and 11,000 patients with pancreatic disease were considered • Current tobacco use was the single most important risk factor for pancreatic diseases
Cavestro et al. (2015)[21]	Cohort	Total (n) = 196 RAP = 40 (of the RAP patients CP = 13)	M, F	40.0-75.0 g/day	13-30 cigarettes/day	• RAP associated with higher cigarette usage • CP associated with cigarette smoking
Prizment, et al. (2015)[16]	Cohort	Total (n) = 36,436 AP (one episode) = 511 CP = 149	F, age ≥65	Not specified	Mild[k] Moderate Heavy	• Alcohol use was not associated with AP or CP • Heavy smoking (40+ pk-y) was associated with 2-fold increase in risk for CP

Abbreviations: ACP = alcoholic chronic pancreatitis; AIP = autoimmune pancreatitis; CP = chronic pancreatitis; Con = controls; DM = diabetes mellitus; ERCP = endoscopic retrograde cholangiopancreatography; F = female; M = male; P = pancreatitis (acute and chronic); PC = pancreatic calcifications; PEP = Post-ERCP pancreatitis; RAP = recurrent acute pancreatitis.

[a] Mild (<20 cigarettes/day), Moderate (20-39 cigarettes/day), Heavy (≥40 cigarettes/day)

[b] Mild (1-14 g/day), Moderate (15-24 g/day), Heavy (>24 g/day)

[c] Never (<100 cigarettes in lifetime); Ever (>100 cigarettes in lifetime) subclassified into Mild, Moderate, and Heavy (<12, 12-35, and >35 pack-years, respectively); Pack-year = average number of cigarettes/day and duration of smoking.

[d] Never (not defined), Former (<20 or ≥ 20 pack-years), Current (<20 or ≥ 20 pack-years)

[e] Ex-daily (<20 pack-years), Current (≥ 20 pack-years)

[f] Not defined

[g] Non-smokers, Current (<10 or ≥ 10 pack-years), Ex-smokers (not specified)

[h] Non-smokers, Current Mild or Heavy (<15 or ≥ 15 pack-years, respectively)

[i] Criteria not clearly specified in the study

[j] Ever smokers were individuals smoking>100 cigarettes (subclassified into: Current, those who had smoked in the month prior to the interview; Former, those who had not smoked in the month prior to the interview), and Never smokers were individuals smoking <100 cigarettes.

[k] Heavy smokers (>40 pack-years)

smoking alone constituted a risk for CP onset. However, the results clearly showed that smoking tobacco increased the occurrence of clinical features associated with the disease. In this study, the incidence of comorbidity with diabetes mellitus and pancreatic calcifications increased significantly in the "never drinking but ever smoking" CP patients compared to the "neither drinking nor smoking" CP patients. These findings imply that smoking poses a risk for developing CP complications independently of alcohol consumption.

Collectively, evidence from clinical studies supports a dose-dependent association between smoking and CP; however, a similar association with acute pancreatitis (AP) has also been revealed.[12,14,21] In a Danish study with a mean follow-up of 20.2 years, a link between smoking and increased risk of AP was observed independent of alcohol consumption. Another novel finding from this study was the risk for developing acute pancreatitis in former-smokers was elevated (1.7, 95% CI 1.0-2.7), compared to "never smokers".[12] However, this study did not account for the level of smoking by former-smokers (e.g., mild, moderate,or heavy) or the extent of smoking abstinence, both of which could alter risk. A subsequent investigation centered on these factors and demonstrated that *duration* of smoking, rather than smoking intensity, was the reason for higher risk in this patient group. Two decades after smoking cessation, the relative risk (RR) was reduced to a level consistent with that seen in never-smokers (RR 1.20, 95% CI 0.66-2.15).[10] Although smoking cessation varied the risk for acute pancreatitis, another study found no significant risk associated with former smoking in terms of CP (OR 0.40, 95% CI 0.14-1.18).[8] In addition to the Danish and American studies, a population-based, cross-sectional analysis of an elderly Chinese population linked tobacco consumption with the risk of AP, particularly in those who had smoked at least 15 pack years.[13] Furthermore, a systematic review and meta-analyses, which included many of the studies detailed here, concluded that current and former smoking are firmly connected with an elevated AP risk.[14,20] A single-center, prospective, cohort study of the natural history of AP found that smoking was a dose-dependent risk factor for *recurrent* acute pancreatitis (RAP).[21] Furthermore they validated the association between cigarette smoking and CP. Therefore, it seems likely that increased levels and/or duration of tobacco consumption could lead to repeat bouts of AP that ultimately evolve into CP.

It should be noted that one Taiwanese population-based cohort study did not find any evidence linking cigarette smoking and the incidence of pancreatitis, although they documented a dose-dependent association between alcohol abuse and pancreatitis.[9] These findings are in sharp contrast to the overwhelming data supporting an independent effect of smoking on pancreatitis development.[4,6-14] The authors reasoned that potential racial differences in nicotine metabolism and susceptibilities to smoking between the Taiwanese populations they examined versus ethnically different populations from the other investigations may explain the discrepancy. However, their study may not have been sufficiently powered to detect a modest association between smoking and pancreatitis given that a small number of subjects developed pancreatitis, follow-up was relatively short, and alcohol and tobacco consumption in Taiwan are much lower compared with Western populations.

In addition to the effects of tobacco smoking on development of AP and CP, the influence of smoking on the course of autoimmune pancreatitis (AIP) and post-endoscopic retrograde cholangiopancreatography (ERCP) pancreatitis (PEP) has been considered.[18-21] The AIP study reported that high smokers (>10 pack years) presented more frequently diabetes (50% vs. 27%) and pancreatic damage on imaging (59% vs. 34%) than low smokers.[19] In addition, there was a trend to observe more pancreatic exocrine insufficiency (41% vs. 29%). These data suggest that smoking could influence the natural course of AIP, similar to that seen with alcoholic CP, although the association between smoking and AIP relapse was not significant. Type 2 AIP is associated with inflammatory bowel disease, especially ulcerative colitis (UC), and although smoking has been shown to have a protective effect in UC, the exact mechanisms are not understood.[22,23] In one study, 22 patients had UC in association with AIP, but a protective effect of smoking on AIP course was not observed. This lack of effect could have been due to an irrelevant statistical analysis owing to small patient numbers. In the study evaluating tobacco's effects on the course of PEP, current smoking was independently *protective* against PEP.[18] That current smoking is protective against PEP apparently contradicts the clinical observation outlined earlier in this review: that smoking is an independent, dose-dependent risk factor for AP and CP. However, the protective effect observed in PEP may occur through nicotine, a major toxic component of tobacco (see section on *Nicotine*) that activates the nicotinic anti-inflammatory pathway and can reduce pancreatic inflammation.[24-27] Nicotine can also relax the sphincter of Oddi in experimental models and might reduce sphincter spasm and obstruction that can cause PEP.[28]

Although numerous clinical studies now substantiate an independent role for smoking in pancreatitis, it is often not acknowledged by physicians as a risk factor for the disease. In a study of 535 patients diagnosed with CP, 382 (71.4%) reported smoking, yet physicians recorded smoking as a risk factor for only 173 (45.3%). There was a greater tendency to do so if the patient was a current smoker, reported elevated levels of smoking, and/or had a concurrent alcohol problem.[15,29] The importance of smoking as an independent risk factor, particularly for CP, is becoming vital for interventional purposes in light of new clinical information. One recent study used a questionnaire to i) investigate patient awareness regarding an association of smoking and pancreatic disease; ii) assess doctor-patient communication regarding smoking in general, and pancreatic disease specifically; and iii) examine the patient's stage of change for quitting smoking.[30] Eighteen patients (mean age 52 years, 85% male) were included in the analysis. The data breakdown revealed that 56% of patients were aware of a connection between smoking and CP, and 72% were conscious of alcohol and its role in pancreatitis. Patients conveyed that physicians were a critical reference source for their knowledge concerning causes of CP, although only 39% stated that their physician had directly referred to the effects that tobacco has on the pancreas. This study highlights that efforts should be directed toward enhancing physicians' knowledge on smoking and pancreatic disease, as well as patient education.

In addition to continuing clinical studies and relating newly relevant information to patients, greater understanding is needed in defining which toxins in tobacco may initiate pancreatic disease at the cellular level. The fundamental biological mechanisms of tobacco-related pancreatitis remain largely uncharted, and further research is necessary to identify potential therapeutic targets. An overview of current scientific findings related to tobacco and pancreatitis follow.

Scientific evidence

In the following section, the effects of tobacco smoke on the pancreas will be explored, and tobacco-specific toxins and their potential for inducing pancreatitis through certain cellular pathways will be considered.

Cigarette smoke

Of the 4,000 chemicals in cigarette smoke, more than 60 have been recognized as prospective carcinogens. Tobacco smoke components, particularly nicotine, 4-(methylnitrosamino)-1-(3-pyridyl)-1-butanone (NNK), and nitrosamines specific to tobacco, have been studied in cells and *in vivo*.[24,31-37] NNK is one of the most potent, as determined by studies in laboratory animals.[37] N'-nitrosonornicotine (NNN) and diethylnitrosamine (DEN) are two more nitrosamines derived from nicotine[38] that are potentially formed via nitrosation during tobacco processing.[39] Approximately 46% of NNN and 26%-37% of NNK in tobacco is preformed, and the remainder is pyrosynthesized from nicotine during smoking.[40] Other harmful constituents of tobacco smoke include polycyclic aromatic hydrocarbons (PAHs), although their role in pancreatic disease remains unclear.[40,41] In the following sections we will report the general effects of tobacco on the pancreas and subsequently focus on nicotine and NNK, since they are the most studied with respect to pancreatic disease.

Effects on human pancreas

In light of the medical evidence linking tobacco smoking and pancreatitis, closer attention has been paid to smoking-induced changes in pancreatic tissue from patients enrolled in such studies.[42-48] Some of those changes are highlighted below.

Pancreatic fibrosis: One study assessed pancreatic fibrosis (PF) in smokers versus non-smokers and found that both total and intralobular PF were significantly more common in smokers (total: 42.9% vs. 26.5%, $P = 0.027$ and intralobular: 39.3% vs. 15.6%, $P = 0.013$).[48] Since pancreatic stellate cells (PSCs) are key players in PF,[42,49] it is highly likely that oxidative stress induced by tobacco components and cigarette smoke could lead to their activation, eventually resulting in PF.

Oxidative stress: Expression of the pro-inflammatory cytokine interleukin-6 (IL-6) and antioxidants in pancreatic fluids and tissues in patients (both smoking and non-smoking) with CP have been measured.[45] Compared to non-smoking patients and healthy subjects, statistically higher levels of IL-6 and metallothionein, as well as increased activities of antioxidants (glutathione peroxidase, copper-zinc superoxide dismutase) are observed in smoking patients with CP. These observations further underscore the role oxidative stress may play in tobacco-related pancreatitis.

Secretion: Several studies have assessed the effects of tobacco smoking on factors that affect both endocrine and exocrine pancreatic secretion in smokers versus non-smokers.[43,46] Numerous publications report decreased insulin secretion in both smoking patients and smokers with CP, and higher blood glucose levels were detected in the latter.[50-52] These changes paralleled adaptations in pancreatic structure and altered endocrine function of the organ resulting from smoking.[51] Another study examined the immunohistochemical localization of somatostatin and pancreatic polypeptide (two hormones that regulate secretion) in the pancreatic tissue of smoking and non-smoking patients with CP and healthy controls.[46] Significantly higher immunostaining of the hormones was detected in samples from smoking patients, suggesting that tobacco smoking may contribute to endocrine disturbances during CP development. Another retrospective study compared pancreatic duct cell function in smokers (current and past) with never-smokers by measuring the secretin-stimulated peak bicarbonate concentration ($[HCO3^-]$) in endoscopically collected pancreatic fluid.[43] Smoking (OR 3.8, 95% CI 1.6-9.1, $P = 0.003$) and definite CP imaging (OR 5.7, 95% CI 2.2-14.8, $P < 0.001$) were determined to be independent predictors of low peak pancreatic fluid $[HCO3^-]$ after controlling for age, sex, and alcohol intake. Furthermore, no interaction between smoking status and alcohol intake was observed in predicting duct cell dysfunction (P = 0.571). Thus, measurement of pancreatic fluid bicarbonate in smokers reveals that cigarette smoking (past and current) is an independent risk factor for pancreatic duct cell secretory dysfunction (low pancreatic fluid [$HCO3^-$]). Furthermore, the risk of duct cell dysfunction in subjects who smoked was approximately doubled (RR 2.2) in never smokers.

Endothelin-1: Endothelin-1 (ET-1) plays a role in blood vessel constriction, and recent evidence indicates that it may be another marker of tobacco-linked pancreatitis.[53,54] Plasma ET-1 levels are nearly two-fold higher in smokers compared to healthy controls. Histopathologic analyses of pancreatic tissue also showed increased ET-1 levels in smokers and smokers suffering from CP. These findings may account for changes in blood flow to the pancreas seen during pancreatitis.

Pancreatic dysfunction/protein catabolism: One study examined levels of creatinine, uric acid, and urea in nonsmoking and smoking patients with CP.[47] Their results showed elevated creatinine and uric acid levels 1.5 times higher in the smoking group compared to healthy controls. These findings suggest that cigarette smoking may be an important factor in potential changes in uric acid levels in patients with CP. In addition, the decreased protein catabolism observed in this study is likely due to progressing exocrine pancreatic dysfunction in both smoking and nonsmoking patients with CP.

Genetic mutations: Chymotrypsinogen C (CTRC) is known to protect the pancreas by degrading the prematurely activated zymogen, trypsinogen. Rare mutations in CRTC prevent it from degrading trypsinogen and are associated with RAP and CP.[55] The occurrence of such mutations in patients was evaluated from the North American Pancreatitis Study cohort II, and it was found that a genetic variant, CTRC Variant G60G (c.180T), acted as a disease modifier and promoted progression of RAP to CP, particularly in the smoking population.[44] The mechanism of how tobacco smoke or toxins interact with variants of CRTC to produce this disease phenotype is not yet clear.

It seems the effects of tobacco exposure on the human pancreas are numerous, and the physical and functional changes it produces are becoming more evident. However, the precise cellular mechanisms and pathways that mediate these events are unclear. Identification of potential disease markers, some of which have been detected by assessing pancreatic tissue from clinical studies, could prove useful in determining which cellular pathways to research and in designing appropriate experimental models for smoking-related pancreatitis. A crucial assumption is that by understanding the disease mechanism, opportunities will arise to develop novel therapeutic strategies.

Effects on pancreas in animal models of cigarette smoke exposure

Cigarette smoke consists of a complex mixture of compounds, making the development of dependable animal models of smoking and pancreatitis challenging. Specific compounds and mixtures that are most likely responsible for human disease have to be considered along with the administration route (i.e., inhalational vs. systemic) and dosing to parallel the human experience. So far, only a small number of reasonable animal models of tobacco-related pancreatitis have been established.[1,24,32,35,56-66]

In one of the earliest animal models, rats were given intravenous ethanol under anesthesia and were exposed to cigarette smoke at 15 and 45 minutes (40 puffs, 2-minute session each time by mechanical ventilation) from the start of ethanol infusion. The investigators determined that this regimen would yield nicotine plasma levels comparable to those found in human smokers (nicotine concentrations 4-72 ng/mL, mean 33 ng/mL). They found that cigarette smoke exacerbated pancreatic ischemia initiated by ethanol. In addition, cigarette smoke by itself elevated leukocyte-endothelium interactions and, in combination with ethanol, augmented pancreatic sequestration.[24]

In another model of rat pancreatitis, tobacco smoke was administered through inhalation for 12 weeks. Animals that received high-dose exposure (160 mg/m^3) developed pancreatic damage consistent with that seen in CP and had increased levels of the pancreatic zymogens trypsinogen and chymotrypsinogen. These rats also developed focal pancreatic lesions with areas of increased extracellular matrix, although the pancreatic damage was reduced compared to that observed in human CP. These differences between the model and human CP might be due to the relatively short experimental time period.[34] Another report concluded that environmental tobacco smoke altered gene expression in the exocrine pancreas by modifying the ratio of trypsinogen to its endogenous inhibitor (pancreas-specific trypsin inhibitor, PSTI). While trypsinogen was elevated in smoke-exposed animals, PSTI expression was not. These modifications rendered smoke-exposed animals prone to pancreatitis.[35]

That these models mimic the features of human pancreatitis is promising, but there is limited information as to which toxins are initiating pancreatitis and what their cellular targets may be. Other approaches have focused on specific toxins in tobacco, which may be likely candidates for initiating pancreatic disease. As mentioned earlier, these include nicotine and the tobacco-specific nitrosamine NNK. Their role in pancreatic and other cancers has been explored and will be discussed later. In the sections that follow, we will describe findings from animal models that explore effects of nicotine and NNK in development of pancreatitis.

Nicotine: Nicotine is a significant toxin in tobacco and cigarettes and may influence the development of pancreatitis and pancreatic cancer. Nicotine is rapidly absorbed in the lungs and is removed from the body within 120-180 minutes.[67] Nicotine metabolism occurs primarily through the cytochrome P450 (CYP) 2A6 pathway along with additional enzymes including aldehyde oxidase 1, UDP-glucuronosyltranferases, flavin-containing monooxygenase 3, and other CYPs (e.g., 2A13 and 2B6). CYP2A6 polymorphisms have been associated with racial and genetic differences in nicotine metabolism, but it is unclear if these impact smoking-related pancreatic disease.[68] Compared to healthy controls, patients with CP and pancreatic cancer have elevated levels of P450 enzyme.[63] Studies in which rats inhaled ^{3}H-nicotine revealed that it accumulates in the pancreas and intestine.[57,63] In addition, elevated levels of nicotine metabolites have been measured in human pancreatic juice from smokers. Cotinine, a primary metabolite, was present at levels around 130 ng/mL, whereas NNK ranged from 1.37 to 600 ng/mL (0.7 μM and 6.6 nM to 3 μM, respectively).[69]

Several studies have established the pathological and functional effects of nicotine on the pancreas. In a rodent model, rats were exposed to graded doses of nicotine either by aerosol, intragastric, or *ad libitum* feeding over a period of 3 to 16 weeks. Exocrine pancreatic cells from these animals exhibited cytoplasmic swelling, vacuolization, pyknotic nuclei, and karyorrhexis. Furthermore, isolated acinar cells either treated with nicotine or harvested from nicotine-exposed animals showed similar cellular damage. These changes reflect those observed in acute or experimental pancreatitis (**Figure 1**).[31,59,62,67] Nicotine also altered pancreatic secretion: it decreased pancreatic amylase secretion in rats, which was accompanied by the retention of pancreatic zymogens.[31,56,59,62,64,66,70] A subsequent study showed that nicotine-induced secretory events in isolated rat acini are abrogated following treatment with the nicotinic receptor antagonist mecamylamine and some calcium channel antagonists.[65] This pharmacologic evidence insinuates that nicotine modulates its responses through a nicotinic acetylcholine receptor (nAChR) and that calcium acts as a downstream effector. Nicotine has also been shown to change circulating levels of the gastrointestinal hormones gastrin and cholecystokinin (CCK) in rats.[60] Fluctuating basal levels of these hormones and serum enzymes such as amylase and lipase have been related to morphological variations in pancreatitis.[56,62] Nicotine can also regulate lipid peroxidation and oxidative stress, although it is undetermined if these processes are involved in pancreatitis pathophysiology.[56]

Nicotine exposure may lead to increased expression of proteins that contribute to pancreatitis and other pancreatic diseases. One study used mass spectrometry-based proteomics to investigate the effects of nicotine on the proteomes of two pancreatic duct cell lines: an immortalized normal cell line (HPNE) and a cancer cell line (PanC1).[71] With more than 5,000 proteins identified per cell line, over 900 were differentially expressed following nicotine treatment, and 57 of these proteins were found in both cell lines. In a prior study, nicotine treatment had been shown to increase expression of amyloid precursor protein (APP) in PSCs,[72] and in this later study, APP upregulation was also observed in both ductal cell lines. Thus nicotine-mediated expression of APP might be linked with inflammatory or fibrotic responses in pancreatitis.

NNK: NNK is a tobacco-specific nitrosamine derived from nicotine and one of the most toxic components in cigarette smoke. The role of NNK as an initiator of and sensitizer to AP was revealed in studies using isolated rat acinar cells and *in vivo* models of pancreatitis.[73] Firstly, NNK was found to induce a key event in the initiation of pancreatitis: premature activation of digestive zymogens (trypsinogen and chymotrypsinogen).

Secondly, the effects of NNK in conjunction with the commonly used "cerulein" model of pancreatitis were determined to see if NNK pretreatment could augment pancreatitis responses. Cerulein is an orthologue of the hormone CCK, and when given at supraphysiologic concentrations (10-100× that required to induce physiological responses), it causes typical pancreatitis responses (zymogen activation, histologic/morphologic changes) in isolated acinar cells or live animals. NNK pretreatment in the cerulein model elevated zymogen activation above that seen with NNK or cerulein treatment alone. [73] Furthermore, NNK triggers cellular injury in the pancreas similar to that typically seen during AP (vacuolization, pyknotic nuclei, and edema). These findings raise the question: how does NNK mediate these pancreatitis responses?

NNK is a high-affinity agonist of β-adrenergic receptors and nAChRs, particularly the α7 isoform, and could influence the development and progression of pancreatic diseases through these receptor-mediated pathways. NNK is structurally similar to classic β-adrenergic agonists and binds with high affinity to human β-1 and β-2 receptors (half maximal effective concentration [EC_{50}] for β1 = 5.8 nM, EC_{50} for β2 = 128 nM).[74] In mammalian cells, β-adrenergic receptor activation triggers adenylate cyclase to generate the second messenger cAMP, although in some cells it can cause arachidonic acid release. Elevations in cAMP may participate in pancreatitis responses.[75] Although one study detected β-adrenergic receptors in rat acinar cells, NNK-mediated zymogen activation was not abrogated when β-adrenergic receptors were inhibited with propranolol.[1] It is possible that NNK mediates arachidonic acid release through phospholipase A2 (PLA2), an important factor in inflammation. Various isoforms, namely phospholipase A2-II and A2-IV, are elevated during human AP and may affect both local disease severity and systemic

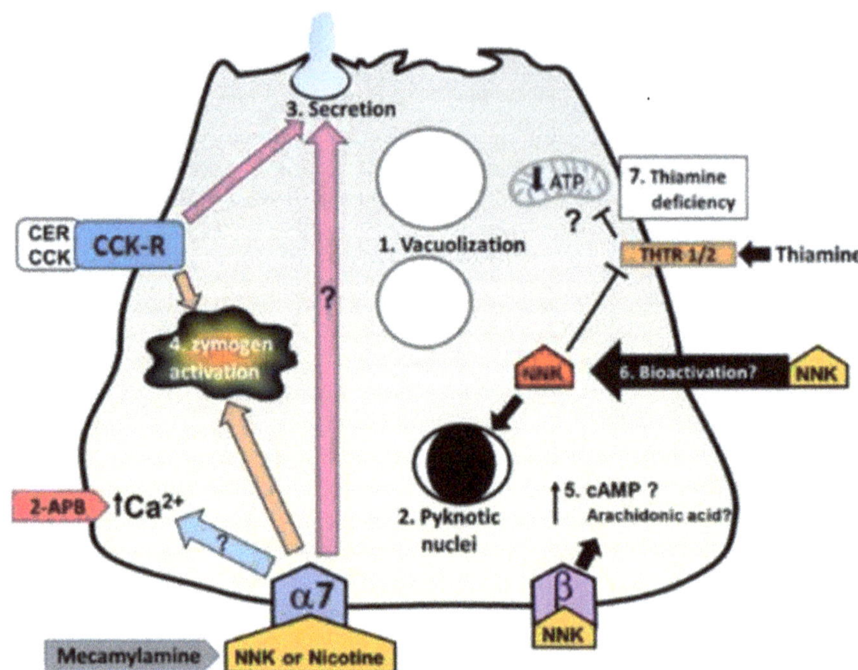

Figure 1. Cellular mechanisms mediated by nicotine and NNK in pancreatic acinar cells. Exposure to nicotine and NNK is known to cause morphological changes comparable to those seen in pancreatitis including 1. vacuolization and 2. pyknotic nuclei. 3. Secretion: nicotine stimulates secretion by itself and augments cholecystokinin-mediated (CCK) secretion at low concentrations (100 μM); at higher concentrations (>1 mM) it inhibits secretion. Pretreatment of pancreatic acinar cells with the nAChR blocker mecamylamine reduces nicotine-mediated effects. The calcium channel antagonist 2-APB also prevents nicotine-stimulated events; this implies that nicotine-sensitive pathways involve the α7 nAChR and intracellular calcium signals. 4. Zymogen activation: NNK induces zymogen activation in acini and augments cerulein (CER)-induced zymogen activation; this effect is abrogated by mecamylamine and in α-$7^{-/-}$ mice. 5. Elevations in cAMP and arachidonic acid through β-adrenergic receptor signaling: NNK binds to β-adrenergic receptors with high affinity. Pre-incubation of acini with the β-blocker propranolol does not block NNK-mediated zymogen activation; therefore, this pathway does not mediate this process. Whether NNK elevates levels of the second messengers cAMP and arachidonic acid to cause other pancreatitis responses is undetermined. 6. Bioactivation: NNK can be taken up by cells and converted to bioactive forms by cytochrome P450 enzymes; this occurs in the pancreas, but it has not been determined if these bioactive forms participate in pancreatitis. Bioactivated NNK can affect cell function at the transcriptional level. 7. Thiamine deficiency and mitochondrial dysfunction. NNK has been shown to inhibit uptake of the vitamin thiamin by reducing levels of thiamin transporters. Whether this is via a bioactivated form of NNK is unclear. Thiamin is crucial for pancreatic function due to its role in metabolism and as a cofactor for multiple enzymes in mitochondrial ATP production. Thiamin deficiency may decrease cellular ATP levels, leaving the pancreas vulnerable to a secondary insult and thus development of pancreatitis.

complications.[76] Whether NNK mediates other pancreatitis responses through these receptors is undetermined.

More recently, attention has focused on the possibility of NNK initiating pancreatitis responses through a non-neuronal form of the α7 isoform of nAChR. These receptors were initially described within the nervous system but have subsequently been identified in non-neuronal cells.[38] Various cancer cell lines, human keratinocytes, and epithelial cells all express α7 nAChR and respond to NNK exposure (EC_{50} for NNK = 0.03 μM). NNK is present in tobacco smoke at concentrations 5,000-10,000 times less than nicotine, yet it exhibits 1,000-fold higher affinity for α7 nAChR. In addition, upregulation of α7 nAchRs are observed in the organs of smokers and in the pancreas and lungs of rodents following chronic experimental exposure to nicotine or NNK.[36,38]

To determine whether NNK mediates pancreatitis through a non-neuronal α7 nAChR, it was first established that the receptor was present in rat pancreatic acini through polymerase chain reaction analysis.[73] Next, a functional role was revealed when isolated acini were pretreated with the nAChR antagonist mecamylamine, which abrogated NNK-induced zymogen activation. These findings were further validated by transgenic mice studies. NNK treatment in acini isolated from α7 $nAChR^{-/-}$ mice failed to elicit zymogen activation compared with wild type animals.[77]

NNK may mediate pancreatitis responses through a direct interaction with α7 nAChR on the acinar cell surface, but it might also influence inflammatory cells during pancreatitis (**Figure 2**). Macrophages express α7 nAChRs, and both NNK and nicotine could potentially modulate immune responses. Nicotine hinders pro-inflammatory cytokine generation from macrophages by inhibiting the nuclear factor-κB (NFκB) pathway, which mediates macrophage activation.[61,78] Furthermore, treating mice with mecamylamine (the general nAChR blocker) decreases neutrophil and macrophage migration to pancreatic tissue and leads to more severe experimental pancreatitis.[25] In addition, prophylactic and delayed therapeutic application of nicotine significantly attenuates the severity of acute experimental pancreatitis in rats through stimulation of the cholinergic anti-inflammatory pathway.[79] Nicotine pretreatment is protective in a model of severe acute pancreatitis (SAP) in which mice are given a retrograde injection of 2% Na-taurocholate into the pancreatic duct.[80] Nicotine (50-300 μg/kg) reduces tissue injury, enzyme production, and pro-inflammatory cytokine generation. Nicotine also upregulates CD4+ CD25+ regulatory T cells (Treg) through increasing the expression of immunoregulatory molecules and secretion of transforming growth factor β1 (TGF-β1).

The notion of nicotine and NNK inducing an anti-inflammatory response and reducing pancreatitis severity may seem contrary to other studies demonstrating that tobacco toxins promoting the disease.[73] However, it has also been shown that prolonged exposure to cigarette smoke results in chronic inflammation in the pancreas. Other studies have indicated that NNK may actually initiate pro-inflammatory effects in macrophages and other cells through its uptake and metabolism. In U937 human macrophages, NNK gets absorbed and metabolized, undergoing a process known as bioactivation.[32] This occurs via the cytochrome P450 (CYP450) enzyme family through three primary pathways: i) carbonyl reduction, ii) pyridine N-oxidation, and iii) alpha-hydroxylation. Following bioactivation, NNK metabolites subsequently *activate* NFκB, inducing TNF-α release while inhibiting IL-10 synthesis. Decreased levels of other cytokines and modulators namely IL-2, IL-6, granulocyte/macrophage-colony-stimulating factor (GM-CSF), and macrophage chemotactic protein 1 (MCP-1) are also seen.[32]

Thus it seems that the effects of NNK and nicotine in pancreatitis are multi-faceted and might appear ambiguous. Early pancreatitis events may consist of a combination of direct interaction of NNK/nicotine with α7 nAChR on acini and a possible anti-inflammatory phase through α7 nAChR localized on macrophages.[25,73,78,79]

The anti-inflammatory phase could be an initial response that ultimately yields to a chronic inflammatory phase with continued exposure to cigarette toxins.[81] Chronic inflammatory responses happen much later, perhaps through macrophage uptake and metabolism (bioactivation) of NNK/nicotine (**Figure 2**).

It is unclear whether NNK bioactivation occurs in pancreatic acinar cells and contributes to tobacco-related pancreatitis. Although P450 enzymes, which are crucial for NNK bioactivation, have been identified in rodents (isoforms 2B6, 3A5, and 2A3), there have been inconsistent

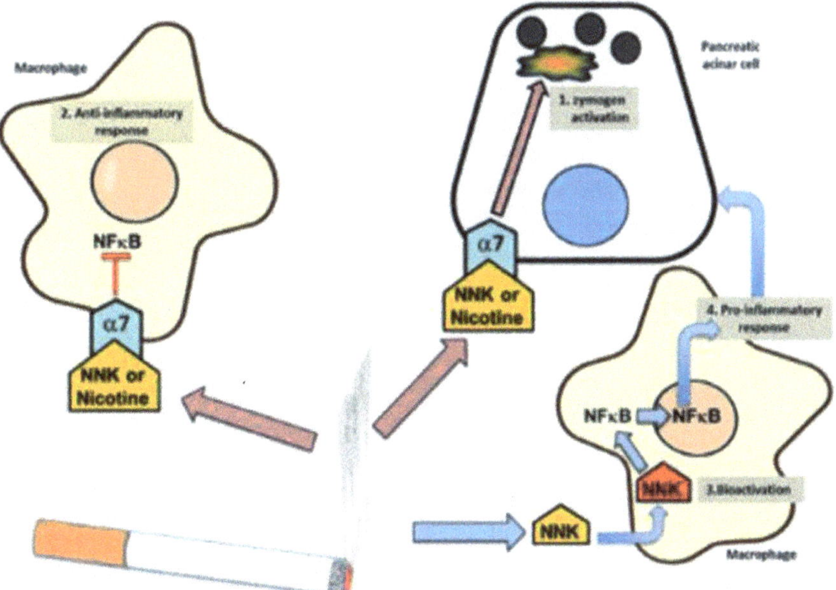

Figure 2. Inflammatory events in smoking-related pancreatitis. Early events in smoking-related pancreatitis include 1. zymogen activation through a direct interaction of NNK with α7 nAChRs on pancreatic acini and 2. stimulation of the cholinergic anti-inflammatory pathway by NNK/nicotine binding to α7 nAChRs localized on macrophages. The anti-inflammatory phase could be an initial response that ultimately yields to a chronic inflammatory phase with continued exposure to cigarette toxins. 3. Bioactivation: NNK is taken up and metabolized by macrophages. 4. Pro-inflammatory response: the "bioactivated" derivatives of NNK can affect gene transcription and lead to activation of pro-inflammatory pathways. Activated macrophages invade damaged pancreatic tissue, giving rise to pancreatic inflammation.

results in the human pancreas.[82] One study using cytochemical detection techniques found no evidence of the P450 enzymes in human pancreatic samples from smokers and non-smokers.[41] However, another study detected CYP450 enzymes in human pancreatic tissue using immunohistochemical methods.[83] Furthermore, the levels of enzymes were elevated in the samples from patients with CP and pancreatic cancer.[83] Thus metabolism of NNK within pancreatic cells may actually be a factor in the development of smoking-related pancreatitis and other pancreatic diseases.

More recent findings have shown that NNK may induce changes within pancreatic acinar cells at the genetic level.[84] Whether this is through a "bioactivated" form of NNK or some other pathway remains unclear. The vitamin thiamin is critical for both exocrine and endocrine functions of the pancreas, and pancreatic cells are known to maintain high levels via uptake from their surroundings. Uptake is achieved through thiamin transporters-1 and -2 (THTR-1 and THTR-2). Protein and mRNA levels of these transporters are significantly reduced when pancreatic acinar 266-6 cells are treated with NNK. These changes are further coupled with decreased thiamin uptake and lower levels of the thiamin transporter promoters SLC19A2 and SLC19A3. Long-term NNK treatment in mice yields similar results.[84] This study highlights that cigarette toxins can cause alterations in pancreatic cells at a genetic level resulting, in this particular case, thiamin deficiency. Thiamin deficiency, followed by a drop in cellular ATP levels, might sensitize the pancreas to a secondary insult, predisposing to pancreatitis.

It is apparent, from all of the scientific studies described here, that tobacco smoke, in particular toxins such as nicotine and NNK, are capable of inducing diverse pancreatitis responses via multiple cellular mechanisms. It is likely, that through similar mechanisms, progression of chronic disease to cancer may occur. In the following sections, we will explore the clinical evidence for a link between smoking and development of pancreatic cancers and describe potential cellular mechanisms.

Role of Tobacco in Development of Pancreatic Disease: Pancreatic Adenocarcinoma

Although there is much debate about the effect of alcohol abuse in causing and/or promoting pancreatic cancer, tobacco smoking is a major established risk factor for the disease.[85,86] Strong evidence indicates that cigarette smoking increases the risk of pancreatic cancer and accelerates its development. Smoking increases the risk of pancreatic cancer up to 6-fold depending on the duration and intensity,[87-89] and nearly one-quarter of all pancreatic cancer deaths are linked to tobacco use.[89] At least two different recent studies recently showed that smokers are diagnosed with pancreatic cancer at ages 6 to 15 years younger than non-smokers.[90,91] Therefore, understanding the mechanisms through which smoking predisposes to pancreatic cancer is important. Such knowledge will help identify patients at high risk for the disease who would benefit from preventive strategies and permit the development of treatment approaches directed at cell signaling pathways involved in smoking-induced pancreatic cancer.

The next sections of this manuscript provide a short review of the clinical evidence for the association between smoking and pancreatic cancer, as well as a more detailed review of the pathways mediating the pro-cancer effects of cigarette smoke compounds in the pancreas.

Clinical evidence

Research on the association between smoking and pancreatic cancer goes back to the mid 1960s. One of the first studies to examine the association was published in 1970 and compared the age-adjusted death rates in the years 1964 and 1965 from cancers of different sites and the annual consumption of cigarettes in data collected from 20 countries. The author found no significant correlation between cigarette smoking and death from pancreatic cancer; although the risk of death from pancreatic cancer in smokers was nonsignificantly increased by an RR of 1.21 in males and 1.15 in females.[92] One possible reason for this result is that the comparison was performed between heavy smokers (smoking a number of cigarettes above the average of cigarettes smoked by the whole population analyzed, which is 3.5 cigarettes per day) and light smokers (smoking a number of cigarettes below the average). Results from the same study showed a nonsignificant increase in deaths from lung cancers in heavy smokers compared to light smokers, confirming that the significance is lost because the threshold between light and heavy smokers was very low at 3.5 cigarettes per day. The first study to show an association between cigarette smoking and pancreatic cancer in humans was published by Wynder et al. in 1973.[93] Two years later, the same author showed an increased risk for pancreatic cancer associated with the number of cigarettes smoked per day. He found that smoking 1 to 10 cigarettes per day significantly increases the RR of pancreatic cancer by 2-fold, while 21-40 cigarettes per day increases it by 3.5-fold, and smoking more than 41 cigarettes per day increases the risk by 5-fold.[94] Another group analyzing 38 case-control studies concluded that the RR for pancreatic cancer among smokers is 2 to 4, making it the third highest smoking-related cancer after lung and upper aero-digestive tract cancers.[95] Depending on the duration and intensity of cigarette smoking, it could increase the risk of pancreatic cancer up to 6-fold.[86,88,96] In addition to these findings, several other studies have assessed the association between smoking and pancreatic cancer and have emphasized cigarette smoking as a major risk factor for the disease.[85,96]

Nearly one-quarter of all pancreatic cancer deaths are linked to tobacco use.[6] Furthermore, two recently published studies highlighted that pancreatic cancer diagnosis occurs 6 to 15 years earlier in smokers compared with non-smokers.[90,91] Compared to non-smokers, smoking less than one and more than two packs a day decreased the age of diagnosis by 3 and 6 years, respectively.[90]

However, the deleterious effect of tobacco smoking is not perpetual. Indeed, a 1986 study showed a strong association between smoking and increased risk for pancreatic cancer, but the effect disappeared after a decade of not smoking.[89] The deleterious effect of smoking did not change in smokers who stopped smoking within <10 years, as the median age of diagnosis was similar to smokers. Conversely, it did completely resolve in patients who had stopped smoking more than 10 years prior, as the age of diagnosis was similar to non-smokers.[90] The same study showed that the proportional hazard ratio among smokers was similar to those who stopped smoking less than 10 years ago (RRs of 1.65 and 1.27, respectively) compared to a relative risk of 0.95 for those who stopped smoking more than 10 years ago.[90]

It is worth noting that animal studies revealed that exposing wild-type mice to cigarette smoke compounds may cause pancreatic lesions, but these rarely reach the pancreatic adenocarcinoma stage, suggesting that smoking cooperates with other environmental and/or genetic factors such as Kras mutation to induce pancreatic cancer. In fact, most rats that consumed NNK and NNAL (0.5, 1, and 5 ppm) in their drinking water for their entire lives did not develop pancreatic ductal adenocarcinoma, except 13% of rats treated with the high dose of 5 ppm NNAL.[37]

Scientific evidence

Smoking and genetic mutations

An analysis of known pancreatic cancer mutations in the pancreatic tissue of patients revealed a significant increase in the number of mutations per tumor in smokers (53.1 mutations per tumor) compared to 38.5 mutations per tumor in never smokers.[97]

Kras mutation is strongly associated with pancreatic cancer and is present in more than 90% of pancreatic cancer patients.[98] A strong association exists between Kras mutation and smoking in lung cancer patients; however, such a link is hard to establish in pancreatic cancer. The meta-analysis performed by Porta et al. showed no significant association between Kras mutations and smoking status in pancreatic and colorectal cancers, whereas a significant association was found in lung cancer.[99] The sequencing of the pancreatic cancer genome revealed that the difference in the total number of mutations between smokers and non-smokers was not driven by mutations of the known driver genes in pancreatic cancer, such as Kras, p53, p16/CDKN2A, and SMAD4, instead changes were predominantly observed in genes mutated at lower frequencies.[97] In addition, no differences were observed in mutations in carcinomas from the head versus tail of the gland. The same study by Porta et al. revealed a very important observation related to the spectrum of mutations of Glycine 12 in the Kras protein in the three cancers. In pancreatic and colon tumors, 85% and 74% of the mutations are Val or Asp in pancreatic and colon cancers, respectively, whereas in lung cancer only 37% are Val or Asp against 49% Cys compared to 3% and 8% Cys in pancreatic and colon cancers, respectively.[99] These data suggest a possible association between the spectrum of mutations and the effect of smoking.

The difference between the spectra of Kras mutations in pancreatic and lung cancers might help differentiate between metastatic pancreatic tumors found in the lung and primary lung tumors. This is extremely important knowing that the treatment approaches and survival rates of these patient groups are significantly different. Kras mutation analysis revealed that the presence of the KRAS G12C mutation had 96% specificity and positive predictive value for lung adenocarcinoma, whereas G12R was 99% specific for pancreatic cancer with a positive predictive value of 86%.[100] However, it is worth nothing that although Kras mutations in the pancreas are not significantly induced by smoking, recent data indicate that nicotine further stimulates mutated Kras activation, leading to more aggressive pancreatic tumors in animal models of the disease.[101] The cell signaling mechanism mediating this effect will be discussed in a subsequent section of this review. Other less common mutations associated with pancreatic cancer include p53, BRAF, Mek, and Cox2, as well as deletion of SMAD4 and p16INK4A.[102]

Analysis of DNA adducts induced in rat lung and pancreas after treatment with different doses of NNK or NNAL showed that both compounds had similar effects in both organs. However, the level of DNA adducts was significantly lower in the pancreas compared to the lung, partially explaining why a higher level of DNA mutations is observed in the lungs of humans and animals exposed to cigarette smoke compared to the pancreas.[103]

Smoking compounds and cell signaling in precancer and cancer cells

As mentioned before, cigarette smoke contains over 4,000 chemicals with at least 60 carcinogens. Of these constituents, nicotine and NNK, in addition to cigarette smoke extracts, are the most studied in the context of cancer and will be reviewed in the following subsections.

Cell signaling pathways affected by nicotine

As mentioned earlier, mass spectrometry-based proteomics analysis of pancreatic ductal and cancer cell lines exposed to nicotine showed that over 900 proteins were significantly abundant following nicotine treatment, and 57 were found in both cell lines. However, most of the proteins regulated by nicotine differed between the two cell types, suggesting that nicotine may play different roles in pancreatic cancer initiation and progression.[72]

Nicotine was shown to stimulate cancer promotion in several animal models of pancreatic cancer. Administration of nicotine accelerates pancreatic cell transformation and tumor formation in both the elastase-Kras (Ela-Kras) and $Kras^{LSL\text{-}G12D/+}$; $Trp53^{LSL\text{-}R172H/+}$; $Pdx^{cre/+}$ (KPC) mice. Nicotine induces dedifferentiation of acinar cells by activating Akt-Erk-Myc signaling; this leads to inhibition of Gata6 promoter activity, decreased GATA6 protein levels, and subsequent loss of acinar differentiation and hyperactivation of oncogenic Kras.[101]

Sustained exposure to nicotine induces activation of Akt and Erk kinases, both important pro-cancer pathways.[104] Adding nicotine to drinking water for 4 weeks significantly reduces the therapeutic response of mouse xenografts to gemcitabine. This is associated with decreased gemcitabine-induced caspase-3 cleavage and inhibition of phosphorylated/activated forms of Akt, Erk, and Src in xenograft tissues.[104]

Nicotine promotes the aggressiveness of established tumors as well as the epithelial–mesenchymal transition (EMT), increasing numbers of circulating cancer cells and their dissemination to the liver compared with mice not exposed to nicotine. Nicotine induces pancreatic cells to acquire the gene expression patterns and functional characteristics of cancer stem cells. These effects are markedly attenuated in KPC mice given metformin, which prevented nicotine-induced pancreatic carcinogenesis and tumor growth by upregulating GATA6 and promoting differentiation toward an acinar cell program.[101] Gata6 ablation renders acinar cells more sensitive to the Kras mutation in a mouse model of pancreatic cancer, thereby accelerating tumor development. Furthermore, Gata6 expression is spontaneously lost in a Kras mouse model of pancreatic cancer in association with altered cell differentiation.[105] Gata6 is a transcription factor that plays a tumor-suppressor role through promoting cell differentiation, suppressing inflammatory pathways, and directly repressing cancer-related pathways. The epidermal growth factor receptor (EGFR) pathway is an example of a pro-cancer pathway inhibited by GATA6 as its activity is upregulated in the normal and pre-neoplastic Gata6-null pancreas.[105]

Trevino et al. showed that stimulation of pancreatic cancer cells with nicotine concentrations within the range of human exposure activates Src kinase and induces the inhibitor of the differentiation-1 (Id1) transcription factor. Depletion of α7-nAChR or Id1 prevents nicotine-mediated induction of pancreatic cancer cell proliferation and invasion *in vitro*.[106,107] In addition, nicotine confers resistance to gemcitabine in pancreatic cancer cells, but Src or Id1 depletion prevents the nicotine-induced resistance. These data show that nicotine promotes pancreatic cancer cell growth and metastasis and confers resistance to gemcitabine *in vivo* in an orthotopic model of pancreatic cancer.[107] Of note, Src kinase plays a major role in promoting pancreatic cancer; it regulates cancer cell proliferation, invasion, and metastasis.[108,109] Clinical analyses of resected pancreatic cancer specimens revealed a statistically significant correlation between phospho-Src, tumor grade/differentiation, and worsening overall patient survival.[107] Another pathway involved in the pro-cancer effect of nicotine is the STAT3/MUC4 pathway.[110] This will be discussed in more detail in the next section.

Figure 3 depicts the important pathways involved in mediating the pro-cancer effects of nicotine in the pancreas.

Cell signaling pathways affected by NNK and cigarette smoke extract

Similar to the effect of nicotine on the Akt pathway, upregulation of Akt kinase phosphorylation/activation is induced by NNK and cigarette smoke extracts (CSE) in pancreatic ductal cells. This effect inhibits apoptosis and is mediated by NADPH oxidase.[111] Chronic exposure to NNK and CSE also inhibit autophagy.[111] NNK also stimulates pancreatic ductal cell proliferation through a mechanism that involves EGFR activation.[112] Both studies demonstrate involvement of the EGFR/Akt pathway in regulating pancreatic ductal cell proliferation and resistance to apoptosis.

Cigarette smoke extract and its major component nicotine significantly upregulate MUC4 in pancreatic cancer cells. MUC-4 plays several roles in cancer progression, especially through its signaling and anti-adhesive properties that contribute to tumor development and metastasis. Smoking-induced MUC4 overexpression was via α7-nAChR stimulation and subsequent activation of the downstream JAK2/STAT3 signaling cascade in cooperation with the MEK/ERK1/2 pathway.[110] MUC4 upregulation promotes pancreatic cancer cell migration, and Src kinase is involved in mediating this pro-metastasis effect. *In vivo*, cigarette smoke exposure significantly stimulates tumor metastasis to various distant organs in an orthotopic model of pancreatic cancer.[110]

The effect of cigarette smoke on promoting pancreatic cancer is observed in the early pre-cancer stages of the disease. Indeed, exposure of the Pdx1-Cre;LSL-Kras (KC) mice to cigarette smoke for 20 weeks significantly accelerates the development of pancreatic intraepithelial neoplasia (PanIN) lesions, the precursors of pancreatic adenocarcinoma. This effect is associated with stimulation of inflammation markers such as IFN-γ and CXCL2, as well as enhanced activation of PSCs.[113]

Data from Edderkaoui et al. show similar up-regulation of PanIN lesion formation, inflammation, fibrosis and stellate cell (SC) activation in the same animal model, but with a shorter exposure to cigarette smoke (6 weeks).[114] Their data further demonstrated significant stimulation of EMT in the PanIN cells of mice exposed to cigarette smoke, suggesting that smoking may cause early metastasis of precancer PanIN cells. Notably, precancer cell EMT was observed in the KPC mouse model of pancreatic cancer. EMT was associated with the expression of cancer stem cell properties, and it was associated with dissemination of these cells to the liver; a phenomenon that preceded pancreatic tumor formation.[115] Very importantly, cancer cell EMT was also associated with an abundant inflammatory response, and treatment with immunosuppressive agents prevented precancer cell dissemination.[115]

Figure 3 depicts important pathways demonstrated to mediate the pro-cancer effects of NNK and cigarette smoke in the pancreas.

Smoking and inflammation

Pancreatic cancer is characterized by strong desmoplasia. Pro-inflammatory mediators have been associated with pancreatic diseases including pancreatitis and pancreatic cancer.

Inflammatory cells, cytokines, chemokines, and their receptors have different biological functions including inflammatory response, angiogenesis, and metastasis. Strong evidence indicates that all of these components are expressed in pancreatic cells and infiltrating immune cells within inflamed pancreatic tissues.[116]

One major mechanism through which smoking induces pancreas inflammation, which may lead to cancer, is through inducing pancreatitis. Mechanisms of smoking-induced pancreatitis were discussed earlier in this review. The next section will discuss the smoking-induced inflammatory pathways independently of pancreatitis.

It is well established that exposure to cigarette smoke stimulates inflammatory cell infiltration. In KC mice, cigarette smoke induces concurrent increase in macrophages and dendritic cells (DCs).[113] NNK treatment significantly increases macrophage infiltration and expression of pro-inflammatory mediators such as macrophage inflammatory protein 1 alpha (MIP-1α, interleukin 1β (IL-1β), and TGF-β in mice neoplastic lesions.[34] Higher infiltration of inflammatory cells including macrophages and mast cells is associated with strong expression of vascular endothelial growth factor (VEGF) and basic fibroblast growth factor (b-FGF) in human pancreatic cancer tissues compared to normal pancreatic tissues.[117]

Cytokines and other pro-inflammatory mediators have been implicated in inflammatory pancreatic diseases including pancreatitis and cancer. Analysis of cytokine gene polymorphisms as risk factors for pancreatic cancer suggests the possibility of interactions between current active smoking and the CCR5-delta32 deletion allele. The age-adjusted interaction ratio (95% CI) for CCR5-delta32 and smoking was 1.4.[118] Of note, macrophages highly express the chemokine (C-C motif) receptor (5CCR5), which is the receptor of the chemokine C-C motif ligand 5 (CCL5). CCL5 is an anti-tumor chemokine that induces immune

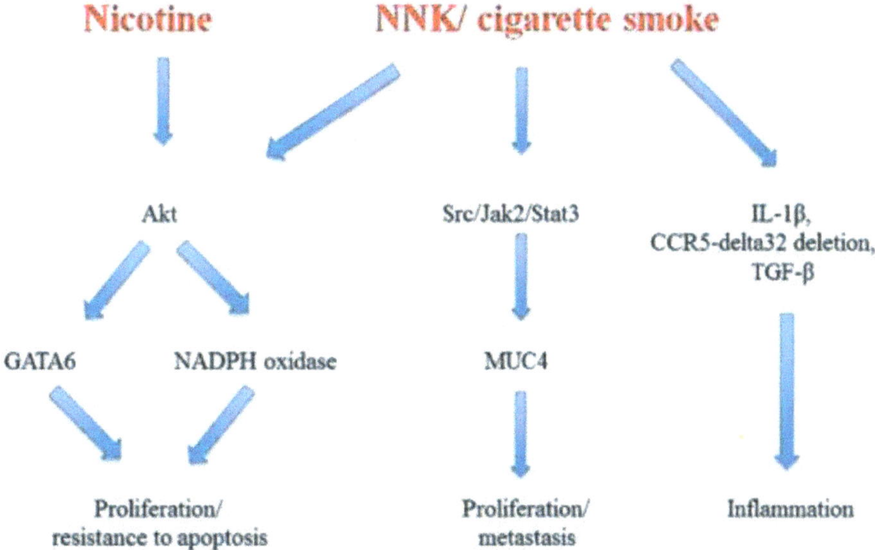

Figure 3. Pancreatic cell pathways regulated by smoking compounds. Nicotine stimulates Akt kinases, leading to activation of the NADPH oxidase and GATA6 pathways, which stimulate proliferation and inhibit apoptosis. NNK and cigarette smoke stimulate the same Akt pathways, the Src/Jak2/Stat3 pathway that leads to proliferation and metastasis, and a pro-inflammation pathway.

cell recruitment.[116,119] The data suggest that intact *CCR5* may protect from smoking-induced pancreatic cancer.[118]

Exposure of elastase-IL-1β transgenic mice (a model of CP) to aqueous CSE for up to 15 months induced a significant flattening of pancreatic ductal epithelial cells and severe glandular atrophy compared with untreated transgenic mice. Ductal epithelial cells displayed a high proliferative index, minimal apoptosis, and COX-2 induction, all markers associated with pancreatic cancer.[120] Notably, Cox2 can induce activation of oncogenic Kras, leading to pancreatic inflammation, fibrosis, and development of pancreatic intraepithelial neoplasia lesions and pancreatic ductal adenocarcinoma.[121]

Another important pathway through which smoking promotes pancreatic cancer is by stimulating oxidative stress. Indeed, nicotine induces oxidative stress in rat pancreas, and this is associated with inflammation and increased IL-6 secretion in the pancreas.[122] Of note, inducible nitric oxide synthase (iNOS) expression is increased during pancreatic cancer development and progression, as well as in inflamed tissues.[123,124]

Lastly, a study by Lazar et al. showed that cigarette smoking and nicotine may contribute to pancreatic cancer inflammation by inducing MCP-1 expression. The authors provided novel insight into a unique role for osteopontin (OPN) in mediating these effects.[125]

Smoking and fibrosis

Published studies show that exposing mice to cigarette smoke activates PSCs as indicated by the level of the marker alpha-smooth muscle actin (α-SMA), and induces extracellular matrix protein expression.[113,114]

In vitro, nicotine at levels found in smokers' blood induces proliferation and upregulates the expression of collagen1-α2 and TGF-β1 in hepatic SCs. This profibrogenic effect of nicotine is exerted through actions on nAChRs expressed on hepatic SCs. Nicotinic receptor antagonists reverse the nicotine-induced profibrogenic effects.[126] Very little data is published on the effect of smoking compounds on pancreatic SCs *in vitro*. A unique 2014 study showed that smoking compounds significantly increase PSC proliferation and migration. It also demonstrated that PSCs express the nAChR isoforms alpha 3, 5, 7 and epsilon.[127]

It is hypothesized that smoking compounds stimulate PSC activation and proliferation and promote extracellular matrix protein deposition. This would result in a microenvironment favorable for proliferation of cancer cells and resistance to apoptosis.

Mouse, rat, and human PSCs have slightly different native morphologies. Following nicotine treatment, PSCs acquire a slightly different morphology and are characterized by a more elongated shape caused by narrow cytoplasmic projections.

Mass spectrometry analysis of nicotine-exposed PSCs showed that of the total proteins identified, 25%-30% were exclusive to either nicotine-treated or untreated cells. Such nicotine-induced proteins include collagen alpha1(III) chain and alpha1(V) chain.[72]

Conclusions

For over four decades, studies have demonstrated that cigarette smoking is a major risk factor for pancreatic cancer. More recently, smoking was found to potentiate alcohol-induced pancreatitis. However, in the last decade, strong evidence suggests an independent effect of smoking in promoting acute and CP. However, despite the vast amount of data indicating an association between smoking and pancreatic diseases, data exploring the cellular mechanisms involved are less accepted. Various well-known pro-pancreatitis pathways (e.g., NFκB) and pro-cancer pathways (e.g., Akt kinase) are shown to be upregulated in pancreatic cells. More comprehensive studies are needed to determine the detailed mechanism of interaction between these pathways and the receptors stimulated by cigarette smoke compounds. Furthermore, the effect of smoking on cells recruited and activated in the pancreatic tumor microenvironment and during acute and CP requires further investigation.

References

1. Alexandre M, Pandol SJ, Gorelick FS, Thrower EC. The emerging role of smoking in the development of pancreatitis. *Pancreatology*. 2011; 11(5): 469-474. PMID: 21986098.
2. Edderkaoui M, Thrower E. Smoking and Pancreatic Disease. *J Cancer Ther*. 2013; 4(10A): 34-40. PMID: 24660091.
3. Bourliere M, Barthet M, Berthezene P, Durbec JP, Sarles H. Is tobacco a risk factor for chronic pancreatitis and alcoholic cirrhosis? *Gut*. 1991; 32(11): 1392-1395. PMID: 1752475.
4. Maisonneuve P, Lowenfels AB, Mullhaupt B, Cavallini G, Lankisch PG, Andersen JR, et al. Cigarette smoking accelerates progression of alcoholic chronic pancreatitis. *Gut*. 2005; 54(4): 510-514. PMID: 15753536.
5. Rebours V, Vullierme MP, Hentic O, Maire F, Hammel P, Ruszniewski P, et al. Smoking and the course of recurrent acute and chronic alcoholic pancreatitis a dose-dependent relationship. *Pancreas*. 2012; 41(8): 1219-1224. PMID: 23086245.
6. Cote GA, Yadav D, Slivka A, Hawes RH, Anderson MA, Burton FR, et al. Alcohol and smoking as risk factors in an epidemiology study of patients with chronic pancreatitis. *Clin Gastroenterol Hepatol*. 2011; 9(3): 266-273. PMID: 21029787.
7. Hirota M, Shimosegawa T, Masamune A, Kikuta K, Kume K, Hamada S, et al. The seventh nationwide epidemiological survey for chronic pancreatitis in Japan: clinical significance of smoking habit in Japanese patients. *Pancreatology*. 2014; 14(6): 490-496. PMID: 25224249.

8. Law R, Parsi M, Lopez R, Zuccaro G, Stevens T. Cigarette smoking is independently associated with chronic pancreatitis. *Pancreatology*. 2010; 10(1): 54-59. PMID: 20332662.
9. Lin HH, Chang HY, Chiang YT, Wu MS, Lin JT, Liao WC. Smoking, drinking, and pancreatitis: a population-based cohort study in Taiwan. *Pancreas*. 2014; 43(7): 1117-1122. PMID: 25083998.
10. Sadr-Azodi O, Andren-Sandberg A, Orsini N, Wolk A. Cigarette smoking, smoking cessation and acute pancreatitis: a prospective population-based study. *Gut*. 2012; 61(2): 262-267. PMID: 21836026.
11. Talamini G, Bassi C, Falconi M, Sartori N, Salvia R, Rigo L, et al. Alcohol and smoking as risk factors in chronic pancreatitis and pancreatic cancer. *Dig Dis Sci*. 1999; 44(7): 1303-1311. PMID: 10489910.
12. Tolstrup JS, Kristiansen L, Becker U, Gronbaek M. Smoking and risk of acute and chronic pancreatitis among women and men: a population-based cohort study. *Arch Intern Med*. 2009; 169(6): 603-609. PMID: 19307524.
13. Yang H, Wang L, Shi YH, Sui GT, Wu YF, Lu XQ, et al. Risk factors of acute pancreatitis in the elderly Chinese population: a population-based cross-sectional study. *J Dig Dis*. 2014; 15(9): 501-507. PMID: 24957953.
14. Yuhara H, Ogawa M, Kawaguchi Y, Igarashi M, Mine T. Smoking and risk for acute pancreatitis: a systematic review and meta-analysis. *Pancreas*. 2014; 43(8): 1201-1207. PMID: 25333404.
15. Yadav D, Hawes RH, Brand RE, Anderson MA, Money ME, Banks PA, et al. Alcohol consumption, cigarette smoking, and the risk of recurrent acute and chronic pancreatitis. *Arch Intern Med*. 2009; 169(11): 1035-1045. PMID: 19506173.
16. Prizment AE, Jensen EH, Hopper AM, Virnig BA, Anderson KE. Risk factors for pancreatitis in older women: the Iowa Women's Health Study. *Ann Epidemiol*. 2015; 25(7): 544-548. PMID: 25656921.
17. Lin Y, Tamakoshi A, Hayakawa T, Ogawa M, Ohno Y. Cigarette smoking as a risk factor for chronic pancreatitis: a case-control study in Japan. Research Committee on Intractable Pancreatic Diseases. *Pancreas*. 2000; 21(2): 109-114. PMID: 10975702.
18. DiMagno MJ, Spaete JP, Ballard DD, Wamsteker EJ, Saini SD. Risk models for post-endoscopic retrograde cholangiopancreatography pancreatitis (PEP): smoking and chronic liver disease are predictors of protection against PEP. *Pancreas*. 2013; 42(6): 996-1003. PMID: 23532001.
19. Maire F, Rebours V, Vullierme MP, Couvelard A, Levy P, Hentic O, et al. Does tobacco influence the natural history of autoimmune pancreatitis? *Pancreatology*. 2014; 14(4): 284-288. PMID: 25062878.
20. Alsamarrai A, Das SL, Windsor JA, Petrov MS. Factors that affect risk for pancreatic disease in the general population: a systematic review and meta-analysis of prospective cohort studies. *Clin Gastroenterol Hepatol*. 2014; 12(10): 1635-1644. PMID: 24509242.
21. Cavestro GM, Leandro G, Di Leo M, Zuppardo RA, Morrow OB, Notaristefano C, et al. A single-centre prospective, cohort study of the natural history of acute pancreatitis. *Dig Liver Dis*. 2015; 47(3): 205-210. PMID: 25475611.
22. Bastida G, Beltran B. Ulcerative colitis in smokers, non-smokers and ex-smokers. *World J Gastroenterol*. 2011; 17(22): 2740-2747. PMID: 21734782.
23. Rosenfeld G, Bressler B. The truth about cigarette smoking and the risk of inflammatory bowel disease. *Am J Gastroenterol*. 2012; 107(9): 1407-1408. PMID: 22951878.
24. Hartwig W, Werner J, Ryschich E, Mayer H, Schmidt J, Gebhard MM, et al. Cigarette smoke enhances ethanol-induced pancreatic injury. *Pancreas*. 2000; 21(3): 272-278. PMID: 11039472.
25. van Westerloo DJ, Giebelen IA, Florquin S, Bruno MJ, Larosa GJ, Ulloa L, et al. The vagus nerve and nicotinic receptors modulate experimental pancreatitis severity in mice. *Gastroenterology*. 2006; 130(6): 1822-1830. PMID: 16697744.
26. McGrath J, McDonald JW, Macdonald JK. Transdermal nicotine for induction of remission in ulcerative colitis. *Cochrane Database Syst Rev*. 2004; 4: CD004722. PMID: 15495126.
27. Tracey KJ. Physiology and immunology of the cholinergic antiinflammatory pathway. *J Clin Invest*. 2007; 117(2): 289-296. PMID: 17273548.
28. Bagcivan I, Kaya T, Turan M, Goktas S, Demirel Y, Gursoy S. Investigation of the mechanism of nicotine-induced relaxation on the sheep sphincter of Oddi. *Can J Physiol Pharmacol*. 2004; 82(11): 935-939. PMID: 15644932.
29. Yadav D, Slivka A, Sherman S, Hawes RH, Anderson MA, Burton FR, et al. Smoking is underrecognized as a risk factor for chronic pancreatitis. *Pancreatology*. 2010; 10(6): 713-719. PMID: 21242712.
30. Haritha J, Wilcox CM. Evaluation of Patients' Knowledge Regarding Smoking and Chronic Pancreatitis: A Pilot Study. *J Gastroenterol Pancreatol Liver Disord*. 2015; 1(2): 1-4. PMID: 25685852.
31. Chowdhury P. An exploratory study on the development of an animal model of acute pancreatitis following nicotine exposure. *Tob Induc Dis*. 2003; 1(3): 213-217. PMID: 19570262.
32. Rioux N, Castonguay A. 4-(methylnitrosamino)-1-(3-pyridyl)-1-butanone modulation of cytokine release in U937 human macrophages. *Cancer Immunol Immunother*. 2001; 49(12): 663-670. PMID: 11258792.
33. Trushin N, Leder G, El-Bayoumy K, Hoffmann D, Beger HG, Henne-Bruns D, et al. The tobacco carcinogen NNK is stereoselectively reduced by human pancreatic microsomes and cytosols. *Langenbecks Arch Surg*. 2008; 393(4): 571-579. PMID: 18259773.
34. Wittel UA, Pandey KK, Andrianifahanana M, Johansson SL, Cullen DM, Akhter MP, et al. Chronic pancreatic inflammation induced by environmental tobacco smoke inhalation in rats. *Am J Gastroenterol*. 2006; 101(1): 148-159. PMID: 16405548.
35. Wittel UA, Singh AP, Henley BJ, Andrianifahanana M, Akhter MP, Cullen DM, et al. Cigarette smoke-induced differential expression of the genes involved in exocrine function of the rat pancreas. *Pancreas*. 2006; 33(4): 364-370. PMID: 17079941.
36. Al-Wadei HA, Schuller HM. Nicotinic receptor-associated modulation of stimulatory and inhibitory neurotransmitters

in NNK-induced adenocarcinoma of the lungs and pancreas. *J Pathol.* 2009; 218(4): 437-445. PMID: 19274673.

37. Rivenson A, Hoffmann D, Prokopczyk B, Amin S, Hecht SS. Induction of lung and exocrine pancreas tumors in F344 rats by tobacco-specific and Areca-derived N-nitrosamines. *Cancer Res.* 1988; 48(23): 6912-6917. PMID: 3180100.
38. Schuller HM. Nitrosamines as nicotinic receptor ligands. *Life Sci.* 2007; 80(24-25): 2274-2280. PMID: 17459420.
39. Hecht SS. Biochemistry, biology, and carcinogenicity of tobacco-specific N-nitrosamines. *Chem Res Toxicol.* 1998; 11(6): 559-603. PMID: 9625726.
40. Ding YS, Zhang L, Jain RB, Jain N, Wang RY, Ashley DL, et al. Levels of tobacco-specific nitrosamines and polycyclic aromatic hydrocarbons in mainstream smoke from different tobacco varieties. *Cancer Epidemiol Biomarkers Prev.* 2008; 17(12): 3366-3371. PMID: 19064552.
41. Anderson KE, Hammons GJ, Kadlubar FF, Potter JD, Kaderlik KR, Ilett KF, et al. Metabolic activation of aromatic amines by human pancreas. *Carcinogenesis.* 1997; 18(5): 1085-1092. PMID: 9163700.
42. Jaster R, Emmrich J. Crucial role of fibrogenesis in pancreatic diseases. *Best Pract Res Clin Gastroenterol.* 2008; 22(1): 17-29. PMID: 18206810.
43. Kadiyala V, Lee LS, Banks PA, Suleiman S, Paulo JA, Wang W, et al. Cigarette smoking impairs pancreatic duct cell bicarbonate secretion. *JOP.* 2013; 14(1): 31-38. PMID: 23306332.
44. LaRusch J, Lozano-Leon A, Stello K, Moore A, Muddana V, O'Connell M, et al. The Common Chymotrypsinogen C (CTRC) Variant G60G (C.180T) Increases Risk of Chronic Pancreatitis But Not Recurrent Acute Pancreatitis in a North American Population. *Clin Transl Gastroenterol.* 2015; 6: e68. PMID: 25569187.
45. Sliwińska-Mossoń M, Milnerowicz H, Jablonowska M, Milnerowicz S, Nabzdyk S, Rabczynski J. The effect of smoking on expression of IL-6 and antioxidants in pancreatic fluids and tissues in patients with chronic pancreatitis. *Pancreatology.* 2012; 12(4): 295-304. PMID: 22898629.
46. Sliwińska-Mossoń M, Milnerowicz H, Milnerowicz S, Nowak M, Rabczynski J. Immunohistochemical localization of somatostatin and pancreatic polypeptide in smokers with chronic pancreatitis. *Acta Histochem.* 2012; 114(5): 495-502. PMID: 22113176.
47. Sliwińska-Mossoń M, Topola M, Milnerowicz S, Milnerowicz H. [Assessment of concentrations of creatinine, uric acid and urea in non-smoking and smoking patients with chronic pancreatitis]. *Przegl Lek.* 2013; 70(10): 809-812. PMID: 24501801.
48. van Geenen EJ, Smits MM, Schreuder TC, van der Peet DL, Bloemena E, Mulder CJ. Smoking is related to pancreatic fibrosis in humans. *Am J Gastroenterol.* 2011; 106(6): 1161-1166; quiz 1167. PMID: 21577244.
49. Shimizu K. Pancreatic stellate cells: molecular mechanism of pancreatic fibrosis. *J Gastroenterol Hepatol.* 2008; 23 Suppl 1: S119-S121. PMID: 18336654.
50. Larsen S, Hilsted J, Tronier B, Worning H. Pancreatic hormone secretion in chronic pancreatitis without residual beta-cell function. *Acta Endocrinol (Copenh).* 1988; 118(3): 357-364. PMID: 2899369.
51. Milnerowicz H, Sliwińska-Mossoń M, Rabczynski J, Nowak M, Milnerowicz S. Dysfunction of the pancreas in healthy smoking persons and patients with chronic pancreatitis. *Pancreas.* 2007; 34(1): 46-54. PMID: 17198182.
52. Wójcik J, Kuska J, Kokot F. [Effect of smoking on the secretion of immunoreactive insulin (IRI) induced by the administration of L-arginine or glucagon]. *Endokrynol Pol.* 1985; 36(5): 263-269. PMID: 3913601.
53. Śliwińska-Mossoń M, Milnerowicz S, Nabzdyk S, Kokot I, Nowak M, Milnerowicz H. The Effect of Smoking on Endothelin-1 in Patients With Chronic Pancreatitis. *Appl Immunohistochem Mol Morphol.* 2015; 23(4): 288-296. PMID: 25203431.
54. Śliwińska-Mossoń M, Sciskalska M, Karczewska-Górska P, Milnerowicz H. The effect of endothelin-1 on pancreatic diseases in patients who smoke. *Adv Clin Exp Med.* 2013; 22(5): 745-752. PMID: 24285461.
55. Zhou J, Sahin-Tóth M. Chymotrypsin C mutations in chronic pancreatitis. *J Gastroenterol Hepatol.* 2011; 26(8): 1238-1246. PMID: 21631589.
56. Chowdhury P, Bose C, Udupa KB. Nicotine-induced proliferation of isolated rat pancreatic acinar cells: effect on cell signalling and function. *Cell Prolif.* 2007; 40(1): 125-141. PMID: 17227300.
57. Chowdhury P, Doi R, Chang LW, Rayford PL. Tissue distribution of [3H]-nicotine in rats. *Biomed Environ Sci.* 1993; 6(1): 59-64. PMID: 8476533.
58. Chowdhury P, Doi R, Tangoku A, Rayford PL. Structural and functional changes of rat exocrine pancreas exposed to nicotine. *Int J Pancreatol.* 1995; 18(3): 257-264. PMID: 8708398.
59. Chowdhury P, Hosotani R, Chang L, Rayford PL. Metabolic and pathologic effects of nicotine on gastrointestinal tract and pancreas of rats. *Pancreas.* 1990; 5(2): 222-229. PMID: 1690423.
60. Chowdhury P, Hosotani R, Rayford PL. Weight loss and altered circulating GI peptide levels of rats exposed chronically to nicotine. *Pharmacol Biochem Behav.* 1989; 33(3): 591-594. PMID: 2587602.
61. Chowdhury P, Hosotani R, Rayford PL. Inhibition of CCK or carbachol-stimulated amylase release by nicotine. *Life Sci.* 1989; 45(22): 2163-2168. PMID: 2481202.
62. Chowdhury P, MacLeod S, Udupa KB, Rayford PL. Pathophysiological effects of nicotine on the pancreas: an update. *Exp Biol Med.* 2002; 227(7): 445-454. PMID: 12094008.
63. Chowdhury P, Rayford PL, Chang LW. Pathophysiological effects of nicotine on the pancreas. *Proc Soc Exp Biol Med.* 1998; 218(3): 168-173. PMID: 9648934.
64. Chowdhury P, Udupa KB. Nicotine as a mitogenic stimulus for pancreatic acinar cell proliferation. *World J Gastroenterol.* 2006; 12(46): 7428-7432. PMID: 17167829.
65. Chowdhury P, Udupa KB. Effect of nicotine on exocytotic pancreatic secretory response: role of calcium signaling. *Tob Induc Dis.* 2013; 11(1): 1. PMID: 23327436.
66. Lindkvist B, Wierup N, Sundler F, Borgstrom A. Long-term nicotine exposure causes increased concentrations of trypsinogens and amylase in pancreatic extracts in the rat. *Pancreas.* 2008; 37(3): 288-294. PMID: 18815551.

67. Chowdhury P, Rayford PL. Smoking and pancreatic disorders. *Eur J Gastroenterol Hepatol.* 2000; 12(8): 869-877. PMID: 10958214.
68. Mwenifumbo JC, Tyndale RF. Molecular genetics of nicotine metabolism. *Handb Exp Pharmacol.* 2009; 192: 235-259. PMID: 19184652.
69. Prokopczyk B, Hoffmann D, Bologna M, Cunningham AJ, Trushin N, Akerkar S, et al. Identification of tobacco-derived compounds in human pancreatic juice. *Chem Res Toxicol.* 2002; 15(5): 677-685. PMID: 12018989.
70. Chowdhury P, Rayford PL, Chang LW. Induction of pancreatic acinar pathology via inhalation of nicotine. *Proc Soc Exp Biol Med.* 1992; 201(2): 159-164. PMID: 1409731.
71. Paulo JA. Nicotine alters the proteome of two human pancreatic duct cell lines. *JOP.* 2014; 15(5): 465-474. PMID: 25262714.
72. Paulo JA, Urrutia R, Kadiyala V, Banks P, Conwell DL, Steen H. Cross-species analysis of nicotine-induced proteomic alterations in pancreatic cells. *Proteomics.* 2013; 13(9): 1499-1512. PMID: 23456891.
73. Alexandre M, Uduman AK, Minervini S, Raoof A, Shugrue CA, Akinbiyi EO, et al. Tobacco carcinogen 4-(methylnitrosamino)-1-(3-pyridyl)-1-butanone initiates and enhances pancreatitis responses. *Am J Physiol Gastrointest Liver Physiol.* 2012; 303(6): G696-G704. PMID: 22837343.
74. Schuller HM, Tithof PK, Williams M, Plummer H 3rd. The tobacco-specific carcinogen 4-(methylnitrosamino)-1-(3-pyridyl)-1-butanone is a beta-adrenergic agonist and stimulates DNA synthesis in lung adenocarcinoma via beta-adrenergic receptor-mediated release of arachidonic acid. *Cancer Res.* 1999; 59(18): 4510-4515. PMID: 10493497.
75. Chaudhuri A, Kolodecik TR, Gorelick FS. Effects of increased intracellular cAMP on carbachol-stimulated zymogen activation, secretion, and injury in the pancreatic acinar cell. *Am J Physiol Gastrointest Liver Physiol.* 2005; 288(2): G235-G243. PMID: 15458924.
76. Friess H, Shrikhande S, Riesle E, Kashiwagi M, Baczako K, Zimmermann A, et al. Phospholipase A2 isoforms in acute pancreatitis. *Ann Surg.* 2001; 233(2): 204-212. PMID: 11176126.
77. Ashat M, Tashkandi N, Sreekumar B, Patel V, Chowdhury AB, Shugrue C, et al. Sa1788 Tobacco Toxin NNK (4-[Methylnitrosamino]-1-[3-Pyridyl]-1-Butanone) Mediates Zymogen Activation in Murine and Human Pancreatic Acini. *Gastroenterology.* 2014; 146(5): S-296.
78. Wang H, Yu M, Ochani M, Amella CA, Tanovic M, Susarla S, et al. Nicotinic acetylcholine receptor alpha7 subunit is an essential regulator of inflammation. *Nature.* 2003; 421(6921): 384-388. PMID: 12508119.
79. Schneider L, Jabrailova B, Soliman H, Hofer S, Strobel O, Hackert T, et al. Pharmacological cholinergic stimulation as a therapeutic tool in experimental necrotizing pancreatitis. *Pancreas.* 2014; 43(1): 41-46. PMID: 24212240.
80. Zheng YS, Wu ZS, Zhang LY, Ke L, Li WQ, Li N, et al. Nicotine ameliorates experimental severe acute pancreatitis via enhancing immunoregulation of CD4+ CD25+ regulatory T cells. *Pancreas.* 2015; 44(3): 500-506. PMID: 25742430.
81. Greer JB, Whitcomb DC. Inflammation and pancreatic cancer: an evidence-based review. *Curr Opin Pharmacol.* 2009; 9(4): 411-418. PMID: 19589727.
82. Akopyan G, Bonavida B. Understanding tobacco smoke carcinogen NNK and lung tumorigenesis. *Int J Oncol.* 2009; 29(4): 745-752. PMID: 16964372.
83. Foster JR, Idle JR, Hardwick JP, Bars R, Scott P, Braganza JM. Induction of drug-metabolizing enzymes in human pancreatic cancer and chronic pancreatitis. *J Pathol.* 1993; 169(4): 457-463. PMID: 8501544.
84. Srinivasan P, Subramanian VS, Said HM. Effect of the cigarette smoke component, 4-(methylnitrosamino)-1-(3-pyridyl)-1-butanone (NNK), on physiological and molecular parameters of thiamin uptake by pancreatic acinar cells. *PLoS One.* 2013; 8(11): e78853. PMID: 24244374.
85. Lowenfels AB, Maisonneuve P. Environmental factors and risk of pancreatic cancer. *Pancreatology.* 2003; 3(1): 1-7. PMID: 12683400.
86. Iodice S, Gandini S, Maisonneuve P, Lowenfels AB. Tobacco and the risk of pancreatic cancer: a review and meta-analysis. *Langenbecks Arch Surg.* 2008; 393(4): 535-545. PMID: 18193270.
87. Raimondi S, Maisonneuve P, Lohr JM, Lowenfels AB. Early onset pancreatic cancer: evidence of a major role for smoking and genetic factors. *Cancer Epidemiol Biomarkers Prev.* 2007; 16(9): 1894-1897. PMID: 17855711.
88. Whittemore AS, Paffenbarger RS Jr, Anderson K, Halpern J. Early precursors of pancreatic cancer in college men. *J Chronic Dis.* 1983; 36(3): 251-256. PMID: 6826689.
89. Mack TM, Yu MC, Hanisch R, Henderson BE. Pancreas cancer and smoking, beverage consumption, and past medical history. *J Natl Cancer Inst.* 1986; 76(1): 49-60. PMID: 3455742.
90. Anderson MA, Zolotarevsky E, Cooper KL, Sherman S, Shats O, Whitcomb DC, et al. Alcohol and tobacco lower the age of presentation in sporadic pancreatic cancer in a dose-dependent manner: a multicenter study. *Am J Gastroenterol.* 2012; 107(11): 1730-1739. PMID: 22929760.
91. Maisonneuve P, Lowenfels AB. Epidemiology of pancreatic cancer: an update. *Dig Dis.* 2010; 28(4-5): 645-656. PMID: 21088417.
92. Stocks P. Cancer mortality in relation to national consumption of cigarettes, solid fuel, tea and coffee. *Br J Cancer.* 1970; 24(2): 215-225. PMID: 5451565.
93. Wynder EL, Mabuchi K, Maruchi N, Fortner JG. Epidemiology of cancer of the pancreas. *J Natl Cancer Inst.* 1973; 50(3): 645-667. PMID: 4350660.
94. Wynder EL. An epidemiological evaluation of the causes of cancer of the pancreas. *Cancer Res.* 1975; 35(8): 2228-2233. PMID: 1149034.
95. Sasco AJ, Secretan MB, Straif K. Tobacco smoking and cancer: a brief review of recent epidemiological evidence. *Lung Cancer.* 2004; 45 Suppl 2: S3-S9. PMID: 15552776.
96. Raimondi S, Lowenfels AB, Morselli-Labate AM, Maisonneuve P, Pezzilli R. Pancreatic cancer in chronic pancreatitis; aetiology, incidence, and early detection. *Best Pract Res Clin Gastroenterol.* 2010; 24(3): 349-358. PMID: 20510834.

97. Blackford A, Parmigiani G, Kensler TW, Wolfgang C, Jones S, Zhang X, et al. Genetic mutations associated with cigarette smoking in pancreatic cancer. *Cancer Res*. 2009; 69(8): 3681-3688. PMID: 19351817.
98. Almoguera C, Shibata D, Forrester K, Martin J, Arnheim N, Perucho M. Most human carcinomas of the exocrine pancreas contain mutant c-K-ras genes. *Cell*. 1988; 53(4): 549-554. PMID: 2453289.
99. Porta M, Crous-Bou M, Wark PA, Vineis P, Real FX, Malats N, et al. Cigarette smoking and K-ras mutations in pancreas, lung and colorectal adenocarcinomas: etiopathogenic similarities, differences and paradoxes. *Mutat Res*. 2009; 682(2-3): 83-93. PMID: 19651236.
100. Krasinskas AM, Chiosea SI, Pal T, Dacic S. KRAS mutational analysis and immunohistochemical studies can help distinguish pancreatic metastases from primary lung adenocarcinomas. *Mod Pathol*. 2014; 27(2): 262-270. PMID: 23887294.
101. Hermann PC, Sancho P, Canamero M, Martinelli P, Madriles F, Michl P, et al. Nicotine promotes initiation and progression of KRAS-induced pancreatic cancer via Gata6-dependent dedifferentiation of acinar cells in mice. *Gastroenterology*. 2014; 147(5): 1119-1133 e1114. PMID: 25127677.
102. Gnoni A, Licchetta A, Scarpa A, Azzariti A, Brunetti AE, Simone G, et al. Carcinogenesis of pancreatic adenocarcinoma: precursor lesions. *Int J Mol Sci*. 2013; 14(10): 19731-19762. PMID: 24084722.
103. Balbo S, Johnson CS, Kovi RC, James-Yi SA, O'Sullivan MG, Wang M, et al. Carcinogenicity and DNA adduct formation of 4-(methylnitrosamino)-1-(3-pyridyl)-1-butanone and enantiomers of its metabolite 4-(methylnitrosamino)-1-(3-pyridyl)-1-butanol in F-344 rats. *Carcinogenesis*. 2014; 35(12): 2798-2806. PMID: 25269804.
104. Banerjee J, Al-Wadei HA, Schuller HM. Chronic nicotine inhibits the therapeutic effects of gemcitabine on pancreatic cancer in vitro and in mouse xenografts. *Eur J Cancer*. 2013; 49(5): 1152-1158. PMID: 23146955.
105. Martinelli P, Madriles F, Cañamero M, Pau EC, Pozo ND, Guerra C, et al. The acinar regulator Gata6 suppresses KrasG12V-driven pancreatic tumorigenesis in mice. *Gut*. 2016; 65(3): 476-486. PMID: 25596178.
106. Dasgupta P, Rizwani W, Pillai S, Kinkade R, Kovacs M, Rastogi S, et al. Nicotine induces cell proliferation, invasion and epithelial-mesenchymal transition in a variety of human cancer cell lines. *Int J Cancer*. 2009; 124(1): 36-45. PMID: 18844224.
107. Trevino JG, Pillai S, Kunigal S, Singh S, Fulp WJ, Centeno BA, et al. Nicotine induces inhibitor of differentiation-1 in a Src-dependent pathway promoting metastasis and chemoresistance in pancreatic adenocarcinoma. *Neoplasia*. 2012; 14(12): 1102-1114. PMID: 23308043.
108. Je DW, O YM, Ji YG, Cho Y and Lee DH. The inhibition of SRC family kinase suppresses pancreatic cancer cell proliferation, migration, and invasion. *Pancreas* 43(5): 768-776, 2014. PMID: 24763074.
109. Macha MA, Rachagani S, Gupta S, Pai P, Ponnusamy MP, Batra SK, et al. Guggulsterone decreases proliferation and metastatic behavior of pancreatic cancer cells by modulating JAK/STAT and Src/FAK signaling. *Cancer Lett*. 2013; 341(2): 166-177. PMID: 23920124.
110. Momi N, Ponnusamy MP, Kaur S, Rachagani S, Kunigal SS, Chellappan S, et al. Nicotine/cigarette smoke promotes metastasis of pancreatic cancer through alpha7nAChR-mediated MUC4 upregulation. *Oncogene*. 2013; 32(11): 1384-1395. PMID: 22614008.
111. Park CH, Lee IS, Grippo P, Pandol SJ, Gukovskaya AS, Edderkaoui M. Akt kinase mediates the prosurvival effect of smoking compounds in pancreatic ductal cells. *Pancreas*. 2013; 42(4): 655-662. PMID: 23271397.
112. Askari MD, Tsao MS, Schuller HM. The tobacco-specific carcinogen, 4-(methylnitrosamino)-1-(3-pyridyl)-1-butanone stimulates proliferation of immortalized human pancreatic duct epithelia through beta-adrenergic transactivation of EGF receptors. *J Cancer Res Clin Oncol*. 2005; 131(10): 639-648. PMID: 16091975.
113. Kumar S, Torres MP, Kaur S, Rachagani S, Joshi S, Johansson SL, et al. Smoking accelerates pancreatic cancer progression by promoting differentiation of MDSCs and inducing HB-EGF expression in macrophages. *Oncogene*. 2015; 34(16): 2052-2060. PMID: 24909166.
114. Edderkaoui M, Grippo PJ, Ouhaddi Y, Benhaddou H, Xu S, Pinkerton K, et al. Mouse models of pancreatic cancer induced by chronic pancreatitis and smoking. *J Clin Oncol*. 2014; 32(3) (Abstract).
115. Rhim AD, Mirek ET, Aiello NM, Maitra A, Bailey JM, McAllister F, et al. EMT and dissemination precede pancreatic tumor formation. *Cell* 148(1-2): 349-361, 2012. PMID: 22265420.
116. Goecke H, Forssmann U, Uguccioni M, Friess H, Conejo-Garcia JR, Zimmermann A, et al. Macrophages infiltrating the tissue in chronic pancreatitis express the chemokine receptor CCR5. *Surgery*. 2000; 128(5): 806-814. PMID: 11056444.
117. Esposito I, Menicagli M, Funel N, Bergmann F, Boggi U, Mosca F, et al. Inflammatory cells contribute to the generation of an angiogenic phenotype in pancreatic ductal adenocarcinoma. *J Clin Pathol*. 2004; 57(6): 630-636. PMID: 15166270.
118. Duell EJ, Casella DP, Burk RD, Kelsey KT, Holly EA. Inflammation, genetic polymorphisms in proinflammatory genes TNF-A, RANTES, and CCR5, and risk of pancreatic adenocarcinoma. *Cancer Epidemiol Biomarkers Prev*. 2006; 15(4): 726-731. PMID: 16614115.
119. Mule JJ, Custer M, Averbook B, Yang JC, Weber JS, Goeddel DV, et al. RANTES secretion by gene-modified tumor cells results in loss of tumorigenicity in vivo: role of immune cell subpopulations. *Hum Gene Ther*. 1996; 7(13): 1545-1553. PMID: 8864755.
120. Song Z, Bhagat G, Quante M, Baik GH, Marrache F, Tu SP, et al. Potential carcinogenic effects of cigarette smoke and Swedish moist snuff on pancreas: a study using a transgenic mouse model of chronic pancreatitis. *Lab Invest*. 2010; 90(3): 426-435. PMID: 20065943.
121. Philip B, Roland CL, Daniluk J, Liu Y, Chatterjee D, Gomez SB, et al. A high-fat diet activates oncogenic Kras and COX2 to induce development of pancreatic ductal adenocarcinoma

in mice. *Gastroenterology.* 2013; 145(6): 1449-1458. PMID: 23958541.

122. Jianyu H, Guang L, Baosen P. Evidence for cigarette smoke-induced oxidative stress in the rat pancreas. *Inhal Toxicol.* 2009; 21(12): 1007-1012. PMID: 19635036.
123. Franco L, Doria D, Bertazzoni E, Benini A, Bassi C. Increased expression of inducible nitric oxide synthase and cyclooxygenase-2 in pancreatic cancer. *Prostaglandins Other Lipid Mediat.* 2004; 73(1-2): 51-58. PMID: 15165031.
124. Vickers SM, MacMillan-Crow LA, Green M, Ellis C, Thompson JA. Association of increased immunostaining for inducible nitric oxide synthase and nitrotyrosine with fibroblast growth factor transformation in pancreatic cancer. *Arch Surg.* 1999; 134(3): 245-251. PMID: 10088562.
125. Lazar M, Sullivan J, Chipitsyna G, Aziz T, Salem AF, Gong Q, et al. Induction of monocyte chemoattractant protein-1 by nicotine in pancreatic ductal adenocarcinoma cells: role of osteopontin. *Surgery.* 2010; 148(2): 298-309. PMID: 20579680.
126. Soeda J, Morgan M, McKee C, Mouralidarane A, Lin C, Roskams T, et al. Nicotine induces fibrogenic changes in human liver via nicotinic acetylcholine receptors expressed on hepatic stellate cells. *Biochem Biophys Res Commun.* 2012; 417(1): 17-22. PMID: 22108052.
127. Xu Z, Lee A, Pothula S, Patel M, Pirola R, Wilson J, et al. The influence of alcohol and cigarette smoke components on pancreatic stellate cell activation: Implications for the progression of chronic pancreatitis. *Pancreatology.* 2014; 14(3): S18-S19 (Abstract).

Chapter 16

Experimental acute pancreatitis models relevant to lipids and obesity

Krutika S. Patel and Vijay P. Singh*

Division of Gastroenterology and Hepatology, Mayo Clinic, Scottsdale, AZ, USA.

Introduction and Background

While severity in conventional animal models of acute pancreatitis (AP) is related to etiology, this is rarely the case in human disease. Most obese individuals do not experience an episode of AP during their lifetime, but those who do are more prone to severe AP (SAP) and associated morbidity and mortality.[1] In this entry, we will discuss the relevance of obesity and lipids as potential modifiers of the course and outcome of AP in the light of limitations posed by conventional models of AP and suggest relevant improvisations with examples in various *in vitro* and *in vivo* systems.

From the perspective of pancreatitis and its experimental models, visceral fat depots can be divided into intra- and peripancreatic fat. Both can contribute to SAP in humans. The human facts relevant to the nature and amounts of lipid used in the sections on experimental models are: 1) adipose tissue may account for >30% of body weight in obese individuals; 2) obesity is associated with SAP[2-5] and is defined as a body mass index (BMI) >30 or >25 kg/m^2 in Western and Eastern countries, respectively; 3) clinical studies from the west[6-11] and Asia[12-15] report increased SAP above the corresponding BMIs; 4) there is greater consumption of polyunsaturated fatty acids (PUFAs) in Asia compared to the west[16-20]; 5) dietary PUFAs accumulate in visceral adipocytes[16]; 6) 80%-90% of adipocyte mass may comprise triglyceride; 7) intrapancreatic fat increases with BMI[21] and account for about 20% of pancreatic area in obese individuals; and 8) peripancreatic fat commonly ranges from 2-9 kg in obese individuals. Intra- and peripancreatic fat may by hydrolyzed in pancreatitis, contributing to SAP. Further details on obesity related human data are provided in the chapter "Relationship between obesity and pancreatitis",[22] but this section focuses on the impact of obesity in animal models of pancreatitis.

Limitations of current animal models in the context of human AP

Current animal models of AP are classified for severity on the basis of an inducer/etiology causing pancreatic necrosis.[23] This is a significant limitation since human AP severity is unrelated to pancreatic necrosis or etiology, with the exception of hypertriglyceridemic pancreatitis.[24-26] Rat cerulein pancreatitis is considered milder due to the lesser pancreatic necrosis,[23,27] while mouse cerulein pancreatitis is considered a SAP model due to the higher amount of acinar necrosis ranging from 5%-30%.[4,23,28] In both models, the pancreas returns to baseline within a few days of inducing AP. Similarly, lung injury is mild and transient with no evidence of impaired gas exchange.

In contrast, development of necrosis during human AP may not result in worse outcomes. While severe pancreatic necrosis is defined as >30% pancreatic parenchymal necrosis during human disease,[29] a prospective human study from the United Kingdom showed no/minimal relationship between the extent of necrosis and outcome.[30] SAP and early mortality in human AP can occur with minimal pancreatic necrosis[2,31,32] due to systemic complications or sustained organ failure.[29] A number of studies have reported that only about half of patients with necrotizing pancreatitis develop organ failure.[5,33,34]

Taurocholate-induced pancreatitis in rats is considered severe due to the extensive pancreatic hemorrhagic necrosis that occurs.[23,27,35] To induce AP, 3% to 5% solutions of bile salts such as sodium taurocholate are injected locally into the biliopancreatic duct to simulate severe biliary AP.[35] This results in a local concentration of 60 to 100 mM, which is 5- to 100- fold above the critical micellar concentration (CMC) that can cause a detergent-like effect on cell membranes in the pancreatic acinar cells.[36] Similarly the monohydroxy bile acid lithocholic acid is commonly injected at 3 mM, which

*Corresponding author. Email: singh.vijay@mayo.edu

is 3-6 times above its CMC. While no published study has verified the relevance of these concentrations of bile salts to human disease, our unpublished data show that bile acid concentrations are in the micromolar range in pancreatic collections from patients with biliary AP. A recent review by Lerch and Gorelick also questioned the injection of bile acids/salts as a model for biliary AP.[23]

Clinically, it is often difficult to establish the causal agents responsible for AP severity in human patients since markers and mediators of disease are indistinguishable. Animal models allow initiation and inhibition of steps relevant to disease pathophysiology and are thus important in establishing causality. Several potential targets like trypsin[37-45] and reactive oxygen species[46] have been considered to have therapeutic relevance since their levels may be increased in AP. However, clinical trials of AP targeting reactive oxygen species,[46] trypsin,[37-45] and inflammatory mediators[3] have shown limited benefits, although these targets seem scientifically sound in animal models. The discord between modifying outcomes and interpreting animal models can be seen in the lack of evidence of clinical improvement despite more than 70 trials of serine protease and trypsin inhibition over the past 60 years.[37-45] Thus, based on the 1) lack of relevance of etiology to outcomes, 2) lack of accurate parameters used to define systemic injury, 3) limited clinical benefits of attractive therapeutic targets in animal models, and 4) overemphasis of pancreatic necrosis in defining AP severity, we need to interpret the relevance of conventional AP models with caution.

Role of Obesity and Lipids in Acute Pancreatitis

Obesity is known to be associated with worse AP outcomes,[7,9,13,47-51] and several clinical and epidemiological studies have shown that patients with increased intra-abdominal fat or higher BMI are at an increased risk for developing SAP.[14,47,52,53] The two other clinical clues to lipids worsening AP outcomes are 1) hypertriglyceridemic pancreatitis generally being severe[24-26,54,55] and 2) AP patients receiving intravenous (IV) total parenteral nutrition including IV lipids having worse outcomes.[56-58] Recent reports from North America show the usage of parenteral nutrition to be as high as 40% to 60% in patients with AP.[59,60] The prevalence of organ failure is reported to be >50% in patients receiving parenteral nutrition containing IV lipid emulsions.[56-58] IV lipids may result in high systemic fatty acid concentrations 6- to 8-fold above normal,[61] consistent with levels found in the serum of patients with SAP.[62,63] These associations of obesity/lipids with worse outcomes suggest that fat is a common modifier of AP outcomes. The following subsections discuss the mechanistic, translational, and potential therapeutic relevance of obesity in the context of *in vitro* and *in vivo* AP models.

In vitro *models of fat-mediated severe acute pancreatitis*

The purpose of an *in vitro* model is to replicate the pathophysiology occurring *in vivo* in a reductionist manner. Therefore, a fat-induced pancreatic damage model should simulate the *in vivo* environment. Several studies show evidence of pancreatic parenchymal necrosis around fat necrosis.[64-67] Physiologically, adipocytes and the neighboring pancreatic acinar cells do not allow their contents to communicate with each other. Acinar cells physiologically secrete digestive enzymes present in zymogen granules from their apical region into the duct lumen; however, an insult that causes pancreatitis can result in basolateral leakage of lipases into the surrounding adipocytes[64,68-72] and consequent lipolysis of adipocyte triglyceride, producing free fatty acids (FFAs). This is seen histologically as positive Von Kossa staining[66,67] and high FFA levels in pancreatic necrosis collections.[67,73,74]

This pathologic *in vivo* lipolytic flux between adipocytes and acinar cells can be simulated *in vitro* using a transwell system that allows macromolecular diffusion between the acinar and adipocyte compartments while preventing cellular contamination (**Figure 1**).[66,67]

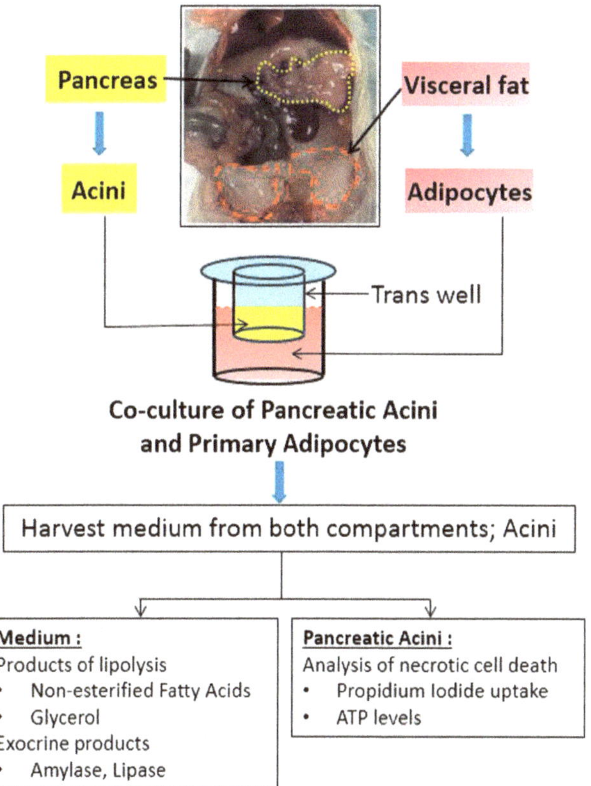

Figure 1. Schematic showing the setup to study *in vitro* lipolytic fluxes. Harvested primary acinar cells are added to the upper compartment of the transwell (with a 3-µm sieve at bottom of insert, yellow), and primary adipocytes are placed in the lower compartment of the well (red). Medium from the individual compartments is analyzed for lipolytic and exocrine products, and the acinar cells are harvested to measure necrotic cell death parameters.

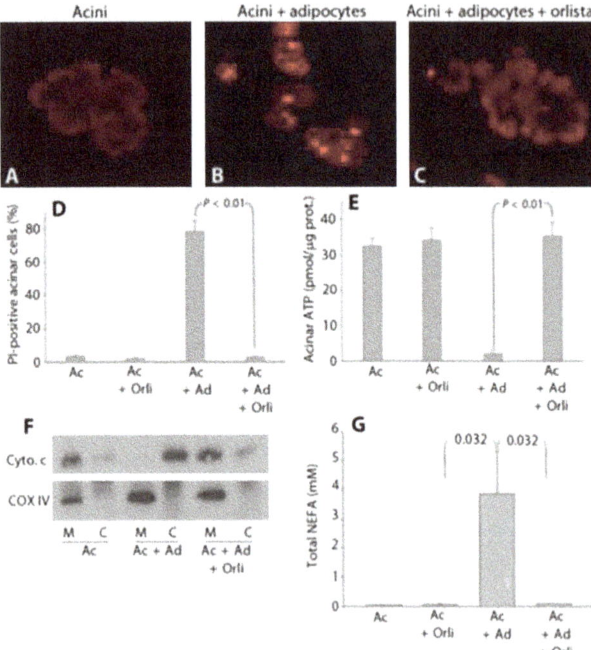

Figure 2. *In vitro* co-culture of acini and adipocytes results in acinar necrosis. A-C show propidium iodide uptake in control acini (A) and acini cocultured with adipocytes (B) or with adipocytes and 50 µM orlistat (C). (D) The percentage of acinar cells positive for PI uptake in coculture with adipocytes (Ac+Ad) was higher compared to acini cultured alone (Ac), with 50 µM orlistat (Ac+Orli), or 50 µM orlistat (Ac+Ad+Orli) in coculture. (E) ATP levels in acinar cells treated as in (D) showed lower ATP levels in coculture. (F) Assessment of cytochrome C (upper panel) in mitochondrial (M) and cytoplasmic (C) fractions of Ac, Ac+Ad, and Ac+Ad+Orli, show its migration from the mitochondrial to cytosolic compartment only in the Ac+Ad group. Levels of the mitochondrial marker COX IV (lower panel) were similar in all groups. (G) Total NEFA concentrations in the medium of acini cells treated as in (D) show increased NEFA in Ac+Ad only. Republished with permission.[67]

The pancreatic lipases released from the acinar compartment diffuse through the transwell into the adipocyte compartment, causing an increase in FFAs that diffuse into the acinar cell compartment resulting in acinar cell necrosis.[66] This is observed as increased propidium iodide uptake, decreased ATP levels, cytochrome C leakage, and increased NEFA levels (**Figure 2**).[67] The lipase inhibitor orlistat prevents all these changes in the coculture system.

In 1992, Mossner et al. showed the direct deleterious effect of long chain unsaturated fatty acids (UFAs) on pancreatic acini.[75] Recently, Navina et al. showed that linoleic, oleic, and linolenic acids were particularly toxic to acinar cells, while the saturated fatty acids palmitic acid and stearic acid were not.[67] Incubation of acinar cells with very low-density lipoprotein also results in an increase in FFAs, resulting in necrotic injury.[76] When acinar cells are stimulated with individual fatty acids, cytosolic calcium concentrations, released from an intracellular pool, are increased only with UFAs (**Figure 3**).[67]

Unsaturated fatty acids also cause leakage of lactate dehydrogenase, leakage of cytochrome C into the cytoplasmic fraction and inhibition of mitochondrial complexes I and V, causing a drop in ATP levels to induce necrotic cell death (**Figure 3**).[67,74] UFAs at sublethal concentrations also upregulate mRNA levels of inflammatory mediators and thus are proinflammatory.[67]

Exposure of peripheral blood mononuclear cells to UFAs at concentrations lower than those in the serum during SAP results in their necroapoptotic cell death.[74]

In vivo *models of obesity-associated severe acute pancreatitis*

Role of intrapancreatic fat in pancreatic necrosis

Several studies have histologically shown that pancreatic acinar necrosis borders fat necrosis.[64,67,77-79] Those studies analyzed intrapancreatic fat in human autopsy samples,[21,64,66,67,78,80] surgically resected samples,[81] and on radiology images[21,82] and found that it increased with BMI. Intrapancreatic fat amounts in obese individuals are typically twice those found in nonobese individuals.[21] Analysis of pancreatic adipocyte triglyceride composition in humans showed increasing amounts of unsaturated triglycerides with higher amounts of fat.[83] Pancreatic necrosis fluid collected from obese patients with necrotizing pancreatitis had higher nonesterfied fatty acid concentrations compared to patients with pseudocysts and cystic neoplasms who had a lower BMI.[63,67,73,74]

Several *in vivo* models have contributed to our understanding of the role of intrapancreatic fat in SAP outcomes.[67,73] Obese mice have increased intrapancreatic fat (about 30% of total pancreatic area), resulting in lethal SAP in response to interleukins (IL)-12 and -18 that are associated with increased acinar necrosis.[67] In these mice, a significant amount of pancreatic acinar necrosis (60%-70% area) occurs in areas surrounding the fat necrosis, which is termed perifat acinar necrosis (PFAN). This contributes to about half the total acinar necrosis in these obese mice.[67] In contrast, lean mice have less intrapancreatic fat and PFAN and have nonlethal SAP.[67] Grossly obese mice have chalky white deposits of saponification, consistent with histologic evidence of fat necrosis.[67] Evaluation of the triglyceride composition of adipose tissue in these obese mice show significantly increased UFAs in obese mice compared to lean mice, with a corresponding relative decrease in saturated fatty acids.[67,77] Normally, visceral fat pads of obese mice have about 70%-80% UFAs, which is significantly more than in lean mice that have about 50%-60% UFA content.[67,77]

The role of acute lipolytic generation of fatty acids on local pancreatic severity was recently studied by

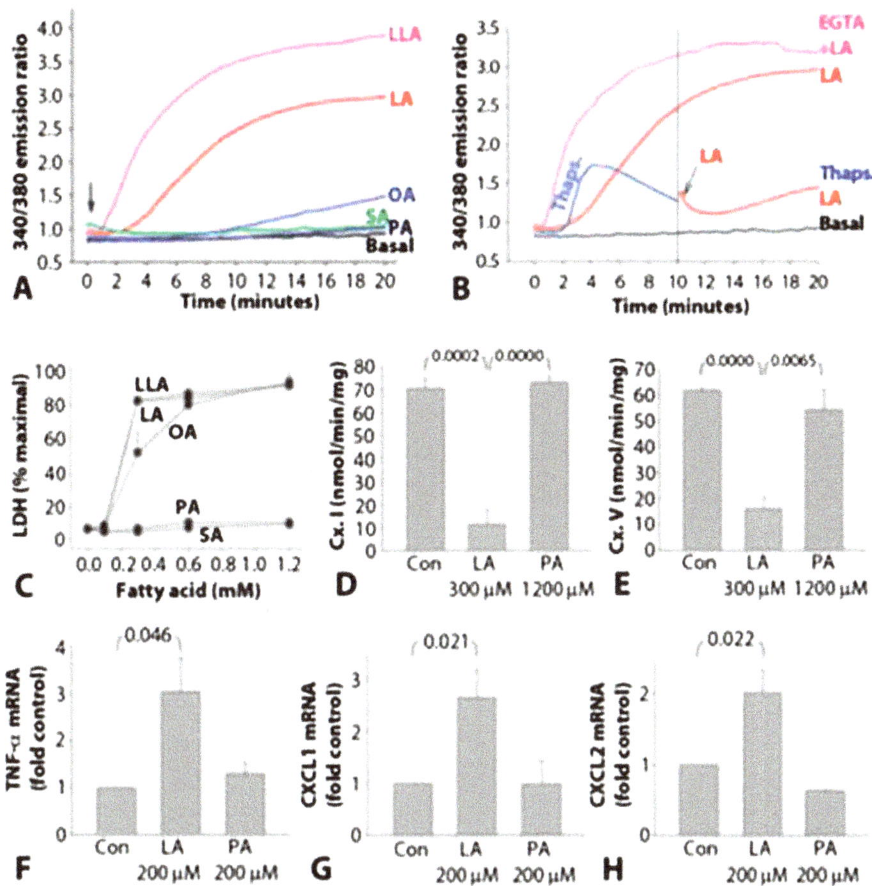

Figure 3. UFAs induce acinar necrosis and inflammatory mediator generation. (A) Intra-acinar calcium concentrations (expressed as a 340/380-nm emission ratio) in response to addition (arrow) of 600 μM fatty acids (LLA, linolenic acid; LA, linoleic acid; OA, oleic acid; SA, stearic acid; PA, palmitic acid), showing release of intracellular calcium only with UFAs (LLA, LA, and OA). (B) Effect of depletion of endoplasmic reticulum calcium with thapsigargin (1 μM) (blue line) and depletion of extracellular calcium by chelation with EGTA (1 mM added 10 min before adding linoleic acid, pink) on 600 μM linoleic acid-induced intracellular calcium increase. (C) Leakage of lactate dehydrogenase (LDH) from acinar cells 5 hours after treatment with fatty acids as in (A). Unsaturated but not saturated fatty acids cause LDH release. (D and E) Effect of linoleic and palmitic acids on the activities of mitochondrial complexes (Cx.) I and V in acini. Linoleic but not palmitic acid paralyzes Cx. I and V. (F-H) Effect of linoleic and palmitic acids on TNF-α (F), CXCL1 (G), and CXCL2 (H) mRNA levels in acini. Linoleic but not palmitic acid increases all three. Republished with permission.[67]

Durgampudi et al. by injecting unsaturated triglyceride into the pancreatobiliary duct to increase intrapancreatic fat.[73] Intraductal triglyceride injection followed by duct ligation allows for triglyceride to be mixed with pancreatic lipases as would occur with basolateral leakage during AP, causing subsequent lipolysis of glyceryl trilinoleate (GTL) mimicking intrapancreatic fat necrosis seen in obese patients with SAP.[66,67] Common biliopancreatic duct ligation results in elevated amylase, lipase, bilirubin and alanine aminotransferase (ALT), fulfilling all the criteria of mild biliary AP. Intraductal injection of the triglyceride GTL in amounts equivalent to about 10% of intrapancreatic fat, along with duct ligation, results in severe hemorrhagic pancreatic necrosis with about 70% necrosis of the pancreatic acinar tissue, multisystem organ failure, and mortality.[73] This acinar parenchymal damage is prevented by inhibition of GTL lipolysis to linoleic acid by orlistat.[73] This inhibition does not affect the increase in serum amylase, bilirubin, or ALT that mark biliary AP. Thus, in an animal model simulating biliary AP (classically regarded as a severe AP model), it was shown that outcomes are unrelated to AP etiology and that intrapancreatic fat is a modifier of outcomes, converting mild AP to SAP.[73] Hence, in obesity-associated SAP, unregulated extracellular basolateral release of pancreatic lipase consequent to an initial insult may cause intrapancreatic fat lipolysis, resulting in an increase in FFAs that directly damage the acinar cells, causing necrosis.

A surge in systemic UFAs also results in significant mortality in these experimental models,[67,73,77] similar to the trend of a rise in FFAs, particularly UFAs in the sera of patients with SAP.[84] Prevention of lipolysis results in reductions in FFAs and systemic inflammatory markers.[67,73,77] As noted in the spectrum of human SAP, obese animals or those with higher UFAs generated by the lipolytic surge are more prone to multisystem organ failure in the form of renal failure and lung injury. Renal injury manifests as fat containing tubular vacuoles, tubular apoptosis and necrosis, mitochondrial swelling, and expression of kidney injury molecule-1 (KIM-1) with associated functional renal injury in the form of high blood urea nitrogen (BUN) levels.[67,73,77] Lung injury is manifested as increased apoptotic cells and lung myeloperoxidase levels.[67,77] Several isolated studies have previously shown intravenous oleic acid to cause acute respiratory distress syndrome with lung myeloperoxidase increase and apoptosis.[85-88] UFAs are also known to elevate serum creatinine and cause renal tubular toxicity.[88] This is also associated with release of proinflammatory cytokines, which have been reported to be increased in human SAP.[89-96] Recent studies from Closa et al. in rats showed unsaturated FFAs generated in peritoneal adipose tissue during pancreatitis to accumulate in ascitic fluid, and cause the release of inflammatory mediators that contribute to the progression of the systemic inflammatory response seen in SAP.[97]

In contrast to the intrapancreatic fat of obesity, pancreatic fat in patients with chronic pancreatitis patients is rarely associated with disease severity.[98-104] A common feature of patients with chronic pancreatitis is fatty replacement of the pancreas after recurrent AP attacks.[105] Secondary fat replacement in chronic pancreatitis is independent of BMI and is associated with fibrosis, which causes a protective walling off effect from the adipocyte-acinar lipolytic flux generated during AP.[66,67] This is supported by observations that chronic pancreatitis patients rarely die from AP or its related complications.[99,102,106] Acharya et al. showed that unlike obesity-associated intrapancreatic fat that worsens AP outcomes, intrapancreatic fat accumulation in chronic pancreatitis is less prone to fat necrosis or surrounding parenchymal damage.[66] In reference to fatty acid ethyl esters (FAEEs), it is noteworthy that the landmark study documenting high FAEE levels in the pancreas of humans at autopsy clearly states that they had no evidence of pancreatitis. The study was done on alcoholics who had died from unrelated causes such as motor vehicle accidents.[107] Criddle and colleagues also demonstrated that it is the conversion of FAEEs to FFAs that results in cell injury.[108] This is supported by our studies in which we note the parent fatty acids to be much more toxic than FAEEs.[109] Thus, while the role and relevance of FAEEs to AP outcomes are unproven, the human and experimental data described above strongly support the lipolytic generation of UFAs to convert AP to SAP in obesity.

Role of peripancreatic fat in severe acute pancreatitis

Visceral adipose tissue such as that surrounding the pancreas contributes to 10% to 30% of the intra-abdominal area.[110] This adipocyte mass can provide a potentially hydrolyzable pool of triglycerides during AP. Adipocytes normally consist of > 80% fat stored in triglyceride form.[111] Unregulated release of pancreatic lipases during an acute attack of pancreatitis can result in the breakdown of these triglycerides and the release of very high amounts of FFAs, resulting in adverse outcomes.

Obesity is considered a proinflammatory state. A recently published study by Patel et al. showed that a traditionally mild model of cerulein AP produces severe outcomes in obese but not lean mice.[77] Mortality in obese mice is associated with fat necrosis and peritoneal saponification, hypocalcemia, an intense cytokine response, lung injury, and renal failure, which are all commonly used markers in AP severity scoring/predicting systems.[77,112] Visceral fat pads of obese mice with AP showed the presence of active pancreatic lipases.[77] The amount of pancreatic necrosis was not significantly different in the lean, obese, and orlistat-treated groups. However, both the lean and orlistat-treated groups had reduced fat necrosis, lack of sustained organ failure, a transient cytokine response, and improved survival. Histologically, the areas of fat necrosis were surrounded by intense accumulation of polymorphonuclear neutrophils and macrophages,[77,97] suggesting that these necrotic areas of adipose tissue generate and release inflammatory mediators that contribute to the progression of the inflammation during SAP.[77]

A recent study by Noel et al. helped distinguish between the acute UFA-mediated lipotoxicity during SAP from the chronic inflammatory state of obesity.[74] For this, the amount of peripancreatic triglyceride was acutely changed in lean rats with cerulein pancreatitis by administering them triolein (the triglyceride of oleic acid, which is the most abundant UFA in visceral fat). This resulted in acute lung and renal injury with minimal pancreatic necrosis and an intense cytokine response, all of which were prevented by inhibiting lipolysis. Conversely, while coadministration of the cytokines IL-8 and IL-1β, which are also increased in pancreatic necrosis collections, did cause pyrexia, they did not lead to any adverse outcomes. Thus, peripancreatic fat necrosis may worsen inflammation and AP outcomes independent of the baseline proinflammatory state of obesity.[74]

In summary, obesity worsens the outcomes of AP due to the acute lipolytic generation of UFAs. This is unrelated to the baseline proinflammatory state of obesity and unrelated to AP etiology. While the hydrolysis of intrapancreatic fat by pancreatic lipases contributes to pancreatic necrosis in obesity, fibrosis in chronic pancreatitis reduces this lipolytic flux and the resulting severity of recurrent AP attacks. Necrosis of large amounts of peripancreatic fat can worsen AP outcomes independent of pancreatic necrosis. These observations mimic human disease, support obesity as an outcome modifier, and also suggest a different way to design and interpret models of AP that are not directly linked to the etiology.

Acknowledgements

This project was supported by Grant Number R01DK092460 (V.P.S.) and a startup package from the department of medicine at Mayo Clinic Arizona (V.P.S.).

References

1. Working Group IAP/APA Acute Pancreatitis Guidelines. IAP/APA evidence-based guidelines for the management of acute pancreatitis. *Pancreatology*. 2013; 13(4 Suppl 2): e1-15. PMID: 24054878.
2. Fu CY, Yeh CN, Hsu JT, Jan YY, Hwang TL. Timing of mortality in severe acute pancreatitis: experience from 643 patients. *World J Gastroenterol*. 2007; 13(13): 1966-1969. PMID: 17461498.
3. Johnson CD, Kingsnorth AN, Imrie CW, McMahon MJ, Neoptolemos JP, McKay C, et al. Double blind, randomised, placebo controlled study of a platelet activating factor antagonist, lexipafant, in the treatment and prevention of organ failure in predicted severe acute pancreatitis. *Gut*. 2001; 48(1): 62-69. PMID: 11115824.
4. Kaiser AM, Saluja AK, Sengupta A, Saluja M, Steer ML. Relationship between severity, necrosis, and apoptosis in five models of experimental acute pancreatitis. *Am J Physiol Cell Physiol*. 1995; 269(5 Pt 1): C1295-C1304. PMID: 7491921.
5. Karimgani I, Porter KA, Langevin RE, Banks PA. Prognostic factors in sterile pancreatic necrosis. *Gastroenterology*. 1992; 103(5): 1636-1640. PMID: 1426885.
6. Hegazi R, Raina A, Graham T, Rolniak S, Centa P, Kandil H, et al. Early jejunal feeding initiation and clinical outcomes in patients with severe acute pancreatitis. *JPEN*. 2011; 35(1): 91-96. PMID: 21224435.
7. Porter KA, Banks PA. Obesity as a predictor of severity in acute pancreatitis. *Int J Pancreatol*. 1991; 10(3-4): 247-252. PMID: 1787336.
8. Brown A, James-Stevenson T, Dyson T, Grunkenmeier D. The panc 3 score: a rapid and accurate test for predicting severity on presentation in acute pancreatitis. *J Clin Gastroenterol*. 2007; 41(9): 855-858. PMID: 17881932.
9. Sempere L, Martinez J, de Madaria E, Lozano B, Sanchez-Paya J, Jover R, et al. Obesity and fat distribution imply a greater systemic inflammatory response and a worse prognosis in acute pancreatitis. *Pancreatology*. 2008; 8(3): 257-264. PMID: 18497538.
10. Johnson CD, Toh SK, Campbell MJ. Combination of APACHE-II score and an obesity score (APACHE-O) for the prediction of severe acute pancreatitis. *Pancreatology*. 2004; 4(1): 1-6. PMID: 14988652.
11. Katuchova J, Bober J, Harbulak P, Hudak A, Gajdzik T, Kalanin R, et al. Obesity as a risk factor for severe acute pancreatitis patients. *Wien Klin Wochenschr*. 2014; 126 (7-8): 223-227. PMID: 24522641.
12. Yang F, Wu H, Li Y, Li Z, Wang C, Yang J, et al. Prevention of severe acute pancreatitis with octreotide in obese patients: a prospective multi-center randomized controlled trial. *Pancreas*. 2012; 41(8): 1206-1212. PMID: 23086244.
13. Shin KY, Lee WS, Chung DW, Heo J, Jung MK, Tak WY, et al. Influence of obesity on the severity and clinical outcome of acute pancreatitis. *Gut Liver*. 2011; 5(3): 335-339. PMID: 21927663.
14. Yashima Y, Isayama H, Tsujino T, Nagano R, Yamamoto K, Mizuno S, et al. A large volume of visceral adipose tissue leads to severe acute pancreatitis. *J Gastroenterol*. 2011; 46(10): 1213-1218. PMID: 21805069.
15. Thandassery RB, Appasani S, Yadav TD, Dutta U, Indrajit A, Singh K, et al. Implementation of the Asia-Pacific guidelines of obesity classification on the APACHE-O scoring system and its role in the prediction of outcomes of acute pancreatitis: a study from India. *Dig Dis Sci*. 2013; 59(6): 1316-1321. PMID: 24374646.
16. Scott RF, Lee KT, Kim DN, Morrison ES, Goodale F. Fatty acids of serum and adipose tissue in six groups eating natural diets containing 7 to 40 per cent fat. *Am J Clin Nutr*. 1964; 14: 280-290. PMID: 14157830.
17. Insull W Jr, Lang PD, Hsi BP, Yoshimura S. Studies of arteriosclerosis in Japanese and American men. I. Comparison of fatty acid composition of adipose tissue. *J Clin Invest*. 1969; 48(7): 1313-1327. PMID: 5794253.
18. Ueshima H, Stamler J, Elliott P, Chan Q, Brown IJ, Carnethon MR, et al. Food omega-3 fatty acid intake of individuals (total, linolenic acid, long-chain) and their blood pressure: INTERMAP study. *Hypertension*. 2007; 50(2): 313-319. PMID: 17548718.
19. Ruixing Y, Qiming F, Dezhai Y, Shuquan L, Weixiong L, Shangling P, et al. Comparison of demography, diet, lifestyle, and serum lipid levels between the Guangxi Bai Ku Yao and Han populations. *J Lipid Res*. 2007; 48(12): 2673-2681. PMID: 17890682.
20. Insull W Jr, Bartsch GE. Fatty acid composition of human adipose tissue related to age, sex, and race. *Am J Clin Nutr*. 1967; 20(1): 13-23. PMID: 6017005.
21. Saisho Y, Butler AE, Meier JJ, Monchamp T, Allen-Auerbach M, Rizza RA, et al. Pancreas volumes in humans from birth to age one hundred taking into account sex, obesity, and presence of type-2 diabetes. *Clin Anat*. 2007; 20(8): 933-942. PMID: 17879305.
22. Navina S, Singh VP. Relationship between obesity and pancreatitis. *The Pancreapedia: Exocrine Pancreas Knowledge Base*. American Pancreatic Association; 2015. DOI: 10.3998/panc.2015.18
23. Lerch MM, Gorelick FS. Models of acute and chronic pancreatitis. *Gastroenterology*. 2013; 144(6): 1180-1193. PMID: 23622127.
24. Lloret Linares C, Pelletier AL, Czernichow S, Vergnaud AC, Bonnefont-Rousselot D, Levy P, et al. Acute pancreatitis in a cohort of 129 patients referred for severe hypertriglyceridemia. *Pancreas*. 2008; 37(1): 13-12. PMID: 18580438.

25. Deng LH, Xue P, Xia Q, Yang XN, Wan MH. Effect of admission hypertriglyceridemia on the episodes of severe acute pancreatitis. *World J Gastroenterol.* 2008; 14(28): 4558-4561. PMID: 18680239.
26. Dominguez-Muñoz JE, Malfertheiner P, Ditschuneit HH, Blanco-Chavez J, Uhl W, Buchler M, et al. Hyperlipidemia in acute pancreatitis. Relationship with etiology, onset, and severity of the disease. *Int J Pancreatol.* 1991; 10(3-4): 261-267. PMID: 1787337.
27. Pandol SJ, Saluja AK, Imrie CW, Banks PA. Acute pancreatitis: bench to the bedside. *Gastroenterology.* 2007; 132(3): 1127-1151. PMID: 17383433.
28. Mareninova OA, Sung KF, Hong P, Lugea A, Pandol SJ, Gukovsky I, et al. Cell death in pancreatitis: caspases protect from necrotizing pancreatitis. *J Biol Chem.* 2006; 281(6): 3370-3381. PMID: 16339139.
29. Forsmark CE, Baillie J. AGA Institute technical review on acute pancreatitis. *Gastroenterology.* 2007; 132(5): 2022-2044. PMID: 17484894.
30. London NJ, Leese T, Lavelle JM, Miles K, West KP, Watkin DF, et al. Rapid-bolus contrast-enhanced dynamic computed tomography in acute pancreatitis: a prospective study. *Br J Surg.* 1991; 78(12): 1452-1456. PMID: 1773324.
31. Carnovale A, Rabitti PG, Manes G, Esposito P, Pacelli L, Uomo G. Mortality in acute pancreatitis: is it an early or a late event? *JOP.* 2005; 6(5): 438-444. PMID: 16186665.
32. Mutinga M, Rosenbluth A, Tenner SM, Odze RR, Sica GT, Banks PA. Does mortality occur early or late in acute pancreatitis? *Int J Pancreatol.* 2000; 28(2): 91-95. PMID: 11128978.
33. Tenner S, Sica G, Hughes M, Noordhoek E, Feng S, Zinner M, et al. Relationship of necrosis to organ failure in severe acute pancreatitis. *Gastroenterology.* 1997; 113(3): 899-903. PMID: 9287982.
34. Perez A, Whang EE, Brooks DC, Moore FD Jr, Hughes MD, Sica GT, et al. Is severity of necrotizing pancreatitis increased in extended necrosis and infected necrosis? *Pancreas.* 2002; 25(3): 229-233. PMID: 12370532.
35. Aho HJ, Koskensalo SM, Nevalainen TJ. Experimental pancreatitis in the rat. Sodium taurocholate-induced acute haemorrhagic pancreatitis. *Scand J Gastroenterol.* 1980; 15(4): 411-416. PMID: 7433903.
36. Spivak W, Morrison C, Devinuto D, Yuey W. Spectrophotometric determination of the critical micellar concentration of bile salts using bilirubin monoglucuronide as a micellar probe. Utility of derivative spectroscopy. *Biochem J.* 1988; 252(1): 275-281. PMID: 3421905.
37. Asang E. [Changes in the therapy of inflammatory diseases of the pancreas. A report on 1 year of therapy and prophylaxis with the kallikrein- and trypsin inactivator trasylol (Bayer)]. *Langenbecks Arch Klin Chir Ver Dtsch Z Chir.* 1960; 293: 645-670. PMID: 13794633.
38. Seta T, Noguchi Y, Shimada T, Shikata S, Fukui T. Treatment of acute pancreatitis with protease inhibitors: a meta-analysis. *Eur J Gastroenterol Hepatol.* 2004; 16(12): 1287-1293. PMID: 15618834.
39. Andriulli A, Caruso N, Quitadamo M, Forlano R, Leandro G, Spirito F, et al. Antisecretory vs. antiprotease drugs in the prevention of post-ERCP pancreatitis: the evidence-based medicine derived from a meta-analysis study. *JOP.* 2003; 4(1): 41-48. PMID: 12555015.
40. Andriulli A, Leandro G, Clemente R, Festa V, Caruso N, Annese V, et al. Meta-analysis of somatostatin, octreotide and gabexate mesilate in the therapy of acute pancreatitis. *Aliment Pharmacol Ther.* 1998; 12(3): 237-245. PMID: 9570258.
41. Büchler M, Malfertheiner P, Uhl W, Schölmerich J, Stöckmann F, Adler G, et al. Gabexate mesilate in human acute pancreatitis. German Pancreatitis Study Group. *Gastroenterology.* 1993; 104(4): 1165-1170. PMID: 8462805.
42. Chen HM, Chen JC, Hwang TL, Jan YY, Chen MF. Prospective and randomized study of gabexate mesilate for the treatment of severe acute pancreatitis with organ dysfunction. *Hepatogastroenterology.* 2000; 47(34): 1147-1150. PMID: 11020900.
43. Park KT, Kang DH, Choi CW, Cho M, Park SB, Kim HW, et al. Is high-dose nafamostat mesilate effective for the prevention of post-ERCP pancreatitis, especially in high-risk patients? *Pancreas.* 2011; 40(8): 1215-1219. PMID: 21775918.
44. Trapnell JE, Rigby CC, Talbot CH, Duncan EH. A controlled trial of Trasylol in the treatment of acute pancreatitis. *Brit J Surg.* 1974; 61(3): 177-182. PMID: 4595174.
45. Trapnell JE, Talbot CH, Capper WM. Trasylol in acute pancreatitis. *Am J Dig Dis.* 1967; 12(4): 409-412. PMID: 5336018.
46. Abbasinazari M, Mohammad Alizadeh AH, Moshiri K, Pourhoseingholi MA, Zali MR. Does allopurinol prevent post endoscopic retrograde cholangio- pancreatography pancreatitis? A randomized double blind trial. *Acta Med Iranica.* 2011; 49(9): 579-583. PMID: 22052140.
47. O'Leary DP, O'Neill D, McLaughlin P, O'Neill S, Myers E, Maher MM, et al. Effects of abdominal fat distribution parameters on severity of acute pancreatitis. *World J Surg.* 2012; 36(7): 1679-1685. PMID: 22491816.
48. Abu Hilal M, Armstrong T. The impact of obesity on the course and outcome of acute pancreatitis. *Obes Surg.* 2008; 18(3): 326-328. PMID: 18202895.
49. Papachristou GI, Papachristou DJ, Avula H, Slivka A, Whitcomb DC. Obesity increases the severity of acute pancreatitis: performance of APACHE-O score and correlation with the inflammatory response. *Pancreatology.* 2006; 6(4): 279-285. PMID: 16636600.
50. Evans AC, Papachristou GI, Whitcomb DC. Obesity and the risk of severe acute pancreatitis. *Minerva Gastroenterol Dietol.* 2010; 56(2): 169-179. PMID: 20485254.
51. Chen SM, Xiong GS, Wu SM. Is obesity an indicator of complications and mortality in acute pancreatitis? An updated meta-analysis. *J Dig Dis.* 2012; 13(5): 244-251. PMID: 22500786.
52. Sadr-Azodi O, Orsini N, Andren-Sandberg A, Wolk A. Abdominal and total adiposity and the risk of acute pancreatitis: a population-based prospective cohort study. *Am J Gastroenterol.* 2013; 108(1): 133-139. PMID: 23147519.
53. Funnell IC, Bornman PC, Weakley SP, Terblanche J, Marks IN. Obesity: an important prognostic factor in acute

pancreatitis. *Br J Surg*. 1993; 80(4): 484-486. PMID: 8495317.
54. Buch A, Buch J, Carlsen A, Schmidt A. Hyperlipidemia and pancreatitis. *World J Surg*. 1980; 4(3): 307-314. PMID: 7415184.
55. Warshaw AL, Lesser PB, Rie M, Cullen DJ. The pathogenesis of pulmonary edema in acute pancreatitis. *Ann Surg*. 1975; 182(4): 505-510. PMID: 1101836.
56. Wu XM, Ji KQ, Wang HY, Li GF, Zang B, Chen WM. Total enteral nutrition in prevention of pancreatic necrotic infection in severe acute pancreatitis. *Pancreas*. 2010; 39(2): 248-251. PMID: 19910834.
57. Petrov MS, Kukosh MV, Emelyanov NV. A randomized controlled trial of enteral versus parenteral feeding in patients with predicted severe acute pancreatitis shows a significant reduction in mortality and in infected pancreatic complications with total enteral nutrition. *Digestive Surg*. 2006; 23 (5-6): 336-344; discussion 344-335. PMID: 17164546.
58. Patel KS, Noel P, Singh VP. Potential influence of intravenous lipids on the outcomes of acute pancreatitis. *Nutr Clin Pract*. 2014; 29(3): 291-294. PMID: 24687866.
59. Sun E, Tharakan M, Kapoor S, Chakravarty R, Salhab A, Buscaglia JM, et al. Poor compliance with ACG guidelines for nutrition and antibiotics in the management of acute pancreatitis: a North American survey of gastrointestinal specialists and primary care physicians. *JOP*. 2013; 14(3): 221-227. PMID: 23669469.
60. Vlada AC, Schmit B, Perry A, Trevino JG, Behrns KE, Hughes SJ. Failure to follow evidence-based best practice guidelines in the treatment of severe acute pancreatitis. *HPB (Oxford)*. 2013; 15(10): 822-827. PMID: 24028271.
61. Hughan KS, Bonadonna RC, Lee S, Michaliszyn SF, Arslanian SA. β-Cell lipotoxicity after an overnight intravenous lipid challenge and free fatty acid elevation in African American versus American white overweight/obese adolescents. *J Clin Endocrinol Metab*. 2013; 98(5): 2062-2069. PMID: 23526462.
62. Domschke S, Malfertheiner P, Uhl W, Buchler M, Domschke W. Free fatty acids in serum of patients with acute necrotizing or edematous pancreatitis. *Int J Pancreatol*. 1993; 13(2): 105-110. PMID: 8501351.
63. Panek J, Sztefko K, Drozdz W. Composition of free fatty acid and triglyceride fractions in human necrotic pancreatic tissue. *Med Sci Monit*. 2001; 7(5): 894-898. PMID: 11535930.
64. Kloppel G, Dreyer T, Willemer S, Kern HF, Adler G. Human acute pancreatitis: its pathogenesis in the light of immunocytochemical and ultrastructural findings in acinar cells. *Virchows Arch A Pathol Anat Histopathol*. 1986; 409(6): 791-803. PMID: 3094241.
65. Nordback IH, Clemens JA, Chacko VP, Olson JL, Cameron JL. Changes in high-energy phosphate metabolism and cell morphology in four models of acute experimental pancreatitis. *Ann Surg*. 1991; 213(4): 341-349. PMID: 2009016.
66. Acharya C, Cline RA, Jaligama D, Noel P, Delany JP, Bae K, et al. Fibrosis Reduces Severity of Acute-on-Chronic Pancreatitis in Humans. *Gastroenterology*. 2013; 145(2): 466-475. PMID: 23684709.
67. Navina S, Acharya C, DeLany JP, Orlichenko LS, Baty CJ, Shiva SS, et al. Lipotoxicity causes multisystem organ failure and exacerbates acute pancreatitis in obesity. *Sci Transl Med*. 2011; 3(107): 107ra110. PMID: 22049070.
68. Fallon MB, Gorelick FS, Anderson JM, Mennone A, Saluja A, Steer ML. Effect of cerulein hyperstimulation on the paracellular barrier of rat exocrine pancreas. *Gastroenterology*. 1995; 108(6): 1863-1872. PMID: 7539388.
69. Gaisano HY, Lutz MP, Leser J, Sheu L, Lynch G, Tang L, et al. Supramaximal cholecystokinin displaces Munc18c from the pancreatic acinar basal surface, redirecting apical exocytosis to the basal membrane. *J Clin Invest*. 2001; 108(11): 1597-1611. PMID: 11733555.
70. Lam PP, Cosen Binker LI, Lugea A, Pandol SJ, Gaisano HY. Alcohol redirects CCK-mediated apical exocytosis to the acinar basolateral membrane in alcoholic pancreatitis. *Traffic*. 2007; 8(5): 605-617. PMID: 17451559.
71. Cosen-Binker LI, Binker MG, Wang CC, Hong W, Gaisano HY. VAMP8 is the v-SNARE that mediates basolateral exocytosis in a mouse model of alcoholic pancreatitis. *J Clin Invest*. 2008; 118(7): 2535-2551. PMID: 18535671.
72. Cosen-Binker LI, Lam PP, Binker MG, Reeve J, Pandol S, Gaisano HY. Alcohol/cholecystokinin-evoked pancreatic acinar basolateral exocytosis is mediated by protein kinase C alpha phosphorylation of Munc18c. *J Biol Chem*. 2007; 282(17): 13047-13058. PMID: 17324928.
73. Durgampudi C, Noel P, Patel K, Cline R, Trivedi RN, DeLany JP, et al. Acute lipotoxicity regulates severity of biliary acute pancreatitis without affecting its initiation. *Am J Pathol*. 2014; 184(6): 1773-1784. PMID: 24854864.
74. Noel P, Patel K, Durgampudi C, Trivedi RN, de Oliveira C, Crowell MD, et al. Peripancreatic fat necrosis worsens acute pancreatitis independent of pancreatic necrosis via unsaturated fatty acids increased in human pancreatic necrosis collections. *Gut*, 2014. PMID: 25500204
75. Mossner J, Bodeker H, Kimura W, Meyer F, Bohm S, Fischbach W. Isolated rat pancreatic acini as a model to study the potential role of lipase in the pathogenesis of acinar cell destruction. *Int J Pancreatol*. 1992; 12(3): 285-296. PMID: 1289421.
76. Siech M, Zhou Z, Zhou S, Bair B, Alt A, Hamm S, et al. Stimulation of stellate cells by injured acinar cells: a model of acute pancreatitis induced by alcohol and fat (VLDL). *Am J Physiol Gastrointest Liver Physiol*. 2009; 297(6): G1163-G1171. PMID: 19779015.
77. Patel K, Trivedi RN, Durgampudi C, Noel P, Cline RA, DeLany JP, et al. Lipolysis of visceral adipocyte triglyceride by pancreatic lipases converts mild acute pancreatitis to severe pancreatitis independent of necrosis and inflammation. *Am J Pathol*. 2015; 185(3): 808-819. PMID: 25579844.
78. Schmitz-Moormann P. Comparative radiological and morphological study of the human pancreas. IV. Acute necrotizing pancreatitis in man. *Pathol Res Pract*. 1981; 171(3-4): 325-335. PMID: 7279784.
79. Nordback I, Lauslahti K. Clinical pathology of acute necrotising pancreatitis. *J Clin Pathol*. 1986; 39: 68-74. PMID: 3950033.

80. Olsen TS. Lipomatosis of the pancreas in autopsy material and its relation to age and overweight. *Acta Pathol Microbiol Scand A*. 1978; 86A(5): 367-373. PMID: 716899.
81. Rosso E, Casnedi S, Pessaux P, Oussoultzoglou E, Panaro F, Mahfud M, et al. The role of "fatty pancreas" and of BMI in the occurrence of pancreatic fistula after pancreaticoduodenectomy. *J Gastrointest Surg*. 2009; 13(10): 1845-1851. PMID: 19639369.
82. Matsumoto S, Mori H, Miyake H, Takaki H, Maeda T, Yamada Y, et al. Uneven fatty replacement of the pancreas: evaluation with CT. *Radiology*. 1995; 194(2): 453-458. PMID: 7824726.
83. Pinnick KE, Collins SC, Londos C, Gauguier D, Clark A, Fielding BA. Pancreatic ectopic fat is characterized by adipocyte infiltration and altered lipid composition. *Obesity (Silver Spring)*. 2008; 16(3): 522-530. PMID: 18239594.
84. Sztefko K, Panek J. Serum free fatty acid concentration in patients with acute pancreatitis. *Pancreatology*. 2001; 1(3): 230-236. PMID: 12120200.
85. Hussain N, Wu F, Zhu L, Thrall RS, Kresch MJ. Neutrophil apoptosis during the development and resolution of oleic acid-induced acute lung injury in the rat. *Am J Respir Cell Mol Biol*. 1998; 19(6): 867-874. PMID: 9843920.
86. Inoue H, Nakagawa Y, Ikemura M, Usugi E, Nata M. Molecular-biological analysis of acute lung injury (ALI) induced by heat exposure and/or intravenous administration of oleic acid. *Leg Med*. 2012; 14(6): 304-308. PMID: 22819303.
87. Lai JP, Bao S, Davis IC, Knoell DL. Inhibition of the phosphatase PTEN protects mice against oleic acid-induced acute lung injury. *Br J Pharmacol*. 2009; 156(1): 189-200. PMID: 19134000.
88. Wu RP, Liang XB, Guo H, Zhou XS, Zhao L, Wang C, et al. Protective effect of low potassium dextran solution on acute kidney injury following acute lung injury induced by oleic acid in piglets. *Chin Med J (Engl)*. 2012; 125(17): 3093-3097. PMID: 22932187.
89. Hirota M, Nozawa F, Okabe A, Shibata M, Beppu T, Shimada S, et al. Relationship between plasma cytokine concentration and multiple organ failure in patients with acute pancreatitis. *Pancreas*. 2000; 21(2): 141-146, 2000. PMID: 10975707.
90. Messmann H, Vogt W, Falk W, Vogl D, Zirngibl H, Leser HG, et al. Interleukins and their antagonists but not TNF and its receptors are released in post-ERP pancreatitis. *Eur J Gastroenterol Hepatol*. 1998; 10(7): 611-617. PMID: 9855088.
91. Brivet FG, Emilie D, Galanaud P. Pro- and anti-inflammatory cytokines during acute severe pancreatitis: an early and sustained response, although unpredictable of death. Parisian Study Group on Acute Pancreatitis. *Crit Care Med*. 1999; 27(4): 749-755. PMID: 10321665.
92. Dambrauskas Z, Giese N, Gulbinas A, Giese T, Berberat PO, Pundzius J, et al. Different profiles of cytokine expression during mild and severe acute pancreatitis. *World J Gastroenterol*. 2010; 16(15): 1845-1853. PMID: 20397261.
93. Aoun E, Chen J, Reighard D, Gleeson FC, Whitcomb DC, Papachristou GI. Diagnostic accuracy of interleukin-6 and interleukin-8 in predicting severe acute pancreatitis: a meta-analysis. *Pancreatology*. 2009; 9(6): 777-785. PMID: 20110745.
94. Daniel P, Lesniowski B, Mokrowiecka A, Jasinska A, Pietruczuk M, Malecka-Panas E. Circulating levels of visfatin, resistin and pro-inflammatory cytokine interleukin-8 in acute pancreatitis. *Pancreatology* 10(4): 477-482, 2010. PMID: 20720449.
95. Ueda T, Takeyama Y, Yasuda T, Matsumura N, Sawa H, Nakajima T, et al. Significant elevation of serum interleukin-18 levels in patients with acute pancreatitis. *J Gastroenterol*. 2006; 41(2): 158-165. PMID: 16568375.
96. Wereszczynska-Siemiatkowska U, Mroczko B, Siemiatkowski A. Serum profiles of interleukin-18 in different severity forms of human acute pancreatitis. *Scand J Gastroenterol*. 2002; 37(9): 1097-1102. PMID: 12374236.
97. Gea-Sorli S, Bonjoch L, Closa D. Differences in the inflammatory response induced by acute pancreatitis in different white adipose tissue sites in the rat. *PloS One*. 2012; 7(8): e41933. PMID: 22870264.
98. Chaudry G, Navarro OM, Levine DS, Oudjhane K. Abdominal manifestations of cystic fibrosis in children. *Pediatr Radiol*. 2006; 36(3): 233-240. PMID: 16391928.
99. Lankisch PG, Breuer N, Bruns A, Weber-Dany B, Lowenfels AB, Maisonneuve P. Natural history of acute pancreatitis: a long-term population-based study. *Am J Gastroenterol*. 2009; 104(11): 2797-2805; quiz 2806. PMID: 19603011.
100. LaRusch J, Whitcomb DC. Genetics of pancreatitis. *Curr Opin Gastroenterol*. 2011; 27(5): 467-474. PMID: 21844754.
101. Nøjgaard C, Becker U, Matzen P, Andersen JR, Holst C, Bendtsen F. Progression from acute to chronic pancreatitis: prognostic factors, mortality, and natural course. *Pancreas*. 2011; 40(8): 1195-1200. PMID: 21926938.
102. Otsuki M. Chronic pancreatitis in Japan: epidemiology, prognosis, diagnostic criteria, and future problems. *J Gastroenterol* . 2003; 38(4): 315-326. PMID: 12743770.
103. Soyer P, Spelle L, Pelage JP, Dufresne AC, Rondeau Y, Gouhiri M, et al. Cystic fibrosis in adolescents and adults: fatty replacement of the pancreas--CT evaluation and functional correlation. *Radiology*. 1999; 210(3): 611-615. PMID: 10207457.
104. Vaughn DD, Jabra AA, Fishman EK. Pancreatic disease in children and young adults: evaluation with CT. *Radiographics*. 1998; 18(5): 1171-1187. PMID: 9747614.
105. Robertson MB, Choe KA, Joseph PM. Review of the abdominal manifestations of cystic fibrosis in the adult patient. *Radiographics*. 2006; 26(3): 679-690. PMID: 16702447.
106. Nøjgaard C, Matzen P, Bendtsen F, Andersen JR, Christensen E, Becker U. Factors associated with long-term mortality in acute pancreatitis. *Scand J Gastroenterol*. 2011; 46(4): 495-502. PMID: 21091094.
107. Laposata EA, Lange LG. Presence of nonoxidative ethanol metabolism in human organs commonly damaged by ethanol abuse. *Science*. 1986; 231(4737): 497-499. PMID: 3941913.
108. Criddle DN, Murphy J, Fistetto G, Barrow S, Tepikin AV, Neoptolemos JP, et al. Fatty acid ethyl esters cause pancreatic calcium toxicity via inositol trisphosphate receptors and loss of ATP synthesis. *Gastroenterology*. 2006; 130(3): 781-793. PMID: 16530519.
109. Patel K, Durgampudi C, Noel P, Trivedi AN, deOliveira C, Singh VP. Fatty acid ethyl esters are less

toxic than their parent fatty acids generated during acute pancreatitis. *Am J Pathol.* 2016; 186(4): 874-884. PMID: 26878214.

110. Camhi SM, Bray GA, Bouchard C, Greenway FL, Johnson WD, Newton RL, et al. The relationship of waist circumference and BMI to visceral, subcutaneous, and total body fat: sex and race differences. *Obesity.* 2011; 19(2): 402-408. PMID: 20948514.

111. Thomas LW. The chemical composition of adipose tissue of man and mice. *Q J Exp Physiol Cogn Med Sci.* 1962; 47: 179-188. PMID: 13920823.

112. Banks PA, Bollen TL, Dervenis C, Gooszen HG, Johnson CD, Sarr MG, et al. Classification of acute pancreatitis--2012: revision of the Atlanta classification and definitions by international consensus. *Gut.* 2013; 62(1): 102-111. PMID: 23100216.

Acute Pancreatitis

Section Editors: Markus M. Lerch and Marc G. Besselink

Chapter 17

Gallstone-related pathogenesis of acute pancreatitis

Markus M. Lerch* and Ali Aghdassi

Department of Medicine A, University Medicine Greifswald, Germany.

Etiology and pathogenesis of pancreatitis

Acute pancreatitis (AP) is an inflammatory disorder of the exocrine pancreas caused in most cases by immoderate alcohol consumption or gallstone passage. Population-based studies indicate that the incidence of AP rose from 14.8 in 100,000 (1990-1994) to 31.2 in 100,000 (2010-2013) among British males.[1] AP is the most frequent reason for hospital admission among all nonmalignant gastrointestinal diseases.[2] It is a lethal disease with an overall mortality of 4.3% within 90 days and a 1-year mortality of 7.9%.[1] Both heavy alcohol consumption and gallstone disease are becoming more common. Population-based studies indicate that the prevalence of gallstones in some western countries surpasses 20% of the adult population.[3] While genetic predispositions clearly play an important role in gallstone formation,[4,5] they cannot explain the continuous rise in gallstone prevalence, which is more likely due to nutritional and lifestyle factors. Once a patient has developed pancreatitis due to gallstones, the disease is likely to recur if the source of migrating bile duct stones is not removed or their impaction at the duodenal papilla is not prevented. In a study involving some 5,000 patients admitted for a first episode of acute gallstone-associated pancreatitis, endoscopic sphincterotomy reduced the recurrence rate from approximately 30% during the first weeks to 6.7%, an elective interval cholecystectomy reduced it to 4.4%, and performing endoscopic sphincterotomy during the same hospital admission combined with elective cholecystectomy reduced it further to 1.2%.[6] Another way to address the problem is the transient insertion of a small plastic stent into the pancreatic duct. Following manipulation of the papilla, (e.g., to remove a gallstone or to perform a spincterotomy), consequent swelling can obstruct the pancreatic duct, an event that triggers pancreatitis in some patients. The inserted plastic stent prevents the prolonged impairment of pancreatic secretion and has been shown to significantly reduce the incidence of ERCP-induced pancreatitis.[7] Taken together these clinical and population-based observations indicate that 1) carrying gallstones increases the risk of developing AP; 2) only gallstones that are small enough to pass through the biliary tract (rather than the ones that remain asymptomatically in the gallbladder), confer a pancreatitis risk; 3) strategies intended to remove the source of migrating gallstone or prevent their impaction near the duodenal papilla reduce the risk of developing pancreatitis in the first place and the risk of pancreatitis recurrence; and 4) preserving the flow from the pancreatic duct is an effective way of preventing ERCP-induced pancreatitis, a clinical entity considered to be caused by pancreatic duct obstruction. The next paragraph will review the century-old discussion regarding the underlying mechanism how a wandering gallstone initiates pancreatitis.

Possible mechanisms of gallstone-induced pancreatitis

A connection between gallbladder stones and pancreatitis has been suspected since at least the 17th century,[8] but how gallstones confer that risk has been the matter of much debate. Claude Bernard discovered in 1856 that bile is an agent that can cause pancreatitis when injected into the pancreatic duct of laboratory animals.[9] Since that time, many studies have been performed to elucidate the underlying mechanisms. It is firmly established today that the initiation of pancreatitis requires the passage of a gallstone from the gallbladder through the biliary tract,[10] and gallstones that remain in the gallbladder will not cause pancreatitis. However, the various hypotheses proposed to explain this association have sometimes been contradictory. In 1901, Eugene Opie postulated that pancreatic outflow impairment due to pancreatic duct obstruction causes pancreatitis.[11] This initial "duct obstruction hypothesis" was somewhat forgotten when Opie published his second

*Corresponding author. Email: Lerch@uni-greifswald.de

A

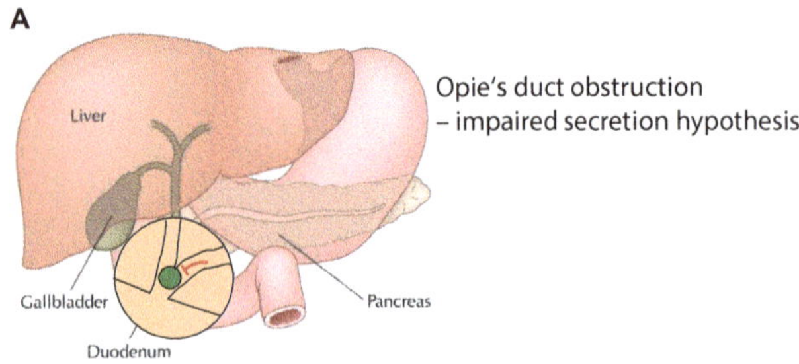

B

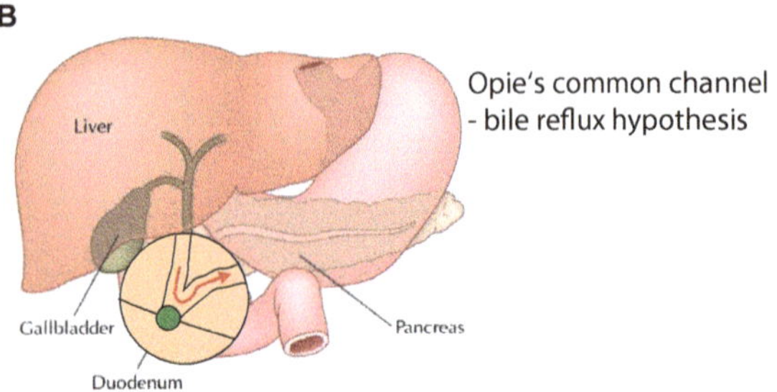

Figure 1. The two "Opie hypotheses" for gallstone-induced pancreatitis pathogenesis, both reported in 1901. A: A gallstone passing through the biliary tract obstructs the pancreatic duct. The impaired flow from the exocrine pancreas triggers acinar or duct cell damage. Whether or not the common bile duct is also obstructed is immaterial to the triggering mechanism of pancreatitis in this scenario. B: A gallstone impacted at the duodenal papilla creates a communication between the pancreatic and common bile ducts. Behind it, bile can flow through this "common channel" into the pancreatic duct and trigger AP onset. Modified from [37].

"common channel" hypothesis in the same year.[12] He predicted that an impacted gallstone at the papilla of Vater creates a communication between the pancreatic and bile ducts (the so called "common channel") through which bile flows into the pancreatic duct and thus causes pancreatitis (**Figure 1**).

Although Opie's "common channel" hypothesis seems rational from a mechanistic point of view and has become one of the most popular theories in the field, considerable experimental and clinical evidence is incompatible with its assumptions.[13,14] Anatomical studies have shown that the communication between the pancreatic duct and common bile duct is much too short (<6 mm) to permit biliary reflux into the pancreatic duct,[15] and an impacted gallstone would most likely obstruct both the common bile and pancreatic ducts.[16] Even in the event of an existing anatomical communication, pancreatic secretory pressure would still exceed biliary pressure, and pancreatic juice would flow into the bile duct rather than bile into the pancreatic duct.[17,18] Late in the course of pancreatitis when necrosis is firmly established, a biliopancreatic reflux due to a loss of barrier function in the damaged pancreatic duct may explain the observation of a bile-stained necrotic pancreas at the time of surgery. However, this should not be regarded as evidence for the assumption that bile reflux into the pancreas is a triggering event for disease onset. Experiments performed on the American opossum, an animal model that is anatomically suited to test the common channel hypothesis, have revealed that neither a common channel nor a biliopancreatic reflux is required for the development of acute necrotizing pancreatitis, but obstruction of the pancreatic duct is required.[14]

In order to overcome the inconsistencies of the "common channel" hypothesis, it was proposed that gallstone passage could damage the duodenal sphincter in a manner that causes sphincter insufficiency. This, in turn, could permit duodenal content including bile and activated pancreatic juice to flow through the incompetent sphincter and into the pancreatitis duct,[19] thus inducing pancreatitis. While this hypothesis would avoid most of the inconsistencies of Opie's "common channel" hypothesis, it is not applicable to the human situation where sphincter stenosis rather than sphincter insufficiency results from gallstone passage through the papilla and pancreatic juice flow into the bile duct, rather than flow of duodenal content into the pancreas.[20]

A final argument against the "common channel" hypothesis is that bile perfusion through the pancreatic duct has been shown to be completely harmless[21] and only a potential influx of infected bile, which might occur after prolonged obstruction at the papilla when the pressure gradient between the pancreatic duct (higher) and the bile duct (lower) is reversed,[22,23] may represent an aggravating factor as opposed to an initiating event for the course of pancreatitis. Taken together, these data suggest that the initial pathophysiologic events during the course of gallstone-induced pancreatitis affect acinar cells[24] and are triggered, in accordance with Opie's initial hypothesis, by obstruction or impairment of flow from the pancreatic duct.[25] Bile reflux into the pancreatic duct—either through a common channel created by an impacted gallstone or through an incompetent sphincter caused by the passage of a gallstone—is neither required nor likely to occur during the initial course of AP.[26]

Cellular events during pancreatic duct obstruction

To investigate the cellular events involved in gallstone-induced pancreatitis, an animal model based on pancreatic duct obstruction in rodents has been employed.[27] In addition to a morphological and biochemical characterization of this experimental disease variety, intracellular calcium (Ca^{2+}) release in response to hormonal stimuli was investigated. Under physiological resting conditions, most cell types including the acinar cells of the exocrine pancreas maintain a Ca^{2+} gradient across the plasma membrane with low intracellular (nanomolar range) facing high extracellular (millimolar range) Ca^{2+} concentrations. Rapid Ca^{2+} release from intracellular stores in response to external and internal stimuli is used by many of these cells as a signaling mechanism that regulates such diverse biological events as growth, proliferation, locomotion, contraction, and the regulated secretion of exportable proteins. An impaired cellular capacity to maintain the Ca^{2+} gradient across the plasma membrane was previously identified as a common pathophysiologic characteristic of vascular hypertension, malignant tumor growth, and cell damage in response to toxins. It was also observed in a secretagogue-induced model of AP,[28,29] where a rapid and sustained rise of intracellular Ca^{2+} caused by release from apical stores and rapid entry of extracellular Ca^{2+} was shown to be involved in the pathogenesis of experimental pancreatitis. Up to 6 hours of pancreatic duct ligation in rats and mice (a condition that mimics the situation in human gallstone-induced pancreatitis) induced leukocytosis, hyperamylasemia, pancreatic edema, and granulocyte immigration into the lungs, none of which were observed in bile duct-ligated controls.[27] It also led to significant intracellular activation of pancreatic proteases such as trypsin, an event discussed in more detail in the next paragraph. While the resting intracellular Ca^{2+} concentration ($[Ca^{2+}]_i$) in isolated acini rose by 45% to 205 ± 7 nM, acetylcholine- and cholecystokinin-stimulated Ca^{2+} peaks and amylase secretion declined. However, pancreatic duct ligation did not impair $[Ca^{2+}]_i$ signaling, amylase output in response to the Ca^{2+}-ATPase inhibitor thapsigargin, or secretin-stimulated amylase release. On the single cell level, pancreatic duct ligation reduced the percentage of cells in which physiological secretagogue stimulation was followed by a physiological response (i.e., Ca^{2+}-oscillations) and increased the percentage of cells with a pathologic response (i.e., peak-plateau or absent Ca^{2+} signal). Moreover, it reduced the frequency and amplitude of Ca^{2+} oscillation and capacitative Ca^{2+} influx in response to secretagogue stimulation.

To test whether these prominent changes in intra-acinar cell Ca^{2+} signaling parallel pancreatic duct obstruction and are directly involved in pancreatitis initiation, animals were systemically treated with the intracellular Ca^{2+} chelator BAPTA-AM. As a consequence, both pancreatitis parameters and intrapancreatic trypsinogen activation induced by duct ligation were significantly reduced. These results suggest that pancreatic duct obstruction, the critical event involved in gallstone-induced pancreatitis, rapidly changes the physiological response of the exocrine pancreas to a pathologic Ca^{2+} signaling pattern. This is associated with premature digestive enzyme activation and the onset of pancreatitis—both of which can be prevented by administering an intracellular Ca^{2+} chelator. A number of preclinical and ongoing clinical trials have employed the dependence of pancreatitis on intracellular Ca^{2+} signaling and have identified magnesium (Mg^{2+}) as a suitable Ca^{2+} antagonist in this context[28,29] in which a Ca^{2+} chelator would be too toxic and have proceeded to test its efficiency in patients.[30]

Whether or not premature intra-acinar cell protease activation provides a sufficient explanation for triggering pancreatitis has recently come under discussion and is covered elsewhere in this volume and in a recent review.[31]

Cellular signaling and sorting mechanisms

Subsequent investigations have focused on the cellular signaling and sorting mechanisms involved in disease onset. Essential events that have been identified are colocalization and transactivation of lysosomal cathepsins with zymogens and the above-mentioned pathologic Ca^{2+}-release from intracellular stores. Both processes were found to be critically important in both supramaximal stimulation-induced models of pancreatitis[32,33] and in clinically more relevant duct obstruction-induced pancreatitis.[34,35]

Two inconsistencies of the duct-ligation models of pancreatitis have renewed interest in the role of bile in the disease onset. The first was that duct-ligation alone, with the notable exception of the opossum, induces mostly mild pancreatitis rather than fully developed necrosis, particularly in the rat.[27] The second inconsistency was that some studies employing the opossum model, while still refuting the common-channel-hypothesis, reported that bile duct ligation, when added to pancreatic duct ligation, increased disease severity.[36] This suggests that elevated bile acids in systemic circulation could aggravate the disease process, and the subsequent line of arguments has previously been summarized.[37]

The first confirmation for this assumption came from studies reporting that bile acids have a direct effect on pancreatic acinar cells and elicit an oscillatory release of Ca^{2+} from intracellular stores.[38] This bile acid effect on $[Ca^{2+}]_i$ is either mediated via bile acid inhibition of the sarco/endoplasmic reticulum Ca^{2+}-ATPase (SERCA) pump with consecutive depletion of ER Ca^{2+}-stores and activation of significant capacitative Ca^{2+}-entry into the cytosol,[39,40] or alternatively by potentiation of Ca^{2+}-release from the ER and apical (vesicular) Ca^{2+}-stores.[38,41,42] Most studies agree that monohydroxy-bile-acids such as taurolithocholic-acid-3–sulfate (TLC-S) have a more potent effect on acinar cells than dihydroxy-bile-acids (i.e., TCDC) or trihydroxy-bile-acids and can cause damage independently of their properties as detergents or ionophores. Most importantly, TLC-S can induce pathologic Ca^{2+} signals and lead to trypsinogen activation at concentrations that correspond to those found in the serum of patients with gallstone-induced biliary obstruction.[41,43] The disease-aggravating effect of common bile duct obstruction in pancreatitis would therefore not require bile reflux into the pancreatic duct but could be readily elicited by bile acids in the serum or interstitial space of jaundiced patients.

The question that remains is to how bile acids enter the acinar cell and whether it is via the basolateral or luminal

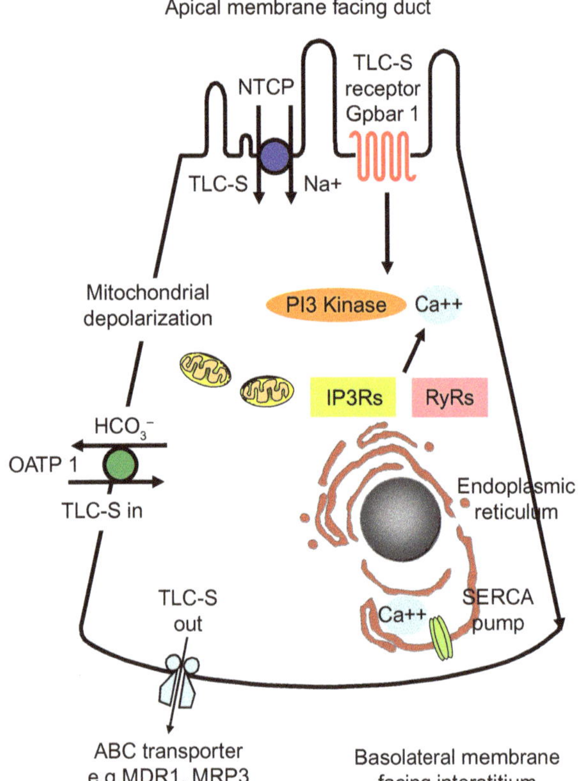

Figure 2: Different cellular mechanisms that can mediate bile acid uptake into duct or acinar cells from either the luminal side of the cell or the interstitial/vascular surface. Modified from[37].

surface. An elegant study by Kim and colleagues identified two potential mechanisms (**Figure 2**).[39] The first involves a Na^+-dependent-co-transporter (Na^+-taurocholate cotransporting-polypeptide, NTCP), that accounts for approximately 25% of bile acid uptake predominantly at the luminal membrane. Bile acid uptake via this transporter would thus require bile reflux to reach the pancreatic acinar cell via the duct. The other uptake mechanism involves an HCO_3^--dependent exchanger (organic-anion-transporting polypeptide, OATP1) that operates from the basolateral acinar cell surface and could thus be supplied with serum or interstitial bile acids.

Perides and coworkers recently identified an additional mechanism for the effects of bile acid on pancreatic acinar cells that 1) seems to require action only at the luminal cell surface; 2) is independent of bile acid uptake mechanisms into the cell; and 3) involves G-protein-receptor-coupled signaling events elicited by TLC-S, which suggests that biliary pancreatitis is a surface-receptor-mediated disease.[44]

Interestingly, only TLC-S injection resulted in pancreatitis in this setting, while Na^+-taurocholate did not. Gpbar1-/- mice were fully protected against TLC-S-induced pancreatitis. These studies have led to renewed interest in events that take place inside the pancreatic duct during the initiating phase of gallstone-induced pancreatitis. Some appear to involve impairment of pancreatic fluid secretion,[47] others require intraductal action of prematurely activated trypsin,[48] intraductal lysosomal enzymes,[35,49] signal transduction events within ductal cells,[44] or intraductal pH changes.[50] While Eugene Opie challenged preconceived theories about the mechanisms that trigger gallstone-induced pancreatitis and set us on the path toward actionable results (e.g., restoring the flow of pancreatic juice or preventing its blockage), clinically relevant information is still accumulating at a rapid pace from laboratories the world over and will hopefully result in better treatment and prevention strategies for this still deadly disease.

References

1. Hazra N, Gulliford M. Evaluating pancreatitis in primary care: a population-based cohort study. *Br J Gen Pract*. 2014; 64: e295-e301. PMID: 24771844.
2. Peery AF, Dellon ES, Lund J, Crockett SD, McGowan CE, Bulsiewicz WJ, et al. Burden of gastrointestinal disease in the United States: 2012 update. *Gastroenterology*. 2012; 143: 1179-1187. PMID: 22885331.
3. Volzke H, Baumeister SE, Alte D, Hoffmann W, Schwahn C, Simon P, et al. Independent risk factors for gallstone formation in a region with high cholelithiasis prevalence. *Digestion*. 2005; 71: 97-105. PMID: 15775677.
4. von Kampen O, Buch S, Nothnagel M, Azocar L, Molina H, Brosch M, et al. Genetic and functional identification of the likely causative variant for cholesterol gallstone disease at the ABCG5/8 lithogenic locus. *Hepatology*. 2013; 57: 2407-2417. PMID: 22898925.
5. Buch S, Schafmayer C, Volzke H, Seeger M, Miquel JF, Sookoian SC, et al. Loci from a genome-wide analysis of bilirubin levels are associated with gallstone risk and composition. *Gastroenterology*. 2010; 139: 1942-1951. PMID: 20837016.
6. Mustafa A, Begaj I, Deakin M, Durkin D, Corless DJ, Wilson R, et al. Long-term effectiveness of cholecystectomy and endoscopic sphincterotomy in the management of gallstone pancreatitis. *Surg Endosc*. 2014; 28: 127-133. PMID: 23982647.
7. Fan JH, Qian JB, Wang YM, Shi RH, Zhao CJ. Updated meta-analysis of pancreatic stent placement in preventing post-endoscopic retrograde cholangiopancreatography pancreatitis. *World J Gastroenterol*. 2015; 21: 7577-7583. PMID: 26140006.
8. Grisellius H. Misc cur Med phys Acad etc. *Ann*. 1681; III: 65.
9. Bernard C. Lecons de physiologie experimentale. *Paris Bailliere*. 1856; 2: 758.
10. Acosta JM, Ledesma CL. Gallstone migration as a cause of acute pancreatitis. *N Engl J Med*. 1974; 290: 484-487. PMID: 4810815.
11. Opie E. The relation of cholelithiasis to disease of the pancreas and to fat necrosis. *Johns Hopkins Hosp Bull*. 1901; 12: 19-21.

12. Opie E. The etiology of acute hemorrhagic pancreatitis. *John Hopkins Hosp Bull.* 1901; 12: 182-188.
13. Neoptolemos JP. The theory of 'persisting' common bile duct stones in severe gallstone pancreatitis. *Ann R Coll Surg Engl.* 1989; 71: 326-331. PMID: 2802482.
14. Lerch MM, Saluja AK, Runzi M, Dawra R, Saluja M, Steer ML. Pancreatic duct obstruction triggers acute necrotizing pancreatitis in the opossum. *Gastroenterology.* 1993; 104: 853-861. PMID: 7680018.
15. DiMagno EP, Shorter RG, Taylor WF, Go VL. Relationships between pancreaticobiliary ductal anatomy and pancreatic ductal and parenchymal histology. *Cancer.* 1982; 49: 361-368. PMID: 7032685.
16. Mann FC, Giordano AS. The bile factor in pancreatitis. *Arch Surg.* 1923; 6: 1-30.
17. Carr-Locke DL, Gregg JA. Endoscopic manometry of pancreatic and biliary sphincter zones in man. Basal results in healthy volunteers. *Dig Dis Sci.* 1981; 26: 7-15. PMID: 7460708.
18. Menguy RB, Hallenbeck GA, Bollman JL, Grindlay JH. Intraductal pressures and sphincteric resistance in canine pancreatic and biliary ducts after various stimuli. *Surg Gynecol Obstet.* 1958; 106: 306-320. PMID: 13519371.
19. McCutcheon AD. Reflux of duodenal contents in the pathogenesis of pancreatitis. *Gut.* 1964; 5: 260-265. PMID: 14178712.
20. Hernandez CA, Lerch MM. Sphincter stenosis and gallstone migration through the biliary tract. *Lancet.* 1993; 341: 1371-1373. PMID: 8098791.
21. Robinson TM, Dunphy JE. Continuous perfusion of bile and protease activators through the pancreas. *JAMA.* 1963; 183: 530-533. PMID: 13974478.
22. Arendt T, Nizze H, Monig H, Kloehn S, Stuber E, Folsch UR. Biliary pancreatic reflux-induced acute pancreatitis--myth or possibility? *Eur J Gastroenterol Hepatol.* 1999; 11: 329-335. PMID: 10333208.
23. Csendes A, Sepúlveda A, Burdiles P, Braghetto I, Bastias J, Schütte H, et al. Common bile duct pressure in patients with common bile duct stones with or without acute suppurative cholangitis. *Arch Surg.* 1988; 123: 697-699. PMID: 3369934.
24. Lerch MM, Saluja AK, Dawra R, Ramarao P, Saluja M, Steer ML. Acute necrotizing pancreatitis in the opossum: earliest morphological changes involve acinar cells. *Gastroenterology.* 1992; 103: 205-213. PMID: 1612327.
25. Lerch MM, Weidenbach H, Hernandez CA, Preclik G, Adler G. Pancreatic outflow obstruction as the critical event for human gall stone induced pancreatitis. *Gut.* 1994; 35: 1501-1503. PMID: 7959214.
26. Pohle T, Konturek JW, Domschke W, Lerch MM. Spontaneous flow of bile through the human pancreatic duct in the absence of pancreatitis: nature's human experiment. *Endoscopy.* 2003; 35: 1072-1075. PMID: 14648423.
27. Mooren F, Hlouschek V, Finkes T, Turi S, Weber IA, Singh J, et al. Early changes in pancreatic acinar cell calcium signaling after pancreatic duct obstruction. *J Biol Chem.* 2003; 278: 9361-9369. PMID: 12522141.
28. Schick V, Scheiber JA, Mooren FC, Turi S, Ceyhan GO, Schnekenburger J, et al. Effect of magnesium supplementation and depletion on the onset and course of acute experimental pancreatitis. *Gut.* 2014; 63: 1469-1480. PMID: 24277728.
29. Mooren FC, Turi S, Gunzel D, Schlue WR, Domschke W, Singh J, et al. Calcium-magnesium interactions in pancreatic acinar cells. *FASEB J.* 2001; 15: 659-672. PMID: 11259384.
30. Fluhr G, Mayerle J, Weber E, Aghdassi A, Simon P, Gress T, et al. Pre-study protocol MagPEP: a multicentre randomized controlled trial of magnesium sulphate in the prevention of post-ERCP pancreatitis. *BMC Gastroenterol.* 2013; 13: 11. PMID: 23320650.
31. Lerch MM, Gorelick FS. Models of acute and chronic pancreatitis. *Gastroenterology.* 2013; 144: 1180-1193. PMID: 23622127.
32. Halangk W, Lerch MM, Brandt-Nedelev B, Roth W, Ruthenbuerger M, Reinheckel T, et al. Role of cathepsin B in intracellular trypsinogen activation and the onset of acute pancreatitis. *J Clin Invest.* 2000; 106: 773-781. PMID: 10995788.
33. Kruger B, Albrecht E, Lerch MM. The role of intracellular calcium signaling in premature protease activation and the onset of pancreatitis. *Am J Pathol.* 2000; 157: 43-50. PMID: 10880374.
34. Lerch MM, Saluja AK, Runzi M, Dawra R, Steer ML. Luminal endocytosis and intracellular targeting by acinar cells during early biliary pancreatitis in the opossum. *J Clin Invest.* 1995; 95: 2222-2231. PMID: 7537759.
35. Hirano T, Saluja A, Ramarao P, Lerch MM, Saluja M, Steer ML. Apical secretion of lysosomal enzymes in rabbit pancreas occurs via a secretagogue regulated pathway and is increased after pancreatic duct obstruction. *J Clin Invest.* 1991; 87: 865-869. PMID: 1705567.
36. Senninger N, Moody FG, Coelho JC, Van Buren DH. The role of biliary obstruction in the pathogenesis of acute pancreatitis in the opossum. *Surgery.* 1986; 99: 688-693. PMID: 2424109.
37. Lerch MM, Aghdassi AA. The role of bile acids in gallstone-induced pancreatitis. *Gastroenterology.* 2010; 138: 429-433. PMID: 20034603.
38. Voronina S, Longbottom R, Sutton R, Petersen OH, Tepikin A. Bile acids induce calcium signals in mouse pancreatic acinar cells: implications for bile-induced pancreatic pathology. *J Physiol.* 2002; 540 Pt 1: 49-55. PMID: 11927668.
39. Kim JY, Kim KH, Lee JA, Namkung W, Sun AQ, Ananthanarayanan M, et al. Transporter-mediated bile acid uptake causes Ca^{2+}-dependent cell death in rat pancreatic acinar cells. *Gastroenterology.* 2002; 122: 1941-1953. PMID: 12055600.
40. Fischer L, Gukovskaya AS, Penninger JM, Mareninova OA, Friess H, Gukovsky I, et al. Phosphatidylinositol 3-kinase facilitates bile acid-induced Ca^{2+} responses in pancreatic acinar cells. *Am J Physiol Gastrointest Liver Physiol.* 2007; 292: G875-G886. PMID: 17158252.
41. Voronina SG, Barrow SL, Gerasimenko OV, Petersen OH, Tepikin AV. Effects of secretagogues and bile acids on mitochondrial membrane potential of pancreatic acinar cells: comparison of different modes of evaluating DeltaPsim. *J Biol Chem.* 2004; 279: 27327-27338. PMID: 15084611.
42. Barrow SL, Voronina SG, da Silva Xavier G, Chvanov MA, Longbottom RE, Gerasimenko OV, et al. ATP depletion inhibits Ca^{2+} release, influx and extrusion in pancreatic acinar cells but not pathological Ca^{2+} responses induced by bile. *Pflugers Arch.* 2008; 455: 1025-1039. PMID: 17952455.

43. Voronina SG, Gryshchenko OV, Gerasimenko OV, Green AK, Petersen OH, Tepikin AV. Bile acids induce a cationic current, depolarizing pancreatic acinar cells and increasing the intracellular Na^+ concentration. *J Biol Chem*. 2005; 280: 1764-1770. PMID: 15536077.
44. Perides G, Laukkarinen JM, Vassileva G, Steer ML. Biliary acute pancreatitis in mice is mediated by the G-protein-coupled cell surface bile acid receptor Gpbar1. *Gastroenterology*. 2010; 138: 715-725. PMID: 19900448.
45. Vassileva G, Golovko A, Markowitz L, Abbondanzo SJ, Zeng M, Yang S, et al. Targeted deletion of Gpbar1 protects mice from cholesterol gallstone formation. *Biochem J*. 2006; 398: 423-430. PMID: 16724960.
46. Wartmann T, Mayerle J, Kahne T, Sahin-Toth M, Ruthenburger M, Matthias R, et al. Cathepsin L inactivates human trypsinogen, whereas cathepsin L-deletion reduces the severity of pancreatitis in mice. *Gastroenterology*. 2010; 138: 726-737. PMID: 19900452.
47. Maleth J, Balazs A, Pallagi P, Balla Z, Kui B, Katona M, et al. Alcohol disrupts levels and function of the cystic fibrosis transmembrane conductance regulator to promote development of pancreatitis. *Gastroenterology*. 2015; 148: 427-439. PMID: 25447846.
48. Pallagi P, Venglovecz V, Rakonczay Z Jr, Borka K, Korompay A, Ozsvari B, et al. Trypsin reduces pancreatic ductal bicarbonate secretion by inhibiting CFTR Cl^- channels and luminal anion exchangers. *Gastroenterology*. 2011; 141: 2228-2239. PMID: 21893120.
49. Lerch MM, Saluja AK, Dawra R, Saluja M, Steer ML. The effect of chloroquine administration on two experimental models of acute pancreatitis. *Gastroenterology*. 1993; 104: 1768-1779. PMID: 8500736.
50. Noble MD, Romac J, Vigna SR, Liddle RA. A pH-sensitive, neurogenic pathway mediates disease severity in a model of post-ERCP pancreatitis. *Gut*. 2008; 57: 1566-1571. PMID: 18625695.

Chapter 18

Alcohol-related mechanisms of acute pancreatitis: The roles of mitochondrial dysfunction and endoplasmic reticulum stress

David N. Criddle[1*], Richard Waldron[2], Aurelia Lugea[2], and Stephen Pandol[2]

[1]*Department of Cellular and Molecular Physiology, Institute of Translational Medicine and NIHR Liverpool Pancreas Biomedical Research Unit, University of Liverpool, UK;*
[2]*Department of Medicine, Cedars-Sinai Medical Center, University of California and Department of Veterans Affairs, Los Angeles, California, USA.*

Introduction

Excessive alcohol consumption is a major contributor to diverse pathologies with an estimated 4 in 100 deaths worldwide caused by alcohol according to the World Health Organization.[1] The close association between alcohol consumption and acute pancreatitis (AP) has been recognized for a long time, with Friedrich first describing the *Drunkard's Pancreas* in 1878, although elevated intake of alcohol had been linked to pancreatic disease a century earlier.[2] More recently, a Danish population-based cohort study reported an increased risk of AP in individuals who consumed in excess of 14 drinks per week, irrespective of beverage type or intake frequency.[3] A subsequent meta-analysis found an elevated risk of AP in those imbibing more than four drinks per day.[4] Despite the recognized risk of AP increasing with alcohol intake, its basis remains incompletely understood, and no specific therapy exists.[5] Intriguingly, some individuals appear more susceptible to developing AP linked to excess alcohol consumption than others, with <10% of heavy drinkers developing clinical disease. However, this phenomenon has no clear explanation and is clearly an important area for investigation. Progress in elucidating the pathophysiology of alcoholic AP has been complicated by the fact that alcohol alone does not reliably induce AP in experimental animal models, with additional factors required to model alcohol-induced pancreatic inflammation and damage, including cerulein, lipopolysaccharide, and ductal obstruction that may not accurately reflect the clinical situation.[6] Direct sensitizing actions of ethanol are thought to contribute to damaging effects including activation of nuclear factor-κB in pancreatic acinar cells via the ε isoform of protein kinase C and activation of cholinergic pathways.[7-9] Recent work has focused on the way in which alcohol metabolism may be involved in mediating pancreatic toxicity.

Ethanol Metabolism

Ethanol is metabolized in the pancreas by both oxidative and nonoxidative routes.[10,11] Current evidence indicates that both pathways are likely to contribute to the detrimental effects of alcohol on the exocrine pancreas via distinct mechanisms that ultimately compromise mitochondrial function.[12-15] Oxidative metabolism proceeds through several nicotinamide adenine dinucleotide (NAD^+)-consuming steps performed by alcohol and aldehyde dehydrogenases (ADH and ALDH) that generate acetaldehyde and acetate, respectively. Recent findings have suggested that ethanol induces mitochondrial dysfunction by reducing the ratio of oxidized to reduced nicotinamide adenine dinucleotide, a mechanism distinct from the effects of cholecystokinin hyperstimulation that are mediated by increasing cytosolic calcium ($[Ca^{2+}]_c$).[13,16]

In contrast to oxidative metabolism of ethanol (OME), nonoxidative metabolism of ethanol (NOME) promotes esterification of fatty acids to yield highly lipophilic fatty acid ethyl esters (FAEEs) via FAEE synthases including carboxylester lipase (CEL). FAEE synthase activity occurs in the human pancreas at rates of up to 54 nmol/min/g tissue, generating high localized levels of FAEEs.[17] An autopsy study showed that individuals who died of acute alcohol intoxication had preferentially elevated FAEEs in the pancreas in contrast to other organs commonly damaged by alcohol such as the heart and lungs,[18] suggesting the importance of NOME in pancreatic damage. In vivo studies in rats subsequently confirmed that saturated FAEEs induced

*Corresponding author. Email: criddle@liverpool.ac.uk

pancreatic damage indicative of AP.[19] Furthermore, administration of ethanol under conditions of OME inhibition generated plasma and tissue FAEEs and AP development.[20] Early (<15 min) redistribution of CEL into the cytosol from a predominantly apical, granular localization within the pancreatic acinar cell occurs following in vivo administration of fat and alcohol to a mouse model of alcoholic AP (FAEE-AP).[21] Furthermore, CEL inhibition blocked FAEE generation and ameliorated the detrimental effects of fat and alcohol.[21] In AP patients, elevated CEL is detectable in necrotic pancreatic lobules and areas of fat necrosis,[22] consistent with localized generation of toxic FAEEs in damaged areas. In pancreatic acinar cells, FAEEs release Ca^{2+} from the endoplasmic reticulum (ER) via stimulation of inositol trisphosphate (IP_3) receptors, depleting internal Ca^{2+} stores that led to store-operated Ca^{2+} entry (SOCE), promoting toxic, sustained elevations of $[Ca^{2+}]_C$ and eventually necrotic cell death.[12,14,23] Furthermore, FAEEs underwent hydrolysis to fatty acids in the mitochondria causing a localized elevation that compromised mitochondrial function.[12,24,25] Pharmacologic inhibition of hydrolase enzymes significantly reduced necrosis induced by a fat and alcohol combination, highlighting the importance of fatty acid release in the mitochondria to cellular damage.[23] Diverse actions of FAEEs have been reported in the pancreas, including increased lysosome fragility and inhibition of serine proteases that may predispose to fibrogenesis and impaired pancreas recovery after organ damage in chronic injury.[26-28]

Recent progress in understanding the basis of alcohol-induced damage has highlighted the importance of organellar dysfunction within the pancreatic acinar cell as central for AP initiation. In particular, the involvement of mitochondria and the ER, two organelles that are intimately linked spatially and functionally together modulate cellular Ca^{2+} homeostasis, energy production, and lipid and protein synthesis (**Figure 1**).[29-31]

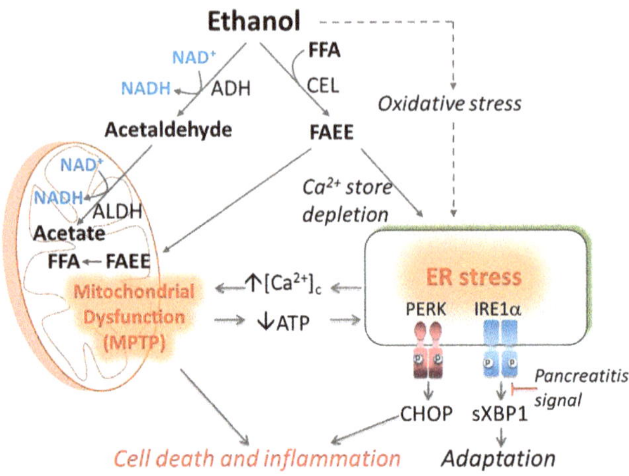

Figure 1. A schematic diagram displaying proposed mechanisms of ethanol-mediated AP. In the pancreatic acinar cell, ethanol can compromise mitochondrial function via two pathways. Oxidative metabolism of ethanol to acetaldehyde, via alcohol dehydrogenase (ADH), and to acetate, via aldehyde dehydrogenase (ALDH) in the mitochondria, decreases cellular NAD^+/NADH balance. Fatty acid ethyl esters (FAEEs) are esterification products of fatty acids and ethanol via FAEE synthases including carboxylester lipase (CEL). FAEE accumulation elicits Ca^{2+} depletion from the endoplasmic reticulum (ER) and other cellular stores leading to sustained elevations of $[Ca^{2+}]_c$ and mitochondrial Ca^{2+} overload. Furthermore, FAEE accumulation in mitochondria leads to the release of fatty acids via the action of hydrolases, which compromises organellar function. Both altered NAD^+/NADH ratios and $[Ca^{2+}]_c$ overload have been proposed to elicit opening of the mitochondrial permeability transition pore (MPTP), which results in mitochondrial depolarization, ATP depletion, and cellular necrosis. Besides ethanol effects on mitochondria, ethanol-induced oxidative stress alters ER redox status (not shown) and elicits chronic ER stress, an effect that can be exacerbated by FAEE-induced ER-Ca^{2+} depletion and compromised ATP production. ER stress is manifested by activation of adaptive IRE1/XBP1 signaling that aids to preserve ER function and protein processing through the secretory pathway. However, severe ethanol-induced cellular damage or additional toxic pancreatitis signaling can compromise cellular adaptation, leading to termination of protective XBP1 signaling and upregulation of cell death pathways downstream of mitochondria and PERK/CHOP signaling, and ultimately to pancreatitis.

Mitochondrial Dysfunction in Alcoholic Acute Pancreatitis

Mitochondria perform a variety of tasks in the pancreatic acinar cell, the most important being provision of energy for cellular processes including the secretion of inactive digestive enzyme precursors. To do this effectively, mitochondria respond to oscillatory rises of $[Ca^{2+}]_C$ induced by hormonal (cholecystokinin) and neuronal (acetylcholine) stimulation,[32-34] by generating NADH via stimulation of Ca^{2+}-dependent dehydrogenases of the Krebs cycle, that feeds into the electron transport chain to promote ATP production. Additionally, mitochondria are thought to constitute a protective perigranular buffer barrier that impedes movement of excessive Ca^{2+} released from the apical pole to the basolateral region where the nucleus resides.[35] However, when sustained rises of $[Ca^{2+}]_C$ occur in pancreatic acinar cells in response to aberrant Ca^{2+} signals induced by diverse AP precipitants including CCK hyperstimulation, bile salts, and ethanol metabolites, mitochondrial dysfunction ensues that leads to rundown of ATP production and induction of cellular necrosis.[23,36-38]

Recent evidence has shown that the trigger for mitochondrial dysfunction in AP is the opening of the mitochondrial permeability transition pore (MPTP),[13,15] which permeabilizes the inner mitochondrial membrane allowing free movement of substances up to 1.5 kDa in and out of the organelle. MPTP formation thus leads to collapse of membrane potential, dissipating the proton gradient necessary for ATP production. Although the exact composition of the pore remains controversial, recent evidence has indicated that it may be a dimer of the F_0/F_1-ATP synthase.[39,40] In response to AP precipitants in both human and murine pancreatic acinar cells, Ca^{2+}-dependent MPTP formation is a consequence of IP_3- and ryanodine receptor-mediated intracellular Ca^{2+} release and subsequent SOCE; diminished ATP production leads to impaired Ca^{2+} clearance, defective autophagy, zymogen activation, cytokine production, phosphoglycerate mutase 5 activation, and necrosis.[15] The crucial role played by compromised intracellular ATP levels as a result of mitochondrial dysfunction has been shown in studies in which the detrimental effects of AP toxins including nonoxidative ethanol metabolites were prevented by intracellular ATP supplementation in isolated pancreatic acinar cells, allowing energy-dependent Ca^{2+} extrusion pumps to reduce $[Ca^{2+}]_C$ and maintain homeostasis.[12,15,41] The mitochondrial matrix protein peptidyl-prolyl cis-trans isomerase cyclophilin D (CypD) plays a pivotal role in modulating the MPTP; all biochemical, immunological and histopathologic responses of AP in four experimental models, including alcoholic (FAEE-AP), were reduced or abolished by genetic deletion or pharmacological modulation of this protein,[15] suggesting the potential of CypD inhibitors for translational therapy.

Endoplasmic Reticulum Responses with Alcohol

The ER of the pancreatic acinar cell plays a predominant role in cellular function as protein synthesis and transport are highly developed in this cell. It is not surprising then that the ER responds to alcohol. A previous study showed that exposure of pancreatic acinar cells to ethanol induced a slow, gradual release of Ca^{2+} from the ER.[23] The ER translates mRNA into newly synthesized proteins in its lumen and performs several posttranslational modifications including disulfide bond formation facilitated by chaperone-mediated protein folding and glycosylation. Correctly folded and otherwise modified proteins are directed to specific cellular organelles. As an example, digestive enzyme proteins are segregated into the secretory pathway and end up in zymogen granules that undergo exocytosis and secretion with neurohormonal stimulation. As another example, acid hydrolases are glycosylated with mannose-6-phosphate, which is necessary for their transport to the lysosome.

In general, protein folding is accomplished in the ER by molecular chaperones and folding enzymes that include disulfide isomerases and oxidoreductases. There is also a quality control mechanism that disposes of improperly processed proteins by proteasomal degradation. This process is called ER-associated degradation (ERAD). Autophagy also participates in the degrading of dysfunctional ER and damaged or misfolded proteins to prevent cellular toxicity that these proteins may cause.[42,43]

To adjust to changing demands encountered by the ER, protein synthesis, and processing machinery including ethanol and its metabolism, eukaryotic cells have developed a complex signaling system referred to as the unfolded protein response (UPR). Activation of the UPR occurs when unfolded or misfolded proteins accumulate in the ER lumen, a phenomenon termed "ER stress".[44] This event has several sources including a physiologic increase in the demand for protein folding, decreased chaperone function, accumulation of permanently misfolded proteins due to mutation, decreases in cellular ATP levels or a fall in Ca^{2+} in the ER ($[Ca^{2+}]_{ER}$), and perturbed ER redox status that occurs with alcohol metabolism.[45,46] Interestingly, the nonoxidative ethanol metabolites palmitoleic acid ethyl ester and palmitoleic acid, which are released by hydrolysis of its parent FAEE,[21] cause complete depletion of $[Ca^{2+}]_{ER}$ and concomitant falls of NADH and cellular ATP (**Figure 1**).[12,23] Also, the folding process itself generates reactive oxygen species that themselves can cause aberrant disulfide bond formation (i.e., misfolding). Thus, in the case of a continuous misfolding stress as occurs with mutation or possibly ethanol metabolism, there will be greater ER stress than would occur during a transient increase in unfolded proteins as a consequence of the need to replenish zymogen stores.

The UPR has three major response systems to ER stress: a global reduction in mRNA translation that attenuates the demand for protein processing, increased expression of chaperones and foldases and greater phospholipid synthesis to expand the functional ER network, and activation of the ERAD and autophagic systems to eliminate misfolded and aberrant proteins.[43,44,47-49] These responses are accomplished by identified sensing and signaling systems including Inositol-requiring protein-1α (IRE1α), activating transcription factor-6 (ATF6), and RNA-activated protein kinase (PKR)-like ER kinase (PERK).[43,44,47-49]

Regarding alcohol-induced ER stress, we found a key role for IRE1α in preventing damage to the exocrine pancreas.[46,50] Upon its activation, endonuclease activity within IRE1α splices X-box binding protein-1 (XBP1) mRNA to yield a shorter mRNA (spliced XBP1, sXBP1 mRNA) that encodes the active transcription factor sXBP1. sXBP1 regulates a broad spectrum of genes involved in protein folding, including chaperones, disulfide isomerases, and oxidoreductases, as well as genes for protein degradation (ERAD), lipid biosynthesis for ER/Golgi biogenesis, vesicular trafficking, and redox metabolism.[49,51] In the exocrine pancreas, sXBP1 is especially necessary for acinar cell homeostasis and function.[51] The critical importance of sXBP1 for pancreatic acinar cell function is supported by studies of *Xbp1*$^{+/-}$ mice[46,52] and acinar cell-specific *Xbp1* null mice.[51,53] XBP1 deficiency results in defective stimulated secretory response, extensive acinar cell loss, and inflammation, as well as severe pathology in the remaining acinar cells as evidenced by reduced levels of ER chaperones, a poorly developed ER network and secretory system, marked reductions in zymogen granules and digestive enzymes, and accumulation of autophagic vacuoles.[52,53]

Ethanol feeding in rodents induces structural changes in the acinar cell consistent with ER stress, such as ER dilation, mitochondrial swelling, and some disorganization of cellular organelles.[46,54,55] However, like humans, chronic ethanol-fed animals do not develop pancreatitis unless challenged with other toxic factors.[56-58] We found that pancreatic mRNA and protein levels of sXBP1 were significantly increased in mouse and rats fed ethanol-containing diets.[46] To determine whether sXBP1 upregulation by alcohol feeding is necessary to maintain homeostasis and prevent pancreatitis, we used *Xbp1* heterozygous mice (*Xbp*$^{+/-}$). Compared to ethanol-fed wild-type mice (*Xbp1*$^{+/+}$), histological analysis of pancreatic tissue in ethanol-fed *Xbp1*$^{+/-}$ mice revealed morphologic features of severe ER stress such as disorganized and dilated ER, accumulation of dense material within the ER, and a reduced number of mature zymogen granules. These features were accompanied by accumulation of autophagic vacuoles and activation of apoptotic signals including upregulation of CHOP (see below) within patchy areas of inflammatory pancreatitis.[46,52] Moreover, recent studies indicate that cerulein-induced AP is more severe in XBP1-deficient mice than controls (unpublished observations). Collectively, the evidence indicates that alcohol feeding activates an adaptive and protective UPR through increased expression of sXBP1 involving activation of the endonuclease activity of IRE1α. Furthermore, these actions of the UPR are necessary to prevent ethanol-induced cellular toxicity.

Whereas IRE1α/XBP1 signaling primarily mediates adaptive responses to protect ER function, it can be prematurely attenuated during severe or prolonged ER stress, resulting in upregulation of proapoptotic cell death mediated through the transcription factor C/EBP homologous protein (CHOP).[59] Also, genetic inhibition of Xbp1 is unequivocally associated with potent upregulation of CHOP and cell death.[46,51] On the other hand, forced and sustained IRE1α/XBP1 activity enhances cell survival in conditions of severe stress,[59] further supporting a protective role for sXBP1 signaling.

The PERK UPR branch has a dual role. Upon activation it rapidly adjusts the cell to ER stress by mediating a general attenuation of protein synthesis.[44,60-62] On the other hand, sustained activation leads to upregulation of the transcription factor activating transcription factor 4 (ATF4) that targets genes involved in antioxidant activities including glutathione synthesis[63] and CHOP, which promotes ER stress-related cell death responses.[64] CHOP also promotes inflammation by regulating cytokine production and promoting inflammatory cell survival.[65,66] In summary, although PERK activation can play a transient protective role, unresolved ER stresses upregulate CHOP and promote inflammation and pancreatitis.

Conclusions

This chapter reviews two bodies of work related to alcohol's effects on the exocrine pancreas. One addresses mitochondrial functional changes and the other ER responses, phenomena that may be interrelated in AP (**Figure 1**). Alcohol-induced disorders of both organelles make the pancreas susceptible to alcohol-induced injury, and recent advances suggest the potential for translational therapy. Interestingly, there are some protective responses from the ER UPR that may be one reason why only a minority of drinkers develops pancreatitis.

Acknowledgement

Support was provided by MRC grant KO12967; the NIHR Biomedical Research Unit funding scheme; NIH grants P01DK098108, P50AA011999, and R01AA019954; and the Department of Veterans Affairs.

References

1. Zarocostas J. Four in 100 deaths worldwide are caused by alcohol, says WHO. *Br Med J*. 2011; 342: d1032. PMID: 2321011.
2. Cawley TA. A singular case of diabetes, consisting entirely in the quantity of urine with an enquiry into the different theories of that disease. *Lond Med J*. 1788; 9: 286.
3. Kristiansen L, Grønbaek M, Becker U, Tolstrup JS. Risk of pancreatitis according to alcohol drinking habits: a population-based cohort study. *Am J Epidemiol*. 2008; 168(8): 932-937. PMID: 18779386
4. Irving HM, Samokhvalov AV, Rehm J. Alcohol as a risk factor for pancreatitis. A systematic review and meta-analysis. *JOP*. 2009; 10(4): 387-392. PMID: 19581740.
5. Pandol SJ, Saluja AK, Imrie CW, Banks PA. Acute pancreatitis: bench to the bedside. *Gastroenterology*. 2007; 133(3): 1056-1056. PMID: 17383433.
6. Lerch MM, Gorelick FS. Models of acute and chronic pancreatitis. *Gastroenterology*. 2013; 144(6): 1180-1193. PMID: 23622127.
7. Pandol SJ, Lugea A, Mareninova OA, Smoot D, Gorelick FS, Gukovskaya AS, et al. Investigating the pathobiology of alcoholic pancreatitis. *Alcohol Clin Exp Res*. 2011; 35(5): 830-837. PMID: 21284675.
8. Satoh A, Gukovskaya AS, Reeve JR Jr, Shimosegawa T, Pandol SJ. Ethanol sensitizes NF-kappaB activation in pancreatic acinar cells through effects on protein kinase C-epsilon. *Am J Physiol Gastrointest Liver Physiol*. 2006; 291(3): G432-G438. PMID: 16574982.
9. Lugea A, Gong J, Nguyen J, Nieto J, French SW, Pandol SJ. Cholinergic mediation of alcohol-induced experimental pancreatitis. *Alcohol Clin Exp Res*. 2010; 34(10): 1768-1781. PMID: 20626730.
10. Criddle DN. The role of fat and alcohol in acute pancreatitis: A dangerous liaison. *Pancreatology*. 2015; 15(4 Suppl): S6-S12. PMID: 25845855.
11. Gukovskaya AS, Mouria M, Gukovsky I, Reyes CN, Kasho VN, Faller LD, et al. Ethanol metabolism and

transcription factor activation in pancreatic acinar cells in rats. *Gastroenterology*. 2002; 122(1): 106-118. PMID: 11781286.

12. Criddle DN, Murphy J, Fistetto G, Barrow S, Tepikin AV, Neoptolemos JP, et al. Fatty acid ethyl esters cause pancreatic calcium toxicity via inositol trisphosphate receptors and loss of ATP synthesis. *Gastroenterology*. 2006; 130(3): 781-793. PMID: 16530519.
13. Shalbueva N, Mareninova OA, Gerloff A, Yuan J, Waldron RT, Pandol SJ, et al. Effects of oxidative alcohol metabolism on the mitochondrial permeability transition pore and necrosis in a mouse model of alcoholic pancreatitis. *Gastroenterology*. 2013; 144(2): 437-446.e6. PMID: 23103769.
14. Criddle DN, Gerasimenko JV, Baumgartner HK, Jaffar M, Voronina S, Sutton R, et al. Calcium signalling and pancreatic cell death: apoptosis or necrosis? *Cell Death Differ*. 2007; 14(7): 1285-1294. PMID: 17431416.
15. Mukherjee R, Mareninova OA, Odinokova IV, Huang W, Murphy J, Chvanov M, et al. Mechanism of mitochondrial permeability transition pore induction and damage in the pancreas: inhibition prevents acute pancreatitis by protecting production of ATP. *Gut*. 2015 Jun 12 [Epub ahead of print]. PMID: 26071131.
16. Raraty M, Ward J, Erdemli G, Vaillant C, Neoptolemos JP, Sutton R, et al. Calcium-dependent enzyme activation and vacuole formation in the apical granular region of pancreatic acinar cells. *Proc Natl Acad Sci U S A*. 2000; 97(24): 13126-13131. PMID: 11087863.
17. Diczfalusy MA, Bjorkhem I, Einarsson C, Hillebrant CG, Alexson SE. Characterization of enzymes involved in formation of ethyl esters of long-chain fatty acids in humans. *J Lipid Res*. 2001; 42(7): 1025-1032. PMID: 11441128.
18. Laposata EA, Lange LG. Presence of nonoxidative ethanol metabolism in human organs commonly damaged by ethanol abuse. *Science*. 1986; 231(4737): 497-499. PMID: 3941913.
19. Werner J, Laposata M, Fernandez-del Castillo C, Saghir M, Iozzo RV, Lewandrowski KB, et al. Pancreatic injury in rats induced by fatty acid ethyl ester, a nonoxidative metabolite of alcohol. *Gastroenterology*. 1997; 113(1): 286-294. PMID: 11850500.
20. Werner J, Saghir M, Warshaw AL, Lewandrowski KB, Laposata M, Iozzo RV, et al. Alcoholic pancreatitis in rats: injury from nonoxidative metabolites of ethanol. *Am J Physiol Gastrointest Liver Physiol*. 2002; 283(1): G65-G73. PMID: 12065293.
21. Huang W, Booth DM, Cane MC, Chvanov M, Javed MA, Elliott VL, et al. Fatty acid ethyl ester synthase inhibition ameliorates ethanol-induced Ca^{2+}-dependent mitochondrial dysfunction and acute pancreatitis. *Gut*. 2014; 63(8): 1313-1324. PMID: 24162590.
22. Aho HJ, Sternby B, Kallajoki M, Nevalainen TJ. Carboxyl ester lipase in human tissues and in acute pancreatitis. *Int J Pancreatol*. 1989; 5(2): 123-134. PMID: 2689525.
23. Criddle DN, Raraty MG, Neoptolemos JP, Tepikin AV, Petersen OH, Sutton R. Ethanol toxicity in pancreatic acinar cells: mediation by nonoxidative fatty acid metabolites. *Proc Natl Acad Sci U S A*. 2004; 101(29): 10738-10743. PMID: 15247419.
24. Huang W, Cash N, Wen L, Szatmary P, Mukherjee R, Armstrong J, et al. Effects of the mitochondria-targeted antioxidant mitoquinone in murine acute pancreatitis. *Mediators Inflamm*. 2015; 2015: 901780. PMID: 25878403.
25. Lange LG, Sobel BE. Mitochondrial dysfunction induced by fatty acid ethyl esters, myocardial metabolites of ethanol. *J Clin Invest*. 1983; 72(2): 724-731. PMID: 6308061.
26. Haber PS, Wilson JS, Apte MV, Pirola RC. Fatty acid ethyl esters increase rat pancreatic lysosomal fragility. *J Lab Clin Med*. 1993; 121(6): 759-764. PMID: 8505587.
27. Lugea A, Gukovsky I, Gukovskaya AS, Pandol SJ. Nonoxidative ethanol metabolites alter extracellular matrix protein content in rat pancreas. *Gastroenterology*. 2003; 125(6): 1845-1859. PMID: 14724836.
28. Lugea A, Nan L, French SW, Bezerra JA, Gukovskaya AS, Pandol SJ. Pancreas recovery following cerulein-induced pancreatitis is impaired in plasminogen-deficient mice. *Gastroenterology*. 2006; 131(3): 885-899. PMID: 16952557.
29. Johnson PR, Dolman NJ, Pope M, Vaillant C, Petersen OH, Tepikin AV, et al. Non-uniform distribution of mitochondria in pancreatic acinar cells. *Cell Tissue Res*. 2003; 313(1): 37-45. PMID: 12838407.
30. Csordas G, Thomas AP, Hajnoczky G. Quasi-synaptic calcium signal transmission between endoplasmic reticulum and mitochondria. *EMBO J*. 1999; 18(1): 96-108. PMID: 9878054.
31. Rizzuto R, Pinton P, Carrington W, Fay FS, Fogarty KE, Lifshitz LM, et al. Close contacts with the endoplasmic reticulum as determinants of mitochondrial Ca^{2+} responses. *Science*. 1988; 280(5370): 1763-1766. PMID: 9624056.
32. Murphy JA, Criddle DN, Sherwood M, Chvanov M, Mukherjee R, McLaughlin E, et al. Direct activation of cytosolic Ca^{2+} signaling and enzyme secretion by cholecystokinin in human pancreatic acinar cells. *Gastroenterology*. 2008; 135(2): 632-641. PMID: 18555802.
33. Criddle DN, Booth DM, Mukherjee R, McLaughlin E, Green GM, Sutton R, et al. Cholecystokinin-58 and cholecystokinin-8 exhibit similar actions on calcium signaling, zymogen secretion, and cell fate in murine pancreatic acinar cells. *Am J Physiol Gastrointest Liver Physiol*. 2009; 297(6): G1085-G1092. PMID: 19815626.
34. Voronina S, Sukhomlin T, Johnson PR, Erdemli G, Petersen OH, Tepikin A. Correlation of NADH and Ca^{2+} signals in mouse pancreatic acinar cells. *J Physiol*. 2002; 539(Pt 1): 41-52. PMID: 11850500.
35. Petersen OH, Tepikin AV. Polarized calcium signaling in exocrine gland cells. *Ann Rev Physiol*. 2008; 70(1): 273-299. PMID: 17850212.
36. Criddle DN, Gerasimenko JV, Baumgartner HK, Jaffar M, Voronina S, Sutton R, et al. Calcium signalling and pancreatic cell death: apoptosis or necrosis? *Cell Death Differ*. 2007; 14(7): 1285-1294. PMID: 17431416.
37. Mukherjee R, Criddle DN, Gukvoskaya A, Pandol S, Petersen OH, Sutton R. Mitochondrial injury in pancreatitis. *Cell Calcium*. 2008; 44(1): 14-23. PMID: 18207570.
38. Gukovsky I, Pandol SJ, Gukovskaya AS. Organellar dysfunction in the pathogenesis of pancreatitis. *Antioxid Redox Signal*. 2011; 15(10): 2699-2710. PMID: 21834686.
39. Giorgio V, von Stockum S, Antoniel M, Fabbro A, Fogolari F, Forte M, et al. Dimers of mitochondrial ATP synthase

form the permeability transition pore. *Proc Natl Acad Sci U S A*. 2013; 110(15): 5887-5892. PMID: 23530243.

40. Bonora M, Bononi A, De Marchi E, Giorgi C, Lebiedzinska M, Marchi S, et al. Role of the c subunit of the FO ATP synthase in mitochondrial permeability transition. *Cell Cycle*. 2013; 12(4): 674-683. PMID: 23343770.
41. Booth DM, Murphy JA, Mukherjee R, Awais M, Neoptolemos JP, Gerasimenko OV, et al. Reactive oxygen species induced by bile acid induce apoptosis and protect against necrosis in pancreatic acinar cells. *Gastroenterology*. 2011; 140(7): 2116-2125. PMID: 21354148.
42. Direnzo D, Hess DA, Damsz B, Hallet JE, Marshall B, Goswami C, et al. Induced mist1 expression promotes remodeling of mouse pancreatic acinar cells. *Gastroenterology*. 2012; 143(2): 469-480. PMID: 22510200.
43. Kim I, Xu W, Reed JC. Cell death and endoplasmic reticulum stress: disease relevance and therapeutic opportunities. *Nat Rev Drug Discov*. 2008; 7(12): 1013-1030. PMID: 19043451.
44. Ron D, Walter P. Signal integration in the endoplasmic reticulum unfolded protein response. *Nat Rev Mol Cell Biol*. 2007; 8(7): 519-529. PMID: 17565364.
45. Pandol SJ, Gorelick FS, Lugea A. Environmental and genetic stressors and the unfolded protein response in exocrine pancreatic function - a hypothesis. *Front Physiol*. 2011; 2: 8. PMID: 21483727.
46. Lugea A, Tischler D, Nguyen J, Gong J, Gukovsky I, French SW, et al. Adaptive unfolded protein response attenuates alcohol-induced pancreatic damage. *Gastroenterology*. 2011; 140(3): 987-997. PMID: 21111739.
47. Rutkowski DT, Kaufman RJ. That which does not kill me makes me stronger: adapting to chronic ER stress. *Trends Biochem Sci*. 2007; 32(10): 469-476. PMID: 17920280.
48. Marciniak SJ, Garcia-Bonilla L, Hu J, Harding HP, Ron D. Activation-dependent substrate recruitment by the eukaryotic translation initiation factor 2 kinase PERK. *J Cell Biol*. 2006; 172(2): 201-209. PMID: 16418533.
49. Kaser A, Lee AH, Franke A, Glickman JN, Zeissig S, Tilg H, et al. XBP1 links ER stress to intestinal inflammation and confers genetic risk for human inflammatory bowel disease. *Cell*. 2008; 134(5): 743-756. PMID: 18775308.
50. Pandol SJ, Gorelick FS, Gerloff A, Lugea A. Alcohol abuse, endoplasmic reticulum stress and pancreatitis. *Dig Dis*. 2010; 28(6): 776-782. PMID: 21525762.
51. Lee AH, Chu GC, Iwakoshi NN, Glimcher LH. XBP-1 is required for biogenesis of cellular secretory machinery of exocrine glands. *EMBO J*. 2005; 24(24): 4368-4380. PMID: 16362047.
52. Lugea A, Waldron RT, French SW, Pandol SJ. Drinking and driving pancreatitis: links between endoplasmic reticulum stress and autophagy. *Autophagy*. 2011; 7(7): 783-785. PMID: 21460613.
53. Hess DA, Humphrey SE, Ishibashi J, Damsz B, Lee AH, Glimcher LH, et al. Extensive pancreas regeneration following acinar-specific disruption of Xbp1 in mice. *Gastroenterology*. 2011; 141(4): 1463-1472. PMID: 21704586.
54. Gukovsky I, Lugea A, Shahsahebi M, Cheng JH, Hong PP, Jung YJ, et al. A rat model reproducing key pathological responses of alcoholic chronic pancreatitis. *Am J Physiol Gastrointest Liver Physiol*. 2008; 294(1): G68-G79. PMID: 17884979.
55. Lam PP, Cosen Binker LI, Lugea A, Pandol SJ, Gaisano HY. Alcohol redirects CCK-mediated apical exocytosis to the acinar basolateral membrane in alcoholic pancreatitis. *Traffic*. 2007; 8(5): 605-617. PMID: 17451559.
56. Pandol SJ, Periskic S, Gukovsky I, Zaninovic V, Jung Y, Zong Y, et al. Ethanol diet increases the sensitivity of rats to pancreatitis induced by cholecystokinin octapeptide. *Gastroenterology*. 1999; 117(3): 706-716. PMID: 10464148.
57. Vonlaufen A, Phillips PA, Xu Z, Zhang X, Yang L, Pirola RC, et al. Withdrawal of alcohol promotes regression while continued alcohol intake promotes persistence of LPS-induced pancreatic injury in alcohol-fed rats. *Gut*. 2011; 60(2): 238-246. PMID: 20870739.
58. Pandol SJ, Gukovsky I, Satoh A, Lugea A, Gukovskaya AS. Animal and in vitro models of alcoholic pancreatitis: role of cholecystokinin. *Pancreas*. 2003; 27(4): 297-300. PMID: 14576490.
59. Lin JH, Li H, Yasumura D, Cohen HR, Zhang C, Panning B, et al. IRE1 signaling affects cell fate during the unfolded protein response. *Science*. 2007; 318(5852): 944-949. PMID: 17991856.
60. Harding HP, Novoa I, Zhang Y, Zeng H, Wek R, Schapira M, et al. Regulated translation initiation controls stress-induced gene expression in mammalian cells. *Mol Cell*. 2000; 6(5): 1099-1108. PMID: 11106749.
61. Scheuner D, Song B, McEwen E, Liu C, Laybutt R, Gillespie P, et al. Translational control is required for the unfolded protein response and in vivo glucose homeostasis. *Mol Cell*. 2001; 7(6): 1165-1176. PMID: 11430820.
62. Han J, Back SH, Hur J, Lin YH, Gildersleeve R, Shan J, et al. ER-stress-induced transcriptional regulation increases protein synthesis leading to cell death. *Nat Cell Biol*. 2013; 15(5): 481-490. PMID: 23624402.
63. Harding HP, Zhang Y, Zeng H, Novoa I, Lu PD, Calfon M, et al. An integrated stress response regulates amino acid metabolism and resistance to oxidative stress. *Mol Cell*. 2003; 11(3): 619-633. PMID: 12667446.
64. Oyadomari S, Mori M. Roles of CHOP/GADD153 in endoplasmic reticulum stress. *Cell Death Differ*. 2004; 11(4): 381-389. PMID: 14685163.
65. Goodall JC, Wu C, Zhang Y, McNeill L, Ellis L, Saudek V, et al. Endoplasmic reticulum stress-induced transcription factor, CHOP, is crucial for dendritic cell IL-23 expression. *Proc Natl Acad Sci U S A*. 2010; 107(41): 17698-17703. PMID: 20876114.
66. Malhi H, Kropp EM, Clavo VF, Kobrossi CR, Han J, Mauer AS, et al. C/EBP Homologous Protein-induced Macrophage Apoptosis Protects Mice from Steatohepatitis. *J Biol Chem*. 2013; 288(26): 18624-18642. PMID: 23720735.

Chapter 19

Genetics of acute pancreatitis

F. Ulrich Weiss* and Markus M. Lerch

Department of Medicine A, University Medicine Greifswald, Ferdinand-Sauerbruch-Strasse, 17489 Greifswald, Germany.

Introduction

It is increasingly apparent that acute pancreatitis (AP), recurrent acute pancreatitis (RAP), and chronic pancreatitis (CP) represent overlapping phenotypes of a single disease entity, and the latter may begin in the guise of the former. Accordingly, genetic risk factors that have been identified for CP have also been found to be of some relevance in AP and RAP. Other inherited factors influence AP severity. The most prominent in this category are genes that regulate cytokines and inflammatory response proteins. This chapter reviews the genetic features that confer disease susceptibility and affect severity in patients with AP.

Definition and diagnosis

AP is a syndrome of a sudden pancreatic inflammation with unpredictable severity, duration, complications and outcome.

The diagnosis of AP requires two of the following three features: 1) abdominal pain consistent with AP (acute onset of a persistent, severe, epigastric pain often radiating to the back), 2) serum lipase activity (or amylase activity) at least three times greater than the upper limit of normal, and 3) characteristic findings of AP on contrast-enhanced computed tomography (CECT) and less commonly magnetic resonance imaging (MRI) or transabdominal ultrasonography.[1]

The main etiologic causes of AP are gallstones and alcohol abuse, but other rare causes include trauma, endoscopic interventions, infections, drugs, and toxins. Conditions such as hypercalcemia or hypertriglyceridemia have also been suggested to increase AP risk. The onset of a "first" AP episode is caused by an acute injury of pancreatic tissue that rapidly disrupts its normal physiologic function and initiates an acute inflammatory response. Histologic damage occurs as a consequence of intra-acinar activation of digestive enzymes and a subsequent infiltration of pancreatic tissue with inflammatory cells. This proinflammatory cascade is normally self-limited and followed by anti-inflammatory responses that may include pancreatic stellate cell activation and the start of fibrosis. Clinical recovery from AP usually occurs within 3-5 days. AP etiology can be established in approximately 75% of patients, leaving one in four patients with so-called idiopathic AP. In contrast to AP as a consequence of environmental factors, inherited forms present with an earlier onset of AP or RAP that eventually progresses to chronic disease. Here we discuss genetic mutations that are associated with AP or influence disease phenotype.

AP, RAP, and CP

CP is a progressive inflammatory disease that may develop from acute to recurrent and chronic disease states. Historically, CP has been associated with alcoholism, and many CP patients are suspected of alcohol abuse, often unjustly.[2] Growing evidence suggests that genetic risk factors also substantially contribute to the pancreatitis risk in CP patients.[3,4] In contrast to sporadic attacks of gallstone or alcohol-induced pancreatitis, hereditary forms of pancreatitis (HP) typically present in childhood with repeated attacks of AP. Over time, HP patients with recurrent episodes of pancreatitis in the absence of precipitating factors may develop the same common complications as alcoholic CP patients, including pancreatic fibrosis, pseudocyst formation, pancreatic exocrine insufficiency (PEI), and diabetes mellitus. Large cohort studies on pancreatitis have established complex interactions between multiple genetic and environmental factors in the progression from RAP to CP. Clinical implications of genetic risk factors have not been established due to prognostic or therapeutic limitations of current genetic testing modalities.

*Corresponding author. Email: ulrich.weiss@uni-greifswald.de

AP in children

There have been several studies in the last years reporting increasing incidences of AP among pediatric patients.[5-8] Current estimates range from 3.6-13.2 cases per 100,000 children, which is close to the incidence of AP in adults.[6] Underlying causes may involve increased testing of amylase and lipase serum levels, more frequent emergency department visits and improved clinical awareness. The rising incidence of obesity in children may also contribute as an independent risk factor for acute biliary pancreatitis, which was previously uncommon among children.[9] A recent national survey of 55,000 hospitalized children (1-20 years old) with AP in the United States revealed that AP occurs more frequently in children older than 5 (62.8% were older than 15 years) and slightly more frequently in girls (63%).[10] Hepatobiliary disease was the comorbid condition with the greatest association with AP in this study, whereas other reports claim that the change in AP incidence is primarily due to an increase of cases with systemic diseases and those with an unidentified (idiopathic) etiology.[8]

Considerable differences exist in AP etiology between adults and children. Whereas 70% of cases in adults can be attributed to gallstones or alcohol abuse, the causes of AP in children are more diverse. In a recent study by Bai et al., the top five etiologies of AP in children were biliary, medications, idiopathic, systemic disease, and trauma, followed by infectious, metabolic, and hereditary causes.[11] Not surprisingly, alcohol was not reported as a common cause of pancreatitis in children, and genetic mutations were identified in about 5%-8% of patients. Mutations were most commonly found in the cationic trypsinogen gene (*PRSS1*), the pancreatic secretory trypsin inhibitor gene (*SPINK1*), and the cystic fibrosis transmembrane conductance regulator gene (*CFTR*). A hereditary etiology is nearly indistinguishable from other causes of AP both clinically and by imaging. Early onset and recurrent events during the first decade of life in combination with a family history may be the best indication for a genetic background of AP.

In a retrospective genetic analysis of 69 children with RAP or CP, Vue et al. identified 48% as a carrier of at least 1 mutation in *PRSS1, CFTR*, or *SPINK1*.[12] Patients with mutations were more likely to have a family history but otherwise could not be identified by any mutation-specific phenotypic differences. Similar results were obtained by Palermo et al. in a genetic analysis of 45 pediatric AP patients, of which 60% carried a least 1 mutation in *PRSS1, SPINK1, CTRC*, or *CFTR*.[13] Even though the study cohort was not completely genotyped, the authors claim that they identified a higher frequency of *CFTR* mutations in CP patients compared to RAP patients. A multinational cross-sectional study of 301 children with RAP and CP was performed by the INSPPIRE consortium.[14] Eighty-four percent of children with CP reported prior recurrent episodes of AP. Sequencing analysis identified at least one mutation in pancreatitis-related genes in 48% of patients with RAP versus 73% of patients with CP. Children with *PRSS1* or *SPINK1* mutations were more likely to develop CP, but ethnic differences also seem to affect disease phenotype and progression. A higher disease burden in CP patients might justify early genetic testing in pediatric AP patients, which may also help to optimize therapeutic strategies to stop disease progression in these patients.

Risk genes

Two decades of worldwide screening efforts have confirmed a complex network of gene-environment interactions that control or influence the development and progression of pancreatic diseases including AP, RAP, and CP. While AP in most cases can be attributed to environmental factors such as gallstones or alcohol abuse, the etiology remains unclear in 20%-25%. In these idiopathic AP patients, genetic risk factors play a major role in disease onset. Most CP patients report prior episodes of AP or RAP, and also hereditary CP starts in most mutation carriers with a first attack of AP. The known genetic risk factors of CP therefore also play a role in the onset of AP and RAP episodes and are identified in genetic association studies of AP patients, albeit at a lower incidence rate compared to patients diagnosed with idiopathic CP. Most identified genetic risk factors to date are involved in regulating protease activity, starting with the initial identification of an autosomal dominant mutation in the cationic trypsinogen (*PRSS1*) in 1996 by Whitcomb and colleagues.[15] Candidate-gene approaches and validation studies in multiple cohorts have increased the number of pancreatitis-related risk genes, which include *CFTR, SPINK1*, and *CTRC*.[16-20] Significant associations with pancreatitis have also been demonstrated for sequence variants in *CPA1, CASR*, and *CEL*.[20-22] Preliminary reports that await further validation include *CLDN2*,[23] *CTSB*,[24] *MYO9B*,[25] and *UBR1*[26] or the association of an increased pancreatitis risk with ABO blood group and the so-called "secretor status," which is determined by a mutation of the fucosyl-transferase gene *FUT2*.[27] With the exception of the dominant *PRSS1* mutations, most variant alleles of these risk genes are not single-factor causes; rather, they predispose to pancreatitis and may lower the threshold for pancreatitis attacks. They also predispose to recurrent episodes and progression to chronic disease. Additional environmental or metabolic factors are operative and relevant in the complex gene-environmental interactions that determine the disease phenotype in each individual patient.

Metabolic causes of pancreatitis are less common, but also constitute an important component of the etiologic factors of AP. They include hypercalcemia, hypertriglyceridemia, diabetes mellitus, and rarely Wilson's disease.[28] Familial hypocalciuric hypercalcemia (FHH) was first described in the 1970s,[29] which led to the subsequent cloning of the calcium-sensing receptor (*CASR*) and the discovery of its pivotal role in disorders of calcium homeostasis like FFH.[30] The CaSR regulates parathyroid hormone (PTH) secretion and calcium reabsorption in the renal tubular system. In 1996, Pearce et al. reported three FHH kindreds with recurrent pancreatitis, and in all patients the disease was associated with missense mutations in the extracellular domain of the CaSR.[31] Low calcium concentrations are prevalent in the cytosol of acinar cells, which constitutes one fail-safe mechanism in preventing intra-acinar trypsinogen activation. Hypercalcemia-related pancreatitis can also be secondary to primary hyper parathyroidism (PHPT) and was first reported by Cope et al. in 1957.[32] PHPT represents a non physiological overproduction of parathyroid hormone, caused by adenoma of the parathyroid gland or multiple endocrine neoplasia (MEN) types 1 and 2A. Genetic studies provide evidence that inherited mutations in pancreatitis-related genes *SPINK1* and *CFTR* but not *CASR* were identified in 36% of hyperparathyroidism patients who developed AP.[33-35] A recent review of the literature by Bai et al. confirmed an association of PHPT with pancreatitis and implicates hypercalcemia,[36] but the functional role of *CaSR* mutations in the context of pancreatitis remains to be elucidated. Apparently PHTP requires multiple genetic and environmental influences to induce pancreatitis.

Another minor but significant etiologic factor of AP are familial disorders including lipoprotein lipase deficiency, apolipoprotein C-II deficiency, and common hypertriglyceridemia that lead to plasma accumulations of chylomicrons or triglycerides. Lipoprotein lipase catalyzes the hydrolysis of triglyceride from chylomicrons and very low-density lipoprotein (VLDL) and therefore plays a central role in regulating energy metabolism. Familial lipoprotein lipase deficiency prevents the enzyme from effectively breaking down triglycerides in the bloodstream and leads to chylomicronemia and consequently very severe hypertriglyceridemia. As a result, triglycerides attached to lipoproteins accumulate in plasma and tissues, leading to inflammation of the pancreas (pancreatitis), enlarged liver and spleen (hepatosplenomegaly), and fatty deposits in the skin (eruptive xanthomas). Triglyceride levels over 2,000 mg/dL should be considered a significant risk factor of developing pancreatitis.[37]

The most common familial disorders associated with chylomicronemia are the type I and type V hyperlipoproteinemias.[38] Hyperlipoproteinemia type I is caused by loss-of-function mutations in the *LPL* gene or in the gene of its co-factor ApoC2[39] and is inherited in an autosomal recessive pattern. The frequency of LPL deficiency in the general population is estimated to be about 1 to 2 per million.[40] More than 100 *LPL* sequence variants have been described, most of them associated with a loss of catalytic activity.[41,42] LPL-deficient patients are homozygous or compound heterozygous for these mutations, and work on a systematic classification of *LPL* gene variants is ongoing.[43] Also, rare mutations in other genes like the apoA5, glycosylphosphatidylinositol-anchored high-density lipoprotein-binding protein 1 (*GPIHBP1*) or lipase maturation factor 1 (*LMF1*) have been reported to affect LPL activity and were found to associate with chylomicronemia.[44,45]

Plasma triglyceride levels are also elevated as a result of hepatic overproduction of VLDL or heterozygous *LPL* deficiency in familial hypertriglyceridemia type IV. This monogenic familial hypertriglyceridemia is associated with only mild hypertriglyceridemia. Additional increases of plasma lipid levels in these predisposed patients may arise from unrelated risk factors like plasmocytoma, systemic lupus erythematosus, and lymphomatous disease and further enhance the risk of developing pancreatitis.

Another very rare autosomal recessive metabolic disorder with associated AP is the congenital lipodystrophy, or Berardinelli-Seip congenital lipodystrophy (BSCL) [OMIM 269700], which has an estimated prevalence of 1 in 10 million. Affected patients have a generalized muscular appearance due to the nearly complete absence of fat tissue[46] and present with tryglyceridemia, hepatomegaly, mental retardation, insulin-resistant diabetes mellitus and hypertrophic cardiomyopathy.[47] Hypertriglyceridemia seems to be the predisposing factor for the development of AP; however, the pathophysiology and genetic background of the disease have not been completely resolved. Linkage analysis identified mutations in the 1-acylglycerol-3-phosphateO-acetyltransferase 2 (*AGPAT2*), a gene encoding a key enzyme in the biosynthesis of triacyglycerol and glycerophospholipids[48] and in a second locus, *BSCL2/seipin* at 11q13,[49] with sequence homology to a murine guanine nucleotide-binding protein γ3-linked gene (Gng3lg). BSCL patients are homozygous or compound heterozygous carriers of loss-of-function mutations.

Disease severity and prognostic markers

AP has an annual incidence of 10-30 per 100,000 population.[50,51] Eighty percent of AP episodes have a mild course without significant morbidity or mortality; however, in 20% of cases the disease is severe with a mortality rate of 25% to 30%.[52,53] In AP patients, increased serum levels of tumor necrosis factor (TNF)-α, interleukin (IL)-1, IL-6, IL-8, and their (soluble) receptors indicate an important role of these major early in mediating the systemic inflammatory response.[54,55] IL secretion is regulated at the transcriptional level, which makes single-nucleotide polymorphisms (SNPs) in the promoter region of these inflammatory mediators likely risk factor candidates for systemic inflammatory response syndrome (SIRS) and organ failure. *TNF*-α variants -238G>A, and -308G>A have been identified as transcriptional enhancers, leading to higher *TNF*-α levels.[56,57] In a recent meta-analysis on more than 1,500 patients and 1,330 controls from 12 published case-control studies, Yang et al. demonstrated that the common *TNF*-α polymorphisms (-238, -308) do not alter the risk of pancreatitis or affect disease severity (shown only for the -308 SNP).[58]

Some polymorphisms in the promoter regions of *IL-1β* (-511C>T, -31C>T, +3954C>T), IL-6 (-634C>G, -174G>C), IL-8 (-251T>A), and IL-10 (-1082A>G, -819C>T, -592C>A) were identified to affect transcriptional activities and therefore were considered as potential risk factors for disease severity.[59-62] The second intron of the IL1Ra gene (*IL1RN*) contains a variable number of tandem repeats (VNTR) of 86 nucleotides, and carriers of allele 2 (containing 2 repeats), have increased IL1Ra protein levels. Some genetic association studies have suggested that different IL1RN alleles are associated with specific disease risks for sepsis[63] and ulcerative colitis[64] or increase the susceptibility to gastric cancer.[65] A number of limited genetic association studies have investigated these polymorphisms in different population cohorts of AP patients, but showed inconclusive results.[66-68] The *IL-1* gene cluster had been implicated in AP by Smithies et al. in 2000, but they found no association of the *IL-1β*+3954C>T polymorphism in a cohort of British AP patients.[69] Also, the *IL-10* -1082A>G, -819C>T and -592C>A polymorphisms did not associate with AP among British AP patients.[70] In contrast, Hofner et al. reported a significant association of the *IL-8*-251T>A polymorphism with AP risk.[71] In a 2013 meta-analysis, Yin and colleagues evaluated 10 studies on *IL* gene polymorphisms and AP susceptibility.[72] Their results suggest that the IL-8-251T>A polymorphism is indeed associated with an increased risk of AP. However, no risk association could be confirmed for any of the polymorphisms in *IL-1β*, *IL-6*, or *IL-10*.

IL-1 actually constitutes a group of cytokines produced by a wide range of cells including macrophages, monocytes, fibroblasts, and dendritic cells and elicits the acute phase response of the body against infection. IL-1α and IL-1β are the most analyzed members that have a natural antagonist (IL1Ra), and they all bind to the same type I IL-1 receptor (IL-1RI). Polymorphisms in *IL-1* genes are associated with some cancers and Grave's disease.[73] In a recent meta-analysis of 37 studies, Ying and colleagues reported that the *IL-1*β-31C>T polymorphism might confer susceptibility to gastric cancer in the presence of *Helicobacter pylori* infection, indicating gene-environment interaction in gastric carcinogenesis.[74] Another analysis of 11 case-control studies by Chen et al. confirmed significant protection of the *IL-1*β-511C>T polymorphism from Grave's disease in Asians but not Caucasians.[75] These results may indicate that the pancreatitis risk evaluation of *IL* polymorphisms is more complex than previously thought, and future studies should be carefully designed to consider genetic background differences, as well as additional gene-environment interactions.

The IL-1 family is also closely linked to the innate immune response, and the cytoplasmic region of the IL-1RI is highly homologous to the cytoplasmic domains of the Toll-like receptors (TLRs).

TLRs play a critical role in the development of pancreatic diseases as they mediate interactions between environmental stimuli and the innate immune response. They belong to a larger family of so-called pattern-recognition receptors (PRRs) that are activated by either pathogen-associated or damage-associated molecular patterns (PAMPs or DAMPs)[76] released by activated or necrotic cells in response to stress or cell damage. TLR signaling involves myeloid differentiation primary response protein (MyD88)-dependent pathways and upregulates the transcription of proinflammatory genes through activation of nuclear factor-κB (NFκB).[77] TLR3 and TLR4 can further activate the TIR-domain-containing adapter-inducing interferon-β (TRIF) pathway, leading to interferon-α/β synthesis.[78]

Sequence variations in *TLR* genes are capable of influencing susceptibility to infectious diseases,[79,80] and the common *TLR4* polymorphisms p.D299G and p.T399I were the first identified risk factors for the development of sepsis in patients.[81] Variant TLR4 receptors show less interaction with lipopolysaccharide, which may result in higher infection with Gram-negative bacteria. A first limited genetic association study by Hofner and colleagues[71] did not reveal an association of these *TLR4* polymorphisms with AP incidence or severity, but several subsequent studies in Caucasian and Asian patient cohorts yielded inconsistent results.[82-85] A meta-analysis by Zhou on 1255 cases and 998 controls did not confirm a risk factor role of *TLR4* D299G and T399I polymorphisms for AP susceptibility.[86] A number of additional genetic analyses have been performed and reported significant association of TLR2 intronic mutation with susceptibility and severity of AP in Japan,[83] and a risk factor role of mannose-binding lectin (MBL) promoter variants with disease severity in Chinese patients.[84] These results await confirmation.

The role of PRRs in the pathophysiology of mucosal barrier failure in AP remains to be resolved. Mucosal barrier disruption plays an essential role in severe AP development as it allows bacterial translocation from the gut into the blood stream, which may trigger infectious complications. Nijmejier et al. performed a candidate gene approach in more than 500 AP patients from the Netherlands and Germany and reported that sequence variants in myosin IXB (MYO9B), a protein that seems to play a role in tight junction assembly, associate with inflammatory bowel disease, celiac disease, and AP.[25] Myosin IXB variants may confer a higher risk of intestinal barrier dysfunction in AP.

Identification of additional risk factors

After the publication of the first pancreatitis-associated risk gene in 1996 by Whitcomb et al., the identification of genetic risk factors in pancreatitis followed mainly candidate gene approaches for two decades. These efforts were successful and significantly contributed to our current understanding of the molecular details of pancreatic pathophysiology. Powerful new screening technologies include genome-wide association (GWA) analyses and next-generation sequencing (NGS) studies. These techniques are rather expensive and require large cohorts of clinically well-defined individuals, but they are ideally suited to identify new risk factors outside the already known or suspected signaling pathways or regulatory mechanisms involved in pancreas physiology. To date, few GWA studies have been performed, mainly in CP and RAP patients, and the study by Whitcomb et al. was able to identify a new susceptibility locus in the claudin-2 gene (*CLDN2*).[23] A second SNP found in the *PRSS1-PRSS2* locus seems to further confirm the importance of this established risk locus for the development of pancreatitis. Derikx and colleagues were able to confirm these findings in a replication GWA study on European patients with alcoholic and nonalcoholic CP.[87] A third GWA was done by Weiss et al. on high serum lipase values in a population-based cohort of healthy individuals.[27] The study reported an association of blood group B and the nonsecretor allele of *FUT2* with elevated lipase activities in asymptomatic individuals. Both loci were also identified to associate with CP. These results await confirmation in larger replication cohorts involving different ethnic populations.

These new findings and upcoming reports from current candidate-free genetic screening approaches may open the route for studies on pathologic mechanisms outside the known protease-antiprotease homeostasis network. More GWA studies and NGS data will significantly expand our current understanding of pancreatic pathophysiology and pancreatic disease and hopefully will help identify new therapeutic strategies.

References

1. Banks PA, Bollen TL, Dervenis C, Gooszen HG, Johnson CD, Sarr MG, et al. Classification of acute pancreatitis-2012: revision of the Atlanta classification and definitions by international consensus. *Gut*. 2012; 62: 102-111. PMID: 23100216.
2. Aghdassi AA, Weiss FU, Mayerle J, Lerch MM, Simon P. Genetic susceptibility factors for alcohol-induced chronic pancreatitis. *Pancreatology*. 2015; 15 4 Suppl: S23-S31. PMID: 26149858.
3. Lerch MM, Mayerle J, Mahajan U, Sendler M, Weiss FU, Aghdassi A, et al. Development of Pancreatic Cancer: Targets for Early Detection and Treatment. *Dig Dis*. 2016; 34: 525-531. PMID: 27332960.
4. Kanth W, Reddy DN. Genetics of acute and chronic pancreatitis: an update. *World J Gastrointest Pathophysiol*. 2014; 5: 427-437. PMID: 25400986.
5. Morinville VD, Barmada MM, Lowe ME. Increasing incidence of acute pancreatitis at an American pediatric tertiary care center: is greater awareness among physicians responsible? *Pancreas*. 2009; 39: 5-8. PMID: 19752770.
6. Pant C, Deshpande A, Sferra TJ, Gilroy R, Olyaee M. Emergency department visits for acute pancreatitis in children: results from the Nationwide Emergency Department Sample 2006-2011. *J Investig Med*. 2015; 63: 646-648. PMID: 25654293.
7. Restrepo R, Hagerott HE, Kulkarni S, Yasrebi M, Lee EY. Acute Pancreatitis in Pediatric Patients: Demographics, Etiology, and Diagnostic Imaging. *Am J Roentgenol*. 2016; 206: 632-644. PMID: 26901022.
8. Nydegger A, Heine RG, Ranuh R, Gegati-Levy R, Crameri J, Oliver MR. Changing incidence of acute pancreatitis: 10-year experience at the Royal Children's Hospital, Melbourne. *J Gastroenterol Hepatol*. 2007; 22: 1313-1316. PMID: 17489962.
9. Ma MH, Bai HX, Park AJ, Latif SU, Mistry PK, Pashankar D, et al. Risk factors associated with biliary pancreatitis in children. *J Pediatr Gastroenterol Nutr.* 54(5): 651-656, 2011. PMID: 22002481.
10. Pant C, Deshpande A, Olyaee M, Anderson MP, Bitar A, Steele MI, et al. Epidemiology of acute pancreatitis in hospitalized children in the United States from 2000-2009. *PLoS One*. 2014; 9: e95552. PMID: 24805879.
11. Bai HX, Lowe ME, Husain SZ. What have we learned about acute pancreatitis in children? *J Pediatr Gastroenterol Nutr*. 2011; 52: 262-270. PMID: 21336157.
12. Vue PM, McFann K, Narkewicz MR. Genetic Mutations in Pediatric Pancreatitis. *Pancreas*. 2015; 45: 992-996. PMID: 26692446.
13. Palermo JJ, Lin TK, Hornung L, Valencia CA, Mathur A, Jackson K, et al. Genophenotypic analysis of pediatric patients with recurrent acute and chronic pancreatitis. *Pancreas.* 2016: In Press. PMID: 27171515.
14. Kumar S, Ooi CY, Werlin S, Abu-El-Haija M, Barth B, Bellin MD, et al. Risk Factors Associated With Pediatric Acute Recurrent and Chronic Pancreatitis: Lessons From INSPPIRE. *JAMA Pediatr*. 2016; 170: 562-569. PMID: 27064572.
15. Whitcomb DC, Gorry MC, Preston RA, Furey W, Sossenheimer MJ, Ulrich CD, et al. Hereditary pancreatitis is caused by a mutation in the cationic trypsinogen gene. *Nat Genet*. 1996; 14: 141-145. PMID: 8841182.
16. Sharer N, Schwarz M, Malone G, Howarth A, Painter J, Super M, et al. Mutations of the cystic fibrosis gene in patients with chronic pancreatitis. *N Engl J Med*. 1998; 339: 645-652. PMID: 9725921.
17. Cohn JA, Friedman KJ, Noone PG, Knowles MR, Silverman LM, Jowell PS. Relation between mutations of the cystic fibrosis gene and idiopathic pancreatitis. *N Engl J Med*. 1998; 339: 653-658. PMID: 9725922.

18. Witt H, Luck W, Hennies HC, Classen M, Kage A, Lass U, et al. Mutations in the gene encoding the serine protease inhibitor, Kazal type 1 are associated with chronic pancreatitis. *Nat Genet*. 2000; 25: 213-216. PMID: 10835640.
19. Rosendahl J, Witt H, Szmola R, Bhatia E, Ozsvari B, Landt O, et al. Chymotrypsin C (CTRC) variants that diminish activity or secretion are associated with chronic pancreatitis. *Nat Genet*. 2008; 40: 78-82. PMID: 18059268.
20. Witt H, Beer S, Rosendahl J, Chen JM, Chandak GR, Masamune A, et al. Variants in CPA1 are strongly associated with early onset chronic pancreatitis. *Nat Genet*. 2013; 45: 1216-1220. PMID: 23955596.
21. Fjeld K, Weiss FU, Lasher D, Rosendahl J, Chen JM, Johansson BB, et al. A recombined allele of the lipase gene CEL and its pseudogene CELP confers susceptibility to chronic pancreatitis. *Nat Genet*. 2015; 47: 518-522. PMID: 25774637.
22. Muddana V, Lamb J, Greer JB, Elinoff B, Hawes RH, Cotton PB, et al. Association between calcium sensing receptor gene polymorphisms and chronic pancreatitis in a US population: role of serine protease inhibitor Kazal 1type and alcohol. *World J Gastroenterol*. 2008; 14: 4486-4491. PMID: 18680227.
23. Whitcomb DC, LaRusch J, Krasinskas AM, Klei L, Smith JP, Brand RE, et al. Common genetic variants in the CLDN2 and PRSS1-PRSS2 loci alter risk for alcohol-related and sporadic pancreatitis. *Nat Genet*. 2012; 44: 1349-1354. PMID: 23143602.
24. Mahurkar S, Idris MM, Reddy DN, Bhaskar S, Rao GV, Thomas V, et al. Association of cathepsin B gene polymorphisms with tropical calcific pancreatitis. *Gut*. 2006; 55: 1270-1275. PMID: 16492714.
25. Nijmeijer RM, van Santvoort HC, Zhernakova A, Teller S, Scheiber JA, de Kovel CG, et al. Association analysis of genetic variants in the myosin IXB gene in acute pancreatitis. *PLoS One*. 2014; 8: e85870. PMID: 24386489.
26. Zenker M, Mayerle J, Lerch MM, Tagariello A, Zerres K, Durie PR, et al. Deficiency of UBR1, a ubiquitin ligase of the N-end rule pathway, causes pancreatic dysfunction, malformations and mental retardation (Johanson-Blizzard syndrome). *Nat Genet*. 2005; 37: 1345-1350. PMID: 16311597.
27. Weiss FU, Schurmann C, Guenther A, Ernst F, Teumer A, Mayerle J, et al. Fucosyltransferase 2 (FUT2) non-secretor status and blood group B are associated with elevated serum lipase activity in asymptomatic subjects, and an increased risk for chronic pancreatitis: a genetic association study. *Gut*. 2015; 64: 646-656. PMID: 25028398.
28. Kota SK, Krishna SV, Lakhtakia S, Modi KD. Metabolic pancreatitis: Etiopathogenesis and management. *Indian J Endocrinol Metab*. 2013; 17: 799-805. PMID: 24083160.
29. Foley TP Jr, Harrison HC, Arnaud CD, Harrison HE. Familial benign hypercalcemia. *J Pediatr*. 1972; 81: 1060-1067. PMID: 4643023.
30. Pollak MR, Brown EM, Chou YH, Hebert SC, Marx SJ, Steinmann B, et al. Mutations in the human Ca^{2+}-sensing receptor gene cause familial hypocalciuric hypercalcemia and neonatal severe hyperparathyroidism. *Cell*. 1993; 75: 1297-1303. PMID: 7916660.
31. Pearce SH, Wooding C, Davies M, Tollefsen SE, Whyte MP, Thakker RV. Calcium-sensing receptor mutations in familial hypocalciuric hypercalcaemia with recurrent pancreatitis. *Clin Endocrinol (Oxf)*. 1996; 45: 675-680. PMID: 9039332.
32. Cope O, Culver PJ, Mixter CG Jr, Nardi GL. Pancreatitis, a diagnostic clue to hyperparathyroidism. *Ann Surg*. 1957; 145: 857-863. PMID: 13425295.
33. LaRusch J, Whitcomb DC. Genetics of pancreatitis. *Curr Opin Gastroenterol*. 2011; 27: 467-474. PMID: 21844754.
34. Felderbauer P, Karakas E, Fendrich V, Bulut K, Horn T, Lebert R, et al. Pancreatitis risk in primary hyperparathyroidism: relation to mutations in the SPINK1 trypsin inhibitor (N34S) and the cystic fibrosis gene. *Am J Gastroenterol*. 2008; 103: 368-374. PMID: 18076731.
35. Felderbauer P, Karakas E, Fendrich V, Bulut K, Werner I, Dekomien G, et al. Pancreatitis in primary hyperparathyroidism-related hypercalcaemia is not associated with mutations in the CASR gene. *Exp Clin Endocrinol Diabetes*. 2007; 115: 527-529. PMID: 17853337.
36. Bai HX, Giefer M, Patel M, Orabi AI, Husain SZ. The association of primary hyperparathyroidism with pancreatitis. *J Clin Gastroenterol*. 2012; 46: 656-661. PMID: 22874807.
37. Berglund L, Brunzell JD, Goldberg AC, Goldberg IJ, Sacks F, Murad MH, et al. Evaluation and treatment of hypertriglyceridemia: an Endocrine Society clinical practice guideline. *J Clin Endocrinol Metab*. 2012; 97: 2969-2989. PMID: 22962670.
38. Beaumont JL, Carlson LA, Cooper GR, Fejfar Z, Fredrickson DS, Strasser T. Classification of hyperlipidaemias and hyperlipoproteinaemias. *Bull World Health Organ*. 1970; 43: 891-915. PMID: 4930042.
39. Cox DW, Wills DE, Quan F, Ray PN. A deletion of one nucleotide results in functional deficiency of apolipoprotein CII (apo CII Toronto). *J Med Genet*. 1988; 25: 649-652. PMID: 3225819.
40. Brunzell JD, Deeb S. Familial lipoprotein lipase deficiency, apo CII deficiency and hepatic lipase deficiency. In: Sciever C, Beaudet A, Sly WS, Valle D, eds. *The Metabolic and Molecular Basis of Inherited Disease*, 8th ed. New York: McGraw-Hill; 2001: 1913-1932.
41. Merkel M, Eckel RH, Goldberg IJ. Lipoprotein lipase: genetics, lipid uptake, and regulation. *J Lipid Res*. 2002; 43: 1997-2006. PMID: 12454259.
42. Rahalkar AR, Giffen F, Har B, Ho J, Morrison KM, Hill J, et al. Novel LPL mutations associated with lipoprotein lipase deficiency: two case reports and a literature review. *Can J Physiol Pharmacol*. 2009; 87: 151-160. PMID: 19295657.
43. Rodrigues R, Artieda M, Tejedor D, Martinez A, Konstantinova P, Petry H, et al. Pathogenic classification of LPL gene variants reported to be associated with LPL deficiency. *J Clin Lipidol*. 2016; 10: 394-409. PMID: 27055971.
44. Adeyo O, Goulbourne CN, Bensadoun A, Beigneux AP, Fong LG, Young SG. Glycosylphosphatidylinositol-anchored high-density lipoprotein-binding protein 1 and the intravascular processing of triglyceride-rich lipoproteins. *J Intern Med*. 2012; 272: 528-540. PMID: 23020258.

45. Kersten S. Physiological regulation of lipoprotein lipase. *Biochim Biophys Acta*. 2014; 1841: 919-933. PMID: 24721265.
46. Berardinelli W. An undiagnosed endocrinometabolic syndrome: report of 2 cases. *J Clin Endocrinol Metab*. 1954; 14: 193-204. PMID: 13130666.
47. Gomes KB, Pardini VC, Fernandes AP. Clinical and molecular aspects of Berardinelli-Seip Congenital Lipodystrophy (BSCL). *Clin Chim Acta*. 2009; 402: 1-6. PMID: 19167372.
48. Agarwal AK, Arioglu E, De Almeida S, Akkoc N, Taylor SI, Bowcock AM, et al. AGPAT2 is mutated in congenital generalized lipodystrophy linked to chromosome 9q34. *Nat Genet*. 2002; 31: 21-23. PMID: 11967537.
49. Magre J, Delepine M, Khallouf E, Gedde-Dahl T Jr, Van Maldergem L, Sobel E, et al. Identification of the gene altered in Berardinelli-Seip congenital lipodystrophy on chromosome 11q13. *Nat Genet*. 2001; 28: 365-370. PMID: 11479539.
50. Andersson R, Andersson B, Haraldsen P, Drewsen G, Eckerwall G. Incidence, management and recurrence rate of acute pancreatitis. *Scand J Gastroenterol*. 2004; 39: 891-894. PMID: 15513389.
51. Eland IA, Sturkenboom MJ, Wilson JH, Stricker BH. Incidence and mortality of acute pancreatitis between 1985 and 1995. *Scand J Gastroenterol*. 2000; 35: 1110-1116. PMID: 11099067.
52. Lankisch PG, Blum T, Maisonneuve P, Lowenfels AB. Severe acute pancreatitis: when to be concerned? *Pancreatology*. 2003; 3: 102-110. PMID: 12748418.
53. Neoptolemos JP, Raraty M, Finch M, Sutton R. Acute pancreatitis: the substantial human and financial costs. *Gut*. 1998; 42: 886-891. PMID: 9691932.
54. de Beaux AC, Goldie AS, Ross JA, Carter DC, Fearon KC. Serum concentrations of inflammatory mediators related to organ failure in patients with acute pancreatitis. *Br J Surg*. 1996; 83: 349-353. PMID: 8665189.
55. Chen CC, Wang SS, Lee FY, Chang FY, Lee SD. Proinflammatory cytokines in early assessment of the prognosis of acute pancreatitis. *Am J Gastroenterol*. 1999; 94: 213-218. PMID: 9934758.
56. Wilson AG, Symons JA, McDowell TL, McDevitt HO, Duff GW. Effects of a polymorphism in the human tumor necrosis factor alpha promoter on transcriptional activation. *Proc Natl Acad Sci U S A*. 1997; 94: 3195-3199. PMID: 9096369.
57. Balog A, Gyulai Z, Boros LG, Farkas G, Tákacs T, Lonovics J, et al. Polymorphism of the TNF-alpha, HSP70-2, and CD14 genes increases susceptibility to severe acute pancreatitis. *Pancreas*. 2005; 30: e46-e50. PMID: 15714129.
58. Yang Z, Qi X, Wu Q, Li A, Xu P, Fan D. Lack of association between TNF-alpha gene promoter polymorphisms and pancreatitis: a meta-analysis. *Gene*. 2012; 503: 229-234. PMID: 22579868.
59. Fishman D, Faulds G, Jeffery R, Mohamed-Ali V, Yudkin JS, Humphries S, et al. The effect of novel polymorphisms in the interleukin-6 (IL-6) gene on IL-6 transcription and plasma IL-6 levels, and an association with systemic-onset juvenile chronic arthritis. *J Clin Invest*. 1998; 102: 1369-1376. PMID: 9769329.
60. Nauck M, Winkelmann BR, Hoffmann MM, Bohm BO, Wieland H, Marz W. The interleukin-6 G(-174)C promoter polymorphism in the LURIC cohort: no association with plasma interleukin-6, coronary artery disease, and myocardial infarction. *J Mol Med (Berl)*. 2002; 80: 507-513. PMID: 12185451.
61. Ohyauchi M, Imatani A, Yonechi M, Asano N, Miura A, Iijima K, et al. The polymorphism interleukin 8 -251 A/T influences the susceptibility of Helicobacter pylori related gastric diseases in the Japanese population. *Gut*. 2005; 54: 330-335. PMID: 15710978.
62. Eskdale J, Gallagher G, Verweij CL, Keijsers V, Westendorp RG, Huizinga TW. Interleukin 10 secretion in relation to human IL-10 locus haplotypes. *Proc Natl Acad Sci U S A*. 1998; 95: 9465-9470. PMID: 9689103.
63. Fang F, Pan J, Li Y, Xu L, Su G, Li G, et al. Association between interleukin 1 receptor antagonist gene 86-bp VNTR polymorphism and sepsis: a meta-analysis. *Hum Immunol*. 2014; 76: 1-5. PMID: 25500257.
64. Mansfield JC, Holden H, Tarlow JK, Di Giovine FS, McDowell TL, Wilson AG, et al. Novel genetic association between ulcerative colitis and the anti-inflammatory cytokine interleukin-1 receptor antagonist. *Gastroenterology*. 1994; 106: 637-642. PMID: 8119534.
65. Zhang Y, Liu C, Peng H, Zhang J, Feng Q. IL1 receptor antagonist gene IL1-RN variable number of tandem repeats polymorphism and cancer risk: a literature review and meta-analysis. *PLoS One*. 2012; 7: e46017. PMID: 23049925.
66. Tukiainen E, Kylanpaa ML, Puolakkainen P, Kemppainen E, Halonen K, Orpana A, et al. Polymorphisms of the TNF, CD14, and HSPA1B genes in patients with acute alcohol-induced pancreatitis. *Pancreas*. 2008; 37: 56-61. PMID: 18580445.
67. de-Madaria E, Martínez J, Sempere L, Lozano B, Sánchez-Payá J, Uceda F, et al. Cytokine genotypes in acute pancreatitis: association with etiology, severity, and cytokine levels in blood. *Pancreas*. 2008; 37: 295-301. PMID: 18815552.
68. Powell JJ, Fearon KC, Siriwardena AK, Ross JA. Evidence against a role for polymorphisms at tumor necrosis factor, interleukin-1 and interleukin-1 receptor antagonist gene loci in the regulation of disease severity in acute pancreatitis. *Surgery*. 2001; 129: 633-640. PMID: 11331456.
69. Smithies AM, Sargen K, Demaine AG, Kingsnorth AN. Investigation of the interleukin 1 gene cluster and its association with acute pancreatitis. *Pancreas*. 2000; 20: 234-240. PMID: 10766448.
70. Sargen K, Demaine AG, Kingsnorth AN. Cytokine gene polymorphisms in acute pancreatitis. *JOP*. 2000; 1: 24-35. PMID: 11852287.
71. Hofner P, Balog A, Gyulai Z, Farkas G, Rakonczay Z, Tákacs T, et al. Polymorphism in the IL-8 gene, but not in the TLR4 gene, increases the severity of acute pancreatitis. *Pancreatology*. 2006; 6: 542-548. PMID: 17124436.
72. Yin YW, Sun QQ, Feng JQ, Hu AM, Liu HL, Wang Q. Influence of interleukin gene polymorphisms on development of acute pancreatitis: a systematic review and meta-analysis. *Mol Biol Rep*. 2013; 40: 5931-5941. PMID: 24072654.

73. El-Omar EM, Carrington M, Chow WH, McColl KE, Bream JH, Young HA, et al. Interleukin-1 polymorphisms associated with increased risk of gastric cancer. *Nature*. 2000; 404: 398-402. PMID: 10746728.
74. Ying HY, Yu BW, Yang Z, Yang SS, Bo LH, Shan XY, et al. Interleukin-1B 31 C>T polymorphism combined with Helicobacter pylori-modified gastric cancer susceptibility: evidence from 37 studies. *J Cell Mol Med*. 2016; 20: 526-536. PMID: 26805397.
75. Chen ML, Liao N, Zhao H, Huang J, Xie ZF. Association between the IL1B (-511), IL1B (+3954), IL1RN (VNTR) polymorphisms and Graves' disease risk: a meta-analysis of 11 case-control studies. *PLoS One*. 2014; 9: e86077. PMID: 24465880.
76. Kawai T, Akira S. Toll-like receptors and their crosstalk with other innate receptors in infection and immunity. *Immunity*. 2011; 34: 637-650. PMID: 21616434.
77. Kawai T, Akira S, Signaling to NF-kappaB by Toll-like receptors. *Trends Mol Med*. 2007; 13: 460-469. PMID: 18029230.
78. O'Neill LA, Bowie AG. The family of five: TIR-domain-containing adaptors in Toll-like receptor signalling. *Nat Rev Immunol*. 2007; 7: 353-364. PMID: 17457343.
79. Schroder NW, Schumann RR. Single nucleotide polymorphisms of Toll-like receptors and susceptibility to infectious disease. *Lancet Infect Dis*. 2005; 5: 156-164. PMID: 15766650.
80. Netea MG, Wijmenga C, O'Neill LA. Genetic variation in Toll-like receptors and disease susceptibility. *Nat Immunol*. 2012; 13: 535-542. PMID: 22610250.
81. Arbour NC, Lorenz E, Schutte BC, Zabner J, Kline JN, Jones M, et al. TLR4 mutations are associated with endotoxin hyporesponsiveness in humans. *Nat Genet*. 2000; 25: 187-191. PMID: 10835634.
82. Guenther A, Aghdassi A, Muddana V, Rau B, Schulz HU, Mayerle J, et al. Toll-like receptor 4 polymorphisms in German and US patients are not associated with occurrence or severity of acute pancreatitis. *Gut*. 2010; 59: 1154-1155. PMID: 20587548.
83. Takagi Y, Masamune A, Kume K, Satoh A, Kikuta K, Watanabe T, et al. Microsatellite polymorphism in intron 2 of human Toll-like receptor 2 gene is associated with susceptibility to acute pancreatitis in Japan. *Hum Immunol*. 2009; 70: 200-204. PMID: 19280717.
84. Zhang D, Zheng H, Zhou Y, Yu B, Li J. TLR and MBL gene polymorphisms in severe acute pancreatitis. *Mol Diagn Ther*. 2008; 12: 45-50. PMID: 18288881.
85. Gao HK, Zhou ZG, Li Y, Chen YQ. Toll-like receptor 4 Asp299Gly polymorphism is associated with an increased risk of pancreatic necrotic infection in acute pancreatitis: a study in the Chinese population. *Pancreas*. 2007; 34: 295-298. PMID: 17414051.
86. Zhou XJ, Cui Y, Cai LY, Xiang JY, Zhang Y. Toll-like receptor 4 polymorphisms to determine acute pancreatitis susceptibility and severity: a meta-analysis. *World J Gastroenterol*. 2014; 20: 6666-6670. PMID: 24914392.
87. Derikx MH, Kovacs P, Scholz M, Masson E, Chen JM, Ruffert C, et al. Polymorphisms at PRSS1-PRSS2 and CLDN2-MORC4 loci associate with alcoholic and non-alcoholic chronic pancreatitis in a European replication study. *Gut*. 2014; 64: 1426-1433. PMID: 25253127.

Chapter 20

Relationship between obesity and pancreatitis

Sarah Navina MD[1] and Vijay P. Singh MD[2*]

[1]*Clin-Path Associates, Tempe, Arizona, USA;*
[2]*Mayo Clinic, Scottsdale, Arizona, USA.*

Acute pancreatitis (AP) has several etiologies and diverse outcomes. The outcomes range from spontaneous resolution of an acute attack that may never recur again to a disease that may progress to severe acute pancreatitis (SAP) over a few days, resulting in prolonged hospitalization for local or systemic complications and sometimes death. Several studies have reported that obese patients with increased visceral fat depots including pancreatic fat are at risk of SAP.[1-11] Repeated AP attacks may result in a clinical picture of recurrent AP that can progress to chronic pancreatitis (CP) with an associated increased in pancreatic fat.[12-14] However, while being potentially debilitating due to pain, exocrine insufficiency, diabetes, or quality of life issues, recurrent acute and CP rarely result in SAP.[13,15,16]

SAP typically occurs during the first or second AP attack.[13,17] The disease spectrum of SAP includes local complications, primarily pancreatic necrosis (PN) and peri-pancreatic necrosis (PPN) that sometimes get infected, and systemic complications including organ failure involving the respiratory and renal systems and a shock-like state. Local complications from extensive PN or PPN or systemic complications lasting >48 hours (sustained organ failure) or more than one organ system (multisystem organ failure, MSOF) can result in prolonged hospitalization or mortality. While obese patients are prone to both local and systemic compilations in AP, no consistent relationship has been reported between an etiology of AP and SAP[18-21] with the exception of hypertriglyceridemic pancreatitis.[22-24] This association and reports that obese patients may have worse outcomes in AP suggest that there is a common lipid-related modifier that can deteriorate the course of AP. Over the last 150 years, investigators have repeatedly broached the role of fat and the cells that contain it (i.e., adipocytes) in pancreatitis. The reports have ranged from gross descriptions of the appearance of the peritoneal cavity in patients dying from severe pancreatitis to the molecular mechanisms by which fatty acids may mediate these outcomes. Within this spectrum are studies of the influence of adipocytes on the histologic appearance of pancreatitis, animal models of obesity and pancreatitis, and cell culture models of lipotoxicity. In this chapter, we will systematically explore the role that fat may play in the outcomes of pancreatitis, especially in the context of obesity.

Historical Perspective

The relevance of obesity to AP was first documented in the 19th century. In 1882, Balser first described the presence of fat necrosis in AP.[25] In 1889, while writing on AP in the *Medical Monographs,* Dr. Reginald Fitz quoted Zenker as stating, "An excessive growth of the fat cells near the pancreas occurs in many men. It may become so excessive, in very fat people, that a large part of the abdominal fat dies, and thus proves fatal, either on account of the quantity destroyed or the associated hemorrhage".[26] Simon Flexner was the first to suggest a role of lipases in pancreatitis-associated fat damage in 1896.[27] Fitz mentioned that Hans Chiari also noted the association between fat and pancreatitis,[26] but Chiari, widely known for the hypothesis of the pancreas autodigesting itself during pancreatitis (thus pioneering the proteolytic hypothesis of pancreatitis), published only later on this topic,[28] as did others.[29] More details of the early observations of fat in pancreatitis are mentioned in the work by Dr. Fitz[26] and are well summarized in more recent reviews.[27]

Chemical analysis of pancreatic fat necrosis was initially performed in the early part of the 20th century and revealed that it involved predominantly free fatty acids with some saponification and calcium soaps.[30] In the 1970s, several independent investigators systematically explored the association between fat and pancreatitis. There were several elegant studies on the lipolytic pathogenesis, morphology, hypocalcemic complications, and therapeutic interventions in animal models of fat necrosis.[31-33] Quantification of fat

*Corresponding author. Email: singh.vijay@mayo.edu

cells in the pancreata of humans at autopsy showed that adipocyte amount increased with body weight.[34,35] Studies in the 1980s by Schmitz-Moormann on pancreatic tissue from patients with AP showed pancreatic parenchymal and vascular damage to be in close proximity to fat cell necrosis.[36] Kloppel made similar observations in the peripancreatic fat of patients with AP, and both investigators hypothesized that fat necrosis was the initiating factor in human pancreatitis.[37] This topic was debated and contrasted to the ubiquitous nature of active proteases in all models of pancreatitis. The earlier use of pharmacologic protease inhibitors like trasylol and gabexate focused attention on proteases preceding the attention paid to lipases.[38-40] However, we have learned that targeting proteases provides no clinically relevant improvement in outcomes.[41-43] The discovery of the lipase inhibitor tetra-hydrolipistatin (THL) in the 1980s (from which orlistat is derived) renewed interest in understanding the role of lipolysis in pancreatitis. In vitro studies by Mossner et al. in the 1990s showed a protective effect of lipase inhibition on pancreatic acinar cells in vitro,[44] but not when pancreatitis was induced by infusing bile salts such as sodium taurocholate into the rat pancreatic duct.[45] Immediately after this work, there were few systematic studies on the role of fat in pancreatitis, but the steady stream of clinical reports repeatedly mentioning intra-abdominal fat/visceral fat/obesity as being risk factors for SAP has revived interest in this topic, as we will discuss below.

Epidemiology of Obesity and Pancreatitis

Several studies have associated obesity or increased intra-abdominal fat with SAP.[1-11] Body mass index (BMI) is commonly used as a measure of body fat amount. Apart from BMI, visceral adipose tissue as measured by waist-to-hip ratio and waist circumference above ideal cut-off value have been proposed as risk factors for worse outcomes in AP.[46,47] Waist circumference has been shown to correlate with intra-abdominal fat volume[48] and is a risk factor for SAP.[9]

Obesity is defined as a BMI >30 kg/m^2 in the western hemisphere or >25 kg/m^2 in the East including countries such as Japan, Korea, China, and India. Studies exploring the association of BMI with SAP from these regions commonly correlate AP severity with these BMI cutoffs. BMIs >30 kg/m^2 are mentioned as being associated with SAP in reports from North America and Europe,[3,6,49-52] while reports from Asia mention BMIs >23-25 kg/m^2 to be associated with SAP.[4,10,53,54] The reason for this relationship is unclear. Previous studies have shown that fat composition in humans is related to the fat in their diets. This observation may link eastern diets and the visceral adipose tissue of the populations that consume them to be richer in unsaturated fatty acids, particularly polyunsaturated fatty acids (PUFAs)[55-58] compared to the west.[55,56,59] An example is that the high PUFA diet of Korean monks was associated with higher PUFA levels in visceral fat compared to American soldiers consuming a diet lower in PUFA.[55] The relevance of this to AP outcomes is supported by the correlation between dietary fatty acid composition and adipose tissue fatty acid composition[55,60] and the findings that unsaturated fatty acids,[61,62] especially PUFAs,[63,64] are relatively more toxic than saturated fatty acids during pancreatitis.

Characteristics of visceral fat in obesity-associated SAP

Total body fat may comprise >30% of body weight in obese individuals.[65] Fat accumulation can occur in the subcutaneous and visceral compartments, and while there are case reports of fat necrosis distant from the pancreas during pancreatitis, including osseous[66,67] and subcutaneous fat[68-70] associated with detectable pancreatic lipases,[70,71] the principal fat depots commonly affected in pancreatitis are the intra-abdominal or visceral ones near the pancreas. The sites of visceral fat deposition include the mesentery, omentum, liver,[72,73] and pancreas and peripancreatic space.[34,35,74-76] Visceral fat averages >3% body weight in obese humans[77,78] and thus contributes a large, potentially hydrolyzable pool for fat necrosis in SAP.

Supporting the human pathologic findings from the 1980s,[36,37] recent studies have noted that both extrapancreatic[79] and intrapancreatic fat necrosis[17,63] are associated with an increase in pancreatitis severity. The evidence comes from both radiologic investigations[79,80] and histologic assessments of postmortem pancreata[17,63] to systematically compare pancreatic parenchymal and fat necrosis with pancreatitis severity. Extrapancreatic fat necrosis is a part of necrotizing pancreatitis,[81,82] the revised Atlanta criteria,[82] and radiographic scoring systems for SAP (e.g., Schroeder and Balthazar)[76,83] and correlates with worse outcomes during AP.[80,84,85]

Fat within the pancreas (intrapancreatic fat, IPF) has been shown to increase with BMI in studies analyzing autopsy samples,[34,35,75] surgically resected samples,[74] and radiologic appearance of the pancreas.[75,86] The distribution of fat is fairly uniform in the dorsal pancreas and is reduced in the ventral pancreas.[35] Uneven fatty replacement in the pancreas is infrequent (3.2%), and the pattern of fat distribution is not influenced by obesity.[86]

White adipocytes are the major cell type comprising visceral fat in obesity and are predominantly composed of triglyceride, which in a pure form has an extremely high concentration of about 1 M and forms 80%-90% of adipocyte mass.[87-89] As we shall note in the section on pathophysiology, the generation of unsaturated fatty acids from the lipolysis of this triglyceride has been mechanistically associated with adverse outcomes in SAP. Recent studies systematically quantifying the amount of IPF in control pancreata and tissue from patients with pancreatitis noted the percentage area occupied by adipocytes correlated with and significantly increased with BMI.[17,63] Patients with a BMI >30 had significantly higher IPF (18.3 ± 2.3%) compared to those with a BMI <30 (10.2 ± 1.9%). These values were similar to AP patients in the respective BMI categories, suggesting that the amount of IPF does not influence the risk of developing AP. Patients who had SAP associated with pancreatic necrosis, however, had higher IPF (23.4 ± 4.3%) and BMI (40.0 ± 2.8 kg/m^2) compared to those with mild disease (7.8 ± 1.9% and 30.3 ± 2.5 kg/m^2, respectively). As we shall see later, the higher amount of IPF may contribute to poorer AP outcomes.

Interestingly, in contrast to obesity-associated IPF, the IPF increase noted in CP,[90-93] is rarely associated with SAP.[13,15,16] Fatty replacement is commonly known to occur in chronic pancreatic diseases over the course of several years, which in some cases may start in utero.[94,95] These diseases include Shwachman-Diamond syndrome,[96] cystic fibrosis[95] and Johannson-Blizzard syndrome.[95] While AP may result in mortality over days,[79,97,98] mortality in CP is rarely attributed to AP over the several years' disease duration.[13,15,16] A recent detailed morphometric analysis comparing AP to CP noted that unlike the IPF associated with obesity which worsens AP, IPF accumulation in CP is independent of BMI.[17,99] Moreover, a large proportion of CP-associated fat is walled off by fibrosis from the rest of the pancreatic parenchyma, resulting in reduced "lipolytic flux" between adipocytes and acinar cells (discussed in more detail in the pathophysiology section), which during AP causes perifat acinar necrosis and contributes to about half of the parenchymal necrosis in obese patients.[17,63]

Chemical analysis of pancreatic fat in normal pancreata revealed an enrichment of unsaturated fatty acids in pancreatic triglyceride from individuals with higher amounts of pancreatic fat compared to those with lower levels.[100] Pancreatic necrosis debridement fluid also has a higher concentration of unsaturated fatty acids.[62-64,101] These observations along with the predisposition of obese patients to have a severe AP attack,[1-11] the higher serum levels of UFAs in patients with SAP,[102] and SAP being reported at lower BMIs from countries with higher UFAs or PUFA in their diets and visceral fat support an association between lipolysis of visceral triglyceride enriched in UFAs with SAP.[4,10,53,54] The mechanisms of this phenomenon are discussed in the next section.

Pathophysiologic Role of Obesity Related Fat in SAP

Adverse outcomes early in the course of the SAP are typically related to distant organ complications such as sustained respiratory or renal failure or shock.[103-105] Those later in the disease course are typically associated with complications of severe pancreatic necrosis, including infection and associated organ failure.[106-109] Here we will systematically explore each of these in the context of obesity.

Role of pancreatic fat in exacerbating pancreatic necrosis

As detailed in the section above, both histologic and radiologic quantification show intrapancreatic adipocyte mass to increase with BMI in the human pancreas.[17,63,75] Unsaturated triglyceride is higher in human pancreata with more adipocytes,[100] and pancreatic necrosis collections from obese patients have higher UFA concentrations than pancreatic fluid from pseudocysts and pancreatic cystic neoplasms,[62] which are typically from patients with lower BMIs compared to patients with necrotic collections. These observations and the epidemiologic data mentioned above associating obesity with SAP support the need for further mechanistic exploration of this area.

The first question these observations raise is how do pancreatic fat and the exocrine pancreas interact in health and disease? Most obese persons will never experience an episode of pancreatitis. While adipocytes that accumulate in obesity are adjacent to cells of the exocrine pancreas (**Figure 1A**), it is the basal surface of the exocrine cells that abuts the adipocytes (red dashed arcs in **Figure 1B**), and the apical lumen into which the exocrine cells secrete (red ovals) is not in contact with the adipocytes. Thus, the two compartments do not normally communicate. Paraffin-embedded sections show that adipocytes in the pancreas have clear cytoplasm, consistent with the wash out of triglycerides from these cells during processing (**Figure 2A**). In contrast, during AP some adipocytes take on an amorphous blue appearance following hematoxylin and eosin staining, consistent with fat necrosis (**Figure 2C**), and there is loss of cellular detail of the surrounding exocrine parenchyma with a morphological appearance of parenchymal necrosis termed perifat acinar necrosis (PFAN).[17,63] Consistent with early 20th century observations of fatty acids generated in fat necrosis being saponified,[30] staining of serial sections of these areas for calcium (e.g., using the Von Kossa method) shows intense brown coloring indicating fat necrosis.

Interestingly, this brown staining is not restricted to fat necrosis; it is also positive in the necrotic parenchyma in close proximity to necrosed fat. It becomes less intense with increasing distance from the fat necrosis, suggestive of spillage of the products of fat necrosis (i.e., free fatty acids, FFAs) into this PFAN.[17,63] The pathophysiologic relevance of this observation is supported by the intense inflammatory reaction and accumulation of CD68-positive macrophages in and around the PFAN, compared to what is normally seen

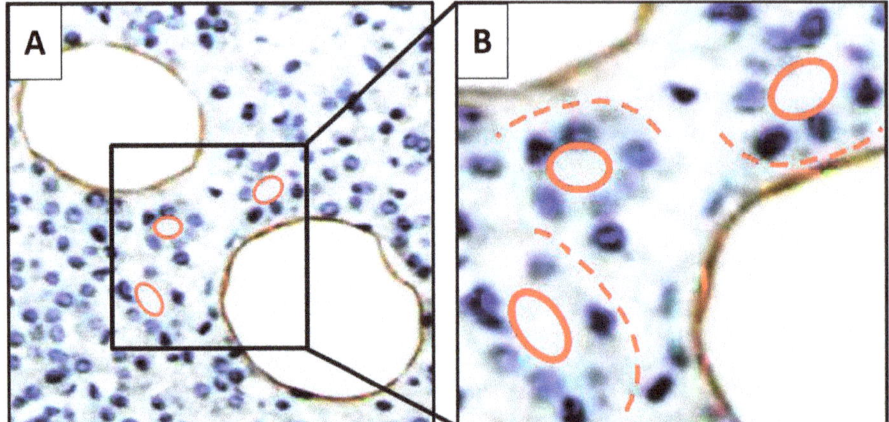

Figure 1.Perilipin1 immunohistochemistry showing brown-staining adipocytes in the human pancreas. A: The apical lumen of the exocrine pancreatic cells (red ovals) into which pancreatic enzymes are secreted face away from the adipocytes. Thebasal surfaces of the exocrine acinar cells (red dashes) abut the adjacent adipocytes.

in pancreatic fat (**Figure 3**). This inflammatory response also supports the antemortem nature of pancreatic fat necrosis in humans. Previous immunohistochemical studies revealed pancreatic lipases in fat necrosis,[110] indicating their mechanistic role in fat necrosis. Basolateral leakage of pancreatic enzymes has been mechanistically studied in detail, and while polarized acinar cells normally pour their exocrine secretions into the lumen, polarity is lost during pancreatitis, resulting in basolateral release of digestive enzymes.[111,112] This phenomenon potentially explains the basolateral leakage of lipases into fat during pancreatitis resulting in the ensuing lipolysis of fat, consequent fat necrosis, and generation of a high concentration of FFAs locally, eventually culminating in PFAN.

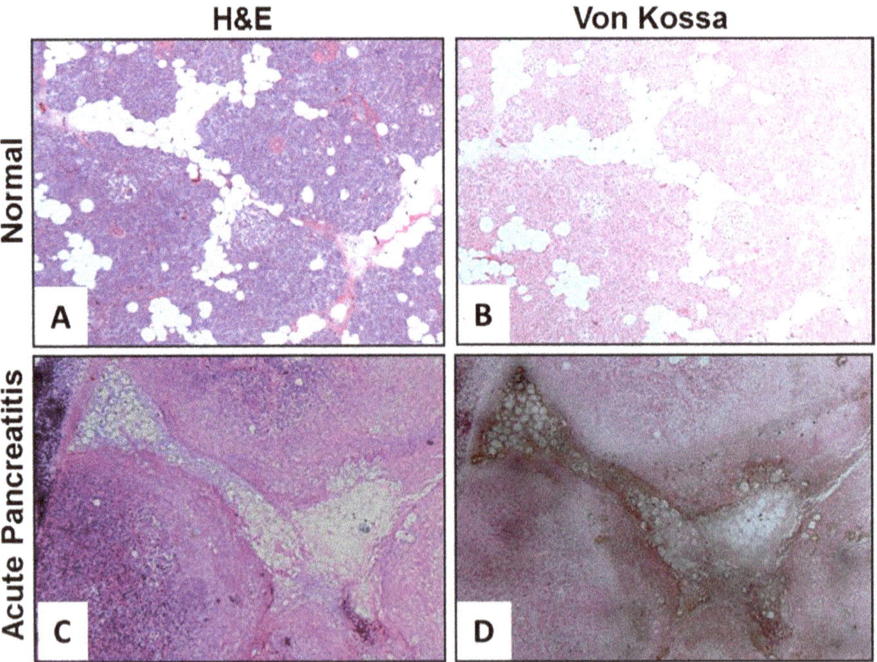

Figure 2. Serial sections of human pancreas stained with hematoxylin and eosin (H&E) and for calcium (von Kossa). Adipocytes normally stain as clear empty round areas, and the exocrine parenchyma adjacent to the adipocytes retains its morphological detail (A) and is von Kossa negative (B). In pancreatitis, fat necrosis of the adipocytes appears as amorphous blue (C), with the adjacent parenchyma losing its morphological detail and appearing diffusely pink consistent with necrosis. This is termed perifat acinar necrosis (PFAN). Von Kossa staining (D) is intensely positive in necrotic fat and adjacent PFAN, with the staining progressively becoming weaker with increasing distance from the fat necrosis. Modified from Acharya et al.[17]

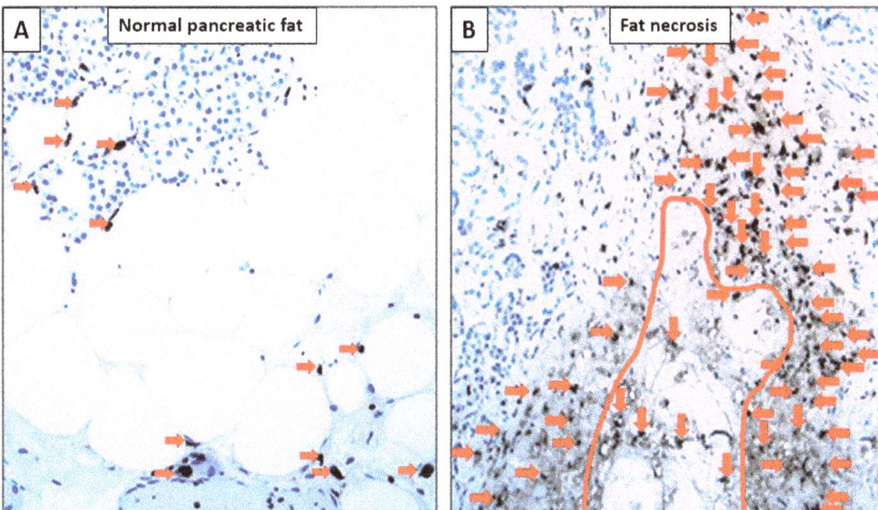

Figure 3. Human pancreas staining for the macrophage marker CD68. While there are a few CD68-positive cells (red arrows) around the adipocytes in a normal pancreas (A), sections from pancreatitis patients (B) show areas of fat necrosis (red polygon) and surrounding PFAN to have a large increase in CD68-positive cells, supporting the proinflammatory and antemortem nature of fat necrosis.

Proof of this "lipolytic flux" between acinar cells and adipocytes being relevant to pancreatic injury during AP is provided by studies using a coculture system of these two cell types. In this system, suspension cultures of acinar cells and adipocytes are physically separated into two different compartments by a 3-μm grid, which allows macromolecular diffusion without contamination of one compartment by the other cell type.[17,63] This system simulating basolateral release allows for pancreatic lipases to increase in the adipocyte compartment and lipolytic products including FFAs and glycerol generated by hydrolysis of adipocyte triglyceride to thereby increase in the adipocyte compartment and diffuse into the acinar compartment. The increase in FAAs in the acinar compartment causes necrosis of these cells as evidenced by prevention of FFA increase and necrosis by the lipase inhibitor orlistat. The pathophysiologic relevance of this in vitro system is supported by the Von-Kossa-positive areas in PFAN noted in histologic sections of human AP (**Figure 2C, D**)[17,63] and is further proven by induction of acinar necrosis following direct exposure to UFAs at concentrations present in human pancreatic necrosis collections.[17,62-64] Further proof is provided by in vivo models in which intraductal injection of the unsaturated triglyceride glyceryl trilinoleate (GTL) results in severe pancreatic necrosis, which is prevented by orlistat-mediated inhibition of its lipolysis to linoleic acid.[64] The mechanism of UFA-induced acinar cell necrosis is the inhibition of mitochondrial complexes I and V, resulting in decreased ATP levels.[63] While the intermediary signaling involved in this lipolytic flux and fatty acid-induced acinar injury remains to be determined, the existing level of evidence regarding the detrimental role of obesity-associated fat necrosis in worsening pancreatic necrosis is extremely strong. Thus, the increase in pancreatic fat during obesity worsens pancreatic necrosis via fat necrosis in those who develop AP.

Role of peripancreatic fat in exacerbating systemic complications during SAP

Early mortality in SAP (i.e., within the first week) may occur from multisystem organ failure (MSOF) with minimal or no evidence of pancreatic necrosis.[103-105] Recent clinical reports and the revised Atlanta criteria mention peripancreatic necrosis as a risk factor for SAP.[79,82-85] Early severe peripancreatic fat stranding is associated with SAP including organ failure, mortality, and longer duration of hospital stay.[80,113,114] While AP associated mortality is currently quoted at 1%-3%,[115-117] recent studies show isolated extrapancreatic necrosis with no radiologic evidence of pancreatic necrosis to have mortality rates of 9%-13%.[79,80]

Extrapancreatic or peripancreatic necrosis is predominantly fat necrosis around the pancreas.[37,118,119] Gross and microscopic pathologic studies of human pancreata surgically resected early in the course of pancreatitis were systematically done in the 1980s by different groups including Nordback et al.,[118] Kloppel et al.,[37,119] and separately by Schmitz-Moormann.[36] Conclusions from these studies supported fat necrosis, specifically peripancreatic fat necrosis, as the earliest lesion in AP. Nordback et al. categorically stated, "The most vulnerable areas seemed to be the peripancreatic adipose tissue, from where the necrosis spread through the septa towards the pancreatic parenchyma".[118] In their series of 78 patients with acute necrotizing pancreatitis, they noted that while all patients had peripancreatic necrosis, 10% had peripancreatic necrosis without acinar necrosis. Peripancreatic necrosis involved >50% of the peripancreatic fat in 23 of the 30 patients operated on within 4 days of presentation, while only 8 of these had >50% of parenchymal necrosis. Supporting the role of systemic injury in SAP-associated early mortality,[103-105] autopsy studies showed patients dying within the first week of AP to have lung injury with a moderate amount of fat necrosis around the pancreas.[120] Overall, this information suggests that peripancreatic fat necrosis is a distinct player in the pathogenesis of MSOF during the first few days of AP.

Various groups have quantified visceral fat, which is the major hydrolyzable pool of triglyceride surrounding the pancreas. It is estimated that this may average >3 kg in subjects with a mean body weight of 84 kg.[77,78] Calculations from imaging studies estimate visceral fat to occupy 10%-30% of the intra-abdominal abdominal area,[48] with intra-abdominal volumes of obese individuals estimated to be 23-30 L,[121] The volume occupied by visceral fat can range from 2-9 L. Since triglyceride comprises 80%-90% of adipocyte volume and each triglyceride molecule can generate three FFA molecules after lipolysis, unregulated leakage of lipases from the pancreas during pancreatitis can potentially generate large amounts of lipotoxic FFAs from these peripancreatic visceral fat depots in a short time and result in adverse outcomes.[87-89]

Recent mechanistic studies have explored the role of peripancreatic fat necrosis in MSOF. Patel et al. noted that a classically self-limited model of pancreatitis in mice (i.e., cerulein pancreatitis) was lethal in obese mice but not lean mice.[61] Interestingly they noted that pancreatic acinar necrosis was no different between the surviving and decreased groups. In contrast, fat necrosis was absent in lean mice and significantly more in obese mice that died, and this was reduced by administering the lipase inhibitor orlistat. The most impressive changes at necropsy were noted in the abdominal fat surrounding the pancreas, with fat necrosis and saponification noted in the mice that died; this resembles human disease. Notably, it was associated with hypocalcemia (an SAP marker/predictor included in Ranson's criteria,[122] the Glasgow criteria,[123] and the Japanese severity score[124]), lung injury, and renal failure (evidenced by elevated BUNs), all of which are commonly used markers or predictors for SAP.[122,123,125,126]

Further proof of the role of peripancreatic fat necrosis in worsening AP outcomes independent of pancreatic necrosis comes from a recent study in which triolein (the triglyceride form of the most abundant UFA in humans, oleic acid) when co-administered during the induction of cerulein pancreatitis in lean rats resulted in MSOF with 97% mortality.[62] This was evidenced by hypoxemic respiratory failure (oxygen saturation <89%) associated with acute lung injury, renal tubular injury along, and elevated serum BUNs, all in the absence of significant pancreatic necrosis. Serum cytokines including interleukin (IL)-1β and IL-8 in the rats with organ failure were more than 10× higher than those with cerulein pancreatitis alone. All of the parameters described above are SAP markers or included in prediction systems.[122-134] To explore this further, the authors exposed peripheral blood mononuclear cells to UFAs or IL-1β + IL-8 and noted that while UFAs at concentrations below those noted in serum resulted in necroapoptotic cell death, cytokines at concentrations above those in the serum did not.[61,62] This is consistent with findings that while UFAs can increase mRNA levels of cytokines and induce cell death,[17,63] cytokines do not induce cell injury and in some cases are hypothesized to have a protective role in AP, possibly by reducing systemic injury.[135-141]

It is worth noting that in the studies mentioned above, triolein was administered to lean rats, and its hydrolysis resulted in high serum levels of its lipolytic product oleic acid (350 ± 294 μM), similar to SAP patients with complications (614 ± 146 μM).[102] These patients also had serum FFA >1,400 μM,[102] which was in the same range as rats dying with MSOF (1,421 ± 851 μM). Thus, it is the acute lipotoxicity from UFAs and not the chronic inflammatory state associated with obesity that leads to adverse AP outcomes. Further proof of the role of UFAs in SAP comes from studies in which pure UFAs were administered to rodents. UFAs caused acute lung injury,[142-145] renal tubular toxicity,[146,147] renal failure,[144,148] and hypocalcemia.[148] This spectrum of endpoints is highly relevant to MSOF associated with SAP, the parameters of which are used in grading AP severity.[122,126,149] Thus, the acute release of large amounts of UFA following lipolysis of large pools of peripancreatic visceral fat can worsen the disease course, even in cases where there is minimal pancreatic necrosis, such as early in the disease course.

Summary

In summary, we studied the mechanisms resulting in excessive pancreatic or visceral fat necrosis during AP in obese patients and how this may exacerbate disease. This occurs due to the lipolysis of the visceral triglyceride by the leaked pancreatic lipases, resulting in large and acute release of UFAs locally or systemically. UFAs inhibit mitochondrial complexes I and V and locally worsen pancreatic necrosis, while systemic UFA release can cause lung and renal injury culminating in MSOF. Thus, unregulated lipolysis of visceral fat in obesity can convert AP to SAP.

Acknowledgement

This work was supported by the National Institutes of Health (NIH) grants RO1DK92460 (V.P.S.) and R01DK100358 (V.P.S.) and the Clinical Translational Science Institute (CTSI) supported by the NIH through Grant Numbers UL1RR024153 and UL1TR000005 (V.P.S. and S.N.).

References

1. Abu Hilal M, Armstrong T. The impact of obesity on the course and outcome of acute pancreatitis. *Obes Surg*. 2008; 18(3): 326-328. PMID: 18202895.
2. Papachristou GI, Papachristou DJ, Avula H, Slivka A, Whitcomb DC. Obesity increases the severity of acute pancreatitis: performance of APACHE-O score and correlation with the inflammatory response. *Pancreatology*. 2006; 6(4): 279-285. PMID: 16636600.
3. Porter KA, Banks PA. Obesity as a predictor of severity in acute pancreatitis. *Int J Pancreatol*. 1991; 10(3-4): 247-252. PMID: 1787336.
4. Shin KY, Lee WS, Chung DW, Heo J, Jung MK, Tak WY, et al. Influence of obesity on the severity and clinical outcome of acute pancreatitis. *Gut Liver*. 2011; 5(3): 335-339. PMID: 21927663.
5. O'Leary DP, O'Neill D, McLaughlin P, O'Neill S, Myers E, Maher MM, et al. Effects of abdominal fat distribution parameters on severity of acute pancreatitis. *World J Surg*. 2012; 36(7): 1679-1685. PMID: 22491816.
6. Sempere L, Martinez J, de Madaria E, Lozano B, Sanchez-Paya J, Jover R, et al. Obesity and fat distribution imply a greater systemic inflammatory response and a worse prognosis in acute pancreatitis. *Pancreatology*. 2008; 8(3): 257-264. PMID: 18497538.
7. Evans AC, Papachristou GI, Whitcomb DC. Obesity and the risk of severe acute pancreatitis. *Minerva Gastroenterol Dietol*. 2010; 56(2): 169-179. PMID: 20485254.
8. Chen SM, Xiong GS, Wu SM. Is obesity an indicator of complications and mortality in acute pancreatitis? An updated meta-analysis. *J Dig Dis* 2012; 13(5): 244-251. PMID: 22500786.
9. Sadr-Azodi O, Orsini N, Andren-Sandberg A, Wolk A. Abdominal and total adiposity and the risk of acute pancreatitis: a population-based prospective cohort study. *Am J Gastroenterol*. 2013; 108(1): 133-139. PMID: 23147519.
10. Yashima Y, Isayama H, Tsujino T, Nagano R, Yamamoto K, Mizuno S, et al. A large volume of visceral adipose tissue leads to severe acute pancreatitis. *Am J Gastroenterol*. 2011; 46(10): 1213-1218. PMID: 21805069.
11. Funnell IC, Bornman PC, Weakley SP, Terblanche J, Marks IN. Obesity: an important prognostic factor in acute pancreatitis. *Br J Surg*. 1993; 80(4): 484-486. PMID: 8495317.
12. Yadav D, O'Connell M, Papachristou GI. Natural history following the first attack of acute pancreatitis. *Am J Gastroenterol*. 2012; 107(7): 1096-1103. PMID: 22613906.
13. Lankisch PG, Breuer N, Bruns A, Weber-Dany B, Lowenfels AB, Maisonneuve P. Natural history of acute pancreatitis: a long-term population-based study. *Am J Gastroenterol*. 2009; 104(11): 2797-2805; quiz 2806. PMID: 19603011.
14. Nojgaard C, Becker U, Matzen P, Andersen JR, Holst C, Bendtsen F. Progression from acute to chronic pancreatitis: prognostic factors, mortality, and natural course. *Pancreas*. 2011; 40(8): 1195-1200. PMID: 21926938.
15. Otsuki M. Chronic pancreatitis in Japan: epidemiology, prognosis, diagnostic criteria, and future problems. *J Gastroenterol*. 2003; 38(4): 315-326. PMID: 12743770.
16. Nøjgaard C, Matzen P, Bendtsen F, Andersen JR, Christensen E, Becker U. Factors associated with long-term mortality in acute pancreatitis. *Scand J Gastroenterol*. 2011; 46(4): 495-502. PMID: 21091094.
17. Acharya C, Cline RA, Jaligama D, Noel P, Delany JP, Bae K, et al. Fibrosis reduces severity of acute-on-chronic pancreatitis in humans. *Gastroenterology*. 2013; 145(2): 466-475. PMID: 23684709.
18. Chen CH, Dai CY, Hou NJ, Chen SC, Chuang WL, Yu ML. Etiology, severity and recurrence of acute pancreatitis in southern taiwan. *J Formosan Med Assoc*. 2006; 105(7): 550-555. PMID: 16877234.
19. Sekimoto M, Takada T, Kawarada Y, Hirata K, Mayumi T, Yoshida M, et al. JPN Guidelines for the management of acute pancreatitis: epidemiology, etiology, natural history, and outcome predictors in acute pancreatitis. *J Hepatobiliary Pancreat Surg*. 2006; 13(1): 10-24. PMID: 16463207.
20. Xin MJ, Chen H, Luo B, Sun JB. Severe acute pancreatitis in the elderly: etiology and clinical characteristics. *World J Gastroenterol*. 2008; 14(16): 2517-2521. PMID: 18442198.
21. Vidarsdottir H, Moller PH, Thorarinsdottir H, Bjornsson ES. Acute pancreatitis: a prospective study on incidence, etiology, and outcome. *Eur J Gastroenterol Hepatol*. 2013; 25(9): 1068-1075. PMID: 23839162.
22. Dominguez-Muñoz JE, Malfertheiner P, Ditschuneit HH, Blanco-Chavez J, Uhl W, Büchler M, et al. Hyperlipidemia in acute pancreatitis. Relationship with etiology, onset, and severity of the disease. *Int J Pancreatol*. 1991; 10(3-4): 261-267. PMID: 1787337.
23. Deng LH, Xue P, Xia Q, Yang XN, Wan MH. Effect of admission hypertriglyceridemia on the episodes of severe acute pancreatitis. *World J Gastroenterol*. 2008; 14(28): 4558-4561. PMID: 18680239.
24. Lloret Linares C, Pelletier AL, Czernichow S, Vergnaud AC, Bonnefont-Rousselot D, Levy P, et al. Acute pancreatitis in a cohort of 129 patients referred for severe hypertriglyceridemia. *Pancreas*. 2008; 37(1): 13-12. PMID: 18580438.
25. Balser W. Ueber Fettnekrose cine zuwcilen todliche Krankheit des Menschen. *Arch Pathol Anat Physiol*. 1882; 90: 520-535.
26. Fitz RH. *Acute pancreatitis: a consideration of pancreatic hemorrhage, hemorrhagic, suppurative, and gangrenous pancreatitis, and of disseminated fat-necrosis*. Boston, MA: Cupples and Hurd; 1889.
27. Pannala R, Kidd M, Modlin IM. Acute pancreatitis: a historical perspective. *Pancreas*. 2009; 38(4): 355-366. PMID: 19390402.
28. Chiari H. Uber die Beziehungen zwischen dem Pankreas und der Fettgewebsnekrose. *Zbl Pathol*. 1906; 17: 798-799.
29. Hotchkiss LW. VIII. Acute Pancreatitis with Very Extensive Fat Necrosis. *Annals Surg*. 1912; 56(1): 111-117. PMID: 17862860.
30. Herbert F. Pancreatic Fat Necrosis: A Chemical Study. *Br J Exp Pathol*. 1928; 9(2): 57-63.
31. Theve NO, Hallberg D, Carlström A. Studies in fat necrosis. I. Lipolysis and calcium content in adipose tissue from rats with experimentally induced fat necrosis. *Acta Chir Scand*. 1973; 139(2): 131-133. PMID: 4718164.
32. Storck G. Experimental fat necrosis in the rat. I. Studies with the vital microscope. *Acta Chir Scand*. 1972; 138(1): 69-77. PMID: 5036400.

33. Theve NO. Studies in fat necrosis. V. Effect of glucose and insulin on fat necrosis in rats with experimental pancreatitis. *Acta Chir Scand.* 1973; 139(6): 507-509. PMID: 4753098.
34. Olsen TS. Lipomatosis of the pancreas in autopsy material and its relation to age and overweight. *Acta Pathol Microbiol Scand A.* 1978; 86A(5): 367-373. PMID: 716899.
35. Schmitz-Moormann P, Pittner PM, Heinze W. Lipomatosis of the pancreas. A morphometrical investigation. *Pathol Res Pract.* 1981; 173(1-2): 45-53. PMID: 7335549.
36. Schmitz-Moormann P. Comparative radiological and morphological study of the human pancreas. IV. Acute necrotizing pancreatitis in man. *Pathol Res Pract.* 1981; 171(3-4): 325-335. PMID: 7279784.
37. Kloppel G, Dreyer T, Willemer S, Kern HF, Adler G. Human acute pancreatitis: its pathogenesis in the light of immunocytochemical and ultrastructural findings in acinar cells. *Virchows Arch A Pathol Anat Histopathol.* 1986; 409(6): 791-803. PMID: 3094241.
38. Trapnell JE, Rigby CC, Talbot CH, Duncan EH. Proceedings: Aprotinin in the treatment of acute pancreatitis. *Gut.* 1973; 14(10): 828. PMID: 4586085.
39. Trapnell JE, Rigby CC, Talbot CH, Duncan EH. A controlled trial of Trasylol in the treatment of acute pancreatitis. *Br J Surg.* 1974; 61(3): 177-182. PMID: 4595174.
40. Trapnell JE, Talbot CH, Capper WM. Trasylol in acute pancreatitis. *Am J Dig Dis.* 1967; 12(4): 409-412. PMID: 5336018.
41. Buchler M, Malfertheiner P, Uhl W, Scholmerich J, Stockmann F, Adler G, et al. Gabexate mesilate in human acute pancreatitis. German Pancreatitis Study Group. *Gastroenterology.* 1993; 104(4): 1165-1170. PMID: 8462805.
42. Andriulli A, Caruso N, Quitadamo M, Forlano R, Leandro G, Spirito F, et al. Antisecretory vs. antiproteasic drugs in the prevention of post-ERCP pancreatitis: the evidence-based medicine derived from a meta-analysis study. *JOP.* 2003; 4(1): 41-48. PMID: 12555015.
43. Seta T, Noguchi Y, Shimada T, Shikata S, Fukui T. Treatment of acute pancreatitis with protease inhibitors: a meta-analysis. *Eur J Gastroenterol Hepatol.* 2004; 16(12): 1287-1293. PMID: 15618834.
44. Mossner J, Bodeker H, Kimura W, Meyer F, Bohm S, Fischbach W. Isolated rat pancreatic acini as a model to study the potential role of lipase in the pathogenesis of acinar cell destruction. *Int J Pancreatol.* 1992; 12(3): 285-296. PMID: 1289421.
45. Kimura W, Meyer F, Hess D, Kirchner T, Fischbach W, Mossner J. Comparison of different treatment modalities in experimental pancreatitis in rats. *Gastroenterology.* 1992; 103(6): 1916-1924. PMID: 1451985.
46. Mery CM, Rubio V, Duarte-Rojo A, Suazo-Barahona J, Pelaez-Luna M, Milke P, et al. Android fat distribution as predictor of severity in acute pancreatitis. *Pancreatology.* 2002; 2(6): 543-549. PMID: 12435867.
47. Martínez J, Sánchez-Payá J, Palazón JM, Aparicio JR, Picó A, Pérez-Mateo M. Obesity: a prognostic factor of severity in acute pancreatitis. *Pancreas.* 1999; 19(1): 15-20. PMID: 10416686.
48. Camhi SM, Bray GA, Bouchard C, Greenway FL, Johnson WD, Newton RL, et al. The relationship of waist circumference and BMI to visceral, subcutaneous, and total body fat: sex and race differences. *Obesity.* 2011; 19(2): 402-408. PMID: 20948514.
49. Hegazi R, Raina A, Graham T, Rolniak S, Centa P, Kandil H, et al. Early jejunal feeding initiation and clinical outcomes in patients with severe acute pancreatitis. *JPEN J Parenter Enteral Nutr.* 2011; 35(1): 91-96. PMID: 21224435.
50. Brown A, James-Stevenson T, Dyson T, Grunkenmeier D. The panc 3 score: a rapid and accurate test for predicting severity on presentation in acute pancreatitis. *J Clin Gastroenterol.* 2007; 41(9): 855-858. PMID: 17881932.
51. Johnson CD, Toh SK, Campbell MJ. Combination of APACHE-II score and an obesity score (APACHE-O) for the prediction of severe acute pancreatitis. *Pancreatology.* 2004; 4(1): 1-6. PMID: 14988652.
52. Katuchova J, Bober J, Harbulak P, Hudak A, Gajdzik T, Kalanin R, et al. Obesity as a risk factor for severe acute pancreatitis patients. *Wien Klin Wochenschr.* 2014; 126(7-8): 223-227. PMID: 24522641.
53. Yang F, Wu H, Li Y, Li Z, Wang C, Yang J, et al. Prevention of severe acute pancreatitis with octreotide in obese patients: a prospective multi-center randomized controlled trial. *Pancreas.* 2012; 41(8): 1206-1212. PMID: 23086244.
54. Thandassery RB, Appasani S, Yadav TD, Dutta U, Indrajit A, Singh K, et al. Implementation of the Asia-Pacific guidelines of obesity classification on the APACHE-O scoring system and its role in the prediction of outcomes of acute pancreatitis: a study from India. *Dig Dis Sci.* 2014; 59(6): 1316-1321. PMID: 24374646.
55. Scott RF, Lee KT, Kim DN, Morrison ES, Goodale F. Fatty acids of serum and adipose tissue in six groups eating natural diets containing 7 to 40 per cent fat. *Am J Clin Nutr.* 1964; 14: 280-290. PMID: 14157830.
56. Insull W Jr, Lang PD, Hsi BP, Yoshimura S. Studies of arteriosclerosis in Japanese and American men. I. Comparison of fatty acid composition of adipose tissue. *J Clin Invest.* 1969; 48(7): 1313-1327. PMID: 5794253.
57. Ueshima H, Stamler J, Elliott P, Chan Q, Brown IJ, Carnethon MR, et al. Food omega-3 fatty acid intake of individuals (total, linolenic acid, long-chain) and their blood pressure: INTERMAP study. *Hypertension.* 2007; 50(2): 313-319. PMID: 17548718.
58. Ruixing Y, Qiming F, Dezhai Y, Shuquan L, Weixiong L, Shangling P, et al. Comparison of demography, diet, lifestyle, and serum lipid levels between the Guangxi Bai Ku Yao and Han populations. *J Lipid Res.* 2007; 48(12): 2673-2681. PMID: 17890682.
59. Insull W Jr, Bartsch GE. Fatty acid composition of human adipose tissue related to age, sex, and race. *Am J Clin Nutr.* 1967; 20(1): 13-23. PMID: 6017005.
60. Hirsch J, Farquhar JW, Ahrens EH Jr., Peterson ML, Stoffel W. Studies of adipose tissue in man. A microtechnic for sampling and analysis. *Am J Clin Nutr.* 1960; 8: 499-511. PMID: 13714574.
61. Patel K, Trivedi RN, Durgampudi C, Noel P, Cline RA, DeLany JP, et al. Lipolysis of visceral adipocyte

triglyceride by pancreatic lipases converts mild acute pancreatitis to severe pancreatitis independent of necrosis and inflammation. *Am J Pathol.* 2015; 185(3): 808-819. PMID: 25579844.

62. Noel P, Patel K, Durgampudi C, Trivedi RN, de Oliveira C, Crowell MD, et al. Peripancreatic fat necrosis worsens acute pancreatitis independent of pancreatic necrosis via unsaturated fatty acids increased in human pancreatic necrosis collections. *Gut.* 2016; 65(1): 100-111. PMID: 25500204.
63. Navina S, Acharya C, DeLany JP, Orlichenko LS, Baty CJ, Shiva SS, et al. Lipotoxicity causes multisystem organ failure and exacerbates acute pancreatitis in obesity. *Sci Transl Med.* 2011; 3(107): 107ra110. PMID: 22049070.
64. Durgampudi C, Noel P, Patel K, Cline R, Trivedi RN, DeLany JP, et al. Acute lipotoxicity regulates severity of biliary acute pancreatitis without affecting its initiation. *Am J Pathol.* 2014; 184(6): 1773-1784. PMID: 24854864.
65. Ehret GB, Munroe PB, Rice KM, Bochud M, Johnson AD, Chasman DI, et al. Genetic variants in novel pathways influence blood pressure and cardiovascular disease risk. *Nature.* 2011; 478(7367): 103-109. PMID: 21909115.
66. Neuer FS, Roberts FF, McCarthy V. Osteolytic lesions following traumatic pancreatitis. *Am J Dis Child.* 1977; 131(7): 738-740. PMID: 879110.
67. Goluboff N, Cram R, Ramgotra B, Singh A, Wilkinson GW. Polyarthritis and bone lesions complicating traumatic pancreatitis in two children. *Canadian Med Assoc J.* 1978; 118(8): 924-928. PMID: 647564.
68. Schrier RW, Melmon KL, Fenster LF. Subcutaneous nodular fat necrosis in pancreatitis. *Arch Intern Med.* 1965; 116(6): 832-836. PMID: 5848214.
69. Blauvelt H. A case of acute pancreatitis with subcutaneous fat necrosis. *Br J Surg.* 1946; 34(134): 207. PMID: 20278132.
70. Cannon JR, Pitha JV, Everett MA. Subcutaneous fat necrosis in pancreatitis. *J Cutan Pathol.* 1979; 6(6): 501-506. PMID: 521541.
71. Wilson HA, Askari AD, Neiderhiser DH, Johnson AM, Andrews BS, Hoskins LC. Pancreatitis with arthropathy and subcutaneous fat necrosis. Evidence for the pathogenicity of lipolytic enzymes. *Arthritis Rheum.* 1983; 26(2): 121-126. PMID: 6337595.
72. Ibrahim MM. Subcutaneous and visceral adipose tissue: structural and functional differences. *Obes Rev.* 2009; 11(1): 11-18. PMID: 19656312.
73. Park BJ, Kim YJ, Kim DH, Kim W, Jung YJ, Yoon JH, et al. Visceral adipose tissue area is an independent risk factor for hepatic steatosis. *J Gastroenterol Hepatol.* 2008; 23(6): 900-907. PMID: 17995942.
74. Rosso E, Casnedi S, Pessaux P, Oussoultzoglou E, Panaro F, Mahfud M, et al. The role of "fatty pancreas" and of BMI in the occurrence of pancreatic fistula after pancreaticoduodenectomy. *J Gastrointest Surg.* 2009; 13(10): 1845-1851. PMID: 19639369.
75. Saisho Y, Butler AE, Meier JJ, Monchamp T, Allen-Auerbach M, Rizza RA, et al. Pancreas volumes in humans from birth to age one hundred taking into account sex, obesity, and presence of type-2 diabetes. *Clin Anat.* 2007; 20(8): 933-942. PMID: 17879305.
76. Balthazar EJ, Robinson DL, Megibow AJ, Ranson JH. Acute pancreatitis: value of CT in establishing prognosis. *Radiology.* 1990; 174(2): 331-336. PMID: 2296641.
77. Choh AC, Demerath EW, Lee M, Williams KD, Towne B, Siervogel RM, et al. Genetic analysis of self-reported physical activity and adiposity: the Southwest Ohio Family Study. *Public Health Nutr.* 2009; 12(8): 1052-1060. PMID: 18778532.
78. Demerath EW, Reed D, Choh AC, Soloway L, Lee M, Czerwinski SA, et al. Rapid postnatal weight gain and visceral adiposity in adulthood: the Fels Longitudinal Study. *Obesity.* 2009; 17(11): 2060-2066. PMID: 19373221.
79. Bakker OJ, van Santvoort H, Besselink MG, Boermeester MA, van Eijck C, Dejong K, et al. Extrapancreatic necrosis without pancreatic parenchymal necrosis: a separate entity in necrotising pancreatitis? *Gut.* 2013; 62(10): 1475-1480. PMID: 22773550.
80. Meyrignac O, Lagarde S, Bournet B, Mokrane FZ, Buscail L, Rousseau H, et al. Acute Pancreatitis: Extrapancreatic Necrosis Volume as Early Predictor of Severity. *Radiology.* 2015; 276(1): 119-128. PMID: 25642743.
81. Freeman ML, Werner J, van Santvoort HC, Baron TH, Besselink MG, Windsor JA, et al. Interventions for necrotizing pancreatitis: summary of a multidisciplinary consensus conference. *Pancreas.* 2012; 41(8): 1176-1194. PMID: 23086243.
82. Banks PA, Bollen TL, Dervenis C, Gooszen HG, Johnson CD, Sarr MG, et al. Classification of acute pancreatitis--2012: revision of the Atlanta classification and definitions by international consensus. *Gut.* 2013; 62(1): 102-111. PMID: 23100216.
83. Schaffler A, Hamer O, Dickopf J, Goetz A, Landfried K, Voelk M, et al. Admission resistin levels predict peripancreatic necrosis and clinical severity in acute pancreatitis. *Am J Gastroenterol.* 2010; 105(11): 2474-2484. PMID: 20648005.
84. Bollen TL, Singh VK, Maurer R, Repas K, van Es HW, Banks PA, et al. A comparative evaluation of radiologic and clinical scoring systems in the early prediction of severity in acute pancreatitis. *Am J Gastroenterol.* 2012; 107(4): 612-619. PMID: 22186977.
85. Singh VK, Bollen TL, Wu BU, Repas K, Maurer R, Yu S, et al. An assessment of the severity of interstitial pancreatitis. *Clin Gastroenterol Hepatol.* 2011; 9(12): 1098-1103. PMID: 21893128.
86. Matsumoto S, Mori H, Miyake H, Takaki H, Maeda T, Yamada Y, et al. Uneven fatty replacement of the pancreas: evaluation with CT. *Radiology.* 1995; 194(2): 453-458. PMID: 7824726.
87. Ren J, Dimitrov I, Sherry AD, Malloy CR. Composition of adipose tissue and marrow fat in humans by 1H NMR at 7 Tesla. *J Lipid Res.* 2008; 49(9): 2055-2062. PMID: 18509197.
88. Thomas LW. The chemical composition of adipose tissue of man and mice. *Q J Exp Physiol Cogn Med Sci.* 1962; 47: 179-188. PMID: 13920823.
89. Garaulet M, Hernandez-Morante JJ, Lujan J, Tebar FJ, Zamora S. Relationship between fat cell size and number and fatty acid composition in adipose tissue from different fat

depots in overweight/obese humans. *Int J Obes*. 2006; 30(6): 899-905. PMID: 16446749.

90. Vaughn DD, Jabra AA, Fishman EK. Pancreatic disease in children and young adults: evaluation with CT. *Radiographics*. 1998; 18(5): 1171-1187. PMID: 9747614.
91. Chaudry G, Navarro OM, Levine DS, Oudjhane K. Abdominal manifestations of cystic fibrosis in children. *Pediatr Radiol*. 2006; 36(3): 233-240. PMID: 16391928.
92. Soyer P, Spelle L, Pelage JP, Dufresne AC, Rondeau Y, Gouhiri M, et al. Cystic fibrosis in adolescents and adults: fatty replacement of the pancreas--CT evaluation and functional correlation. *Radiology*. 1999; 210(3): 611-615. PMID: 10207457.
93. LaRusch J, Whitcomb DC. Genetics of pancreatitis. *Curr Opin Gastroenterol*. 2011; 27(5): 467-474. PMID: 21844754.
94. Jackson WD. Pancreatitis: etiology, diagnosis, and management. *Curr Opin Pediatr*. 2001; 13(5): 447-451. PMID: 11801891.
95. Robertson MB, Choe KA, Joseph PM. Review of the abdominal manifestations of cystic fibrosis in the adult patient. *Radiographics*. 2006; 26(3): 679-690. PMID: 16702447.
96. Toiviainen-Salo S, Raade M, Durie PR, Ip W, Marttinen E, Savilahti E, et al. Magnetic resonance imaging findings of the pancreas in patients with Shwachman-Diamond syndrome and mutations in the SBDS gene. *J Pediatr*. 2008; 152(3): 434-436. PMID: 18280855.
97. Vege SS, Gardner TB, Chari ST, Munukuti P, Pearson RK, Clain JE, et al. Low mortality and high morbidity in severe acute pancreatitis without organ failure: a case for revising the Atlanta classification to include "moderately severe acute pancreatitis". *Am J Gastroenterol*. 2009; 104(3): 710-715. PMID: 19262525.
98. Omdal T, Dale J, Lie SA, Iversen KB, Flaatten H, Ovrebo K. Time trends in incidence, etiology, and case fatality rate of the first attack of acute pancreatitis. *Scand J Gastroenterol*. 2011; 46(11): 1389-1398. PMID: 21830851.
99. Acharya C, Navina S, Singh VP. Role of pancreatic fat in the outcomes of pancreatitis. *Pancreatology*. 2014; 14(5): 403-408. PMID: 25278311.
100. Pinnick KE, Collins SC, Londos C, Gauguier D, Clark A, Fielding BA. Pancreatic ectopic fat is characterized by adipocyte infiltration and altered lipid composition. *Obesity (Silver Spring)*. 2008; 16(3): 522-530. PMID: 18239594.
101. Panek J, Sztefko K, Drozdz W. Composition of free fatty acid and triglyceride fractions in human necrotic pancreatic tissue. *Med Sci Monit*. 2001; 7(5): 894-898. PMID: 11535930.
102. Sztefko K, Panek J. Serum free fatty acid concentration in patients with acute pancreatitis. *Pancreatology*. 2001; 1(3): 230-236. PMID: 12120200.
103. Mofidi R, Duff MD, Wigmore SJ, Madhavan KK, Garden OJ, Parks RW. Association between early systemic inflammatory response, severity of multiorgan dysfunction and death in acute pancreatitis. *Br J Surg*. 2006; 93(6): 738-744. PMID: 16671062.
104. McKay CJ, Evans S, Sinclair M, Carter CR, Imrie CW. High early mortality rate from acute pancreatitis in Scotland, 1984-1995. *Br J Surg*. 1999; 86(10): 1302-1305. PMID: 10540138.
105. Johnson CD, Abu-Hilal M. Persistent organ failure during the first week as a marker of fatal outcome in acute pancreatitis. *Gut*. 2004; 53(9): 1340-1344. PMID: 15306596.
106. Carnovale A, Rabitti PG, Manes G, Esposito P, Pacelli L, Uomo G. Mortality in acute pancreatitis: is it an early or a late event? *JOP*. 2005; 6(5): 438-444. PMID: 16186665.
107. Fu CY, Yeh CN, Hsu JT, Jan YY, Hwang TL. Timing of mortality in severe acute pancreatitis: experience from 643 patients. *World J Gastroenterol*. 2007; 13(13): 1966-1969. PMID: 17461498.
108. Mutinga M, Rosenbluth A, Tenner SM, Odze RR, Sica GT, Banks PA. Does mortality occur early or late in acute pancreatitis? *Int J Pancreatol*. 2000; 28(2): 91-95. PMID: 11128978.
109. Gloor B, Muller CA, Worni M, Martignoni ME, Uhl W, Buchler MW. Late mortality in patients with severe acute pancreatitis. *Br J Surg*. 2001; 88(7): 975-979. PMID: 11442530.
110. Fallon MB, Gorelick FS, Anderson JM, Mennone A, Saluja A, Steer ML. Effect of cerulein hyperstimulation on the paracellular barrier of rat exocrine pancreas. *Gastroenterology*. 1995; 108(6): 1863-1872. PMID: 7539388.
111. Cosen-Binker LI, Binker MG, Wang CC, Hong W, Gaisano HY. VAMP8 is the v-SNARE that mediates basolateral exocytosis in a mouse model of alcoholic pancreatitis. *J Clin Invest*. 2008; 118(7): 2535-2551. PMID: 18535671.
112. Cosen-Binker LI, Lam PP, Binker MG, Reeve J, Pandol S, Gaisano HY, Alcohol/cholecystokinin-evoked pancreatic acinar basolateral exocytosis is mediated by protein kinase C alpha phosphorylation of Munc18c. *J Biol Chem*. 2007; 282(17): 13047-13058. PMID: 17324928.
113. King NK, Powell JJ, Redhead D, Siriwardena AK. A simplified method for computed tomographic estimation of prognosis in acute pancreatitis. *Scand J Gastroenterol*. 2003; 38(4): 433-436. PMID: 12739717.
114. Eatock FC, Brombacher GD, Steven A, Imrie CW, McKay CJ, Carter R. Nasogastric feeding in severe acute pancreatitis may be practical and safe. *Int J Pancreatol*. 2000; 28(1): 23-29. PMID: 11185707.
115. Yadav D, Lowenfels AB. The epidemiology of pancreatitis and pancreatic cancer. *Gastroenterology*. 2013; 144(6): 1252-1261. PMID: 23622135.
116. Peery AF, Dellon ES, Lund J, Crockett SD, McGowan CE, Bulsiewicz WJ, et al. Burden of gastrointestinal disease in the United States: 2012 update. *Gastroenterology*. 2012; 143(5): 1179-1187 e1171-e1173. PMID: 22885331.
117. Wormer BA, Swan RZ, Williams KB, Bradley JF 3rd, Walters AL, Augenstein VA, et al. Outcomes of pancreatic debridement in acute pancreatitis: analysis of the nationwide inpatient sample from 1998 to 2010. *Am J Surg*. 2014; 208(3): 350-362. PMID: 24933665.
118. Nordback I, Lauslahti K. Clinical pathology of acute necrotising pancreatitis. *J Clin Path*. 1986; 39(1): 68-74. PMID: 3950033.
119. Klöppel G, von Gerkan R, Dreyer T. Pathomorphology of acute pancreatitis. Analysis of 367 autopsy cases and 3 surgical specimens. In: Gyr KE, Singer MV, Sarles H, editors. *Pancreatitis - concepts and classification*. New York, NY: Elsevier; 1984.

120. Renner IG, Savage WT 3rd, Pantoja JL, Renner VJ. Death due to acute pancreatitis. A retrospective analysis of 405 autopsy cases. *Dig Dis Sci.* 1985; 30(10): 1005-1018. PMID: 3896700.
121. Guerrero-Romero F, Rodríguez-Morán M. Abdominal volume index. An anthropometry-based index for estimation of obesity is strongly related to impaired glucose tolerance and type 2 diabetes mellitus. *Arch Med Res.* 2003; 34(5): 428-432. PMID: 14602511.
122. Ranson JH, Rifkind KM, Roses DF, Fink SD, Eng K, Spencer FC. Prognostic signs and the role of operative management in acute pancreatitis. *Surg Gynecol Obstet.* 1974; 139(1): 69-81. PMID: 4834279.
123. Blamey SL, Imrie CW, O'Neill J, Gilmour WH, Carter DC. Prognostic factors in acute pancreatitis. *Gut.* 1984; 25(12): 1340-1346. PMID: 6510766.
124. Ueda T, Takeyama Y, Yasuda T, Kamei K, Satoi S, Sawa H, et al. Utility of the new Japanese severity score and indications for special therapies in acute pancreatitis. *J Gastroenterol.* 2009; 44(5): 453-459. PMID: 19308309.
125. Wu BU, Johannes RS, Sun X, Tabak Y, Conwell DL, Banks PA. The early prediction of mortality in acute pancreatitis: a large population-based study. *Gut.* 2008; 57(12): 1698-1703. PMID: 18519429.
126. Harrison DA, D'Amico G, Singer M. The Pancreatitis Outcome Prediction (POP) Score: a new prognostic index for patients with severe acute pancreatitis. *Crit Care Med.* 2007; 35(7): 1703-1708. PMID: 17522578.
127. Hirota M, Nozawa F, Okabe A, Shibata M, Beppu T, Shimada S, et al. Relationship between plasma cytokine concentration and multiple organ failure in patients with acute pancreatitis. *Pancreas* 21(2): 141-146, 2000. PMID: 10975707.
128. Messmann H, Vogt W, Falk W, Vogl D, Zirngibl H, Leser HG, et al. Interleukins and their antagonists but not TNF and its receptors are released in post-ERP pancreatitis. *Eur J Gastroenterol Hepatol.* 1998; 10(7): 611-617. PMID: 9855088.
129. Brivet FG, Emilie D, Galanaud P. Pro- and anti-inflammatory cytokines during acute severe pancreatitis: an early and sustained response, although unpredictable of death. Parisian Study Group on Acute Pancreatitis. *Crit Care Med.* 1999; 27(4): 749-755. PMID: 10321665.
130. Dambrauskas Z, Giese N, Gulbinas A, Giese T, Berberat PO, Pundzius J, et al. Different profiles of cytokine expression during mild and severe acute pancreatitis. *World J Gastroenterol.* 2010; 16(15): 1845-1853. PMID: 20397261.
131. Aoun E, Chen J, Reighard D, Gleeson FC, Whitcomb DC, Papachristou GI. Diagnostic accuracy of interleukin-6 and interleukin-8 in predicting severe acute pancreatitis: a meta-analysis. *Pancreatology.* 2009; 9(6): 777-785. PMID: 20110745.
132. Daniel P, Lesniowski B, Mokrowiecka A, Jasinska A, Pietruczuk M, Malecka-Panas E. Circulating levels of visfatin, resistin and pro-inflammatory cytokine interleukin-8 in acute pancreatitis. *Pancreatology.* 2010; 10(4): 477-482. PMID: 20720449.
133. Ueda T, Takeyama Y, Yasuda T, Matsumura N, Sawa H, Nakajima T, et al. Significant elevation of serum interleukin-18 levels in patients with acute pancreatitis. *J Gastroenterol.* 2006; 41(2): 158-165. PMID: 16568375.
134. Regnér S, Appelros S, Hjalmarsson C, Manjer J, Sadic J, Borgstrom A. Monocyte chemoattractant protein 1, active carboxypeptidase B and CAPAP at hospital admission are predictive markers for severe acute pancreatitis. *Pancreatology.* 2008; 8(1): 42-49. PMID: 18235216.
135. Guice KS, Oldham KT, Remick DG, Kunkel SL, Ward PA. Anti-tumor necrosis factor antibody augments edema formation in caerulein-induced acute pancreatitis. *J Surg Res.* 1991; 51(6): 495-499. PMID: 1943086.
136. Cuzzocrea S, Mazzon E, Dugo L, Centorrino T, Ciccolo A, McDonald MC, et al. Absence of endogenous interleukin-6 enhances the inflammatory response during acute pancreatitis induced by cerulein in mice. *Cytokine.* 2002; 18(5): 274-285. PMID: 12161103.
137. Borjesson A, Norlin A, Wang X, Andersson R, Folkesson HG. TNF-alpha stimulates alveolar liquid clearance during intestinal ischemia-reperfusion in rats. *Am J Physiol Lung Cell Mol Physiol.* 2000; 278(1): L3-L12. PMID: 10645884.
138. Rezaiguia S, Garat C, Delclaux C, Meignan M, Fleury J, Legrand P, et al. Acute bacterial pneumonia in rats increases alveolar epithelial fluid clearance by a tumor necrosis factor-alpha-dependent mechanism. *J Clin Invest.* 1997; 99(2): 325-335. PMID: 9006001.
139. Kida H, Yoshida M, Hoshino S, Inoue K, Yano Y, Yanagita M, et al. Protective effect of IL-6 on alveolar epithelial cell death induced by hydrogen peroxide. *Am J Physiol Lung Cell Mol Physiol.* 2005; 288(2): L342-349. PMID: 15475383.
140. Yan C, Naltner A, Martin M, Naltner M, Fangman JM, Gurel O. Transcriptional stimulation of the surfactant protein B gene by STAT3 in respiratory epithelial cells. *J Biol Chem.* 2002; 277(13): 10967-10972. PMID: 11788590.
141. Xing Z, Gauldie J, Cox G, Baumann H, Jordana M, Lei XF, et al. IL-6 is an antiinflammatory cytokine required for controlling local or systemic acute inflammatory responses. *J Clin Invest.* 1998; 101(2): 311-320. PMID: 9435302.
142. Hussain N, Wu F, Zhu L, Thrall RS, Kresch MJ. Neutrophil apoptosis during the development and resolution of oleic acid-induced acute lung injury in the rat. *Am J Respir Cell Mol Biol.* 1998; 19(6): 867-874. PMID: 9843920.
143. Inoue H, Nakagawa Y, Ikemura M, Usugi E, Nata M. Molecular-biological analysis of acute lung injury (ALI) induced by heat exposure and/or intravenous administration of oleic acid. *Legal Med.* 2012; 14(6): 304-308. PMID: 22819303.
144. Wu RP, Liang XB, Guo H, Zhou XS, Zhao L, Wang C, et al. Protective effect of low potassium dextran solution on acute kidney injury following acute lung injury induced by oleic acid in piglets. *Chin Med Sci J.* 2012; 125(17): 3093-3097. PMID: 22932187.
145. Lai JP, Bao S, Davis IC, Knoell DL. Inhibition of the phosphatase PTEN protects mice against oleic acid-induced acute lung injury. *Br J Pharmacol.* 2009; 156(1): 189-200. PMID: 19134000.
146. Moran JH, Nowak G, Grant DF. Analysis of the toxic effects of linoleic acid, 12,13-cis-epoxyoctadecenoic acid,

and 12,13-dihydroxyoctadecenoic acid in rabbit renal cortical mitochondria. *Toxicol Appl Pharmacol.* 2001; 172(2): 150-161. PMID: 11298501.

147. Ishola DA, Jr., Post JA, van Timmeren MM, Bakker SJ, Goldschmeding R, Koomans HA, et al. Albumin-bound fatty acids induce mitochondrial oxidant stress and impair antioxidant responses in proximal tubular cells. *Kidney Int.* 2006; 70(4): 724-731. PMID: 16837928.
148. Dettelbach MA, Deftos LJ, Stewart AF. Intraperitoneal free fatty acids induce severe hypocalcemia in rats: a model for the hypocalcemia of pancreatitis. *J Bone Miner Res.* 1990; 5(12): 1249-1255. PMID: 2075838.
149. Wu BU, Johannes RS, Sun X, Conwell DL, Banks PA. Early changes in blood urea nitrogen predict mortality in acute pancreatitis. *Gastroenterology.* 2009; 137(1): 129-135. PMID: 19344722.

Chapter 21

Drug-induced acute pancreatitis

Maria Cristina Conti Bellocchi, Pietro Campagnola, and Luca Frulloni*

Department of Medicine, Pancreas Center, University of Verona, Verona, Italy.

Introduction

Acute pancreatitis (AP) is a heterogeneous disease ranging from a clinically mild form to a more severe forms associated with high morbidity and mortality.[1] A correct diagnosis of AP should be made within 48 hours of admission. Understanding the etiology and severity assessment are essential as they may affect the acute management of the disease.[2]

The most common etiologies for AP are gallstones and alcohol abuse. Other causes include iatrogenic injury (e.g., following endoscopic retrograde cholangiopancreatography), metabolic and autoimmune disorders, inherited disorders, neoplasia (e.g., intraductal papillary mucinous neoplasia, IPMN), anatomic abnormalities, infections, ischemia, trauma, and drugs.[3] Additional investigations after recovery from the acute episode are recommended in patients with an episode of AP classified as idiopathic.[4]

Drugs may be considered a potential cause of disease in patients who take medications that have been associated with AP. Drug-induced pancreatitis (DIP) is assumed to be a relatively rare entity, and its reported incidence ranges from 0.1% to 2% of AP cases.[5] However, the true incidence of DIP is still unknown since little evidence has been obtained from clinical trials, and most incidences have been documented as case reports and are generally limited by the absence or inadequacy of diagnostic criteria for AP, failure to rule out common etiologies of AP, and lack of a rechallenge test.[5]

The main problem in DIP identification is the absence of a clear and largely accepted definition of the disease. The diagnosis is difficult to establish since it is rarely accompanied by clinical or laboratory evidence of a drug reaction, and many patients admitted for AP are already taking a medication. Therefore, criteria to diagnose DIP should include evidence for drug intake shortly preceding AP, an increased risk for AP in patients taking the drug, a direct correlation between increased risk and dose, the presence of a plausible biological mechanism, evidence in clinical trials using the specific drug, and a rechallenge test. However, we lack a definition for each of these potential diagnostic criteria for DIP (i.e., elapsed time between drug intake and AP).

The World Health Organization database includes 525 different drugs suspected to cause AP.[6] The majority of the data was derived from case reports, case series, or summaries of them. Furthermore, the causality for many of these drugs remains elusive, and a definitely causality has only been established for about 30 of them.[6] Another methodological problem is the evaluation of other potential causes of AP. Some definitions exclude the presence of other etiologies of AP, primarily biliary lithiasis and alcohol abuse. The presence of other causes of AP does not exclude DIP, but it certainly decreases the probability.

The rechallenge test under the same conditions as in the first episode of suspected DIP is probably the best diagnostic criterion, but its use in clinical practice is limited particularly in patients with a severe attack of pancreatitis. The consequence is a dramatic decrease in the number of drugs shown to induce pancreatitis using the rechallenge test. However, this test cannot be considered as a definitive criterion for the diagnosis since stopping and restarting a drug with a recurrence of pancreatitis may be a coincidence and not a demonstration of a cause and effect. This is probably the reason why Tenner raised the question about the real existence of DIP in a recent review.[7]

A consequence of all these problems for the definition of DIP is its classification. Many have been proposed. More recent critical reviews used classification systems of the published case reports based on the level of evidence.[5,8] A larger number of case reports and/or a consistent latency among the reports for a particular drug were evaluated. Badalov et al. created a new DIP classification based on the features of case reports and the presence or absence of a rechallenge test.[9] However, a classification in definite, probable, and possible association between drugs and pancreatitis is the most preferred (**Table 1**)[6,10] based

*Corresponding author. Email: luca.frulloni@univr.it

Table 1. Classification of evidence according to Karch and Lasagna.[10]

DEFINITIVE	Drug reaction that follows a reasonable temporal sequence from administration of the drug, follows a known response pattern that is confirmed by stopping the drug (dechallenge), and is confirmed by symptom reappearance upon repeated exposure to the drug (rechallenge).
PROBABLE	Drug reaction that follows a reasonable temporal sequence from administration of the drug, follows a known response pattern, is confirmed by de-challenge, and cannot not be explained by the known characteristics of the patient's clinical state.
POSSIBLE	Drug reaction that follows a reasonable temporal sequence from administration of the drug and follows a known response pattern but that could have been produced by the patient's clinical state or other modes of therapy.

on evaluation of the re-/dechallenge test and temporal sequence and exclusion of other causes of pancreatitis. The Naranjo score could be useful to establish the association of a drug with pancreatitis (**Table 2**).[11]

A list of drugs classified in definitive and probable is listed on **Table 3**.[6]

Drugs More Commonly Associated with AP

Azathioprine and 6-mercaptopurine

Azathioprine (AZA) and its metabolite 6-mercaptopurine (6-MP) were first reported to induce pancreatitis in 1980.[12] The incidence is reported between 1 and 6% of exposed individuals. A Danish study demonstrated a 7- to 8-fold increase in the risk of developing AP comparing ever- with never-takers.[13] Despite the large size of the sample of study, the uniformly organized health care system, and the use of appropriate population controls, the study was limited by the incomplete registration of confounders (e.g., risk factors like alcohol or gallstones) and included potential association between inflammatory bowel disease (IBD) and autoimmune pancreatitis.[14] Indeed, previous case reports have suggested that IBD is associated with a liability to develop pancreatitis, especially for Crohn's disease, because of common pathogenic mechanisms, diminished enterohepatic circulation of bile acids in patients with ileal involvement or who underwent surgical ileal resection,[14] mechanic factors in duodenal localizations of disease (papilla of Oddi dysfunction), and concomitant therapy with other drugs involved in DIP like mesalamine, glucocorticoids, or metronidazole.[15]

The mechanism of how azathioprine causes pancreatitis is not well elucidated, and the development of pancreatitis

Table 2. Score of probability of association between drugs and adverse effect, modified from Naranjo et al.[11]

QUESTION	Yes	No	Don't know	SCORE
1. Are there previous conclusive reports on this reaction?	+ 1	0	0	
2. Did the adverse event appear after the suspected drug was administered?	+ 2	- 1	0	
3. Did the adverse reaction improve when the drug was discontinued or a specific antagonist was administered?	+ 1	0	0	
4. Did the adverse reaction reappear when the drug was readministered?	+ 2	- 1	0	
5. Are there alternative causes (other than the drug) that could on their own have caused the reaction?	- 1	+ 2	0	
6. Did the reaction reappear when a placebo was given?	- 1	+1	0	
7. Was the drug detected in the blood (or other fluids) in concentrations known to be toxic?	+ 1	0	0	
8. Was the reaction more severe when the dose was increased, or less severe when the dose was decreased?	+ 1	0	0	
9. Did the patient have a similar reaction to the same or similar drug in any previous exposure?	+ 1	0	0	
10. Was the adverse event confirmed by any objective evidence?	+ 1	0	0	
			Total score*	

*Total score is the sum of all subcategory scores. The relationship is categorized as *definite* if the score is > 8, *probable* if the score is 5 to 8, *possible* if the score is 1 to 4, and *doubtful* if the score is 0.

Table 3. Drugs with definite or probable association to pancreatitis as reported in the summary of Nitsche et al.[6] and other case reports until 2014.

CAUSALITY	MEDICATION	n	RECHALLANGE
Definite	Acetaminophen	13	1
	Asparaginase	177	2
	Azathioprine	87	16
	Bortezomib	2	2
	Capecitabine	1	1
	Carbamazepine	15	1
	Cisplatin	11	1
	Cytarabine	26	4
	Didanosine	883	9
	Enalapril	12	2
	Erythromycin	11	1
	Estrogens	42	11
	Furosemide	22	3
	Hydrochlorothiazide	12	1
	Ifosphamid	2	1
	Interferon α2b	12	2
	Isoniazide	8	4
	Itroconazol	4	2
	Lamivudine	19	1
	Mercaptopurine	69	10
	Mesalamine/olsalazine	60	12
	Metronidazole	15	3
	Octreotide	16	4
	Olanzepine	1	1
	Opiates	42	5
	Pentamidine	79	2
	Pentavalent antimonials	80	14
	Phenformin	13	1
	Steroids	25	1
	Sulfasalazine	23	5
	Sulfmethaxazole/Tmp	24	1
	Sulindac	21	8
	Tamoxifen	1	1
	Tetracycline	36	2
	Valproic acid	82	11
	Vemurafenib	1	1
Probable	Atorvastatine	2	0
	Bezafibrate	1	1
	Carboplatin/docetaxel	1	0
	Ceftriaxon	1	0
	Cyclopenthiazide	11	0
	Liraglutide/DPP4 inhibitors	5	1
	Orlistat	9	0
	Rifampin	6	0
	Simvastatin	25	0
	Tyrosine kinase inhibitor	1	0

Abbreviations: DPP-4 = dipeptidyl peptidase-4; Tmp = trimethoprim.

does not appear to be dose related.[16] Therefore, it may be better classified as allergic or idiosyncratic. Although some authors have suggested the utility of thiopurine methyltransferase (TPMT) heterozygosity and enzyme activity as predictive tests for the development of azathioprine-related adverse effects (AEs), the role in predicting AP has not been studied.[17] Even if some authors have communicated that MP could safely be used after an AZA-induced episode of AP,[18] most authors agree that a cross reaction after reexposure of the related drug is probable.

Angiotensin-converting enzyme inhibitors

Angiotensin-converting enzyme (ACE) inhibitors are one of the most commonly prescribed classes of medications; they are used in hypertension, heart failure, and proteinuria.[19] The first reported case of ACE inhibitor-induced pancreatitis was with enalapril.[20-22] Case reports about pancreatitis induced by lisinopril,[23-26] captopril,[27] ramipril,[28] and perindopril[29] have also been published.

In one case-control study, the use of ACE inhibitor was associated with an increased risk of AP, with an odds ratio of 1.5. The risk increased with higher daily doses and was highest during the first 6 months of therapy.[30]

Pancreatitis associated with ACE inhibitors is thought to reflect localized angioedema of the gland, probably linked to an increase of bradykinin secondary to its decreased degradation. Angiotensin II receptors regulate pancreatic secretion and microcirculation, and these effects may contribute to the pathogenesis of ACE inhibitor-induced pancreatitis.[31] However, ACE inhibitors, in particular captopril, showed an important role in attenuating vascular permeability in experimental severe AP in rats, reducing matrix metalloproteinase 9 expression. No human studies are available to confirm this experimental evidence and develop a target therapy. In summary, there are controversies on the role of ACE inhibitors in DIP since they may induce mild pancreatitis in humans but may reduce experimental AP severity in animals.

Antidiabetic drugs

Metformin, a biguanide commonly used in type 2 diabetes, is considered to be a safe drug with minimal side effects; only a few case reports suggest metformin as associated with DIP. Among these publications, the postulated mechanisms are drug overdose, drug accumulation, and acute renal failure triggered by vomiting.[32-34] Therefore, metformin has been classified as possible DIP.

Incretin-based therapies such as glucagon-like peptide-1 agonists (GLP-1) and dipeptidyl peptidase-4 (DPP-4) inhibitors have become important therapeutic options for type 2 diabetes. Proposed mechanisms of action include enhanced glucose-dependent insulin secretion from pancreatic cells, restoration of the first-phase insulin response, suppression of glucagon secretion, and delay of gastric emptying. AP has been reported with both GLP-1 agonists[35-39] and DPP-4 inhibitors.[40,41] Over the last several years, postmarketing reporting of this AE to the FDA resulted in manufacturers emphasizing the risk of AP and, later, in contraindications for incretin-based therapies in patients with a history of pancreatitis.[42]

Recently, several meta-analyses and cohort studies demonstrated that the incidence of pancreatitis in patients taking incretins is low and that these drugs do not increase the risk of pancreatitis.[43-50] Li et al. found no association between the use of GLP-1-based therapies and pancreatitis in a self-controlled case series analysis in a large observational database from dispensing data on 1.2 million patients.[49] Even animal research demonstrated no evidence of AP in GLP-1 agonist/DPP-4 inhibitors.[51-55] A recent meta-analysis of randomized and nonrandomized studies confirmed that the risk of AP under incretin-based therapy is not increased.[56]

Statins

While statins are generally well tolerated, they have been known to be associated with pancreatitis.

DIP is a rare AE of statin therapy and has mainly been documented in case reports involving atorvastatin,[57,58] fluvastatin,[59] rosuvastatin,[60,61] simvastatin,[62-64] and pravastatin,[65,66] leading to the conclusion that statin-induced pancreatitis may be a class effect.[67] An immune-mediated inflammatory response, direct cellular toxicity, and metabolic effects have all been postulated, even though the mechanism of action remains ill-defined. Statin-induced pancreatitis can occur at any time but seems to be very uncommon early in treatment and is more likely after months of therapy. Singh and Loke postulated that differences exist in the safety profiles of the various statins that may correlate with the degree to which they inhibit cytochrome P450 CYPA4, as well as the degree of their lipophilicity.[68]

Recently, larger studies have challenged the correlations made by earlier case reports, and demonstrate instead a mild protective effect in statin users, as previously shown in animal models of AP,[69] where statins appear to reduce inflammatory cytokines and pulmonary neutrophilic activation in a severe AP model.[70]

5-ASA and derivatives

Mesalamine-induced pancreatitis has been described since 1989.[71] Several oral and enema mesalamine preparations have been implicated in causing pancreatitis, as has sulfasalazine. A hypersensitivity mechanism seems to be involved, and pancreatitis occurs usually after few days or weeks (short latency).

A higher frequency of pancreatitis has been proposed for new mesalamine formulations including multi-matrix release (MMX). However, a recent pharmacoepidemiologic study showed a similar incidence compared to delayed or controlled release, warranting a formal postmarketing safety assessment. It has been well established that newer drugs are monitored more closely for AEs and that those AEs are more likely to be reported than for medications that have been in long-term use.[72]

Antibiotics

Metronidazole has been reported to have a probable association with AP,[73-78] although the mechanism of DIP is still unknown. Possible pathways include free radical production, immune-mediated inflammatory response, and metabolic effects.[78] The association is based on case reports, 3 of them with positive rechallenge tests (latency time 1-7 days).[73,74,77] In a population-based case-control study, Nørgaard et al. showed that metronidazole was associated to a threefold increased risk of AP.[76] Furthermore, the use of metronidazole in combination with other drugs used for *Helicobacter pylori* (proton pump inhibitors, antibiotics) within 30 days before admission was associated with an eightfold increased risk of AP.

Tetracyclines have been implicated as causative agents for AP. Early reports of AP after tetracycline administration were associated with liver dysfunction attributed to the drug's ability to induce fatty degeneration of this organ.[79] In the following years, case reports about tetracycline induced pancreatitis even in patients without evidence of liver abnormalities have been described. A large Swedish pharmacoepidemiologic study reported a 1.6 odds ratio among current users of tetracycline after adjustment for potential confounders.[80]

With regard to the new drug tygecycline, an analogue of the semisynthetic tetracycline minocycline, McGovern et al. defined the pancreatitis as uncommon in treated patients, with an occurrence of <1% in Phase 3 and 4 clinical studies. Caution should be exercised with close monitoring in patients with past acute or chronic pancreatitis, although there is documented safety even in these patients.[81]

Valproic acid

Since the 1979 introduction of valproic acid (VPA), a drug commonly prescribed for generalized and focal epilepsy, migraine, neuropathic pain, and bipolar disorder, cases of coincident pancreatitis have been reported,[82-86] often involving children. AP is rarely seen in children, and, in contrast to adult cases, it is more commonly associated with drugs. The common side effects associated with VPA are typically benign, but more serious adverse effects may occur. These include hepatotoxicity, hyperammonemic encephalopathy, coagulation disorders, and pancreatitis. The possible association between VPA and pancreatitis led the U.S. Food and Drug Association to issue a box warning for all VPA products in 2000. In a recent systematic review, Pellock et al. reported that there were several confounding elements and possible alternative etiologies in many of the trials and case reports, leading to the conclusion that VPA-coincident AP is an uncommon but definite and idiosyncratic event.[87] It is most common during the first year of therapy and during dosage increases.

Conclusions

DIP is a rare, difficult-to-diagnose entity. Only a minority of cases associated with AP are linked to drugs, and the clinical presentation and mechanisms of injury to the pancreas are not well understood or controversial. The diagnosis of DIP remains possible or probable in many patients. Several of these drugs are used for diseases associated with pancreatitis (i.e., inflammatory bowel diseases, dyslipidemia). The resolution of pancreatitis after drug discontinuation (dechallenge test) could improve the diagnosis of DIP. However, it is difficult to establish the direct correlation between symptom resolution and drug withdrawal. Rechallenge tests may be performed in some cases, but it is strictly dependent on the severity of the index pancreatitis.

Clinically, it is important to exclude any alternative possible etiology to avoid unnecessary drug withdrawal. However, drugs suspected to induce pancreatitis should be discontinued or exchanged with an alternative drug when possible. Drugs even probably associated with pancreatitis should be avoided in patients with previous episode(s) of pancreatitis. The knowledge of drugs commonly linked to AP (**Table 3**) may lead to earlier suspicion of the diagnosis of DIP and faster discontinuation of drug administration in patients for whom a cause of AP cannot be found.

References

1. Steinberg W, Tenner S. Acute pancreatitis. *N Engl J Med.* 1994; 330(17): 1198-1210. PMID: 7811319.
2. Banks PA, Freeman ML; Practice Parameters Committee of the American College of Gastroenterology. Practice guidelines in acute pancreatitis. *Am J Gastroenterol.* 2006; 101(10): 2379-2400. PMID: 17032204.
3. Wang GJ, Gao CF, Wei D, Wang C, Ding SQ. Acute pancreatitis: etiology and common pathogenesis. *World J Gastroenterol.* 2009; 15(12): 1427-1430. PMID: 19322914.
4. Pezzilli R, Zerbi A, Di Carlo V, Bassi C, Delle Fave GF; Working Group of the Italian Association for the Study of the Pancreas on Acute Pancreatitis. Practical guidelines for acute pancreatitis. *Pancreatology.* 2010; 10(5): 523-535. PMID: 20975316.

5. Nitsche CJ, Jamieson N, Lerch MM, Mayerle JV. Drug induced pancreatitis. *Best Pract Res Clin Gastroenterol.* 2010; 24(2): 143-155. PMID: 20227028.
6. Nitsche C, Maertin S, Scheiber J, Ritter CA, Lerch MM, Mayerle J. Drug-induced pancreatitis. *Curr Gastroenterol Rep.* 2012; 14(2): 131-138. PMID: 22314811.
7. Tenner S. Drug induced acute pancreatitis: does it exist? *World J Gastroenterol.* 2014; 20(44): 16529-16534. PMID: 25469020.
8. Trivedi CD, Pitchumoni CS. Drug-induced pancreatitis: an update. *J Clin Gastroenterol.* 2005; 39(8): 709-716. PMID: 16082282.
9. Badalov N, Baradarian R, Iswara K, Li J, Steinberg W, Tenner S. Drug-induced acute pancreatitis: an evidence-based review. *Clin Gastroenterol Hepatol.* 2007; 5(6): 648-661; quiz 644. PMID: 17395548.
10. Karch FE, Lasagna L. Adverse drug reactions. A critical review. *JAMA.* 1975; 234(12): 1236-1241. PMID: 1242749.
11. Naranjo CA, Busto U, Sellers EM, Sandor P, Ruiz I, Roberts EA, et al. A method for estimating the probability of adverse drug reactions. *Clin Pharmacol Ther.* 1981; 30(2): 239-245. PMID: 7249508.
12. Guillaume P, Grandjean E, Male PJ. Azathioprine-associated acute pancreatitis in the course of chronic active hepatitis. *Dig Dis Sci.* 1984; 29(1): 78-79. PMID: 6692736.
13. Floyd A, Pedersen L, Nielsen GL, Thorlacius-Ussing O, Sorensen HT. Risk of acute pancreatitis in users of azathioprine: a population-based case-control study. *Am J Gastroenterol.* 2003; 98(6): 1305-1308. PMID: 12818274.
14. Fraquelli M, Losco A, Visentin S, Cesana BM, Pometta R, Colli A, et al. Gallstone disease and related risk factors in patients with Crohn disease: analysis of 330 consecutive cases. *Arch Intern Med.* 2001; 161(18): 2201-2204. PMID: 11575976.
15. Hegnhøj J, Hansen CP, Rannem T, Søbirk H, Andersen LB, Andersen JR. Pancreatic function in Crohn's disease. *Gut.* 1990; 31(9): 1076-1079. PMID: 1698692.
16. Inoue H, Shiraki K, Okano H, Deguchi M, Yamanaka T, Sakai T, et al. Acute pancreatitis in patients with ulcerative colitis. *Dig Dis Sci.* 2005; 50(6): 1064-1067. PMID: 15986855.
17. Heckmann JM, Lambson EM, Little F, Owen EP. Thiopurine methyltransferase (TPMT) heterozygosity and enzyme activity as predictive tests for the development of azathioprine-related adverse events. *J Neurol Sci.* 2005; 231(1-2): 71-80. PMID: 15792824.
18. Alexander S, Dowling D. Azathioprine pancreatitis in inflammatory bowel disease and successful subsequent treatment with mercaptopurine. *Intern Med J.* 2005; 35(9): 570-571. PMID: 16105163.
19. Grendell JH. Editorial: drug-induced acute pancreatitis: uncommon or commonplace? *Am J Gastroenterol.* 2003; 106(12): 2189-2191. PMID: 22138943.
20. Carnovale A, Esposito P, Bassano P, Russo L, Uomo G. Enalapril-induced acute recurrent pancreatitis. *Dig Liver Dis.* 2003; 35(1): 55-57. PMID: 12725609.
21. González Ramallo VJ, Muiño Miguez A, Torres Segovia FJ. Necrotizing pancreatitis and enalapril. *Eur J Med.* 1992; 1(2): 123. PMID: 1342370.
22. Maringhini A, Termini A, Patti R, Ciambra M, Biffarella P, Pagliaro L. Enalapril-associated acute pancreatitis: recurrence after rechallenge. *Am J Gastroenterol.* 1997; 92(1): 166-167. PMID: 8995963.
23. Brown KV, Khan AZ, Paterson IM. Lisinopril-induced acute pancreatitis. *J R Army Med Corps.* 2007; 153(3): 191-192. PMID: 18200917.
24. Gershon T, Olshaker JS. Acute pancreatitis following lisinopril rechallenge. *Am J Emerg Med.* 1998; 16(5): 523-524. PMID: 9725973.
25. Kanbay M, Selcuk H, Yilmaz U, Boyacioglu S. Recurrent acute pancreatitis probably secondary to lisinopril. *South Med J.* 2006; 99(12): 1388-1389. PMID: 17233197.
26. Marinella MA, Billi JE. Lisinopril therapy associated with acute pancreatitis. *West J Med.* 1995; 163(1): 77-78. PMID: 7667995.
27. Jeandidier N, Klewansky M, Pinget M. Captopril-induced acute pancreatitis. *Diabetes Care.* 1995; 18(3): 410-411. PMID: 7555489.
28. Kanbay M, Korkmaz M, Yilmaz U, Gur G, Boyacioglu S. Acute pancreatitis due to ramipril therapy. *Postgrad Med J.* 2004; 80(948): 617-618. PMID: 15467001.
29. Gallego-Rojo FJ, Gonzalez-Calvin JL, Guilarte J, Casado-Caballero FJ, Bellot V. Perindopril-induced acute pancreatitis. *Dig Dis Sci.* 1997; 42(8): 1789-1791. PMID: 9286249.
30. Eland IA, van Puijenbroek EP, Sturkenboom MJ, Wilson JH, Stricker BH. Drug-associated acute pancreatitis: twenty-one years of spontaneous reporting in The Netherlands. *Am J Gastroenterol.* 1999; 94(9): 2417-2422. PMID: 10484002.
31. Singh S. Angiotensin-converting enzyme (ACE) inhibitor-induced acute pancreatitis: in search of the evidence. *South Med J.* 2006; 99(12): 1327-1328. PMID: 17233187.
32. Ben MH, Thabet H, Zaghdoudi I, Amamou M. Metformin associated acute pancreatitis. *Vet Hum Toxicol.* 2002; 44(1): 47-48. PMID: 11824780.
33. Fimognari FL, Corsonello A, Pastorell R, Antonelli-Incalzi R. Metformin-induced pancreatitis: A possible adverse drug effect during acute renal failure. *Diabetes Care.* 2006; 29(5): 1183. PMID: 16644670.
34. Mallick S. Metformin induced acute pancreatitis precipitated by renal failure. *Postgrad Med J.* 2004; 80(942): 239-240. PMID: 15082849.
35. Anderson SL, Trujillo JM. Association of pancreatitis with glucagon-like peptide-1 agonist use. *Ann Pharmacother.* 2010; 44(5): 904-909. PMID: 20371755.
36. Knezevich E, Crnic T, Kershaw S, Drincic A. Liraglutide-associated acute pancreatitis. *Am J Health Syst Pharm.* 2012; 69(5): 386-389. PMID: 22345417.
37. Lee PH, Stockton MD, Franks AS. Acute pancreatitis associated with liraglutide. *Ann Pharmacother.* 2011; 45(4): e22. PMID: 21487080.
38. Singh S, Chang HY, Richards TM, Weiner JP, Clark JM, Segal JB. Glucagonlike peptide 1-based therapies and risk of hospitalization for acute pancreatitis in type 2 diabetes mellitus: a population-based matched case-control study. *JAMA Intern Med.* 2013; 173(7): 534-539. PMID: 23440284.
39. Tripathy NR, Basha S, Jain R, Shetty S, Ramachandran A. Exenatide and acute pancreatitis. *J Assoc Physicians India.* 2008; 56: 987-988. PMID: 19322980.
40. Girgis CM, Champion BL. Vildagliptin-induced acute pancreatitis. *Endocr Pract.* 2011; 17(3): e48-e50. PMID: 21324812.
41. Kunjathaya P, Ramaswami PK, Krishnamurthy AN, Bhat N. Acute necrotizing pancreatitis associated with vildagliptin. *JOP.* 2013; 14(1): 81-84. PMID: 23306341.

42. Iyer SN, Tanenberg RJ, Mendez CE, West RL, Drake AJ 3rd. Pancreatitis associated with incretin-based therapies. *Diabetes Care*. 2013; 36(4): e49. PMID: 23520376.
43. Alves C, Batel-Marques F, Macedo AF. A meta-analysis of serious adverse events reported with exenatide and liraglutide: acute pancreatitis and cancer. *Diabetes Res Clin Pract*. 2012; 98(2): 271-284. PMID: 23010561.
44. Dore DD, Bloomgren GL, Wenten M, Hoffman C, Clifford CR, Quinn SG, et al. A cohort study of acute pancreatitis in relation to exenatide use. *Diabetes Obes Metab*. 2011; 13(6): 559-566. PMID: 21320263.
45. Dore DD, Hussein M, Hoffman C, Pelletier EM, Smith DB, Seeger JD. A pooled analysis of exenatide use and risk of acute pancreatitis. *Curr Med Res Opin*. 2013; 29(12): 1577-1586. PMID: 23981106.
46. Funch D, Gydesen H, Tornoe K, Major-Pedersen A, Chan KA. A prospective, claims-based assessment of the risk of pancreatitis and pancreatic cancer with liraglutide compared to other antidiabetic drugs. *Diabetes Obes Metab*. 2014; 16(3): 273-275. PMID: 24199745.
47. Giorda CB, Picariello R, Nada E, Tartaglino B, Marafetti L, Costa G, et al. Incretin therapies and risk of hospital admission for acute pancreatitis in an unselected population of European patients with type 2 diabetes: a case-control study. *Lancet Diabetes Endocrinol*. 2014; 2(2): 111-115. PMID: 24622714.
48. Jespersen MJ, Knop FK, Christensen M. GLP-1 agonists for type 2 diabetes: pharmacokinetic and toxicological considerations. *Expert Opin Drug Metab Toxicol*. 2013; 9(1): 17-29. PMID: 23094590.
49. Li X, Zhang Z, Duke J. Glucagon-like peptide 1-based therapies and risk of pancreatitis: a self-controlled case series analysis. *Pharmacoepidemiol Drug Saf*. 2014; 23(3): 234-239. PMID: 24741695.
50. Monami M, Dicembrini I, Nardini C, Fiordelli I, Mannucci E. Glucagon-like peptide-1 receptor agonists and pancreatitis: a meta-analysis of randomized clinical trials. *Diabetes Res Clin Pract*. 2014; 103(2): 269-275. PMID: 24485345.
51. Aston-Mourney K, Subramanian SL, Zraika S, Samarasekera T, Meier DT, Goldstein LC, et al. One year of sitagliptin treatment protects against islet amyloid-associated beta-cell loss and does not induce pancreatitis or pancreatic neoplasia in mice. *Am J Physiol Endocrinol Metab*. 2013; 305(4): E475-484. PMID: 23736544.
52. Koehler JA, Baggio LL, Lamont BJ, Ali S, Drucker DJ. Glucagon-like peptide-1 receptor activation modulates pancreatitis-associated gene expression but does not modify the susceptibility to experimental pancreatitis in mice. *Diabetes*. 2009; 58(9): 2148-2161. PMID: 19509017.
53. Tatarkiewicz K, Belanger P, Gu G, Parkes D, Roy D. No evidence of drug-induced pancreatitis in rats treated with exenatide for 13 weeks. *Diabetes Obes Metab*. 2013; 15(5): 417-426. PMID: 23163898.
54. Tatarkiewicz K, Smith PA, Sablan EJ, Polizzi CJ, Aumann DE, Villescaz C, et al. Exenatide does not evoke pancreatitis and attenuates chemically induced pancreatitis in normal and diabetic rodents. *Am J Physiol Endocrinol Metab*. 2010; 299(6): E1076-E1086. PMID: 20923958.
55. Vrang N, Jelsing J, Simonsen L, Jensen AE, Thorup I, Søeborg H, et al. The effects of 13 wk of liraglutide treatment on endocrine and exocrine pancreas in male and female ZDF rats: a quantitative and qualitative analysis revealing no evidence of drug-induced pancreatitis. *Am J Physiol Endocrinol Metab*. 2012; 303(2): E253-E264. PMID: 22589391.
56. Li L, Shen J, Bala MM, Busse JW, Ebrahim S, Vandvik PO, et al. Incretin treatment and risk of pancreatitis in patients with type 2 diabetes mellitus: systematic review and meta-analysis of randomised and non-randomised studies. *BMJ*. 2014; 348: g2366. PMID: 24736555.
57. Belaïche G, Ley G, Slama JL. Acute pancreatitis associated with atorvastatine therapy [Article in French]. *Gastroenterol Clin Biol*. 2000; 24(4): 471-472. PMID: 10844297.
58. Singh S, Nautiyal A, Dolan JG. Recurrent acute pancreatitis possibly induced by atorvastatin and rosuvastatin. Is statin induced pancreatitis a class effect? *JOP*. 2004; 5(6): 502-504. PMID: 15536291.
59. Tysk C, Al-Eryani AY, Shawabkeh AA. Acute pancreatitis induced by fluvastatin therapy. *J Clin Gastroenterol*. 2002; 35(5): 406-408. PMID: 12394230.
60. Chintanaboina J, Gopavaram D. Recurrent acute pancreatitis probably induced by rosuvastatin therapy: a case report. *Case Rep Med*. 2012; 2012: 973279. PMID: 22536267.
61. Lai SW, Lin CL, Liao KF. Rosuvastatin and risk of acute pancreatitis in a population-based case-control study. *Int J Cardiol*. 2015; 187: 417-420. PMID: 25841139.
62. Johnson JL, Loomis IB. A case of simvastatin-associated pancreatitis and review of statin-associated pancreatitis. *Pharmacotherapy*. 2006; 26(3): 414-422. PMID: 16503723.
63. Pezzilli R, Ceciliato R, Corinaldesi R, Barakat B. Acute pancreatitis due to simvastatin therapy: increased severity after rechallenge. *Dig Liver Dis*. 2004; 36(9): 639-640. PMID: 15460851.
64. Ramdani M, Schmitt AM, Liautard J, Duhamel O, Legroux P, Gislon J, et al. Simvastatin-induced acute pancreatitis: two cases [Article in French]. *Gastroenterol Clin Biol*. 1991; 15(12): 986. PMID: 1783260.
65. Anagnostopoulos GK, Tsiakos S, Margantinis G, Kostopoulos P, Arvanitidis D. Acute pancreatitis due to pravastatin therapy. *JOP*. 2003; 4(3): 129-132. PMID: 12743419.
66. Becker C, Hvalic C, Delmore G, Krahenbuhl S, Schlienger R. Recurrent acute pancreatitis during pravastatin-therapy [Article in German]. *Praxis (Bern 1994)*. 2006; 95(4): 111-116. PMID: 16485606.
67. Singh S. Drug induced pancreatitis might be a class effect of statin drugs. *JOP*. 2005; 6(4): 380; author reply 380-381. PMID: 16006693.
68. Singh S, Loke YK. Statins and pancreatitis: a systematic review of observational studies and spontaneous case reports. *Drug Saf*. 2006; 29(12): 1123-1132. PMID: 17147459.
69. Choi OS, Park SJ, Seo SW, Park CS, Cho JJ, Ahn HJ. The 3-hydroxy-3-methylglutaryl coenzyme A (HMG-CoA) reductase inhibitor, lovastatin (statin) ameliorates CCK-induced acute pancreatitis in rats. *Biol Pharm Bull*. 2005; 28(8): 1394-1397. PMID: 16079481.
70. Almeida JL, Sampietre SN, Mendonça Coelho AM, Trindade Molan NA, Machado MC, Monteiro da Cunha JE, et al. Statin pretreatment in experimental acute pancreatitis. *JOP*. 2008; 9(4): 431-439. PMID: 18648134.
71. Sachedina B, Saibil F, Cohen LB, Whittey J. Acute pancreatitis due to 5-aminosalicylate. *Ann Intern Med*. 1989; 110(6): 490-492. PMID: 2465715.

72. Russo L, Schneider G, Gardiner MH, Lanes S, Streck P, Rosen S. Role of pharmacoepidemiology studies in addressing pharmacovigilance questions: a case example of pancreatitis risk among ulcerative colitis patients using mesalazine. *Eur J Clin Pharmacol*. 2014; 70(6): 709-717. PMID: 24609467.
73. Celifarco A, Warschauer C, Burakoff R. Metronidazole-induced pancreatitis. *Am J Gastroenterol*. 1989; 84(8): 958-960. PMID: 2756988.
74. de Jongh FE, Ottervanger JP, Stuiver PC. Acute pancreatitis caused by metronidazole [Article in Dutch]. *Ned Tijdschr Geneeskd*. 1996; 140(1): 37-38. PMID: 8569910.
75. Nigwekar SU, Casey KJ. Metronidazole-induced pancreatitis. A case report and review of literature. *JOP*. 2004; 5(6): 516-519. PMID: 15536294.
76. Nørgaard M, Ratanajamit C, Jacobsen J, Skriver MV, Pedersen L, Sørensen HT. Metronidazole and risk of acute pancreatitis: a population-based case-control study. *Aliment Pharmacol Ther*. 2005; 21(4): 415-420. PMID: 15709992.
77. O'Halloran E, Hogan A, Mealy K. Metronidazole-induced pancreatitis. *HPB Surg*. 2010; 2010: 523468. PMID: 20862338.
78. Sura ME, Heinrich KA, Suseno M. Metronidazole-associated pancreatitis. *Ann Pharmacother*. 2000; 34(10): 1152-1155. PMID: 11054984.
79. Nicolau DP, Mengedoht DE, Kline JJ. Tetracycline-induced pancreatitis. *Am J Gastroenterol*. 1991; 86(11): 1669-1671. PMID: 1951248.
80. Ljung R, Lagergren J, Bexelius TS, Mattsson F, Lindblad M. Increased risk of acute pancreatitis among tetracycline users in a Swedish population-based case-control study. *Gut*. 2012; 61(6): 873-876. PMID: 21957155.
81. McGovern PC, Wible M, Korth-Bradley JM, Quintana A. Pancreatitis in tigecycline Phase 3 and 4 clinical studies. *J Antimicrob Chemother*. 2014; 69(3): 773-778. PMID: 24216769.
82. Batalden PB, Van Dyne BJ, Cloyd J. Pancreatitis associated with valproic acid therapy. *Pediatrics*. 1979; 64(4): 520-522. PMID: 114966.
83. Camfield PR, Bagnell P, Camfield CS, Tibbles JA. Pancreatitis due to valproic acid. *Lancet*. 1979; 1(8127): 1198-1199. PMID: 86928.
84. Murphy MJ, Lyon IW, Taylor JW, Mitts G. Valproic acid associated pancreatitis in an adult. *Lancet*. 1981; 1(8210): 41-42. PMID: 6109073.
85. Parker PH, Helinek GL, Ghishan FK, Greene HL. Recurrent pancreatitis induced by valproic acid. A case report and review of the literature. *Gastroenterology*. 1981; 80(4): 826-828. PMID: 6162706.
86. Sasaki M, Tonoda S, Aoki Y, Katsumi M. Pancreatitis due to valproic acid. *Lancet*. 1980; 1(8179): 1196. PMID: 6104020.
87. Pellock JM, Wilder BJ, Deaton R, Sommerville KW. Acute pancreatitis coincident with valproate use: a critical review. *Epilepsia*. 2002; 43(11): 1421-1424. PMID: 12423394.

Chapter 22

Imaging assessment of etiology and severity of acute pancreatitis

Thomas L. Bollen*

Department of Radiology, St Antonius Hospital, Nieuwegein, the Netherlands.

Introduction

The incidence of acute pancreatitis (AP) continues to increase worldwide, in parallel with an increasing demand on imaging resources to evaluate the severity of disease. Imaging modalities available for assessment of AP include conventional radiography, abdominal ultrasound (US), multidetector computed tomography (CT), and magnetic resonance imaging (MRI). Of these, CT has become the standard of choice and worldwide the most commonly used imaging modality for the initial evaluation of AP and its sequelae.[1-5] This chapter reviews the role of imaging in the evaluation of patients with AP. Emphasis will be on the use of imaging to assess the etiology and stage the severity of AP. This review applies only to cases of AP, not to chronic pancreatitis, flair-ups of chronic pancreatitis (i.e., acute-on-chronic pancreatitis), groove pancreatitis, auto-immune pancreatitis and other forms of pancreatitis (e.g., tuberculous, hereditary pancreatitis), which all differ considerably in clinical presentation, imaging findings, prognosis, therapy, and clinical outcome.

Imaging modalities

The need for imaging in patients suspected of having AP largely depends on the severity of disease and clinical presentation. In patients with mild AP, imaging is rarely necessary for patient management, except for identifying the cause of AP. Conversely, those with severe AP often demand imaging for reasons stated in **Table 1**. Of all imaging modalities available, contrast-enhanced CT (CECT) is the standard technique for overall assessment of AP and its sequelae.[6-11] Other adjunctive imaging modalities include US, MRI, and angiography.[11,12] Angiography is primarily used to help diagnose the vascular complications of AP. This section will review the imaging techniques of US, CT, and MRI along with their advantages and disadvantages.

Role of US in AP

In the initial phase of AP, abdominal US is the primary imaging technique for assessment of biliary stones as the cause of AP and to examine the biliary tract.[6,13] Abdominal US is about 95% sensitive for the detection of cholecystolithiasis compared to just 50% for the detection of choledocholithiasis.[14] At this stage, US enables the allocation of patients that may benefit from a cholecystectomy (to prevent future attacks) and those requiring an endoscopic retrograde cholangiopancreatography (ERCP). US may also be used to detect and monitor pancreatic collections. Furthermore, US is useful for characterizing pancreatic collections by demonstrating necrotic debris within pancreatic collections, thus differentiating fluid from nonliquid material.[11] With Doppler techniques, vascular structures can be evaluated, particularly the presence of arterial pseudoaneurysms. US can serve as an imaging guide during diagnostic or therapeutic interventions. Finally, US is the imaging technique of choice in children. US has various advantages: it is inexpensive, widely available, quick and easy to perform at the bedside or in an intensive care environment, and able to examine the pancreas in a variety of anatomical planes. US does not expose the patient to ionizing radiation and requires no potential hazardous intravenous contrast agents. Despite these advantages, there are several significant disadvantages that preclude US from being the primary imaging modality. The major disadvantage of US remains the limited visibility of the pancreas and peripancreatic region in a large proportion of patients with severe AP because of the presence of overlying bowel gas, particularly in the case of the ileus. The body habitus may also limit acoustic wave penetration in obese patients. Additionally, abdominal US is less accurate in delineating extrapancreatic inflammatory spread within retroperitoneal spaces and detecting intrapancreatic necrosis. Finally, US is operator dependent and displayed on a limited number of images which are not easy to comprehend and convey to practicing clinicians.

*Corresponding author. Email: t.bollen@antoniusziekenhuis.nl

Table 1. Indications for cross-sectional imaging in AP

Early phase (<1 week)
- To establish the correct diagnosis or provide an alternative diagnosis
- To elucidate the etiology
- To stage the morphologic severity
- To assess for complications for those who deteriorate clinically or fail to improve

Late phase (>1 week)
- To monitor established pancreatic collections
- To delineate the presence of symptomatic and asymptomatic complications
- To guide interventional procedures

Role of CT in AP

CT is at present the best imaging technique for the initial assessment and follow-up of patients with AP (**Table 1**).[1-5] Advantageous features of currently available multislice CT scanners are the high speed of acquisition with narrow collimation, high image resolution, possibility of multiplanar imaging and reformats using volume data. Even in severely ill patients, CT will yield data of diagnostic quality that can be acquired during quiet respiration. Furthermore, CT is widely available, easily accessible in most institutions, less costly than MRI, highly sensitive for detecting gas bubbles and calcification, highly accurate, reproducible, and relatively easy to read by both radiologists and clinicians (**Figures 1, 2**). Indications to perform a CT varies considerably among institutions in different geographic areas and is largely dictated by local preferences and cost factors. Some advocate performing CT on admission for staging purposes and triaging patients to different levels of care.[15,16] Others defer CT for the first week for several legitimate reasons.[5,6,8,9] First, early CT may underestimate the final morphologic severity of disease, as parenchymal necrosis may not be visible on CECT within 24-48 h after symptom onset (**Figure 3**).[17-19] On the other hand, a small number of patients will have a false-positive diagnosis for parenchymal necrosis due to interstitial edema and vasoconstriction of the vascular arcades. Repeat CT within a few days may show normal pancreatic enhancement. Second, CT at this stage will not have an impact on patient decision-making, unless the diagnosis is unclear. Third, only one out of four to five patients with AP will develop parenchymal necrosis (i.e., the majority will have morphologically mild findings).[7,8] Finally, the presence and extent of parenchymal necrosis shows no linear correlation with the development of systemic complications, such as organ failure.[20-23] However, urgent CT is indicated if an early complication of pancreatitis is suspected, primarily bowel ischemia or perforation. Conversely, at a later stage (after 3-7 days of hospitalization) patients who present with severe AP or who present initially with mild to moderate AP but fail to response to supportive treatment should undergo abdominal CT.[24] Serial CT enables following the evolution of pancreatic collections and will delineate the extent of extrapancreatic inflammatory changes that will serve as a roadmap for interventional procedures like endoscopic, transabdominal, or minimally invasive surgical approaches. Imaging protocols vary in practice worldwide, but the common opinion is to obtain thin section images during the pancreatic (delay of 40-50 seconds) or portal venous phase (delay 60-70 seconds).[2-4,11,12] The use of intravenous contrast material is essential for detecting parenchymal necrosis and vascular complications. Yet, noncontrast CT still allows for ascertaining the diagnosis and depicting pancreatic collections. Typically, the entire abdomen and pelvis are scanned to fully evaluate the extent of pancreatic

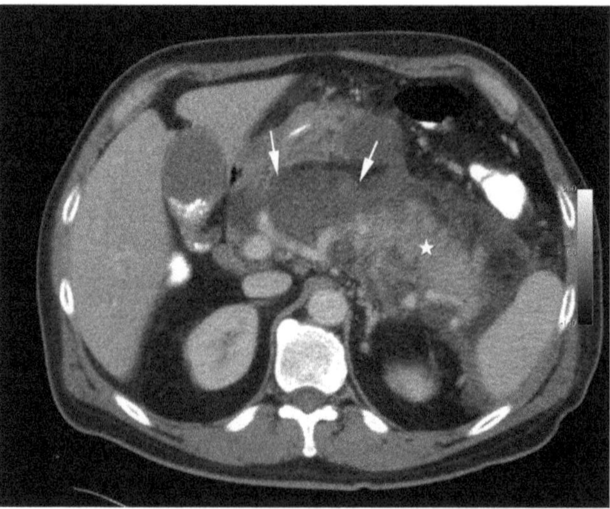

Figure 2. Acute necrotizing pancreatitis. CT shows nonenhancing parts of the pancreatic head, neck, and body (arrows) with normal enhancing tail (asterisk). Note stones in the gallbladder.

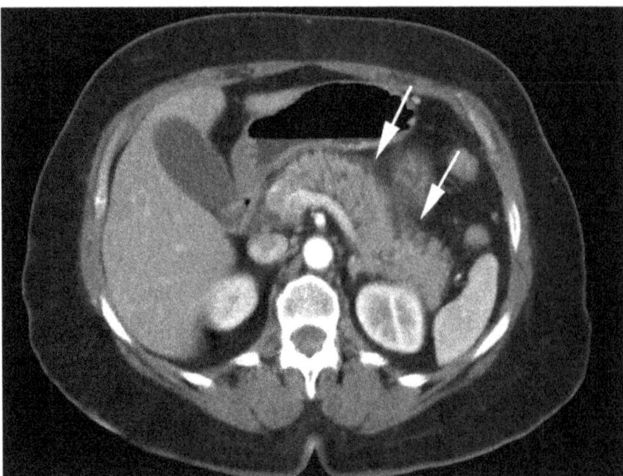

Figure 1. Acute interstitial pancreatitis. Normal enhancing pancreas with swelling and little peripancreatic fat stranding (arrows).

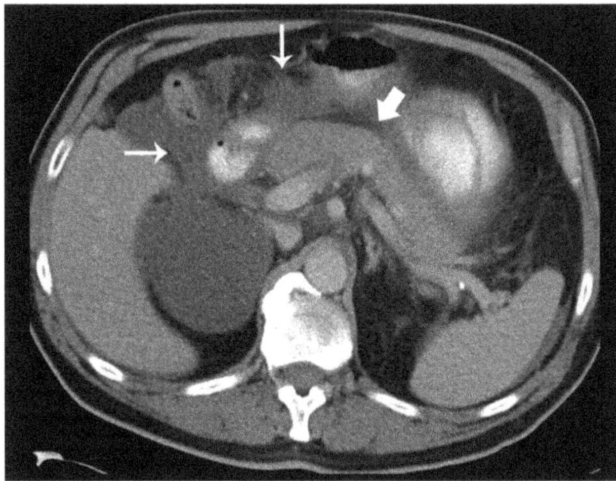

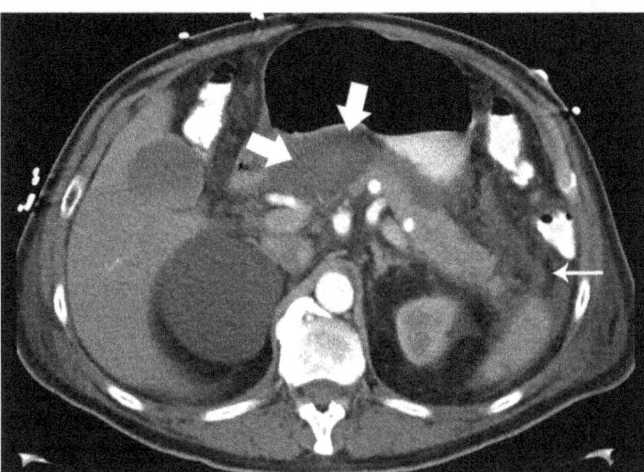

Figure 3. Pancreatic necrosis on day 1 (top) and day 5 (bottom). CT performed on the day of admission (top) shows a normal enhancing pancreatic parenchyma (thick arrow) with little peripancreatic fluid (thin arrows). Follow-up CT on day 5 (bottom) shows necrosis of the pancreatic head and neck (thick arrows) and an acute necrotic collection in the left retroperitoneal space (thin arrow).

collections and extrapancreatic abnormalities. A monophasic CT protocol after intravenous contrast administration is usually sufficient for the diagnosis, severity assessment, and monitoring the progression of AP. Dual-phase studies are recommended in case of hemorrhage, mesenteric ischemia, or suspicion of an arterial pseudoaneurysm or underlying pancreatic mass. CT has some important limitations. CECT is contraindicated in patients who have intravenous contrast allergy or renal insufficiency. In addition, CECT is less sensitive than US in identifying gallstones or biliary duct stones, a common cause of AP. Therefore, US is required if gallstones are not depicted on CT. The radiation dose may be significant in those requiring multiple CT examinations. Finally, although CT elegantly documents the extent of the pancreatic inflammatory process, it has limited capability of differentiating fluid from nonliquid material within peripancreatic collections.[25] However, the

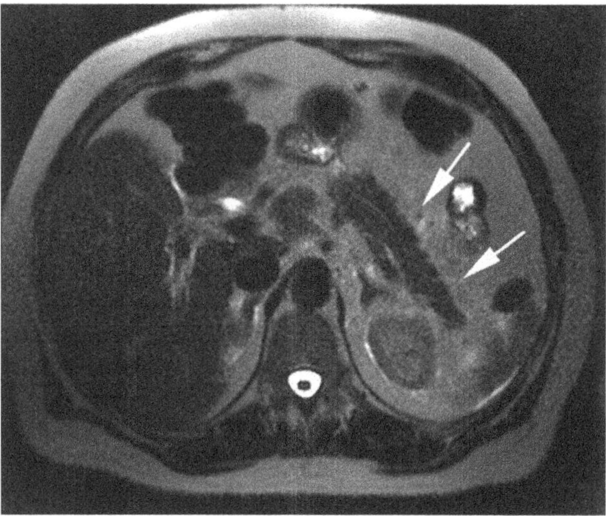

Figure 4. MRI of interstitial pancreatitis. T2-weighted sequence depicts little peripancreatic edema (arrows) around the pancreatic body and tail.

aforementioned advantages of CECT clearly outweigh its limitations.

Role of MRI in AP

Over the years, MRI has gained a more prominent role in the assessment of AP. The presence and extent of pancreatic necrosis and peripancreatic collections can be evaluated with equal accuracy compared with CECT. In fact, MRI is better in detecting mild AP and elucidating the cause of AP with high sensitivity and specificity for choledocholithiasis and congenital pancreatic anomalies (**Figure 4**).[26-30] Due to its inherent tissue contrast resolution capability, MRI is superior to CECT in internal characterization of pancreatic collections (i.e., delineating the presence and extent of necrotic material).[25] Indeed, MRI findings have been shown to accurately predict collection drainability (**Figures 5, 6**). In addition, MRI is capable of detecting pancreatic duct disruption by using MR cholangiopancreatography (MRCP).[31] In approximately 30% of patients with severe AP, disruption of the pancreatic duct is observed, which heralds important prognostic and therapeutic information.[32,33] Finally, MRI is an excellent alternative imaging modality in the setting of renal failure, young patients, and pregnant women. The major disadvantages of MRI include the longer scanning time (which can pose a problem for very ill patients), motion artefacts, the need for specialized MRI- compatible monitoring equipment in critically ill patients, lack of general availability (especially in urgent settings), and high costs if routinely used. Moreover, MRI is not as sensitive as CECT in detecting gas bubbles, whereas image-guided percutaneous intervention is easier to perform with CT. Finally, MRI is more difficult to read

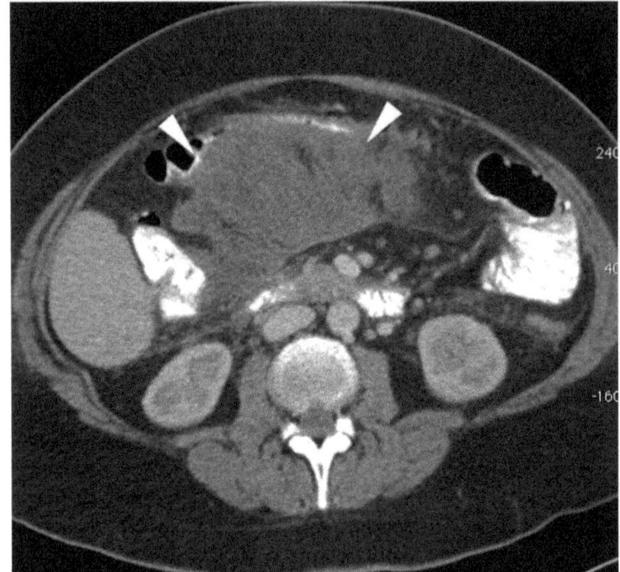

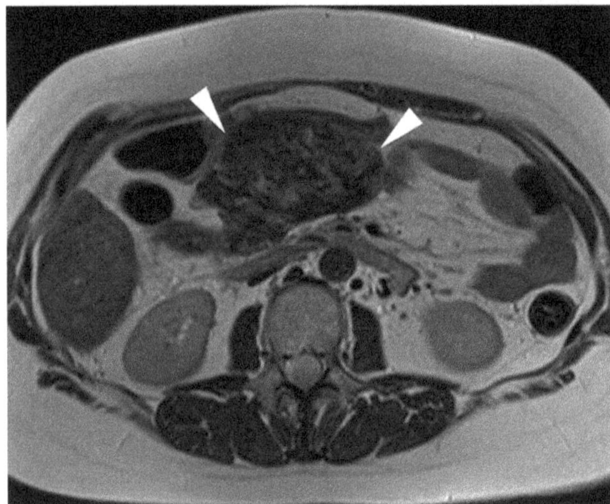

Figure 5. CT versus MRI in AP. CT (top) shows a heterogeneous collection in the transverse mesocolon with predominantly fluid density and fat density (arrowheads pointing at the borders). MRI (bottom) more accurately depicts the contents of T2-weighted hypointense necrotic material without any significant amount of fluid (arrowheads pointing at the borders).

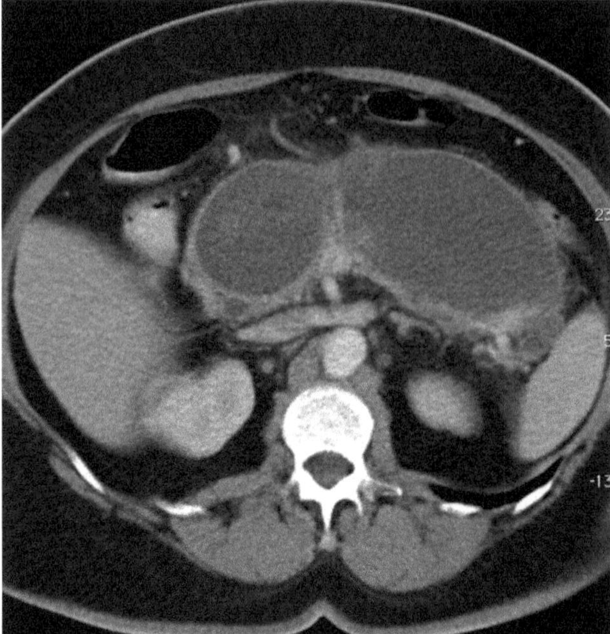

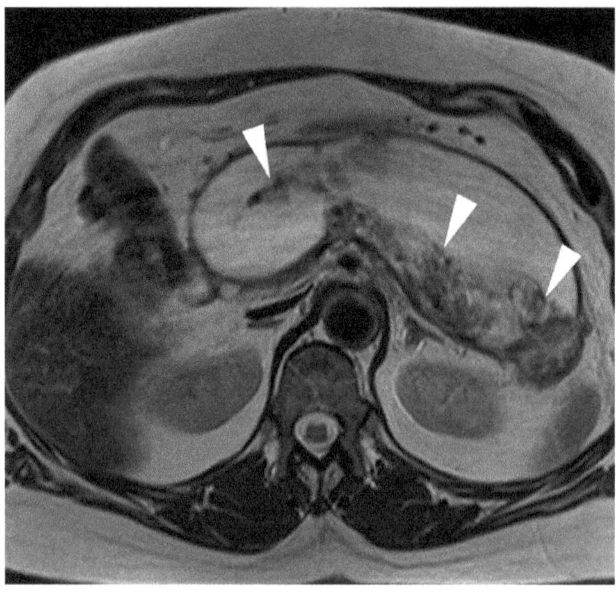

Figure 6. CT versus MRI of walled-off necrosis. CT (top) shows walled-off necrosis replacing a large part of the pancreatic parenchyma. Corresponding T2-weighted MRI (bottom) accurately depicts necrotic material (arrowheads) within the collection.

and understand for non-radiologists (compared with CT) given the multitude of sequences generally required for full evaluation. Therefore, at present, MRI is mainly used as problem solving tool in AP.

Imaging & etiology

Determining the cause is essential in the assessment of all patients presenting with AP. First, elucidation of the cause may significantly affect patient management. An etiologic diagnosis may result in removal of the provocative factor and prevention of repeated insults (i.e., discontinuation of medication causing drug-induced pancreatitis). Second, some causes of AP have long-term consequences (i.e., acute alcoholic pancreatitis may result in recurrent and chronic pancreatitis with increased risk of pancreatic cancer, especially in those with a smoking history).[34] Third, different etiologies have different natural courses with different complications (i.e., acute biliary pancreatitis requires a cholecystectomy or endoscopic intervention).[35-37]

Despite a wide variety of etiologies of AP, gallstones and alcohol abuse account for about 75%-80% of all causes.[7,8,38] The relative rate of gallstones versus alcoholism as the cause of pancreatitis highly depends on patient's age and the geographic area. Other causes include hypercalcemic states (of which the most commonly recognized condition is hyperparathyroidism), hypertriglyceridemia, hereditary pancreatitis, trauma including postprocedural trauma (i.e., ERCP) or surgery, drug induced pancreatitis (i.e., thiazide diuretics, steroids, and azathioprine), and rare causes like scorpion venom. With thorough evaluation the cause of AP can be identified in 85%-90% of cases, leaving about 10%-15% of cases as idiopathic applying to patients with confirmed pancreatitis in whom a causative agent cannot be identified.[38]

While many causes of AP require a detailed assessment of clinical history and biochemical evaluation, some causes are suggested or identified by imaging. In the following section, causes of AP depicted by imaging will be outlined.

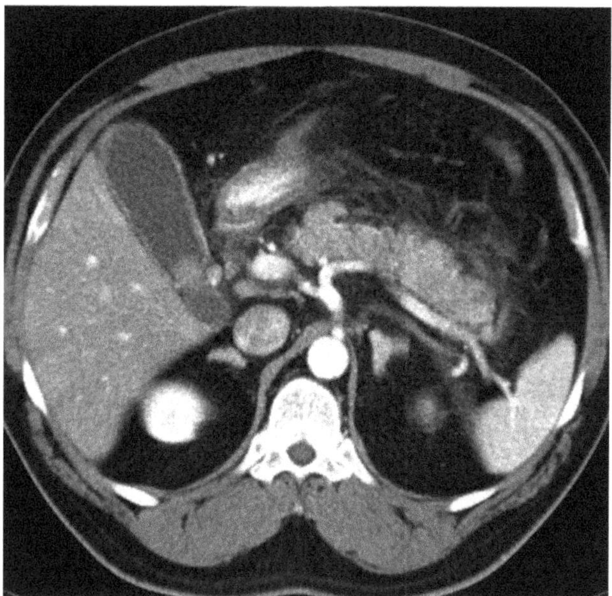

Figure 7. Biliary pancreatitis. Hyperdense stone is present in the gallbladder in a patient with interstitial pancreatitis.

Biliary

The diagnosis of biliary lithiasis is straightforward when gallstones are seen at abdominal US; gallstones appear as intraluminal, echogenic, mobile foci that are gravity-dependent and create a clean acoustic shadow. US has a sensitivity and specificity of around 95% for depicting gallstones and is the preferred imaging modality as CT shows significant lower sensitivity (of around 75%).[14] A repeat abdominal US is advised in those with "idiopathic" AP as gallstones may be missed on the initial evaluation.[39] Because of the superior sensitivity, an abdominal US should be performed in every patient presenting with AP early in the disease course to rule out gallstones as possible etiology. However, acute biliary pancreatitis may also be due to microlithiasis or biliary sludge (defined as stones smaller than 2 mm), which can be difficult to diagnose by abdominal US, but may be responsible for recurrent episodes of AP.[14,40] Biliary sludge is a viscous suspension of bile fluid that includes small stones, cholesterol monohydrate crystals, or calcium bilirubinate particles. Most patients who have biliary sludge are asymptomatic. Yet, biliary sludge is detected with increasing frequency in patients who have acute, otherwise idiopathic, pancreatitis.[41] Although controversial, many institutions perform cholecystectomy for repeated episodes of otherwise idiopathic pancreatitis associated with biliary sludge. On CT gallstones appear as single or multiple filling defects within the gallbladder. Gallstones may have varying densities on CT depending on the composition (**Figures 7, 8**). Stones may be densely calcified, rim calcified, laminated, or have a central nidus of calcification. Stones also may present as a soft-tissue density or a lucent filling defect within the bile. Some stones may contain gas. In about 25% of cases, stones are isodense to fluid and therefore not identifiable on CT.[14] MRI is an excellent, but costly alternative for US for depicting stones (larger than 4-5 mm) in the gallbladder or common bile duct (**Figure 9**). If a biliary etiology of AP is not diagnosed, the risk of pancreatitis recurrence is about 30% after 6 months follow-up with variable severity.[42] Hence, current guidelines advocate performing cholecystectomy during hospitalization in those with mild AP.[13]

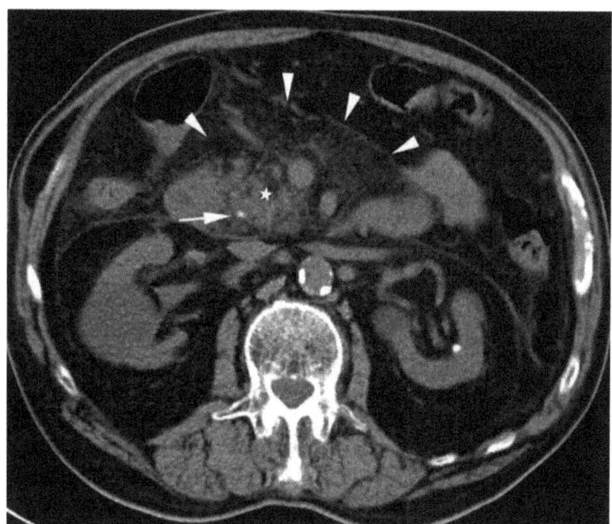

Figure 8. CT of choledocholithiasis. Unenhanced CT depicts a calcified stone in the common bile duct (arrow) at the level of pancreatic head (asterisk) with little peripancreatic fat stranding (arrowheads) compatible with interstitial pancreatitis.

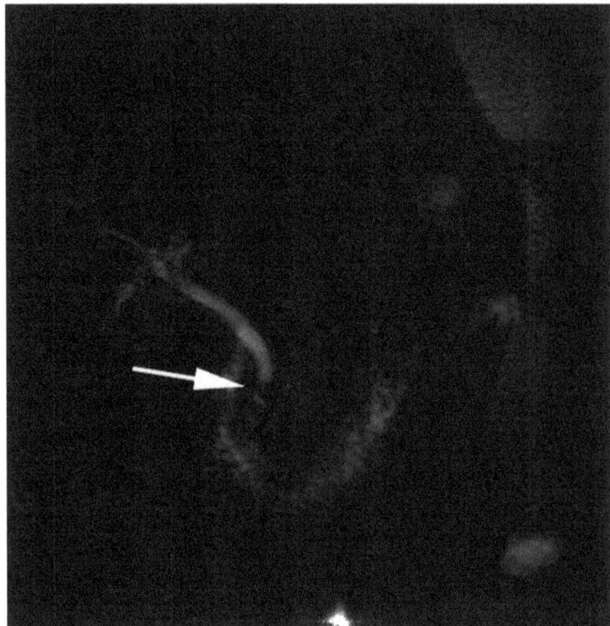

Figure 9. MRCP of choledocholithiasis. Heavily T2-weighted 3D sequence depicts two filling defects in the distal part of the common bile duct (arrow) representing stones.

Cross-sectional imaging may show secondary findings suggesting a biliary cause of pancreatitis. The "choledochal ring" sign, defined as hyperenhancement of the common bile duct wall relative to the pancreatic parenchyma (difference of more than 15 HU), has been reported to be indicative for a biliary cause of acute pancreatitis.[43] However, the sensitivity of this finding was not significant in the study by Yie et al[44] and needs to be validated in large-scale studies. In this study, some other CT features were significantly associated with biliary pancreatitis, including pericholecystic fluid or fat stranding, pericholecystic increased attenuation of the liver, increased gallbladder wall enhancement, and gallbladder wall thickening.[44,45] Further study is needed to validate these results.

Traumatic

Pancreatic injury is more commonly seen in children than in adults and occurs in less than 2% of all abdominal injuries with associated mortality ranging from 9%-34%.[46-50] Early mortality is caused by massive hemorrhage (often due to concomitant organ injuries) and late mortality by multi-organ dysfunction and/or sepsis.[46,47] The low rate of pancreatic injury after abdominal trauma is related to its retroperitoneal location. Isolated pancreatic injury is less commonly seen than concomitant duodenal and pancreatic injury. Coexisting injuries are often present owing to the central location of the pancreas and the close relationship with surrounding organs and vessels. Injury to the pancreas can cause AP (posttraumatic pancreatitis) that may present with equivocal clinical symptoms and laboratory findings, often masked by other organ injuries.[46-48] Posttraumatic pancreatitis should be considered when patients present with abdominal pain, nausea, and vomiting associated with increased serum amylase levels after blunt abdominal trauma. Contrast-enhanced CT is the primary imaging modality in abdominal trauma as it may diagnose posttraumatic pancreatitis and readily depicts accompanying traumatic injuries to other parenchymal organs, vessels, and bony structures.[49,50] Posttraumatic pancreatitis is likely in the right clinical setting combined with imaging features of pancreatitis. CT features of posttraumatic pancreatitis vary with the impact and severity of abdominal trauma and ranges from normal findings, mild pancreatic swelling, and exudate or soft tissue infiltration in the retroperitoneal spaces and mesenteries to hypo-enhancement of pancreatic parenchyma (representing contusion) or frank pancreatic transection with associated hemorrhage, fluid exudate, and duct disruption. Most CT findings in posttraumatic pancreatitis lack specificity and are often indistinguishable from pancreatitis of other etiologies, except for transection or laceration (depicted as a hypoattenuating linear density perpendicular oriented to the long axis of the pancreas) and fracture of the pancreas (clear separation of pancreatic fragments). Similar to findings of nontraumatic pancreatitis, CT findings of traumatic pancreatitis are time dependent: CT may show near normal findings in 20%-40% of cases during the first 12 hours after trauma with progressive changes on serial CT.[49,50] These subtle findings may be overlooked initially especially when coexistent organ injuries are present. Therefore, repeated imaging (CT or MRI) is warranted in those with sustained abdominal pain despite normal findings at index CT.[49,50] A diligent search for ductal injury should be undertaken in every patient with blunt abdominal trauma and posttraumatic pancreatitis as its integrity dictates clinical management: when intact, a conservative management is maintained, whereas a disrupted duct necessitates urgent surgical intervention. Delays in diagnosis and treatment of ductal injury results in subsequent increases in morbidity and mortality.[46-50] The main pancreatic duct is most prone to injury from blunt trauma at the pancreatic neck or body as it traverses the vertebral column. Minor or major pancreatic duct rupture can cause pancreatic ascites from leakage of pancreatic fluid into the lesser and greater peritoneal compartments. Ductal injury can be diagnosed non-invasively by CT or MRCP and semi-invasively by ERCP. On CT, ductal injury can be inferred when a pancreatic laceration of more than one-half the pancreatic diameter is observed or in case of a complete transection or pancreatic fracture along the expected course of the pancreatic duct. A characteristic telltale sign of ductal injury is the presence of a posttraumatic pancreatic collection or pseudocyst. Occasionally, MRCP may be a helpful noninvasive adjunct to emergency abdominal CT to better assess pancreatic duct integrity. A long-term complication of posttraumatic pancreatitis is ductal scarring and stenosis, which may cause obstructive pancreatitis proximal to the stricture.

Pancreatic neoplasms

Obstructive causes of AP due to pancreatic neoplasms involve periampullary tumors, cystic and solid pancreatic tumors, of which pancreatic adenocarcinoma is the most frequent and challenging diagnosis given the narrow therapeutic window for curative surgery. The incidence of solitary or recurrent attacks of AP associated with pancreatic adenocarcinoma is estimated to be 3%-5%.[51-55] Pancreatic cancer may cause pancreatitis because of pancreatic duct obstruction. Yet, the triggering mechanism of acute inflammation is incompletely understood as a minority of patients with pancreatic adenocarcinoma develop pancreatitis. Fortunately, pancreatitis resulting from underlying malignancy is usually mild (interstitial pancreatitis) such that curative resection is still possible (**Figure 10**). Necrotizing pancreatitis caused by pancreatic adenocarcinoma is rarely reported and notoriously difficult to diagnose and treat, as the extensive peripancreatic changes associated with necrotizing pancreatitis would likely render curative resection impossible in the majority of cases.[56] Pancreatic adenocarcinoma as the cause of pancreatitis is surrounded by pitfalls in clinical presentation and diagnostic imaging features leading to delays in correct diagnosis and appropriate treatment.[51-54] Often, the diagnosis of an occult pancreatic adenocarcinoma is masked by the clinical presentation of signs and symptoms of AP. Also, on imaging, features of the inflammatory process may hamper the visualization of a pancreatic mass. On CT, primary diagnostic signs for pancreatic adenocarcinoma are an infiltrating irregular hypovascular mass, signs of invasion of surrounding organs and vascular structures, necrotic regional lymph nodes, and metastases in liver or peritoneum.[51] Suspicious secondary imaging findings are an abrupt stop of the pancreatic duct with upstream duct dilation (whether or not with associated atrophy of pancreatic parenchyma), as this is rarely, if at all, seen in AP of benign cause. In most published reports, pancreatic adenocarcinoma has not been suspected clinically with a delay of diagnosis up to 12-24 months.[51-54] In patients with worrisome clinical symptoms such as new-onset of diabetes, jaundice, high bilirubin levels, recurrent attacks of "idiopathic" pancreatitis (unknown or uncertain etiologies), and weight loss, complimentary tests are warranted to rule out pancreatic cancer.[53,54] Also, in patients with suspicious findings on regular CT, a short interval (2-3 weeks) follow-up study is needed to ascertain the right diagnosis. Complementary imaging by means of EUS and/or MRI (depending on availability and expertise) is excellent in defining the morphology of pancreatic duct, the nature of obstructive lesion, and depicting the presence of a pancreatic mass in case of equivocal CT findings.

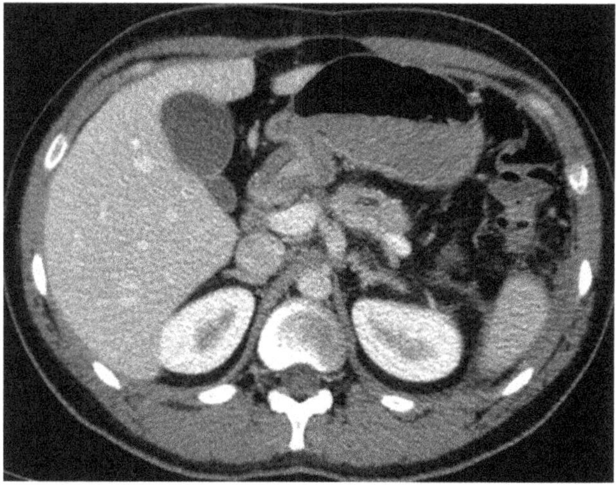

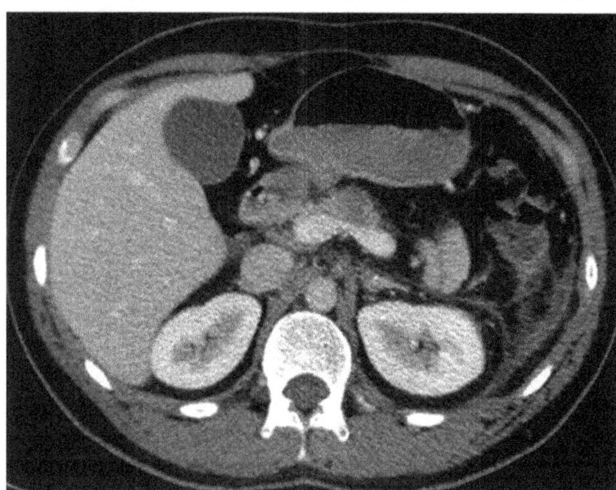

Figure 10. Interstitial pancreatitis due to pancreatic adenocarcinoma. A slightly dilated pancreatic duct (top) is noted that ends abruptly due to a hypovascular mass in the body of the pancreas (bottom). Mild exudate is present in the left retroperitoneal space. The patient underwent surgery and pancreatic adenocarcinoma was confirmed at pathology.

Congenital pancreatic anomalies

The following two etiologies (pancreas divisum and annular pancreas) occasionally cause AP. The association between these congenital pancreatic anomalies and AP remains, however, controversial.

Pancreas divisum is the most common congenital pancreatic duct anomaly with a reported prevalence of 2%-14% in the normal population.[57-62] Pancreas divisum represents a fusion anomaly in which the dorsal (containing the Santorini duct) and ventral (containing the Wirsung duct) pancreatic anlagen fail to fuse. Accordingly, the ventral (Wirsung) duct drains only the pancreatic head via the major papilla, whereas the majority of the pancreas drains via the minor papilla through the dorsal (Santorini) duct. It is assumed that drainage via the smaller caliber minor papilla into the duodenum may result in structural and functional outflow obstruction leading to pain and/or pancreatitis. Pancreas divisum is a definite cause of AP only when associated with ductal hypertension from increased resistance to flow through a proximally narrowed pancreatic duct and delayed clearance of injected contrast during ERCP.[60,61] Pancreas divisum is usually asymptomatic and the clinical relevance has been the subject of considerable debate. However, it is undoubtedly more frequently diagnosed in patients with repeated episodes of AP and chronic pancreatitis than in the general population. Yet, the incidence of pancreatitis in patients with pancreas divisum is low (about 5%) as ductal narrowing at the papillary origin is infrequently observed.[60,61] Pancreatic divisum can be confidently diagnosed semi-invasively by ERCP and non-invasively by MRCP. MRCP with secretin stimulation may depict inadequate outflow of pancreatic secretions through the minor papilla. In the normal population, multidetector CT (with its high spatial resolution and thin collimation) also allows for accurate assessment of pancreas divisum when the dorsal (Santorini) duct courses directly from the tail and body of the pancreas through the anterior part of the pancreatic head draining into the minor papilla without evident connection with the ventral duct. However, inflammatory changes of the pancreas (e.g., pancreatic edema, swelling, and necrosis) often preclude accurate CT assessment of ductal anatomy in patients with AP.[63] Recognition of cross-sectional findings suggestive for pancreatic divisum can guide patient management by recommending ERCP evaluation and assessment of minor papilla function. Possible treatments include stent placement in the minor papilla or minor papillotomy.

Annular pancreas is an uncommon congenital migration anomaly (1/20,000) where a ring of pancreatic tissue most commonly encircles the second part of the duodenum.[64] Annular pancreas is usually diagnosed during infancy (with severe duodenal obstruction requiring urgent surgery), but clinical manifestations may develop at any age. Pancreatitis due to annular pancreas is often focal, confined to the pancreatic head and likely relates to the obstruction of pancreatic secretions through the annular duct (Santorini duct). In infants, the diagnosis is usually made by upper gastrointestinal double-contrast studies (with the classic "double-bubble" sign, i.e., proximal dilation of both duodenum and stomach) or gastroduodenoscopy (with concentric narrowing and prestenotic duodenal dilatation). In adults presenting with pancreatitis, annular pancreas can be depicted on CT as a ring of inflammatory tissue (isodense with pancreatic parenchyma) surrounding the descending duodenum. Sometimes CT may show an annular duct (Santorini) also encircling the duodenum. EUS and MRI can be valuable for the diagnosis too.

Ischemic and postoperative

Ischemic and postoperative pancreatitis are rare etiologies of acute pancreatitis.[38,61] Although their mechanisms in inducing acute pancreatitis are intimately intermingled, independently they may account for an acute episode of pancreatitis. The common denominator in the pathogenesis of both etiologies is the disturbance of pancreatic microcirculation (i.e., the decrease of capillary perfusion and hemoglobin desaturation) which relates to the durations of both ischemia and reperfusion. The pancreas is highly susceptible to ischemia/reperfusion injury as established by experimental studies and in clinical settings such as cardiopulmonary bypass surgery and hemorrhagic shock.[65-68] Important components in the pathophysiology of ischemia-/reperfusion-induced AP include release of oxygen free radicals, activation of polymorphonuclear leukocytes, cellular acidosis, disturbance of intracellular homeostasis, and compromised pancreatic microvascular perfusion. These factors both induce and propagate premature intracellular activation of autodigestive pancreatic proteases and the resultant inflammatory response. Pancreatic ischemia may occur as a secondary event and, as such, may aggravate AP severity caused by other etiologies, but may also be the primary initiator of AP.[65-68]

Postoperative pancreatitis may occur after a variety of surgical procedures, including intra-abdominal procedures (e.g., common bile duct exploration, sphincteroplasty, distal gastrectomy, splenectomy, and organ transplantation) and operations distant from the gastrointestinal tract. It can occur after major surgery like cardiovascular surgery, spinal, vascular, and esophageal surgery, but also after relatively minor procedures that do not involve manipulations near the pancreas, such as thyroidectomy, parathyroidectomy, and inguinal hernia repair.[69-71]

Possible factors linking these surgical procedures with AP include drugs (medication during cardiopulmonary bypass surgery, immunosuppressive drugs in organ transplantation), intra- or postoperative periods of low flow or hypotension resulting in reduced splanchnic flow and impaired pancreatic vascularization, thromboembolic events, mechanical factors (direct pancreatic, duodenal or biliary manipulation), and metabolic factors.

The spectrum of symptoms associated with ischemia-induced AP may vary from asymptomatic hyperamylasemia (e.g., after cardiopulmonary bypass) to clinically severe disease as in hemorrhagic shock. The definition and diagnosis of ischemia-induced AP are difficult to determine and often delayed.[65-71] Clinical symptoms of AP may be masked after major surgery in patients who are mechanically ventilated, sedated, and/or receive narcotic analgesics. Ischemic AP should be considered in patients who develop abdominal pain and signs of sepsis after an episode of prolonged hypotension and/or visceral hypoperfusion, especially in those after cardiac or major surgery or who unexpectedly deteriorate rapidly postoperatively.[68-71] Imaging studies are necessary when the diagnosis of AP is uncertain. CT is a valuable objective imaging modality for the evaluation of patients with suspected ischemic or postoperative pancreatitis. In postoperative patients, CT may show findings of AP (with or without parenchymal necrosis) with peripancreatic collections that show varying degrees of encapsulation due to the often delayed diagnosis. Also, it is important to bear in mind that in patients with ischemic AP, a possible coexistence of intestinal ischemia may occur, in particular of the right hemicolon, transverse colon, or gallbladder. Furthermore, special attention should be paid to the patency of the portomesenteric venous structures, as well as the celiac trunk and superior mesenteric artery (i.e., high-grade stenosis, occlusion, or emboli).[68-71]

In conclusion, the diagnosis of ischemic or postoperative pancreatitis requires a high index of suspicion. Increased perioperative clinical awareness appears to be the most effective strategy for early diagnosis and timely treatment of acute ischemic pancreatitis following cardiac or major vascular surgery. Liberal use of diagnostic imaging modalities, primarily CT, to establish an early diagnosis and institution of appropriate therapy is therefore warranted.

Miscellaneous findings

Steatosis of the liver may be seen in patients with an alcoholic etiology or metabolic disturbances such as hypertriglyceridemia, but may also be a pre-existing condition (in case of obesity or medication use) and, therefore, lacks specificity (**Figure 11**). The presence of liver abnormalities characteristic for cirrhosis (caudate lobe hypertrophy, lobularity of liver contour, venous collaterals, splenomegaly) may however suggest an alcoholic etiology.

Diagnostic algorithm for assessing etiology

The standard work-up of the cause of AP may vary significantly among different centers based on personal experience and acquired skills, available equipment, and institutional strengths and weaknesses. Timing and the individual contribution of available imaging tests (US, EUS, CT, MRI/MRCP, and ERCP) are subject to debate and mainly driven by individual preferences. However, based on current available evidence and recommendations according to established guidelines, an abdominal US is advised in all patients presenting with AP, both at first presentation and in recurrent episodes of otherwise idiopathic pancreatitis.[6,9,60,61] Depending on expertise, availability, and local practices, further testing by means of EUS or MRCP is indicated as a next step if US is negative but the clinical suspicion for a biliary etiology is high. Additional imaging (i.e., state-of-the-art multidetector CT, EUS, and/or MRI/MRCP) is especially warranted in patients over 40-50 years of age with "idiopathic" AP or repeated episodes of AP to exclude a pancreatic neoplasm as a possible cause of the pancreatitis.

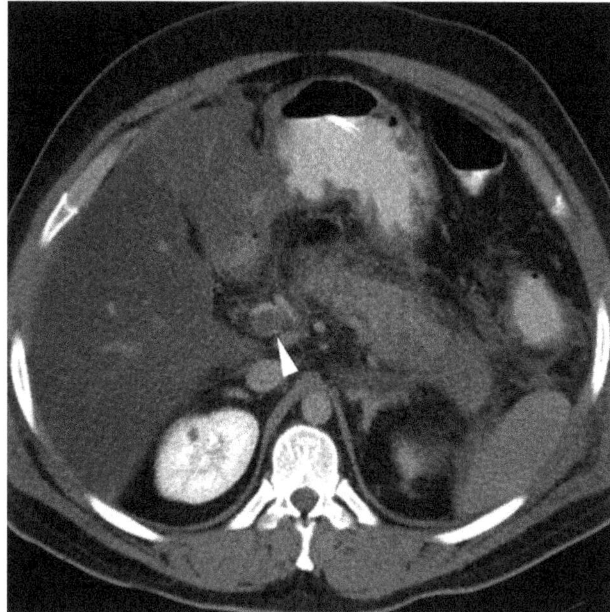

Figure 11. Hepatic steatosis in drug-induced pancreatitis. Markedly hypodense liver parenchyma is seen indicating severe hepatic steatosis in a patient with necrotizing pancreatitis and a thrombus in the portal vein (arrowhead).

Imaging & severity

AP is a serious disease with varying severity. The recently revised Atlanta Classification 2012 on AP (RAC) classified the severity of AP clinically (on the basis of presence or absence of organ failure) and morphologically (on the basis of presence or absence of tissue necrosis).[1] Morphologically (i.e., on imaging), two types of pancreatitis are discriminated: interstitial pancreatitis (no tissue necrosis) and necrotizing pancreatitis (tissue necrosis).

Interstitial pancreatitis

Interstitial pancreatitis is usually a self-limiting disease with a short hospitalization stay and represents the most common form of AP.[7,8] These patients typically recover uneventfully without complications. On imaging, interstitial pancreatitis may reveal a minimal increase in size of the pancreas, focally or diffusely (**Figure 12**). The pancreatic contour becomes irregular with inflammatory changes;

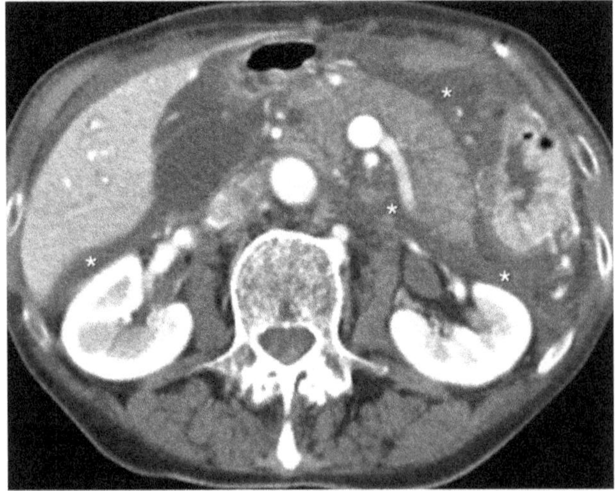

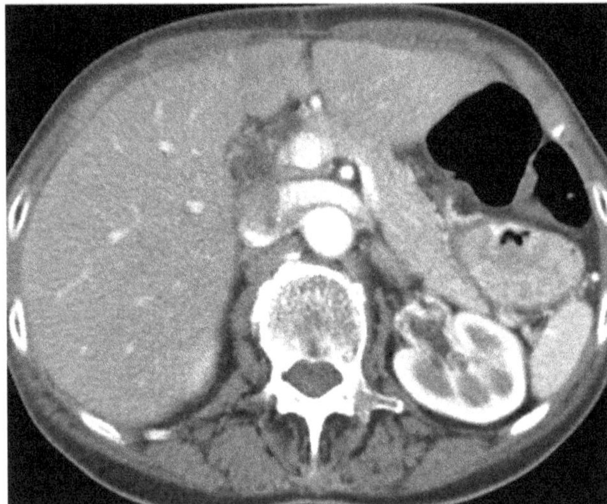

Figure 12. Interstitial pancreatitis. CT (top) depicts a swollen and slightly heterogeneous enhancing pancreatic parenchyma with fluid in the peripancreatic and retroperitoneal spaces (asterisks). Follow-up CT (bottom) 9 days later shows resolution of fluid and normalization of the pancreatic parenchyma.

the peripancreatic fat planes become blurred with increased attenuation values. Peripancreatic extension of the inflammatory process is relatively common because the pancreas lacks a well-defined capsule. Thickening of the small bowel mesentery, renal fascia, and lateroconal fascia are common. More severe forms of interstitial pancreatitis can result in moderate amounts of peripancreatic fluid.[2-4] Morbidity from interstitial disease ranges about 10% with mortality less than 3%, primarily due to comorbid disease.[72]

Necrotizing pancreatitis

Necrotizing pancreatitis is associated with a protracted clinical course, long hospital stay with a high morbidity (30%-80%), and a mortality rate up to 20%-30%.[73] The 2012 revised Atlanta Classification distinguishes three subtypes

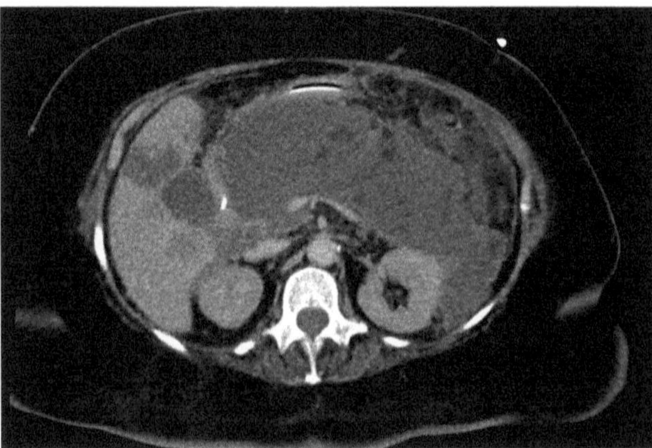

Figure 13. Acute necrotizing pancreatitis. CT shows extensive necrosis involving more than 90% of pancreatic parenchyma with associated acute necrotic collections.

of necrosis depending on involvement of pancreatic parenchyma alone (rare), peripancreatic tissues (extrapancreatic necrosis or EXPN, more common), or the combination of both (combined necrosis, most common).[1] Pancreatic parenchymal necrosis tends to occur early in the course of the disease, within the first 48-72 h after symptom onset. CT criteria for the diagnosis of pancreatic parenchymal necrosis are dependent on the detection of areas lacking enhancement, which may be focal or diffuse **(Figure 13)**. Lack of pancreatic enhancement corresponds with decreased blood perfusion of the pancreatic gland and correlates well with necrosis. Accuracy for depicting areas of pancreatic parenchymal necrosis is excellent when the region measures at least 3 cm or larger in diameter or involves more than one-third of the gland. Caution in defining pancreatic parenchymal necrosis is important as areas of intrapancreatic fluid or reversible ischemia can simulate areas of necrosis. Pancreatic parenchymal necrosis is ideally detected on scans performed >72 h after the onset of an attack of AP.[2-5] Scans done within this timeframe may be falsely negative or equivocal. EXPN is a relatively new subtype of necrotizing pancreatitis that has received increasing attention in the literature over the past years.[74-76] Its diagnosis hinges on the detection of heterogeneous peripancreatic collections with preserved pancreatic parenchyma perfusion. On CT, EXPN is determined when a normally perfused pancreatic parenchyma is noted surrounded by collections composed of various densities (fat, fluid, and nonliquid Hounsfield units) (**Figure 14**). In general, EXPN heralds a better prognosis than combined necrosis when sterile, but there is a similar prognosis when infection of necrotic tissue develops.[75,76]

Scoring systems for predicting severity

The clinical course of AP is highly variable ranging from mild self-limiting symptoms to rapidly progressive organ

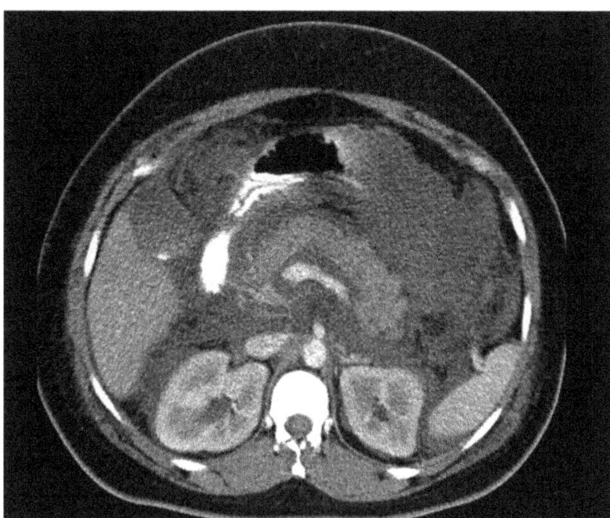

Figure 14. Extrapancreatic necrosis. CT depicts a normal enhancing pancreatic parenchyma surrounded by acute necrotic collections. Note, calcified stone in the gallbladder.

dysfunction potentially culminating in death if not treated appropriately. Proper initial management includes transfer of patients to specialized centers or admission to intensive care units for supportive treatment or for targeted therapy (i.e., institution of tailored fluid resuscitation, endoscopic intervention, enteral nutrition, or new therapies as they become available). Besides the need from a clinical management perspective, there are other potential benefits for early severity prediction of AP. Accurate stratification is essential for reliable comparison of clinical outcomes among institutions, for evaluation of novel therapeutic strategies, and for inclusion of patients in randomized controlled clinical trials.[1] Hence, considerable efforts have been targeted over the past decades to the early identification of those who will develop persistent organ failure in the early stages and infected necrosis and sepsis in the later phase.

Prediction of disease severity can be done using thorough clinical evaluation including detailed assessment of established risk factors (e.g., age, obesity, and comorbid disease). However, based on clinical evaluation alone, even experienced physicians fail to diagnose those with severe AP in 30%-50% of cases. Other means of determining severity include the use of single prognostic indicators (e.g., serum blood urea nitrogen, creatinine, hematocrit, levels of C-reactive protein, procalcitonin) and the utilization of multiple clinical scoring systems that incorporate physiologic and laboratory parameters (among these are the Ranson score, Systemic Inflammatory Response Syndrome [SIRS], Bedside Index of Severity in AP [BISAP], and Acute Physiology and Chronic Health Evaluation [APACHE]-II score). In a large dual-center study, the accuracies of all available clinical scoring systems in predicting the development of persistent organ failure (signifying severe AP) on the day of admission were prospectively studied using comparative effectiveness analysis. This study found that all clinical scoring systems failed to perform with high performance characteristics and revealed only modest and comparable predictive accuracy.[77] Finally, since the introduction of CT for diagnosis and assessment of AP some four decades ago, several imaging-based scoring systems have been proposed to predict the severity of AP.

Imaging-based scoring systems related to CT are the most studied and widely used because CT is regarded the frontline imaging modality for the overall assessment of AP. Determinants of most CT-based scoring systems include pancreatic, peripancreatic and extrapancreatic features. Pancreatic changes include the subjective or objective enlargement of the pancreatic gland and presence and extent of parenchymal necrosis. Peripancreatic features include fat stranding or edema, (fluid) collection(s) (presence, number, and volume), perirenal edema, mesenteric inflammation, and retroperitoneal extension. Extrapancreatic features include the presence of ascites, pleural effusion, vascular, gastrointestinal, and/or extrapancreatic parenchymal organ complications. Over the past four decades, at least 10 different radiographic scoring systems have been developed (**Table 2**) using incremental numerical scores or grades with higher scores or grades correlating with increasing morbidity and mortality.[17,78-86] Two of these evaluate the presence and extent of parenchymal necrosis (i.e., CT Severity Index [CTSI] and Modified CT Severity Index [MCTSI]) for which the use of intravenous contrast material is indispensable.[17,82] The remainder of scoring systems can be assessed on unenhanced CT scans. **Table 2** provides an overview of existing imaging-based scoring systems in order of year of development with the parameters evaluated and their respective advantages and limitations.

Among all radiographic scoring systems available, the CTSI is the most commonly used and studied.[17] The CTSI combines the Balthazar grade (0-4 points) with the extent of pancreatic necrosis (0-6 points) on a 10-point severity scale (**Figure 15, Table 3**). The calculated CTSI can then be subdivided in three categories (CTSI 0-3, 4-6, and 7-10; corresponding to predicted mild, moderate, and severe disease, respectively) that have subsequent increases in morbidity and mortality.[17] The main advantage of the CTSI is its intuitive design as it accurately depicts the order of increasing morphologic AP severity. Interstitial pancreatitis is reflected by CTSI of 0 (normal pancreas), 1 (swelling of the pancreatic gland), and 2 (peripancreatic fat stranding). Extrapancreatic necrosis is potentially reflected by CTSI of 3 and 4 (1 or more pancreatic collections, respectively). In general, CTSI greater than 4 (5-10) denotes the presence of pancreatic collections and parenchymal necrosis with more points accredited with increasing extent of necrosis.

Table 2. Radiographic scoring systems in AP

Radiographic scoring system	Year of development	CECT	CT parameters	Advantage(s)	Disadvantage(s)
Extrapancreatic score (EP or Schroeder index, range 0-7)	1985	-	Edema in part or entire pancreas, ascites, pleural effusion, perirenal fat edema, mesenteric fat edema, and bowel paralysis.	Relatively easy to assess; does not require intravenous contrast	Not validated for early use*; presence of ascites and perirenal edema can be a normal finding; not extensively studied¶
Balthazar Grade (A-E)	1985	-	Pancreatic swelling, peripancreatic fat stranding, presence and number of associated pancreatic collections	Relatively easy to assess; does not require intravenous contrast	Variable interobserver agreement (i.e., counting the number of collections)
Pancreatic size index (PSI, cut-off 10 cm^2)	1989	-	Multiplying the maximum anteroposterior measurement of the head and body of the pancreas	Measurement of single parameter; does not require intravenous contrast	Normal size may vary depending on age and previous attack; not extensively studied¶
CT Severity Index (CTSI, range 0-10)	1990	+	Balthazar grade + presence and extent of parenchymal necrosis	Most used and studied Depicts the order of morphologic severity in AP	Variable interobserver agreement for counting pancreatic collections and assessing % of necrosis
MOP score (range 0-2)	2003	-	Mesenteric edema and peritoneal fluid (ascites)	Measurement of just two parameters; simple and easy to assess; does not require intravenous contrast	Not validated for early use*; ascites can be physiologic in female and elderly; not extensively studied¶
Modified CTSI (MCTSI, range 0-10)	2004	+	Pancreatic swelling or fat stranding, pancreatic collection(s), presence and extent of parenchymal necrosis, extrapancreatic complications including vascular, parenchymal, gastrointestinal organs and pleural effusion and ascites	Inherent simplifications; easier to assess for unexperienced readers	Does not outperform the original CTSI
Retroperitoneal Extension Grade (I-V)	2006	-	Extension of peripancreatic inflammation to retroperitoneal spaces	Does not require intravenous contrast	Advanced interpretative skills required; not extensively studied¶
EPIC score (range 0-7)	2007	-	Pleural effusion, ascites, retroperitoneal and mesenteric inflammation	Relatively easy to assess; does not require intravenous contrast	Original study biased towards severe disease; not extensively studied¶
Renal Rim Grade (A-C)	2010	-	Extension of peripancreatic inflammation to pararenal and/or perirenal space	Easy to assess; does not require intravenous contrast	Not extensively studied¶
EXPN Volume (cut-off 100 mL)	2014	-	Volume of extrapancreatic exudate or fluid	Objective; does not require intravenous contrast	Not validated for early use*; additional software required for calculating volume; not extensively studied¶

*: within 24 hours of admission; ¶: fewer than 5 studies in English literature.

Table 3. Balthazar Grade and CT Severity Index (CTSI)

Characteristics	Balthazar Grade	CTSI
Pancreatic inflammation		
Normal pancreas	A	0
Focal or diffuse enlargement of the pancreas	B	1
Peripancreatic inflammation/fat stranding	C	2
Single acute fluid collection	D	3
Two or more acute fluid collections	E	4
Pancreatic parenchymal necrosis		
None		0
Less than 30%		2
Between 30% and 50%		4
More than 50%		6

However, patients with less than 30% parenchymal necrosis without associated collections also have CTSI of 4, although this is a rare event.

Despite the profound heterogeneity in study design and the variable endpoints used among the different studies, all reports on the discriminatory power of radiographic scoring systems show a modestly positive correlation between the scoring system studied and patient outcome. Two recent studies compared the accuracy of several radiographic scoring systems, including the CTSI, and found comparable performance characteristics among the CT scoring systems studied in the prediction of disease severity and overall mortality.[19,87] Also, these studies show that CT scoring systems did not perform better than commonly used clinical scoring systems, such as BISAP and APACHE II score.

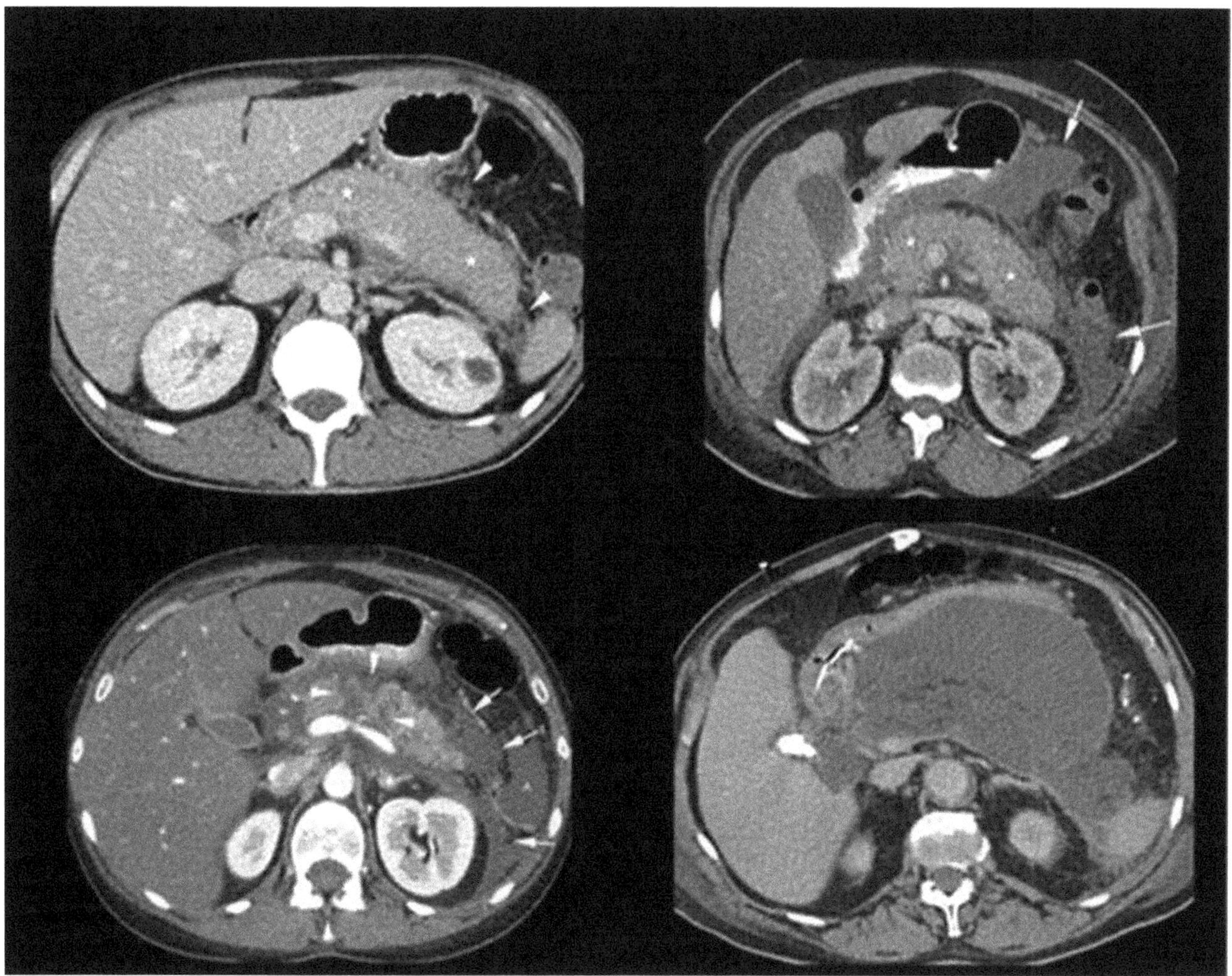

Figure 15. CT severity index. CTSI of 2 (top left): swollen but normal enhancing pancreas (asterisks) with little peripancreatic fat stranding (arrowheads). CTSI of 4 (top right): normal enhancing pancreatic parenchyma (asterisks) with more than 2 collections (arrows). CTSI of 6 (bottom left): less than 30% nonenhancing pancreatic parenchyma at the level of pancreatic body (arrowheads) with associated necrotic collections (arrows). CTSI of 10 (bottom right): extensive necrosis of more than 50% of pancreatic parenchyma with associated necrotic collections. Note, calcified stones in the gallbladder.

There are several explanations for the moderate performance characteristics of imaging-based scoring systems. First, the degree of morphologic abnormalities is largely influenced by the time interval between symptom onset and performance of the imaging study with increasing changes seen with increasing time interval (with correspondent higher scores or, grades). Second, radiographic scoring systems do not account for well-known risk factors, such as obesity, age, and pre-existent comorbid disease. Third, in a small but definite percentage of patients with AP, there is a non-linear relationship between morphologic findings and clinical severity. Also, some 30%-40% of patients with parenchymal necrosis will have a relatively benign clinical course (without organ dysfunction or systemic complications).[19-23] Fourth, radiographic scoring systems correlate better with local complications (infected necrosis and need for intervention) than with systemic complications (primarily persistent organ failure, which signifies severe disease). Fifth, radiographic scoring systems are biased towards more severe disease as those with very mild symptoms often do not need or undergo cross-sectional imaging. Sixth, the use of most CT-based systems is confounded as reliable predictor by the subjective nature of its interpretation with variable interobserver agreement, which likely relates to readers' expertise and familiarity of imaging findings of AP. Seventh, as opposed to clinical scoring systems, radiographic scoring systems are not repeated routinely within a short time period such that an interval change in significant morphology may go unnoticed (e.g., interval detection of parenchymal necrosis on serial CT not visible on the index CT). Eighth, scoring systems (radiographic and clinical systems) do not correlate with the risk of specific extrapancreatic complications (e.g., abdominal compartment syndrome, bowel ischemia or perforation, or arterial pseudoaneurysm). Therefore, they fail to provide detailed information that instantly affects patient management on an individual basis. Finally, the fallacy of linking one imaging feature or a constellation of imaging features to severe clinical outcome falls short simply because of the intrinsic morbidity and mortality, albeit low in numbers, in patients with interstitial pancreatitis.[72] Typically, grave imaging features in interstitial pancreatitis are absent to foretell a dismal outcome. It is therefore unlikely that radiographic scoring systems will ever serve as an accurate means of correctly identifying all those with severe pancreatitis early on in the disease process. The limited efficacy of radiographic scoring systems for prognostication reflects the complexity, variability, and heterogeneity of AP with its myriad possible clinical expressions.

Clinicians need a powerful, simple, and easy-to-use predictive system early on in the disease process, preferably within several hours after admission, for directing patients to different levels of care or tailored therapy measures. Cross-sectional imaging studies performed within this timeframe will not likely surpass clinical scoring systems, as has been shown in the aforementioned reports comparing the various radiographic scoring systems on the day of admission. In view of the abovementioned limitations of radiographic scoring systems, the added costs, efforts, and radiation burden associated with CT,[88-91] and the ease of use of some of the clinical scoring systems, it is the author's opinion that the initial severity assessment should be based on clinical scoring systems rather than relying on imaging parameters. The decision about if and when to perform CT therefore depends on the overall clinical presentation. Undeniably, CT has its greatest merits in the later phase of the disease in those who have predicted severe AP by clinical assessment or those who do not improve clinically despite appropriate therapy when local complications (most commonly infection of necrotic tissue) largely direct clinical decision-making.[24,92]

Prognostic cross-sectional imaging findings

Irrespective of the etiologic factor, the degree of morphologic findings in AP depends on the severity of the attack and the time interval between onset of symptoms and imaging. In general, morphologic findings are well-established 5-7 days after symptom onset. Mild disease presents with only mild pancreatic and peripancreatic abnormalities that resolve spontaneously. Severe disease presents with extensive peripancreatic abnormalities (including necrotic collections) and parenchymal necrosis, which may become infected and give rise to various extrapancreatic parenchymal, vascular, or visceral complications, potentially with significant impacts on patient management.

Pancreatic collections

In moderate to severe AP, pancreatic collections can accumulate in and around the pancreas. These collections may be single or multiple, vary in size, and lack a well-defined capsule initially, only confined by the anatomic space in which they arise. Many collections resolve spontaneously, but a certain percentage goes on to develop a complete wall, which usually takes 4-5 weeks to develop. These collections may become symptomatic due to persistent pain, secondary infection or hemorrhage or by exerting mass-effect on surrounding structures (e.g., extrinsic biliary obstruction).[5-12] Other complications include compression and occlusion of the splenic vein, which can result in extensive collateralization around the spleen and stomach. This may in time become a source of gastrointestinal bleeding. The most common sites of pancreatic collections are the lesser sac and left anterior pararenal space.[2-5] Larger collections can extend retroperitoneally over the psoas muscles to enter the pelvis and groin. Pancreatic

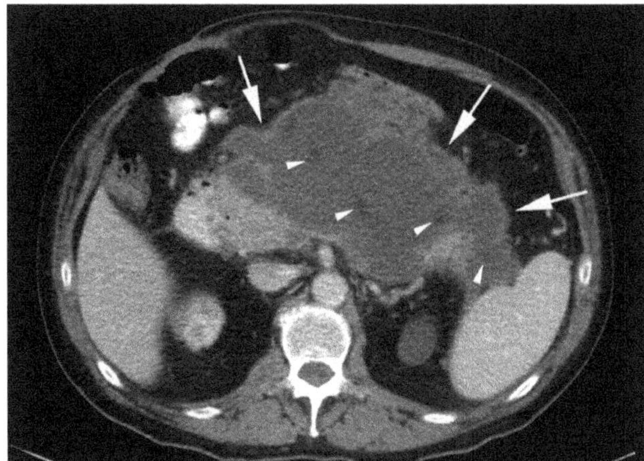

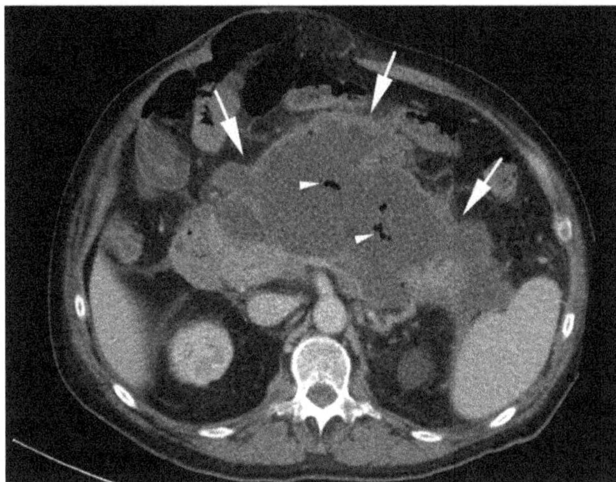

Figure 16. Walled-off necrosis (WON). (Top) CT shows a fully encapsulated heterogeneous collection replacing a large part of pancreatic parenchyma (arrows pointing at the borders). Collection consist of fluid and non-liquid (fat) densities (small arrowheads). (Bottom) Follow-up CT performed 1 week later because of fever now shows gas bubbles (small arrowheads) within the WON (arrows pointing at the borders), representing infected necrosis.

collections may also involve the posterior pararenal space, perirenal space, transverse mesocolon, and small bowel mesentery. Notably, pancreatic collections should not be mistaken for areas where ascites reside, such as in the perihepatic and perisplenic areas, in the paracolic gutters, and pelvis. Management of pancreatic collections depend on the patient's clinical condition and whether they cause symptoms (**Figures 16, 17**).

Pancreatic necrosis

Pancreatic parenchymal necrosis represents a severe form of AP. In addition to the presence of parenchymal necrosis, its extent (particularly when more than 30% is involved in the necrotic process) has also been correlated with worse

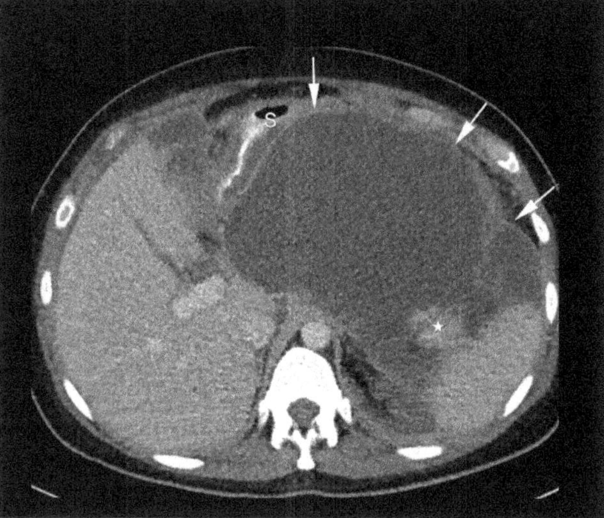

Figure 17. Gastric outlet obstruction due to large walled-off necrosis. CT shows a large fully encapsulated pancreatic collection (arrows pointing at the borders) which exerts mass effect on the stomach (S). Note, little preserved pancreatic parenchyma at the tail (asterisk).

clinical outcome in some[19-22] but not all reports.[93-95] The site of necrosis is deemed equally important, especially when the central part of the gland is involved with a viable pancreatic tail (**Figure 18**). Full thickness necrosis of the midgland (neck and/or body of the pancreas) may lead to pancreatic duct disruption with increased need for intervention and definitive therapies to control the continuing secretion of pancreatic juice.[96,97] Isolated parenchymal necrosis is a rare event. In the majority of cases, the necrosis is not confined to the pancreatic parenchyma alone, it often also involves the peripancreatic tissues. Necrotic tissue or necrotic collections are prone to bacterial colonization from adjacent bowel structures with development of infected necrosis. Infected necrosis is regarded as one of the most feared local complications of AP, responsible for prolonged hospitalization, need for invasive intervention with high demand of health care resources.[7,73] Infected pancreatic necrosis is recognized at CT as bubbles of gas within areas of the pancreas or as a collection of gas and tissue within the retroperitoneum (**Figure 19**). Infected necrosis carries a grave prognosis compared with sterile necrosis, with a two- to threefold increase of mortality.[6,9,73]

Vascular complications

Vascular complications arising from AP include portosplenomesenteric venous thrombosis, arterial pseudoaneurysms, and hemorrhage due to vessel wall erosion by extravasated proteolytic pancreatic enzymes. Splenic vein thrombosis occurs most common and may often result in

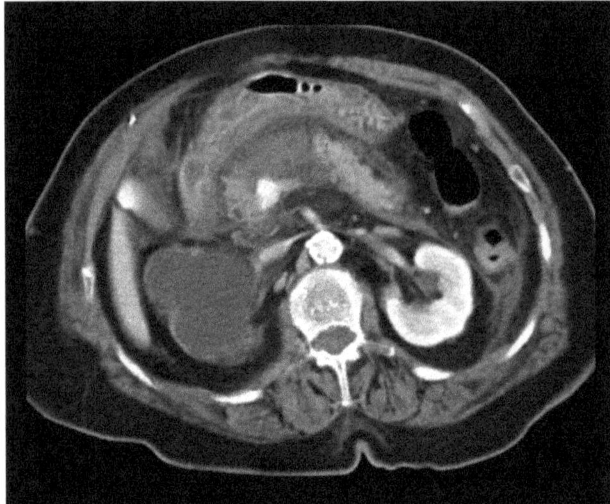

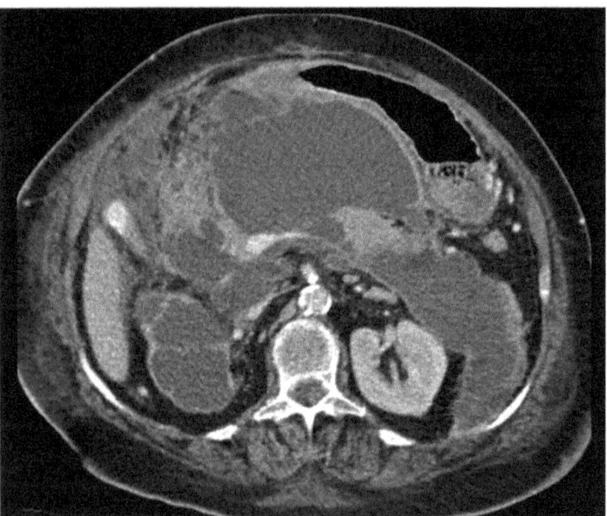

Figure 18. Central gland necrosis. CT 3 days after symptom onset (top) shows nonenhancement of the midgland with preserved pancreatic body and tail. Note, severe and longstanding ureteropelvic junction obstruction of the right kidney with loss of renal parenchyma. Follow-up CT 3 weeks later (bottom) shows a marked increase in the size of necrotic collections exerting a mass effect on the stomach and extending to the left retroperitoneal space.

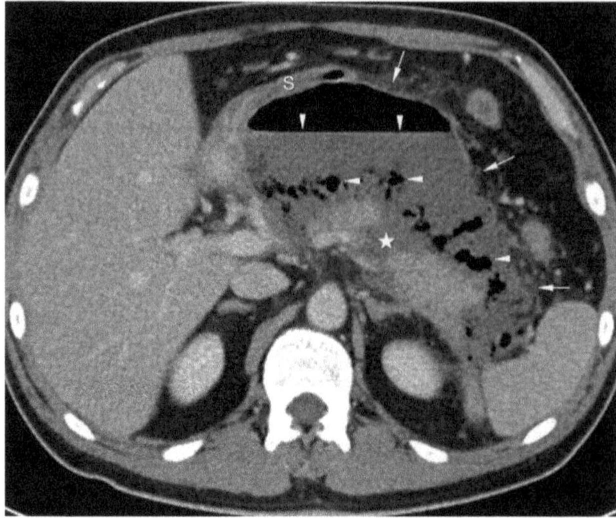

Figure 19. Infected pancreatic necrosis. CT shows a necrotic area at the junction of pancreatic body and tail (asterisk) with associated necrotic collections (small arrowheads pointing at the borders) that contains impacted gas bubbles (small horizontal arrowheads) in the retroperitoneal compartment and a gas-fluid level (small vertical arrowheads) in the lesser sac, signifying infection of necrosis. S: stomach.

complications such as gastric or esophageal varices and splenomegaly (left-sided portal hypertension) (**Figure 20**). Multiphasic CT accurately depicts sites of vascular thrombosis and demonstrates collateral vascular pathways.[98-100] Erosion of arterial vessel wall initially results in a confined perivascular blood leak with subsequent arterial pseudoaneurysm formation. Injuries commonly involve the splenic artery, the pancreaticoduodenal or the gastroduodenal arteries, which are closely related to the pancreas. An arterial pseudoaneurysm is often the underlying etiology in cases of massive haemorrhage.[101-103] CT with arterial phase multidetector CT or 3D CT angiography can routinely detect the presence and specific site of such pseudoaneurysms. Bleeding may also occur into a preexisting pancreatic collection, often in areas of necrosis. Cross-sectional imaging is helpful in identifying the source of hemorrhage. Massive acute hemorrhage secondary to

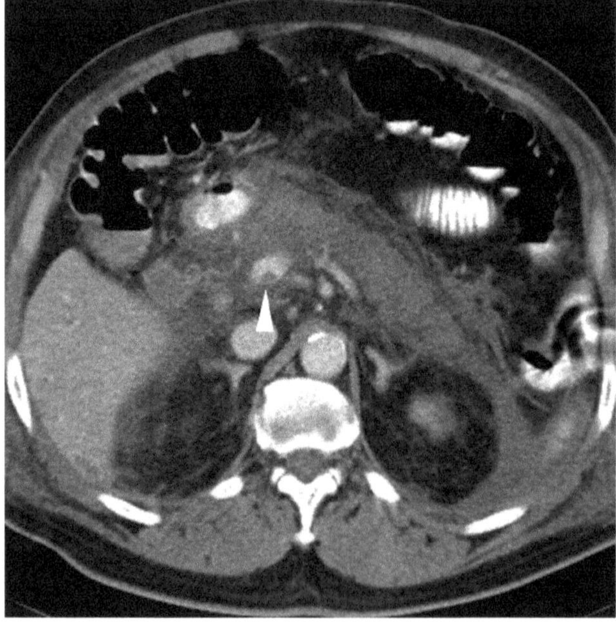

Figure 20. Portal vein thrombus in necrotizing pancreatitis. Small intraluminal filling defect is noted in the portal vein (arrowhead) in a patient with necrotizing pancreatitis.

bleeding pancreatic collections or arterial pseudoaneurysm has an associated mortality rate of 10%-35%.[101-103] An easily overlooked complication on abdominal CT in patients who are bedridden because of their illness (i.e., not unique to AP) is the occurrence of deep vein thrombosis in the iliacofemoral veins that may lead to pulmonary emboli. In contrast to portosplenomesenteric vein thrombosis, this finding urgently necessitates the initiation of anticoagulant treatment.

Involvement of extrapancreatic organs

Typically, AP is a disease process where the inflammatory spread is not limited by adjacent organs, mesenteries, omentum, or peritoneal and retroperitoneal fascial planes. While pancreatitis most commonly involves the pararenal spaces and lesser sac, it can extend to and involve adjacent organs.

Renal involvement is typically due to inflammatory extension into the anterior and sometimes posterior pararenal space. The left pararenal space is most commonly involved. Occasionally, a pancreatic collection can extend into the perirenal space and even beneath the renal capsule, potentially resulting in a Page kidney due to compressive forces on the renal parenchyma requiring percutaneous drainage. Other unusual complications include renal vascular abnormalities such as narrowing of the renal vein, renal vein thrombosis, perirenal varices and obstructive hydroneprosis due to extrinsic ureteral compression.[104-106]

Splenic involvement by pancreatitis is not uncommon given the close relationship of the pancreatic tail and splenic hilum. In addition to vascular complications ranging from splenic artery pseudoaneurysm to splenic vein occlusion, pancreatic collection may extend deep into the spleen. This can result in complications including intrasplenic collections, splenic infarction, splenic abscess, and intrasplenic hemorrhage. Intrasplenic collections render the organ vulnerable to rupture with even minor trauma.[107,108] Similar complications may occur in the liver.

Biliary complications during the course of AP include cholecystitis, biliary obstruction, or rarely gallbladder perforation.[109-111]

Gastrointestinal complications in severe necrotizing pancreatitis are not uncommon because the extravasated pancreatic enzymes may directly extend into the mesenteries of bowel structures. Besides the risk of bacterial translocation, other catastrophic and life-threatening complications are bowel ischemia and perforation that demand emergent surgery.[112-114] Another complication is abdominal compartment syndrome (ACS), which is increasingly recognized in necrotizing pancreatitis (see Chapter 32).[115-117] ACS is an important cause of multi-organ dysfunction associated with high mortality if left untreated. Although ACS is a clinical diagnosis, at times the diagnosis is suggested on CT in patients who exhibit the "round-belly sign," defined as abdominal distension with an increased ratio of anteroposterior-to-transverse abdominal diameter (ratio >0.80).[118,119] Particularly, the change in girth compared with prior CT scans may suggest ACS in the appropriate clinical setting. Finally, multiple pulmonary complications may be seen during the course of severe AP that includes the presence of pleural effusions, pulmonary infiltrates, pulmonary emboli and associated infarction, and, more rarely, pulmonary empyema and pneumothorax.[120,121]

Conclusion

Imaging is an indispensable tool that is increasingly utilized in the care of patients with AP by providing critical information for clinicians, especially those with severe disease. Multidetector CT is the imaging modality of choice that allows for a quick and accurate overall assessment of AP and its complications with (E)US and MRI reserved for elucidating the etiology of the pancreatitis or as problem-solving tools. Imaging-based predictive systems are useful for identifying groups of patients at risk for local complications or comparing outcomes of different groups in clinical research. However, for the individual patient, providing a radiographic grading score will not directly affect clinical management as opposed to some specific cross-sectional imaging findings. Among these are the presence of extended necrosis (more than 30%), especially when the midgland is involved (associated with increased need for intervention), signs of infected necrosis (requiring empirical antibiotics or invasive intervention), massive hemorrhage or detection of an arterial pseudoaneurysm (indication for angiographic coiling or surgery), deep vein thrombosis or detection of pulmonary emboli (indication for anticoagulant therapy), acute cholecystitis (amenable for percutaneous drainage or cholecystectomy), bowel ischemia or perforation (indication for emergent surgery), and findings of ACS (requiring percutaneous drainage of ascites or surgery). Most of these complications are not included in any radiographic scoring system but will help guide individual patient management.

References

1. Banks PA, Bollen TL, Dervenis C, Gooszen HG, Johnson CD, Sarr MG, et al. Classification of acute pancreatitis--2012: revision of the Atlanta classification and definitions by international consensus. *Gut*. 2013; 62: 102-111. PMID: 23100216.
2. Thoeni RF. The revised Atlanta classification of acute pancreatitis: its importance for the radiologist and its effect on treatment. *Radiology*. 2012; 262: 751-764. PMID: 22357880.

3. Thoeni RF. Imaging of Acute Pancreatitis. *Radiol Clin North Am*. 2015; 53: 1189-1208. PMID: 26526433.
4. Bollen TL. Imaging of acute pancreatitis: update of the revised Atlanta classification. *Radiol Clin North Am*. 2012; 50: 429-445. PMID: 22560690.
5. Bollen TL. Acute pancreatitis: international classification and nomenclature. *Clin Radiol*. 2016; 71: 121-133. PMID: 26602933.
6. Tenner S, Baillie J, DeWitt J, Vege SS; American College of Gastroenterology. American College of Gastroenterology guideline: management of acute pancreatitis. *Am J Gastroenterol*. 2013; 108: 1400-1415; 1416. PMID: 23896955.
7. Lankisch PG, Apte M, Banks PA. Acute pancreatitis. *Lancet*. 2015; 386: 85-96. PMID: 25616312.
8. Johnson CD, Besselink MG, Carter R. Acute pancreatitis. *BMJ*. 2014; 349 g4859. PMID: 25116169.
9. Wu BU, Banks PA. Clinical management of patients with acute pancreatitis. *Gastroenterology*. 2013; 144: 1272-1281. PMID: 23622137.
10. Fisher JM, Gardner TB. The "golden hours" of management in acute pancreatitis. *Am J Gastroenterol*. 2012; 107: 1146-1150. PMID: 22858994.
11. Zhao K, Adam SZ, Keswani RN, Horowitz JM, Miller FH. Acute Pancreatitis: Revised Atlanta Classification and the Role of Cross-Sectional Imaging. *AJR Am J Roentgenol*. 2015; 205: W32-W41. PMID: 26102416.
12. Shyu JY, Sainani NI, Sahni VA, Chick JF, Chauhan NR, Conwell DL, et al. Necrotizing pancreatitis: diagnosis, imaging, and intervention. *Radiographics*. 2014; 34: 1218-1239. PMID: 25208277.
13. Working Group IAP/APA Acute Pancreatitis Guidelines. IAP/APA evidence-based guidelines for the management of acute pancreatitis. *Pancreatology*. 2013; 13 4 Suppl 2: e1-e15. PMID: 24054878.
14. Surlin V, Saftoiu A, Dumitrescu D. Imaging tests for accurate diagnosis of acute biliary pancreatitis. *World J Gastroenterol*. 2014; 20: 16544-16549. PMID: 25469022.
15. Vriens PW, van de Linde P, Slotema ET, Warmerdam PE, Breslau PJ. Computed tomography severity index is an early prognostic tool for acute pancreatitis. *J Am Coll Surg*. 2005; 201: 497-502. PMID: 16183486.
16. Pocard M, Soyer P. CT of acute pancreatitis: a matter of time. *Diagn Interv Imaging*. 2015; 96: 129-131. PMID: 25617113.
17. Balthazar EJ, Robinson DL, Megibow AJ, Ranson JH. Acute pancreatitis: value of CT in establishing prognosis. *Radiology*. 1990; 174: 331-336. PMID: 2296641.
18. Balthazar EJ. Acute pancreatitis: assessment of severity with clinical and CT evaluation. *Radiology*. 2002; 223: 603-613. PMID: 12034923.
19. Bollen TL, Singh VK, Maurer R, Repas K, van Es HW, Banks PA, et al. A comparative evaluation of radiologic and clinical scoring systems in the early prediction of severity in acute pancreatitis. *Am J Gastroenterol*. 2012; 107: 612-619. PMID: 22186977.
20. Casas JD, Diaz R, Valderas G, Mariscal A, Cuadras P. Prognostic value of CT in the early assessment of patients with acute pancreatitis. *AJR Am J Roentgenol*. 2004; 182: 569-574. PMID: 14975947.
21. Lankisch PG, Pflichthofer D, Lehnick D. No strict correlation between necrosis and organ failure in acute pancreatitis. *Pancreas*. 2000; 20: 319-322. PMID: 10766460.
22. Perez A, Whang EE, Brooks DC, Moore FD Jr, Hughes MD, Sica GT, et al. Is severity of necrotizing pancreatitis increased in extended necrosis and infected necrosis? *Pancreas*. 2002; 25: 229-233. PMID: 12370532.
23. Isenmann R, Runzi M, Kron M, Kahl S, Kraus D, Jung N, et al. Prophylactic antibiotic treatment in patients with predicted severe acute pancreatitis: a placebo-controlled, double-blind trial. *Gastroenterology*. 2004; 126: 997-1004. PMID: 15057739.
24. Brand M, Gotz A, Zeman F, Behrens G, Leitzmann M, Brunnler T, et al. Acute necrotizing pancreatitis: laboratory, clinical, and imaging findings as predictors of patient outcome. *AJR Am J Roentgenol*. 2014; 202: 1215-1231. PMID: 24848818.
25. Morgan DE, Baron TH, Smith JK, Robbin ML, Kenney PJ. Pancreatic fluid collections prior to intervention: evaluation with MR imaging compared with CT and US. *Radiology*. 1997; 203: 773-778. PMID: 9169703.
26. Xiao B, Zhang XM. Magnetic resonance imaging for acute pancreatitis. *World J Radiol*. 2010; 2: 298-308. PMID: 21160684.
27. Xiao B, Zhang XM, Tang W, Zeng NL, Zhai ZH. Magnetic resonance imaging for local complications of acute pancreatitis: a pictorial review. *World J Gastroenterol*. 2010; 16: 2735-2742. PMID: 20533593.
28. Manikkavasakar S, AlObaidy M, Busireddy KK, Ramalho M, Nilmini V, Alagiyawanna M, et al. Magnetic resonance imaging of pancreatitis: an update. *World J Gastroenterol*. 2014; 20: 14760-14777. PMID: 25356038.
29. Arvanitakis M, Delhaye M, De Maertelaere V, Bali M, Winant C, Coppens E, et al. Computed tomography and magnetic resonance imaging in the assessment of acute pancreatitis. *Gastroenterology*. 2004; 126: 715-723. PMID: 14988825.
30. Stimac D, Miletić D, Radić M, Krznarić I, Mazur-Grbac M, Perković D, et al. The role of nonenhanced magnetic resonance imaging in the early assessment of acute pancreatitis. *Am J Gastroenterol*. 2007; 102: 997-1004. PMID: 17378903.
31. Sandrasegaran K, Tann M, Jennings SG, Maglinte DD, Peter SD, Sherman S, et al. Disconnection of the pancreatic duct: an important but overlooked complication of severe acute pancreatitis. *Radiographics*. 2007; 27: 1389-1400. PMID: 17848698.
32. Pelaez-Luna M, Vege SS, Petersen BT, Chari ST, Clain JE, Levy MJ, et al. Disconnected pancreatic duct syndrome in severe acute pancreatitis: clinical and imaging characteristics and outcomes in a cohort of 31 cases. *Gastrointest Endosc*. 2008; 68: 91-97. PMID: 18378234.
33. Fischer TD, Gutman DS, Hughes SJ, Trevino JG, Behrns KE. Disconnected pancreatic duct syndrome: disease classification and management strategies. *J Am Coll Surg*. 2014; 219: 704-712. PMID: 25065360.

34. Munigala S, Kanwal F, Xian H, Scherrer JF, Agarwal B. Increased risk of pancreatic adenocarcinoma after acute pancreatitis. *Clin Gastroenterol Hepatol*. 2014; 12: 1143-1150. PMID: 24440214.
35. van Baal MC, Besselink MG, Bakker OJ, van Santvoort HC, Schaapherder AF, Nieuwenhuijs VB, et al. Timing of cholecystectomy after mild biliary pancreatitis: a systematic review. *Ann Surg*. 2012; 255: 860-866. PMID: 22470079.
36. Kulvatunyou N, Watt J, Friese RS, Gries L, Green DJ, Joseph B, et al. Management of acute mild gallstone pancreatitis under acute care surgery: should patients be admitted to the surgery or medicine service? *Am J Surg*. 2014; 208: 981-987; discussion 986-987. PMID: 25312841.
37. Bakker OJ, van Santvoort HC, Hagenaars JC, Besselink MG, Bollen TL, Gooszen HG, et al. Timing of cholecystectomy after mild biliary pancreatitis. *Br J Surg*. 2011; 98: 1446-1454. PMID: 21710664.
38. Bank S, Indaram A. Causes of acute and recurrent pancreatitis. Clinical considerations and clues to diagnosis. *Gastroenterol Clin North Am*. 1999; 28: 571-589. PMID: 10503137.
39. Signoretti M, Baccini F, Piciucchi M, Iannicelli E, Valente R, Zerboni G, et al. Repeated transabdominal ultrasonography is a simple and accurate strategy to diagnose a biliary etiology of acute pancreatitis. *Pancreas*. 2014; 43: 1106-1110. PMID: 25003222.
40. Venneman NG, Buskens E, Besselink MG, Stads S, Go PM, Bosscha K, et al. Small gallstones are associated with increased risk of acute pancreatitis: potential benefits of prophylactic cholecystectomy? *Am J Gastroenterol*. 2005; 100: 2540-2550. PMID: 16279912.
41. Venneman NG, van Brummelen SE, van Berge-Henegouwen GP and van Erpecum KJ. Microlithiasis: an important cause of "idiopathic" acute pancreatitis? *Ann Hepatol*. 2003; 2: 30-35. PMID: 15094703.
42. Testoni PA, Mariani A, Curioni S, Zanello A, Masci E. MRCP-secretin test-guided management of idiopathic recurrent pancreatitis: long-term outcomes. *Gastrointest Endosc*. 2008; 67: 1028-1034. PMID: 18179795.
43. Delabrousse E, Di Martino V, Aubry S, Fein F, Sarlieve P, Carbonnel F, et al. The choledochal ring sign: a specific finding in acute biliary pancreatitis. *Abdom Imaging*. 2008; 33: 337-341. PMID: 17435981.
44. Yie M, Jang KM, Kim MJ, Lee Y, Choi D. Diagnostic value of CT features of the gallbladder in the prediction of gallstone pancreatitis. *Eur J Radiol*. 2011; 80: 208-212. PMID: 20576384.
45. Ji YF, Zhang XM, Li XH, Jing ZL, Huang XH, Yang L, et al. Gallbladder patterns in acute pancreatitis: an MRI study. *Acad Radiol*. 2012; 19: 571-578. PMID: 22366559.
46. Kao LS, Bulger EM, Parks DL, Byrd GF, Jurkovich GJ. Predictors of morbidity after traumatic pancreatic injury. *J Trauma*. 2003; 55: 898-905. PMID: 14608163.
47. Bradley EL 3rd, Young PR Jr, Chang MC, Allen JE, Baker CC, Meredith W, et al. Diagnosis and initial management of blunt pancreatic trauma: guidelines from a multiinstitutionalreview.*AnnSurg*.1998;227:861-869.PMID: 9637549.
48. Debi U, Kaur R, Prasad KK, Sinha SK, Sinha A, Singh K. Pancreatic trauma: a concise review. *World J Gastroenterol*. 2013; 19: 9003-9011. PMID: 24379625.
49. Linsenmaier U, Wirth S, Reiser M, Korner M. Diagnosis and classification of pancreatic and duodenal injuries in emergency radiology. *Radiographics*. 2008; 28: 1591-1602. PMID: 18936023.
50. Melamud K, LeBedis CA, Soto JA. Imaging of Pancreatic and Duodenal Trauma. *Radiol Clin North Am*. 2015; 53: 757-771, viii. PMID: 26046509.
51. Balthazar EJ. Pancreatitis associated with pancreatic carcinoma. Preoperative diagnosis: role of CT imaging in detection and evaluation. *Pancreatology*. 2005; 5: 330-344. PMID: 16015017.
52. Mujica VR, Barkin JS, Go VL. Acute pancreatitis secondary to pancreatic carcinoma. Study Group Participants. *Pancreas*. 2000; 21: 329-332. PMID: 11075985.
53. Tummala P, Tariq SH, Chibnall JT, Agarwal B. Clinical predictors of pancreatic carcinoma causing acute pancreatitis. *Pancreas*. 2013; 42: 108-113. PMID: 22722258.
54. Dzeletovic I, Harrison ME, Crowell MD, Pannala R, Nguyen CC, Wu Q, et al. Pancreatitis before pancreatic cancer: clinical features and influence on outcome. *J Clin Gastroenterol*. 2014; 48: 801-805. PMID: 24153158.
55. Federico E, Falconi M, Zuodar G, Falconieri G, Puglisi F. B-cell lymphoma presenting as acute pancreatitis. *Pancreatology*. 2011; 11: 553-556. PMID: 22205036.
56. Zyromski NJ, Haidenberg J, Sarr MG. Necrotizing pancreatitis caused by pancreatic ductal adenocarcinoma. *Pancreas*. 2001; 22: 431-432. PMID: 11345146.
57. Mortele KJ, Rocha TC, Streeter JL, Taylor AJ. Multimodality imaging of pancreatic and biliary congenital anomalies. *Radiographics*. 2006; 26: 715-731. PMID: 16702450.
58. Borghei P, Sokhandon F, Shirkhoda A, Morgan DE. Anomalies, anatomic variants, and sources of diagnostic pitfalls in pancreatic imaging. *Radiology*. 2013; 266: 28-36. PMID: 23264525.
59. Turkvatan A, Erden A, Turkoglu MA, Yener O. Congenital variants and anomalies of the pancreas and pancreatic duct: imaging by magnetic resonance cholangiopancreaticography and multidetector computed tomography. *Korean J Radiol*. 2013; 14: 905-913. PMID: 24265565.
60. Levy MJ, Geenen JE. Idiopathic acute recurrent pancreatitis. *Am J Gastroenterol*. 2001; 96: 2540-2555. PMID: 11569674.
61. Cappell MS. Acute pancreatitis: etiology, clinical presentation, diagnosis, and therapy. *Med Clin North Am*. 2008; 92: 889-923, ix-x. PMID: 18570947.
62. Ng WK, Tarabain O. Pancreas divisum: a cause of idiopathic acute pancreatitis. *CMAJ*. 2009; 180: 949-951. PMID: 19398743.
63. Asayama Y, Fang W, Stolpen A, Kuehn D. Detectability of pancreas divisum in patients with acute pancreatitis on multi-detector row computed tomography. *Emerg Radiol*. 2012; 19: 121-125. PMID: 22167339.

64. Sandrasegaran K, Patel A, Fogel EL, Zyromski NJ, Pitt HA. Annular pancreas in adults. *AJR Am J Roentgenol.* 2009; 193: 455-460. PMID: 19620443.
65. Sakorafas GH, Tsiotos GG, Sarr MG. Ischemia/Reperfusion-Induced pancreatitis. *Dig Surg.* 2000; 17: 3-14. PMID: 10720825.
66. Piton G, Barbot O, Manzon C, Moronval F, Patry C, Navellou JC, et al. Acute ischemic pancreatitis following cardiac arrest: a case report. *JOP.* 2010; 11: 456-459. PMID: 20818115.
67. Mast JJ, Morak MJ, Brett BT, van Eijck CH. Ischemic acute necrotizing pancreatitis in a marathon runner. *JOP.* 2009; 10: 53-54. PMID: 19129616.
68. Hackert T, Hartwig W, Fritz S, Schneider L, Strobel O, Werner J. Ischemic acute pancreatitis: clinical features of 11 patients and review of the literature. *Am J Surg.* 2009; 197: 450-454. PMID: 18778810.
69. Perez A, Ito H, Farivar RS, Cohn LH, Byrne JG, Rawn JD, et al. Risk factors and outcomes of pancreatitis after open heart surgery. *Am J Surg.* 2005; 190: 401-405. PMID: 16105526.
70. Blom RL, van Heijl M, Busch OR, van Berge Henegouwen MI. Acute Pancreatitis in the Postoperative Course after Esophagectomy: A Major Complication Described in 4 Patients. *Case Rep Gastroenterol.* 2009; 3: 382-388. PMID: 21103258.
71. Burkey SH, Valentine RJ, Jackson MR, Modrall JG, Clagett GP. Acute pancreatitis after abdominal vascular surgery. *J Am Coll Surg.* 2000; 191: 373-380. PMID: 11030242.
72. Singh VK, Bollen TL, Wu BU, Repas K, Maurer R, Yu S, et al. An assessment of the severity of interstitial pancreatitis. *Clin Gastroenterol Hepatol.* 2011; 9: 1098-1103. PMID: 21893128.
73. van Santvoort HC, Bakker OJ, Bollen TL, Besselink MG, Ahmed Ali U, Schrijver AM, et al. A conservative and minimally invasive approach to necrotizing pancreatitis improves outcome. *Gastroenterology.* 2011; 141: 1254-1263. PMID: 21741922.
74. Sakorafas GH, Tsiotos GG, Sarr MG. Extrapancreatic necrotizing pancreatitis with viable pancreas: a previously under-appreciated entity. *J Am Coll Surg.* 1999; 188: 643-648. PMID: 10359357.
75. Bakker OJ, van Santvoort H, Besselink MG, Boermeester MA, van Eijck C, Dejong K, et al. Extrapancreatic necrosis without pancreatic parenchymal necrosis: a separate entity in necrotising pancreatitis? *Gut.* 2013; 62: 1475-1480. PMID: 22773550.
76. Rana SS, Sharma V, Sharma RK, Chhabra P, Gupta R, Bhasin DK. Clinical significance of presence and extent of extrapancreatic necrosis in acute pancreatitis. *J Gastroenterol Hepatol.* 2015; 30: 794-798. PMID: 25251298.
77. Mounzer R, Langmead CJ, Wu BU, Evans AC, Bishehsari F, Muddana V, et al. Comparison of existing clinical scoring systems to predict persistent organ failure in patients with acute pancreatitis. *Gastroenterology.* 2012; 142: 1476-1482; quiz e1415-1476. PMID: 22425589.
78. Schroder T, Kivisaari L, Somer K, Standertskjold-Nordenstam CG, Kivilaakso E, Lempinen M. Significance of extrapancreatic findings in computed tomography (CT) of acute pancreatitis. *Eur J Radiol.* 1985; 5: 273-275. PMID: 3878784.
79. Balthazar EJ, Ranson JH, Naidich DP, Megibow AJ, Caccavale R, Cooper MM. Acute pancreatitis: prognostic value of CT. *Radiology.* 1985; 156: 767-772. PMID: 4023241.
80. London NJ, Neoptolemos JP, Lavelle J, Bailey I, James D. Contrast-enhanced abdominal computed tomography scanning and prediction of severity of acute pancreatitis: a prospective study. *Br J Surg.* 1989; 76: 268-272. PMID: 2720324.
81. King NK, Powell JJ, Redhead D, Siriwardena AK. A simplified method for computed tomographic estimation of prognosis in acute pancreatitis. *Scand J Gastroenterol.* 2003; 38: 433-436. PMID: 12739717.
82. Mortele KJ, Wiesner W, Intriere L, Shankar S, Zou KH, Kalantari BN, et al. A modified CT severity index for evaluating acute pancreatitis: improved correlation with patient outcome. *AJR Am J Roentgenol.* 2004; 183: 1261-1265. PMID: 15505289.
83. Ishikawa K, Idoguchi K, Tanaka H, Tohma Y, Ukai I, Watanabe H, et al. Classification of acute pancreatitis based on retroperitoneal extension: application of the concept of interfascial planes. *Eur J Radiol.* 2006; 60: 445-452. PMID: 16891082.
84. De Waele JJ, Delrue L, Hoste EA, De Vos M, Duyck P, Colardyn FA. Extrapancreatic inflammation on abdominal computed tomography as an early predictor of disease severity in acute pancreatitis: evaluation of a new scoring system. *Pancreas.* 2007; 34: 185-190. PMID: 17312456.
85. Imamura Y, Hirota M, Ida S, Hayashi N, Watanabe M, Takamori H, et al. Significance of renal rim grade on computed tomography in severity evaluation of acute pancreatitis. *Pancreas.* 2010; 39: 41-46. PMID: 19745776.
86. Meyrignac O, Lagarde S, Bournet B, Mokrane FZ, Buscail L, Rousseau H, et al. Acute Pancreatitis: Extrapancreatic Necrosis Volume as Early Predictor of Severity. *Radiology.* 2015; 276: 119-128. PMID: 25642743.
87. Sharma V, Rana SS, Sharma RK, Kang M, Gupta R, Bhasin DK. A study of radiological scoring system evaluating extrapancreatic inflammation with conventional radiological and clinical scores in predicting outcomes in acute pancreatitis. *Ann Gastroenterol.* 2015; 28: 399-404. PMID: 26129965.
88. Fagenholz PJ, Fernandez-del Castillo C, Harris NS, Pelletier AJ, Camargo CA Jr. Direct medical costs of acute pancreatitis hospitalizations in the United States. *Pancreas.* 2007; 35: 302-307. PMID: 18090234.
89. Smith-Bindman R, Lipson J, Marcus R, Kim KP, Mahesh M, Gould R, et al. Radiation dose associated with common computed tomography examinations and the associated lifetime attributable risk of cancer. *Arch Intern Med.* 2009; 169: 2078-2086. PMID: 20008690.

90. Mortele KJ, Ip IK, Wu BU, Conwell DL, Banks PA, Khorasani R. Acute pancreatitis: imaging utilization practices in an urban teaching hospital--analysis of trends with assessment of independent predictors in correlation with patient outcomes. *Radiology*. 2011; 258: 174-181. PMID: 20980450.
91. Spanier BW, Nio Y, van der Hulst RW, Tuynman HA, Dijkgraaf MG, Bruno MJ. Practice and yield of early CT scan in acute pancreatitis: a Dutch Observational Multicenter Study. *Pancreatology*. 2010; 10: 222-228. PMID: 20484959.
92. Sharma V, Rana SS, Sharma RK, Gupta R, Bhasin DK. Clinical outcomes and prognostic significance of early vs. late computed tomography in acute pancreatitis. *Gastroenterol Rep (Oxf)*. 2015; 3: 144-147. PMID: 25305375.
93. Simchuk EJ, Traverso LW, Nukui Y, Kozarek RA. Computed tomography severity index is a predictor of outcomes for severe pancreatitis. *Am J Surg*. 2000; 179: 352-355. PMID: 10930478.
94. Isenmann R, Rau B, Beger HG. Bacterial infection and extent of necrosis are determinants of organ failure in patients with acute necrotizing pancreatitis. *Br J Surg*. 1999; 86: 1020-1024. PMID: 10460637.
95. Gotzinger P, Sautner T, Kriwanek S, Beckerhinn P, Barlan M, Armbruster C, et al. Surgical treatment for severe acute pancreatitis: extent and surgical control of necrosis determine outcome. *World J Surg*. 2002; 26: 474-478. PMID: 11910483.
96. Kemppainen E, Sainio V, Haapiainen R, Kivisaari L, Kivilaakso E, Puolakkainen P. Early localization of necrosis by contrast-enhanced computed tomography can predict outcome in severe acute pancreatitis. *Br J Surg*. 1996; 83: 924-929. PMID: 8813776.
97. Ocampo C, Zandalazini H, Kohan G, Silva W, Szelagowsky C, Oria A. Computed tomographic prognostic factors for predicting local complications in patients with pancreatic necrosis. *Pancreas*. 2009; 38: 137-142. PMID: 19002019.
98. Harris S, Nadkarni NA, Naina HV, Vege SS. Splanchnic vein thrombosis in acute pancreatitis: a single-center experience. *Pancreas*. 2013; 42: 1251-1254. PMID: 24152951.
99. Easler J, Muddana V, Furlan A, Dasyam A, Vipperla K, Slivka A, et al. Portosplenomesenteric venous thrombosis in patients with acute pancreatitis is associated with pancreatic necrosis and usually has a benign course. *Clin Gastroenterol Hepatol*. 2014; 12: 854-862. PMID: 24161350.
100. Thatipelli MR, McBane RD, Hodge DO, Wysokinski WE. Survival and recurrence in patients with splanchnic vein thromboses. *Clin Gastroenterol Hepatol*. 2010; 8: 200-205. PMID: 19782767.
101. Balthazar EJ, Fisher LA. Hemorrhagic complications of pancreatitis: radiologic evaluation with emphasis on CT imaging. *Pancreatology*. 2001; 1: 306-313. PMID: 12120209.
102. Kirby JM, Vora P, Midia M, Rawlinson J. Vascular complications of pancreatitis: imaging and intervention. *Cardiovasc Intervent Radiol*. 2008; 31: 957-970. PMID: 17680304.
103. Mortele KJ, Mergo PJ, Taylor HM, Wiesner W, Cantisani V, Ernst MD, et al. Peripancreatic vascular abnormalities complicating acute pancreatitis: contrast-enhanced helical CT findings. *Eur J Radiol*. 2004; 52: 67-72. PMID: 15380848.
104. Mortele KJ, Mergo PJ, Taylor HM, Ernst MD, Ros PR. Renal and perirenal space involvement in acute pancreatitis: spiral CT findings. *Abdom Imaging*. 2000; 25: 272-278. PMID: 10823450.
105. Li XH, Zhang XM, Ji YF, Jing ZL, Huang XH, Yang L, et al. Renal and perirenal space involvement in acute pancreatitis: An MRI study. *Eur J Radiol*. 2012; 81: e880-e887. PMID: 22613509.
106. Takeyama Y, Ueda T, Hori Y, Takase K, Fukumoto S, Kuroda Y. Hydronephrosis associated with acute pancreatitis. *Pancreas*. 2001; 23: 218-220. PMID: 11484926.
107. Fishman EK, Soyer P, Bliss DF, Bluemke DA, Devine N. Splenic involvement in pancreatitis: spectrum of CT findings. *Am J Roentgenol*. 1995; 164: 631-635. PMID: 7863884.
108. Mortele KJ, Mergo PJ, Taylor HM, Ernst MD, Ros PR. Splenic and perisplenic involvement in acute pancreatitis: determination of prevalence and morphologic helical CT features. *J Comput Assist Tomogr*. 2001; 25: 50-54. PMID: 11176293.
109. Perera M, Pham T, Toshniwal S, Lennie Y, Chan S, Houli N. A case of concomitant perforated acute cholecystitis and pancreatitis. *Case Rep Surg*. 2013; 2013: 263046. PMID: 23956917.
110. Chaudhary A, Sachdev A, Negi S. Biliary complications of pancreatic necrosis. *Int J Pancreatol*. 2001; 29: 129-131. PMID: 12067215.
111. Brar R, Singh I, Brar P, Prasad A, Doley RP, Wig JD. Pancreatic choledochal fistula complicating acute pancreatitis. *Am J Case Rep*. 2012; 13: 47-50. PMID: 23569486.
112. Ho HS, Frey CF. Gastrointestinal and pancreatic complications associated with severe pancreatitis. *Arch Surg*. 1995; 130: 817-822; discussion 822-823. PMID: 7632140.
113. Van Minnen LP, Besselink MG, Bosscha K, Van Leeuwen MS, Schipper ME, Gooszen HG. Colonic involvement in acute pancreatitis. A retrospective study of 16 patients. *Dig Surg*. 2004; 21: 33-38; discussion 39-40. PMID: 14707391.
114. Mohamed SR, Siriwardena AK. Understanding the colonic complications of pancreatitis. *Pancreatology*. 2008; 8: 153-158. PMID: 18382101.
115. Kirkpatrick AW, Roberts DJ, De Waele J, Jaeschke R, Malbrain ML, De Keulenaer B, et al. Intra-abdominal hypertension and the abdominal compartment syndrome: updated consensus definitions and clinical practice guidelines from the World Society of the Abdominal Compartment Syndrome. *Intensive Care Med*. 2013; 39: 1190-1206. PMID: 23673399.
116. Boone B, Zureikat A, Hughes SJ, Moser AJ, Yadav D, Zeh HJ, et al. Abdominal compartment syndrome is an early, lethal complication of acute pancreatitis. *Am Surg*. 2013; 79: 601-607. PMID: 23711270.

117. van Brunschot S, Schut AJ, Bouwense SA, Besselink MG, Bakker OJ, van Goor H, et al. Abdominal compartment syndrome in acute pancreatitis: a systematic review. *Pancreas*. 2014; 43: 665-674. PMID: 24921201.
118. Al-Bahrani AZ, Abid GH, Sahgal E, O'Shea S, Lee S, Ammori BJ. A prospective evaluation of CT features predictive of intra-abdominal hypertension and abdominal compartment syndrome in critically ill surgical patients. *Clin Radiol*. 2007; 62: 676-682. PMID: 17556037.
119. Patel A, Lall CG, Jennings SG, Sandrasegaran K. Abdominal compartment syndrome. *AJR Am J Roentgenol*. 2007; 189: 1037-1043. PMID: 17954637.
120. Raghu MG, Wig JD, Kochhar R, Gupta D, Gupta R, Yadav TD, et al. Lung complications in acute pancreatitis. *JOP*. 2007; 8: 177-185. PMID: 17356240.
121. Deiss R, Young P, Yeh J, Reicher S. Pulmonary embolism and acute pancreatitis: case series and review. *Turk J Gastroenterol*. 2014; 25: 575-577. PMID: 25417623.

Chapter 23

Classification systems for the severity of acute pancreatitis

Rupjyoti Talukdar[1] and Santhi Swaroop Vege[2*]

[1]Asian Institute of Gastroenterology/Asian Healthcare Foundation 6-3-661, Somajiguda Hyderabad-500082 Telangana, India;
[2]Division of Gastroenterology and Hepatology, Mayo Clinic, 200 First Street SW, Rochester, MN 55905, USA.

Introduction

Several attempts have been made over decades to establish a clinically relevant classification of acute pancreatitis (AP) severity, and the quest for such a system continues. A uniform severity classification is essential for efficient therapeutic decision making, communication with patients and relatives, and uniform research design and data reporting. One of the earliest proposals came in the late 19th century wherein the terms pancreatic hemorrhage, hemorrhagic, suppurative and gangrenous pancreatitis, and disseminated fat necrosis were suggested. The subsequent proposal of defining severity was the Marseilles classification in 1963,[1] which was subsequently revised in 1984.[2] At the same time (1983), the Cambridge classification was also published,[3] which bore several similarities with the 1984 Marseilles classification. Both the Cambridge and Marseilles 1984 classifications recognized the possibility of a variable systemic response in AP and identified complications such as necrosis, hemorrhage and pseudocysts.

In addition, the Marseilles 1984 classification defined mild and severe AP based on morphologic features, namely peripancreatic fat necrosis and interstitial edema that characterized mild disease, and extensive peri- and intrapancreatic fat necrosis, parenchymal necrosis, and hemorrhage that marked severe disease. There were further modifications of the Marseilles 1984 classification in the form of the Marseilles-Rome classification published in 1988.[4]

These classifications were followed by the Atlanta classification in 1992,[5] which was a great improvement and became clinically useful for many years. However, several limitations of the Atlanta classification were recognized in the following years with increasing use of imaging and the introduction of new nomenclature.[6,7] These finally led to a revision that was made through a web-based multiply iterative process that resulted in the revised Atlanta classification of 2013.[8] Another system called the determinant-based classification was also proposed in parallel, which was based on actual factors that determines mortality.[9] **Figure 1** depicts the timeline for the development of severity classification systems from the Atlanta Classification onwards.

In this chapter, we elaborate on these classification systems and discuss their relevance, utility, and limitations. **Table 1** summarizes the recent classifications of severity of AP.

Severity Classification Systems

Atlanta classification

Genesis

The 1992 Atlanta classification was the result of an international symposium that included 40 internationally recognized experts on AP across 6 medical disciplines and 15 countries. The primary intent of the symposium was to develop a clinically useful classification of AP that would provide a consensus on AP terminologies and facilitate comparison of interinstitutional data. The development of this classification was a major step at the time and a clear improvement over the previously described Marseilles classification, which was primarily dependent on imaging-based morphologic changes.

The Atlanta classification permitted a working definition of AP severity based on clinical, biochemical, and imaging data obtained within the first 1-2 days of hospitalization and can further be redefined based on new data available during the hospitalization period.

Components

The Atlanta classification defined severity based on the presence of organ failure and/or local complications and/or ≥3 Ranson's criteria, or ≥8 APACHE II criteria. Organ

*Corresponding author. Email: vege.santhi@mayo.edu

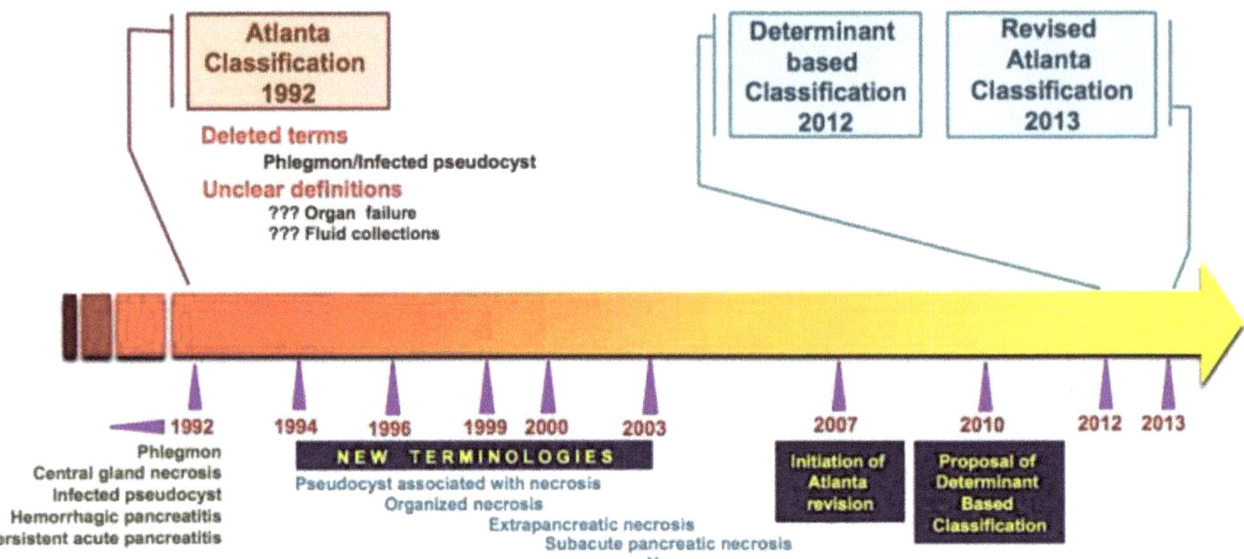

Figure 1. Timeline depicting the development of the recent classification systems for AP severity.

failure was defined as shock (systolic blood pressure <90 mmHg), pulmonary insufficiency (partial pressure of oxygen [PaO_2] <60 mmHg), renal failure (serum creatinine level >2 mg/dL after rehydration), or gastrointestinal bleeding (>500 mL/24 h). Local complications included necrosis, abscess, or (acute) pseudocyst. The presence of peripancreatic fat necrosis was considered in the definition of necrosis. An acute pseudocyst was defined as fluid collection with a definite wall in association with AP that emanates from acute fluid collections that persists for ≥ 4 weeks. Even though pancreatic abscess had been defined as a local complication of AP, it was also appreciated that the mortality risk of infected pancreatic necrosis was higher than for pancreatic abscess and that the treatment modalities for the two entities differ. Terms such as phlegmon and infected pseudocyst were discarded, and the use of terms such as hemorrhagic pancreatitis was suggested to be restricted to descriptions of operative or postmortem appearances of the gland.

Revised Atlanta classification

Genesis

The revised Atlanta classification was initiated as an international, web-based process that began in a clinical symposium in 2007 at the Digestive Diseases Week.[10] The process

Table 1. Definition of severity of acute pancreatitis according to different classification systems.

Atlanda Classification	Revised Atlanda Classification	Determinant based classification
Mild AP	**Mild AP**	**Mild AP**
- Minimal organ dysfunction and uneventful recovery	- No organ failure	- No organ failure
- Absence of organ failure and/or local complications	- No local or systemic complications	- No (peri)pancreatic necrosis
Severe AP	**Moderately severe AP**	**Moderate AP**
- Organ failure and/or local complications	- Transient organ failure AND/OR local or systemic complication OR exacerbation of pre-existing co-morbidities.	- Sterile (peri)pancreatic necrosis AND/OR transient organ failure
	Severe AP	**Severe AP**
	- Persistent organ failure (single or multiple)	- Infected (peri)pancreatic necrosis OR persistent organ failure
		Critical AP
		- Infected (peri)pancreatic necrosis AND persistent organ failure

was initiated with a meeting of 40 selected pancreatologists and pancreatic surgeons to decide on the process and revision areas. Following this, a working group with two pancreatic surgeons, two pancreatologists, and one pancreatic radiologist prepared an initial draft. This document was circulated among the 40 participants. After suggested revisions, the first working draft was e-mailed to all members of 11 national and international organizations interested in AP. A second working draft was prepared based on the modifications suggested in the first draft and resent to the members. The process was repeated, and a third draft with minor modifications was generated. After this, the final revision was made wherein the three-tier severity classification was incorporated.[11,12]

Revision of the Atlanta classification was made with an intent to address areas of confusion in the original Atlanta classification, incorporate modern concepts of the disease, improve clinical assessment of severity, enable standardized data reporting, assist objective evaluation of new treatments, and facilitate communication among treating physicians and different institutions.

Components

The revised Atlanta classification dealt primarily with two broad areas: 1) discrete definitions of organ failure and local complications (including necrosis) and 2) classification of disease severity.

The revised classification categorizes AP into interstitial edematous pancreatitis (IEP) and necrotizing pancreatitis based on contrast-enhanced computed tomography (CECT) imaging. IEP constitutes 80%-90% of AP, in which the pancreas appears relatively homogenously enhanced on CECT with or without mild peripancreatic stranding or peripancreatic fluid collection. On the other hand, necrotizing pancreatitis is characterized by lack of enhancement of the pancreas and/or (peri)pancreatic tissues on CECT. Both the pancreatic parenchyma and peripancreatic tissues are involved more frequently than either alone. Recognition of the degree of necrosis (pancreatic alone, peripancreatic alone, or both) is important since the prognosis varies. For instance, peripancreatic necrosis alone results in a less severe disease course compared to pancreatic parenchymal and peripancreatic necrosis, but higher morbidity compared to IEP. Pure pancreatic necrosis is a rare event. Pancreatic and peripancreatic necrosis usually evolves over the first week of the disease and might not be mature enough for early imaging (<72 h). Necrotizing AP is detectable on CECT after 72 h and more definitely by 7 days, when the low attenuation of necrosis on CECT becomes more apparent. (Peri)pancreatic necrosis is prone to infection, which is usually seen after the first week. Infected necrosis should be strongly suspected in the presence of signs of sepsis in a patient with necrotizing pancreatitis. Even though gram stain and culture of fine-needle aspiration (FNA) were recommended in earlier guidelines, they may be falsely negative. Therefore, FNA is not routinely recommended in the diagnosis of infected (peri)pancreatic necrosis but may become necessary in patients who are not responding to antibiotics to guide therapy based on susceptibility information. Presence of extraluminal gas bubbles on CECT strongly suggests the presence of infected necrosis.

According to the revised Atlanta classification, complications of AP can be organ failure and local and systemic complications. Organ failure, which needs to be evaluated by the Modified Marshall Scoring System,[13] is considered to be present if the Marshall Score is ≥ 2. Organ failure may be transient (resolves within 48 h of onset) or persistent (persists for >48 h). Local complications include fluid collections, gastric outlet dysfunction, splenic and portal vein thrombosis, and colonic necrosis. Four discrete types of collections have been described: acute peripancreatic fluid collection (APFC), pancreatic pseudocyst (PP), acute necrotic collection (ANC), and walled-off necrosis (WON). **Table 2** presents the definitions and characteristics of the different types of fluid collections.

Severity has been categorized into mild, moderately severe, and severe AP. This is based on the presence or absence of local complications and organ failure. Mild AP is defined as AP without organ failure and local/systemic complications. This usually resolves within the first week after onset and has minimal morbidity and rare mortality. Patients will usually be discharged within a week. Moderately severe AP is defined as AP with transient organ failure and/or local complications and/or systemic complications. Systemic complication is defined as exacerbation of a pre-existing condition like coronary artery disease, congestive cardiac failure, chronic obstructive pulmonary disease, diabetes, or chronic liver disease as a result of AP. Patients with moderately severe AP may run a protracted course and develop further complications such as infected necrosis and bleeding from pseudoaneurysms. The management of moderately severe AP is guided by the type of local complications, presence of symptoms, and development of issues related to the defining local complications. Mortality is significantly less compared to that of severe AP. Severe AP is defined by the presence of persistent organ failure irrespective of the time of development in relation to disease onset.

Determinant-based classification

Genesis

The primary highlight of the determinant-based classification was the introduction of the group called critical AP. This category and thereby the determinant-based

Table 2. Definition and characteristics of local collections in acute pancreatitis according to the Revised Atlanta Classification.

Terminology	Definitions and characteristics
APFC (acute peripancreatic fluid collection)	• Associated with interstitial edematous pancreatitis • Appear as peripancreatic fluid seen within the first 4 weeks after disease onset. • Does not have a definable wall. • Confined to normal peripancreatic fascial planes. • Does not have intrapancreatic extensions.
Pancreatic pseudocyst	• An encapsulated collection of fluid with a well-defined wall. • Usually located outside the pancreas. • Usually requires more than 4 weeks after onset to mature. • Does not contain non-liquid component.
ANC (acute necrotic collection)	• Contains variable amount of both fluid and necrosis. • Associated with necrotizing pancreatitis. • Appear as heterogeneous and non-liquid density of varying degrees in different locations. • Does not have a definable wall. • Necrosis can involve the pancreatic parenchyma and/or the peripancreatic tissues
WON (walled-off necrosis)	• Heterogeneous with liquid and non-liquid density with varying degrees of loculations • Usually occurs 4 weeks after onset of necrotizing pancreatitis. • Appear as an encapsulated collection in pancreatic and/or peripancreatic areas of necrosis. • Contains a well-defined inflammatory wall.

classification stemmed from the results of a meta-analysis of 14 studies involving 1,478 patients that evaluated the pooled effect of organ failure and infected pancreatic necrosis on mortality.[14] The results demonstrated that the mortality rate among patients who had both organ failure and infected pancreatic necrosis was 43%. This was significantly higher than that of patients with organ failure alone (22%) or infected pancreatic necrosis alone (11%). The mortality rates between patients with either condition alone were not statistically different. However, the authors did acknowledge a few limitations in their study. Most notably, the individual studies in the meta-analysis were observational, definitions used for organ failure varied across different studies, and most did not address the dynamic nature of organ failure. Nevertheless, based on these results, patients with both organ failure and infected necrosis were categorized into the new group of critical AP and the four-tier severity classification was proposed. Once the proposal was published,[15] 525 pancreatologists from 55 countries were invited by e-mail for a web-based survey, of which 240 pancreatologists from 49 countries agreed to participate. The result of the web-based global consultation led to publication of the determinant-based classification in English, which was eventually published in German, Italian, Spanish, and Chinese.[16-19] Issues regarding the classification and its development and the conduct of the web-based survey were noted by several authors and highlighted in letters to editors.[20,21]

Components

The determinant-based classification primarily centers on causally associated factors (or determinants) for mortality. The determinants could be local (i.e., (peri) pancreatic necrosis) or systemic (i.e., organ failure). (Peri) pancreatic necrosis is defined as nonviable tissue located in the pancreas alone, in the pancreas and peripancreatic tissues, or in the peripancreatic tissues alone. (Peri)pancreatic necrosis could be sterile or infected. Infected (peri)pancreatic necrosis is defined by the presence of either gas bubbles within necrotic areas on CT, a positive culture of (peri)pancreatic necrosis obtained by image-guided FNA, or positive culture of (peri)pancreatic necrosis obtained during the first drainage and/or necrosectomy. Organ failure is defined as a score ≥ 2 according to the Sequential Organ Failure Assessment (SOFA) system[22] or if there is a need for inotropic support, and/or serum creatinine of >2 mg/dL, and/or PaO_2/fraction of inspired oxygen (FiO_2) <300 mm Hg. Organ failure less than or greater than 48 h is defined as transient or persistent, respectively. This is similar to the definitions proposed in the revised Atlanta classification.

The four categories in the determinant-based classification include mild, moderate, severe, and critical AP. Mild AP is defined as the absence of both (peri)pancreatic necrosis and organ failure, moderate AP is defined as sterile (peri)pancreatic necrosis and/or transient organ failure, severe AP is defined as the presence of either infected (peri)pancreatic necrosis or persistent organ failure, and critical AP is defined as the presence of both infected (peri)pancreatic necrosis and persistent organ failure.

Utility and Limitations

Table 3 depicts the similarities and differences between different classifications of AP severity.

Even though the 1992 Atlanta classification was initially greeted with substantial enthusiasm, over time it turned out that several descriptions pertaining to the disease such as definition of local complications and definition and duration of organ failure were either not addressed elaborately or lacked clarity.[6] In the past two decades, terminologies from the Atlanta classification were inappropriately used, and several new terms were introduced as more data on the natural history and pathophysiology of the disease emerged.[7,23] This was complemented by technical developments in cross-sectional imaging. Terms such as pancreatic phlegmon and infected pseudocyst found continued use, and terms such as organized pancreatic necrosis, subacute pancreatic necrosis, necroma, and pseudocyst associated with necrosis came into existence (**Figure 1**). There were even alterations in the definitions of organ failure in clinical practice and studies, and reliance on the Atlanta classification diminished with time. This mandated revision of the classification system that culminated in the revised Atlanta classification.

The revised Atlanta and determinant-based classifications were published almost simultaneously and have since been validated and compared in several studies. The determinant-based classification was initially validated in a cohort of 151 patients in a 2-year prospective study in which 13.9%, 41.7%, 39.1%, and 5.3% had mild, moderate, severe, and critical AP, respectively. [24] The study outcomes were length of hospital stay, CT severity index scores, occurrence of bloodstream infections, incidence of infected necrosis, requirements for percutaneous catheter drain, numbers of operations, and mortality, all of which had step-wise increases in frequency across the groups. Another recent small study from China that included 92 consecutive patients evaluated in the moderate category of the determinant-based classification category and concluded that this is a distinct group compared to the severe and critical groups.[25] However, this group was not compared with the moderately severe group in the revised Atlanta classification. Furthermore, evaluation of the

Table 3. Similarities and differences between different classifications of severity of acute pancreatitis.

	Atlanta Classification	Revised Atlanta Classification	Determinant based Classification
Description of the natural course of the disease (early and late phases)	• No	• Yes	• No
Distiction of organ failure depending on duration	• No	• Yes (Transient and persistent organ failure)	• Yes (Transient and persistent organ failure)
Definition of organ failure	• Non-uniform	• Uniform (use of Modified Marshall Scoring system).	• Uniform (use of Sequential Organ Failure Assessment system).
Definition of local complications	• No distinction of (peri) pancreatic collections with and without necrotic debris. • Local complications included necrosis, abscess and pseudocyst.	• Defines pancreatic and peripancreatic necrosis. • Discrete definitions of fluid collections [acute (peri) pancreatic fluid collections, pancreatic pseudocyst, acute necrotic collection and walled off necrosis]. • Included gastric outlet dysfunction, portal and splenic vein thrombosis, and colonic necrosis.	• Defines pancreatic and peripancreatic necrosis. • No definitions of fluid collections. • Does not consider gastric outlet dysfunction, portal and splenic vein thrombosis, and colonic necrosis as local complications.
Systemic complications	• Not considered in classification of severity.	• Defined as exacerbation of pre-existing conditions such as coronary artery disease, congestive cardiac failure, chronic obstructive pulmonary disease, diabetes, and chronic liver disease.	• Not considered in classification of severity.

critical group according to the determinant-based classification would have been more meaningful in view of the emphasis on critical AP in this classification.

The study by Nawaz et al. was the first report to compare the revised Atlanta and the determinant based classifications.[26] This post-hoc analysis of 256 prospectively admitted patients (49% transferred) used both classifications to predict mortality, need for intensive care unit (ICU) admission, need for interventions, length of stay in the ICU, and total hospital stay. According to the revised Atlanta classification, 49% patients in this study had mild disease, 25.5% moderately severe, and 25.5% severe disease. According to the determinant-based classification, 67% patients had mild AP, 7% moderate, 19% severe, and 7% critical. The revised Atlanta classification appeared to predict length of hospital stay better than the determinant-based classification, while the latter better predicted the need for intervention. However, it is important to note that the two classification systems are meant to categorize disease severity once certain severity criteria are reached. This is different from prediction, which is performed before severity criteria are reached. Furthermore, using different systems to predict different outcomes is unlikely to be appealing in clinical practice.

The next comparison between the two classifications came from Spain in a retrospective, community-based study of 459 patients who had 543 episodes of AP over 5 years.[27] According to the revised Atlanta classification, 66.9%, 29.5%, and 3.7% of the patients had mild, moderately severe, and severe AP. respectively. With the determinant-based classification, 71.1%, 24.1%, 4.2%, and 0.6% patients has mild, moderate, severe, and critical AP, respectively. Interestingly, unlike Nawaz et al., this group did not observe any significant differences in frequencies or outcomes between the two classifications.

A recent retrospective study of 7 years of data from China evaluated 553 patients for outcomes according to the severity categories proposed in the revised Atlanta classification.[28] The authors observed that mortality was significantly higher in patients with infected necrosis and organ failure compared to organ failure alone (32.2% vs. 8%). Mortality was similar in patients who had infected necrosis without organ failure compared to patients with organ failure alone (7.1% vs. 8%). Infected necrosis either preceded or developed concurrently in 45.8% of patients with persistent organ failure.

In a prospective study of 163 directly admitted consecutive patients with AP, 44.4% of those with SAP developed persistent organ failure within the first week of disease onset, and mortality within this group of patients was as high as 37.5%.[29] This entity was not addressed in the revised Atlanta or determinant based classifications. Previous studies have also shown that persistent organ failure in the early phase of disease can result in a mortality rate of 36%-50%.[30-31] Early organ failure usually results from severe and persistent systemic inflammatory response syndrome. The high mortality rate among these patients makes it a discrete group; it was previously named early severe AP but has not been considered in the two recent classifications.[32-34]

Future Directions

It needs to be reiterated that both the revised Atlanta and determinant-based classification were meant to classify severity (i.e., categorize a patient into a predefined set of characteristics once the patient had developed those). Based on the dynamic progression of the disease, the categorization could progressively change according to the classification system utilized. Even though both classifications can guide patient management, neither has the provision to track the progression from one severity category to the other. It is understandable that classification and prediction of severity are different aspects, but incorporation of some provision of prediction would make the utility of either classification system more meaningful. This is particularly important for patients managed in the community setting, when prompt referral to a higher center becomes important. On the other hand, classification systems could guide patient management in the tertiary care setting. For example, the management strategies for ANC and WON (as per the revised Atlanta classification) would be different in the presence or absence of mechanical symptoms and/or infections. Classification and guidelines in AP are based mostly on studies from tertiary care academic centers; while a substantial proportion of patients initially present to primary and community level healthcare facilities. It is the latter group of patients that need to be studied to improve our understanding of the dynamic progression of the disease and evaluate the utility of classification and predicting systems.

Even though both recent classifications have certain merits, there is substantial room for improvement. Concerted efforts should be made to address the dynamics of the disease in both the classification systems, and the individual categories need to be validated in large, prospective, population-based studies. An ideal classification system would incorporate all attributes of the disease pathophysiology, track the disease dynamics, and allow prediction of transition from one category to another. These would make the system applicable at all levels of healthcare and accurately guide clinical decision making.

References

1. Fitz RH. Acute pancreatitis: a consideration of pancreatic hemorrhage, hemorrhagic suppurative, and gangrenous

pancreatitis and of disseminated fat necrosis. *Boston Med Surg J.* 1889; 120: 181-187, 205-207, 229-235.
2. Singer MV, Gyr K, Sarles H. Revised classification of pancreatitis. Report of the Second International Symposium on the Classification of Pancreatitis in Marseille, France, March 28-30, 1984. *Gastroenterology*. 1985; 89: 683-685. PMID: 4018507.
3. Singer MV. Classification of pancreatitis-comparison of the revised 1984 Marseille Classification and the 1983 Cambridge classification [Article in German]. *Z Gastroenterol Verh.* 1991; 26: 39-42. PMID: 1714203.
4. Sarles H. Classification and definition of pancreatitis. Marseilles-Rome 1988 [Article in French]. *Gastroenterol Clin Biol.* 1989; 13: 857-859. PMID: 2612829.
5. Bradley EL III. A clinically based classification system for acute pancreatitis. Summary of the International Symposium on Acute Pancreatitis, Atlanta, GA, September 11 through 13, 1992. *Arch Surg*. 1993; 128: 586-590. PMID: 8489394.
6. Banks PA, Freeman ML. Practice guidelines in acute pancreatitis. *Am J Gastroenterol*. 2006; 101: 2379-2400. PMID: 17032204.
7. Bollen TL, van Santvoort HC, Besselink MG, van Leeuwen MS, Horvath KD, Freeny PC, et al. The Atlanta classification of acute pancreatitis revisited. *Br J Surg*. 2008; 95: 6-21. PMID: 17985333.
8. Banks PA, Bollen TL, Dervenis C, Gooszen HG, Johnson CD, Sarr MG, et al. Classification of Acute Pancreatitis-2102: revision of the Atlanta classification and definitions by international consensus. *Gut*. 2013; 62: 102-111. PMID: 23100216.
9. Dellinger EP, Forsmark CE, Layer P, Lévy P, Maraví-Poma E, Petrov MS, et al. Determinant-based classification of acute pancreatitis severity: an international multidisciplinary consultation. *Ann Surg*. 2012; 256: 875-880. PMID: 22735715.
10. Vege SS, Chari ST. Organ failure as an indicator of severity of acute pancreatitis: time to revisit the Atlanta classification. *Gastroenterology*. 2005; 128: 1133-1135. PMID: 15825098.
11. Vege SS, Gardner TB, Chari ST, Munukuti P, Pearson RK, Clain JE, et al. Low mortality and high morbidity in severe acute pancreatitis without organ failure: a case for revising the Atlanta classification to include "moderately severe acute pancreatitis". *Am J Gastroenterol*. 2009; 104: 710-715. PMID: 19262525.
12. Talukdar R, Clemens M, Vege SS. Moderately severe acute pancreatitis: prospective validation of this new subgroup of acute pancreatitis. *Pancreas*. 2012; 41: 306-309. PMID: 22015971.
13. Marshall JC, Cook DJ, Christou NV, Bernard GR, Sprung CL, Sibbald WJ. Multiple organ dysfunction score: a reliable descriptor of a complex clinical outcome. *Crit Care Med.* 1995; 23: 1638-1652. PMID: 7587228.
14. Petrov MS, Shanbhag S, Chakraborty M, Phillips AR, Windsor JA. Organ failure and infection of pancreatic necrosis as determinants of mortality in patients with acute pancreatitis. *Gastroenterology*. 2010; 139: 813-820. PMID: 20540942.
15. Petrov MS, Windsor JA. Classification of the severity of acute pancreatitis: how many categories make sense? *Am J Gastroenterol.* 2010; 105: 74-76. PMID: 19844203.
16. Uomo G, Patchen Dellinger E, Forsmark CE, Layer P, Lévy P, Maravì-Poma E, et al. Multidisciplinar international classification of the severity of acute pancreatitis: Italian version 2013 [Article in Italian]. *Minerva Med.* 2013; 104: 649-657. PMID: 24316918.
17. Maraví-Poma E, Patchen Dellinger E, Forsmark CE, Layer P, Lévy P, Shimosegawa T, et al. International multidisciplinary classification of acute pancreatitis severity: the 2013 Spanish edition [Article in Spanish]. *Med Intensiva.* 2014; 38: 211-217. PMID: 23747189.
18. Layer P, Dellinger EP, Forsmark CE, Lévy P, Maraví-Poma E, Shimosegawa T, et al. Determinant-based classification of acute pancreatitis severity. International multidisciplinary classification of acute pancreatitis severity: the 2013 German edition [Article in German]. *Z Gastroenterol.* 2013; 51: 544-550. PMID: 23740353.
19. Li W, Zhang L, Li J, Dellinger EP, Forsmark CE, Layer P, et al. Determinant-based classification of acute pancreatitis severity: an international multidisciplinary consultation: the 2013 Chinese edition [Article in Chinese]. *Zhonghua Wai Ke Za Zhi.* 2014; 52: 321-324. PMID: 25034735.
20. Talukdar R, Rau BM. Determinant-based classification of severity of acute pancreatitis: have we really reached consensus? *Ann Surg.* 2015; 261: e22. PMID: 24441802.
21. Thomson A. Fulminant acute pancreatitis. *Ann Surg.* 2015; 261: e23. PMID: 24646557.
22. Vincent JL, Moreno R, Takala J, Willatts S, De Mendonça A, Bruining H, et al. The SOFA (Sepsis-related Organ Failure Assessment) score to describe organ dysfunction/failure. On behalf of the Working Group on Sepsis-Related Problems of the European Society of Intensive Care Medicine. *Intensive Care Med.* 1996; 22: 707-710. PMID: 8844239.
23. Bollen TL, Besselink MG, van Santvoort HC, Gooszen HG, van Leeuwen MS. Toward an update of the Atlanta classification on acute pancreatitis: review of new and abandoned terms. *Pancreas.* 2007; 35: 107-113. PMID: 17632315.
24. Thandassery RB, Yadav TD, Dutta U, Appasani S, Singh K, Kochhar R. Prospective validation of 4-category classification of acute pancreatitis severity. *Pancreas.* 2013; 42: 392-396. PMID: 23429498.
25. Jin T, Huang W, Yang XN, Xue P, Javed MA, Altaf K, et al. Validation of the moderate severity category of acute pancreatitis defined by determinant-based classification. *Hepatobiliary Pancreat Dis Int.* 2014; 13: 323-327. PMID: 24919617.
26. Nawaz H, Mounzer R, Yadav D, Yabes JG, Slivka A, Whitcomb DC, et al. Revised Atlanta and determinant-based classification: application in a prospective cohort of acute pancreatitis patients. *Am J Gastroenterol.* 2013; 108: 1911-1917. PMID: 24126632.
27. Acevedo-Piedra NG, Moya-Hoyo N, Rey-Riveiro M, Gil S, Sempere L, Martínez J, et al. Validation of the determinant-based classification and revision of the Atlanta classification systems for acute pancreatitis. *Clin Gastroenterol Hepatol.* 2014; 12: 311-316. PMID: 23958561.
28. Choi JH, Kim MH, Oh D, Paik WH, Park do H, Lee SS, et al. Clinical relevance of the revised Atlanta classification focusing on severity stratification system. *Pancreatology.* 2014; 14: 324-329. PMID: 25174301.

29. Talukdar R, Bhattacharrya A, Rao B, Sharma M, Nageshwar Reddy D. Clinical utility of the revised Atlanta classification of acute pancreatitis in a prospective cohort: have all loose ends been tied? *Pancreatology*. 2014; 14: 257-262. PMID: 25062873.
30. Buter A, Imrie CW, Carter CR, et al. Dynamic nature of early organ dysfunction determines outcome in acute pancreatitis. *Br J Surg*. 2002; 89: 298-302. PMID: 11872053.
31. Johnson CD, Abu-Hilal M. Persistent organ failure during the first week as a marker of fatal outcome in acute pancreatitis. *Gut*. 2004; 53: 1340-1344. PMID: 15306596.
32. Sharma M, Banerjee D, Garg PK. Characterization of newer subgroups of fulminant and subfulminant pancreatitis associated with a high early mortality. *Am J Gastroenterol*. 2007; 102: 2688-2695. PMID: 17662103.
33. Isenmann R, Rau B, Beger HG. Early severe acute pancreatitis: characteristics of a new subgroup. *Pancreas*. 2001; 22: 274-278. PMID: 11291929.
34. Talukdar R, Vege SS. Classification of the severity of acute pancreatitis. *Am J Gastroenterol*. 2011; 106: 1169-1170. PMID: 21637274.

Chapter 24

Fluid resuscitation in acute pancreatitis

Georg Beyer*, Julia Mayerle, Peter Simon, and Markus M. Lerch

Department of Medicine A, University Medicine Greifswald, Germany.

Pathophysiological Considerations

Alterations of the pancreatic microperfusion are an early event in the course of pancreatitis irrespective of the underlying etiology.[1] They result in reduced blood flow, capillary leakage, pancreatic and peripancreatic edema, and transmigration of inflammatory cells. The sources of proinflammatory mediators leading to these events have not been fully identified, but studies indicate that acinar and stellate cells, as well as resident immune cells, can all respond to pancreatic injury by secreting proinflammatory cytokines such as interleukin (IL)-1b, IL-6, and tumor necrosis factor (TNF)-α.[2] Ultimately, endothelial activation and decreased microperfusion will also lead to hypercoagulability which, in turn, aggravates pancreatic hypoperfusion and hypoxia. Both the lack of oxygen and reperfusion damage will lead to pancreatic necrosis with sometimes catastrophic consequences such as infected pancreatic collections, sepsis, bleeding, and death.[3] Systemically, multiorgan failure due to systemic inflammatory response syndrome, hypoperfusion, and shock are common events in severe forms of acute pancreatitis, leading to mortality rates close to 50% in some patient cohorts.[4]

Early fluid resuscitation could help to restore local pancreatic perfusion, counteract systemic hypotension, and thus prevent secondary organ failure due to fluid sequestration. The critical question in this context is how much fluid replacement is optimal to improve outcome and how much will lead to fluid overload with negative consequences such as abdominal compartment syndrome.[5,6]

Estimation of Fluid Requirement

Early and adequate fluid resuscitation remains the cornerstone of initial treatment in acute pancreatitis and probably has the most detrimental consequences if not properly administered. An observational study including 403 patients from two prospectively collected cohorts showed an association between early fluid deficit and the development of pancreatic fluid collections, pancreatic necrosis, persistent organ failure, and hospital stay length.[7] In a smaller cohort, Scottish patients who died from acute pancreatitis received significantly less fluids within 48 h of admission than survivors.[8] In a small pooled analysis of 44 patients with and without necrotizing pancreatitis, only those with a high hematocrit after 24 h developed necrosis during their subsequent course of pancreatitis, even though similar amounts of fluid were given to both groups.[9]

Although the need for fluid resuscitation in these patients is widely accepted, it remains challenging to predict the extent of fluid sequestration and thus the clinical outcome. Clinically used scoring systems and recently published studies focus on surrogates for fluid sequestration as predictors of outcome and indicators for goal-directed fluid administration in the early phase. These include hematocrit, blood urea nitrogen (BUN), creatinine, heart rate, mean arterial pressure (MAP), and central venous pressure (CVP).[8,10-14]

Choice of Fluids

Based on the current evidence from pancreatitis-specific and general critical care studies, balanced crystalloid solutions such as Ringers' lactate should be used for fluid resuscitation in acute pancreatitis patients. In a randomized controlled trial including 40 North American patients, Wu et al. showed that patients randomly assigned to receive lactated Ringers' had a significant reduction in systemic inflammatory response syndrome (SIRS; 84% reduction vs. 0%; χ^2 $P = 0.035$) and CRP levels (mean 51 vs. 104 mg/L; analysis of variance $P = 0.018$) compared to patients receiving normal saline.[15] One advantage of balanced solutions is their favorable effect on acid-base metabolism.

*Corresponding author. Email: georg.beyer@uni-greifswald.de

Experimental animal studies suggest that lactate has a direct anti-inflammatory effect via the GPR81 receptor and the cellular inflammasome.[16,17] Studies outside the pancreatitis field have also shown that hyperchloremic acidosis induced by infusing large amounts of saline can lead to a worse outcome with an increased risk for kidney injury, thus leaving normal saline to be the second fluid choice for critically ill patients.[18] In pancreatitis patients, resuscitation with Ringers' lactate led to a significantly reduced rate of acidosis with a reverse correlation of bicarbonate to CRP levels.[15]

Hydroxyethyl starch (HES) is a colloid fluid that has been widely used for plasma expansion in critically ill patients. A large randomized, blinded intensive care patient trial not specific for pancreatitis analyzed the outcome of 798 ICU patients receiving either HES or crystalloids. The use of HES was associated with higher mortality than Ringers' acetate (201/398, 51% vs. 172/400, 43%; P = 0.03) and increased the risk for renal failure and the need for renal replacement therapy (87/398, 22% vs. 65/400, 16%; P = 0.04).[19] The unfavorable effect of HES did not reach significance in the long-term mortality after 6 month or 1 year, which may be due to insufficient power of the study for this endpoint. However, HES failed to show any long-term superiority.[20] A previous study by Brunkhorst and colleagues reported similar results.[21] For pancreatitis patients, Mole et al. observed increased use of HES in a group of patients that had died from acute pancreatitis.[8] One small study showed that a combination of Ringers' lactate and HES reduced the mean intra-abdominal pressure and the need for mechanical ventilation within the first week of acute pancreatitis compared to Ringers' lactate alone.[22] However, due to the small sample sizes, the grade of evidence remains too low to currently recommend the use of HES in acute pancreatitis in the light of the larger ICU studies. In summary, balanced, full electrolyte crystalloid solutions are currently recommended for initial fluid resuscitation in acute pancreatitis, with the limitation that only Ringers' lactate has been investigated for this purpose to date. In patients with hypercalcemia, calcium-free normal saline serves as an alternative.

Course of Fluid Resuscitation

Earlier observational studies on pancreatitis patients concluded that early and aggressive fluid therapy improved outcome and prevented necrosis.[8,23,24] The first randomized controlled trial to investigate this question originated from China and, somewhat unexpectedly, showed that overly aggressive fluid administration can be harmful when compared to controlled fluid expansion. The rapid fluid expansion group received crystalloids or colloids at a rate 10-15 ml/kg body weight/h and was at higher risk for mechanical ventilation (94.4% vs. 65%) and death (30.6% vs. 10%) compared to the controlled fluid expansion

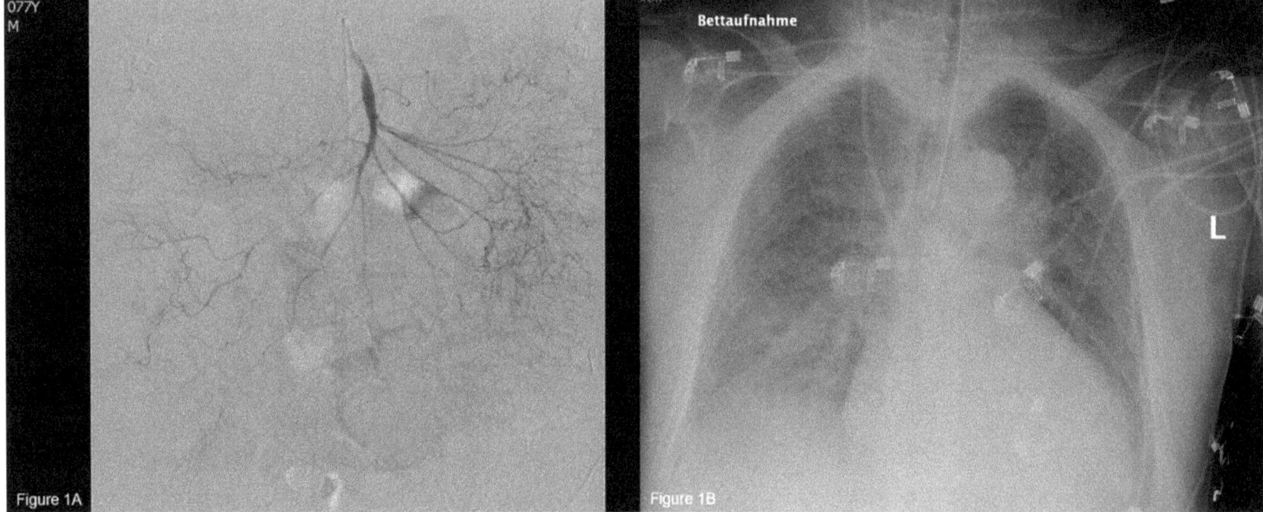

Figure 1. Complications of fluid overload in severe acute pancreatitis. A 77-year-old male patient with biliary pancreatitis and pre-existing congestive heart failure due to chronic arterial hypertension and aortic valve stenosis was resuscitated with a total of 2,500 mL balanced crystalloid infusion over the first 24 h. Within 48 h of admission, he developed respiratory failure with increasing oxygen requirements and was consequently admitted to the intensive care unit. He developed severe ARDS due to fluid overload and cardiac decompensation and was intubated and ventilated (Figure 1B). Later in his course he also developed increased intra-abdominal pressure and abdominal compartment syndrome with central venous congestion followed by nonocclusive mesenteric ischemia. Figure 1A shows the angiogram of the superior mesenteric artery with narrowing of all vessels and distal hypoperfusion. A papaverin catheter was inserted, but the patient died of multiorgan failure and sepsis despite maximal escalation of treatment.

group with 5-10 mL/kg body weight/h. The amounts of fluid given only differed over the first 24 h but were similar over the subsequent 4 days. The same applied to hematocrit levels, which were also transiently lower in the aggressive fluid treatment group on the first day.[25] In a subsequent, larger, randomized trial from the same institution, patients were assigned to meet a resuscitation goal above or below 35% hematocrit within 48 h. Again, patients with more aggressive treatment receiving more fluids in the early course had a worse outcome with higher APACHE II scores and higher risks of sepsis and death.[26] Taken together, these results suggest that fluids should be given at moderate rates of 5-10 mL/kg of body weight over the first 24 h aiming for a total volume of 2,500 to 4,000 mL. Recently, the concept of goal-directed fluid resuscitation has been more heavily investigated both in and outside the pancreatitis field. Parameters that have been investigated are BUN, hematocrit, CVP, blood pressure, heart rate, and urine output.

Wu et al. performed a small randomized trial and concluded that BUN, despite its prognostic values, does not help guide fluid resuscitation because the total amount of fluid administered and the prevalence of SIRS and CRP values were similar between the group receiving BUN-guided fluids and the control arm.[15] An observational study concluded that CVP might be a misleading parameter to guide fluid administration because patients with high values were more likely to receive vasopressors and were at a higher risk for death.[8] Lately, the most controversial parameter is hematocrit. A retrospective study by Brown and colleagues showed that all 12 patients with persistently high hematocrit >44% after 24 h died, whereas Mao et al. convincingly showed that rapid hemodilution to a hematocrit <35% within 48 h also puts the patient at higher risk for pancreatitis-related death.[26] Pathophysiologically, these effects could be explained by kidney damage and tissue hypoperfusion in cases of high hematocrit, and impaired oxygen delivery, coagulation failure, and decreased migration of inflammatory cells in the presence of low hematocrit.

In general, the physician in charge needs to consider coexisting conditions such as congestive heart failure or pulmonary disease that drastically limit a patient's tolerance towards fluid administration and thus adjust fluid management. The study by Mao further suggests that a heart rate <120 bpm, a mean arterial pressure of 65-85 mmHg, and urine output of 0.5-1 mL/kg/h can be used to noninvasively estimate fluid requirements. However, low urine output can also be a consequence of acute tubular necrosis in which case more fluid administration will lead to fluid overload and respiratory failure. Three large multicenter randomized trials conducted in Australia/New Zealand, the United States, and the United Kingdom uniformly concluded that early goal-directed fluid therapy was not superior to usual care protocols.[27-29] This supports the conclusion that predictive factors that can guide fluid treatment in acute pancreatitis patients remain to be identified. Whether modern hemodynamic monitoring using, for example, thermodilution methods, can be of benefit for a subset of patients is currently under investigation.[30]

IAP/APA Guideline Recommendations

During the 2012 APA annual meeting, an expert panel developed new evidence-based guidelines for the management of acute pancreatitis.[31] The following was recommended for fluid resuscitation.

- Ringer´s lactate is recommended for initial fluid resuscitation in acute pancreatitis (GRADE 1B, strong agreement).
- Goal-directed intravenous fluid therapy with 5-10 mL/kg/h should be used initially until resuscitation goals are reached (GRADE 1B, weak agreement).
- The preferred approach to assessing the response to fluid resuscitation should be based on one or more of the following: (1) noninvasive clinical targets of heart rate <120/min, mean arterial pressure between 65 and 85 mmHg (8.7-11.3 kPa), and urinary output >0.5-1 mL/kg/h; (2) invasive clinical targets of stroke volume variation and intrathoracic blood volume determination; and (3) biochemical target of hematocrit 35%-44% (GRADE 2B, weak agreement).

References

1. Lerch MM, Weidenbach H, Gress TM, Adler G. Effect of kinin inhibition in experimental acute pancreatitis. *Am J Physiol Gastrointest Liver Physiol*. 1995; 269: G490-G499. PMID: 7485500.
2. Sendler M, Dummer A, Weiss FU, Krüger B, Wartmann T, Scharffetter-Kochanek K, et al. Tumour necrosis factor α secretion induces protease activation and acinar cell necrosis in acute experimental pancreatitis in mice. *Gut*. 2013; 62(3): 430-439. PMID: 26228362.
3. Lankisch PG, Apte M, Banks PA. Acute pancreatitis. *Lancet*. 2015; 386 85-96. PMID: 25616312.
4. Banks PA, Bollen TL, Dervenis C, Gooszen HG, Johnson CD, Sarr MG, et al. Classification of acute pancreatitis–2012: revision of the Atlanta classification and definitions by international consensus. *Gut*. 2013; 62(1): 102-111. PMID: 23100216.
5. Holodinsky JK, Roberts DJ, Ball CG, Blaser AR, Starkopf J, Zygun DA, et al. Risk factors for intraabdominal hypertension and abdominal compartment syndrome among adult intensive care unit patients: a systematic review and metaanalysis. *Crit Care*. 2013; 17: R249. PMID: 24144138.
6. Trikudanathan G, Vege SS. Current concepts of the role of abdominal compartment syndrome in acute pancreatitis - an opportunity or merely an epiphenomenon. *Pancreatology*. 2014; 14: 238-243. PMID: 25062870.
7. de-Madaria E, Banks PA, Moya-Hoyo N, Wu BU, Rey-Riveiro M, Acevedo-Piedra NG, et al. Early factors associated with

fluid sequestration and outcomes of patients with acute pancreatitis. *Clin Gastroenterol Hepatol.* 2014; 12: 997-1002. PMID: 24183957.

8. Mole DJ, Hall A, McKeown D, Garden OJ, Parks RW. Detailed fluid resuscitation profiles in patients with severe acute pancreatitis. *HPB.* 2011; 13: 51-58. PMID: 21159104.
9. Brown A, Baillargeon JD, Hughes MD, Banks PA. Can fluid resuscitation prevent pancreatic necrosis in severe acute pancreatitis? *Pancreatology.* 2002; 2: 104-107. PMID: 12123089.
10. Mounzer R, Langmead CJ, Wu BU, Evans AC, Bishehsari F, Muddana V, et al. Comparison of existing clinical scoring systems to predict persistent organ failure in patients with acute pancreatitis. *Gastroenterology.* 2012; 142: 1476-1482; quiz e15-16. PMID: 22425589.
11. Muddana V, Whitcomb DC, Khalid A, Slivka A, Papachristou GI. Elevated serum creatinine as a marker of pancreatic necrosis in acute pancreatitis. *Am J Gastroenterol.* 2009; 104: 164-170. PMID: 19098865.
12. Trikudanathan G, Navaneethan U, Vege SS. Current controversies in fluid resuscitation in acute pancreatitis: a systematic review. *Pancreas.* 2012; 41: 827-834. PMID: 22781906.
13. Wu BU, Bakker OJ, Papachristou GI, Besselink MG, Repas K, van Santvoort HC, et al. Blood urea nitrogen in the early assessment of acute pancreatitis: an international validation study. *Arch Intern Med.* 2011; 171: 669-676. PMID: 21482842.
14. Wu BU, Johannes RS, Sun X, Conwell DL, Banks PA. Early changes in blood urea nitrogen predict mortality in acute pancreatitis. *Gastroenterology.* 2009; 137: 129-135. PMID: 19344722.
15. Wu BU, Hwang JQ, Gardner TH, Repas K, Delee R, Yu S, et al. Lactated Ringer's solution reduces systemic inflammation compared with saline in patients with acute pancreatitis. *Clin Gastroenterol Hepatol.* 2011; 9: 710-717.e1. PMID: 21645639.
16. Hoque R, Farooq A, Ghani A, Gorelick F, Mehal WZ. Lactate reduces liver and pancreatic injury in Toll-like receptor- and inflammasome-mediated inflammation via GPR81-mediated suppression of innate immunity. *Gastroenterology.* 2014; 146(7): 1763-1774. PMID: 24657625.
17. Lerch MM, Conwell DL, Mayerle J. The anti-inflammasome effect of lactate and the lactate GPR81-receptor in pancreatic and liver inflammation. *Gastroenterology.* 2014; 146(7): 1602-1605. PMID: 24780214.
18. Lobo DN, Awad S. Should chloride-rich crystalloids remain the main-stay of fluid resuscitation to prevent "pre-renal" acute kidney injury? *Kidney Int.* 2014; 86: 1096-1105. PMID: 24717302.
19. Perner A, Haase N, Guttormsen AB, Tenhunen J, Klemenzson G, Åneman A, et al. Hydroxyethyl starch 130/0.42 versus Ringer's acetate in severe sepsis. *N Engl J Med.* 2012; 367: 124-134. PMID: 22738085.
20. Perner A, Haase N, Winkel P, Guttormsen AB, Tenhunen J, Klemenzson G, et al. Long-term out-comes in patients with severe sepsis randomised to resuscitation with hydroxyethyl starch 130/0.42 or Ringer's acetate. *Intensive Care Med.* 2014; 40: 927-934. PMID: 24807084.
21. Brunkhorst FM, Engel C, Bloos F, Meier-Hellmann A, Ragaller M, Weiler N, et al. Intensive insulin therapy and pentastarch resuscitation in severe sepsis. *N Engl J Med.* 2008; 358: 125-139. PMID: 18184958.
22. Du XJ, Hu WM, Xia Q, Huang ZW, Chen GY, Jin XD, et al. Hydroxyethyl starch resuscitation reduces the risk of intra-abdominal hypertension in severe acute pancreatitis. *Pancreas.* 2011; 40: 1220-1225. PMID: 21775917.
23. Gardner TB, Vege SS, Chari ST, Petersen BT, Topazian MD, Clain JE, et al. Faster rate of initial fluid resuscitation in severe acute pancreatitis diminishes in-hospital mortality. *Pancreatology.* 2009; 9: 770-776. PMID: 20110744.
24. Wall I, Badalov N, Baradarian R, Iswara K, Li JJ, Tenner S. Decreased mortality in acute pancreatitis related to early aggressive hydration. *Pancreas.* 2011; 40: 547-550. PMID: 21499208.
25. Mao E, Tang Y, Fei J, Qin S, Wu J, Li L, et al. Fluid therapy for severe acute pancreatitis in acute response stage. *Chin Med J (Engl).* 2009; 122: 169-173. PMID: 19187641.
26. Mao EQ, Fei J, Peng YB, Huang J, Tang YQ, Zhang SD. Rapid hemodilution is associated with increased sepsis and mortality among patients with severe acute pancreatitis. *Chin Med J (Engl).* 2010; 123: 1639-1644. PMID: 20819621.
27. ARISE Investigators, ANZICS Clinical Trials Group, Peake SL, Delaney A, Bailey M, Bellomo R, Cameron PA, et al. Goal-directed resuscitation for patients with early septic shock. *N Engl J Med.* 2014; 371: 1496-1506. PMID: 25272316.
28. Mouncey PR, Osborn TM, Power GS, Harrison DA, Sadique MZ, Grieve RD, et al. Trial of early, goal-directed resuscitation for septic shock. *N Engl J Med.* 2015; 372: 1301-1311. PMID: 25776532.
29. ProCESS Investigators, Yealy DM, Kellum JA, Huang DT, Barnato AE, Weissfeld LA, et al. A randomized trial of protocol-based care for early septic shock. *N Engl J Med.* 2014; 370: 1683-1693. PMID: 24635773.
30. Early Goal-directed Volume Resuscitation in Severe Acute Pancreatitis - Full Text View - ClinicalTrials.gov [Online]. https://clinicaltrials.gov/ct2/show/NCT00894907 [25 Oct. 2015].
31. Working Group IAP/APA Acute Pancreatitis Guidelines. IAP/APA evidence-based guidelines for the management of acute pancreatitis. *Pancreatology.* 2013; 13: e1-15. PMID: 24054878.

Chapter 25

Pain management in acute pancreatitis

Stephan Schorn, Güralp O. Ceyhan, Elke Tieftrunk, Helmut Friess, and Ihsan Ekin Demir*

Department of Surgery, Klinikum rechts der Isar, Technische Universität München, Munich, Germany.

Introduction

Severe abdominal pain is a hallmark of acute pancreatitis (AP). AP-associated pain is often described by patients as a deep and penetrating pain with an acute onset and without any prodrome. Typically, AP patients locate the maximal pain in the upper abdomen and report that it radiates like a belt around the trunk into their back. Pain reaches its maximum severity within hours after its onset and can last from hours up to days or even months.[1-5] Therefore, it is not surprising that the presence of persistent epigastric pain dictates the diagnostic workup of patients suffering from AP in the clinical routine.[1-3,6,7] Interestingly, beside its diagnostic aid,[2] recent studies suggest that pain can serve as a prognostic tool to predict AP severity and patient outcome.[5,8] Nevertheless, adequate pain therapy after hospital admission is often a challenging task that requires interdisciplinary management. In clinical practice, pain treatment ranges and escalates from low-dose nonopioid analgesics to high-dose opioid analgesics and even to interventional and surgical approaches. Over 80% of all cases of acute pancreatitis (AP) are due to gallstones or alcohol abuse.[9-11]

In AP, the most common localization of acute pain is the epigastric region.[3,4,12,13] Due to the retroperitoneal localization of the pancreas, it is not unusual that patients describe AP-associated pain as deep and penetrating. Pain in AP is often associated with nausea and vomiting. Physical examination reveals pronounced tenderness of the upper abdomen with guarding, which can in occur in combination with other unspecific symptoms like fever or tachycardia. Maximum pain is typically in the upper epigastric region and radiates like a belt around the trunk into the back.[1,2,13] Pain detection is a well-accepted diagnostic tool in AP. According to the modified Atlanta consensus guidelines,[2,13] AP can be diagnosed if at least two of the following criteria are fulfilled:

1. The occurrence of abdominal pain that is characterized by an acute onset and radiates to the back
2. Serum pancreatic enzymes (lipase or amylase) elevated at least threefold over the normal serum enzyme level
3. Characteristic findings of AP in imaging (contrast-enhanced-computed tomography, magnetic resonance imaging, transabdominal ultrasound)

Role of pain in diagnosis and prognosis of patients with AP

Pain is increasingly recognized as a diagnostic and prognostic factor in AP.[2,5,8,14,15] Interestingly, beside its role in AP diagnosis, more recent studies described the interval between onset of pain and hospitalization as an adequate prognostic factor for estimating AP severity.[5,8,12] In a study by Phillip et al., patients with severe pain had shorter median pain-to-admission time compared to patients with only moderate pain.[5,8,12] Interestingly, pain and AP severity also correlated in these two cohorts, and together with serum lipase and C-reactive protein levels, pain was identified as a predictor of AP.[12] The severity may also allow determinations of the cause of AP.[3,16] Here, a genuinely severe abdominal pain preferentially occurs in biliary AP, whereas alcoholic AP and especially autoimmune pancreatitis are predominantly accompanied by milder abdominal pain.[17-19]

Main arms of pain management in AP

The successful treatment of patients with AP has three prerequisites: 1) adequate and early fluid resuscitation,[10,20-22] 2) proper nutritional support,[10,23,24] and 3) adequate pain management.[10,25,26] The effective treatment of pain in AP ranges from administering simple analgesic drugs, which might be sufficient for patients with mild AP, up to potent opioid drugs, high doses of antibiotics for infected pancreatic necrosis, and even surgical or interventional procedures in cases of severe AP.[1,3,4,7,10,14,27-31]

The full spectrum of medical, interventional, and surgical possibilities raises the question on how to treat rather

*Corresponding author. Email: ekin.demir@tum.de

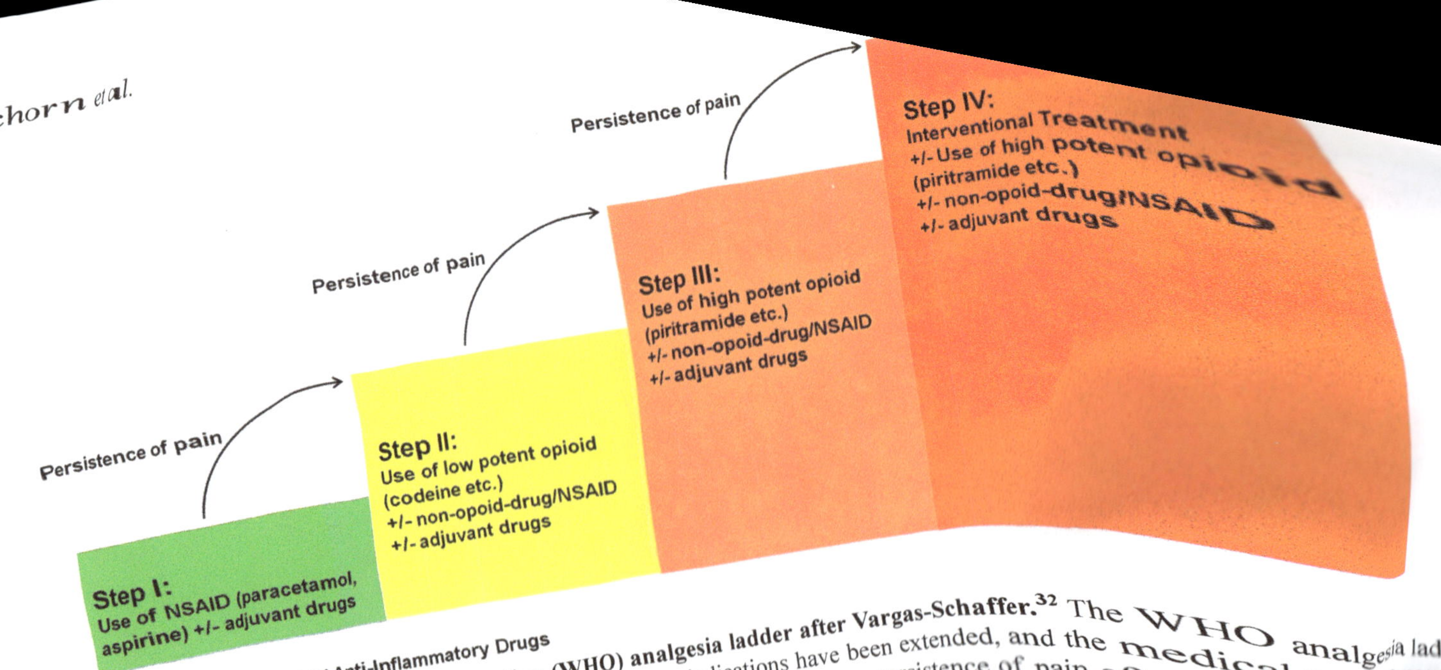

Figure 1. The modified World Health Organization (WHO) analgesia ladder after Vargas-Schaffer.[32] The WHO analgesia ladder was originally developed to treat pain due to cancer. Over time, the indications have been extended, and the medical management of pain in AP can similarly be grounded on a modified version of the WHO ladder. Here, persistence of pain after implementation of a low-potency measure warrants escalation of analgesia to a more potent substance, which, if there is ongoing need, can be adjuvantly combined with any measure/agent from the lower step. This modified ladder includes interventional procedures that can be indicated once medical measures have failed to provide adequate analgesia.

than overtreat AP. Treatment of pain may seem to be a simple clinical task routine. Besides the World Health Organization (WHO) analgesic ladder (**Figure 1**), which includes the use of nonsteroidal anti-inflammatory drugs (NSAIDs) or their combination with highly potent opioid analgesics in an escalating regime,[1,14,30-33] abdominal pain management also includes interventional strategies depending on AP-related complication occurrence.[3,6,7,11,16,27,34-38] In fact, adequate pain treatment is much more complex and often requires interdisciplinary action. One reason for the challenge behind pain management is the high complexity of AP itself. Whereas mild to moderate epigastric pain is often the single symptom of edematous pancreatitis, patients with necrotizing AP often suffer from severe pain attacks, pleural effusion, ascites, and even multiple organ failure. Importantly, whereas mild AP is rarely lethal,[39] the lethality of AP reaches up to at least 30% in patients with necrotizing AP and persistent multiple organ failure.[40-42] As discussed later in this chapter, novel analgesic interventions like thoracic spinal analgesia are receiving more attention for treating pain in patients with AP.[43,44]

Role of medical treatment in pain management during AP

In 1986, the WHO presented the analgesia ladder as a framework to treat severe pain due to cancer.[33] Later, the analgesic pain regime was also used to treat pain due to other causes.[1,32] According to the WHO regime, pain treatment begins with low-potency NSAIDs, which may be sufficient in patients with mild or moderate pain due to AP,[10,20,26,45] and increases up to highly potent NSAIDs alone or in combination with opioids.[32,33] In the past, the WHO analgesic ladder was only partially useful for treating AP patients because opioid analgesics, especially morphine, were long blamed to cause dysfunction of the sphincter of Oddi after systemic administration.[46] However, several studies showed that morphine has no proven significantly unfavorable influence on the course of AP.[47] In a comparative study on metamizole (2 g/8 h intravenous [i.v.]) versus morphine (10 mg/4 h subcutaneous [s.c.]), metamizole resulted in somewhat more frequent and quicker pain relief.[47] Earlier studies postulated pethidine as the analgesic of choice in pain due to AP.[48] However, Blamey et al. showed that buprenorphine is a longer-acting analgesic with a similar analgesic capacity as pethidine but a lower potential to cause physical opioid dependence.[48]

Indeed, the latest studies including systematic reviews convincingly demonstrated that opioid analgesics could be safely administered with major benefit in AP, and that the dogma of "no opioids in AP" should be considered obsolete. To this end, Jakobs et al. treated 40 patients with AP or chronic pancreatitis with either buprenorphine or procaine administered via continuous i.v. infusion and additional analgesics on demand.[49] Those who received buprenorphine had significantly less demand after additional analgesics and had lower visual analogue scale pain scores than procaine-receiving patients, especially during the first 2 days of treatment.[49] In another open, randomized, controlled trial including 107 AP patients, subjects were randomized to receive either procaine (2 g/ 24 has continuous i.v. infusion) or pentazocine (bolus i.v. every 6 h).[50] Those treated with procaine were more likely to demand additional analgesics compared to patients receiving pentazocine alone (98% versus 44%).[50] Furthermore, the pain scores were much lower in the pentazocine group during the first 3 days of analgesic treatment.[50] These studies therefore provided evidence for the lack of effectiveness of procaine in AP-associated pain.[45]

Overall, there seems to be no difference in the risk of pancreatitis-associated complications or clinically serious adverse events between opioids and other analgesic agents.[30,49,51,52] Opioid analgesics may be considered an appropriate choice in the treatment of AP-associated pain, and importantly, they may decrease the need for supplementary analgesia.[30]

Role of nutrition in pain management during AP

One interesting feature of AP-associated pain is potential pain exacerbation after ingestion of food or fluids.[7,16] This food-dependent progression of abdominal pain raises the question as to how far adequate nutrition therapy also contributes to pain management. In contrast to the long-believed paradigm on the benefits of total parenteral nutrition in AP, Sax et al. clearly showed that early, total parenteral feeding of patients with AP does not provide any benefit with regard to the number of days to oral intake, total hospital stay, or number of AP-associated complications.[53] Current literature supports the notion that appropriate management of nutrition is strongly dependent on AP severity. Importantly in patients with mild to moderate AP, nasogastric feeding seems to be well tolerated and might reduce abdominal pain intensity and duration, the need of pain medication, and the risk of oral food intolerance.[54] However, there is no evidence that it might also reduce the length of hospital stay in these patients.[54,55]

An interesting question regarding the interaction between pain and nutrition in AP is related to pain relapse after oral refeeding during AP. In different studies, the incidence of pain onset or exacerbation after refeeding ranged from 21%-25% and reached a maximum of 50%-100% of cases within 48 h of refeeding.[56] Therefore, the incidence of pain relapse after oral refeeding during AP seems to be quite high.[56] Current evidence suggests that nutrition support should only be performed in patients with severe pancreatitis, whereas nutrition support is generally not needed in patients with mild or moderate disease for whom oral feeding should be started as soon as possible and as tolerated by patients. If nutrition support is needed, enteral nutrition should be preferred over parenteral nutrition.[57] However, a clear consensus on how and when oral refeeding should be initiated has not yet been reached. In this context, Teich et al. reported in their prospective, randomized study that patients who could decide to start oral refeeding were able to start 1 day earlier compared to patients who received oral nutrition based on the serum lipase.[55] Interestingly, in the self-selected eating group, oral feeding had no impact on postprandial pain or hospital stay compared to the lipase-directed decision to oral refeeding.

Role of endoscopic retrograde cholangiopancreatography in pain due to AP

Gallstones are the most common cause of AP in Western and Asian countries with an incidence reaching up to at least 40% of all AP cases.[16,58,59] An important question is how far the removal of pancreatitis-associated gallstones by endoscopic retrograde cholangiopancreatography (ERCP) affects pain sensation and AP patient morbidity and mortality. It is conceivable that ERCP contributes to adequate pain management in AP due to removal of the etiologic agent. The role of ERCP in pain management for AP patients is barely described in the current medical literature.

In 2009, Chen et al. demonstrated that patients undergoing ERCP for AP may still benefit from pain management.[60] Still, because of its potential complications, there is a clear consensus on the indication of ERCP in patients with AP. The single indication for primary therapy via ERCP in AP is suspected remaining pancreatic or bile duct obstructions or existing cholangitis.[10,16,20,36,61,62] ERCP should only be used for clearance of proven bile duct stones, especially in patients who suffer from severe AP, with clear evidence of cholangitis, in those who are poor candidates for cholecystectomy, those who are postcholecystectomy, and those with strong evidence of persistent biliary obstructions (**Table 1**). In contrast, ERCP should be avoided in

Table 1. Indications of ERCP with endoscopic papillotomy and stenting in AP.

Clear indications of ERCP in AP (must-do)	• Bile duct stones in patients with severe pancreatitis • Cholangitis • Poor candidates for cholecystectomy • Postcholecystectomy • Strong evidence of persistent biliary obstruction
Intermediate indication of ERCP in AP (can-do)	• High suspicion of bile duct stones and indication of therapy
Contraindication of ERCP in AP	• Low to intermediate suspicion of retained bile duct stones, • Cholecystectomy planned

Bases on Banks, Freeman et al (20).

patients with low or intermediate suspicion of retracted bile duct stones.[10,16,20,36,61] A large meta-analysis by Tse et al. plainly demonstrated that early ERCP has no clear benefit for patients with AP compared to early conservative medical treatment.[62]

In conclusion, in the analgesic regime of AP, other non- or less invasive procedures than ERCP should be preferred to treat pain in AP. Because of its morbidity and mortality, ERCP should be avoided as a single analgesic procedure and only performed if there is strong evidence for remaining bile duct stones or coexisting cholangitis.

Role of minimally-invasive necrosectomy and decompressive laparotomy in pain due to AP

The management of necrotizing AP has witnessed considerable progress in recent years. Traditionally, infected pancreatic necrosis as a result of AP was considered an indication for open surgical necrosectomy. However, in recent years, an increasing number of minimally invasive approaches have emerged that could effectively limit local and systemic damage without the need for open invasive surgery, thus effectively contributing to prognostic improvement comparable to open necrosectomy. These approaches including repetitive percutaneous drainage via large-caliber catheters,[63] endoscopic transluminal necrosectomy,[64] retroperitoneal approach with percutaneous insertion of endoscopic material,[65] and especially a "step-up approach"[66] have been convincingly shown to decrease the complication rate associated with necrotic AP. Still, the long-term outcomes of these minimally invasive approaches have not been sufficiently investigated. In the GEPARD trial that studied the long-term outcome of AP patients with endoscopic necrosectomy, 81% of the patients could be freed from pancreatic necrosis and associated complications during the first hospital stay.[64] Among the long-term survivors, 16% suffered from secondary clinical recurrence of necrosis or pseudocyst emergence. Importantly, all 11 patients with recurrence were dependent on regular intake of analgesic medication, whereas in 6 out of 11 cases, analgesic intake was only occasional.[64] In a study that recently described the long-term outcomes of combined percutaneous and endoscopic approaches for symptomatic and infected walled-off necrosis, Ross et al. reported that only 2 out of 117 patients required late surgery for persistent pain.[67] However, this study did not report on pain severity and frequency or the analgesic intake of patients who did not require surgery for pain.[67] Overall, these observations imply that treating pain in necrotic AP via interventional techniques is also dependent on the overall success of the intervention to resolve AP-associated complications such as necrosis. On the other hand, persistent pain despite these minimally invasive approaches seems to guide the decision toward surgical intervention.[68] Patients who have persistent necrotic collections or pseudocysts seem to be prone to develop chronic abdominal pain, but the long-term results of these interventional approaches are lacking. Moreover, the impact of these promising procedures on pain sensation does not seem to be systematically recorded or reported.[69]

An approach that was put forward to deal with AP-associated abdominal hypertension is decompressive laparotomy.[70] Abdominal hypertension is assumed to result from a combination of pancreatic and visceral edema, acute peripancreatic fluid collections, capillary leakage, ascites, and paralytic ileus and is encountered around 27%-38% of severe AP cases.[70] Abdominal hypertension is defined by the World Society of Abdominal Compartment Syndrome as a "life-threatening sustained elevation of the intra-abdominal pressure (IAP) that is associated with new onset organ failure or acute worsening of existing organ failure".[71] Thus, elevated IAP is frequently associated with kidney dysfunction and increased peak airway pressure. However, the question whether elevated IAP is a direct cause of multiorgan failure or a consequence of organ dysfunction has not yet been answered.[72] Furthermore, when and how to escalate percutaneous drainage to an aggressive decompressive laparotomy is also yet unclear.[70] The DECOMPRESS trial as a multicenter study will compare percutaneous catheter drainage with decompressive laparotomy in patients with elevated IAP during severe AP.[73] Until the results of this study are available, decompressive laparotomy should be considered to represent a major invasive intervention with no convincingly proven benefit for treating elevated IAP to date.[70,72,74] Accordingly, the long-term pain outcomes of patients who undergo this aggressive surgical intervention should be addressed in future studies.

Novel pain management strategies in AP

Besides the common methods of pain management in AP described above, clinical researchers are devising novel analgesic techniques that affect the interaction between the nervous system and pancreatitis (**Figure 2**). In an interdisciplinary setting, such interventions have been recently shown to be beneficial for both pain and the overall disease course.

To this end, Bachmann et al. recently reported improved survival with thoracic epidural analgesia (TEA) in a porcine AP model based on the infusion of glycodeoxycholic acid into the pancreatic duct.[43] The 7-day-survival rate of animals that received bupivacaine as TEA was 82%,compared to a mere 29% in the control group.This difference was largely attributable to the improved microcirculation, tissue oxygenation, and consequently preserved microscopic tissue architecture in the group of pigs treated with TEA, with similar results previously reported for murine AP.[75,76] In a study on 121 patients admitted to the intensive care unit

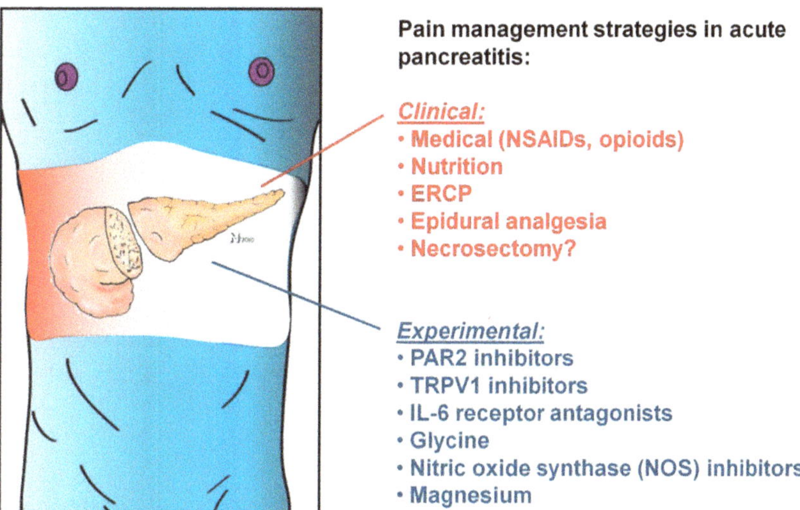

Pain management strategies in acute pancreatitis:
Clinical:
• Medical (NSAIDs, opioids)
• Nutrition
• ERCP
• Epidural analgesia
• Necrosectomy?
Experimental:
• PAR2 inhibitors
• TRPV1 inhibitors
• IL-6 receptor antagonists
• Glycine
• Nitric oxide synthase (NOS) inhibitors
• Magnesium

Figure 2. Pain management in AP. Analgesic measures to treat AP-associated pain can be classified into clinical methods that are in widespread use in daily clinical practice and experimental measures shown to be effective in numerous studies with murine or porcine AP models that have not been translated into clinical practice.

with AP, Bernhardt et al. reported excellent analgesia on 72% of observation days during which no systemic use of other analgesics was necessary.[77] The rate of hemodynamic instability was also low (8%). The time to normalization of serum amylase and lipase was 17.4 days (minimum 1 day, maximum 19 days), and the overall lethality was 2.5%. In this prospective single cohort study, epidural analgesia produced a considerable analgesic effect without a large complication rate.[77] Based on these promising observations, the results of the three clinical trials that are currently investigating the effect epidural analgesia on the course of AP are eagerly awaited.[78]

Looking at the potential benefits of analgesia on the course of AP, especially epidural analgesia with its peripheral neurolytic effects, it is essential to remember the contribution of "neurogenic inflammation" in AP pathogenesis. In this context, different noxious substances released from damaged acini (i.e., zymogens, trypsin, proteases, and ions such as hydrogen or potassium) can activate peripheral nociceptive sensory nerve endings. These activated sensory neurons signal centrally toward the spinal cord and can also cross-activate other neurons in the neighboring spinal cord regions that then signal into the periphery in an antidromic fashion. This antidromic reflex leads to the release of substance P and calcitonin-gene-related-peptide from the peripheral nociceptive nerve endings.

These neuropeptides have the intriguing ability to chemoattract immune cells, cause vasodilatation, and thereby augment local inflammation. Neurogenic inflammation is recognized as a central pathophysiological event in AP.[79] Based on this premise, it is not surprising to see an analgesic and overall beneficial effect of epidural anesthesia on the course of AP. In accordance with this strategy, inhibitors of the proteinase-activated-receptor-2 (PAR2) or the transient receptor potential vanilloid-1 (TRPV1) have been shown to be beneficial for treating pain during experimental AP in mice.[80] During experimental AP in rats, intrathecal administration of gabapentin was reported to enhance the analgesic effects of subtherapeutic doses of morphine.[81] Other neuronal targets to treat both the inflammation in AP and AP-associated pain are nitric oxide (NO) signaling and glycine. Treatment of rats with NO synthase (NOS) inhibitors or glycine reduced abdominal hyperalgesia and AP-associated histologic alterations during AP in rats.[82,83] Recently, blockade of interleukin-6 (IL-6) signaling by an orally available, small-molecule IL-6 receptor inhibitor was shown to diminish abdominal hyperalgesia during AP.[84] However, these promising neuronal targets have not yet been studied in early phase clinical trials. Based on its promising effects during experimental AP in rats, a promising and inexpensive agent that may be clinically useful as a novel analgesic agent is magnesium.[85] The MagPEP study as a multicenter randomized controlled trial of magnesium sulfate in the prevention of post-ERPC pancreatitis shall provide data on the impact of magnesium on pain sensation during post-ERCP pancreatitis.[86] Once shown to be effective, beyond its preventive usage, magnesium may be considered a novel analgesic alternative to treat pain in AP.[86] Overall, the interaction between the nervous system and pancreatic inflammation may offer numerous clues for more effective treatment of both the disease itself and the associated pain. Therefore, efforts toward translating this axis into the clinical practice need to become more visible in the near future.

Table 2. Different Facets of Pain management in patients with AP.

Analgesic drugs	• According to the WHO analgesic ladder • No evidence of higher morality or morbidity due to opioids • Administration of procain has no benefit for patients with AP
Supplement of nutrition	• Oral refeeding should be begun as fast as possible • No evidence that normalization of serum pancreatic enzymes was needed • No benefit for parenteral nutrition supplement in patients with mild or moderate pancreatitis
ERCP	• Only indicated if there is clear evidence of persistent biliary obstruction
Thoracic Epidural Analgesia	• Only few data available • Yet evidence of rapid pain relief and of reduction of the need for opiates

Conclusion

Abdominal pain is the earliest and a leading symptom of patients with AP. There is solid evidence that pain severity may also predict the clinical course of AP. Treatment of pain during AP continues to be challenging task in the clinicand involves a combination of medical treatment according to the WHO analgesic ladder, adequate nutritional support and, in some cases, interventional therapy (e.g., ERCP) (**Table 2**). Novel studies also suggest that severe abdominal pain in AP could be effectively treated with thoracic epidural anesthesia because it can improve pancreatic microcirculation and preserve tissue architecture. Disruption of neurogenic inflammation in AP holds great promise as a novel analgesic and therapeutic strategy for AP, but this approach needs to be tested in early phase clinical trials. The development of inhibitors directed against selected targets on pancreatic afferents is likely to open new paths toward more effective pain management as an interdisciplinary challenge.

Acknowledgements

The authors thank Dr. Matthias Maak for his valuable assistance with figure generation.

References

1. Flasar MH, Goldberg E. Acute abdominal pain. *Med Clin North Am.* 2006; 90(3): 481-503. PMID: 16473101.
2. Banks PA, Bollen TL, Dervenis C, Gooszen HG, Johnson CD, Sarr MG, et al. Classification of acute pancreatitis--2012: revision of the Atlanta classification and definitions by international consensus. *Gut.* 2013; 62(1): 102-111. PMID: 23100216.
3. Whitcomb DC. Clinical practice. Acute pancreatitis. *N Engl J Med.* 2006; 354(20): 2142-2150. PMID: 16707751.
4. Swaroop VS, Chari ST, Clain JE. Severe acute pancreatitis. *JAMA.* 2004; 291(23): 2865-2868. PMID: 15199038.
5. Phillip V, Schuster T, Hagemes F, Lorenz S, Matheis U, Preinfalk S, et al. Time period from onset of pain to hospital admission and patients' awareness in acute pancreatitis. *Pancreas.* 2013; 42(4): 647-654. PMID: 23303202.
6. Frossard JL, Steer ML, Pastor CM. Acute pancreatitis. *Lancet.* 2008; 371(9607): 143-152. PMID: 18191686.
7. Lankisch PG, Apte M, Banks PA. Acute pancreatitis. *Lancet.* 2015; 386(9988): 85-96. PMID: 25616312.
8. Kapoor K, Repas K, Singh VK, Conwell DL, Mortele KJ, Wu BU, et al. Does the duration of abdominal pain prior to admission influence the severity of acute pancreatitis? *JOP.* 2013; 14(2): 171-175. PMID: 23474564.
9. Halangk W, Lerch MM. Early events in acute pancreatitis. *Gastroenterol Clin North Am.* 2004; 33(4): 717-731. PMID: 15528014.
10. Mayerle J, Hlouschek V, Lerch MM. Current management of acute pancreatitis. *Nat Clin Pract Gastroenterol Hepatol.* 2005; 2(10): 473-483. PMID: 16224479.
11. Kadakia SC. Biliary tract emergencies. Acute cholecystitis, acute cholangitis, and acute pancreatitis. *Med Clin North Am.* 1993; 77(5): 1015-1036. PMID: 8371614.
12. Phillip V, Steiner JM, Algül H. Early phase of acute pancreatitis: Assessment and management. *World J Gastrointest Pathophysiol.* 2014; 5(3): 158-168. PMID: 25133018.
13. Bradley EL 3rd. A clinically based classification system for acute pancreatitis. Summary of the International Symposium on Acute Pancreatitis, Atlanta, Ga, September 11 through 13, 1992. *Arch Surg.* 1993; 128(5): 586-590. PMID: 8489394.
14. American Society of Anesthesiologists Task Force on Acute Pain Management. Practice guidelines for acute pain management in the perioperative setting: an updated report by the American Society of Anesthesiologists Task Force on Acute Pain Management. *Anesthesiology.* 2004; 100(6): 1573-1581. PMID: 15166580.
15. American Society of Anesthesiologists Task Force on Acute Pain Management. Practice guidelines for acute pain management in the perioperative setting: an updated report by the American Society of Anesthesiologists Task Force on Acute Pain Management. *Anesthesiology.* 2012; 116(2): 248-273. PMID: 22227789.
16. Cappell MS. Acute pancreatitis: etiology, clinical presentation, diagnosis, and therapy. *Med Clin North Am.* 2008; 92(4): 889-923, ix-x. PMID: 18570947.
17. Kloppel G, Luttges J, Lohr M, Zamboni G, Longnecker D. Autoimmune pancreatitis: pathological, clinical, and immunological features. *Pancreas.* 2003; 27(1): 14-19. PMID: 12826900.
18. Kim KP, Kim MH, Song MH, Lee SS, Seo DW, Lee SK. Autoimmune chronic pancreatitis. *Am J Gastroenterol.* 2004; 99(8): 1605-1616. PMID: 15307882.
19. Finkelberg DL, Sahani D, Deshpande V, Brugge WR. Autoimmune pancreatitis. *N Engl J Med.* 2006; 355(25): 2670-2676. PMID: 17182992.
20. Banks PA, Freeman ML; Practice Parameters Committee of the American College of Gastroenterology. Practice guidelines in acute pancreatitis. *Am J Gastroenterol.* 2006; 101(10): 2379-2400. PMID: 17032204.

21. Gardner TB, Vege SS, Chari ST, Petersen BT, Topazian MD, Clain JE, et al. Faster rate of initial fluid resuscitation in severe acute pancreatitis diminishes in-hospital mortality. *Pancreatology*. 2009; 9(6): 770-776. PMID: 20110744.
22. Gardner TB, Vege SS, Pearson RK, Chari ST. Fluid resuscitation in acute pancreatitis. *Clin Gastroenterol Hepatol.* 2008; 6(10): 1070-1076. PMID: 18619920.
23. Li JY, Yu T, Chen GC, Yuan YH, Zhong W, Zhao LN, et al. Enteral nutrition within 48 hours of admission improves clinical outcomes of acute pancreatitis by reducing complications: a meta-analysis. *PLoS One*. 2013; 8(6): e64926. PMID: 23762266.
24. Yi F, Ge L, Zhao J, Lei Y, Zhou F, Chen Z, et al. Meta-analysis: total parenteral nutrition versus total enteral nutrition in predicted severe acute pancreatitis. *Intern Med*. 2012; 51(6): 523-530. PMID: 22449657.
25. Lankisch PG. Acute and chronic pancreatitis. An update on management. *Drugs*. 1984; 28(6): 554-564. PMID: 6083859.
26. Banks PA. Practice guidelines in acute pancreatitis. *Am J Gastroenterol*. 1997; 92(3): 377-386. PMID: 9068455.
27. Folsch UR, Nitsche R, Ludtke R, Hilgers RA, Creutzfeldt W. Early ERCP and papillotomy compared with conservative treatment for acute biliary pancreatitis. The German Study Group on Acute Biliary Pancreatitis. *N Engl J Med*. 1997; 336(4): 237-242. PMID: 8995085.
28. Banks PA, Conwell DL, Toskes PP. The management of acute and chronic pancreatitis. *Gastroenterol Hepatol (N Y)*. 2010; 6(2 Suppl 3): 1-16. PMID: 20567557.
29. Kaw M, Al-Antably Y, Kaw P. Management of gallstone pancreatitis: Cholecystectomy or ERCP and endoscopic sphincterotomy. *Gastrointestinal Endoscopy*. 2002; 56(1): 61-65. PMID: 12085036.
30. Basurto Ona X, Rigau Comas D, Urrútia G. Opioids for acute pancreatitis pain. *Cochrane Database Syst Rev*. 2013; 7: CD009179. PMID: 23888429.
31. Meng W, Yuan J, Zhang C, Bai Z, Zhou W, Yan J, et al. Parenteral analgesics for pain relief in acute pancreatitis: a systematic review. *Pancreatology*. 2013; 13(3): 201-206. PMID: 23719588.
32. Vargas-Schaffer G. Is the WHO analgesic ladder still valid? Twenty-four years of experience. *Can Fam Physician*. 2010; 56(6): 514-517, e202-e515. PMID: 20547511.
33. World Health Organization. *Traitement de la douleur cancéreuse.* Geneva, Switzerland: World Health Organization; 1987.
34. Carroll JK, Herrick B, Gipson T, Lee SP. Acute pancreatitis: diagnosis, prognosis, and treatment. *Am Fam Physician*. 2007; 75(10): 1513-1520. PMID: 17555143.
35. Rodriguez JR, Razo AO, Targarona J, Thayer SP, Rattner DW, Warshaw AL, et al. Debridement and closed packing for sterile or infected necrotizing pancreatitis: insights into indications and outcomes in 167 patients. *Ann Surg*. 2008; 247(2): 294-299. PMID: 18216536.
36. Tenner S. Initial management of acute pancreatitis: critical issues during the first 72 hours. *Am J Gastroenterol*. 2004; 99(12): 2489-2494. PMID: 15571599.
37. Tsiotos GG, Luque-de León E, Sarr MG. Long-term outcome of necrotizing pancreatitis treated by necrosectomy. *Br J Surg*. 1998; 85(12): 1650-1653. PMID: 9876068.
38. Heyries L, Barthet M, Delvasto C, Zamora C, Bernard JP, Sahel J. Long-term results of endoscopic management of pancreas divisum with recurrent acute pancreatitis. *Gastrointest Endosc*. 2002; 55(3): 376-381. PMID: 11868012.
39. Singh VK, Bollen TL, Wu BU, Repas K, Maurer R, Yu S, et al. An assessment of the severity of interstitial pancreatitis. *Clin Gastroenterol Hepatol*. 2011; 9(12): 1098-1103. PMID: 21893128.
40. Buter A, Imrie CW, Carter CR, Evans S, McKay CJ. Dynamic nature of early organ dysfunction determines outcome in acute pancreatitis. *Br J Surg*. 2002; 89(3): 298-302. PMID: 11872053.
41. Johnson CD, Abu-Hilal M. Persistent organ failure during the first week as a marker of fatal outcome in acute pancreatitis. *Gut*. 2004; 53(9): 1340-1344. PMID: 15306596.
42. Mofidi R, Duff MD, Wigmore SJ, Madhavan KK, Garden OJ, Parks RW. Association between early systemic inflammatory response, severity of multiorgan dysfunction and death in acute pancreatitis. *Br J Surg*. 2006; 93(6): 738-744. PMID: 16671062.
43. Bachmann KA, Trepte CJ, Tomkötter L, Hinsch A, Stork J, Bergmann W, et al. Effects of thoracic epidural anesthesia on survival and microcirculation in severe acute pancreatitis: a randomized experimental trial. *Crit Care*. 2013; 17(6): R281. PMID: 24314012.
44. Harper D, McNaught CE. The role of thoracic epidural anesthesia in severe acute pancreatitis. *Crit Care*. 2014; 18(1): 106. PMID: 24502591.
45. Lerch MM. No more intravenous procaine for pancreatitis pain? *Digestion*. 2004; 69(1): 2-4. PMID: 14755146.
46. Helm JF, Venu RP, Geenen JE, Hogan WJ, Dodds WJ, Toouli J, et al. Effects of morphine on the human sphincter of Oddi. *Gut*. 1988; 29(10): 1402-1407. PMID: 3197985.
47. Peiró AM, Martínez J, Martínez E, de Madaria E, Llorens P, Horga JF, et al. Efficacy and tolerance of metamizole versus morphine for acute pancreatitis pain. *Pancreatology*. 2008; 8(1): 25-29. PMID: 18235213.
48. Blamey SL, Finlay IG, Carter DC, Imrie CW. Analgesia in acute pancreatitis: comparison of buprenorphine and pethidine. *Br Med J (Clin Res Ed)*. 1984; 288(6429): 1494-1495. PMID: 6426616.
49. Jakobs R, Adamek MU, von Bubnoff AC, Riemann JF. Buprenorphine or procaine for pain relief in acute pancreatitis. A prospective randomized study. *Scand J Gastroenterol*. 2000; 35(12): 1319-1323. PMID: 11199374.
50. Kahl S, Zimmermann S, Pross M, Schulz HU, Schmidt U, Malfertheiner P. Procaine hydrochloride fails to relieve pain in patients with acute pancreatitis. *Digestion*. 2004; 69(1): 5-9. PMID: 14755147.
51. Thompson DR. Narcotic analgesic effects on the sphincter of Oddi: a review of the data and therapeutic implications in treating pancreatitis. *Am J Gastroenterol*. 2001; 96(4): 1266-1272. PMID: 11316181.
52. Stevens M, Esler R, Asher G. Transdermal fentanyl for the management of acute pancreatitis pain. *Appl Nurs Res*. 2002; 15(2): 102-110. PMID: 11994827.
53. Sax HC, Warner BW, Talamini MA, Hamilton FN, Bell RH Jr, Fischer JE, et al. Early total parenteral nutrition in acute

pancreatitis: lack of beneficial effects. *Am J Surg*. 1987; 153(1): 117-124. PMID: 3099588.

54. Petrov MS, McIlroy K, Grayson L, Phillips AR, Windsor JA. Early nasogastric tube feeding versus nil per os in mild to moderate acute pancreatitis: a randomized controlled trial. *Clin Nutr*. 2013; 32(5): 697-703. PMID: 23340042.
55. Teich N, Aghdassi A, Fischer J, Walz B, Caca K, Wallochny T, et al. Optimal timing of oral refeeding in mild acute pancreatitis: results of an open randomized multicenter trial. *Pancreas*. 2010; 39(7): 1088-1092. PMID: 20357692.
56. Petrov MS,van Santvoort HC, Besselink MG, Cirkel GA, Brink MA, Gooszen HG. Oral refeeding after onset of acute pancreatitis: a review of literature. *Am J Gastroenterol*. 2007; 102(9): 2079-2084; quiz 2085. PMID: 17573797.
57. Mirtallo JM, Forbes A, McClave SA, Jensen GL, Waitzberg DL, Davies AR, et al. International consensus guidelines for nutrition therapy in pancreatitis. *J Parenter Enteral Nutr*. 2012; 36(3): 284-291. PMID: 22457421.
58. Steinberg W, Tenner S. Acute pancreatitis. *N Engl J Med*. 1994; 330(17): 1198-1210. PMID: 7811319.
59. Corfield AP, Cooper MJ, Williamson RC. Acute pancreatitis: a lethal disease of increasing incidence. *Gut*. 1985; 26(7): 724-729. PMID: 4018637.
60. Chen WX, Li YM, Gao DJ, Xiang Z, Yu CH, Xu GQ, et al. Application of endoscopic sphincterotomy in acute pancreatitis with fluid collection: a prospective study. *World J Gastroenterol*. 2005; 11(23): 3636-3639. PMID: 15962392.
61. Neoptolemos JP, Carr-Locke DL, London NJ, Bailey IA, James D, Fossard DP. Controlled trial of urgent endoscopic retrograde cholangiopancreatography and endoscopic sphincterotomy versus conservative treatment for acute pancreatitis due to gallstones. *Lancet*. 1988; 2(8618): 979-983. PMID: 2902491.
62. Tse F, Yuan Y. Early routine endoscopic retrograde cholangiopancreatography strategy versus early conservative management strategy in acute gallstone pancreatitis. *Cochrane Database Syst Rev*. 2012; 5: CD009779. PMID: 22592743.
63. da Costa DW, Boerma D, van Santvoort HC, Horvath KD, Werner J, Carter CR, et al. Staged multidisciplinary step-up management for necrotizing pancreatitis. *Br J Surg*. 2014; 101(1): e65-e79. PMID: 24272964.
64. Seifert H, Biermer M, Schmitt W, Jurgensen C, Will U, Gerlach R, et al. Transluminal endoscopic necrosectomy after acute pancreatitis: a multicentre study with long-term follow-up (the GEPARD Study). *Gut*. 2009; 58(9): 1260-1266. PMID: 19282306.
65. Cirocchi R, Trastulli S, Desiderio J, Boselli C, Parisi A, Noya G, et al. Minimally invasive necrosectomy versus conventional surgery in the treatment of infected pancreatic necrosis: a systematic review and a meta-analysis of comparative studies. *Surg Laparosc Endosc Percutan Tech*. 2013; 23(1): 8-20. PMID: 23386143.
66. van Santvoort HC, Besselink MG, Bakker OJ, Hofker HS, Boermeester MA, Dejong CH, et al. A step-up approach or open necrosectomy for necrotizing pancreatitis. *N Engl J Med*. 2010; 362(16): 1491-1502. PMID: 20410514.
67. Ross AS, Irani S, Gan SI, Rocha F, Siegal J, Fotoohi M, et al. Dual-modality drainage of infected and symptomatic walled-off pancreatic necrosis: long-term clinical outcomes. *Gastrointest Endosc*. 2014; 79(6): 929-935. PMID: 24246792.
68. Puli SR, Graumlich JF, Pamulaparthy SR, Kalva N. Endoscopic transmural necrosectomy for walled-off pancreatic necrosis: a systematic review and meta-analysis. *Can J Gastroenterol Hepatol*. 2014; 28(1): 50-53. PMID: 24212912.
69. Bang JY, Holt BA, Hawes RH, Hasan MK, Arnoletti JP, Christein JD, et al. Outcomes after implementing a tailored endoscopic step-up approach to walled-off necrosis in acute pancreatitis. *Br J Surg*. 2014; 101(13): 1729-1738. PMID: 25333872.
70. van Brunschot S, Schut AJ, Bouwense SA, Besselink MG, Bakker OJ, van Goor H, et al. Abdominal compartment syndrome in acute pancreatitis: a systematic review. *Pancreas*. 2014; 43(5): 665-674. PMID: 24921201.
71. Kirkpatrick AW, Roberts DJ, De Waele J, Jaeschke R, Malbrain ML, De Keulenaer B, et al. Intra-abdominal hypertension and the abdominal compartment syndrome: updated consensus definitions and clinical practice guidelines from the World Society of the Abdominal Compartment Syndrome. *Intensive Care Med*. 2013; 39(7): 1190-1206. PMID: 23673399.
72. Trikudanathan G, Vege SS. Current concepts of the role of abdominal compartment syndrome in acute pancreatitis - an opportunity or merely an epiphenomenon. *Pancreatology*. 2014; 14(4): 238-243. PMID: 25062870.
73. Radenkovic DV, Bajec D, Ivancevic N, Bumbasirevic V, Milic N, Jeremic V, et al. Decompressive laparotomy with temporary abdominal closure versus percutaneous puncture with placement of abdominal catheter in patients with abdominal compartment syndrome during acute pancreatitis: background and design of multicenter, randomised, controlled study. *BMC Surg*. 2010; 10: 22. PMID: 20624281.
74. De Waele JJ, Leppaniemi AK. Intra-abdominal hypertension in acute pancreatitis. *World J Surg*. 2009; 33(6): 1128-1133. PMID: 19350318.
75. Demirag A, Pastor CM, Morel P, Jean-Christophe C, Sielenkämper AW, Güvener N, et al. Epidural anaesthesia restores pancreatic microcirculation and decreases the severity of acute pancreatitis. *World J Gastroenterol*. 2006; 12(6): 915-920. PMID: 16521220.
76. Freise H, Lauer S, Anthonsen S, Hlouschek V, Minin E, Fischer LG, et al. Thoracic epidural analgesia augments ileal mucosal capillary perfusion and improves survival in severe acute pancreatitis in rats. *Anesthesiology*. 2006; 105(2): 354-359. PMID: 16871070.
77. Bernhardt A, Kortgen A, Niesel HCh, Goertz A. [Using epidural anesthesia in patients with acute pancreatitis--prospective study of 121 patients] [article in German]. *Anaesthesiol Reanim*. 2002; 27(1): 16-22. PMID: 11908096.
78. Siniscalchi A, Gamberini L, Laici C, Bardi T, Faenza S. Thoracic epidural anesthesia: Effects on splanchnic circulation and implications in Anesthesia and Intensive care. *World J Crit Care Med*. 2015; 4(1): 89-104. PMID: 25685727.
79. Liddle RA, Nathan JD. Neurogenic inflammation and pancreatitis. *Pancreatology*. 2004; 4(6): 551-559; discussion 559-560. PMID: 15550764.

80. Nishimura S, Ishikura H, Matsunami M, Shinozaki Y, Sekiguchi F, Naruse M, et al. The proteinase/proteinase-activated receptor-2/transient receptor potential vanilloid-1 cascade impacts pancreatic pain in mice. *Life Sci.* 2010; 87(19-22): 643-650. PMID: 20932849.
81. Smiley MM, Lu Y, Vera-Portocarrero LP, Zidan A, Westlund KN. Intrathecal gabapentin enhances the analgesic effects of subtherapeutic dose morphine in a rat experimental pancreatitis model. *Anesthesiology.* 2004; 101(3): 759-765. PMID: 15329602.
82. Camargo EA, Santana DG, Silva CI, Teixeira SA, Toyama MH, Cotrim C, et al. Inhibition of inducible nitric oxide synthase-derived nitric oxide as a therapeutical target for acute pancreatitis induced by secretory phospholipase A2. *Eur J Pain.* 2014; 18(5): 691-700. PMID: 24166730.
83. Ceyhan GO, Timm AK, Bergmann F, Gunther A, Aghdassi AA, Demir IE, et al. Prophylactic glycine administration attenuates pancreatic damage and inflammation in experimental acute pancreatitis. *Pancreatology.* 2011; 11(1): 57-67. PMID: 21474970.
84. Vardanyan M, Melemedjian OK, Price TJ, Ossipov MH, Lai J, Roberts E, et al. Reversal of pancreatitis-induced pain by an orally available, small molecule interleukin-6 receptor antagonist. *Pain.* 2010; 151(2): 257-265. PMID: 20599324.
85. Schick V, Scheiber JA, Mooren FC, Turi S, Ceyhan GO, Schnekenburger J, et al. Effect of magnesium supplementation and depletion on the onset and course of acute experimental pancreatitis. *Gut.* 2004; 63(9): 1469-1480. PMID: 24277728.
86. Fluhr G, Mayerle J, Weber E, Aghdassi A, Simon P, Gress T, et al. Pre-study protocol MagPEP: a multicentre randomized controlled trial of magnesium sulphate in the prevention of post-ERCP pancreatitis. *BMC Gastroenterol.* 2013; 13: 11. PMID: 23320650.

Chapter 26

Prophylaxis and treatment with antibiotics or probiotics in acute pancreatitis

Stefan A. Bouwense[1*], Mark C. van Baal[2], Hjalmar C. van Santvoort[3], Harry van Goor[1], and Marc G. Besselink[4]
for the Dutch Pancreatitis Study Group

[1]*Department of Surgery, Radboud University Medical Center, Nijmegen, The Netherlands;*
[2]*Department of Surgery, Tweesteden Hospital, Tilburg, The Netherlands;*
[3]*Department of Surgery, St. Antonius Hospital, Nieuwegein, The Netherlands;*
[4]*Department of Surgery, Academic Medical Center, Amsterdam, The Netherlands.*

Introduction

Acute pancreatitis (AP) is the most common gastrointestinal disease requiring acute hospitalization, and its incidence is rising.[1] Approximately 20% of patients develop necrotizing pancreatitis,[2,3] which is defined by either pancreatic parenchymal necrosis and/or peripancreatic tissue necrosis.[2,4] These patients are at risk for (multiple) organ failure often due to a persisting systemic inflammatory response syndrome. If the (peri)pancreatic collections with necrosis remain sterile, the majority of patients will recover with conservative measures without the need for invasive intervention.[3] Secondary infection of necrosis develops in 30% of patients with necrotizing pancreatitis, which substantially increases morbidity and mortality.[5,6] Overall, necrotizing pancreatitis mortality (15% to 30%) is much higher than for mild pancreatitis (0% to 1%).[7,8]

Secondary infection of the peripancreatic collections or pancreas necrosis is considered to be caused by bacterial translocation. In this phenomenon, enteral bacteria cross the gastrointestinal mucosal barrier and invade the systemic compartment or move by hematogenous spread from other sites in the body.[9] Experimental and clinical studies indicate that bacterial translocation is the result of a cascade of events dependent on a disturbance of host-bacterial interactions on three levels: 1) the presence of impaired small bowel motility and bacterial overgrowth in the intestinal lumen, 2) structural mucosal barrier failure leading to increased gut permeability in the intestinal epithelium,[10] and 3) dysregulation in the balance of pro- and anti-inflammatory factors of the immune system.[11] Another possible pathway of transmission by mesenteric lymphatics was described in an experimental rat study.[12]

Two treatment strategies have been suggested to prevent secondary infection of peripancreatic collections and pancreas necrosis early in the disease course of necrotizing pancreatitis:

1. Prophylactic antibiotics
2. Therapeutic probiotics

Antibiotics

Multiple studies have studied the prophylactic use of systemic antibiotics in AP over the last several decades.[13,14] The rationale for prophylactic treatment is to diminish the potential hematogenous spread of pathogens after bacterial translocation has occurred.

Fourteen randomized controlled trials have studied the effect of systemic antibiotic prophylaxis on preventing the infection of pancreatic necrosis.[13,14] In the 1990s, enthusiasm for antibiotic prophylaxis was expressed in a number of small case series and editorials.[15-18] As a result, many surgeons started using antibiotic prophylaxis.[19] The studies at that time were underpowered and generated variable results, but the meta-analysis at that time suggested reductions in morbidity and mortality. There were also concerns about selection of multidrug-resistant bacteria and opportunistic fungal infections.[19]

A 2006 Cochrane review by Villatoro and colleagues suggested a survival benefit and a decrease in pancreatic sepsis associated with the prophylactic use of beta-lactam antibiotics.[20] However, the conclusion on prophylactic antibiotics changed with the publication of two double-blinded randomized clinical trials.[21,22] The Villatoro group included those trials in their 2010 Cochrane review, which included 7 studies with 404 randomized patients. They found no statistically significant effect on mortality (8.4% vs. 14.4%) or the presence of infected pancreatic

*Corresponding author. Email: Stefan.Bouwense@pancreatitis.nl

necrosis (19.7% vs. 24.4%). The rate of other infections (not related to necrosis) was also not significantly reduced by prophylactic antibiotics. A nonsignificant trend was shown with beta-lactam antibiotics toward lower mortality and fewer infected pancreatic necrosis. Interestingly, this effect was stronger for imipenem, which showed no reduction in mortality but a lower risk of pancreatic infections (relative risk 0.34, 95% confidence interval 0.13-0.84).[13] Study quality has been a major concern throughout the years, and all were underpowered. The main conclusion was that there is no evidence for the prophylactic use of antibiotics in AP.[13] This was confirmed by a second review that suggested that further research is needed to identify subpopulations that may benefit from prophylactic antibiotics.[14]

Selective digestive tract decontamination (SDD) is used on many intensive care units, particularly in ventilated patients. The goal of decontamination of the upper respiratory and digestive tracts is to reduce infections by decreasing microorganism colonization at these sites. Both selective decontamination of the oropharyngeal tract (SOD) and digestive tract (SDD) with nonabsorbable antibiotics have shown modest decreases in mortality and reduced rates of bacteremia.[23] The only trial of SDD in patients with severe AP demonstrated a significant reduction of gram-negative bacterial colonization of the digestive tract and significant reductions of morbidity and mortality.[24] Due to the moderate methodological quality (a nonblinded, underpowered study lacking clear definitions) and the overall scarceness of evidence in severe AP, SDD is not considered standard practice in severe AP.

Conclusion

Current evidence does not support routine antibiotic prophylaxis or SDD in patients with severe AP.[3] However, this does not imply that antibiotic treatment (rather than prophylaxis) is ineffective and should not be started as soon as evidence for superinfection of (peri)pancreatic necrosis emerges. In these cases antibiotics are useful in controlling sepsis and in some cases, infected (peri)pancreatic necrosis can be successfully treated solely with antibiotics.

Probiotics

Probiotics are defined as "living micro-organisms which, when administered in adequate amounts, confer a health benefit on the host."[25] They can be administered together with prebiotics (synbiotics), which are nondigestible fibers that enhance probiotic activity. Probiotics have been suggested to reduce bacterial translocation (in AP) through beneficial effects on three levels of host-bacterial interactions: the intestinal lumen, the intestinal epithelium, and the immune system.

Bacterial overgrowth of potential pathogens in the intestinal lumen is prevented by a direct antimicrobial effect and competitive growth.[26] At the intestinal epithelium, probiotics prevent bacterial adherence to the epithelial surface by competitive exclusion and inhibition of a pathogen-induced increase of epithelial permeability. They also regulate enterocyte gene expression involved in maintaining the mucosal barrier and thus may preserve epithelial function.[10,27] Selected probiotic strains have been found to inhibit local proinflammatory reactions in enterocytes after pathogenic bacterial adhesion or ischemia.[27] Finally, in vitro probiotic strains have been shown to induce production of the anti-inflammatory cytokine interleukin-10. A similar effect is thought to regulate the mucosal and systemic immune systems in humans.[28]

The prophylactic role of probiotics in AP has been examined in experimental studies. In rats with pancreatitis, probiotics reduced the overgrowth of potential pathogens in the duodenum, resulting in reduced bacterial translocation to extraintestinal sites and lower mortality.[29]

The prophylactic use of probiotics was also examined in several randomized controlled trials. In patients undergoing major abdominal surgery, the administration of pre- and probiotics significantly reduced the incidence of postoperative infections, although there were some methodological issues in these studies.[30-32]

Initially, two small randomized controlled trials, both from Hungary, studied probiotic prophylaxis in AP. The first trial showed in 45 patients with predicted mild and severe pancreatitis that probiotics reduced pancreatic sepsis and the need for surgical intervention.[33] The second trial studied 62 patients with severe pancreatitis and concluded that nasojejunal feeding with synbiotics may prevent organ dysfunction in the late phase of severe AP.[34] Given the weak evidence, a larger randomized controlled multicenter trial was performed (PROPATRIA) in which probiotics were compared with placebo in 298 patients with predicted severe pancreatitis. No probiotic effect was found in reducing infectious complications. There was, however, a surprisingly higher rate of bowel ischemia (9 vs. 0) and mortality (16% vs. 6%) in the probiotics group.[35] The mechanism underlying this adverse effect remains unclear, even after post hoc research in experimental animals.[36,37]

Conclusion

There is currently no place for probiotic treatment in patients with AP. Further research on probiotic prophylaxis in patients with organ failure has been returned to the experimental stage to study the possible mechanism(s) of adverse events such as those observed in the PROPATRIA study.

Summary

Based on the current literature and in accordance with IAP/APA Acute Pancreatitis Guidelines[3]:

1. Intravenous antibiotic prophylaxis is not recommended for the prevention of infectious complications in AP. (GRADE 1B, strong agreement)
2. Probiotic prophylaxis is not recommended for the prevention of infectious complications in AP. (GRADE 1B, strong agreement)
3. Intravenous antibiotics should be given in case of suspected infection of necrotizing pancreatitis and further intervention considered

References

1. Peery AF, Dellon ES, Lund J, Crockett SD, McGowan CE, Bulsiewicz WJ, et al. Burden of gastrointestinal disease in the United States: 2012 update. *Gastroenterology*. 2012; 143: 1179-1187. PMID: 22885331.
2. Banks PA, Bollen TL, Dervenis C, Gooszen HG, Johnson CD, Sarr MG, et al. Classification of acute pancreatitis--2012: revision of the Atlanta classification and definitions by international consensus. *Gut*. 2013; 62: 102-111. PMID: 23100216.
3. Working Group IAP/APA Acute Pancreatitis Guidelines. IAP/APA evidence-based guidelines for the management of acute pancreatitis. *Pancreatology*. 2013; 13 4 Suppl 2: e1-15. PMID: 24054878.
4. Bakker OJ, van Santvoort H, Besselink MG, Boermeester MA, van Eijck C, Dejong K, et al. Extrapancreatic necrosis without pancreatic parenchymal necrosis: a separate entity in necrotising pancreatitis? *Gut*. 2013; 62: 1475-1480. PMID: 22773550.
5. van Santvoort HC, Bakker OJ, Bollen TL, Besselink MG, Ahmed Ali U, Schrijver AM, et al. A conservative and minimally invasive approach to necrotizing pancreatitis improves outcome. *Gastroenterology*. 2011; 141: 1254-1263. PMID: 21741922.
6. Petrov MS, Shanbhag S, Chakraborty M, Phillips AR, Windsor JA. Organ failure and infection of pancreatic necrosis as determinants of mortality in patients with acute pancreatitis. *Gastroenterology*. 2010; 139: 813-820. PMID: 20540942.
7. Johnson CD, Abu-Hilal M. Persistent organ failure during the first week as a marker of fatal outcome in acute pancreatitis. *Gut*. 2004; 53: 1340-1344. PMID: 15306596.
8. Mofidi R, Duff MD, Wigmore SJ, Madhavan KK, Garden OJ, Parks RW. Association between early systemic inflammatory response, severity of multiorgan dysfunction and death in acute pancreatitis. *Br J Surg*. 2006; 93: 738-744. PMID: 16671062.
9. Guarner F, Malagelada JR. Gut flora in health and disease. *Lancet*. 2003; 361: 512-519. PMID: 12583961.
10. Lutgendorff F, Nijmeijer RM, Sandström PA, Trulsson LM, Magnusson KE, Timmerman HM, et al. Probiotics prevent intestinal barrier dysfunction in acute pancreatitis in rats via induction of ileal mucosal glutathione biosynthesis. *PLoS One*. 2009; 4: e4512. PMID: 19223985.
11. Ammori BJ, Fitzgerald P, Hawkey P, McMahon MJ. The early increase in intestinal permeability and systemic endotoxin exposure in patients with severe acute pancreatitis is not associated with systemic bacterial translocation: molecular investigation of microbial DNA in the blood. *Pancreas*. 2003; 26: 18-22. PMID: 12499912.
12. Mittal A, Phillips AR, Middleditch M, Ruggiero K, Loveday B, Delahunt B, et al. The proteome of mesenteric lymph during acute pancreatitis and implications for treatment. *JOP*. 2009; 10: 130-142. PMID: 19287105.
13. Villatoro E, Mulla M, Larvin M. Antibiotic therapy for prophylaxis against infection of pancreatic necrosis in acute pancreatitis. *Cochrane Database Syst Rev*. 2010; 5: CD002941. PMID: 20464721.
14. Jiang K, Huang W, Yang XN, Xia Q. Present and future of prophylactic antibiotics for severe acute pancreatitis. *World J Gastroenterol*. 2012; 18: 279-284. PMID: 22294832.
15. Bradley EL 3rd. Antibiotics in acute pancreatitis. Current status and future directions. *Am J Surg*. 1989; 158: 472-477. PMID: 2683821.
16. Johnson CD. Antibiotic prophylaxis in severe acute pancreatitis. *Br J Surg*. 1996; 83: 883-884. PMID: 8813769.
17. Golub R, Siddiqi F, Pohl D. Role of antibiotics in acute pancreatitis: A meta-analysis. *J Gastrointest Surg*. 1998; 2: 496-503. PMID: 10457308.
18. Powell JJ, Miles R, Siriwardena AK. Antibiotic prophylaxis in the initial management of severe acute pancreatitis. *Br J Surg*. 1998; 85: 582-587. PMID: 9635800.
19. Powell JJ, Campbell E, Johnson CD, Siriwardena AK. Survey of antibiotic prophylaxis in acute pancreatitis in the UK and Ireland. *Br J Surg*. 1999; 86: 320-322. PMID: 10201771.
20. Villatoro E, Bassi C, Larvin M. Antibiotic therapy for prophylaxis against infection of pancreatic necrosis in acute pancreatitis. *Cochrane Database Syst Rev*. 2006; 4: CD002941. PMID: 17054156.
21. Dellinger EP, Tellado JM, Soto NE, Ashley SW, Barie PS, Dugernier T, et al. Early antibiotic treatment for severe acute necrotizing pancreatitis: a randomized, double-blind, placebo-controlled study. *Ann Surg*. 2007; 245: 674-683. PMID: 17457158.
22. Røkke O, Harbitz TB, Liljedal J, Pettersen T, Fetvedt T, Heen LØ, et al. Early treatment of severe pancreatitis with imipenem: a prospective randomized clinical trial. *Scand J Gastroenterol*. 2007; 42: 771-776. PMID: 17506001.
23. Roquilly A, Marret E, Abraham E, Asehnoune K. Pneumonia prevention to decrease mortality in intensive care unit: a systematic review and meta-analysis. *Clin Infect Dis*. 2015; 60: 64-75. PMID: 25252684.
24. Luiten EJ, Hop WC, Lange JF, Bruining HA. Controlled clinical trial of selective decontamination for the treatment of severe acute pancreatitis. *Ann Surg*. 1995; 222: 57-65. PMID: 7618970.
25. FAO/WHO. *Health and Nutritional Properties of Probiotics in Food including Powder Milk with Live Lactic Acid Bacteria. Report of a Joint FAO/WHO Expert Consultation*

on Evaluation of Health and Nutritional Properties of Probiotics in Food Including Powder Milk with Live Lactic Acid Bacteria. Rome, Italy: FAO; 2001.

26. Servin AL. Antagonistic activities of lactobacilli and bifidobacteria against microbial pathogens. *FEMS Microbiol Rev.* 2004; 28: 405-440. PMID: 15374659.
27. Marco ML, Pavan S, Kleerebezem M. Towards understanding molecular modes of probiotic action. *Curr Opin Biotechnol.* 2006; 17: 204-210. PMID: 16510275.
28. Niers LE, Timmerman HM, Rijkers GT, van Bleek GM, van Uden NO, Knol EF, et al. Identification of strong interleukin-10 inducing lactic acid bacteria which down-regulate T helper type 2 cytokines. *Clin Exp Allergy.* 2005; 35: 1481-1489. PMID: 16297146.
29. van Minnen LP, Timmerman HM, Lutgendorff F, Verheem A, Harmsen W, Konstantinov SR, et al. Modification of intestinal flora with multispecies probiotics reduces bacterial translocation and improves clinical course in a rat model of acute pancreatitis. *Surgery.* 2007; 141: 470-480. PMID: 17383524.
30. Nomura T, Tsuchiya Y, Nashimoto A, Yabusaki H, Takii Y, Nakagawa S, et al. Probiotics reduce infectious complications after pancreaticoduodenectomy. *Hepatogastroenterology.* 2007; 54: 661-663. PMID: 17591036.
31. Rayes N, Seehofer D, Hansen S, Boucsein K, Muller AR, Serke S, et al. Early enteral supply of lactobacillus and fiber versus selective bowel decontamination: a controlled trial in liver transplant recipients. *Transplantation.* 2002; 74: 123-127. PMID: 12134110.
32. Sugawara G, Nagino M, Nishio H, Ebata T, Takagi K, Asahara T, et al. Perioperative synbiotic treatment to prevent postoperative infectious complications in biliary cancer surgery: a randomized controlled trial. *Ann Surg.* 2006; 244: 706-714. PMID: 17060763.
33. Olah A, Belagyi T, Issekutz A, Gamal ME, Bengmark S. Randomized clinical trial of specific lactobacillus and fibre supplement to early enteral nutrition in patients with acute pancreatitis. *Br J Surg.* 2002; 89: 1103-1107. PMID: 12190674.
34. Olah A, Belagyi T, Poto L, Romics L Jr, Bengmark S. Synbiotic control of inflammation and infection in severe acute pancreatitis: a prospective, randomized, double blind study. *Hepatogastroenterology.* 2007; 54: 590-594. PMID: 17523328.
35. Besselink MG, Van Santvoort HC, Buskens E, Boermeester MA, van GH,Timmerman HM, et al. Probiotic prophylaxis in predicted severe acute pancreatitis: a randomised, double-blind, placebo-controlled trial. *Lancet.* 2008; 371: 651-659. PMID: 18279948.
36. van Baal MC, Kohout P, Besselink MG, van Santvoort HC, Benes Z, Zazula R, et al. Probiotic treatment with Probioflora in patients with predicted severe acute pancreatitis without organ failure. *Pancreatology.* 2012; 12: 458-462. PMID: 23127536.
37. van Baal MC, van Rens MJ, Geven CB, van de Pol FM, van den Brink IW, Hannink G, et al. Association between probiotics and enteral nutrition in an experimental acute pancreatitis model in rats. *Pancreatology.* 2014; 14: 470-477. PMID: 25458667.

Chapter 27

Role of enteral and parenteral nutrition

Vinciane Rebours*

Pôle des Maladies de l'Appareil Digestif, Service de Pancréatologie, INSERM UMR1149. Hôpital Beaujon, 100 Boulevard du Général Leclerc, 92110 Clichy, France.

Introduction

Acute pancreatitis (AP) can be regarded as a hypercatabolic situation, and nutrition plays a key role in the treatment of this disease. When a patient's food intake is limited because of pancreatic pain, organ failure, or other complications, adapted nutrition support should be initiated early in AP management to decrease mortality and morbidity. Numerous studies and meta analysis are now available and the most appropriate modalities for artificial nutrition are well established.[1,2]

Pathophysiology

The importance of providing nutritional support in patients with severe AP has been well demonstrated and leads to decreased morbidity and mortality rates.[3,4] The main objectives are to provide adequate calories in this hypercatabolic condition and to decrease pancreatic necrosis infection.

The concept of "pancreatic rest" was developed many decades ago to decrease pancreatic inflammation. It suggests prolonged fasting in cases of mild pancreatitis and parenteral nutrition in case of severe pancreatitis to prevent stimulation of exocrine function and proteolytic enzyme release. However, it is now well known that parenteral nutrition leads to electrolyte and metabolic disturbances, gut barrier alterations, and increased intestinal permeability. Moreover, parenteral nutrition is not cost effective and may increase the risk of sepsis complications.[5-8]

Pancreatic infection and organ failure are determinants of AP severity. Gut barrier dysfunction and increased bacterial translocation are implicated in the development of secondary infection, sepsis, multiple organ failure, and death in AP. Studies have shown that microorganisms responsible for sepsis and pancreatic infection originate mainly from the digestive tract. Moreover, gut barrier dysfunction and the translocation of digestive bacteria into the portal venous system may cause multiple organ failure. Gut barrier dysfunction is characterized by damages of the gut epithelium and intestinal cell junctions, resulting in increased intestinal permeability.[9-12] Splanchnic hypoperfusion and ischemia/reperfusion injury have been postulated as possible causes. A decrease in splanchnic perfusion results in a concomitant decrease in oxygen delivery to the intestinal mucosa; this coupled with the consequences of reperfusion leads to histologic evidence of mucosal ischemia.[13,14] Loss of cell membrane integrity and cytoskeletal alterations during hypoperfusion result in cytoplasmic protein leakage. In the literature, only enteral nutrition has been shown to have significant clinical benefits in patients with AP in reducing the risks of developing pancreatic infections and multiple organ failure. Enteral nutrition may attenuate mucosal barrier breakdown and subsequent bacterial translocation. It also may increase intestinal motility and decrease bacterial overgrowth by facilitating bacteria clearance in the digestive tract.[15]

Indications of artificial nutrition

Artificial nutrition is often not initiated in mild pancreatitis;oral nutrition can be indicated after pain relief. Patients usually recover and are discharged after a few days. The recently published International Association of Pancreatology guidelines recommend oral feeding in predicted mild pancreatitis once abdominal pain is decreasing and inflammatory markers are improving.[1] A clinical trial showed that immediate oral refeeding with a normal diet is safe in predicted mild pancreatitis and leads to a shorter hospital stay (4 vs. 6 days).[16] Feeding can be started with a full solid diet without needing to first start with a liquid or soft diet.[17] Normalization of lipase levels is not required before restarting oral feeding.[18] Finally, international guidelines from gastroenterologic and pancreatic societies state that nutrition support is indicated when patients are

*Corresponding author. Email: vinciane.rebours@bjn.aphp.fr

not able to tolerate oral food for up to 7 days, regardless of disease severity.[1,19]

Patients who can eat do not require additional enteral nutrition via a feeding tube. However, artificial nutrition support can be supplemented in the specific situation of mild pancreatitis, notably in the setting of severe malnutrition, which is frequent in alcoholic patients. This nutrition support must be performed by nasoenteric tube feeding to minimize intravenous catheter infections and should be added to oral intake.

In patients with predicted severe pancreatitis, nutritional support should be the primary therapy and may begin within 48 hours. A recent clinical trial of 60 patients reported improved outcomes when nutrition was started within 48 h as compared to after 7 days of fasting.[20]

Type of artificial nutrition: parenteral versus enteral nutrition

Parenteral nutrition used to be the preferred option for the treatment of AP. This approach places patients on strict bowel rest and bypasses the stimulatory effects of oral feeding, leading to gastrointestinal atrophy with decreased villous thickness in the intestinal tract, which results in bacterial translocation across the gut barrier, sepsis, and organ failure.

The comparison of total parenteral nutrition and total enteral nutrition in patients with predicted severe AP was studied in more than eight randomized controlled trials.[21-28] Several meta-analyses have demonstrated the benefits of enteral over parenteral nutrition: a significant 2-twofold reduction in the risk of systemic and pancreatic infectious complications, a decrease of multiorgan failure, a reduction of the need for surgical interventions, and finally a 2.5-fold reduction in mortality risk in patients receiving exclusively enteral nutrition.[29-34]

Regarding the recently published international guidelines, parenteral nutrition can be used in AP as second-line therapy if nasojejunal tube feeding is not tolerated and nutritional support is required.[1] However, the authors proposed that parenteral nutrition should only be started if the nutritional goals cannot be reached with oral or enteral feeding. A delay up to 5 days in initiation of parenteral nutrition may be appropriate to allow for restarting of oral or enteral feeding.[34,35]

Optimal route of enteral nutrition delivery

This issue has been debated regarding the "pancreatic rest" theory. It was suggested that prepyloric delivery would stimulate pancreatic secretion and consequently increase AP severity. However, a postpyloric tube (mainly nasojejunal location) usually requires an endoscopic or radiologic procedure. This may delay nutritional support and can impact the clinical outcome. In contrast, a nasogastric feeding tube can be immediately inserted in everyday practice and does not require specific assistance. A prepyloric feeding (gastric location) can be started without delay.[3]

Pancreatic exocrine function and route of enteral nutrition delivery

Studies in healthy subjects have demonstrated that all types of oral feeding stimulate exocrine pancreatic secretion. In enteral nutrition,the exocrine pancreatic response varies depending on the nutrition delivery route. Trypsin and lipase secretion was significantly lower in response to nutrition delivered into the jejunum in comparison with the duodenum; this secretion was not different in subjects with distal jejunum delivery or the fasting group.[3,36]

Pancreatic exocrine function is not normal in AP, and the level of pancreatic secretions is decreased compared with healthy subjects. This pancreatic "stunning" is correlated with pancreatitis severity, and lower secretions of trypsin and lipase were found in patients with severe pancreatitis. These data suggest that acinar cells are not able to respond normally to a secretory stimulus during AP. This explains why no study has demonstrated that nasogastric tube can increase inflammation and AP severity.[37]

Safety and tolerance of enteral nutrition delivery route

Several randomized controlled trials and the latest published meta-analyses have demonstrated the equivalence of nasogastric and nasojejunal tube feeding regarding safety and tolerance.[27,38-46] A recently published review compared nasogastric and nasojejunal tube feeding. Four randomized controlled trials and a cohort study were included and represented 131 patients who received nasogastric tube feeding for severe pancreatitis. In 107/131 (82%) patients, total nasogastric nutrition was administered without withdrawal. In 18% of the patients, enteral nutrition was stopped because of gastric ileus, diarrhea, or repeatedly dislocated feeding tubes. A meta-analysis restricted to randomized studies included 82 and 75 patients with nasogastric and nasojejunal feeding, respectively. The risks of mortality and numbers of nutrition-associated adverse events were similar between the two groups. In that review, nasogastric tube feeding was not associated with an increased risk of aspiration pneumonia.[38]

A recent meta-analysis reported data from 3 randomized controlled trials including a total of 157 patients.

There were no significant differences in mortality, tracheal aspiration, diarrhea, pain exacerbation, or energy balance between the two groups. Nasogastric feeding was not inferior to nasojejunal feeding.[46]

The international guidelines recommend that enteral nutrition in AP can be administered via either the nasojejunal or nasogastric route.[1] The choice of the location should not delay the nutritional support. Nasogastric tube feeding is probably easier than nasojejunal tube feeding, however some patients will not tolerate nasogastric feeding because of delayed gastric emptying. It is known that patients with severe AP frequently present with gastric ileus because the pancreatic inflammation is close to the stomach. In addition, inflammation can lead to a transient duodenal stenosis (partial or complete). In this specific case, a nasojejunal tube feeding can be used and the tube should be placed endoscopically.

Enteral nutrition formulations

More than 100 different enteral nutrition formulations are available in 3 categories: elemental/semielemental, polymeric, and immunoenhanced (immunonutrition and probiotics). In AP, (semi)elemental nutrition is usually preferred over the polymeric formulation because it is supposed to have superior absorption from the intestine, less stimulation of pancreatic secretions,and a better tolerance.[47] A meta-analysis compared the safety and tolerance of different enteral nutrition formulations used in AP; 20 randomized controlled trials including 1,070 patients were selected. No significant difference was observed between the formulations regarding feeding tolerance, including the use of (semi)elemental versus polymeric formulation or versus supplementation of enteral nutrition with probiotics or immunonutrition. The risk of infectious complications and death did not differ significantly in any of the comparisons. The relatively inexpensive polymeric feeding formulations were associated with similar feeding tolerance and appeared as beneficial as the more expensive (semi)elemental formulations in reducing the risks of infectious complications and mortality.[48,49] Probiotics should not be used in acute pancreatitis because they were associated with a higher complication rate and mortality in one randomized trial.[50] International published guidelines recommend that either elemental or polymeric enteral nutrition formulations can be used in acute pancreatitis.[1]

Conclusion

Nutrition plays a key role in AP treatment. When food intake is impaired, an adapted nutritional support is required early in disease management to decrease mortality and morbidity. Several meta-analyses have been published, and the most appropriate modalities of artificial nutrition are well-established.Compared to parenteral nutrition, the enteral route has been shown to have a greater clinical benefit in patients with AP, reducing the risks of both pancreatic infection and multiple organ failure. The international guidelines recommend that enteral nutrition in AP can be administered via either the nasojejunal or nasogastric route, but the choice of administration route should not delay nutritional support. Either elemental or polymeric enteral nutrition formulations can be used in AP.

References

1. Working Group IAP/APA Acute Pancreatitis Guidelines. IAP/APA evidence-based guidelines for the management of acute pancreatitis. *Pancreatology*. 2013; 13(4 Suppl 2): e1-e15. PMID: 24054878.
2. Loveday BP, Srinivasa S, Vather R, Mittal A, Petrov MS, Phillips AR, et al. High quantity and variable quality of guidelines for acute pancreatitis: a systematic review. *Am J Gastroenterol*. 2010; 105(7): 1466-1476. PMID: 20606652.
3. O'Keefe SJ, McClave SA. Feeding the injured pancreas. *Gastroenterology*. 2005; 129(3): 1129-1130. PMID: 16143153.
4. Ioannidis O, Lavrentieva A, Botsios D. Nutrition support in acute pancreatitis. *JOP*. 2008; 9(4): 375-390. PMID: 18648127.
5. Wu LM, Sankaran SJ, Plank LD, Windsor JA, Petrov MS. Meta-analysis of gut barrier dysfunction in patients with acute pancreatitis. *Br J Surg*. 2014; 101(13): 1644-1656. PMID: 25334028.
6. Brandtzaeg P, Halstensen TS, Kett K, Krajci P, Kvale D, Rognum TO, et al. Immunobiology and immunopathology of human gut mucosa: humoral immunity and intraepithelial lymphocytes. *Gastroenterology*. 1989; 97(6): 1562-1584. PMID: 2684725.
7. Liu H, Li W, Wang X, Li J, Yu W. Early gut mucosal dysfunction in patients with acute pancreatitis. *Pancreas*. 2008; 36(2): 192-196. PMID: 18376312.
8. Capurso G, Zerboni G, Signoretti M, Valente R, Stigliano S, Piciucchi M, et al. Role of the gut barrier in acute pancreatitis. *J Clin Gastroenterol*. 2012; 46 Suppl: S46-S51. PMID: 22955357.
9. Ammori BJ. Gut barrier dysfunction in patients with acute pancreatitis. *J Hepatobiliary Pancreat Surg*. 2002; 9(4): 411-412. PMID: 12483261.
10. Ammori BJ, Leeder PC, King RF, Barclay GR, Martin IG, Larvin M, et al. Early increase in intestinal permeability in patients with severe acute pancreatitis: correlation with endotoxemia, organ failure, and mortality. *Gastrointest Surg*. 1999; 3(3): 252-262. PMID: 10481118.
11. Ralls MW, Demehri FR, Feng Y, Woods Ignatoski KM, Teitelbaum DH. Enteral nutrient deprivation in patients leads to a loss of intestinal epithelial barrier function. *Surgery*. 2015; 157(4): 732-742. PMID: 25704423.
12. Rahman SH, Ammori BJ, Holmfield J, Larvin M, McMahon MJ. Intestinal hypoperfusion contributes to gut barrier failure

in severe acute pancreatitis. *J Gastrointest Surg*. 2003; 7(1): 26-35; discussion 35-36. PMID: 12559182.
13. Kovacs GC, Telek G, Hamar J, Furesz J, Regoly-Merei J. Prolonged intestinal mucosal acidosis is associated with multiple organ failure in human acute pancreatitis: gastric tonometry revisited. *World J Gastroenterol*. 2006; 12(30): 4892-2896. PMID: 16937476.
14. Zou XP, Chen M, Wei W, Cao J, Chen L, Tian M. Effects of enteral immunonutrition on the maintenance of gut barrier function and immune function in pigs with severe acute pancreatitis. *J Parenter Enteral Nutr*. 2010; 34(5): 554-566. PMID: 20852186.
15. Powell JJ, Murchison JT, Fearon KC, Ross JA, Siriwardena AK. Randomized controlled trial of the effect of early enteral nutrition on markers of the inflammatory response in predicted severe acute pancreatitis. *Br J Surg*. 2000; 87(10): 1375-1381. PMID: 11044164.
16. Eckerwall GE, Tingstedt BB, Bergenzaun PE, Andersson RG. Immediate oral feeding in patients with mild acute pancreatitis is safe and may accelerate recovery--a randomized clinical study. *Clin Nutr*. 2007; 26(6): 758-763. PMID: 17719703.
17. Moraes JM, Felga GE, Chebli LA, Franco MB, Gomes CA, Gaburri PD, et al. A full solid diet as the initial meal in mild acute pancreatitis is safe and result in a shorter length of hospitalization: results from a prospective, randomized, controlled, double-blind clinical trial. *J Clin Gastroenterol*. 2010; 44(7): 517-522. PMID: 20054282.
18. Teich N, Aghdassi A, Fischer J, Walz B, Caca K, Wallochny T, et al. Optimal timing of oral refeeding in mild acute pancreatitis: results of an open randomized multicenter trial. *Pancreas*. 2010; 39(7): 1088-1092. PMID: 20357692.
19. Banks PA, Freeman ML; Practice Parameters Committee of the American College of Gastroenterology. Practice guidelines in acute pancreatitis. *Am J Gastroenterol*. 2006; 101(10): 2379-2400. PMID: 17032204.
20. Sun JK, Mu XW, Li WQ, Tong ZH, Li J, Zheng SY. Effects of early enteral nutrition on immune function of severe acute pancreatitis patients. *World J Gastroenterol*. 2013; 19(6): 917-922. PMID: 23431120.
21. Windsor AC, Kanwar S, Li AG, Barnes E, Guthrie JA, Spark JI, et al. Compared with parenteral nutrition, enteral feeding attenuates the acute phase response and improves disease severity in acute pancreatitis. *Gut*. 2005; 42(3): 431-435. PMID: 9577354.
22. Pupelis G, Austrums E, Jansone A, Sprucs R, Wehbi H. Randomised trial of safety and efficacy of postoperative enteral feeding in patients with severe pancreatitis: preliminary report. *Eur J Surg*. 2000; 166(5): 383-387. PMID: 10881949.
23. Pupelis G, Selga G, Austrums E, Kaminski A. Jejunal feeding, even when instituted late, improves outcomes in patients with severe pancreatitis and peritonitis. *Nutrition*. 2001; 17(2): 91-94. PMID: 11240334.
24. Kalfarentzos F, Kehagias J, Mead N, Kokkinis K, Gogos CA. Enteral nutrition superior to parenteral nutrition in severe acute pancreatitis: results of a randomized prospective trial. *Br J Surg*. 1997; 84(12): 1665-1669. PMID: 9448611.
25. Gupta R, Patel K, Calder PC, Yaqoob P, Primrose JN, Johnson CD. A randomised clinical trial to assess the effect of total enteral and total parenteral nutritional support on metabolic, inflammatory and oxidative markers in patients with predicted severe acute pancreatitis (APACHE II $\geq$ 6). *Pancreatology*. 2003; 3(5): 406-413. PMID: 14526151.
26. Eckerwall GE, Axelsson JB, Andersson RG. Early nasogastric feeding in predicted severe acute pancreatitis: A clinical, randomized study. *Ann Surg*. 2006; 244(6): 959-965. PMID: 17122621.
27. Jiang K, Chen XZ, Xia Q, Tang WF, Wang L. Early nasogastric enteral nutrition for severe acute pancreatitis: a systematic review. *World J Gastroenterol*. 2007; 13(39): 5253-5260. PMID: 17876897.
28. Abou-Assi S, Craig K, O'Keefe SJ. Hypocaloric jejunal feeding is better than total parenteral nutrition in acute pancreatitis: results of a randomized comparative study. *Am J Gastroenterol*. 2002; 97(9): 2255-2262. PMID: 12358242.
29. McClave SA, Chang WK, Dhaliwal R, Heyland DK. Nutrition support in acute pancreatitis: a systematic review of the literature. *J Parenter Enteral Nutr*. 2006; 30(2): 143-156. PMID: 16517959.
30. Petrov MS, van Santvoort HC, Besselink MG, van der Heijden GJ, Windsor JA, Gooszen HG. Enteral nutrition and the risk of mortality and infectious complications in patients with severe acute pancreatitis: a meta-analysis of randomized trials. *Arch Surg*. 2008; 143(11): 1111-1117. PMID: 19015471.
31. Yi F, Ge L, Zhao J, Lei Y, Zhou F, Chen Z, et al. Meta-analysis: total parenteral nutrition versus total enteral nutrition in predicted severe acute pancreatitis. *Intern Med*. 2012; 51(6): 523-530. PMID: 22449657.
32. Quan H, Wang X, Guo C. A meta-analysis of enteral nutrition and total parenteral nutrition in patients with acute pancreatitis. *Gastroenterol Res Pract*. 2011; 2011: 698248. PMID: 21687619.
33. Petrov MS, Whelan K. Comparison of complications attributable to enteral and parenteral nutrition in predicted severe acute pancreatitis: a systematic review and meta-analysis. *Br J Nutr*. 2010; 103(9): 1287-1295. PMID: 20370944.
34. Al-Omran M, Albalawi ZH, Tashkandi MF, Al-Ansary LA. Enteral versus parenteral nutrition for acute pancreatitis. *Cochrane Database Syst Rev*. 2010; (1): CD002837. PMID: 20091534.
35. Mirtallo JM, Forbes A, McClave SA, Jensen GL, Waitzberg DL, Davies AR. International Consensus Guideline Committee Pancreatitis Task Force. International consensus guidelines for nutrition therapy in pancreatitis. *J Parenter Enteral Nutr*. 2012; 36(3): 284-291. PMID: 22457421.
36. O'Keefe SJ, Lee RB, Anderson FP, Gennings C, Abou-Assi S, Clore J, et al. Physiological effects of enteral and parenteral feeding on pancreaticobiliary secretion in humans. *Am J Physiol Gastrointest Liver Physiol*. 2003; 284(1): G27-G36. PMID: 12488233.
37. Boreham B, Ammori BJ. A prospective evaluation of pancreatic exocrine function in patients with acute pancreatitis: correlation with extent of necrosis and pancreatic endocrine insufficiency. *Pancreatology*. 2003; 3(4): 303-308. PMID: 12890992.
38. Nally DM, Kelly EG, Clarke M, Ridgway P. Nasogastric nutrition is efficacious in severe acute pancreatitis: a systematic review and meta-analysis. *Br J Nutr*. 2014; 112(11): 1769-1778. PMID: 25333639.

39. Petrov MS, Correia MI, Windsor JA. Nasogastric tube feeding in predicted severe acute pancreatitis. A systematic review of the literature to determine safety and tolerance. *JOP*. 2008; 9(4): 440-448. PMID: 18648135.
40. Eatock FC, Brombacher GD, Steven A, Imrie CW, McKay CJ, Carter R. Nasogastric feeding in severe acute pancreatitis may be practical and safe. *Int J Pancreatol*. 2000; 28(1): 23-29. PMID: 11185707.
41. Jiyong J, Tiancha H, Huiqin W, Jingfen J. Effect of gastric versus post-pyloric feeding on the incidence of pneumonia in critically ill patients: observations from traditional and Bayesian random-effects meta-analysis. *Clin Nutr*. 2013; 32(1): 8-15. PMID: 22853861.
42. Eatock FC, Chong P, Menezes N, Murray L, McKay CJ, Carter CR, et al. A randomized study of early nasogastric versus nasojejunal feeding in severe acute pancreatitis. *Am J Gastroenterol*. 2005; 100(2): 432-439. PMID: 15667504.
43. Kumar A, Singh N, Prakash S, Saraya A, Joshi YK. Early enteral nutrition in severe acute pancreatitis: a prospective randomized controlled trial comparing nasojejunal and nasogastric routes. *J Clin Gastroenterol*. 2006; 40(5): 431-434. PMID: 16721226.
44. Singh N, Sharma B, Sharma M, Sachdev V, Bhardwaj P, Mani K, et al. Evaluation of early enteral feeding through nasogastric and nasojejunal tube in severe acute pancreatitis: a noninferiority randomized controlled trial. *Pancreas*. 2012; 41(1): 153-159. PMID: 21775915.
45. Marik PE, Zaloga GP. Gastric versus post-pyloric feeding: a systematic review. *Crit Care*. 2003; 7(3): R46-R51. PMID: 12793890.
46. Chang YS, Fu HQ, Xiao YM, Liu JC. Nasogastric or nasojejunal feeding in predicted severe acute pancreatitis: a meta-analysis. *Crit Care*. 2013; 17(3): R118. PMID: 23786708.
47. Duerksen DR, Bector S, Parry D, Yaffe C, Vajcner A, Lipschitz J. A comparison of the effect of elemental and immune-enhancing polymeric jejunal feeding on exocrine pancreatic function. *J Parenter Enteral Nutr*. 2002; 26(3): 205-208. PMID: 12005463.
48. Petrov MS, Loveday BP, Pylypchuk RD, McIlroy K, Phillips AR, Windsor JA. Systematic review and meta-analysis of enteral nutrition formulations in acute pancreatitis. *Br J Surg*. 2009; 96(11): 1243-1252. PMID: 19847860.
49. Tiengou LE, Gloro R, Pouzoulet J, Bouhier K, Read MH, Arnaud-Battandier F, et al. Semi-elemental formula or polymeric formula: is there a better choice for enteral nutrition in acute pancreatitis? Randomized comparative study. *J Parenter Enteral Nutr*. 2006; 30(1): 1-5.
50. Besselink MG, van Santvoort HL, Buskens E, Boermeester MA, van Goor H, Timmerman HM, et al. Probiotic prophylaxis in predicted severe acute pancreatitis: a randomised, double-blind, Placebo-controlled trial. *Lancet*. 2008; 371: 651-659. PMID: 18279948.

Chapter 28

Endoscopic treatment of infected necrosis

Robbert A. Hollemans[1,2], Martin L. Freeman[3], and Hjalmar C. van Santvoort[1,2*]

[1]*Dept. of Surgery, Academic Medical Center, Amsterdam, The Netherlands;*
[2]*Dept. of Surgery, St Antonius Hospital, Nieuwegein, The Netherlands;*
[3]*Division of Gastroenterology, Department of Medicine, University of Minnesota, Minneapolis, Minnesota, USA.*

Introduction

Acute pancreatitis is complicated by necrosis of the pancreas or peripancreatic tissue in around 20% of patients.[1,2] Necrotizing pancreatitis can often be treated successfully with a conservative approach, without the need for invasive intervention.[3-5] In a subset of patients, however, there is a need for a more aggressive regimen that includes invasive intervention. The primary indication for this is bacterial infection of peripancreatic collections with walled-off necrosis, which occurs in around 30% of patients with necrotizing pancreatitis.[3-5] Indications for invasive intervention in sterile necrosis include mechanical obstruction of the biliary or gastrointestinal tract, persisting abdominal discomfort, and failure to thrive caused by persisting necrotic collections beyond 8 weeks after acute attack onset.[3,5]

The traditional approach to infected walled-off necrosis has long been primary laparotomy with complete debridement of pancreatic and peripancreatic necrosis. This surgical approach of primary "open necrosectomy" is associated with a high risk of complications and death.[6] In the last decade, minimally invasive procedures have gained popularity. Recent guidelines now advocate the use of a step-up approach, consisting of catheter drainage, followed only if necessary by necrosectomy.[3,5] The aim of catheter drainage as a first step is to temporize sepsis by releasing infected fluid from the peripancreatic collections. This may improve the patient's clinical condition and thereby postpone or even obviate the need for further intervention.[7,8] Catheter drainage can be performed percutaneously under guidance of ultrasound or computed tomography or endoscopically through the wall of the stomach or duodenum.[3-5]

If the patient's clinical condition does not improve after catheter drainage, necrosectomy can be performed through laparotomy, laparoscopy, a minimally invasive retroperitoneal approach, or by an endoscopic transluminal approach. This chapter focuses on the technique and the results of published studies on endoscopic drainage and necrosectomy.

Technical aspects

Endoscopic drainage and necrosectomy can be performed under conscious sedation using midazolam or propofol and fentanyl. As a first step, linear-array endoscopic ultrasound is performed to visualize the walled-off necrosis and identify the optimal route for puncture through the posterior wall of the stomach or duodenum. This is facilitated by finding the collection bulging into the stomach or duodenum. Under endoscopic ultrasound guidance, the collection is punctured using a 19-gauge needle. The stylette is withdrawn, and the content of the collection is aspirated to confirm the correct position. A guidewire is then advanced through the needle under fluoroscopic guidance. The outer sheath of a cystgastrostomy is advanced using electrocautery, and balloon dilatation of the puncture tract is performed up to 15 mm. The aspirate is sent for microbiological culturing, after which rigorous irrigation of the collection is performed using normal saline. As a next step, for the traditional approach, two or more double-pigtail plastic stents (size varying from 5 to 10 French [Fr]) are placed in the cystgastrostomy. A nasocystic catheter may be positioned in the space of the walled-off necrosis, which can be used for continuous irrigation of the collection with at least 1 L normal saline/24 hours to secure cystgastrostomy patency. Although obvious, it must be stressed that flushing with large amounts of fluid is not possible as the nasocystic catheter is only for inflow (i.e., all fluids are considered as intake and must be accounted for as such). Many centers do not routinely place nasocystic drains; rather, they perform

*Corresponding author. Email: h.vansantvoort@pancreatitis.nl

repeated endoscopic intervention or flushing via an adjunctive retroperitoneal percutaneous catheter, which allows "one-way" irrigation through the endoscopic cystenterostomy into the stomach or duodenum.[9]

The effects of endoscopic drainage on the clinical condition of the patient are followed for the next 72 hours. A new endoscopic procedure is planned if there is no clinical improvement (i.e., decreased need for organ supportive therapy, disappearance of fever and improvement of vital signs, or decreased serum C-reactive protein and white blood cell count).[8]

If a subsequent endoscopic procedure is performed and a traditional style of double pigtail stents is utilized, the endoluminal access site is dilated up to 15 to 20 mm using a dilatation balloon. A forward-viewing endoscope is advanced in the collection, and the necrosectomy is performed. The pancreatic and peripancreatic necrotic tissue can be evacuated with several instruments such as a basket, polypectomy snare, or grasping forceps. At the end of the procedure, several double-pigtail plastic stents (5 to 10 Fr) are placed in the collection, and irrigation is continued. Endoscopic necrosectomy is repeated as needed in the subsequent days, depending on the amount of necrosis left in the collection and the patient's clinical condition. The steps of transgastric necrosectomy are illustrated in **Figure 1**, and a video of the procedure is available at http://www.jama.com.[10]

Results from published studies

Case series

Since endoscopic necrosectomy was introduced to treat necrotizing pancreatitis, numerous case series have been published. Two systematic reviews on endoscopic necrosectomy including these cohorts stated that it is an effective and safe treatment option.[11,12] The more recent systematic review included 14 studies published up to June 2013, with a total of 455 patients.[11] The primary intervention was endoscopic drainage of the necrotic collection in 92% of patients at a mean of 57 days after the diagnosis of acute pancreatitis. Drainage was followed by endoscopic necrosectomy at a mean of 7 days. Complications occurred in 36% of patients, with bleeding (18%), perforation of a hollow organ other than the stomach or duodenum due to the intervention itself (4%), and pancreatic fistulae (5%) being the most predominant. Endoscopic necrosectomy was clinically successful, i.e. the condition was treated by endoscopic procedures alone in 81% of patients with a mean of four endoscopic procedures per patient.

The remaining patients needed additional percutaneous or surgical intervention to treat the pancreatic necrosis or complications from endoscopic necrosectomy. Overall mortality was 6% (range 0%-15%).[11] More recent and relatively large case series (n = 57 and 176) on the endoscopic treatment of necrotizing pancreatitis reported similar results regarding the number of endoscopic procedures (2 to 5), clinical success rate (76%-94%) and mortality (0%-11%) to those reported in the systematic review.[13-17] The types of complications in these newer series are also similar and include bleeding, pneumoperitoneum, perforation of a hollow organ, and infection, but their occurrence seemed to decrease with a reported incidence of 3% to 33%.[13-17]

Selection bias is a limitation of most case series. Endoscopic necrosectomy series often only include patients felt to be suitable for endoscopic drainage and necrosectomy, such as those with well-demarcated necrotic collections in close apposition to the gastric or duodenal lumen and without deep retroperitoneal or pelvic extension.

Comparative studies

Few studies compare endoscopic treatment with percutaneous/surgical treatment for necrotizing pancreatitis, and the indications for interventions are diverse. A retrospective analysis of 20 patients undergoing endoscopic necrosectomy compared with 20 patients undergoing surgical necrosectomy for symptomatic sterile pancreatic necrosis showed no significant differences in mortality or complications.[18] Patients in the endoscopic group underwent more reinterventions (9 vs. 3 patients), had a shorter length of hospital stay (3 vs. 7 days) and a longer time to resolution of the necrotic collection (3.6 vs. 0.4 months). Another retrospective analysis included 62 patients (30 open necrosectomy, 14 minimally invasive retroperitoneal necrosectomy, and 18 endoscopic necrosectomy) and showed lower severe complication and mortality rates for endoscopic necrosectomy.[19] However, significant baseline differences on disease severity and necrosis infection were evident, which restricts judgment on comparisons.

One prospective registry study matched 12 patients undergoing endoscopic necrosectomy with 12 patients undergoing the surgical step-up approach for suspected or confirmed infected walled-off necrosis.[20] In the surgical step-up group, three patients only required catheter drainage, and nine underwent subsequent minimally invasive surgical necrosectomy. One patient in the endoscopic group needed additional percutaneous drainage of an endoscopically inaccessible necrotic collection. Patients in the endoscopic necrosectomy group experienced fewer severe complications (1 vs. 7) and less postprocedural new-onset organ failure. Furthermore, endocrine insufficiency was less frequent in the endoscopically treated group during follow-up (0 vs. 7). One patient in the surgical group died.[20]

A randomized trial that included 20 patients and compared endoscopic necrosectomy with surgical necrosectomy

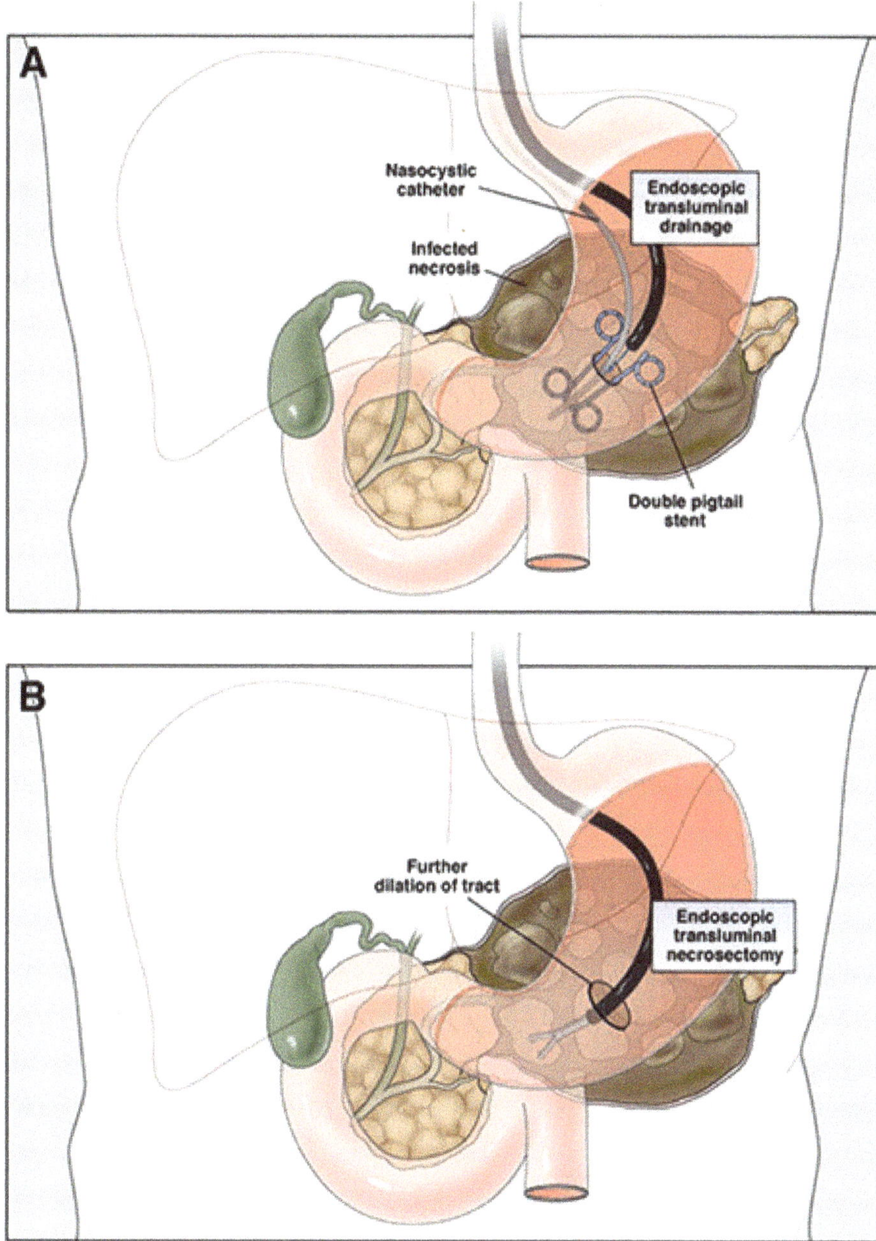

Figure 1. Endoscopic drainage and necrosectomy. The image depicts a peripancreatic collection of walled-off fluid and necrosis. The collection is identified behind the posterior gastric wall through bulging into the gastric lumen and endoscopic ultrasound. (A) Endoscopic drainage: The collection is punctured, and the balloon is dilated. Double pigtail stents and a nasocystic catheter drain are placed for continuous irrigation and to secure cystgastrostomy patency. (B) Endoscopic necrosectomy: The tract is dilated by 15-20 mm, and endoscopic necrosectomy is performed with grasping forceps (shown) or other endoscopic necrosectomy instruments. (From ref 36).

for infected walled-off necrosis showed that the primary endpoint of postprocedural proinflammatory response measured by serum interleukin 6 was significantly lower in the endoscopically treated group. The trial also reported lower incidence rates of post procedural new-onset organ failure (0% vs. 50%) and pancreatic fistulae (10% vs. 70%) in the endoscopic group.[21]

Innovation

The endoscopic techniques are subject to rapid development. Recently, several series have been published using single, lumen-apposing, self-expandable metal stents as a substitute for the multiple 5- to 10-Fr pigtail stents that are placed in the cystgastrostomy.[22-26] The stents are saddle shaped and equipped with bilateral double-walled

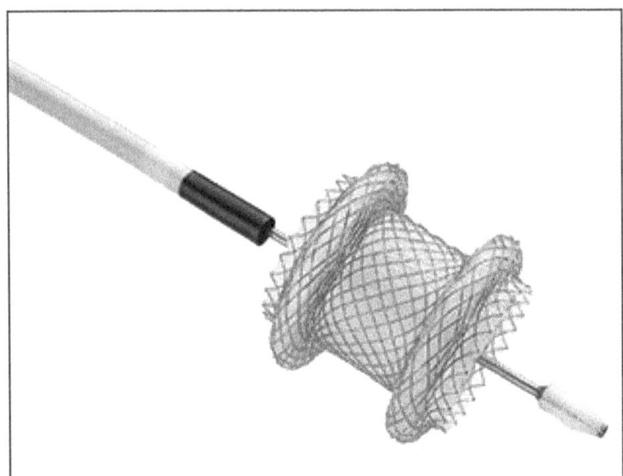

Figure 2. Lumen-apposing self-expandable metal stent.

anchoring flanges designed to hold the gastrointestinal wall in direct apposition to the wall of the pancreatic collection (**Figure 2**).[25,27] Their length is 10 mm and they are available in 10- or 15-mm diameters, the latter being more suitable if necrosectomy is anticipated. These stents, specifically designed to be delivered via endoscopic ultrasound, are easily deployed, and direct endoscopic necrosectomy can be performed through the stent after primary drainage of the pancreatic collection, if necessary. The stent can be left in situ for additional necrosectomies in the following days or weeks.[24,25] Clinical outcomes are similar to recent studies using a traditional endoscopic approach, with a 86%-88% clinical success rate with endoscopic intervention alone.

Major complications include bleeding, infection, stent migration and stent occlusion and occur in 7%-13% of patients. Two large retrospective studies (n = 124 and 68) reported no mortality.[24,25] The advantages of metallic stents are of particular interest for treating necrotizing pancreatitis in children. Specifically this young and fragile patient group may benefit from the high patency of the stent, easy access to the collection, possible need for less interventions, and the absence of external fistulae.[28] Given the fact that these interventions are infrequently performed in children, treatment is reserved for specialist centers.[28]

Another alternative to the traditional approach of endoscopic drainage and double pigtail stent placement is the use of a fully covered, large-bore, esophageal metal stent. The stent is placed directly following primary endoscopic ultrasound-guided drainage of large necrotic collections. The flares at both ends limit migration, and the large diameter (up to 23 mm) facilitates drainage and instrumental access for necrosectomy. Due to its size, the stent is limited to transgastric (as opposed to transduodenal) drainage and necrosectomy. Results of case series are preliminary but suggest that these stents are particularly useful for larger necrotic collections when the need for repeated endoscopic intervention is expected.[29,30]

Discussion

In this chapter we presented an overview of the indication, technique, and primary structured results of the latest and most innovative invasive treatment strategy for necrotizing pancreatitis. The endoscopic approach appears to measure up to surgical techniques in terms of choice of primary and definitive treatment, number of complications, healthcare utilization, and cost.[11,18,20,31] Available studies even suggest lower mortality rates and a lower incidence of new onset endocrine insufficiency.[11,13-17,20]

Endoscopic intervention carries a number of advantages over surgical techniques. First, the procedure can be performed under conscious sedation, obviating the need for general anesthesia, which is known to induce or prolong systemic inflammatory response syndrome in critically ill patients.[32] Second, a lumbotomy or laparotomy is avoided by creating an internal fistula between the necrotic collection and gastrointestinal lumen as a drainage and necrosectomy gateway. External fistulae, which can be cumbersome to reverse, are thereby nonexistent if endoscopic therapy is successful without additional percutaneous or surgical interventions. There is special interest for the endoscopic approach for treatment of disconnected pancreatic duct syndrome with pancreatic fluid collections obstructing the biliary tree or gastrointestinal tract. By internally bypassing the disrupted natural drainage canal of the exocrine pancreas to the stomach or duodenum, the pancreatic juices are not lost, bothersome external fistulae from percutaneous catheters are prevented, and extensive surgery with alteration of the intestinal anatomy and loss of functional pancreatic tissue is avoided.[33] It must be stressed however, that interventions for sterile collections after necrotizing pancreatitis are preferably delayed to more than 8 weeks after the acute attack as symptoms are known to spontaneously regress over time.[5] Third, with endoscopic intervention, the integrity of the abdominal wall remains intact, which prevents wound infections, debilitating incisional hernias, and unsightly scars. As opposed to surgical procedures such as video-assisted retroperitoneal debridement and sinus tract necrosectomy, endoscopic treatment of necrotizing pancreatitis can therefore be called "truly minimally invasive."

A limitation of the endoscopic approach is that, in order for the endoscopist to safely enter, the necrotic collection must adjoin the lumen of the stomach or duodenum. Not every patient with necrotizing pancreatitis in need for invasive intervention is therefore suited for this treatment. However, due to the anatomic relation of the pancreas with the stomach and duodenum, it is likely that the vast majority of necrotic collections can be reached endoscopically. The positive side of this limitation is that in some cases the endoscopic route is preferred, as large vessels and the kidney, spleen, stomach, and intestine can complicate the surgical route toward the centrally located walled-off necrosis. A second limitation of the endoscopic technique is that complications such as perforations and bleeding can be difficult to manage. Perforation often requires additional surgical intervention that partly nullifies the benefits of primary endoscopic treatment.[11,13] Small bleeds can often be controlled endoscopically by clipping, thermal coagulation, or local epinephrine injection. Persistent bleeding requires more definite treatment, in which angiographic coiling of the artery is the treatment of choice, and emergency laparotomy with its associated surgical disadvantages is the last resort.[11] Thirdly, endoscopic drainage and necrosectomy are challenging due to the small anatomical space in which the endoscopist must operate, indirect vision, and limited options for simultaneous tool use. The procedure can therefore only be executed by an experienced endoscopist with access to advanced instruments. This, combined with the fact that necrotizing pancreatitis is relatively rare and invasive interventions are not performed frequently, means that the endoscopic approach is reserved for specialist centers. Finally, for treatment success with endoscopic necrosectomy, an average of four procedures per patient are necessary as opposed to one to three for minimally invasive surgical and open necrosectomy.[8,11,31] Although not necessarily associated with higher costs, this can be a significant burden on the patient and their relatives, as well as on healthcare resources.

Advantages and options for improving technical aspects of the endoscopic approach are evident and outcomes in treatment of necrotizing pancreatitis are promising.[9] This seems to justify the increasing role of endoscopy in treating this condition. However, reports on endoscopic treatment for necrotizing pancreatitis included patients that are generally less ill than patients treated in studies reporting on surgical procedures. This is indicated by lower Acute Physiology and Chronic Health Evaluation (APACHE)-II scores, less organ failure, and less infected necrosis in the endoscopic studies.[11,31] These differences may partly explain the more favorable outcomes of endoscopy. On the other hand, it is likely that less invasive interventions in necrotizing pancreatitis induce less surgical, proinflammatory stress and could thereby lead to better outcomes. A decreased proinflammatory response after less invasive intervention was already shown in a randomized trial comparing endoscopic with surgical necrosectomy.[21] This trial also reported fewer complications for the endoscopy group but was not powered for clinical endpoints. Another randomized controlled multicenter trial, adequately powered for clinical endpoints, compared a minimally invasive surgical step-up approach with primary open necrosectomy in infected necrotizing pancreatitis. Patients in the (less invasive) step-up group experienced less postprocedural new-onset organ failure, underwent fewer operations, and had fewer incisional hernias and less new-onset endocrine and exocrine insufficiency at the 6-month follow-up.[2] It could be that the less invasive nature of endoscopic treatment translates to equal or even better outcomes than minimally invasive surgical necrosectomy. Comparative studies on this matter are scarce and include small numbers of patients, and bias is likely due to the mostly retrospective study design.[18-21] A randomized controlled multicenter (TENSION) trial in the Netherlands is comparing the transluminal endoscopic step-up approach and minimally invasive surgical step-up approach (controlled trials ISRCTN09186711).[34] This direct comparison in 98 patients with infected necrotizing pancreatitis will answer the question whether endoscopic step-up treatment is superior to surgical step-up treatment on the combined endpoint of death/major complications. A randomized controlled trial on the outcome death alone will most likely never be performed due to the complexity and rarity of the disease. Therefore an international collaboration between pancreatic specialist centers worldwide was founded to pool the results of individual participant data undergoing necrosectomy for necrotizing pancreatitis. The protocol for this study is prospectively registered at the PROSPERO registry for systematic reviews (CRD42014008995) and is available online.[35] Both the randomized TENSION trial and individual participant data meta-analysis are being finalized, and results are expected by the end of 2016.

Conclusion

In conclusion, endoscopic transluminal drainage and necrosectomy is a rapidly developing and increasingly popular technique in the treatment of necrotizing pancreatitis. Results from numerous case series and small comparative studies are promising, but evidence from adequately powered trials or studies with robust methodological quality are needed. Results of a large multicenter randomized controlled trial and an international meta-analysis of individual participant data are pending.

References

1. Banks PA, Bollen TL, Dervenis C, Gooszen HG, Johnson CD, Sarr MG, et al. Classification of acute pancreatitis--2012: revision of the Atlanta classification and definitions by international consensus. *Gut*. 2013; 62: 102-111. PMID: 23100216.
2. van Santvoort HC, Bakker OJ, Bollen TL, Besselink MG, Ahmed Ali U, Schrijver AM, et al. A conservative and minimally invasive approach to necrotizing pancreatitis improves outcome. *Gastroenterology*. 2011; 141: 1254-1263. PMID: 21741922.
3. Tenner S, Baillie J, DeWitt J, Vege SS; American College of Gastroenterology. American College of Gastroenterology guideline: management of acute pancreatitis. *Am J Gastroenterol*. 2013; 108: 1400-1415; 1416. PMID: 23896955.

4. Whitcomb DC. Clinical practice. Acute pancreatitis. *N Engl J Med*. 2006; 354: 2142-2150. PMID: 16707751.
5. Working Group IAP/APA Acute Pancreatitis Guidelines. IAP/APA evidence-based guidelines for the management of acute pancreatitis. *Pancreatology*. 2013; 13 4 Suppl 2: e1-e15. PMID: 24054878.
6. Mier J, Leon EL, Castillo A, Robledo F, Blanco R. Early versus late necrosectomy in severe necrotizing pancreatitis. *Am J Surg*. 1997; 173: 71-75. PMID: 9074366.
7. van Baal MC,van Santvoort HC, Bollen TL, Bakker OJ, Besselink MG, Gooszen HG, et al. Systematic review of percutaneous catheter drainage as primary treatment for necrotizing pancreatitis. *Br J Surg*. 2011; 98: 18-27. PMID: 21136562.
8. van Santvoort HC, Besselink MG, Bakker OJ, Hofker HS, Boermeester MA, Dejong CH, et al. A step-up approach or open necrosectomy for necrotizing pancreatitis. *N Engl J Med*. 2010; 362: 1491-1502. PMID: 20410514.
9. Trikudanathan G, Attam R, Arain MA, Mallery S, Freeman ML. Endoscopic interventions for necrotizing pancreatitis. *Am J Gastroenterol*. 2014; 109: 969-981; quiz 982. PMID: 24957157.
10. Endoscopic Transgastric Necrosectomy. Available at: http://jama.jamanetwork.com/multimediaPlayer.aspx?mediaid=2522044. Accessed July 12, 2016.
11. van Brunschot S, Fockens P, Bakker OJ, Besselink MG, Voermans RP, Poley JW, et al. Endoscopic transluminal necrosectomy in necrotising pancreatitis: a systematic review. *Surg Endosc*. 2014; 28: 1425-1438. PMID: 24399524.
12. Haghshenasskashani A, Laurence JM, Kwan V, Johnston E, Hollands MJ, Richardson AJ, et al. Endoscopic necrosectomy of pancreatic necrosis: a systematic review. *Surg Endosc*. 2011; 25: 3724-3730. PMID: 21656324.
13. Bang JY, Holt BA, Hawes RH, Hasan MK, Arnoletti JP, Christein JD, et al. Outcomes after implementing a tailored endoscopic step-up approach to walled-off necrosis in acute pancreatitis. *Br J Surg*. 2014; 101: 1729-1738. PMID: 25333872.
14. Jagielski M, Smoczyński M, Jabłońska A, Marek I, Dubowik M, Adrych K. The role of endoscopic ultrasonography in endoscopic debridement of walled-off pancreatic necrosis--A single center experience. *Pancreatology*. 2015; 15: 503-507. PMID: 26122305.
15. Schmidt PN, Novovic S, Roug S, Feldager E. Endoscopic, transmural drainage and necrosectomy for walled-off pancreatic and peripancreatic necrosis is associated with low mortality--a single-center experience. *Scand J Gastroenterol*. 2015; 50: 611-618. PMID: 25648776.
16. Thompson CC, Kumar N, Slattery J, Clancy TE, Ryan MB, Ryou M, et al. A standardized method for endoscopic necrosectomy improves complication and mortality rates. *Pancreatology*. 2016; 16: 66-72. PMID: 26748428.
17. Yasuda I, Nakashima M, Iwai T, Isayama H, Itoi T, Hisai H, et al. Japanese multicenter experience of endoscopic necrosectomy for infected walled-off pancreatic necrosis: The JENIPaN study. *Endoscopy*. 2013; 45: 627-634. PMID: 23807806.
18. Khreiss M, Zenati M, Clifford A, Lee KK, Hogg ME, Slivka A, et al. Cyst Gastrostomy and Necrosectomy for the Management of Sterile Walled-Off Pancreatic Necrosis: a Comparison of Minimally Invasive Surgical and Endoscopic Outcomes at a High-Volume Pancreatic Center. *J Gastrointest Surg*. 2015; 19: 1441-1448. PMID: 26033038.
19. Bausch D, Wellner U, Kahl S, Kuesters S, Richter-Schrag HJ, Utzolino S, et al. Minimally invasive operations for acute necrotizing pancreatitis: comparison of minimally invasive retroperitoneal necrosectomy with endoscopic transgastric necrosectomy. *Surgery*. 2012; 152 3 Suppl 1: S128-S134. PMID: 22770962.
20. Kumar N, Conwell DL, Thompson CC. Direct endoscopic necrosectomy versus step-up approach for walled-off pancreatic necrosis: comparison of clinical outcome and health care utilization. *Pancreas*. 2014; 43: 1334-1339. PMID: 25083997.
21. Bakker OJ, van Santvoort HC, van Brunschot S, Geskus RB, Besselink MG, Bollen TL, et al. Endoscopic transgastric vs surgical necrosectomy for infected necrotizing pancreatitis: a randomized trial. *JAMA*. 2012; 307: 1053-1061. PMID: 22416101.
22. Rinninella E, Kunda R, Dollhopf M, Sanchez-Yague A, Will U, Tarantino I, et al. EUS-guided drainage of pancreatic fluid collections using a novel lumen-apposing metal stent on an electrocautery-enhanced delivery system: a large retrospective study (with video). *Gastrointest Endosc*. 2015; 82: 1039-1046. PMID: 26014960.
23. Shah RJ, Shah JN, Waxman I, Kowalski TE, Sanchez-Yague A, Nieto J, et al. Safety and efficacy of endoscopic ultrasound-guided drainage of pancreatic fluid collections with lumen-apposing covered self-expanding metal stents. *Clin Gastroenterol Hepatol*. 2015; 13: 747-752. PMID: 25290534.
24. Sharaiha RZ, Tyberg A, Khashab MA, Kumta NA, Karia K, Nieto J, et al. Endoscopic Therapy With Lumen-apposing Metal Stents Is Safe and Effective for Patients With Pancreatic Walled-off Necrosis. *Clin Gastroenterol Hepatol*. 2016 May 14. [Epub ahead of print]PMID: 27189914.
25. Siddiqui AA, Adler DG, Nieto J, Shah JN, Binmoeller KF, Kane S, et al. EUS-guided drainage of peripancreatic fluid collections and necrosis by using a novel lumen-apposing stent: a large retrospective, multicenter U.S. experience (with videos). *Gastrointest Endosc*. 2016; 83: 699-707. PMID: 26515956.
26. Walter D, Will U, Sanchez-Yague A, Brenke D, Hampe J, Wollny H, et al. A novel lumen-apposing metal stent for endoscopic ultrasound-guided drainage of pancreatic fluid collections: a prospective cohort study. *Endoscopy*. 2015; 47: 63-67. PMID: 25268308.
27. Boston Scientific. AXIOS Electrocautery Enhanced System. Available at: http://www.bostonscientific.com/content/gwc/en-US/products/stents--gastrointestinal/axios-stent-and-electrocautery-enhanced-delivery-system/_jcr_content/maincontent-par/image_1.img.axios-electrocautery-deployed-400x248.jpg. Accessed July 13, 2016.
28. Trikudanathan G, Arain M, Mallery S, Freeman M, Attam R. Endoscopic necrosectomy in children. *J Pediatr Gastroenterol Nutr*. 2014; 59: 270-273. PMID: 24796802.
29. Attam R, Trikudanathan G, Arain M, Nemoto Y, Glessing B, Mallery S, et al. Endoscopic transluminal drainage and

necrosectomy by using a novel, through-the-scope, fully covered, large-bore esophageal metal stent: preliminary experience in 10 patients. *Gastrointest Endosc*. 2014; 80: 312-318. PMID: 24721519.

30. Sarkaria S, Sethi A, Rondon C, Lieberman M, Srinivasan I, Weaver K, et al. Pancreatic necrosectomy using covered esophageal stents: a novel approach. *J Clin Gastroenterol*. 2014; 48: 145-152. PMID: 23751853.
31. van Brunschot S, Besselink MG, Bakker OJ, Boermeester MA, Gooszen HG, Horvath KD, et al. Video-Assisted Retroperitoneal Debridement (VARD) of Infected Necrotizing Pancreatitis: An Update. *Curr Surg Rep*. 2013; 1: 121-130.
32. Strøm T, Martinussen T, Toft P. A protocol of no sedation for critically ill patients receiving mechanical ventilation: a randomised trial. *Lancet*. 2010; 375: 475-480. PMID: 20116842.
33. Nadkarni NA, Kotwal V, Sarr MG, Swaroop Vege S. Disconnected Pancreatic Duct Syndrome: Endoscopic Stent or Surgeon's Knife? *Pancreas*. 2015; 44: 16-22. PMID: 25493375.
34. van Brunschot S,van Grinsven J, Voermans RP, Bakker OJ, Besselink MG, Boermeester MA, et al. Transluminal endoscopic step-up approach versus minimally invasive surgical step-up approach in patients with infected necrotising pancreatitis (TENSION trial): design and rationale of a randomised controlled multicenter trial [ISRCTN09186711]. *BMC Gastroenterol*. 2013; 13: 161. PMID: 24274589.
35. van Brunschot S, All International Collaborators, van Santvoort HC. "International mortality after pancreatic necrosectomy: a meta-analysis of individual patient data." Available at: http://www.crd.york.ac.uk/PROSPERO/display_record.asp?ID=CRD42014008995. Updated April 2, 2014. Accessed July 12, 2016.
36. van Brunschot S, Bakker OJ, Besselink MG, Bollen TL, Fockens P, Gooszen HG, et al. Treatment of necrotizing pancreatitis. *Clin Gastroenterol Hepatol*. 2012; 10: 1190-1201. PMID: 22610008.

Chapter 29

Treatment of pancreatic necrosis: The multimodal Glasgow algorithm

C. Ross Carter*, Euan J. Dickson, and Colin J. McKay

West of Scotland Pancreatico-Biliary Unit, Glasgow Royal Infirmary, 84 Castle Street, Glasgow, United Kingdom, G4 0SF.

Introduction

The 2013 American Pancreatic Association/International Association of Pancreatology (APA/IAP) consensus document outlined the principles of early targeted organ support, nutritional (enteral) optimization, avoidance of antibiotic prophylaxis/endoscopic retrograde cholangio pancreatography (ERCP) (in the absence of jaundice), and delayed minimally invasive intervention embedded within a "step-up" framework where possible.[1] An in-depth discussion of the evidence supporting these principles is beyond the scope of this chapter and will be dealt with elsewhere. This chapter will focus on the indications and rationale for intervention, and the options available within a multimodal management algorithm.

Revised Atlanta classification of acute pancreatitis

The original Atlanta classification of acute pancreatitis (AP) characterized clinical behavior as mild or severe AP and intervention for necrosis was often focused on early removal of sterile or infected necrosis usually by open necrosectomy.[2] This simplistic dichotomization proved inadequate in clinical practice until the revised Atlanta Criteria recognized the importance of early systemic organ dysfunction and multiple organ failure in determining disease severity and outcome.[3] The management of local complications is heavily influenced by the degree of systemic disturbance, and this is reflected in an additional category of "moderately severe" pancreatitis (**Table 1**). In addition to disease severity, mortality is strongly associated with age, comorbidity and the presence of infection, which has been recognized in an addendum adding a category of "critical" recognizing those patients with sepsis and organ failure are associated with the highest mortality.[4]

Furthermore, this classification further categorizes local complications on the basis of time from presentation (< or >4 weeks) and on the presence of necrosis, leading to definitions aimed at permitting comparison of case series (**Table 2**). The "early" phase is characterized by the initial host response to the pancreatitis, the severity being determined by the magnitude or organ disturbance/failure, and a "late" phase typified by the persistence of organ dysfunction and the management of local or systemic complications. The vast majority of acute fluid collections without necrosis will resolve within 4 weeks, and a persistent fluid collection with minimal or no necrotic component ("pseudocyst") is very rare. Collections may be sterile or infected. The majority of clinically significant peripancreatic complications are therefore related to either acute necrotic collections (<4 weeks) or walled-off necrosis (WON) (>4 weeks). This temporal separation is somewhat arbitrary as the clinical management and surgical approach is determined by multifactorial individual patient factors. However, this does serve to provide a timeline beyond which, if appropriate, intervention should be delayed (**Figure 1**).

Indications for intervention for pancreatic necrosis: the biphasic model

Two distinct phases of mortality are seen in AP: early death (arbitrarily defined as within 2 weeks of onset) is usually

Table 1. Grades of severity for acute pancreatitis[3] (based on the clinical parameters of the presence or absence of organ failure and / or complications).

Mild acute pancreatitis
- No organ failure
- No local or systemic complications

Moderately severe acute pancreatitis
- Organ failure that resolves within 48 h (transient organ failure) and/or
- Local or systemic complications without persistent organ failure

Severe acute pancreatitis
- Persistent organ failure (>48 h)
  - Single organ failure
  - Multiple organ failure

*Corresponding author. Email: ross.carter@ggc.scot.nhs.uk

Table 2. Local complications in AP (2012 revised Atlanta classification).[3]

Time scale	Necrosis absent	Necrosis present
<4 weeks	**Acute peripancreatic fluid collection** (peripancreatic fluid associated with interstitial edematous pancreatitis with no associated peripancreatic necrosis)	**Acute necrotic collection** (a collection containing variable amounts of both fluid and necrosis; the necrosis can involve the pancreatic parenchyma or the extrapancreatic tissues)
>4 weeks	**Pancreatic pseudocyst** (an encapsulated collection of fluid with a well-defined inflammatory wall usually outside the pancreas with minimal or no necrosis)	**Walled-off necrosis** (a mature, encapsulated collection of pancreatic or extrapancreatic necrosis that has developed a well-defined inflammatory wall)
Infection	May be sterile or infected	May be sterile or infected

a consequence of progressive multiple organ failure.[5] Late mortality is usually a consequence of local pancreatic complications related to pancreatic or peripancreatic necrosis. Whereas intervention during the early phase of illness is usually counterproductive, timely and appropriate intervention for specific local complications can be lifesaving.[6] Although the incidence of AP has been increasing, the overall case mortality has been falling for several decades. Mortality in the subgroup with severe AP is also decreasing, and this is attributed to improvements in intensive care management, minimally invasive approaches to management, advances in vascular intervention, nutritional support,and the development of specialist centers. The IAP/APA consensus document provides a broad framework on which to structure management of what are invariably complex and individual management algorithms. The main impact of these improvements has been to better support patients for longer through the early phase of illness, allowing interventions for local complications to be carried out later with less invasive methods.

Surgical intervention for necrosis in the first 2 weeks carries a high risk of morbidity and mortality and should

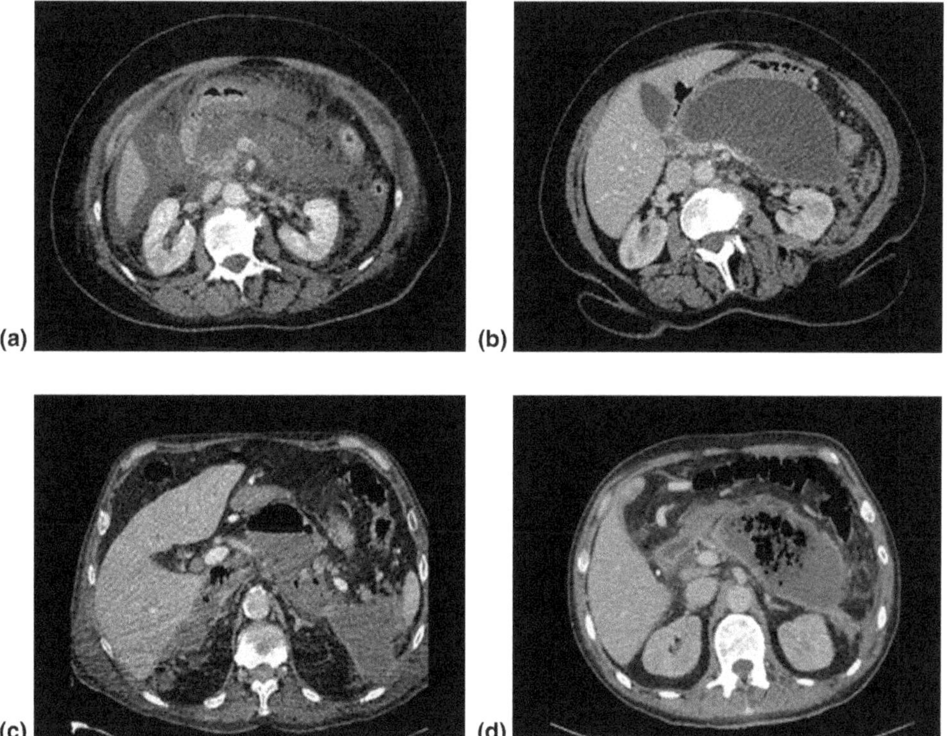

Figure 1. Contrast-enhanced computed tomography in a 69-year-old female with severe acute gallstone pancreatitis (a) showing an acute necrotic collection (ANC) at 5 days and (b) WON at 7 weeks subsequently managed by laparoscopic cystgastrotomy and cholecystectomy. The fluid level in an acute necrotic collection suggestive of spontaneous fistulation (c) (clinically well) and (d) loculated gas within an infected acute necrotic collection suggestive of bacterial contamination (clinical sepsis).

therefore to be avoided in the absence of specific complications such as bleeding or mesenteric ischemia.[7] While intervention may eventually be required for a persistent WON collection, intervention for an acute necrotic collection before it has sufficiently matured to become encapsulated is usually only indicated in the presence of secondary infection as evidenced by a secondary clinical and biochemical deterioration coupled with computed tomography (CT) evidence of infection such as small gas pockets.[8] Gas within a collection is not in itself an indication for intervention as spontaneous enteric discharge of a collection may be associated with clinical improvement. In such situations there is often a gas/fluid level; therefore, any imaging result needs to be interpreted in the overall clinical context.

Once a decision is made that intervention is required, these poorly demarcated pancreatic (and peripancreatic) collections can be managed by a variety of approaches. In the 1990s, Freeny and colleagues showed that aggressive percutaneous sepsis control would promote recovery in the absence of formal necrosectomy, although a number required subsequent surgical intervention.[9] Several minimally invasive approaches have since been described, including percutaneous necrosectomy (MIRP),[10] video-assisted retroperitoneal debridement (VARD),[11] endoscopic cystgastrostomy,[12] and laparoscopic cystgastrostomy.[13] Laparoscopic direct necrosectomy was described in the 1990s but has failed to gain popularity due to technical difficulty,[14] and so far there are only two recent retrospective studies describing laparoscopic necrosectomy alone with a total of 29 highly selected patients, and no follow-up was available for either study.[15,16]

There is evidence that minimal access techniques may pose less of a challenge to the patient's systemic inflammatory response, and in our own experience, patients have reduced requirements for postoperative intensive care management.[17] The choice of approach in worldwide clinical practice is often influenced by local resource limitations and familiarity with a particular technique, but most now have foundation within a "step-up framework."

Management techniques for sepsis associated with acute necrotic collections

Initial "step-up" drainage

Whereas a number of differing minimally invasive techniques had been described in cohort series showing benefit over historical controls, the PANTER trial from the Dutch Pancreatitis Study Group provided good quality randomized data regarding the management of infected pancreatic necrosis.[18] Patients requiring surgical intervention for pancreatic necrosis were randomized to either primary open necrosectomy or a "step-up" approach based on percutaneous drainage as the initial intervention, with progression to retroperitoneal debridement (VARD) with lavage if no improvement was observed. The composite endpoint of death or major complication demonstrated a significant benefit with the "step-up" approach. Indeed, 35% were successfully managed with percutaneous drainage alone and did not require subsequent debridement. There is now a consensus advocating a principle of early organ support and nutritional optimization, followed ideally by delayed and selective minimally invasive intervention if required.

The choice between initial percutaneous or endoscopic drainage is based on the position of the collection relative to the stomach, colon, liver, spleen, and kidney. Furthermore, the ability to perform endoscopic ultrasound (EUS)-guided puncture within an intensive therapy unit setting, without the need for patient transfer to the radiology department for CT-guided drainage, may influence the management decision when a patient is in extremis, and unstable to transfer. In general, our practice has been to approach lateral collections and those extending behind the colon from the left or right flank by a percutaneous approach, preferring endoscopic drainage for medial retrogastric collections where a percutaneous route may be compromised by overlying bowel, spleen, or liver. Improved delivery devices to enable rapid deployment of self-expanding metal stents (SEMs) may represent a significant advance by allowing adequate and rapid initial drainage while minimizing the risk of hemorrhage due to lateral compression of the drain tract by the SEMS.[19] The route of percutaneous drainage should ideally consider the probability of subsequent "step-up" escalation, siting the drain as lateral and inferior as possible to avoid the costal margin, but the initial priority must be sepsis control. If the initial drainage route is suboptimal, alternative secondary access can be obtained, sometimes resulting in a combination of percutaneous and endoscopic techniques.

The choice of one approach over another is determined by the patient's clinical condition, local experience and expertise, anatomical position/content of the collection, and the time from presentation/maturation of the collection wall. There is an acceptance that due to the complexity of presentation, no single technique will be suitable for all patients, and the aim should be to provide a multimodal, multidisciplinary approach. Our current management algorithm has emerged from a process of continuous evolution based on increased experience of the "step-up" concepts, the approach in the last decade being for solid predominant or infected necrotic collections to be managed percutaneously by MIRP or VARD, and for late, well-organized and predominantly fluid collections to be managed by endoscopic or laparoscopic transgastric drainage, but these concepts are now being assessed in randomized trials.[20,21]

Secondary "step-up" management following primary drainage (Figure 2)

Enhanced catheter drainage (± lavage)

The "step-up" concept is based on the stabilization of patients in organ failure and sepsis, as a bridge to surgery or as definitive treatment in a proportion of patients. Some authors have promoted secondary "upsizing" or insertion of multiple drains if immediate sepsis resolution is delayed, rather than proceeding to one of the necrosectomy techniques described below. Freeny et al. first described a series of 34 patients with infected acute necrotizing pancreatitis primarily treated with image guided percutaneous drain (PCD) as an alternative to primary surgical necrosectomy.[9] They focused on the placement of multiple large-bore catheters and vigorous irrigation and successfully avoided the need for surgical necrosectomy in 47% of patients. Lee and his colleagues routinely undertook stepwise dilation to 20FG along with twice weekly lavage.[22] They reported resolution in 83% of subjects, but two prospective studies have suggested a more realistic primary success rate of 33% to 35% for PCD.[18,23] Early PCD placement before 3 weeks is associated with a prolonged course and more frequent drain exchanges,[24,25] underscoring the importance of maturation of WON before intervention. Persistent external fistulae occur in up to one-third of patients.

The Dutch Pancreatitis Study Group compared the success of further upsizing of PCD versus VARD as the initial enhanced step-up procedure if immediate resolution does not occur. More than 50% of patients will settle without formal necrosectomy in the dilatation alone group. Drawbacks include limited ability to remove necrotic debris, prolonged hospitalization, and the need for multiple procedures. The use of grasping forceps to extract the debris after sequential tract dilatation has been described in a small series,[26] as has the use of assist devices such as stone retrieval baskets,[27] but these techniques are seldom performed in clinical practice. A dedicated team of surgeons/radiologists willing to perform meticulous catheter care, with frequent upsizing of drainage catheters and frequent imaging to localize loculated undrained areas, is critical for successful percutaneous management of necrotizing pancreatitis.[9]

Percutaneous necrosectomy/VARD

Both MIRP and VARD retroperitoneal techniques are modifications of the open lateral approach initially described in the 1980s by Fagniez et al.[28] They utilized a loin/subcostal and retrocolic approach to allow debridement of pancreatic and peripancreatic necroses. This open approach was associated with major morbidity (enteric fistula 45%, hemorrhage 40%, and colonic necrosis 15%) and failed to gain popularity.

For both minimally invasive techniques, a left-sided small diameter percutaneous drain is ideally placed into the acute necrotic collection between the spleen, kidney, and colon. Right-sided or transperitoneal drainage are also possible. In those who fail to respond adequately to simple drainage, this access drain is then used as a guide to gain enhanced drainage of the collection.

Minimally invasive pancreatic necrosectomy

For percutaneous necrosectomy, the catheter is exchanged for a radiological guidewire, and a low-compliance balloon dilator is inserted into the collection and dilated to 34 FG. Access to the cavity is then maintained by an Amplatz sheath through which is passed an operating nephroscope, allowing debridement under direct vision. The nephroscope has an operating channel that permits standard (5 mm) laparoscopic graspers, as well as an irrigation/suction channel. The directed, high-flow lavage promotes rapid evacuation of pus and liquefied necrotic material, revealing black or grey devascularized pancreatic tissue and peripancreatic fat which, if loose, is extracted in a piecemeal fashion until a cavity lined by viable tissue or granulating pancreas is created after several procedures. At the end of each procedure, an 8-FG catheter sutured to a 24-FG drain is passed

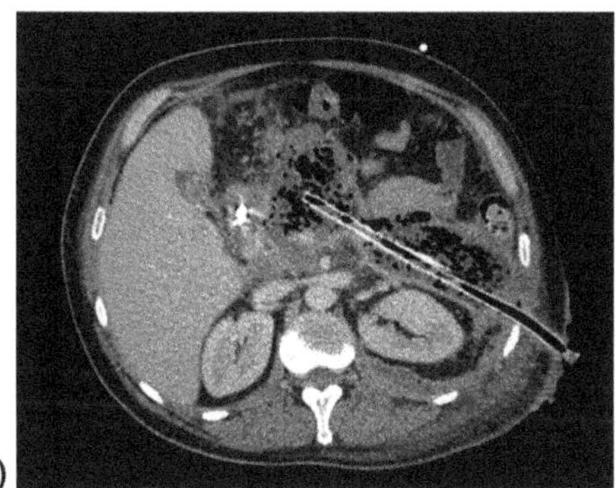

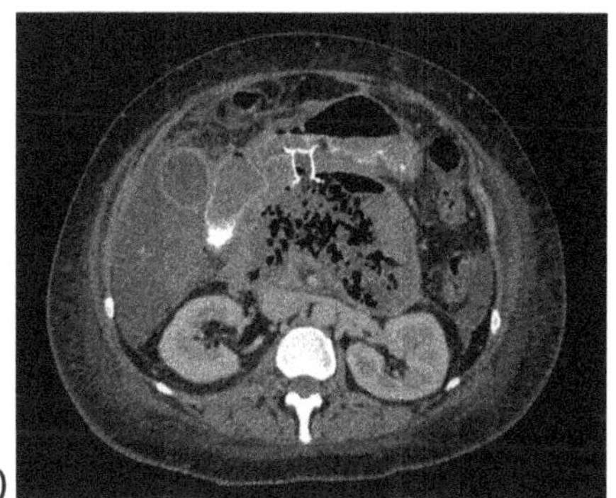

Figure 2. Initial "step-up" drainage using (a) MIRP percutaneous lavage drain and (b) EUS-guided transgastric cystgastrostomy with SEMS.

into the cavity to allow continuous postoperative lavage of warmed fluid, initially at 250 mL/hour. Subsequent conversion of the lavage system to simple drainage may be all that is required prior to recovery, or the procedure may be repeated until sepsis control is achieved and interval CT confirms resolution.

Video-assisted retroperitoneal debridement

A video-assisted retroperitoneal debridement (VARD) procedure is performed with the patient placed in a supine position with the left side 30 to 40° elevated. A 5-cm subcostal incision is placed in the left flank at the midaxillary line, close to the exit point of the percutaneous drain. Using the *in situ* percutaneous drain as a guide, the retroperitoneal collection is entered. The cavity is cleared of purulent material using a standard suction device. Visible necrosis is carefully removed with the use of long grasping forceps, deeper access under direct vision is facilitated using a 0° laparoscope, and further debridement performed with laparoscopic forceps. As with a percutaneous necrosectomy, complete necrosectomy is not the aim of this procedure;only loosely adherent pieces of necrosis are removed, minimizing the risk of hemorrhage. Two large-bore, single-lumen drains are positioned in the cavity, and the fascia is closed to facilitate a closed continuous postoperative lavage system.

Endoscopic necrosectomy

Endoscopic cystgastrostomy was initially reported for the management of a mature pancreatic abscess with minimal necrosis,[29] but the technique has evolved in the last 10 years to become an established Natural Orifice (NOTES) procedure, with endoscopic transmural exploration and debridement of the retroperitoneum. Single-step drainage under EUS guidance may be carried out by either a transgastric or less commonly a transduodenal route. This is preferred to "blind" drainage as EUS allows for identification of the collection when there is no obvious bulge and helps identify a safe route for puncture, free of intervening vessels.[30,31] The presence of significant WON is no longer considered a contraindication, but concerns do remain regarding the adequacy of endoscopic drainage, particularly in solid predominant or larger collections. The principles are similar to those discussed above, with initial simple drainage of a collection under pressure, followed by subsequent "step-up" tract dilatation and potential necrosectomy.

The procedure involves puncture of the collection with either a 19-G needle or cystotome, with dilatation of the track followed by placement of two or more plastic pigtail stents. Increasingly, metallic stents may be used which facilitate subsequent endoscopic access to the cyst cavity for debridement of necrosis. Where there is evidence of infection or systemic sepsis it is our practice to use a nasocystic catheter, which can be used for continuous lavage of the cavity. Factors associated with a failure of resolution are large size and retrocolic extension of the collections. In these cases, other approaches or combinations of approaches should be considered.[25,32] Other options include the multiple gateway technique,[31] where two or three transmural stents are placed under EUS guidance, one of which is used for nasocystic cavity lavage and the others to facilitate drainage of necrotic debris.

Delayed endoscopic necrosectomy may be required where there is extensive necrosis.[33] It is our practice to defer this for a week following the initial drainage procedure to allow the fluid component to drain and any associated sepsis to improve. A recent systematic review of 14 studies with 455 patients found an overall success rate of 81% and mortality of 6%, but these studies included highly selected patients, and all but one was retrospective.[34] One small randomized trial compared endoscopic with surgical drainage and found a reduction in significant complications with the endoscopic approach.[20]

Endoscopic necrosectomy is a challenging procedure and not without risk. Major complications including fatal air embolism, bleeding, and perforation occurred in 26% of patients in the multicenter GEPARD study.[35] The use of carbon dioxide insufflation is therefore now recommended. A persistent problem is the lack of availability of suitable endoscopic devices to facilitate necrosectomy. Although endoscopic access to the cyst cavity is now facilitated by metallic stents, piecemeal necrosectomy using standard graspers, baskets, and snares is a time-consuming and painstaking process.[21] One possible modification is the use of intracavity hydrogen peroxide to facilitate necrosectomy, although further experience is required before this can be recommended for routine practice.[36]

Despite these limitations, the initial experience has been promising,[35] and an early randomized pilot study exploring the outcome of endoscopic transmural drainage versus minimally invasive intervention (VARD, the PENGUIN trial) suggested at least equivalence, if not benefit, from endoscopic drainage.[20] This study has been criticized due to very small numbers and excessive mortality (40%) within the VARD arm compared to historical results. The results of the on-going TENSION trial are awaited with interest.[21]

Open surgical necrosectomy

Open necrosectomy is still employed but increasingly has been replaced by the procedures described above. Three general variations of open necrosectomy are currently practiced and remain widespread while experience with minimally invasive approaches increases. These can also be used within a step-up framework with preoperative percutaneous drainage, allowing control of sepsis prior to intervention. Although the procedures are broadly similar in terms of the necrosectomy, they differ in terms of how they prevent recurrence of an infected collection within the debridement cavity: 1) open necrosectomy with open or closed packing, 2) open necrosectomy with continuous closed postoperative lavage, and 3) programmed open necrosectomy.

In all approaches, the abdomen is entered though a midline or preferably a bilateral subcostal incision, as this minimizes contamination of the lower abdomen and allows bilateral paracolic access. The pancreas is exposed by dividing the gastrocolic omentum or gastrohepatic omentum to access the pancreas through the lesser sac. Open transgastric debridement has recently been proposed to minimize postoperative peritoneal contamination.[37]

Open necrosectomy with open packing

Bradley described this technique in 1987,[38] with sepsis control achieved by leaving the abdomen open following debridement and packing the cavity as a laparostomy.[38] Planned reintervention with sequential pack changes allows resolution with healing by secondary intention. Drains may be placed in addition to the packing. Open packing techniques have been reported to have higher incidences of fistulae, bleeding, and incisional hernias as well as a slightly higher mortality rate.[39]

Open necrosectomy with closed packing

Following necrosectomy to achieve sepsis control,[40] primary closure of the abdomen over gauze-stuffed Penrose drains is performed with the intention to fill the cavity and provide some compression.[41] Additional silicone drains (Jackson-Pratt) may be placed in the pancreatic bed and lesser sac for fluid drainage. The drains are removed sequentially starting 5 to 7 days postoperatively, allowing gradual involution of the cavity.

Open necrosectomy with continuous closed postoperative lavage

When possible after debridement, a closed peripancreatic compartment is reconstituted by suturing the gastrocolic and duodenocolic ligaments over large-bore drains allowing flank to flank continuous lavage.[42] Postoperative continuous lavage is instituted at 1 to 10 L per day and continued until the effluent is clear and the patient shows improvement in clinical and laboratory parameters.[43] No evidence is available to suggest the best irrigation fluid, the optimal number or caliber of drains, or the duration of irrigation.

Programmed open necrosectomy

In response to the bleeding and fistulation that can arise following aggressive necrosectomy, this approach attempts to initially perform a more conservative debridement, with the intention of performing repeat procedures every 48 hours until debridement is no longer required. This mimics the "minimal hit" concept associated with the step-up approaches. The pancreatic bed is drained or packed, and the abdomen is closed by suturing mesh or a zipper to the fascial edges of the wound.[44] The addition of intra-abdominal vacuum dressings may encourage granulation of the pancreatic bed, and it has been suggested they may reduce the number of operations and mortality, but there is little data to support this and they have been associated with enteric fistulation.[45]

Management for late WON

Indications for intervention for WON are: 1) infection, 2) nutritional failure, and 3) persistent abdominal pain. The decision on when to intervene and the choice of intervention are made within a multidisciplinary environment with consideration of all available options. Spontaneous resolution of even large acute WON collections are not infrequent, and continued nonintervention is often the best approach, particularly where continued maturation of a collection may be anticipated and where the clinical picture is improving. In any individual case, the choice of intervention may be guided by factors including the clinical picture, the position of the collection in relation to the stomach and duodenum, and available expertise.

Laparoscopic cystgastrostomy

For many years, the conventional approach to the management of late WON was open pancreatic cystgastrostomy with necrosectomy. This procedure can now be safely and effectively carried out using a laparoscopic approach and is the main alternative to endoscopic cystgastrostomy. Our current technique for laparoscopic cystgastrostomy begins with an open subumbilical cut down. Further 12- and 5-mm ports are inserted on the patient's left and right sides, with the specific port site placement being determined by the anatomical position of the retrogastric collection. Adhesions are divided to expose the anterior gastric wall. An anterior gastrotomy (5-10-cm long) is then performed using the harmonic scalpel (Ethicon Endo-Surgery, Inc, Cincinnati, OH, USA). The superior leaf of the opened stomach is lifted toward the anterior abdominal wall to maximize access and delineate the area of adherence between the cyst and the posterior aspect of the stomach. This is achieved by passing a straight needle 2/0 suture through the abdominal wall, anterior stomach wall, and back out of the abdomen. A key advance has been the use of a "Step" dilatation port system (Covidien plc, Dublin, Ireland) to achieve initial cyst puncture, allow tract dilatation, and maintain access until insertion of the initial staple device. Following aspiration of the collection contents to relative dryness, the port is withdrawn, leaving the suction instrument within the collection to maintain access, and a stapled cystgastrostomy is performed using four to five firings of the angulating Universal Endo GIA stapler (Covidien plc). Necrotic debris within the cavity is removed and placed in the fundus of the stomach. Once adequate debridement and hemostasis have been assured, the anterior gastrotomy is closed using a running 3/0 monofilament suture (BiosynTM, Covidien plc), with the integrity of the closure then tested by insufflating the stomach through an orogastric tube while the anastomosis is held under lavage fluid. Postoperative fluid and diet is allowed as tolerated. In this complex cohort of patients, suitability for hospital discharge is often multifactorial, but it may be within 36 hours of surgery when dietary intake is adequate. A simultaneous laparoscopic cholecystectomy is performed when gallstones are present. Our initial results have been presented elsewhere, and we are currently undertaking a randomized trial of EUS-guided endoscopic versus laparoscopic cystgastrostomy for WON.[13]

EUS-guided cystgastrostomy/necrosectomy

The technique of EUS-guided drainage is as described above, the principle difference being the indication of failure to thrive rather than sepsis control. Many reports in the literature describe EUS-guided drainage of "pseudocysts" but is now recognized that true pancreatic pseudocysts are rare following AP, as some degree of necrosis is usually present where collections persist. The revised Atlanta criteria define these collections as WON, but there is still a spectrum of clinical presentations. WON may have varying degrees of fluid content, and infection may be present with or without systemic disturbance or organ failure. EUS-guided drainage of these collections is now an established technique in specialist units, and several different modifications have been described. The frequent requirement for repeated endoscopic procedures, particularly in the presence of significant necrosis, have led to a former preference to select fluid-predominant WON collections for this approach, but this assumption is being currently challenged in a randomized trial in our unit.

Management of complications

Early procedure-related complications: SIRS/bacteremia requiring critical care support

For patients with established organ failure, drainage has an unpredictable effect,and the clinical picture may improve or worsen, at least temporarily. Evidence now supports a "step-up" approach in the presence of organ failure, so initial management in these patients should be either percutaneous or endoscopic drainage, with more definitive intervention deferred until organ failure stabilizes or improves.

Following any intervention, however minimal, it is not unusual for patients to show signs of significant SIRS or postprocedure bacteremia, and this may necessitate critical care admission for organ support. Our experience has been that minimally invasive approaches are less likely to cause the development of new organ failure, and this has been confirmed in randomized trials.[18] More significant deterioration is common following open necrosectomy, so it is no longer the preferred approach.

Acute or delayed hemorrhage

Periprocedural hemorrhage following initial drainage may be due to bleeding from submucosal or perigastric vessels during endoscopic or percutaneous drainage and is usually self-limiting. Bleeding from the cavity itself is more likely during necrosectomy, particularly if it is carried out too early or aggressively. Venous bleeding is more common in this situation and may occur intra- or postoperatively. It will usually resolve with correction of any coagulopathy, but tamponade may be required, either by simply clamping the percutaneous drain, insertion of a modified Sengstaken-Blakemore tube (having amputated the gastric balloon), or gauze packing if there is sufficient cutaneous access following a VARD procedure.

Secondary hemorrhage is occasionally sudden and massive, but there is usually a prelude with a self-terminating "herald bleed," presenting clinically with hemorrhage into a retroperitoneal drain or by a gastrointestinal bleed following transluminal drainage. Secondary hemorrhage is usually of arterial origin and is often a consequence of persistent local sepsis. This is now the major cause of death in patients with infected pancreatic collections and rapid intervention may be life-saving. Initial controlled volume support of the circulation and a simultaneous emergency CT angiogram is followed by angiography and embolization if appropriate. Upper gastrointestinal endoscopy in this setting is usually nondiagnostic and should therefore not delay radiological assessment that allows definitive management. The increased intracavity pressure associated with hemorrhage into an infected cavity may escalate organ dysfunction through bacteremia and sepsis. Timely consideration of further intervention to improve surgical drainage is important once bleeding has been arrested.

Enteric fistulation

Spontaneous discharge of a pancreatic collection into the gastrointestinal tract is common and may occur in the presence or absence of infection. This should be suspected when a collection contains gas, particularly where a gas/fluid level is present, in a patient who is not systemically unwell. Indeed, discharge of a collection into the stomach or duodenum can be associated with improvement in a patient's condition. In our experience, foregut fistulation will usually resolve without the need for intervention (other than adequate drainage of a collection by percutaneous or endoscopic means), but fistulation into the colon is often associated with clinical deterioration and persistent sepsis. Some form of defunctioning procedure is usually required, and formal colonic resection with exteriorization may be required in occasional cases.

Late complications

Pancreatic fistulation

Persistent pancreatic fistula is a common sequel of percutaneous necrosectomy or VARDS. Pancreatic duct disruption is common in the presence of extensive necrosis, and although resolution is the norm, persistent fistulae can be a challenging management problem. If a pancreatic fistula persists once sepsis resolves and CT has confirmed any significant collection, pancreatic duct stent insertion at ERCP is the management of choice. Failure of resolution thereafter is often associated with more extensive parenchymal loss or a disconnected pancreatic tail with loss of continuity of the main pancreatic duct. Prolonged catheter drainage will lead to maturation of the fistula tract, and planned interval drain removal may result in spontaneous resolution or development of a late pseudocyst, which can often be resolved by transmural endoscopic cystgastrostomy. The avoidance of pancreatic fistula is one of the main advantages of endoscopic (or laparoscopic) drainage of pancreatic collections.

Disconnected pancreatic tail

Following extensive necrosis or complete necrosis of a section of the pancreas neck or body, complete separation of the main pancreatic duct in the pancreatic tail may occur leading to a persistent fistula and "disconnected duct syndrome." This may lead to persistence of a pancreatic fistula or a late "pseudocyst" following initial successful management of a pancreatic collection. Ductal occlusion at the pancreatic neck precludes transpapillary access but if this has not occurred, intracystic transpapillary stenting or a stent bridging the defect into the tail may result in resolution. If transpapillary access is not possible, the preferred option is transmural EUS-guided drainage with placement of long-term pigtail stents, although distal pancreatectomy may be required in some patients. This is a challenging procedure, particularly when patients have undergone previous interventions.

Conclusion

Clinical complexity and diversity precludes algorithm driven management in severe AP. Three phases of management exist: (1) organ support, (2) sepsis control, and (3) failure to thrive.Based on an understanding of the evolution of necrosis/collections and the dynamic nature of the physiological response in AP, the rationale and interventional approach chosen will differ depending on the specific issues that need to be addressed. Maintaining nutritional competence throughout is essential. Individual patient management within a step-up framework remains key, utilizing a multimodal approach focused on delayed minimally invasive intervention when possible.

References

1. Working Group IAPAPAAPG. IAP/APA evidence-based guidelines for the management of acute pancreatitis. *Pancreatology*. 2013; 13(4 Suppl 2): e1-15. PMID: 24054878.
2. Bradley EL 3rd. A clinically based classification system for acute pancreatitis. Summary of the International Symposium on Acute Pancreatitis, Atlanta, Ga, September 11 through 13, 1992. *Arch Surg*. 1993; 128(5): 586-590. PMID: 8489394.
3. Banks PA, Bollen TL, Dervenis C, Gooszen HG, Johnson CD, Sarr MG, et al. Classification of acute pancreatitis--2012: revision of the Atlanta classification and definitions by international consensus. *Gut*. 2013; 62(1): 102-111. PMID: 23100216.
4. Petrov MS, Shanbhag S, Chakraborty M, Phillips AR, Windsor JA. Organ failure and infection of pancreatic necrosis as determinants of mortality in patients with acute pancreatitis. *Gastroenterology*. 2010; 139(3): 813-820. PMID: 20540942.
5. McKay CJ, Evans S, Sinclair M, Carter CR, Imrie CW. High early mortality rate from acute pancreatitis in Scotland, 1984-1995. *Br J Surg*. 1999; 86(10): 1302-1305. PMID: 10540138.
6. Aldridge MC, Francis ND, Glazer G, Dudley HA. Colonic complications of severe acute pancreatitis. *Br J Surg*. 1989; 76(4): 362-367. PMID: 2655821.
7. Mier J, Leon EL, Castillo A, Robledo F, Blanco R.Early versus late necrosectomy in severe necrotizing pancreatitis. *Am J Surg*. 1997; 173(2): 71-75. PMID: 9074366.
8. Buchler M, Uhl W, Beger HG. Acute pancreatitis: when and how to operate. *Dig Dis*. 1992; 10(6): 354-362. PMID: 1473288.
9. Freeny PC, Hauptmann E, Althaus SJ, Traverso LW, Sinanan M. Percutaneous CT-guided catheter drainage of infected acute necrotizing pancreatitis: techniques and results. *Am J Roentgenol*. 1998; 170(4): 969-975. PMID: 9530046.
10. Carter CR, McKay CJ, Imrie CW. Percutaneous necrosectomy and sinus tract endoscopy in the management of infected pancreatic necrosis: an initial experience. *Ann Surg*. 2000; 232(2): 175-180. PMID: 10903593.

11. Horvath KD, Kao LS, Wherry KL, Pellegrini CA, Sinanan MN. A technique for laparoscopic-assisted percutaneous drainage of infected pancreatic necrosis and pancreatic abscess. *Surg Endosc*. 2001; 15(10): 1221-1225. PMID: 11727105.
12. Wiersema MJ, Baron TH, Chari ST. Endosonography-guided pseudocyst drainage with a new large-channel linear scanning echoendoscope. *Gastrointest Endosc*. 2001; 53(7): 811-813. PMID: 11375600.
13. Gibson SC, Robertson BF, Dickson EJ, McKay CJ, Carter CR. 'Step-port' laparoscopic cystgastrostomy for the management of organized solid predominant post-acute fluid collections after severe acute pancreatitis. *HPB (Oxford)*. 2014; 16(2): 170-176. PMID: 23551864.
14. Gagner M. Laparoscopic Treatment of Acute Necrotizing Pancreatitis. *Semin Laparosc Surg*. 1996; 3(1): 21-28. PMID: 10401099.
15. Parekh D. Laparoscopic-assisted pancreatic necrosectomy: A new surgical option for treatment of severe necrotizing pancreatitis. *Arch Surg*. 2006; 141(9): 895-902; discussion 902-893. PMID: 16983033.
16. Zhu JF, Fan XH, Zhang XH. Laparoscopic treatment of severe acute pancreatitis. *Surg Endosc*. 2001; 15(2): 146-148. PMID: 11285957.
17. Elgammal S MC, Imrie CW, Carter CR. Does surgical approach affect outcome in patients with infected pancreatic necrosis requiring necrosectomy. *Br J Surg*. 2003; 90: 93.
18. van Santvoort HC, Besselink MG, Bakker OJ, Hofker HS, Boermeester MA, Dejong CH, et al. A step-up approach or open necrosectomy for necrotizing pancreatitis. *N Engl J Med*. 2010; 362(16): 1491-1502. PMID: 20410514.
19. Shah RJ, Shah JN, Waxman I, Kowalski TE, Sanchez-Yague A, Nieto J, et al. Safety and efficacy of endoscopic ultrasound-guided drainage of pancreatic fluid collections with lumen-apposing covered self-expanding metal stents. *Clin Gastroenterol Hepatol*. 2015; 13(4): 747-752. PMID: 25290534.
20. Bakker OJ, van Santvoort HC, van Brunschot S, Geskus RB, Besselink MG, Bollen TL, et al. Endoscopic transgastric vs surgical necrosectomy for infected necrotizing pancreatitis: a randomized trial. *JAMA*. 2012; 307(10): 1053-1061. PMID: 22416101.
21. van Brunschot S,van Grinsven J, Voermans RP, Bakker OJ, Besselink MG, Boermeester MA, et al. Transluminal endoscopic step-up approach versus minimally invasive surgical step-up approach in patients with infected necrotising pancreatitis (TENSION trial): design and rationale of a randomised controlled multicenter trial [ISRCTN09186711]. *BMC Gastroenterol*. 2013; 13: 161. PMID: 24274589.
22. Lee JK, Kwak KK, Park JK, Yoon WJ, Lee SH, Ryu JK, et al. The efficacy of nonsurgical treatment of infected pancreatic necrosis. *Pancreas*. 2007; 34(4): 399-404. PMID: 17446837.
23. Hollemans RA, Bollen TL, van Brunschot S, Bakker OJ, Ahmed Ali U, van Goor H, et al. Predicting Success of Catheter Drainage in Infected Necrotizing Pancreatitis. *Ann Surg*. 2016; 263(4): 787-792. PMID: 25775071.
24. Ramesh H, Prakash K, Lekha V, Jacob G, Venugopal A. Are some cases of infected pancreatic necrosis treatable without intervention? *Dig Surg*. 2003; 20(4): 296-299; discussion 300. PMID: 12789025.
25. Ross A, Gluck M, Irani S, Hauptmann E, Fotoohi M, Siegal J, et al. Combined endoscopic and percutaneous drainage of organized pancreatic necrosis. *Gastrointest Endosc*. 2010; 71(1): 79-84. PMID: 19863956.
26. Bala M, Almogy G, Klimov A, Rivkind AI, Verstandig A. Percutaneous "stepped" drainage technique for infected pancreatic necrosis. *Surg Laparosc Endosc Percutan Tech*. 2009; 19(4): e113-e118. PMID: 19692859.
27. Echenique AM, Sleeman D, Yrizarry J, Scagnelli T, Guerra JJ Jr, Casillas VJ, et al. Percutaneous catheter-directed debridement of infected pancreatic necrosis: results in 20 patients. *J Vasc Interv Radiol*. 1998; 9(4): 565-571. PMID: 9684824.
28. Fagniez PL, Rotman N, Kracht M. Direct retroperitoneal approach to necrosis in severe acute pancreatitis. *Br J Surg*. 1989; 76(3): 264-267. PMID: 2720323.
29. Baron TH, Thaggard WG, Morgan DE, Stanley RJ. Endoscopic therapy for organized pancreatic necrosis. *Gastroenterology*. 1996; 111(3): 755-764. PMID: 8780582.
30. Giovannini M, Bernardini D, Seitz JF. Cystogastrotomy entirely performed under endosonography guidance for pancreatic pseudocyst: results in six patients. *Gastrointest Endosc*. 1998; 48(2): 200-203. PMID: 9717789.
31. Varadarajulu S, Phadnis MA, Christein JD, Wilcox CM. Multiple transluminal gateway technique for EUS-guided drainage of symptomatic walled-off pancreatic necrosis. *Gastrointest Endosc*. 2011; 74(1): 74-80. PMID: 21612778.
32. Takahashi N, Papachristou GI, Schmit GD, Chahal P, LeRoy AJ, Sarr MG, et al. CT findings of walled-off pancreatic necrosis (WOPN): differentiation from pseudocyst and prediction of outcome after endoscopic therapy. *Eur Radiol*. 2008; 18(11): 2522-2529. PMID: 18563416.
33. Seifert H, Wehrmann T, Schmitt T, Zeuzem S, Caspary WF. Retroperitoneal endoscopic debridement for infected peripancreatic necrosis. *Lancet*. 2000; 356(9230): 653-655. PMID: 10968442.
34. van Brunschot S, Fockens P, Bakker OJ, Besselink MG, Voermans RP, Poley JW, et al. Endoscopic transluminal necrosectomy in necrotising pancreatitis: a systematic review. *Surg Endosc*. 2014; 28(5): 1425-1438. PMID: 24399524.
35. Seifert H, Biermer M, Schmitt W, Jurgensen C, Will U, Gerlach R, et al. Transluminal endoscopic necrosectomy after acute pancreatitis: a multicentre study with long-term follow-up (the GEPARD Study). *Gut*. 2009; 58(9): 1260-1266. PMID: 19282306.
36. Siddiqui AA, Easler J, Strongin A, Slivka A, Kowalski TE, Muddana V, et al. Hydrogen peroxide-assisted endoscopic necrosectomy for walled-off pancreatic necrosis: a dual center pilot experience. *Dig Dis Sci*. 2014; 59(3): 687-690. PMID: 24282052.
37. Sasnur P, Nidoni R, Baloorkar R, Sindgikar V, Shankar B. Extended Open Transgastric Necrosectomy (EOTN) as a Safer Procedure for Necrotizing Pancreatitis. *J Clin Diagn Res*. 2014; 8(7): NR01-NR02. PMID: 25177603.
38. Bradley EL 3rd. Management of infected pancreatic necrosis by open drainage. *Ann Surg*. 1987; 206(4): 542-550. PMID: 3662663.

39. Heinrich S, Schäfer M, Rousson V, Clavien PA. Evidence-based treatment of acute pancreatitis: a look at established paradigms. *Ann Surg*. 2006; 243(2): 154-168. PMID: 16432347.
40. Pezzilli R, Uomo G, Gabbrielli A, Zerbi A, Frulloni L, De Rai P, et al. A prospective multicentre survey on the treatment of acute pancreatitis in Italy. *Dig Liver Dis*. 2007; 39(9): 838-846. PMID: 17602904.
41. Fernández-del Castillo C, Rattner DW, Makary MA, Mostafavi A, McGrath D, Warshaw AL. Débridement and closed packing for the treatment of necrotizing pancreatitis. *Ann Surg*. 1998; 228(5): 676-684. PMID: 9833806.
42. Beger HG. Operative management of necrotizing pancreatitis--necrosectomy and continuous closed postoperative lavage of the lesser sac. *Hepatogastroenterology*. 1991; 38(2): 129-133. PMID: 1855769.
43. Wig JD, Mettu SR, Jindal R, Gupta R, Yadav TD. Closed lesser sac lavage in the management of pancreatic necrosis. *J Gastroenterol Hepatol*. 2004; 19(9): 1010-1015. PMID: 15304118.
44. Radenkovic DV, Bajec DD, Tsiotos GG, Karamarkovic AR, Milic NM, Stefanovic BD, et al. Planned staged reoperative necrosectomy using an abdominal zipper in the treatment of necrotizing pancreatitis. *Surg Today*. 2005; 35(10): 833-840. PMID: 16175464.
45. Olejnik J, Vokurka J, Vician M. Acute necrotizing pancreatitis: intra-abdominal vacuum sealing after necrosectomy. *Hepato-gastroenterology*. 2008; 55(82-83): 315-318. PMID: 18613356.

Chapter 30

Endoscopic assessment and treatment of biliary pancreatitis

Nora D. L. Hallensleben[1,2*], Nicolien J. Schepers[1,3], Marco J. Bruno[1], and Djuna L. Cahen[1,4]; on behalf of the Dutch Pancreatitis Study Group

[1]*Dept. of Gastroenterology and Hepatology, Erasmus University Medical Center, Rotterdam, the Netherlands;*
[2]*Dept. of Surgery, St. Antonius Hospital, Nieuwegein, the Netherlands;*
[3]*Dept. of Gastroenterology and Hepatology, St. Antonius Hospital Nieuwegein, the Netherlands;*
[4]*Dept. of Gastroenterology and Hepatology, Amstelland Medical Center, Amstelveen, the Netherlands.*

Introduction

Acute pancreatitis is the most common gastro-intestinal cause for acute hospital admission in the United States and is associated with substantial costs.[1] The reported incidence varies from 5 to 73 per 100,000 persons in different populations.[2,3] The overall mortality rate is 4% to 8%, which increases to 33% in patients with infected necrosis.[1,4-6] As the incidence of acute pancreatitis rises, the burden for patients and society will further increase.[3,7] An ageing population and abdominal obesity, which confers a concomitant increased risk of gallstone formation, are likely to play important roles. [3,7,8]

"Sludge" or gallstones, particularly small common bile duct stones, are the cause of acute pancreatitis in approximately 32% to 40% of cases.[9-12] Although the pathogenesis of acute biliary pancreatitis is not fully understood, transient or persistent obstruction of the ampulla that compromises the outflow of pancreatic juices and bile is thought to be the initiating event.[13] Either an obstructing stone or mucosal edema after spontaneous gallstone passage can result in ampullary obstruction. The etiology of acute pancreatitis should be determined on admission, as biliary obstruction may require duct clearance in the early phase. This chapter gives an overview of the available diagnostic tests and imaging modalities. Subsequently, the role of endoscopic retrograde cholangiography (ERC) will be discussed.

Establishing a Biliary Etiology

Acute pancreatitis is diagnosed when two of the following three criteria are fulfilled: 1) typical abdominal pain, 2) more than three times elevated serum amylase/lipase, and 3) signs of acute pancreatitis on imaging. Determining the etiology is important for clinical decision-making. A history of gallstone disease or biliary colics points towards a biliary etiology. Biochemical markers can be helpful in the early disease phase. In the absence of alcohol abuse, an alanine transaminase (ALT) >150 IU/L has a predictive value of 88 to 100% in establishing biliary etiology.[14-16] Other elevated biochemical markers such as serum alkaline phosphatase, bilirubin, gammaglutamyl-transferase, and aspartate aminotransferase are also suggestive of a biliary origin. However, 15% to 20% of patients with acute biliary pancreatitis have normal liver function tests at presentation.[17]

Recent guidelines advocate abdominal ultrasonography on admission to identify cholelithiasis because of its high sensitivity of 92% to 95%.[18,19] However, sensitivity is lower in patients with acute pancreatitis (67% to 87%) due to bowel distension, and it decreases even further in obese patients.[20,21] Nevertheless, the combination of cholelithiasis on abdominal ultrasonography and elevated liver biochemistry has a positive predictive value of 100% for biliary pancreatitis.[21,22] Predicting disease course severity is desirable to determine whether intensive monitoring or early interventions are needed. Although several scoring systems exist, they lack accuracy and are generally cumbersome to use.[23] Due to the simplicity, familiarity, and comparable performance, recent IAP/APA guidelines recommend using persistent (>48 hours) systemic inflammatory response syndrome (SIRS) as a predictor for disease severity.[19]

Endoscopic Ultrasonography or Magnetic Resonance Cholangiopancreatography?

If the etiology of pancreatitis remains unclear, endoscopic ultrasonography (EUS) or magnetic resonance cholangiopancreatography (MRCP) is the next step in the diagnostic pathway (**Figure 1**). Both modalities have a higher accuracy

*Corresponding author. Email: n.hallensleben@pancreatitis.nl

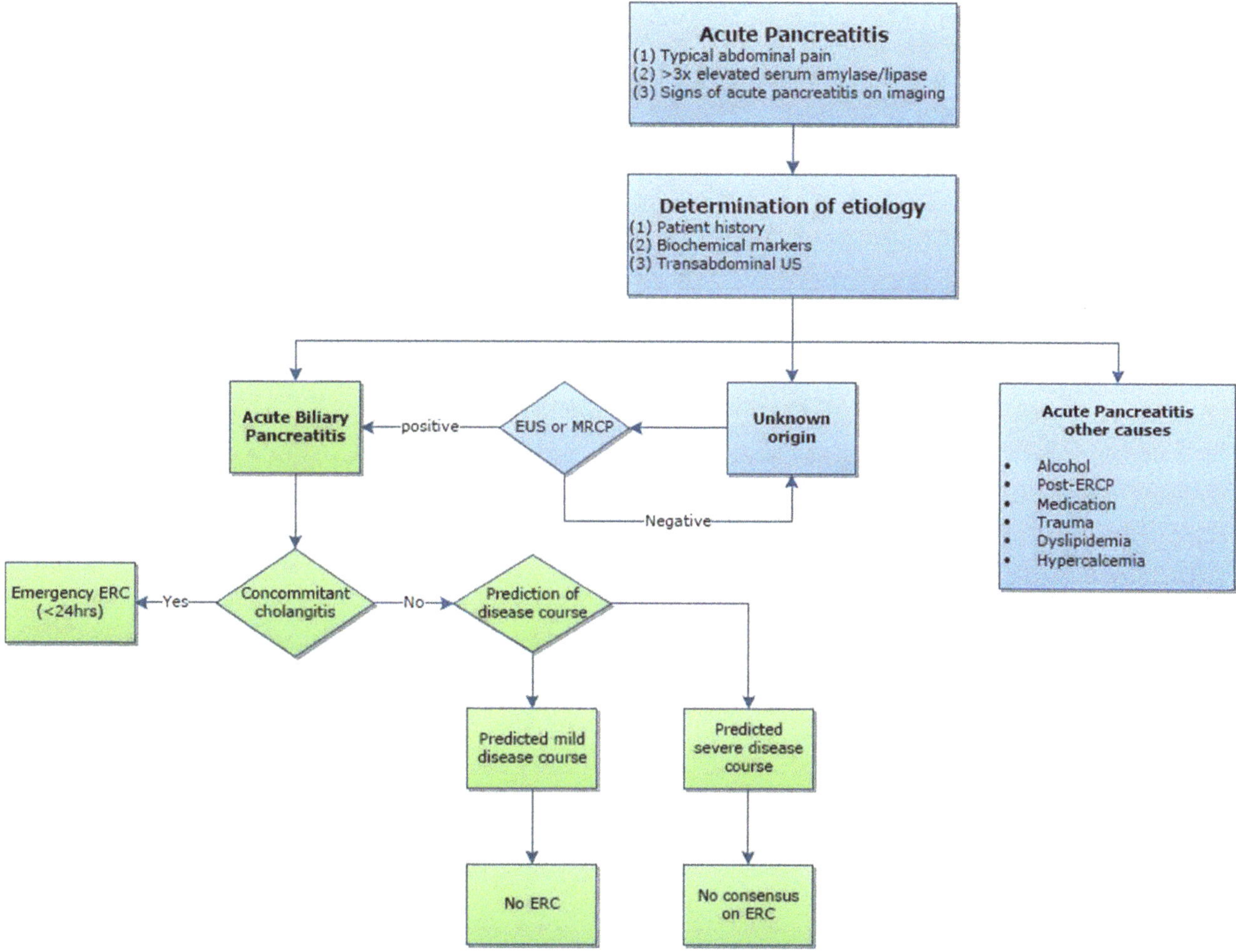

Figure 1. Diagnosis and management in the early phase of acute (biliary) pancreatitis.

in detecting common bile duct (CBD) stones compared to laboratory tests and transabdominal ultrasound.[24]

For EUS, a recent meta-analysis showed a sensitivity and specificity for detecting choledocholithiasis of 0.95 (95% confidence interval [CI] 0.91-0.97) and 0.97 (95% CI 0.94-0.99), respectively.[25] In patients with pancreatitis, data are limited, but the accuracy of EUS does not seem to drop, with a reported sensitivity of 91% to 100% and specificity of 85% to 100%.[26]

An advantage of EUS over MRCP is the possibility of conversion to ERC, in case common bile duct (CBD) stones are detected, provided the procedures are done in the same setting and by investigators trained in both techniques. Thus, in the hands of a trained physician with access to the appropriate equipment, diagnosis and treatment can be combined into a single procedure, with minimal additional burden for the patient. In patients with a contraindication for MRCP (e.g., claustrophobia, metal implants, or cardiac pacemaker), EUS is the only semi-invasive technique available before intraoperative cholangiography or ERC.

The advantage of the MRCP over EUS is that it is non-invasive and not operator dependent. Although small gallstones (<5 mm) and sludge may be missed, the sensitivity and specificity of MRCP were 0.93 (95% CI 0.87-0.96) and 0.96 (95% CI 0.89-0.98) in a meta-analysis.[25,27,28] Data regarding the accuracy of MRCP in the acute phase of pancreatitis are lacking.

In conclusion, the diagnostic accuracies of both EUS and MRCP are excellent, and these modalities can prevent unnecessary invasive procedures by preselecting patients for ERC.[29] In clinical practice, factors such as availability, cost, and experience will determine the choice between these two modalities.[30]

Endoscopic Retrograde Cholangiography

In biliary pancreatitis, ampullary obstruction results in pancreatic inflammation and complications. Accordingly, early biliary decompression using endoscopic sphincterotomy and, if necessary, stone extraction, may ameliorate disease severity and prevent complications. On the other hand, CBD stones pass spontaneously in up to 80% of cases, in which case ERC might be redundant and even unhelpful.[31] This is important, as ERC is associated with a complication rate of around 10% and a resultant mortality of 0.3% to 1%.[32,33] The most common complications are perforation and bleeding. Furthermore, contrast injection or cannulation of the pancreatic duct may aggravate the disease course.[34]

Recent guidelines state that emergency ERC is warranted in patients with acute biliary pancreatitis and concomitant cholangitis.[18,19] Urgent biliary decompression has been proven to reduce mortality and complications.[35] However, diagnosing cholangitis can be challenging in this group, as the clinical signs of cholangitis are often not easily differentiated from an SIRS reaction due to pancreatitis. Evidence-based diagnostic criteria for cholangitis in patients with acute pancreatitis are currently not available.

In patients with predicted mild disease, the potential benefits of ERC do not outweigh the risks for complications. Therefore, ERC is not advocated in this group.[18,19] The indication for ERC in patients with an acute biliary pancreatitis and a predicted severe disease course is controversial. Recent international guidelines state that early ERC with sphincterotomy may be beneficial but acknowledge the limited evidence.[18,19] A recent systematic review drew a similar conclusion; despite the publication of multiple randomized trials and systematic reviews on this subject, there is no consensus on the use of ERC in this group of patients.[36] Study heterogeneity is a possible source of contradiction. Some included patients with predicted mild disease or nonbiliary etiology, and different scoring systems for identifying patients at high risk for complications were used. Also, patients with cholangitis or signs of biliary obstruction were not separately analyzed. Furthermore, the pooled sample size of patients with a predicted severe disease course was too small and statistically underpowered to draw conclusions. Finally, the definition of "early" ERC differed between trials and varied between 24 to 72 hours after symptom onset or after hospital admission. Timing may be important as the duration of biliary obstruction seems to correlate with disease severity. Therefore, some suggest that ERC should be performed as early as possible.[37]

Currently, an adequately powered, randomized multicenter superiority trial is being conducted by the Dutch Pancreatitis Study Group to study the role of early ERC with sphincterotomy in patients with predicted severe biliary pancreatitis without cholangitis. (APEC trial, Current Controlled Trials number, ISRCTN97372133).

Conclusion

Acute pancreatitis is a common and potentially fatal disease. Establishing its etiology on admission is paramount for adequate treatment. In about half of cases, acute pancreatitis is caused by gallstones or "sludge." The first steps in establishing a biliary origin are obtaining a detailed history and performing laboratory tests and transabdominal ultrasound. In the acute phase, elevated ALT (>150 IU/L) is the most sensitive biomechanical marker. MRCP and EUS both have excellent diagnostic accuracy in detecting choledocholithiasis and can be used as second-line diagnostic tools. Early ERC is only indicated in patients with proven biliary pancreatitis and concomitant cholangitis. It is not indicated in patients with a predicted mild disease course and its role is currently under investigation in those with a predicted severe disease course. A flow sheet on the diagnosis and management of acute biliary pancreatitis is provided in **Figure 1**.

Funding

N.D.L. Hallensleben and N.J. Schepers are sponsored by The Netherlands Organisation for Health Research and Development (ZonMW, grant number 837002008) and the Foundation for Health Care Subsidies (Fonds NutsOhra, grant number 1203-052) to perform a clinical trial of acute pancreatitis.

References

1. Peery AF, Dellon ES, Lund J, Crockett SD, McGowan CE, Bulsiewicz WJ, et al. Burden of Gastrointestinal Disease in the United States: 2012 Update. *Gastroenterology.* 2012; 143: 1179-1187.e1-3. PMID: 22885331.
2. Fagenholz PJ, Castillo CF, Harris NS, Pelletier AJ, Camargo CA Jr. Increasing United States hospital admissions for acute pancreatitis, 1988-2003. *Ann Epidemiol.* 2007; 17: 491-497. PMID: 17448682.
3. Yadav D, Lowenfels AB. Trends in the epidemiology of the first attack of acute pancreatitis: a systematic review. *Pancreas.* 2006; 33: 323-330. PMID: 17079934.
4. Banks PA, Freeman ML. Practice guidelines in acute pancreatitis. *Am J Gastroenterol.* 2006; 101: 2379-2400. PMID: 17032204.
5. Gullo L, Migliori M, Olah A, Farkas G, Levy P, Arvanitakis C, et al. Acute pancreatitis in five European countries: etiology and mortality. *Pancreas.* 2002; 24: 223-227. PMID: 11893928.
6. van Santvoort HC, Bakker OJ, Bollen TL, Besselink MG, Ahmed Ali U, Schrijver AM, et al. A conservative and minimally invasive approach to necrotizing pancreatitis improves outcome. *Gastroenterology.* 2011; 141: 1254-1263. PMID: 21741922.
7. Spanier B, Bruno MJ, Dijkgraaf MG. Incidence and mortality of acute and chronic pancreatitis in the Netherlands: A nationwide record-linked cohort study for the years 1995-2005. *World J Gastroenterol.* 2013; 19: 3018-3026. PMID: 23716981.
8. Torgerson JS, Lindroos AK, Naslund I, Peltonen M. Gallstones, gallbladder disease, and pancreatitis: cross-sectional and 2-year data from the Swedish Obese Subjects (SOS) and SOS reference studies. *Am J Gastroenterol.* 2003; 98: 1032-1041. PMID: 12809825.
9. Frey CF, Zhou H, Harvey DJ, White RH. The incidence and case-fatality rates of acute biliary, alcoholic, and idiopathic pancreatitis in California, 1994-2001. *Pancreas.* 2006; 33: 336-344. PMID: 17079936.

10. Toh SK, Phillips S, Johnson CD. A prospective audit against national standards of the presentation and management of acute pancreatitis in the South of England. *Gut*. 2000; 46: 239-243. PMID: 10644319.
11. Venneman NG, Buskens E, Besselink MG, Stads S, Go PM, Bosscha K, et al. Small gallstones are associated with increased risk of acute pancreatitis: potential benefits of prophylactic cholecystectomy? *Am J Gastroenterol*. 2005; 100: 2540-2550. PMID: 16279912.
12. Yadav D, Lowenfels AB. The epidemiology of pancreatitis and pancreatic cancer. *Gastroenterology*. 2013; 144: 1252-1261. PMID: 23622135.
13. Acosta JM, Ledesma CL. Gallstone migration as a cause of acute pancreatitis. *N Engl J Med*. 1974; 290: 484-487. PMID: 4810815.
14. Liu CL, Fan ST, Lo CM, Tso WK, Wong Y, Poon RT, et al. Clinico-biochemical prediction of biliary cause of acute pancreatitis in the era of endoscopic ultrasonography. *Aliment Pharmacol Ther*. 2005; 22: 423-431. PMID: 16128680.
15. Moolla Z, Anderson F, Thomson SR. Use of amylase and alanine transaminase to predict acute gallstone pancreatitis in a population with high HIV prevalence. *World J Surg*. 2013; 37: 156-161. PMID: 23015223.
16. Tenner S, Dubner H, Steinberg W. Predicting gallstone pancreatitis with laboratory parameters: a meta-analysis. *Am J Gastroenterol*. 1994; 89: 1863-1866. PMID: 7942684.
17. Dholakia K, Pitchumoni CS, Agarwal N. How often are liver function tests normal in acute biliary pancreatitis? *J Clin Gastroenterol*. 2004; 38: 81-83. PMID: 22341094.
18. Tenner S, Baillie J, DeWitt J, Vege SS, American College of Gastroenterology. American College of Gastroenterology guideline: management of acute pancreatitis. *Am J Gastroenterol*. 2013; 108: 1400-1415. PMID: 23896955.
19. Working Group IAPAPAAPG. IAP/APA evidence-based guidelines for the management of acute pancreatitis. *Pancreatology*. 2013; 13: e1-e15. PMID: 24054878.
20. Goodman AJ, Neoptolemos JP, Carr-Locke DL, Finlay DB, Fossard DP. Detection of gall stones after acute pancreatitis. *Gut*. 1985; 26: 125-132. PMID: 2578422.
21. Neoptolemos JP, Hall AW, Finlay DF, Berry JM, Carr-Locke DL, Fossard DP. The urgent diagnosis of gallstones in acute pancreatitis: a prospective study of three methods. *Br J Surg*. 1984; 71: 230-233. PMID: 6141833.
22. Ammori BJ, Boreham B, Lewis P, Roberts SA. The biochemical detection of biliary etiology of acute pancreatitis on admission: a revisit in the modern era of biliary imaging. *Pancreas*. 2003; 26: e32-e35. PMID: 12604925.
23. Mounzer R, Langmead CJ, Wu BU, Evans AC, Bishehsari F, Muddana V, et al. Comparison of existing clinical scoring systems to predict persistent organ failure in patients with acute pancreatitis. *Gastroenterology*. 2012; 142: 1476-1482. PMID: 22425589.
24. van Santvoort HC, Bakker OJ, Besselink MG, Bollen TL, Fischer K, Nieuwenhuijs VB, et al. Prediction of common bile duct stones in the earliest stages of acute biliary pancreatitis. *Endoscopy*. 2011; 43: 8-13. PMID: 20972954.
25. Giljaca V, Gurusamy KS, Takwoingi Y, Higgie D, Poropat G, Stimac D, et al. Endoscopic ultrasound versus magnetic resonance cholangiopancreatography for common bile duct stones. *Cochrane Database Syst Rev*. 2015; 2: CD011549. PMID: 25719224.
26. Kotwal V, Talukdar R, Levy M, Vege SS. Role of endoscopic ultrasound during hospitalization for acute pancreatitis. *World J Gastroenterol*. 2010; 16: 4888-4891. PMID: 20954274.
27. Kondo S, Isayama H, Akahane M, Toda N, Sasahira N, Nakai Y, et al. Detection of common bile duct stones: comparison between endoscopic ultrasonography, magnetic resonance cholangiography, and helical-computed-tomographic cholangiography. *Eur J Radiol*. 2005; 54: 271-275. PMID: 15837409.
28. Polistina FA, Frego M, Bisello M, Manzi E, Vardanega A, Perin B. Accuracy of magnetic resonance cholangiography compared to operative endoscopy in detecting biliary stones, a single center experience and review of literature. *World J Radiol*. 2015; 7: 70-78. PMID: 25918584.
29. Liu CL, Fan ST, Lo CM, Tso WK, Wong Y, Poon RT, et al. Comparison of early endoscopic ultrasonography and endoscopic retrograde cholangiopancreatography in the management of acute biliary pancreatitis: a prospective randomized study. *Clin Gastroenterol Hepatol*. 2005; 3: 1238-1244. PMID: 16361050.
30. Verma D, Kapadia A, Eisen GM, Adler DG. EUS vs MRCP for detection of choledocholithiasis. *Gastrointest Endosc*. 2006; 64: 248-254. PMID: 16860077.
31. Tranter SE, Thompson MH. Spontaneous passage of bile duct stones: frequency of occurrence and relation to clinical presentation. *Ann R Coll Surg Engl*. 2003; 85: 174-177. PMID: 12831489.
32. Andriulli A, Loperfido S, Napolitano G, Niro G, Valvano MR, Spirito F, et al. Incidence rates of post-ERCP complications: a systematic survey of prospective studies. *Am J Gastroenterol*. 2007; 102: 1781-1788. PMID: 17509029.
33. Committee ASGE, Anderson MA, Fisher L, Jain R, Evans JA, Appalaneni V, et al. Complications of ERCP. *Gastrointest Endosc*. 2012; 75: 467-473. PMID: 22341094.
34. Uy MC, Daez ML, Sy PP, Banez VP, Espinosa WZ, Talingdan-Te MC. Early ERCP in acute gallstone pancreatitis without cholangitis: a meta-analysis. *JOP*. 2009; 10: 299-305. PMID: 19454823.
35. Tse F, Yuan Y. Early routine endoscopic retrograde cholangiopancreatography strategy versus early conservative management strategy in acute gallstone pancreatitis. *Cochrane Database Syst Rev*. 2012; 5: CD009779. PMID: 22592743.
36. Burstow MJ, Yunus RM, Hossain MB, Khan S, Memon B, Memon MA. Meta-Analysis of Early Endoscopic Retrograde Cholangiopancreatography (ERCP) +/- Endoscopic Sphincterotomy (ES) Versus Conservative Management for Gallstone Pancreatitis (GSP). *Surg Laparosc Endosc Percutan Tech*. 2015; 25: 185-203. PMID: 25799261.
37. Runzi M, Saluja A, Lerch MM, Dawra R, Nishino H, Steer ML. Early ductal decompression prevents the progression of biliary pancreatitis: an experimental study in the opossum. *Gastroenterology*. 1993; 105: 157-164. PMID: 8514033.

Chapter 31

Timing of cholecystectomy after acute biliary pancreatitis

Stefan A. Bouwense[1*], Mark C. van Baal[2], David da Costa[3], and Marc G. Besselink[4]

[1]*Department of Surgery, Radboud University Medical Center, Nijmegen, The Netherlands;*
[2]*Department of Surgery, Tweesteden Hospital, Tilburg, The Netherlands;*
[3]*Department of Surgery, St. Antonius Hospital, Nieuwegein, The Netherlands;*
[4]*Department of Surgery, Academic Medical Center, Amsterdam, The Netherlands.*

Introduction

Acute pancreatitis (AP) is a common gastrointestinal disorder, and in the majority of patients the etiology is either alcohol-associated or biliary (i.e., caused by gallstones or sludge).[1,2] The incidence of acute biliary pancreatitis is increasing worldwide, possibly because of the increased risk of gallstone disease due to nutritional and lifestyle factors and obesity.[3,4] The economic burden of AP is high; in the United States alone, the annual costs currently exceed $2.2 billion.[5] The majority (80%) of patients with AP have a mild disease course, but 20% develop severe pancreatitis, which is associated with high morbidity and mortality.[6] Once biliary pancreatitis is resolved, cholecystectomy is indicated to reduce the risk of recurrent gallstone-related complications such as AP, cholecystitis, cholangitis, or gallstone colics.[7,8] A much discussed question is when the gallbladder should be removed in the course of pancreatitis.

High complication and mortality rates after early cholecystectomy in patients with severe pancreatitis have prompted guidelines recommending delaying cholecystectomy until all signs of inflammation have resolved (i.e., interval cholecystectomy).[7,9,10] After mild biliary pancreatitis, early cholecystectomy is advised by current guidelines.[7,11,12] However, no consensus exists between these guidelines about the exact definition of "early." The British Society of Gastroenterology recommend cholecystectomy within 2 weeks after discharge, whereas the International Association of Pancreatology and American Gastroenterological Association recommend that all patients with mild biliary pancreatitis should undergo cholecystectomy as soon as the patient has recovered from the attack.[7,8,11] However, in contrast with these guidelines, cholecystectomy after mild biliary pancreatitis is often postponed for several weeks after hospital discharge (interval cholecystectomy). Nationwide audits from Europe and the United States have shown that laparoscopic cholecystectomy is usually performed around 6 weeks after discharge from hospital admission for mild biliary pancreatitis.[13-21] The main reason for delaying cholecystectomy is a perceived danger of perioperative complications in early cholecystectomy after AP.[13,22] It is believed that distortion of biliary tract anatomy by inflammation and edema may complicate dissection and confer a higher risk of conversion and surgical complications such as bile duct injury.[10,23,24] Another reason is that a delayed approach facilitates surgical scheduling, as emergency operating capacity is often limited.[22]

In patients with mild biliary pancreatitis, the role of endoscopic sphincterotomy is limited when cholangitis is not present.[7] However, large nationwide studies from the United Kingdom and United States still show relatively high percentages of patients with mild biliary pancreatitis undergoing endoscopic sphincterotomy.[13,24,25] Several retrospective studies have suggested that patients do not need to undergo early cholecystectomy after sphincterotomy.[26] However, a recent meta-analysis on prophylactic cholecystectomy after sphincterotomy for gallstone-related complications other than pancreatitis still suggested that a cholecystectomy should be performed even after sphincterotomy to further reduce recurrent biliary events.[27] Some have advocated the use of endoscopic sphincterotomy as a bridge to cholecystectomy in patients with severe pancreatitis.[26,28] This issue has not been addressed in prospective trials and needs further study in patients with severe biliary pancreatitis.

The drawback of the present practice of postponing cholecystectomy until several weeks after discharge is that during this period patients are at risk of developing recurrent biliary events (e.g., recurrent biliary pancreatitis, cholecystitis, symptomatic choledocholithiasis, and biliary colics). This risk is substantial and has been reported to occur in up to 60% of patients in observational studies.[29,30] It is thought

*Corresponding author. Email: Stefan.Bouwense@radboudumc.nl

that the lack of high-quality evidence may be attributable to the reported low adherence to guidelines.[13-15,24,25]

Three main questions will be discussed in this review:

1) Does early cholecystectomy reduce recurrent biliary events compared to interval cholecystectomy?
2) Is early cholecystectomy technically more difficult to perform than interval cholecystectomy?
3) Are patients in whom early cholecystectomy is performed more at risk for complications than patients who undergo interval cholecystectomy?

In the next paragraphs we will discuss available studies on cholecystectomy timing and try to answer these three questions.

Studies addressing the timing of cholecystectomy in mild biliary pancreatitis

In 2011, Bakker et al. published a retrospective multicenter study that evaluated recurrent biliary events as a consequence of delayed cholecystectomy following mild biliary pancreatitis.[21] Patients with mild biliary pancreatitis who were candidates for cholecystectomy were registered prospectively in 15 Dutch hospitals from 2004 to 2007. Recurrent biliary events requiring admission were evaluated before and after cholecystectomy, as well as for a subgroup of patients who underwent endoscopic sphincterotomy. Of 308 patients with mild biliary pancreatitis, 267 had an indication for cholecystectomy. Early and late (after a median of 6 weeks) cholecystectomy were performed in 18 (7%) and 188 (76%) patients, respectively. Before cholecystectomy was performed, 34 (14%) patients were readmitted for biliary events, including 24 with recurrent biliary pancreatitis. During the initial admission, endoscopic sphincterotomy had been performed in 108 patients. Among these, eight (7%) suffered from recurrent biliary events after endoscopic sphincterotomy and before cholecystectomy. In the group of patients who did not undergo endoscopic sphincterotomy, 26 of 141 (18%) had recurrent biliary events, which was significant compared to the group of patients who did undergo endoscopic sphincterotomy (risk ratio 0.51, 95% confidence interval 0.27 to 0.94; $P = 0.015$). It was concluded that an interval cholecystectomy after mild biliary pancreatitis carries a substantial risk of recurrent biliary events. Endoscopic sphincterotomy reduces the risk of recurrent biliary pancreatitis but not of other biliary events. The shortcomings of this study were that it was not primarily designed to analyze cholecystectomy safety, and it was not a randomized clinical trial comparing early versus interval cholecystectomy.

In 2012, van Baal et al. published a systematic review on the timing of cholecystectomy after mild biliary pancreatitis.[31] The objective was to determine the risk of recurrent biliary events in the period after mild biliary pancreatitis but before interval cholecystectomy and to determine the safety of cholecystectomy during the index admission. A systematic search in PubMed, Embase, and Cochrane for studies published from January 1992 to July 2010 was performed. Cohort studies of patients with mild biliary pancreatitis reporting on the timing of cholecystectomy, number of readmissions for recurrent biliary events before cholecystectomy, operative complications (e.g., bile duct injury, bleeding), and mortality were included. Study quality and risks of bias were also assessed. From 2,413 screened studies, 8 cohort studies and 1 randomized trial were included,

Table 1. Patient outcomes in cholecystectomy after mild biliary pancreatitis.

	Number of patients		Time between discharge and cholecystectomy (days)		Readmissions for biliary events		Complications	
Study	Early	Interval	Early	Interval	Early	Interval	Early	Interval
Schachter et al.[32]	-	19	-	Mean >56	-	0	-	0
McCullough et al.[33]	74	90	0	Mean 40	0	18 (20%)	11	16
Cameron et al.[34]	-	58	-	Mean 93, Median 68	-	11 (19%)	-	0
Griniatsos et al.[35]*	-	20	-	Median 14	-	0	-	1
Griniatsos et al.[35]*	-	24	-	Median 60	-	1 (4%)	-	1
Clarke et al.[36]	110	92	0	Mean 23	0	8 (9%)	4	5
Ito et al.[37]	162	119	0	Median45	0	39 (33%)	37	34
Nebiker et al.[38]	32	67	0	Mean >14	0	15 (22%)	2	5
Sinha et al.[39]	81	26	0	Mean >42	0	3 (12%)	0	0
Aboulian et al.[40]	24	-	0	-	0	-	0	-
Total	483	515	0	Median 40	0	95 (18%)	17 (4%)	29 (6%)

This table was adapted from the original manuscript of van Baal et al.[31]

*In one study, two different interval cholecystectomy groups were described.

in total describing 998 patients. An early cholecystectomy was performed in 483 (48%) patients without any reported readmissions (**Table 1**). An interval cholecystectomy was performed in 515 (52%) patients after a median of 40 days (interquartile range 19-58 days). Before the interval cholecystectomy was performed 95 patients (18%) were readmitted for recurrent biliary events (0% vs. 18%; $P < 0.0001$). Forty-three (8%) patients were readmitted due to recurrent biliary pancreatitis, 17 (3%) with acute cholecystitis, and 35 (7%) with biliary colics. Fewer recurrent biliary events were present in patients who had an endoscopic sphincterotomy (10% vs. 24%; $P = 0.001$), with especially less recurrent biliary pancreatitis (1% vs. 9%). No differences were found in operative complications or the conversion (7%) or mortality (0%) rates between early and interval cholecystectomy. Baseline characteristics were often missing (reported in 26% of patients), so subgroups could not be compared. It was concluded that interval cholecystectomy after mild biliary pancreatitis is associated with a high risk of readmission for recurrent biliary events, especially recurrent biliary pancreatitis. Furthermore, early cholecystectomy for mild biliary pancreatitis appears to be safe. The main shortcomings of this systematic review were that the included studies were of relatively low quality and selection bias could not be excluded.

In 2010, a randomized clinical trial on the timing of cholecystectomy after mild biliary pancreatitis was published by Aboulian et al.[40] The authors hypothesized that performing laparoscopic cholecystectomy within 48 hours after admission for mild biliary pancreatitis would result in shorter hospital stays. Patients with mild pancreatitis (defined as a Ranson score ≤3) were randomized to early laparoscopic cholecystectomy (within 48 hours of admission) or to control laparoscopic cholecystectomy performed after resolution of abdominal pain and normalizing trends of laboratory enzymes. In this single-center study with interim analyses, 25 patients were randomized to early cholecystectomy, and 25 were included in a control group and underwent cholecystectomy after resolution of abdominal pain and normalization of laboratory values. The median duration of symptoms was 2 days upon presentation with a median Ranson score of 1. The hospital stay duration was 1 day shorter in the early cholecystectomy group with a median of 3 days (interquartile range 2-4) compared with the control group with a median of 4 days (interquartile range 4-6, $P = 0.0016$). There were no statistically significant differences between the groups for conversions to an open procedure or perioperative complications. It was concluded that a laparoscopic cholecystectomy performed within 48 hours after admission (very early cholecystectomy) results in shorter hospital stay and appears to be safe and not more technical demanding. This study was not powered to detect differences in clinically relevant outcomes such as recurrent biliary events. Moreover, cholecystectomy within 48 hours after admission in gallstone pancreatitis is controversial because patients may still develop pancreatic necrosis or organ failure during this phase of the disease, both of which are considered contraindications for early surgery.

These three studies all show a benefit of early cholecystectomy in mild biliary pancreatitis, which appears a safe strategy without an increase in cholecystectomy difficulty. However, the design and evidence quality of these studies were not particularly high. It appeared that a well-designed randomized clinical trial was needed to resolve the issue of timing of cholecystectomy in mild biliary pancreatitis.

In 2012, the study protocol for a randomized controlled trial titled pancreatitis of biliary origin, optimal timing of cholecystectomy (PONCHO) was published by Bouwense et al.[41] The hypothesis for this trial is that early laparoscopic cholecystectomy minimizes the risk of recurrent biliary events in patients with mild biliary pancreatitis without increasing the difficulty of dissection or surgical complication rate compared with interval laparoscopic cholecystectomy. PONCHO is a randomized controlled superiority multicenter trial in which patients are randomly allocated to undergo early laparoscopic cholecystectomy within 72 hours after randomization or interval laparoscopic cholecystectomy 25 to 30 days after randomization. Patients are randomized during their index admission when all signs of the disease have resolved and patients are expected to be discharged within 1 to 2 days. A total of 266 patients in 18 Dutch hospitals were enrolled. The primary endpoint is a composite endpoint of mortality and acute readmissions for biliary events (e.g., recurrent biliary pancreatitis, acute cholecystitis, symptomatic/obstructive choledocholithiasis requiring endoscopic retrograde cholangiopancreaticography including cholangitis [with/without endoscopic sphincterotomy], and uncomplicated biliary colics) occurring within 6 months following randomization. Secondary endpoints include the individual endpoints of the composite endpoint, surgical and other complications, technical difficulty of cholecystectomy and costs.The PONCHO trial results are expected to be published at the end of 2015. This trial will provide the high level of evidence needed to finally close the debate on cholecystectomy timing in mild biliary pancreatitis.

Conclusion

In patients with severe biliary pancreatitis, it is generally acceptable to perform an interval cholecystectomy. Although advocated by current guidelines, patients with mild biliary pancreatitis frequently do not undergo an early cholecystectomy, resulting in a high percentage of hospital readmissions due to recurrent biliary events. All published studies are of medium to low methodological quality, and the results of the first randomized controlled clinical trial comparing early versus interval cholecystectomy in patients with mild biliary pancreatitis are expected at the end of 2015. The role of endoscopic sphincterotomy remains under debate, although it is generally accepted that it is not indicated in patients without cholangitis. It is thought that endoscopic sphincterotomy will reduce the number of recurrent biliary events but will not prevent all events.

References

1. Yadav D, Lowenfels AB. The epidemiology of pancreatitis and pancreatic cancer. *Gastroenterology*. 2013; 144(6): 1252-1261. PMID: 23622135.
2. Venneman NG,van Brummelen SE,van Berge-Henegouwen GP,van Erpecum KJ. Microlithiasis: an important cause of "idiopathic" acute pancreatitis? *Ann Hepatol*. 2003; 2(1): 30-35. PMID: 15094703.
3. Yadav D, Lowenfels AB. Trends in the epidemiology of the first attack of acute pancreatitis: a systematic review. *Pancreas*. 2006; 33(4): 323-330. PMID: 17079934.
4. Torgerson JS, Lindroos AK, Naslund I, Peltonen M. Gallstones, gallbladder disease, and pancreatitis: cross-sectional and 2-year data from the Swedish Obese Subjects (SOS) and SOS reference studies. *Am J Gastroenterol*. 2003; 98(5): 1032-1041. PMID: 12809825.
5. Fagenholz PJ, Fernandez-del Castillo C, Harris NS, Pelletier AJ, Camargo CA. Direct medical costs of acute pancreatitis hospitalizations in the United States. *Pancreas*. 2007; 35(4): 302-307. PMID: 18090234.
6. Banks PA, Freeman ML; Practice Parameters Committee of the American College of Gastroenterology. Practice guidelines in acute pancreatitis. *Am J Gastroenterol*. 2006; 101(10): 2379-2400. PMID: 17032204.
7. Working Group IAP/APA Acute Pancreatitis Guidelines. IAP/APA evidence-based guidelines for the management of acute pancreatitis. *Pancreatology*. 2013; 13(4 Suppl 2): e1-e15. PMID: 24054878.
8. Tenner S, Baillie J, Dewitt J, Vege SS; American College of Gastroenterology. American College of Gastroenterology Guidelines: management of acute pancreatitis. *Am J Gastroenterol*. 2013. PMID: 23896955.
9. Nealon WH, Bawduniak J, Walser EM. Appropriate timing of cholecystectomy in patients who present with moderate to severe gallstone-associated acute pancreatitis with peripancreatic fluid collections. *Ann Surg*. 2004; 239(6): 741-749. PMID: 15166953.
10. Kelly TR, Wagner DS. Gallstone pancreatitis: a prospective randomized trial of the timing of surgery. *Surgery*. 1988; 104(4): 600-605. PMID: 3175860.
11. Working Party of the British Society of Gastroenterology; Association of Surgeons of Great Britain and Ireland; Pancreatic Society of Great Britain and Ireland; Association of Upper GI Surgeons of Great Britain and Ireland. UK guidelines for the management of acute pancreatitis. *Gut*. 2005; 54 Suppl 3: iii1-iii9. PMID: 15831893.
12. Forsmark CE, Baillie J. AGA Institute Technical Review on Acute Pancreatitis. *Gastroenterology*. 2007; 132(5): 2022-2044. PMID: 17484894.
13. Nguyen GC, Boudreau H, Jagannath SB. Hospital volume as a predictor for undergoing cholecystectomy after admission for acute biliary pancreatitis. *Pancreas*. 2010; 39(1): e42-e47. PMID: 19910833.
14. Lankisch PG, Weber-Dany B, Lerch MM. Clinical perspectives in pancreatology: compliance with acute pancreatitis guidelines in Germany. *Pancreatology*. 2005; 5(6): 591-593. PMID: 16110257.
15. El-Dhuwaib Y, Deakin M, David GG, Durkin D, Corless DJ, Slavin JP. Definitive management of gallstone pancreatitis in England. *Ann R Coll Surg Engl*. 2012; 94(6): 402-406. PMID: 22943329.
16. Sandzén B, Haapamäki MM, Nilsson E, Stenlund HC, Oman M. Cholecystectomy and sphincterotomy in patients with mild acute biliary pancreatitis in Sweden 1988 - 2003: a nationwide register study. *BMC Gastroenterol*. 2009; 9: 80. PMID: 19852782.
17. Pezzilli R, Uomo G, Gabbrielli A, Zerbi A, Frulloni L, De Rai P, et al. A prospective multicentre survey on the treatment of acute pancreatitis in Italy. *Dig Liver Dis*. 2007; 39(9): 838-846. PMID: 17602904.
18. Barnard J, Siriwardena AK. Variations in implementation of current national guidelines for the treatment of acute pancreatitis: implications for acute surgical service provision. *Ann R Coll Surg Engl*. 2002; 84(2): 79-81. PMID: 11995768.
19. Senapati PS, Bhattarcharya D, Harinath G, Ammori BJ. A survey of the timing and approach to the surgical management of cholelithiasis in patients with acute biliary pancreatitis and acute cholecystitis in the UK. *Ann R Coll Surg Engl*. 2003; 85(5): 306-312. PMID: 14594533.
20. Toh SK, Phillips S, Johnson CD. A prospective audit against national standards of the presentation and management of acute pancreatitis in the South of England. *Gut*. 2000; 46(2): 239-243. PMID: 10644319.
21. Bakker OJ, Van Santvoort HC, Hagenaars JC, Besselink MG, Bollen TL, Gooszen HG, et al. Timing of cholecystectomy after mild biliary pancreatitis. *Br J Surg*. 2011; 98(10): 1446-1454. PMID: 21710664.
22. Monkhouse SJ, Court EL, Dash I, Coombs NJ. Two-week target for laparoscopic cholecystectomy following gallstone pancreatitis is achievable and cost neutral. *Br J Surg*. 2009; 96(7): 751-755. PMID: 19526610.
23. Tate JJ, Lau WY, Li AK. Laparoscopic cholecystectomy for biliary pancreatitis. *Br J Surg*. 1994; 81(5): 720-722. PMID: 8044561.
24. Johnstone M, Marriott P, Royle TJ, Richardson CE, Torrance A, Hepburn E, et al. The impact of timing of cholecystectomy following gallstone pancreatitis. *Surgeon*. 2014; 12(3): 134-140. PMID: 24210949.
25. Hwang SS, Li BH, Haigh PI. Gallstone pancreatitis without cholecystectomy. *JAMA Surg*. 2013; 148(9): 867-872. PMID: 23884515.
26. Heider TR, Brown A, Grimm IS, Behrns KE. Endoscopic sphincterotomy permits interval laparoscopic cholecystectomy in patients with moderately severe gallstone

pancreatitis. *J Gastrointest Surg*. 2006; 10(1): 1-5. PMID: 16368484.
27. McAlister VC, Davenport E, Renouf E. Cholecystectomy deferral in patients with endoscopic sphincterotomy. *Cochrane Database Syst Rev*. 2007;(4): CD006233. PMID: 17943900.
28. Sanjay P, Yeeting S, Whigham C, Judson H, Polignano FM, Tait IS. Endoscopic sphincterotomy and interval cholecystectomy are reasonable alternatives to index cholecystectomy in severe acute gallstone pancreatitis (GSP). *Surg Endosc*. 2008; 22(8): 1832-1837. PMID: 18071797.
29. Alimoglu O, Ozkan OV, Sahin M, Akcakaya A, Eryilmaz R, Bas G. Timing of cholecystectomy for acute biliary pancreatitis: outcomes of cholecystectomy on first admission and after recurrent biliary pancreatitis. *World J Surg*. 2003; 27(3): 256-259. PMID: 12607047.
30. van Geenen EJ,van der Peet DL, Mulder CJ, Cuesta MA, Bruno MJ. Recurrent acute biliary pancreatitis: the protective role of cholecystectomy and endoscopic sphincterotomy. *Surg Endosc*. 2009; 23(5): 950-956. PMID: 19266236.
31. van Baal MC, Besselink MG, Bakker OJ,van Santvoort HC, Schaapherder AF, Nieuwenhuijs VB, et al. Timing of cholecystectomy after mild biliary pancreatitis: a systematic review. *Ann Surg*. 2012; 255(5): 860-866. PMID: 22470079.
32. Schachter P, Peleg T, Cohen O. Interval laparoscopic cholecystectomy in the management of acute biliary pancreatitis. *HPB Surg*. 2000; 11(5): 319-322. PMID: 10674747.
33. McCullough LK, Sutherland FR, Preshaw R, Kim S. Gallstone pancreatitis: does discharge and readmission for cholecystectomy affect outcome? *HPB*. 2003; 5(2): 96-99. PMID: 18332964.
34. Cameron DR, Goodman AJ. Delayed cholecystectomy for gallstone pancreatitis: re-admissions and outcomes. *Ann R Coll Surg Engl*. 2004; 86(5): 358-362. PMID: 15333174.
35. Griniatsos J, Karvounis E, Isla A. Early versus delayed single-stage laparoscopic eradication for both gallstones and common bile duct stones in mild acute biliary pancreatitis. *Am Surg*. 2005; 71(8): 682-686. PMID: 16217952.
36. Clarke T, Sohn H, Kelso R, Petrosyan M, Towfigh S, Mason R. Planned early discharge-elective surgical readmission pathway for patients with gallstone pancreatitis. *Arch Surg*. 2008; 143(9): 901-905; discussion 905-906. PMID: 18794429.
37. Ito K, Ito H, Whang EE. Timing of cholecystectomy for biliary pancreatitis: do the data support current guidelines? *J Gastrointest Surg*. 2008; 12(12): 2164-2170. PMID: 18636298.
38. Nebiker CA, Frey DM, Hamel CT, Oertli D, Kettelhack C. Early versus delayed cholecystectomy in patients with biliary acute pancreatitis. *Surgery*. 2009; 145(3): 260-264. PMID: 19231577.
39. Sinha R. Early laparoscopic cholecystectomy in acute biliary pancreatitis: the optimal choice? *HPB (Oxford)*. 2008; 10(5): 332-335. PMID: 18982148.
40. Aboulian A, Chan T, Yaghoubian A, Kaji AH, Putnam B, Neville A, et al. Early cholecystectomy safely decreases hospital stay in patients with mild gallstone pancreatitis: a randomized prospective study. *Ann Surg*. 2010; 251(4): 615-619. PMID: 20101174.
41. Bouwense SA, Besselink MG,van Brunschot S, Bakker OJ,van Santvoort HC, Schepers NJ, et al. Pancreatitis of biliary origin, optimal timing of cholecystectomy (PONCHO trial): study protocol for a randomized controlled trial. *Trials*. 2012; 13: 225. PMID: 23181667.

Chapter 32

Management of abdominal compartment syndrome in acute pancreatitis

Jan J. De Waele*

Department of Critical Care Medicine, Ghent University Hospital De Pintelaan 185, 9000 Gent, Belgium.

Introduction

Insights in the diagnosis and management of acute pancreatitis are evolving with many treatment strategies that were once considered the standard of care eventually being discarded as non- beneficial or even harmful.[1] Both medical treatment and surgery have advanced significantly, but the morbidity and mortality of severe acute pancreatitis remain high, and the course of the disease is often protracted in severe cases.

Intra-abdominal hypertension (IAH) and abdominal compartment syndrome (ACS) have been found to be significant contributors to organ dysfunction in a variety of critically ill patients, and several strategies have been developed to prevent and treat ACS.[2]

Patients with severe acute pancreatitis appear to be at an increased risk of IAH due to the several mechanisms that occur in pancreatitis, as well as the treatment they receive. Our understanding of both the development of IAH and ACS in SAP has advanced significantly, and ACS has evolved from an incompletely understood and poorly managed complication in SAP to a preventable and treatable condition that should be understood by all physicians involved in the care of these patients.

Definitions

IAH has been defined as an intra-abdominal pressure (IAP) ≥12 mmHg or higher.[3] This is the threshold at which organ dysfunction may set in, although it is often undetectable unless specifically sought for. Oxygen exchange for instance may be impaired, but compensatory mechanisms may be effective, and oxygen saturation may not be changed.

In case of ACS, the IAP is ≥20 mmHg with clinically evident new organ dysfunction; acute kidney injury, cardiovascular instability, and respiratory insufficient are the most commonly encountered organ dysfunctions in ACS. A complete review of IAH and ACS and how it affects organ function falls beyond the scope of this chapter.[4]

Pathophysiology

IAH and ACS are typically early phenomena in SAP; in most reports IAH develops in the first 3-5 days after hospital admission.[5] Several mechanisms lead to increased IAP in these patients (**Table 1**), with pancreatic and peripancreatic inflammation probably only of minor importance as the increase in intra-abdominal volume from local edema is often minimal.[6] The ileus that often accompanies this disease process, as well as the development of ascites, may further increase the intra-abdominal volume, but a major contributor is undoubtedly the fluid resuscitation often initiated in patients with severe pancreatitis to compensate for central hypovolemia due to third spacing. Early aggressive fluid resuscitation is still considered the standard of care in many guidelines; however, fluid overload (although variably defined) has been found to be a major risk factor in several studies and different patient categories.[7] Also, in studies that specifically looked into ACS in pancreatitis, fluid resuscitation was consistently reported as contributing to both increased intra-abdominal volume and reduced abdominal wall compliance.[8]

In the context of acute pancreatitis, the effects of IAH may have an important impact, not only on organ function as a whole, but on pancreatic perfusion in particular. Animal studies have found that pancreatic perfusion is decreased in IAH,[9] which may further increase the risk of pancreatic necrosis. Also bacterial translocation—the presumed pathway for pancreatic infection in SAP—is frequent in IAH; there is a dose-dependent relationship with the extent of bacterial infection. As a result, IAH may impact both pancreatic necrosis and subsequent infection.

*Corresponding author. Email: Jan.DeWaele@UGent.be

Table 1. Contributors to IAH and ACS in acute pancreatitis.

Intra-abdominal volume increase
Pancreatic and peripancreatic edema (often fueled by fluid resuscitation)
Ascites
Ileus
Abdominal wall compliance decrease
Abdominal wall edema
Abdominal pain

Epidemiology

SAP is one of the conditions where IAH and ACS are consistently reported. Using the original Atlanta criteria, the incidence of IAH was between 60% and 80%, and ACS developed in roughly 25%-50% of the patients according to one study.[6] Using the new criteria, the incidence in severe disease may be even higher, as some patients with what is now considered moderate pancreatitis were in the original severe category. Acute pancreatitis itself has been identified as a risk factor for IAH in a recent systematic review, but several other factors are also often present in patients with SAP.[10]

IAH and especially ACS have been associated with a worse outcome in all reports on this problem.[5,11-14] Rosas et al. even proposed using an IAP of 14 mmHg or higher as a marker of severity in SAP; in their analysis, the receiver operating characteristic curve of IAP was higher compared to the Ranson and Imrie score, which could make IAP measurement a simple tool.[15] Unfortunately, no other studies have evaluated IAP for this purpose.

Diagnosis of IAH

Diagnosing IAH and ACS in SAP is simple. Clinical examination is notoriously unreliable in these patients, but IAP measurement should be now in the armamentarium of all contemporary intensive care units. The bladder is used as a window to the abdomen, and multiple methods for reproducible IAP measurement are now available. Several reviews describing IAP measurement techniques have been published.[16] In brief: 25 mL sterile saline is instilled in the urinary bladder and the hydrostatic pressure is subsequently measured in mmHg (>12 mmHg IAH, >20 mmHg ACS) IAH grade I 12-15 mmHg, grade II 16-20 mmHg, grade III (ACS) 21-25 mmHg, grade IV >25 mmHg.[17] Small studies have investigated computed tomography features of ACS patients and found that signs such as vena cava narrowing and an increased anteroposterior diameter and bowel wall thickening were associated with ACS.[18] These are late signs, and IAP measurement should be implemented before they occur.

Prevention of IAH in SAP

Now that the contributors to IAH have been better described, several options for prevention can be devised. As in other critically ill patients, fluid resuscitation is one of the key iatrogenic contributors to IAH and ACS, and the concept of vigorous fluid resuscitation should be urgently re-evaluated in many of these conditions. Several studies have linked overly positive fluid balances to worse outcomes including ACS.[14] In this context, studies have found that patients who were resuscitated less aggressively had a lower incidence of ACS and better clinical outcomes. Whether the type of resuscitation fluid impacts this phenomenon remains unclear, and given the ban on starches in many countries, crystalloids remain the primary resuscitation fluid. However, Zhao et al. found that patients resuscitated with normal saline only had higher IAP and ACS more often than those treated with a combination of colloids and crystalloids.[19]

It is difficult to recommend an appropriate resuscitation endpoint in SAP; conventional parameters such as central venous pressure are not recommended as they are not predictive of fluid responsiveness, especially in IAH. Urinary output also has drawbacks as it is a typical early indicator of IAH, and further fluid loading as a response to oliguria may aggravate rather than solve the problem. Dynamic indices such as stroke volume variation may be better tools,[20] but they can also be affected by IAH, so judicious use of any parameter is advisable, and at all points, the requirement for fluids should be balanced against its side effects.

Treatment

The World Society of the Abdominal Compartment Syndrome recently updated the guidelines for managing IAH and ACS, which suggest a stepwise approach to decreasing IAP in patients (**Figure 1**).[3] In the context of SAP, a number of specifically relevant interventions are discussed below. It is very important to realize that there are different nonsurgical strategies available, and although surgical intervention remains a definite treatment modalities, it should be reserved for therapy-resistant ACS.

Medical therapy is the first step for most patients, and when applied consistently, this will dramatically reduce the need for decompressive laparotomy. In any case, early and repeated IAP measurement is the first step towards recognition of the problem and therapy.

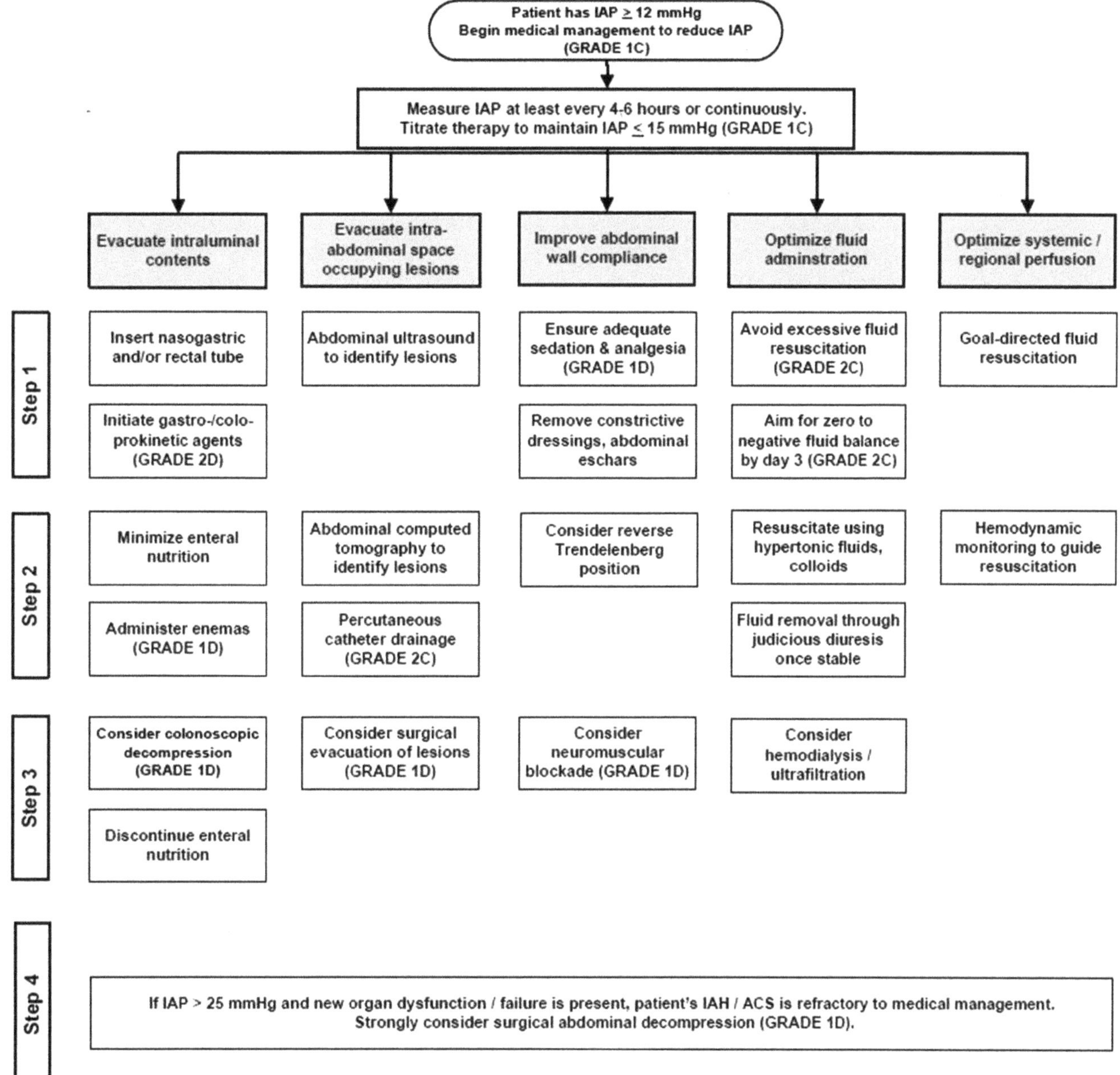

Figure 1. Medical management of IAH and ACS.[3]

Nasogastric decompression

As ileus and gastroparesis are often present, reducing the intraluminal volume of the gastrointestinal tract is a logical first step. In case of gastric dilatation, nasogastric decompression is easily performed and may have an important impact on IAP. The role of prokinetic drugs remains unclear.

Percutaneous drainage

Percutaneous drainage of ascites is a more useful, minimally invasive treatment option that can be done at the bedside under ultrasound guidance. In the largest study to date in AP, Sun et al. described a decrease in IAP from 29 to 14 mmHg after draining a median of 1,800 mL of ascites.[21] Percutaneous drainage of retroperitoneal fluid collections or pseudocysts may also reduce IAP and improve organ function.[22]

Neuromuscular blockers

As in other conditions associated with IAH, improving abdominal wall compliance through neuromuscular blockers

(NMBs) may be used.[23] Although often used as a bridge to abdominal decompression, this may be continued for a short time (2-3 days) when necessary.

Fluid removal and hemofiltration

Small studies have focused on extracorporeal techniques to remove fluid overload. In a retrospective analysis Pupelis et al. found that hemofiltration was effective in removing fluid overload and reducing IAH, and was associated with improved outcomes.[24] Also Oda et al. claimed improved outcomes after early hemofiltration to prevent IAH,[25] but its exact role remains to be defined. Diuretics may be ineffective as patients often suffer from acute kidney injury with oligo- or anuria.

Surgical decompression and open abdomen therapy

Surgical decompression—usually through a full midline laparotomy—may be required in deteriorating patients with ACS who do not respond to medical therapy. Decompressive laparotomy is very effective in reducing the IAP in patients with ACS irrespective of the underlying cause,[26] and this has also been documented in SAP. The role of decompressive laparotomy remains controversial, and many surgeons are reluctant to operate in patients with SAP early in the course of the disease as many studies have reported that early debridement is harmful. It is crucial that the pancreas is not touched during decompressive laparotomy.

Alternatives to median laparotomy have been described for patients with SAP. Leppäniemi et al. introduced the subcutaneous linea alba fasciotomy through small skin incisions on the anterior abdominal wall.[27] Although an effective approach for avoiding median laparotomy in many patients,[28] the resulting giant hernia is definitely a downside of the technique. Fascial closure rates after open laparotomy are increasing because of improved temporary abdominal closure techniques. In the context of SAP, some surgeons may prefer a transverse incision to facilitate access to the pancreas later.[29]

The timing of surgical decompression is a particularly interesting topic. In a series of patients treated with decompression in Finland, the authors reported a 100% mortality rate in those who were decompressed more than 5 days after symptom onset.[30] It should not be surprising that organ dysfunction-induced damage is irreversible in cases of prolonged exposure to high IAP. Still, the exact time frame within which decompressive laparotomy can be successful is difficult to determine. In an animal study, Ke et al. found that early intervention (as soon 6 hours after ACS) was more effective.[31]

The resulting open abdomen should be managed appropriately. Whereas this was once a surgeon's nightmare, negative pressure therapy has become the standard of care for the open abdomen, with the lowest complications and highest primary fascial closure rates.[32] This method has also been effective in patients with SAP.[33,34] A mesh-based technique is most successful method in achieving early abdominal closure and can also be applied in SAP.[34,35]

Conclusions

IAH and ACS are frequent findings in patients with SAP, and as in other settings, relevant contributors to organ dysfunction. IAP monitoring allows early detection of IAH and is recommended in all patients with severe disease. Fluid overload is an important risk factor for IAH and should be avoided. When IAH develops, percutaneous drainage of fluid collections is an effective strategy to reduce IAP, but other medical treatment options can be considered and should be used selectively. If medical therapy fails, decompressive laparotomy may be an appropriate option to reduce IAP and restore organ function.

Acknowledgements and disclosures

Financial support and sponsorship: Jan J. De Waele is a Senior Clinical Researcher with the Research Foundation Flanders (Belgium).

Conflicts of interest: Jan J. De Waele has served as a consultant to Smith & Nephew, and Kinetic Concepts Inc.

References

1. De Waele JJ. Acute pancreatitis. *Curr Opin Crit Care*. 2014; 20: 189-195. PMID: 24553339.
2. De Keulenaer B, Regli A, De Laet I, Roberts D, Malbrain ML. What's new in medical management strategies for raised intra-abdominal pressure: evacuating intra-abdominal contents, improving abdominal wall compliance, pharmacotherapy, and continuous negative extra-abdominal pressure. *Anaesthesiol Intensive Ther*. 2015; 47(1): 54-62. PMID: 25421926.
3. Kirkpatrick AW, Roberts DJ, De Waele J, Jaeschke R, Malbrain ML, De Keulenaer B, et al. Intra-abdominal hypertension and the abdominal compartment syndrome: updated consensus definitions and clinical practice guidelines from the World Society of the Abdominal Compartment Syndrome. *Intensive Care Med*. 2013; 39: 1190-1206. PMID: 23673399.
4. De Waele JJ, De Laet I, Kirkpatrick AW, Hoste E. Intra-abdominal Hypertension and Abdominal Compartment Syndrome. *Am J Kidney Dis*. 2011; 57: 159-169. PMID: 21184922.

5. De Waele JJ, Hoste E, Blot SI, Decruyenaere J, Colardyn F. Intra-abdominal hypertension in patients with severe acute pancreatitis. *Crit Care*. 2005; 9: R452-R457. PMID: 16137360.
6. De Waele JJ, Leppäniemi AK. Intra-abdominal hypertension in acute pancreatitis. *World J Surg*. 2009; 33: 1128-1133. PMID: 19350318.
7. Malbrain ML, Marik PE, Witters I, Cordemans C, Kirkpatrick AW, Roberts DJ, et al. Fluid overload, de-resuscitation, and outcomes in critically ill or injured patients: a systematic review with suggestions for clinical practice. *Anaesthesiol Intensive Ther*. 2014; 46: 361-380. PMID: 25432556.
8. Blaser AR, Björck M, De Keulenaer B, Regli A. Abdominal compliance: A bench-to-bedside review. *J Trauma Acute Care Surg*. 2015; 78: 1044-1053. PMID: 25909429.
9. Endo K, Sasaki T, Sata N, Hishikawa S, Sugimoto H, Lefor AT, et al. Elevation of intra-abdominal pressure by pneumoperitoneum decreases pancreatic perfusion in an in vivo porcine model. *Surg Laparosc Endosc Percutan Tech*. 2014; 24: 221-225. PMID: 24710250.
10. Holodinsky JK, Roberts DJ, Ball CG, Blaser AR, Starkopf J, Zygun DA, et al. Risk factors for intra-abdominal hypertension and abdominal compartment syndrome among adult intensive care unit patients: a systematic review and meta-analysis. *Crit Care*. 2013; 17: R249. PMID: 24144138.
11. Aitken E, Gough V, Jones A, Macdonald A. Observational study of intra-abdominal pressure monitoring in acute pancreatitis. *Surgery*. 2013; 155(5): 910-918. PMID: 24630146.
12. Bhandari V, Jaipuria J, Singh M, Chawla AS. Intra-abdominal pressure in the early phase of severe acute pancreatitis: canary in a coal mine? Results from a rigorous validation protocol. *Gut Liver*. 2013; 7: 731-738. PMID: 24312716.
13. Chen H, Li F, Sun JB, Jia JG. Abdominal compartment syndrome in patients with severe acute pancreatitis in early stage. *World J Gastroenterol*. 2008; 14: 3541-3548. PMID: 18567084.
14. Ke L, Ni HB, Sun JK, Tong ZH, Li WQ, Li N, et al. Risk factors and outcome of intra-abdominal hypertension in patients with severe acute pancreatitis. *World J Surg*. 2012; 36: 171-178. PMID: 21964817.
15. Rosas JM, Soto SN, Aracil JS, Cladera PR, Borlan RH, Sanchez AV, et al. Intra-abdominal pressure as a marker of severity in acute pancreatitis. *Surgery*. 2007; 141: 173-178. PMID: 17263972.
16. Sugrue M, De Waele JJ, De Keulenaer BL, Roberts DJ, Malbrain ML. A user's guide to intra-abdominal pressure measurement. *Anaesthesiol Intensive Ther*. 2015; 47(3): 241-251. PMID: 25973661.
17. Working Group IAP/APA Acute Pancreatitis Guidelines. IAP/APA evidence-based guidelines for the management of acute pancreatitis. *Pancreatology*. 2013; 13(4 Suppl 2): e1-e15. PMID: 24054878.
18. Al-Bahrani AZ, Abid GH, Sahgal E, O'shea S, Lee S, Ammori BJ. A prospective evaluation of CT features predictive of intra-abdominal hypertension and abdominal compartment syndrome in critically ill surgical patients. *Clin Radiol*. 2007; 62: 676-682. PMID: 17556037.
19. Zhao G, Zhang JG, Wu HS, Tao J, Qin Q, Deng SC, et al. Effects of different resuscitation fluid on severe acute pancreatitis. *World J Gastroenterol*. 2013; 19: 2044-2052. PMID: 23599623.
20. Trepte CJ, Bachmann KA, Stork JH, Friedheim YJ, Hinsch A, Goepfert MS, et al. The impact of early goal-directed fluid management on survival in an experimental model of severe acute pancreatitis. *Intensive Care Med*. 2013; 39: 717-726. PMID: 23287870.
21. Sun ZX, Huang HR, Zhou H. Indwelling catheter and conservative measures in the treatment of abdominal compartment syndrome in fulminant acute pancreatitis. *World J Gastroenterol*. 2006; 12: 5068-5070. PMID: 16937509.
22. Papavramidis TS, Duros V, Michalopoulos A, Papadopoulos VN, Paramythiotis D, Harlaftis N. Intra-abdominal pressure alterations after large pancreatic pseudocyst transcutaneous drainage. *BMC Gastroenterol*. 2009; 9: 42. PMID: 19500396.
23. De Laet I, Hoste E, Verholen E, De Waele JJ. The effect of neuromuscular blockers in patients with intra-abdominal hypertension. *Intensive Care Med*. 2007; 33: 1811-1814. PMID: 17594072.
24. Pupelis G, Plaudis H, Zeiza K, Drozdova N, Mukans M, Kazaka I. Early continuous veno-venous haemofiltration in the management of severe acute pancreatitis complicated with intra-abdominal hypertension: retrospective review of 10 years' experience. *Ann Intensive Care*. 2012; 2 Suppl 1: S21. PMID: 23281603.
25. Oda S, Hirasawa H, Shiga H, Matsuda K, Nakamura M, Watanabe E, et al. Management of intra-abdominal hypertension in patients with severe acute pancreatitis with continuous hemodiafiltration using a polymethyl methacrylate membrane hemofilter. *Ther Apher Dial*. 2005; 9: 355-361. PMID: 16076382.
26. De Waele JJ, Hoste EA, Malbrain ML. Decompressive laparotomy for abdominal compartment syndrome--a critical analysis. *Crit Care*. 2006; 10: R51. PMID: 16569255.
27. Leppäniemi AK, Hienonen PA, Siren JE, Kuitunen AH, Lindström OK, Kemppainen EA. Treatment of abdominal compartment syndrome with subcutaneous anterior abdominal fasciotomy in severe acute pancreatitis. *World J Surg*. 2006; 30: 1922-1924. PMID: 16983467.
28. Leppäniemi A, Hienonen P, Mentula P, Kemppainen E. Subcutaneous linea alba fasciotomy, does it really work? *Am Surg*. 2011; 77: 99-102. PMID: 21396315.
29. Leppäniemi A, Mentula P, Hienonen P, Kemppainen E. Transverse laparostomy is feasible and effective in the treatment of abdominal compartment syndrome in severe acute pancreatitis. *World J Emerg Surg*. 2008; 3: 6.
30. Mentula P, Hienonen P, Kemppainen E, Puolakkainen P, Leppäniemi A. Surgical decompression for abdominal compartment syndrome in severe acute pancreatitis. *Arch Surg*. 2010; 145: 764-769. PMID: 20713929.
31. Ke L, Ni HB, Sun JK, Tong ZH, Li WQ, Li N, et al. The importance of timing of decompression in severe acute pancreatitis combined with abdominal compartment syndrome. *J Trauma Acute Care Surg*. 2013; 74: 1060-1066. PMID: 23511145.
32. Atema JJ, Gans SL, Boermeester MA. Systematic Review and Meta-analysis of the Open Abdomen and Temporary Abdominal Closure Techniques in Non-trauma Patients. *World J Surg*. 2014; 39(4): 912-925. PMID: 25446477.

33. Plaudis H, Rudzats A, Melberga L, Kazaka I, Suba O, Pupelis G. Abdominal negative-pressure therapy: a new method in countering abdominal compartment and peritonitis - prospective study and critical review of literature. *Ann Intensive Care*. 2012; 2 Suppl 1: S23. PMID: 23281649.
34. Rasilainen SK, Mentula PJ, Leppäniemi AK. Vacuum and mesh-mediated fascial traction for primary closure of the open abdomen in critically ill surgical patients. *Br J Surg*. 2012; 99: 1725-1732. PMID: 23034811.
35. Acosta S, Bjarnason T, Petersson U, Pålsson B, Wanhainen A, Svensson M, et al. Multicentre prospective study of fascial closure rate after open abdomen with vacuum and mesh-mediated fascial traction. *Br J Surg*. 2011; 98: 735-743. PMID: 21462176.

Chapter 33

Prevention of ERCP-induced pancreatitis

B. Joseph Elmunzer*

Division of Gastroenterology & Hepatology, Medical University of South Carolina, 114 Doughty St., Suite 249 Charleston, SC 29425.

Introduction

Despite important advances over the last several decades, postendoscopic retrograde cholangiopancreatography (ERCP) pancreatitis (PEP) remains the most frequent complication of ERCP, occurring in 2%-15% of cases, and accounting for substantial morbidity, occasional mortality, and increased healthcare expenditures.[1,2] Approximately 10% of those who develop PEP will follow a severe clinical course that results in prolonged hospitalization and/or additional interventions, leading to significant patient suffering.[1,2] It's been estimated that >700,000 ERCPs are performed annually in the United States. Assuming a midrange post-ERCP pancreatitis rate of 5%, more than 35,000 cases of PEP occur in the U.S. each year; the average Medicare reimbursement for PEP is approximately $6,000, resulting in an estimated annual cost burden in excess of $200 million.[3] Furthermore, PEP is a source of significant endoscopist stress and has been the most common reason for malpractice lawsuits relating to ERCP.[4,5] Given the magnitude of this problem, prevention of PEP remains a major clinical and research priority.

Definition

PEP is most frequently diagnosed according to consensus criteria originally established in 1991: 1) new or increased abdominal pain that is clinically consistent with a syndrome of acute pancreatitis; 2) associated pancreatic enzyme elevation at least three times the upper limit of normal 24 hours after the procedure; *and* 3) resultant hospitalization (or prolongation of existing hospitalization) of at least 2 nights.[2,6] This definition is straightforward and widely accepted but is primarily limited by its subjective nature. Specifically, the interpretation of post-ERCP pain and the decision to hospitalize a patient after the procedure—both central to the consensus diagnosis of PEP—are nonobjective and variable across practice styles and institutional policies. Indeed, practitioners with a lower threshold to hospitalize patients after ERCP may observe a higher rate of PEP, and vice versa. Thus, between-study and between-center comparisons of PEP rates must be interpreted with caution, and blinding to treatment allocation is particularly important in PEP prevention trials.

A proposed alternative to the consensus definition is the standard clinical definition of acute pancreatitis, which mandates the presence of two of the three following features: 1) abdominal pain typical of acute pancreatitis, 2) at least a 3-fold elevation in serum amylase or lipase levels, and 3) evidence of pancreatitic inflammation on cross-sectional imaging.[7] A prospective comparative study demonstrated that the clinical definition is more sensitive than the consensus definition,[8] however the clinical impact of this more sensitive diagnostic approach—which may only capture additional mild (self-limited) cases—is unclear. Further, the radiation exposure and costs of systematic computed tomography (CT) scanning are not justified in all patients with post-ERCP pain.

Given the limitations of both definitions, additional research aiming to elucidate a practical and accurate diagnostic tool for PEP is of substantial importance. Ideally, this tool would be objective, applicable early in the course of disease, and reliably diagnose patients destined to develop a clinically important adverse course for whom hospitalization (and other interventions) is likely to be beneficial.

Pathophysiology

Our understanding of the mechanisms underlying PEP has evolved slowly and remains limited. As the only true human model for the study of acute pancreatitis, fully elucidating the pathophysiology of PEP is of substantial importance,

*Corresponding author. Email: elmunzer@musc.edu

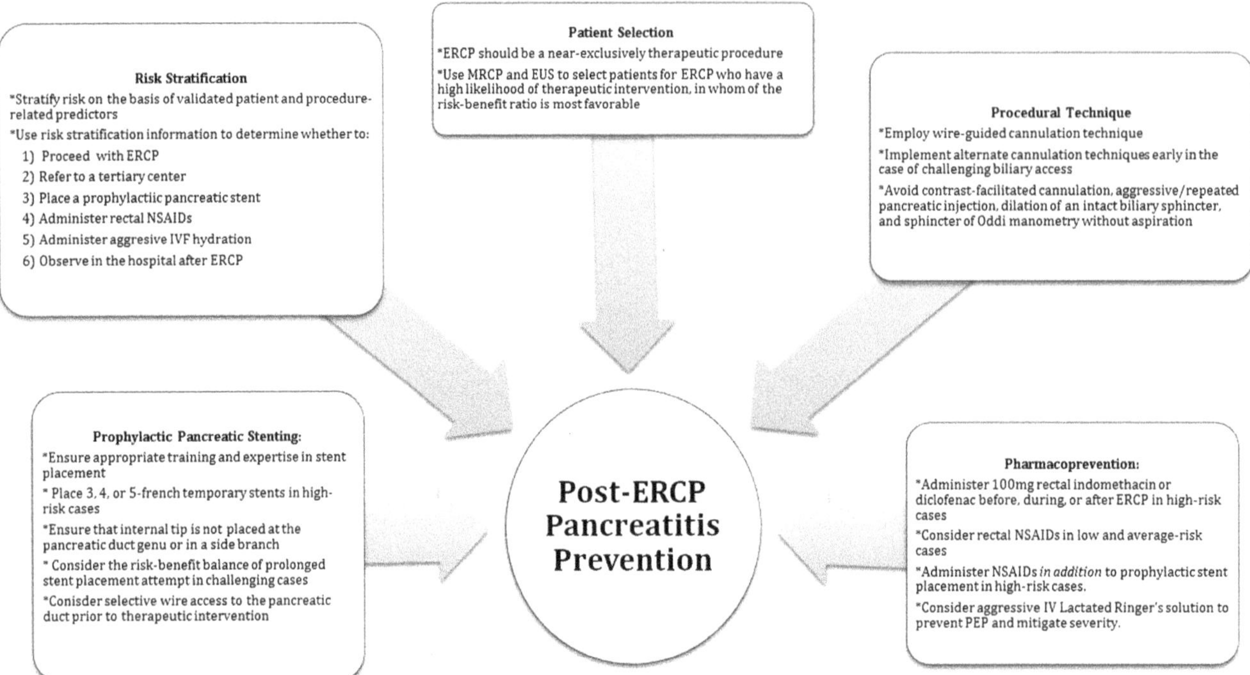

Figure 1. Framework for a comprehensive approach to post-ERCP pancreatitis prevention.

not only to guide the development of novel pharmacologic interventions, but also to expand our understanding of pancreatitis in general. It is hypothesized that PEP results from some combination of mechanical, thermal, chemical, allergic, or infectious injury, and/or increased pancreatic duct (PD) hydrostatic pressure. This initial injury leads to premature intrapancreatic activation of trypsinogen,[9] which incites the inflammatory cascade in patients with genetic or environmental predisposition. The relative contribution of each of these injurious factors remains unclear and is probably variable, but no single factor appears dominant. Thus, a multifactorial approach involving several complementary pharmacologic and mechanical prophylactic measures addressing different mechanisms of injury may be the most effective approach to PEP prevention. Alternatively, interventions that impact downstream inflammatory targets (e.g., zymogen activation or the early inflammatory cascade) or patient predisposition (e.g., microbiome) may prove most effective. A principal objective of an upcoming large-scale comparative effectiveness trial of indomethacin and prophylactic stent placement is to develop a robust repository of biological specimens from study participants to drive translational research elucidating the pathophysiology of PEP and pancreatitis in general.

Framework for a Comprehensive Approach to PEP Prevention

Since PEP is potentially preventable, a comprehensive approach to risk reduction should be employed by all who perform ERCP (**Figure 1**). Preventive strategies can be broadly divided into five areas: 1) appropriate patient selection, 2) risk stratification of patients undergoing ERCP and meaningful use of this information in clinical decision-making, 3) atraumatic and efficient procedural technique, 4) prophylactic pancreatic stent placement, and 5) pharmacoprevention.

All five strategy areas should be considered in every case, and the latter two implemented when appropriate.

Patient Selection

Thoughtful patient selection prior to ERCP remains the most important strategy in reducing the incidence of PEP. Endoscopic ultrasound (EUS) and magnetic resonance cholangiopancreatography (MRCP) allow highly accurate pancreaticobiliary imaging while avoiding the significant risks of ERCP.[10-12] Two large meta-analyses have demonstrated that EUS is highly sensitive and specific in the detection of bile duct stones (sensitivity 89%-94%, specificity 94%-95%).[13,14] Similarly, MRCP has a sensitivity of 85% to 92% and a specificity of 93% to 97% for the same indication,[12,15] although magnetic resonance imaging (MRI) appears less sensitive than EUS for stones <6 mm.[16,17] Additionally, EUS, MRI, and other noninvasive modalities such as radionucleotide-labeled scanning and percutaneous drain fluid analysis are very accurate in diagnosing a multitude of other pancreaticobiliary processes (e.g., chronic pancreatitis, malignancy, and leaks), often obviating the need for ERCP.[18-20]

Indeed, the utilization of ERCP as a diagnostic procedure has steadily declined in favor of less invasive but equally accurate alternative tests, and ERCP has appropriately become a near-exclusively therapeutic procedure reserved for patients with a high pretest probability of intervention.[21,22] This trend is consistent with recent clinical practice guidelines on the role of endoscopy in the evaluation of choledocholithiasis and the National Institutes of Health consensus statement on ERCP for diagnosis and therapy, both favoring less invasive tests over ERCP in the *diagnosis* of biliary disease.[23,24]

An exception to the widespread practice of reserving ERCP for patients with a high likelihood of therapeutic intervention has been the evaluation of patients with suspected sphincter of Oddi dysfunction (SOD), for which an accurate, less invasive alternative to ERCP-guided sphincter of Oddi manometry (SOM) remains elusive.[25,26] Even when considering patients for SOM, thoughtful clinical judgment is necessary to select those who are most likely to benefit from the procedure. A recent multicenter randomized trial (the EPISOD study) demonstrated that there appears to be no role for ERCP in patients with suspected SOD but no laboratory or radiographic abnormalities (previously known as type 3 SOD).[27] Additional studies are necessary to determine whether diagnostic ERCP with SOM is truly beneficial in cases of suspected type 2 biliary or pancreatic SOD (recurrent unexplained pancreatitis). Pending such studies, many experts believe ERCP remains reasonable in such cases after careful assessment of the risk-benefit ratio and detailed informed consent. Another possible exception to the therapeutic ERCP trend may be the evaluation of biliary complications in liver transplant recipients, for whom a recent retrospective study suggested that *diagnostic* ERCP is a reasonable and efficient clinical approach in this patient population based on a high likelihood of therapeutic intervention and a very low rate of complications, in particular PEP.[28]

Recognizing Patients at Increased Risk for PEP

A substantial amount of research over the last two decades has contributed to our understanding of the independent risk factors for post-ERCP pancreatitis. These risk factors can be divided into patient- and procedure-related characteristics. The definite and probable patient-related risk factors that predispose to PEP are a clinical suspicion of sphincter of SOD (regardless of whether or not SOM is performed),[2,29-34] a history of prior PEP,[29,35-37] a history of recurrent pancreatitis,[30] normal bilirubin,[29,38] younger age,[35,39-41] and female sex.[29,30,41] The definite and probable procedure-related risk factors for PEP are difficult cannulation,[2,29,37] pancreatic sphincterotomy,[29,35] ampullectomy,[42,43] repeated or aggressive pancreatography,[2,29,30,39] and short-duration balloon dilation of an intact biliary sphincter.[44-46] Two recent systematic reviews have affirmed that most of these factors are independently associated with PEP.[47,48] Additional risk factors that have been implicated but are not concretely accepted as independent predictors of PEP are precut (access) sphincterotomy (see below),[2,30,37] PD wire passage (see below), biliary sphincterotomy, self-expanding metal stent placement, nondilated bile duct, intraductal papillary mucinous neoplasm, and Billroth 2 anatomy.

Operator (endoscopist)-dependent characteristics have also been implicated in the risk of PEP. Endoscopist procedure volume is suggested to be a risk factor for PEP, although multicenter studies have not confirmed this trend, presumably because low-volume endoscopists tend to perform lower-risk cases.[2,29,39,49] Nevertheless, potentially dangerous cases (based on either patient-related factors or anticipated high-risk interventions) are best referred to expert medical centers where a high-volume endoscopist with expertise in prophylactic pancreatic stent placement can perform the case, and where more experience with rescue from serious complications may improve clinical outcomes.[50,51] Similarly, trainee involvement in ERCP is a possible independent risk factor for PEP, although results of existing multivariable analyses are conflicting.[29,35] It stands to reason that inexperienced trainees may augment procedure-related risk factors (e.g., prolonging a difficult cannulation, delivering excess electrosurgical current during an inefficient pancreatic sphincterotomy, etc.). Therefore, an improved understanding of the process of ERCP training is necessary to minimize the contribution of trainee involvement to PEP development. Future research focused on defining ERCP training metrics and developing an evidence-based list of appropriate fellow cases based on stage of training and skill level is needed. Further, defining the optimal parameters that guide trainee-attending scope exchange during any particular case or intervention is necessary to maximize learning potential while minimizing patient risk.

Several additional points regarding clinical risk stratification are worth considering. First, predictors of PEP appear synergistic in nature.[29] For example, a widely referenced multicenter study by Freeman et al., predating prophylactic pancreatic stent placement, showed that a young female with a clinical suspicion of SOD, normal bilirubin, and a difficult cannulation has a risk of PEP in excess of 40%.[29] Second, patients with a clinical suspicion of SOD, particularly women, are not only at increased risk for PEP in general, but appear more likely to develop severe pancreatitis and death.[2,29,52] When considering the risk-benefit ratio of ERCP in this patient population, the patient's overall risk of PEP and their probability of experiencing a more dramatic clinical course should be considered and discussed. Additionally, several clinical characteristics are thought to significantly reduce PEP risk.

First, biliary interventions in patients with a pre-existing biliary sphincterotomy probably confer a very low risk of PEP. Prior sphincterotomy will have generally separated the biliary and pancreatic orifices, allowing avoidance of the pancreas, and making pancreatic sphincter or duct trauma unlikely. Further, patients with chronic pancreatitis, in particular those with calcific pancreatitis, are at low risk for PEP because of gland atrophy, fibrosis, and consequent decrease in exocrine enzymatic activity.[29] Similarly, the progressive decline in pancreatic exocrine function associated with aging may protect older patients from pancreatic injury.[53] Lastly, perhaps due to postobstructive parenchymal atrophy, patients with pancreatic head malignancy also appear to be relatively protected.[54]

While understanding these aforementioned risk factors and incorporating them into clinical decision-making are important aspects of preventing PEP, additional research focused on developing more robust risk-stratification tools based upon existing literature and future multicenter studies is important. Such risk stratification instruments are unlikely to be developed using conventional statistical models (i.e., multivariable regression analysis), and may require the use of novel, more advanced prediction methods involving artificial intelligence, such as machine learning—a technique that has already been successfully utilized in both business and medicine.[55] In addition, a more specific understanding of how these tools' outputs should concretely direct clinical management is necessary.

Meaningful Use of Risk-Stratification Information

Armed with risk assessment information, clinicians can better inform patients about adverse events and tailor costly and potentially dangerous risk-reducing strategies. For example, prophylactic pancreatic stent placement and consideration of postprocedure hospital observation are appropriate for a patient predicted to be at high risk for PEP, but they are not justified in low-risk cases.

Patient-related characteristics are not modifiable, but can be used (at least in part) to predict the risk of PEP prior to ERCP, allowing appropriate case selection and a meaningful discussion with the patient regarding the procedure's risk-benefit ratio. For example, a young female with suspected biliary SOD but moderate symptoms that are partially responsive to pain-modulating therapy may elect to forgo ERCP after understanding her elevated risk of severe PEP. Procedural risk factors may occasionally be modified during the case (see below), but in combination with patient-related factors, they allow global assessment of a patient's overall risk profile, guiding clinical management. Indeed, the ability to risk-stratify patients can concretely influence the decision-making process that surrounds 1) proceeding with ERCP, 2) referral to a tertiary center, 3) fluid resuscitation, 4) prophylactic stent placement, 5) pharmacoprevention, and 6) postprocedural hospital observation.

Procedure Technique

Efficient and atraumatic technical practices during ERCP are central to minimizing the risk of pancreatitis. Many of the procedure-related risk factors listed above, while predisposing to PEP, are mandatory elements of a successful case. Even though these high-risk interventions are unavoidable for execution of the clinical objective, certain strategies can be utilized to minimize procedure-related risk.

As mentioned, difficult cannulation and PD injection are independent risk factors for PEP. As such, interventions that improve cannulation efficiency and limit contrast injection into the pancreas are likely to decrease the risk of pancreatitis. Guidewire-assisted cannulation accomplishes both, representing a major paradigm shift in ERCP practice. Unlike conventional contrast-assisted cannulation, which may lead to inadvertent injection of the PD or contribute to papillary edema, guidewire-assisted cannulation employs a small-diameter wire with a hydrophilic tip that is initially advanced into the duct, subsequently guiding passage of the catheter. Because the wire is thinner and more maneuverable than the cannula, it is easier to advance across a potentially narrow and off-angle orifice. Moreover, this process limits the likelihood of an inadvertent pancreatic or intramural papillary injection. A recent Cochrane Collaboration meta-analysis that included 12 randomized controlled trials (RCTs) involving 3,450 subjects confirmed that guidewire-assisted cannulation reduces the risk of PEP by approximately 50% (relative risk [RR] 0.51, 95% confidence interval [CI] 0.32 to 0.82).[56] A more recent prospective cohort study and RCT revealed no difference in PEP between the contrast and guidewire-assisted groups.[57,58] However the results of these studies have been questioned for a multitude of reasons, including small sample sizes and selection bias.

When initial cannulation attempts are unsuccessful, alternative techniques to facilitate biliary access include precut sphincterotomy, needle-knife fistulotomy, transpancreatic septomotomy, double-wire cannulation, and wire cannulation alongside a pancreatic stent.[59,60] While these techniques can be immensely helpful in gaining biliary access during challenging cases, some have been implicated as procedure-related risk factors for PEP. In many cases, however, the risk of PEP is actually driven by the preceding prolonged cannulation time that leads to increasing papillary trauma/edema. Therefore, implementing alternate cannulation techniques early in the case and in rapid succession is an important aspect of reducing PEP. This principle is best demonstrated by a meta-analysis of six randomized trials which showed that early precut sphincterotomy significantly reduced the risk of PEP compared to repeated standard cannulation attempts (2.5% vs. 5.3%, odds ratio [OR] 0.47).[61] Additional observational and randomized data have also suggested that precut sphincterotomy, especially if successful, is not an independent risk factor for PEP.[62-64] Further studies are needed to help define the exact point at which the risk-benefit ratio favors precut sphincterotomy over repeated cannulation attempts, although the natural tendency to continue standard cannulation attempts beyond 5-10 minutes should be controlled, and alternative strategies should be attempted early in a difficult case.

The double wire technique is a common second-line approach when initial cannulation attempts result in repeated unintentional passage of the wire into the pancreas. The wire can be left in the PD thereby straightening the common channel and partially occluding the pancreatic orifice, allowing subsequent biliary cannulation alongside the existing pancreatic wire. The double wire technique has been shown to improve cannulation success compared to standard methods,[65] although some data suggest a higher incidence of PEP when a wire is passed into the PD.[66-68] Furthermore, a recent RCT of difficult cannulation cases requiring double wire technique demonstrated that prophylactic pancreatic stent placement reduced the incidence of PEP in this patient population.[69] On this basis, some experts believe that a prophylactic pancreatic stent should be placed in all patients requiring double wire cannulation or when the wire inadvertently passes more than once into the pancreas. Others, including the author, believe that wire placement in the pancreas does not independently predispose to PEP, and that pancreatitis in this context is generally related to the preceding difficult cannulation. If the double wire technique is employed early in a low-risk patient (within 2-3 cannulation attempts), and the wire advances seamlessly into the PD in a typical pancreatic trajectory, pancreatic stent placement may not be necessary, particularly if rectal indomethacin is administered.

Other technical strategies that reduce the risk of PEP include limiting PD injection frequency and vigor, performing SOM using the aspiration technique,[70] and avoiding short-duration balloon dilation of an intact sphincter, especially without prophylactic pancreatic stent placement.[71] In coagulopathic patients with choledocholithiasis and native papillae, balloon dilation can be avoided by providing real-time decompression with an endobiliary stent and repeating the ERCP with sphincterotomy and stone extraction when coagulation parameters have been restored. If this is not possible, and balloon dilation is mandatory, longer duration dilation (2-5 minutes) appears to result in lower rates of pancreatitis compared with 1-minute dilation.[71] Of note, is that balloon dilation *after* biliary sphincterotomy to facilitate large stone extraction does not appear to increase the risk of PEP.[72,73]

Procedure Equipment

Recent advances in ERCP equipment have increased technical success rates but have unfortunately not reduced the risk of post-ERCP pancreatitis.[74] In particular, the use of a sphincterotome has been shown to improve cannulation success compared with a standard cannula, but it does not result in lower PEP rates.[75] Similarly, comparative effectiveness studies evaluating sphincterotomes of various diameters have shown no difference in the risk of PEP.[76,77] There are no comparative effectiveness data evaluating the effect of various guidewires on pancreatitis risk.[78]

Along these same lines, the type of contrast medium used during pancreatography does not appear to affect the incidence of PEP,[79] and it remains unclear (but unlikely) that the now commonly used microprocessor controlled electrosurgical generators offer any protection over the previously popular pure-cut current for thermal injury-induced pancreatitis.[80]

Overall, it appears that equipment has little to no impact on post-ERCP pancreatitis. Therefore practitioners should use the devices with which they are most comfortable for any particular indication to maximize technical success and efficiency, the latter of which is likely inversely related to PEP risk.

Prophylactic Pancreatic Stent Placement

One of many proposed mechanisms of PEP implicates impaired PD drainage caused by trauma-induced edema of the papilla. Pancreatic stent placement (PSP) is therefore thought to reduce the risk of PEP by relieving PD hypertension that develops as a result of transient procedure-induced stenosis of the pancreatic orifice. Twelve published RCTs and as at least as many nonrandomized trials have consistently demonstrated that PSP reduces the risk of PEP by approximately 60%.[81,82] Equally importantly, prophylactic pancreatic stents appear to profoundly reduce the likelihood of severe and necrotizing pancreatitis.[81,82]

It is important to keep in mind that the demonstrated benefits of PSP must be weighed against several potential disadvantages. First, attempting to place a PD stent with subsequent failure actually increases the risk of PEP above baseline by inducing injury to the pancreatic orifice but providing no subsequent ductal decompression.[83] Second, significant nonpancreatitis complications induced by PSP, such as stent migration and duct perforation, occur in ~4% of cases.[81] Further, prolonged stent retention may induce ductal changes that resemble chronic pancreatitis,[84] although the long term clinical relevance of these changes remains unclear. Finally, PSP is associated with some patient inconvenience and increased costs by mandating follow-up abdominal radiography to ensure spontaneous passage of the stent and additional upper endoscopy to retrieve retained stents in 5%-10% of cases.[85,86]

Despite these considerations, PSP is widely regarded as an effective means of preventing PEP, is commonly used in academic medical centers in the United States,[87] and is recommended by the European Society of Gastrointestinal Endoscopy.[42] In light of the aforementioned concerns and the associated costs, PSP should be reserved for high-risk cases.[42,88] Based on the known independent patient and procedure-related risk factors for PEP, experts have suggested that the following cases are appropriate for prophylactic PD stent placement: 1) clinical suspicion of SOD (whether or not manometry or therapeutic intervention performed), 2) prior PEP, 3) difficult cannulation, 4) precut (access) sphincterotomy, 5) pancreatic sphincterotomy (major or minor papilla), 6) endoscopic ampullectomy, 7) aggressive instrumentation or injection of the PD, and 8) balloon dilation of an intact biliary sphincter.[87,89] Furthermore, preliminary studies have suggested that "salvage" PSP may be beneficial early in the course of PEP for patients who did not originally receive a stent or in the case of early stent dislodgement.[90,91] Additional studies that include a control group are necessary to fully evaluate PSP for this indication.

Several questions surrounding PSP remain. First, the true magnitude of benefit of PSP remains unclear as none of the RCTs evaluating this intervention were blinded. Studies without treatment allocation blinding are often biased in favor of the intervention and exaggerate perceived effects. Second, there is limited consensus regarding the optimal stent length and caliber.[87] An early study suggested improved outcomes with 3- or 4-French stents,[92] while a subsequent trial showed no difference in PEP rates but a higher insertion success rate with 5-Fr stents,[86] and a recent network meta-analysis comprising the broader prophylaxis literature suggests that 5-Fr stents are most effective.[93] Similarly, there is little consensus regarding optimal stent length. Most experts agree that the intrapancreatic tip of the stent should not rest at the pancreatic genu or in a side branch,[89] however whether short stents (ending in the pancreatic head) or longer stents (ending in the body or tail) are preferable is unknown, and comparative effectiveness studies in this area are needed.

Finally, the acceptable amount of time that can be spent on the insertion process in cases of difficult pancreatic access is unknown. While the merits of PSP have been clearly presented above, if achieving pancreatic access proves difficult, there is presumably a point of diminishing returns when the risk of additional attempts outweighs the benefit of stent placement, especially if insertion eventually proves unsuccessful. Future clinical studies are unlikely to answer this question in a methodologically rigorous fashion; therefore, endoscopists should be aware of this important clinical balance and use their best judgment regarding the acceptable duration of time for stent insertion. One potential approach to circumvent this problem in cases of anticipated stent placement (e.g., ampullectomy or SOD cases) is to place and maintain a guidewire in the PD early in the case to guarantee access later on, avoiding the occasional phenomenon of failing to identify the pancreatic orifice due to the anatomic distortion that develops as a consequence of trauma, edema, or bleeding. Another approach is to place the prophylactic pancreatic stent prior to therapeutic intervention.

Pharmacoprevention

Pharmacoprevention for PEP has been a major research priority in the last three decades. Since 1977, nearly 100 RCTs have evaluated over 35 pharmacologic agents, with largely disappointing results. Unfortunately, clinical trials in this area have suffered from inadequate sample sizes; low methodological quality; and negative, conflicting, or inconclusive results. Moreover, the pessimism surrounding PEP pharmacoprevention had been amplified by prior positive meta-analyses of agents that were subsequently disproved by further clinical investigation.[94,95] Until recently, no medication for the prevention of PEP had been adopted into widespread clinical use.

Nonsteroidal anti-inflammatory drugs

In the last decade, research focusing on rectal nonsteroidal anti-inflammatory drugs (NSAIDs) has provided renewed hope for pharmacoprevention. Four studies evaluating the protective effects of single-dose rectal indomethacin or diclofenac were reported between 2003 and 2008 and demonstrated conflicting, but generally encouraging results.[96-99] A meta-analysis of these RCTs, involving 912 patients, demonstrated a robust 64% reduction in PEP associated with rectal NSAIDs (RR 0.36, 95% CI 0.22 to 0.60) and no increase in associated adverse events.[100]

Despite this meta-analysis, however, NSAIDs were seldom used in clinical practice due to the absence of conclusive RCT evidence.[101] Moreover, it remained unclear whether NSAIDs provide incremental benefit over temporary pancreatic stent placement in high-risk cases. A large-scale, multicenter, methodologically rigorous RCT was conducted to definitively evaluate the efficacy of prophylactic rectal indomethacin for preventing PEP in high-risk cases.[102] In this study, rectal indomethacin was associated with a 7.7% absolute risk reduction (number needed to treat = 13) and a 46% RR reduction in PEP (P = 0.005). Additional RCTs of low-dose rectal diclofenac,[103] the combination of rectal diclofenac plus infusion somatostatin,[104] and the combination of indomethacin plus sublingual nitroglycerin[105] also demonstrated benefit. To date, eight RCTs of rectal NSAIDs have been published, and recent meta-analyses have refined our estimates of effectiveness.[106,107] On the basis of these data, 100 mg rectal indomethacin or diclofenac can be recommended immediately before or after ERCP in all high-risk cases.

Controversy remains within the advanced endoscopy community regarding the role of NSAIDs in low-risk cases. The aforementioned large-scale RCT, which represents the most definitive study of rectal NSAIDs to date, only enrolled subjects at elevated risk for pancreatitis, leading to the perception that these medications may only be effective in high-risk cases. A post hoc analysis of this RCT, however, demonstrated that the benefit associated with indomethacin was consistent across the entire spectrum of enrolled subjects' PEP risk. In other words, among study subjects, those at mildly elevated risk (e.g., difficult cannulation) derived similar benefit to those at more substantially elevated risk (e.g., suspicion of SOD and pancreatic sphincterotomy), suggesting that indomethacin's RR reduction may be equivalent in all risk groups, including average risk cases (unpublished data). This observation is corroborated by data from other published RCTs, which have demonstrated that rectal NSAIDs are effective in both high- and average-risk cases.[106,107] In light of the very low cost of a single NSAID dose, its highly favorable safety profile, and the above-mentioned data supporting its efficacy in low-risk cases, it is reasonable to consider these medications in all patients undergoing ERCP. The European Society of Gastrointestinal Endoscopy recommends rectal indomethacin or diclofenac for *all* patients undergoing ERCP as a grade A recommendation.[108]

RCTs evaluating NSAIDs administered via nonrectal routes have demonstrated a lack of efficacy in preventing PEP. Specifically, single RCTs of intravascular valdecoxib,[109] oral diclofenac,[110] and intramuscular diclofenac[111] have all yielded negative results. Even though these studies were underpowered and prone to type II statistical error, there are no existing data to support administration of prophylactic NSAIDs via any nonrectal route. Practitioners may be tempted to administer intravenous NSAIDs because of their widespread availability on anesthesia carts, their relative ease of delivery compared to suppository insertion, and the perception that their efficacy is a class effect. Endoscopists, however, should resist this temptation because of the above-mentioned data suggesting that intravenous NSAIDs are not effective, as well as the absence of proof of a class effect. Indeed, indomethacin and diclofenac are postulated to be specifically effective because they are particularly potent inhibitors of phospholipase A2 compared to other NSAIDs.

Available data indicate that rectal NSAIDs are effective *in addition* to PSP in high-risk cases, but to date, there are no clinical trial data examining whether indomethacin is effective when administered *instead* of PSP. Since PSP is technically challenging, potentially dangerous, time consuming, and costly,[85,112-114] major clinical and cost benefits in ERCP practice could be realized if rectal NSAIDs were to obviate the need for pancreatic stent placement. A post hoc, hypothesis-generating analysis of the aforementioned indomethacin RCT suggested that subjects who received indomethacin alone were less likely to develop PEP than those who received a pancreatic stent alone or the combination of indomethacin and stent, even after adjusting for imbalances in PEP risk between groups.[115] Additionally, a recent network meta-analysis comparing the data supporting PSP with those supporting prophylactic NSAIDs suggested that the combination of NSAIDs and PSP is not superior to rectal NSAIDs alone.[116] Confirmatory research focusing on whether PSP remains necessary in the era of indomethacin prophylaxis is critical. To this end, a multicenter randomized noninferiority trial comparing rectal indomethacin alone versus the combination of indomethacin and prophylactic stent placement is in its final planning phase, should begin enrolling subjects late 2015, and will hopefully provide concrete guidance for this critical management issue. Until the results of this trial are available, however, the combination of rectal indomethacin and prophylactic stent placement should remain the standard approach to preventing PEP in high-risk patients.

Other agents

A recent systematic review of PEP pharmacoprevention aiming to provide an evidence-based research roadmap in this area identified bolus-administration somatostatin, sublingual nitroglycerin, and nafamostat as promising agents for which there is a high priority of additional confirmatory research. Topical epinephrine, aggressive intravenous administration of lactated Ringer's solution, gabexate, ulinastatin, secretin, and antibiotics were identified as warranting exploratory research to justify a confirmatory RCT.[117]

Somatostatin

Somatostatin is a potent inhibitor of pancreatic exocrine function and may therefore prevent or mitigate the pathophysiologic processes that lead to pancreatic inflammation. Six of the 12 RCTs comparing somatostatin to placebo have yielded positive results. Benefit has been demonstrated more consistently with bolus administration (4/6 published studies positive) than infusion (3/8 published studies positive). All four published meta-analyses have suggested benefit associated with somatostatin, especially when delivered as a bolus, with a number needed to treat of approximately 12.[94,118-120] An RCT of somatostatin in combination with diclofenac also demonstrated benefit.[104] Given these inconclusive but promising results, a high-quality confirmatory RCT of bolus somatostatin (the most practical and likely cost-effective approach) is necessary.

Nitroglycerin

Nitroglycerin is a smooth muscle relaxant that may lower sphincter of Oddi (SO) pressure and increase pancreatic parenchymal blood flow.[121] Seven placebo-controlled RCTs have examined the effect of nitroglycerin on PEP. Three of these studies demonstrated a significant reduction in PEP,[122-124] while the remaining four showed no benefit.[125-128] The two RCTs that used sublingual administration yielded positive results.[122,124] However, these results have been questioned because neither study defined pancreatitis according to the consensus definition,[6] which may have contributed to the higher than expected event rates (18% and 25%).[122,124] Transdermal administration of nitroglycerin has yielded conflicting results, with three RCTs showing no benefit,[125-127] and one achieving a positive outcome.[123] One RCT evaluating the role of intravenous nitroglycerin in preventing PEP in moderate- to high-risk cases was prematurely terminated because of an interim analysis suggesting futility and a concerning frequency of adverse hemodynamic events.[128] Five meta-analyses have demonstrated an approximately 30%-40% reduction in risk associated with the use of nitroglycerin in PEP prevention.[129-133] Since nitroglycerin is postulated to work by reducing SO pressure, it is unclear whether it would provide incremental benefit over pancreatic stent placement. Nevertheless, sublingual nitroglycerin may have a role in lower-risk cases, in resource-limited environments, or in place of pancreatic stent insertion. A recent small comparative effectiveness RCT demonstrated that the combination of sublingual nitroglycerin plus rectal indomethacin was more effective than indomethacin alone in a study sample that largely did not receive pancreatic stents.[105] Another methodologically rigorous large-scale multicenter RCT is warranted to confirm the effectiveness of combined sublingual nitroglycerin and rectal indomethacin in the appropriate patient population (high-risk cases in environments where stenting is not widely available). In the interim, sublingual nitroglycerin may be reasonable to consider in patients with a NSAID allergies or as an adjunct to rectal NSAIDs in high-risk cases that do not receive a prophylactic pancreatic stent.

Nafamostat mesylate

Nafamostat mesylate is a low molecular weight protease inhibitor that inhibits trypsin, a proteolytic enzyme considered to play an initial role in the pathogenesis of pancreatitis. It has a half-life 20-times longer and a potency 10 to 100-times greater than gabexate mesylate, another protease inhibitor that has been the focus of much prior research and has been utilized in clinical practice in parts of the world.[108] Three RCTs have identified a significant reduction in PEP associated with nafamostat: Yoo et al. 2011, n = 266 (2.8% vs. 9.1% in the nafamostat group vs. control group, $P = 0.03$),[134] Choi et al. 2009, n = 704 (3.3% vs. 7.4% in the nafamostat vs. group control, $P = .018$),[135] and Park et al. n = 608 (three arms: 13.0% in control group vs. 4.0% in 20 mg nafamostat group vs. 5.1% in 50 mg nafamostat group, $P < 0.0001$).[136] A recent meta-analysis demonstrated an approximately 60% benefit associated with nafamostat (RR = 0.41; 95% CI 0.28-0.59).[137] Major concerns related to the use of nafamostat are its high cost, need for a prolonged intravenous infusion (7-25 hours), and apparent absence of benefit in high-risk cases. In light of these potentially prohibitive disadvantages, statistical modeling analyses are necessary to determine whether a confirmatory RCT could show a magnitude of benefit large enough to justify use of nafamostat in clinical practice.

Epinephrine

Epinephrine sprayed directly upon the papilla at the time of ERCP has been postulated to prevent PEP through direct relaxation of the SO and reduction of papillary edema by decreasing capillary permeability.[138] Two RCTs have been conducted to evaluate the effect of topical epinephrine application on the papilla. In the study by Matsushita et al., patients were randomized to 10 mL of either 0.02% epinephrine or saline sprayed on the papilla after diagnostic ERCP.[139] PEP occurred in 4 of 185 subjects in the control group compared to 0 of 185 subjects in the epinephrine group; however, this difference did not reach statistical significance ($P = 0.12$). In a subsequent study by Hua et al., a total of 941 subjects undergoing diagnostic ERCP were randomized to 20 mL 0.02% epinephrine or saline sprayed upon the papilla after ERCP.[140] The incidence of pancreatitis was higher in the control group (31/480, 6.45%) than in the epinephrine group (9/461, 1.95%) ($P = 0.009$). Limitations of this study include the exclusion of all "therapeutic" ERCP and the atypical definition of PEP (elevated serum amylase levels associated with at least two clinical symptoms 6-24 hours after ERCP), reducing the external validity of the results in this era of high-quality diagnostic pancreaticobiliary imaging. Because it works primarily by SO relaxation, the impact of topical epinephrine in addition to pancreatic stent placement is unclear, but this agent may be effective as a "surrogate" stent, or in situations that do not warrant prophylactic stent placement. Given topical epinephrines potential benefit, safety, low cost, and widespread availability, a large-scale confirmatory RCT in the appropriate patient population (high-risk therapeutic ERCP, limited availability of pancreatic stents) may be warranted.[141]

Aggressive intravenous fluid

Mechanistically, aggressive intravenous fluid (IVF) hydration with lactated Ringer's solution, which attenuates the acidosis that appears to promote zymogen activation and pancreatic inflammation, may be an effective intervention for PEP by favorably affecting physiologic (pH) and microanatomic (pancreatic parenchymal perfusion) parameters. Recently, two observational studies and a pilot RCT have suggested the potential benefit of IVF in reducing PEP incidence and severity.[142-144] This RCT had a very small sample size, defined PEP atypically (abdominal pain and pancreatic enzyme elevation 2 or 8 hours after ERCP; no hospitalization requirement), and administered IVF over 8-10 hours, a schedule that is likely unrealistic in the U.S.

Because IVF administration can be dangerous in older persons or those with sodium retaining states, and the fact that the volume of infusion at which the risk-benefit ratio of IVF is optimized remains unknown, additional research is necessary to establish an evidence-based approach. Since data supporting its use in non-ERCP pancreatitis are robust and many practitioners already administer IVF for PEP prevention, large-scale RCTs may be warranted despite the absence of robust preliminary PEP data.

Future Directions

Despite the approaches outlined above, up to 15% of high-risk patients will still develop PEP. Appropriate patient selection, sound procedural technique, NSAIDs, and pancreatic stents have been effective in *improving* the problem; however, additional research in multiple areas is necessary to achieve the goal of *eliminating* PEP. To this end there are at least 13 active registered pharmacoprevention RCTs evaluating topical epinephrine, hemin, magnesium, antibiotics, NSAIDs, and aggressive IVF hydration, among others. There are also ongoing comparative effectiveness trials assessing the optimal timing and dose of rectal NSAIDs. As mentioned, an RCT comparing rectal indomethacin alone versus indomethacin + PSP is in the final planning phase. These and future studies should aim to improve the quality of PEP prevention research, embracing adequate sample sizes, strict patient follow-up, adherence to the intention-to-treat principle, blinding (especially in prophylactic stent trials), strict use of the consensus definition (until more accurate diagnostic criteria or tests are validated), and involvement of a data and safety monitoring board to ensure methodologic rigor and study data integrity.

References

1. Kochar B, Akshintala VS, Afghani E, Elmunzer BJ, Kim KJ, Lennon AM, et al. Incidence, severity, and mortality of post-ERCP pancreatitis: a systematic review by using randomized, controlled trials. *Gastrointest Endosc.* 2015; 81(1): 143-149.e9. PMID: 25088919.
2. Freeman ML, Nelson DB, Sherman S, Haber GB, Herman ME, Dorsher PJ, et al. Complications of endoscopic biliary sphincterotomy. *N Engl J Med.* 1996; 335(13): 909-918. PMID: 8782497.
3. "Healthcare Cost and Utilization Project 2012". Available at http://hcupnet.ahrq.gov.).
4. Keswani RN, Taft TH, Cote GA, Keefer L. Increased levels of stress and burnout are related to decreased physician experience and to interventional gastroenterology career choice: findings from a US survey of endoscopists. *Am J Gastroenterol.* 2011; 106(10): 1734-1740. PMID: 21979198.
5. Cotton PB. Analysis of 59 ERCP lawsuits; mainly about indications. *Gastrointest Endosc.* 2006; 63(3): 378-382; quiz 464. PMID: 16500382.
6. Cotton PB, Lehman G, Vennes J, Geenen JE, Russell RC, Meyers WC, et al. Endoscopic sphincterotomy complications and their management: an attempt at consensus. *Gastrointest Endosc.* 1991; 37(3): 383-393. PMID: 2070995.
7. Banks PA, Bollen TL, Dervenis C, Gooszen HG, Johnson CD, Sarr MG, et al. Classification of acute pancreatitis–2012: revision of the Atlanta classification and definitions by international consensus. *Gut.* 2013; 62(1): 102-111. PMID: 23100216.
8. Artifon EL, Chu A, Freeman M, Sakai P, Usmani A, Kumar A. A comparison of the consensus and clinical definitions of pancreatitis with a proposal to redefine post-endoscopic retrograde cholangiopancreatography pancreatitis. *Pancreas.* 2010; 39(4): 530-535. PMID: 20093992.
9. Rinderknecht H. Activation of pancreatic zymogens. Normal activation, premature intrapancreatic activation, protective mechanisms against inappropriate activation. *Dig Dis Sci.* 1986; 31(3): 314-321. PMID: 2936587.
10. Hawes RH. The evolution of endoscopic ultrasound: improved imaging, higher accuracy for fine needle aspiration and the reality of endoscopic ultrasound-guided interventions. *Curr Opin Gastroenterol.* 2010; 26(5): 436-444. PMID: 20703111.
11. Petrov MS, Savides TJ. Systematic review of endoscopic ultrasonography versus endoscopic retrograde cholangiopancreatography for suspected choledocholithiasis. *Br J Surg.* 2009; 96(9): 967-974. PMID: 19644975.
12. Romagnuolo J, Bardou M, Rahme E, Joseph L, Reinhold C, Barkun AN. Magnetic resonance cholangiopancreatography: a meta-analysis of test performance in suspected biliary disease. *Ann Intern Med.* 2003; 139(7): 547-557. PMID: 14530225.
13. Garrow D, Miller S, Sinha D, Conway J, Hoffman BJ, Hawes RH, et al. Endoscopic ultrasound: a meta-analysis of test performance in suspected biliary obstruction. *Clin Gastroenterol Hepatol.* 2007; 5(5): 616-623. PMID: 17478348.
14. Tse F, Liu L, Barkun AN, Armstrong D, Moayyedi P. EUS: a meta-analysis of test performance in suspected choledocholithiasis. *Gastrointest Endosc.* 2008; 67(2): 235-244. PMID: 18226685.
15. Verma D, Kapadia A, Eisen GM, Adler DG. EUS vs MRCP for detection of choledocholithiasis. *Gastrointest Endosc.* 2006; 64(2): 248-254. PMID: 16860077.
16. Boraschi P, Neri E, Braccini G, Gigoni R, Caramella D, Perri G, et al. Choledocolithiasis: diagnostic accuracy of MR cholangiopancreatography. Three-year experience. *Magn Reson Imaging.* 1999; 17(9): 1245-1253. PMID: 10576709.

17. Zidi SH, Prat F, Le Guen O, Rondeau Y, Rocher L, Fritsch J, et al. Use of magnetic resonance cholangiography in the diagnosis of choledocholithiasis: prospective comparison with a reference imaging method. *Gut*. 1999; 44(1): 118-122. PMID: 9862837.
18. Gardner TB, Levy MJ. EUS diagnosis of chronic pancreatitis. *Gastrointest Endosc*. 2010; 71(7): 1280-1289. PMID: 20598255.
19. Lambie H, Cook AM, Scarsbrook AF, Lodge JP, Robinson PJ, Chowdhury FU. Tc99m-hepatobiliary iminodiacetic acid (HIDA) scintigraphy in clinical practice. *Clin Radiol*. 2011; 66(11): 1094-1105. PMID: 21861996.
20. Darwin P, Goldberg E, Uradomo L. Jackson Pratt drain fluid-to-serum bilirubin concentration ratio for the diagnosis of bile leaks. *Gastrointest Endosc*. 2010; 71(1): 99-104. PMID: 19945100.
21. Mazen Jamal M, Yoon EJ, Saadi A, Sy TY, Hashemzadeh M. Trends in the utilization of endoscopic retrograde cholangiopancreatography (ERCP) in the United States. *Am J Gastroenterol*. 2007; 102(5): 966-975. PMID: 17319932.
22. Moffatt DC, Yu BN, Yie W, Bernstein CN. Trends in utilization of diagnostic and therapeutic ERCP and cholecystectomy over the past 25 years: a population-based study. *Gastrointest Endosc*. 2014; 79(4): 615-622. PMID: 24119510.
23. ASGE Standards of Practice Committee, Maple JT, Ben-Menachem T, Anderson MA, Appalaneni V, Banerjee S, et al. The role of endoscopy in the evaluation of suspected choledocholithiasis. *Gastrointest Endosc*. 2010; 71: 1-9. PMID: 20105473.
24. NIH state-of-the-science statement on endoscopic retrograde cholangiopancreatography (ERCP) for diagnosis and therapy. *NIH Consens State Sci Statements*. 2002; 19(1); 1-26.
25. Rosenblatt ML, Catalano MF, Alcocer E, Geenen JE. Comparison of sphincter of Oddi manometry, fatty meal sonography, and hepatobiliary scintigraphy in the diagnosis of sphincter of Oddi dysfunction. *Gastrointest Endosc*. 2001; 54(6): 697-704. PMID: 11726844.
26. Di Francesco V, Brunori MP, Rigo L, Toouli J, Angelini G, Frulloni L, et al. Comparison of ultrasound-secretin test and sphincter of Oddi manometry in patients with recurrent acute pancreatitis. *Dig Dis Sci*. 1999; 44(2): 336-340. PMID: 10063920.
27. Cotton PB, Durkalski V, Romagnuolo J, Pauls Q, Fogel E, Tarnasky P, et al. Effect of endoscopic sphincterotomy for suspected sphincter of Oddi dysfunction on pain-related disability following cholecystectomy: the EPISOD randomized clinical trial. *JAMA*. 2014; 311(20): 2101-2109. PMID: 24867013.
28. Elmunzer BJ, Debenedet AT, Volk ML, Sonnenday CJ, Waljee AK, Fontana RJ, et al. Clinical yield of diagnostic endoscopic retrograde cholangiopancreatography in orthotopic liver transplant recipients with suspected biliary complications. *Liver Transpl*. 2012; 18(12): 1479-1484. PMID: 22888069.
29. Freeman ML, Guda NM. ERCP cannulation: a review of reported techniques. *Gastrointest Endosc*. 2005; 61(1): 112-125. PMID: 15672074.
30. Masci E, Mariani A, Curioni S, Testoni PA. Risk factors for pancreatitis following endoscopic retrograde cholangiopancreatography: a meta-analysis. *Endoscopy*. 2003; 35(10): 830-834. PMID: 14551860.
31. Cotton PB, Garrow DA, Gallagher J, Romagnuolo J. Risk factors for complications after ERCP: a multivariate analysis of 11,497 procedures over 12 years. *Gastrointest Endosc*. 2009; 70(1): 80-88. PMID: 19286178.
32. Singh P, Gurudu SR, Davidoff S, Sivak MV Jr, Indaram A, Kasmin FE, et al. Sphincter of Oddi manometry does not predispose to post-ERCP acute pancreatitis. *Gastrointest Endosc*. 2004; 59(4): 499-505. PMID: 15044885.
33. Fogel EL, Eversman D, Jamidar P, Sherman S, Lehman GA. Sphincter of Oddi dysfunction: pancreaticobiliary sphincterotomy with pancreatic stent placement has a lower rate of pancreatitis than biliary sphincterotomy alone. *Endoscopy*. 2002; 34(4): 280-285. PMID: 11932782.
34. Maldonado ME, Brady PG, Mamel JJ, Robinson B. Incidence of pancreatitis in patients undergoing sphincter of Oddi manometry (SOM). *Am J Gastroenterol*. 1999; 94(2): 387-390. PMID: 10022634.
35. Cheng CL, Sherman S, Watkins JL, Barnett J, Freeman M, Geenen J, et al. Risk factors for post-ERCP pancreatitis: a prospective multicenter study. *Am J Gastroenterol*. 2006; 101(1): 139-147. PMID: 16405547.
36. Friedland S, Soetikno RM, Vandervoort J, Montes H, Tham T, Carr-Locke DL. Bedside scoring system to predict the risk of developing pancreatitis following ERCP. *Endoscopy*. 2002; 34(6): 483-488. PMID: 12048633.
37. Vandervoort J, Soetikno RM, Tham TC, Wong RC, Ferrari AP Jr, Montes H, et al. Risk factors for complications after performance of ERCP. *Gastrointest Endosc*. 2002; 56(5): 652-656. PMID: 12397271.
38. Mehta SN, Pavone E, Barkun JS, Bouchard S, Barkun AN. Predictors of post-ERCP complications in patients with suspected choledocholithiasis. *Endoscopy*. 1998; 30(5): 457-463. PMID: 9693893.
39. Loperfido S, Angelini G, Benedetti G, Chilovi F, Costan F, De Berardinis F, et al. Major early complications from diagnostic and therapeutic ERCP: a prospective multicenter study. *Gastrointest Endosc*. 1998; 48(1): 1-10. PMID: 9684657.
40. Masci E, Toti G, Mariani A, Curioni S, Lomazzi A, Dinelli M, et al. Complications of diagnostic and therapeutic ERCP: a prospective multicenter study. *Am J Gastroenterol*. 2001; 96(2): 417-423. PMID: 11232684.
41. Williams EJ, Taylor S, Fairclough P, Hamlyn A, Logan RF, Martin D, et al. Risk factors for complication following ERCP; results of a large-scale, prospective multicenter study. *Endoscopy*. 2007; 39(9): 793-801. PMID: 17703388.
42. Dumonceau JM, Andriulli A, Elmunzer BJ, Mariani A, Meister T, Deviere J, et al. Prophylaxis of post-ERCP pancreatitis: European Society of Gastrointestinal Endoscopy (ESGE) Guideline - updated June 2014. *Endoscopy*. 2014; 46(9): 799-815. PMID: 25148137.
43. Patel R, Varadarajulu S, Wilcox CM. Endoscopic ampullectomy: techniques and outcomes. *J Clin Gastroenterol*. 2012; 46(1): 8-15. PMID: 22064552.

44. Disario JA, Freeman ML, Bjorkman DJ, Macmathuna P, Petersen BT, Jaffe PE, et al. Endoscopic balloon dilation compared with sphincterotomy for extraction of bile duct stones. *Gastroenterology*. 2004; 127(5): 1291-1299. PMID: 15520997.
45. Baron TH, Harewood GC. Endoscopic balloon dilation of the biliary sphincter compared to endoscopic biliary sphincterotomy for removal of common bile duct stones during ERCP: a metaanalysis of randomized, controlled trials. *Am J Gastroenterol*. 2004; 99(8): 1455-1460. PMID: 15307859.
46. Weinberg BM, Shindy W, Lo S. Endoscopic balloon sphincter dilation (sphincteroplasty) versus sphincterotomy for common bile duct stones. *Cochrane Database Syst Rev*. 2006;(4): CD004890. PMID: 17054222.
47. Ding X, Zhang F, Wang Y. Risk factors for post-ERCP pancreatitis: A systematic review and meta-analysis. *Surgeon*. 2015; 13(4): 218-229. PMID: 25547802.
48. Chen JJ, Wang XM, Liu XQ, Li W, Dong M, Suo ZW, et al. Risk factors for post-ERCP pancreatitis: a systematic review of clinical trials with a large sample size in the past 10 years. *Eur J Med Res*. 2014; 19: 26. PMID: 24886445.
49. Rabenstein T, Schneider HT, Bulling D, Nicklas M, Katalinic A, Hahn EG, et al. Analysis of the risk factors associated with endoscopic sphincterotomy techniques: preliminary results of a prospective study, with emphasis on the reduced risk of acute pancreatitis with low-dose anticoagulation treatment. *Endoscopy*. 2000; 32(1): 10-19. PMID: 10691266.
50. Ghaferi AA, Birkmeyer JD, Dimick JB. Variation in hospital mortality associated with inpatient surgery. *N Engl J Med*. 2009; 361(14): 1368-1375. PMID: 19797283.
51. Ghaferi AA, Birkmeyer JD, Dimick JB. Hospital volume and failure to rescue with high-risk surgery. *Med Care*. 2011; 49(12): 1076-1081. PMID: 22002649.
52. Trap R, Adamsen S, Hart-Hansen, Henriksen M. Severe and fatal complications after diagnostic and therapeutic ERCP: a prospective series of claims to insurance covering public hospitals. *Endoscopy*. 1999; 31(2): 125-130. PMID: 10223360.
53. Laugier R, Bernard JP, Berthezene P, Dupuy P. Changes in pancreatic exocrine secretion with age: pancreatic exocrine secretion does decrease in the elderly. *Digestion*. 1991; 50(3-4): 202-211. PMID: 1812045.
54. Banerjee N, Hilden K, Baron TH, Adler DG. Endoscopic biliary sphincterotomy is not required for transpapillary SEMS placement for biliary obstruction. *Dig Dis Sci*. 2011; 56(2): 591-595. PMID: 20632105.
55. Waljee AK, Higgins PD. Machine learning in medicine: a primer for physicians. *Am J Gastroenterol*. 2010; 105(6): 1224-1226. PMID: 20523307.
56. Tse F, Yuan Y, Moayyedi P, Leontiadis GI. Guidewire-assisted cannulation of the common bile duct for the prevention of post-endoscopic retrograde cholangiopancreatography (ERCP) pancreatitis. *Cochrane Database Syst Rev*. 2012; 12: CD009662. PMID: 23235679.
57. Kawakami H, Maguchi H, Mukai T, Hayashi T, Sasaki T, Isayama H, et al. A multicenter, prospective, randomized study of selective bile duct cannulation performed by multiple endoscopists: the BIDMEN study. *Gastrointest Endosc*. 2012; 75(2): 362-372. PMID: 22248605.
58. Mariani A, Giussani A, Di Leo M, Testoni S, Testoni PA. Guidewire biliary cannulation does not reduce post-ERCP pancreatitis compared with the contrast injection technique in low-risk and high-risk patients. *Gastrointest Endosc*. 2012; 75(2): 339-346. PMID: 22075192.
59. Testoni PA, Testoni S, Giussani A. Difficult biliary cannulation during ERCP: how to facilitate biliary access and minimize the risk of post-ERCP pancreatitis. *Dig Liver Dis*. 2011; 43(8): 596-603. PMID: 21377432.
60. Bourke MJ, Costamagna G, Freeman ML. Biliary cannulation during endoscopic retrograde cholangiopancreatography: core technique and recent innovations. *Endoscopy*. 2009; 41(7): 612-617. PMID: 19588290.
61. Cennamo V, Fuccio L, Zagari RM, Eusebi LH, Ceroni L, Laterza L, et al. Can early precut implementation reduce endoscopic retrograde cholangiopancreatography-related complication risk? Meta-analysis of randomized controlled trials. *Endoscopy*. 2010; 42(5): 381-388. PMID: 20306386.
62. Navaneethan U, Konjeti R, Lourdusamy V, Lourdusamy D, Mehta D, Sanaka MR, et al. Precut sphincterotomy: efficacy for ductal access and the risk of adverse events. *Gastrointest Endosc*. 2015; 81(4): 924-931. PMID: 25440676.
63. Swan MP, Alexander S, Moss A, Williams SJ, Ruppin D, Hope R, et al. Needle knife sphincterotomy does not increase the risk of pancreatitis in patients with difficult biliary cannulation. *Clin Gastroenterol Hepatol*. 2013; 11(4): 430-436 e431. PMID: 23313840.
64. Gong B, Hao L, Bie L, Sun B, Wang M. Does precut technique improve selective bile duct cannulation or increase post-ERCP pancreatitis rate? A meta-analysis of randomized controlled trials. *Surg Endosc*. 2010; 24(11): 2670-2680. PMID: 20414680.
65. Ito K, Fujita N, Noda Y, Kobayashi G, Obana T, Horaguchi J, et al. Pancreatic guidewire placement for achieving selective biliary cannulation during endoscopic retrograde cholangio-pancreatography. *World J Gastroenterol*. 2008; 14(36): 5595-5600; discussion 5599. PMID: 18810780.
66. Herreros de Tejada A, Calleja JL, Diaz G, Pertejo V, Espinel J, Cacho G, et al. Double-guidewire technique for difficult bile duct cannulation: a multicenter randomized, controlled trial. *Gastrointest Endosc*. 2009; 70(4): 700-709. PMID: 19560764.
67. Wang P, Li ZS, Liu F, Ren X, Lu NH, Fan ZN, et al. Risk factors for ERCP-related complications: a prospective multicenter study. *Am J Gastroenterol*. 2009; 104(1): 31-40. PMID: 19098846.
68. Nakai Y, Isayama H, Sasahira N, Kogure H, Sasaki T, Yamamoto N, et al. Risk factors for post-ERCP pancreatitis in wire-guided cannulation for therapeutic biliary ERCP. *Gastrointest Endosc*. 2015; 81(1): 119-126. PMID: 25442080.
69. Ito K, Fujita N, Noda Y, Kobayashi G, Obana T, Horaguchi J, et al. Can pancreatic duct stenting prevent post-ERCP pancreatitis in patients who undergo pancreatic duct guidewire placement for achieving selective biliary cannulation? A prospective randomized controlled trial. *J Gastroenterol*. 2010; 45(11): 1183-1191. PMID: 20607310.

70. Sherman S, Troiano FP, Hawes RH, Lehman GA. Sphincter of Oddi manometry: decreased risk of clinical pancreatitis with use of a modified aspirating catheter. *Gastrointest Endosc*. 1990; 36(5): 462-466. PMID: 1699837.
71. Liao WC, Tu YK, Wu MS, Wang HP, Lin JT, Leung JW, et al. Balloon dilation with adequate duration is safer than sphincterotomy for extracting bile duct stones: a systematic review and meta-analyses. *Clin Gastroenterol Hepatol*. 2012; 10(10): 1101-1109. PMID: 22642953.
72. Misra SP, Dwivedi M. Large-diameter balloon dilation after endoscopic sphincterotomy for removal of difficult bile duct stones. *Endoscopy*. 2008; 40(3): 209-213. PMID: 18264886.
73. Heo JH, Kang DH, Jung HJ, Kwon DS, An JK, Kim BS, et al. Endoscopic sphincterotomy plus large-balloon dilation versus endoscopic sphincterotomy for removal of bile-duct stones. *Gastrointest Endosc*. 2007; 66(4): 720-726; quiz 768, 771. PMID: 17905013.
74. Freeman ML, DiSario JA, Nelson DB, Fennerty MB, Lee JG, Bjorkman DJ, et al. Risk factors for post-ERCP pancreatitis: a prospective, multicenter study. *Gastrointest Endosc*. 2001; 54(4): 425-434. PMID: 11577302.
75. Schwacha H, Allgaier HP, Deibert P, Olschewski M, Allgaier U, Blum HE. A sphincterotome-based technique for selective transpapillary common bile duct cannulation. *Gastrointest Endosc*. 2000; 52(3): 387-391. PMID: 10968855.
76. Abraham NS, Williams SP, Thompson K, Love JR, MacIntosh DG. 5F sphincterotomes and 4F sphincterotomes are equivalent for the selective cannulation of the common bile duct. *Gastrointest Endosc*. 2006; 63(4): 615-621. PMID: 16564862.
77. García-Cano J, González-Martín JA. Bile duct cannulation: success rates for various ERCP techniques and devices at a single institution. *Acta Gastroenterol Belg*. 2006; 69(3): 261-267. PMID: 17168121.
78. Somogyi L, Chuttani R, Croffie J, Disario J, Liu J, Mishkin D, et al. Guidewires for use in GI endoscopy. *Gastrointest Endosc*. 2007; 65(4): 571-576. PMID: 17383455.
79. George S, Kulkarni AA, Stevens G, Forsmark CE, Draganov P. Role of osmolality of contrast media in the development of post-ERCP pancreatitis: a metanalysis. *Dig Dis Sci*. 2004; 49(3): 503-508. PMID: 15139506.
80. Freeman ML. Complications of endoscopic retrograde cholangiopancreatography: avoidance and management. *Gastrointest Endosc Clin N Am*. 2012; 22(3): 567-586. PMID: 22748249.
81. Mazaki T, Mado K, Masuda H, Shiono M. Prophylactic pancreatic stent placement and post-ERCP pancreatitis: an updated meta-analysis. *J Gastroenterol*. 2014; 49(2): 343-355. PMID: 23612857.
82. Choudhary A, Bechtold ML, Arif M, Szary NM, Puli SR, Othman MO, et al. Pancreatic stents for prophylaxis against post-ERCP pancreatitis: a meta-analysis and systematic review. *Gastrointest Endosc*. 2011; 73(2): 275-282. PMID: 21295641.
83. Choksi NS, Fogel EL, Cote GA, Romagnuolo J, Elta GH, Scheiman JM, et al. The risk of post-ERCP pancreatitis and the protective effect of rectal indomethacin in cases of attempted but unsuccessful prophylactic pancreatic stent placement. *Gastrointest Endosc*. 2015; 81(1): 150-155. PMID: 25527053.
84. Bakman YG, Safdar K, Freeman ML. Significant clinical implications of prophylactic pancreatic stent placement in previously normal pancreatic ducts. *Endoscopy*. 2009; 41(12): 1095-1098. PMID: 19904701.
85. Zolotarevsky E, Fehmi SM, Anderson MA, Schoenfeld PS, Elmunzer BJ, Kwon RS, et al. Prophylactic 5-Fr pancreatic duct stents are superior to 3-Fr stents: a randomized controlled trial. *Endoscopy*. 2011; 43(4): 325-330. PMID: 21455872.
86. Chahal P, Tarnasky PR, Petersen BT, Topazian MD, Levy MJ, Gostout CJ, et al. Short 5Fr vs long 3Fr pancreatic stents in patients at risk for post-endoscopic retrograde cholangiopancreatography pancreatitis. *Clin Gastroenterol Hepatol*. 2009; 7(8): 834-839. PMID: 19447196.
87. Brackbill S, Young S, Schoenfeld P, Elta G. A survey of physician practices on prophylactic pancreatic stents. *Gastrointest Endosc*. 2006; 64(1): 45-52. PMID: 16813802.
88. Das A, Singh P, Sivak MV Jr, Chak A. Pancreatic-stent placement for prevention of post-ERCP pancreatitis: a cost-effectiveness analysis. *Gastrointest Endosc*. 2007; 65(7): 960-968. PMID: 17331513.
89. Freeman ML. Pancreatic stents for prevention of post-endoscopic retrograde cholangiopancreatography pancreatitis. *Clin Gastroenterol Hepatol*. 2007; 5(11): 1354-1365. PMID: 17981248.
90. Madacsy L, Kurucsai G, Joo I, Godi S, Fejes R, Szekely A. Rescue ERCP and insertion of a small-caliber pancreatic stent to prevent the evolution of severe post-ERCP pancreatitis: a case-controlled series. *Surg Endosc*. 2009; 23(8): 1887-1893. PMID: 19057957.
91. Kerdsirichairat T, Attam R, Arain M, Bakman Y, Radosevich D, Freeman M. Urgent ERCP with pancreatic stent placement or replacement for salvage of post-ERCP pancreatitis. *Endoscopy*. 2014; 46(12): 1085-1094. PMID: 25216326.
92. Rashdan A, Fogel EL, McHenry L Jr, Sherman S, Temkit M, Lehman GA. Improved stent characteristics for prophylaxis of post-ERCP pancreatitis. *Clin Gastroenterol Hepatol*. 2004; 2(4): 322-329. PMID: 15067627.
93. Afghani E, Akshintala VS, Khashab MA, Law JK, Hutfless SM, Kim KJ, et al. 5-Fr vs. 3-Fr pancreatic stents for the prevention of post-ERCP pancreatitis in high-risk patients: a systematic review and network meta-analysis. *Endoscopy*. 2014; 46(7): 573-580. PMID: 24830399.
94. Andriulli A, Leandro G, Niro G, Mangia A, Festa V, Gambassi G, et al. Pharmacologic treatment can prevent pancreatic injury after ERCP: a meta-analysis. *Gastrointest Endosc*. 2000; 51(1): 1-7. PMID: 10625786.
95. Andriulli A, Leandro G, Federici T, Ippolito A, Forlano R, Iacobellis A, et al. Prophylactic administration of somatostatin or gabexate does not prevent pancreatitis after ERCP: an updated meta-analysis. *Gastrointest Endosc*. 2007; 65(4): 624-632. PMID: 17383459.
96. Sotoudehmanesh R, Khatibian M, Kolahdoozan S, Ainechi S, Malboosbaf R, Nouraie M. Indomethacin may reduce the

incidence and severity of acute pancreatitis after ERCP. *Am J Gastroenterol.* 2007; 102(5): 978-983. PMID: 17355281.

97. Montaño Loza A, Rodríguez Lomeli X, García Correa JE, Dávalos Cobián C, Cervantes Guevara G, Medrano Muñoz F, et al. [Effect of the rectal administration of indomethacin on amylase serum levels after endoscopic retrograde cholangiopancreatography, and its impact on the development of secondary pancreatitis episodes] [Article in Spanish]. *Rev Esp Enferm Dig.* 2007; 99(6): 330-336. PMID: 17883296.
98. Murray B, Carter R, Imrie C, Evans S, O'Suilleabhain C. Diclofenac reduces the incidence of acute pancreatitis after endoscopic retrograde cholangiopancreatography. *Gastroenterology.* 2003; 124(7): 1786-1791. PMID: 12806612.
99. Khoshbaten M, Khorram H, Madad L, Ehsani Ardakani MJ, Farzin H, Zali MR. Role of diclofenac in reducing post-endoscopic retrograde cholangiopancreatography pancreatitis. *J Gastroenterol Hepatol.* 2008; 23(7 Pt 2): e11-e16. PMID: 17683501.
100. Elmunzer BJ, Waljee AK, Elta GH, Taylor JR, Fehmi SM, Higgins PD. A meta-analysis of rectal NSAIDs in the prevention of post-ERCP pancreatitis. *Gut.* 2008; 57(9): 1262-1267. PMID: 18375470.
101. Dumonceau JM, Rigaux J, Kahaleh M, Gomez CM, Vandermeeren A, Devière J. Prophylaxis of post-ERCP pancreatitis: a practice survey. *Gastrointest Endosc.* 2010; 71(6): 934-939. PMID: 20226455.
102. Elmunzer BJ, Scheiman JM, Lehman GA, Chak A, Mosler P, Higgins PD, et al. A randomized trial of rectal indomethacin to prevent post-ERCP pancreatitis. *N Engl J Med.* 2012; 366(15): 1414-1422. PMID: 22494121.
103. Otsuka T, Kawazoe S, Nakashita S, Kamachi S, Oeda S, Sumida C, et al. Low-dose rectal diclofenac for prevention of post-endoscopic retrograde cholangiopancreatography pancreatitis: a randomized controlled trial. *J Gastroenterol.* 2012; 47(8): 912-917. PMID: 22350703.
104. Katsinelos P, Fasoulas K, Paroutoglou G, Chatzimavroudis G, Beltsis A, Terzoudis S, et al. Combination of diclofenac plus somatostatin in the prevention of post-ERCP pancreatitis: a randomized, double-blind, placebo-controlled trial. *Endoscopy.* 2012; 44(1): 53-59. PMID: 22198776.
105. Sotoudehmanesh R, Eloubeidi MA, Asgari AA, Farsinejad M, Khatibian M. A Randomized Trial of Rectal Indomethacin and Sublingual Nitrates to Prevent Post-ERCP Pancreatitis. *Am J Gastroenterol.* 2014; 109(6): 903-909. PMID: 24513806.
106. Sun HL, Han B, Zhai HP, Cheng XH, Ma K. Rectal NSAIDs for the prevention of post-ERCP pancreatitis: A meta-analysis of randomized controlled trials. *Surgeon.* 2014; 12(3): 141-147. PMID: 24332479.
107. Sethi S, Sethi N, Wadhwa V, Garud S, Brown A. A meta-analysis on the role of rectal diclofenac and indomethacin in the prevention of post-endoscopic retrograde cholangiopancreatography pancreatitis. *Pancreas.* 2014; 43(2): 190-197. PMID: 24518496.
108. Dumonceau JM, Andriulli A, Deviere J, Mariani A, Rigaux J, Baron TH, et al. European Society of *Gastrointestinal Endoscopy* (ESGE) Guideline: prophylaxis of post-ERCP pancreatitis. *Endoscopy.* 2010; 42(6): 503-515. PMID: 20506068.
109. Bhatia V, Ahuja V, Acharya SK, Garg PK. Randomized controlled trial of valdecoxib and glyceryl trinitrate for the prevention of post-ERCP pancreatitis. *J Clin Gastroenterol.* 2011; 45(2): 170-176. PMID: 20717044.
110. Cheon YK, Cho KB, Watkins JL, McHenry L, Fogel EL, Sherman S, et al. Efficacy of diclofenac in the prevention of post-ERCP pancreatitis in predominantly high-risk patients: a randomized double-blind prospective trial. *Gastrointest Endosc.* 2007; 66(6): 1126-1132. PMID: 18061712.
111. Senol A, Saritas U, Demirkan H. Efficacy of intramuscular diclofenac and fluid replacement in prevention of post-ERCP pancreatitis. *World J Gastroenterol.* 2009; 15(32): 3999-4004. PMID: 19705494.
112. Das A, Singh P, Sivak MV Jr, Chak A. Pancreatic-stent placement for prevention of post-ERCP pancreatitis: a cost-effectiveness analysis. *Gastrointest Endosc.* 2007; 65(7): 960-968. PMID: 17331513.
113. Tarnasky PR, Palesch YY, Cunningham JT, Mauldin PD, Cotton PB, Hawes RH. Pancreatic stenting prevents pancreatitis after biliary sphincterotomy in patients with sphincter of Oddi dysfunction. *Gastroenterology.* 1998; 115(6): 1518-1524. PMID: 9834280.
114. Fazel A, Quadri A, Catalano MF, Meyerson SM, Geenen JE. Does a pancreatic duct stent prevent post-ERCP pancreatitis? A prospective randomized study. *Gastrointest Endosc.* 2003; 57(3): 291-294. PMID: 12612504.
115. Elmunzer BJ, Higgins PD, Saini SD, Scheiman JM, Parker RA, Chak A, et al. Does rectal indomethacin eliminate the need for prophylactic pancreatic stent placement in patients undergoing high-risk ERCP? Post hoc efficacy and cost-benefit analyses using prospective clinical trial data. *Am J Gastroenterol.* 2013; 108(3): 410-415. PMID: 23295278.
116. Akbar A, Abu Dayyeh BK, Baron TH, Wang Z, Altayar O, Murad MH. Rectal nonsteroidal anti-inflammatory drugs are superior to pancreatic duct stents in preventing pancreatitis after endoscopic retrograde cholangiopancreatography: a network meta-analysis. *Clin Gastroenterol Hepatol.* 2013; 11(7): 778-783. PMID: 23376320.
117. Kubiliun NM, Adams MA, Akshintala VS, Conte ML, Cote GA, Cotton PB, et al. Evaluation of Pharmacologic Prevention of Pancreatitis Following Endoscopic Retrograde Cholangiopancreatography: a Systematic Review. *Clin Gastroenterol Hepatol.* 2015; 13(7): 1231-1239. PMID: 25579870.
118. Andriulli A, Leandro G, Federici T, Ippolito A, Forlano R, Iacobellis A, et al. Prophylactic administration of somatostatin or gabexate does not prevent pancreatitis after ERCP: an updated meta-analysis. *Gastrointest Endosc.* 2007; 65(4): 624-632. PMID: 17383459.
119. Rudin D, Kiss A, Wetz RV, Sottile VM. Somatostatin and gabexate for post-endoscopic retrograde cholangiopancreatography pancreatitis prevention: Meta-analysis of randomized placebo-controlled trials. *J Gastroenterol Hepatol.* 2007; 22(7): 977-983. PMID: 17559376.
120. Omata F, Deshpande G, Tokuda Y, Takahashi O, Ohde S, Carr-Locke DL, et al. Meta-analysis: somatostatin or its long-acting analogue, octreotide, for prophylaxis against

post-ERCP pancreatitis. *J Gastroenterol.* 2010; 45(8): 885-895. PMID: 20373114.

121. Staritz M, Poralla T, Ewe K, Meyer zum Büschenfelde KH. Effect of glyceryl trinitrate on the sphincter of Oddi motility and baseline pressure. *Gut.* 1985; 26(2): 194-197. PMID: 3917965.
122. Sudhindran S, Bromwich E, Edwards PR. Prospective randomized double-blind placebo-controlled trial of glyceryl trinitrate in endoscopic retrograde cholangiopancreatography-induced pancreatitis. *Br J Surg.* 2001; 88(9): 1178-1182. PMID: 11531863.
123. Moretó M, Zaballa M, Casado I, Merino O, Rueda M, Ramírez K, et al. Transdermal glyceryl trinitrate for prevention of post-ERCP pancreatitis: a randomized double-blind trial. *Gastrointest Endosc.* 2003; 57(1): 1-7. PMID: 12518122.
124. Hao JY, Wu DF, Wang YZ, Gao YX, Lang HP, Zhou WZ. Prophylactic effect of glyceryl trinitrate on post-endoscopic retrograde cholangiopancreatography pancreatitis: a randomized placebo-controlled trial. *World J Gastroenterol.* 2009; 15(3): 366-368. PMID: 19140238.
125. Kaffes AJ, Bourke MJ, Ding S, Alrubaie A, Kwan V, Williams SJ..A prospective, randomized, placebo-controlled trial of transdermal glyceryl trinitrate in ERCP: effects on technical success and post-ERCP pancreatitis. *Gastrointest Endosc.* 2006; 64(3): 351-357. PMID: 16923481.
126. Nøjgaard C, Hornum M, Elkjaer M, Hjalmarsson C, Heyries L, Hauge T, et al. Does glyceryl nitrate prevent post-ERCP pancreatitis? A prospective, randomized, double-blind, placebo-controlled multicenter trial. *Gastrointest Endosc.* 2009; 69(6): e31-37. PMID: 19410035.
127. Bhatia V, Ahuja V, Acharya SK, Garg PK. A randomized controlled trial of valdecoxib and glyceryl trinitrate for the prevention of post-ERCP pancreatitis. *J Clin Gastroenterol.* 2011; 45(2): 170-176. PMID: 20717044.
128. Beauchant M, Ingrand P, Favriel JM, Dupuychaffray JP, Capony P, Moindrot H, et al. Intravenous nitroglycerin for prevention of pancreatitis after therapeutic endoscopic retrograde cholangiography: a randomized, double-blind, placebo-controlled multicenter trial. *Endoscopy.* 2008; 40(8): 631-636. PMID: 18680075.
129. Bai Y, Xu C, Yang X, Gao J, Zou DW, Li ZS, Glyceryl trinitrate for prevention of pancreatitis after endoscopic retrograde cholangiopancreatography: a meta-analysis of randomized, double-blind, placebo-controlled trials. *Endoscopy.* 2009; 41(8): 690-695. PMID: 19670137.
130. Bang UC, Nøjgaard C, Andersen PK, Matzen P. Meta-analysis: Nitroglycerin for prevention of post-ERCP pancreatitis. *Aliment Pharmacol Ther.* 2009; 29(10): 1078-1085. PMID: 19236312.
131. Chen B, Fan T, Wang CH. A meta-analysis for the effect of prophylactic GTN on the incidence of post-ERCP pancreatitis and on the successful rate of cannulation of bile ducts. *BMC Gastroenterol.* 2010; 10: 85. PMID: 20673365.
132. Shao LM, Chen QY, Chen MY, Cai JT. Nitroglycerin in the prevention of post-ERCP pancreatitis: a meta-analysis. *Dig Dis Sci.* 2010; 55(1): 1-7. PMID: 19160042.
133. Ding J, Jin X, Pan Y, Liu S, Li Y. Glyceryl trinitrate for prevention of post-ERCP pancreatitis and improve the rate of cannulation: a meta-analysis of prospective, randomized, controlled trials. *PLoS One.* 2013; 8(10): e75645. PMID: 24098392.
134. Yoo KS, Huh KR, Kim YJ, Kim KO, Park CH, Hahn T, et al. Nafamostat mesilate for prevention of post-endoscopic retrograde cholangiopancreatography pancreatitis a prospective, randomized, double-blind, controlled trial. *Pancreas.* 2011; 40(2): 181-186. PMID: 21206331.
135. Choi CW, Kang DH, Kim GH, Eum JS, Lee SM, Song GA, et al. Nafamostat mesylate in the prevention of post-ERCP pancreatitis and risk factors for post-ERCP pancreatitis. *Gastrointest Endosc.* 2009; 69(4): e11-e18. PMID: 19327467.
136. Park KT, Kang DH, Choi CW, Cho M, Park SB, Kim HW, et al. Is high-dose nafamostat mesilate effective for the prevention of post-ERCP pancreatitis, especially in high-risk patients? *Pancreas.* 2011; 40(8): 1215-1219. PMID: 21775918.
137. Yuhara H, Ogawa M, Kawaguchi Y, Igarashi M, Shimosegawa T, Mine T. Pharmacologic prophylaxis of post-endoscopic retrograde cholangiopancreatography pancreatitis: protease inhibitors and NSAIDs in a meta-analysis. *J Gastroenterol.* 2014; 49(3): 388-399. PMID: 23720090.
138. Ohno T, Katori M, Nishiyama K, Saigenji K. Direct observation of microcirculation of the basal region of rat gastric mucosa. *J Gastroenterol.* 1995; 30(5): 557-564. PMID: 8574325.
139. Matsushita M, Takakuwa H, Shimeno N, Uchida K, Nishio A, Okazaki K. Epinephrine sprayed on the papilla for prevention of post-ERCP pancreatitis. *J Gastroenterol.* 2009; 44(1): 71-75. PMID: 19159075.
140. Hua XL, Bo QJ, Gen GL, Wei QJ, Ming GZ, Fei L, et al. Prevention of post-endoscopic retrograde cholangiopancreatography pancreatitis by epinephrine sprayed on the papilla. *J Gastroenterol Hepatol.* 2011; 26(7): 1139-1144. PMID: 21392105.
141. Singh VK. A Randomized Trial of Rectal Indomethacin and Papillary Spray of Epinephrine Versus Rectal Indomethacin to Prevent Post-ERCP Pancreatitis in High Risk Patients. NCT02116309.
142. DiMagno MJ, Wamsteker EJ, Maratt J, Rivera MA, Spaete JP, Ballard DD, et al. Do larger periprocedural fluid volumes reduce the severity of post-endoscopic retrograde cholangiopancreatography pancreatitis? *Pancreas.* 2014; 43(4): 642-647. PMID: 24713841.
143. Sagi SV, Schmidt S, Fogel E, Lehman GA, McHenry L, Sherman S, et al. Association of greater intravenous volume infusion with shorter hospitalization for patients with post-ERCP pancreatitis. *J Gastroenterol Hepatol.* 2014; 29(6): 1316-1320. PMID: 24372871.
144. Buxbaum J, Yan A, Yeh K, Lane C, Nguyen N, Laine L. Aggressive hydration with lactated ringer's solution reduces pancreatitis after endoscopic retrograde cholangiopancreatography. *Clin Gastroenterol Hepatol.* 2014; 12(2): 303-307.e1. PMID: 23920031.

Chapter 34

Timing of oral refeeding after acute pancreatitis

Simone Gärtner*, Antje Steveling, and Peter Simon

University Medicine Greifswald, Department of Medicine A, Ferdinand-Sauerbruch-Straße 17475 Greifswald, Germany

Introduction

The onset of acute pancreatitis (AP) involves the early activation of digestive enzymes followed by a systemic inflammatory response mediated by cytokines. Treatment depends on the degree of severity.[1]

Even though nutritional deficits are common in AP, nutritional therapy—orally or by tube feeding—was long believed to have a negative effect on the outcome of the disease due to assumed stimulation of exocrine pancreatic secretion and consequent worsening of the autodigestive processes within the pancreas.[2] The goal of fasting as a traditional AP therapy was to "put the pancreas at rest." Much of this belief is derived from physiological studies and is not supported by evidence from prospective clinical trials.

Meta-analyses of clinical trials has revealed that enteral nutrition in AP is superior to parenteral nutrition in terms of associated complications and cost. For enteral nutrition there is a benefit in terms of risk reduction of infectious complication and mortality.[3-7] Meta-analyses demonstrate significantly lower mortality rates in AP when enteral nutrition was started within 24 h of admission compared with between 24 and 72 h,[8] a finding somewhat disputed by a recently completed Dutch study that found no benefit of early refeeding.[9]

In mild AP, traditional treatment still includes initial fasting for 2 or 3 days. From this time forward, oral nutrition is gradually increased from clear liquids to soft solids, and hospital discharge is planned on the basis of the patient's tolerance to solid food.[10] Studies on optimal timing and oral refeeding diet in AP are still rare.

When to start oral refeeding

Patients with mild AP normally do not have an elevated nutrient or energy requirement.[2] In those patients, enteral nutrition is unnecessary if the patient can consume normal food orally after 5-7 days. Enteral nutrition within 5-7 days has no beneficial effect on the disease course and is therefore not recommended.[2]

For mild and severe AP, the ESPEN Guidelines on Enteral Nutrition recommend that oral feeding (normal food and/or nutritional supplements) can be actively attempted once gastric outlet obstruction has resolved, given that it does not result in pain and complications are under control. Tube feeding can therefore be gradually reduced as oral intake improves.[2]

Different approaches in timing of the normal oral food intake after AP have been investigated in clinical studies. The prospective study by Lévy et al. showed that patients can be fed orally after a short period of starvation if pain ceased and amylase and lipase values are decreasing.[11] Pain relapse after oral refeeding occurred in 21% of patients on the first and second refeeding days.[12] A threefold higher than the upper limit of normal lipase level and a higher Balthazar computed tomography score at refeeding onset were identified as risk factors for pain relapse.[11,13]

Teich et al. investigated the optimal timing of oral refeeding in mild AP.[10] They compared a self-selected group in whom the patients were allowed to restart eating as they chose and a lipase-directed group in whom patients were not allowed to eat until lipase had fallen below a value twofold the upper limit of the reference range. They showed that the self-selected group was not superior to the lipase-directed group but also generated no additional risk in comparison with traditional fasting. They also showed a trend towards a shorter length of hospital stay in the self-selected refeeding group and no exacerbation of pain or higher relapse rates.[10]

The study by Li and colleagues similarly analyzed two groups of mild AP.[8] One started eating as soon as they felt hungry and the second started eating when they fulfilled the following criteria: 1) absence of abdominal pain, 2) decrease of serum amylase and lipase to less than

*Corresponding author. Email: simone.gaertner@uni-greifswald.de

twofold the upper limit of the reference range, 3) normal bowel sounds, and 4) subjective feeling of hunger. There were no differences in abdominal pain relapse, transitional abdominal distension, serum amylase or lipase activities higher than the upper limit of normal, or hyperglycemia after oral refeeding between these groups.[8] This study provides evidence that the best time to restart oral refeeding is when the patient feels hungry; this approach is safe and shortens the length of hospital stay. It is not necessary to delay oral refeeding until abdominal pain has resolved or serum pancreatic enzymes have normalized.

The same question was investigated in patients with moderate and severe AP, which often cause complications and lead to high catabolic, hypermetabolic, and hyperdynamic stress with higher morbidity and mortality. Optimal nutritional support has become a key element in the treatment of these patients. Data on the reinitiating of oral feeding in moderate or severe AP are mostly lacking. Li et al. showed equivalent results for refeeding on the basis of hunger for moderate and severe AP.[8] Zhao et al. showed that refeeding based on the patient feeling hunger is safe. Although it increases the risk of hyperglycemia, which could be minimized by a strict glucose-control protocol, there were no differences between the two groups in terms of abdominal pain, relapse of abdominal distension, organ failure, or occurrence of local or systemic complications before hospital discharge.[14]

Eckerwall et al. performed a clinical randomized study and demonstrated the efficacy and feasibility of immediate oral feeding ad libitum as compared to traditional fasting and stepwise reintroduction of oral intake in patients with mild AP.[15] They showed that patients with immediate oral feeding started earlier with solid food and needed fewer days of intravenous fluids. There were no signs of exacerbation of the disease process, increased abdominal pain, or the number of gastrointestinal symptoms as a result of immediate oral feeding. They also showed an association with a significant decrease in length of hospital stay from 6 to 4 days compared to the fasting group.[15]

Lariño-Noia et al. likewise found that early refeeding, as soon as bowel sounds were present, decreased the length of hospital stay by 2 days compared with a standard refeeding protocol.[16]

Type of oral nutrition formulation

In a typical oral refeeding protocol, the diet is gradually reintroduced, starting with small amounts of clear liquids for the first 24 h. If tolerated, the diet is stepwise changed to a soft, low-fat regime followed by a solid diet. Hospital discharge is then contingent on tolerance of a low-fat, solid diet.[17]

Jacobson et al. investigated the initiation of oral nutrition within 3 days of hospitalization with a clear liquid diet (588kcal, 2g fat) or a low-fat, solid diet (1,200kcal, 35g fat) in patients after mild AP. They found no significant difference in the proportions of patients failing to tolerate oral refeeding, suggesting that both practices are safe.[18]

Standard refeeding with a stepwise increasing caloric intake is not needed as shown by Lariño-Noia et al.[16] Early refeeding using a low-fat 1,800 kcal diet from the first day bowel sounds were present was demonstrated to be well tolerated and safe. Gastrointestinal complaints were registered with no significant difference to the standard refeeding group.[16] Similar results were found between a hypocaloric clear liquid diet, an intermediate hypocaloric soft diet, and a full solid diet in patients with mild AP. There were no differences in pain relapse or length of hospital stay.[19,20]

Based on existing evidence, the German Society for Nutritional Medicine in Cooperation with the Society for Clinical Nutrition of Switzerland, the Austrian Consortium for Clinical Nutrition and the German Society for Gastroenterology recommend in their S3-guideline that depending on the clinical course, nutrition can be changed to a light full diet.[21] There is no special need for a stepwise progression to a normal full diet. An indication of clinical relevant malabsorption during the course of severe AP can result in pancreatic enzyme substitution.[21] Oral refeeding with a diet rich in carbohydrates and protein and low in fat (<30% of total energy intake) is recommended, but no clinical trials have shown it to be superior to other food compositions. If the diet is well tolerated, oral nutrition can be continuously increased, and special products are not needed.[2]

Enzyme supplementation in early oral refeeding

Pancreatic exocrine insufficiency is a relevant problem after AP. Exocrine insufficiency severity is directly related to disease severity.[22-25] Even in patients with mild AP, exocrine function is impaired in the early course after an acute attack but recovers in the majority of patients.[23] Some of these patients experience abdominal symptoms during oral refeeding (i.e., flatulence, diarrhea, and pain). This may be due to pancreatic exocrine insufficiency when refeeding starts.[26] The effect of early supplementation of pancreatic enzymes during the refeeding period after AP was evaluated by Kahl et al.[26] They showed a trend towards a faster recovery from exocrine pancreatic insufficiency under enzyme supplementation versus placebo (14 vs. 23 days, P=0.641) and no relevant differences in safety or tolerability. Airey et al. also showed a significant improvement in exocrine pancreatic function after 5 days of refeeding with pancreatic enzyme supplementation.[27]

Conclusion

A small number of studies have been conducted in order to determine the optimal timing, schedule, and oral nutrition type in AP. They show that normalization of pancreatic enzyme levels is not a precondition for starting oral refeeding. To let the patient choose when to restart oral refeeding irrespective of serum enzyme levels might be the most appropriate option. Furthermore, early refeeding can shorten the length of hospital stay. There still appears no consensus about the definition of "early refeeding."

Oral intake generally started with clear liquids followed by solid low-fat meals with increasing caloric content over a period of 3-6 days seems to have no advantage over starting with regular light meals. Early oral refeeding with a solid diet might therefore provide better outcomes and is safe for mild and moderate AP patients. However, the best randomized study to date failed to show a benefit of early refeeding over on-demand refeeding of patients,[9] whenever the patient feels ready to take regular food by mouth. None of the previously published studies observed any increased risk of refeeding intolerance or other adverse events related to a more active refeeding protocol. Few studies indicate that pancreatic enzyme supplementation when oral refeeding starts can be beneficial in terms of pain relapse prevention, but further investigations are needed to confirm this potential benefit.

References

1. Halangk W, Lerch MM. Early events in acute pancreatitis. *Gastroenterol Clin North Am.* 2004; 33: 717-731. PMID: 15528014.
2. Meier R, Ockenga J, Pertkiewicz M, Pap A, Milinic N, Macfie J, et al. ESPEN Guidelines on Enteral Nutrition: Pancreas. *Clin Nutr.* 2006; 25: 275-284. PMID: 16678943.
3. Marik PE, Zaloga GP. Meta-analysis of parenteral nutrition versus enteral nutrition in patients with acute pancreatitis. *BMJ.* 2004; 328: 1407. PMID: 15175229.
4. McClave SA, Chang WK, Dhaliwal R, Heyland DK. Nutrition support in acute pancreatitis: a systematic review of the literature. *J Parenter Enteral Nutr.* 2006; 30: 143-156. PMID: 16517959.
5. Petrov MS, Pylypchuk RD, Emelyanov NV. Systematic review: nutritional support in acute pancreatitis. *Aliment Pharmacol Ther.* 2008; 28: 704-712. PMID: 19145726.
6. Petrov MS, van Santvoort HC, Besselink MG, van der Heijden GJ, Windsor JA, Gooszen HG. Enteral nutrition and the risk of mortality and infectious complications in patients with severe acute pancreatitis: a meta-analysis of randomized trials. *Arch Surg.* 2008; 143: 1111-1117. PMID: 19015471.
7. Dervenis C. Enteral nutrition in severe acute pancreatitis: future development. *JOP.* 2004; 5: 60-63. PMID: 15007186.
8. Li X, Ma F, Jia K. Early enteral nutrition within 24 hours or between 24 and 72 hours for acute pancreatitis: evidence based on 12 RCTs. *Med Sci Monit.* 2014; 20: 2327-2335. PMID: 25399541.
9. Bakker OJ, van Brunschot S, van Santvoort HC, Besselink MG, Bollen TL, Boermeester MA, et al. Early versus on-demand nasoenteric tube feeding in acute pancreatitis. *N Engl J Med* 371(21): 1983-1993,2014. PMID: 25409371.
10. Teich N, Aghdassi A, Fischer J, Walz B, Caca K, Wallochny T, et al. Optimal timing of oral refeeding in mild acute pancreatitis: results of an open randomized multicenter trial. *Pancreas.* 2010; 39: 1088-1092. PMID: 20357692.
11. Lévy P, Heresbach D, Pariente EA, Boruchowicz A, Delcenserie R, Millat B, et al. Frequency and risk factors of recurrent pain during refeeding in patients with acute pancreatitis: a multivariate multicentre prospective study of 116 patients. *Gut.* 1997; 40: 262-266. PMID: 9071942.
12. Chebli JM, Gaburri PD, De Souza AF, Junior EV, Gaburri AK, Felga GE, et al. Oral refeeding in patients with mild acute pancreatitis: prevalence and risk factors of relapsing abdominal pain. *J Gastroenterol Hepatol.* 2005; 20: 1385-1389. PMID: 16105125.
13. Petrov MS, van Santvoort HC, Besselink MG, Cirkel GA, Brink MA, Gooszen HG. Oral refeeding after onset of acute pancreatitis: a review of literature. *Am J Gastroenterol.* 2007; 102: 2079-2084; quiz 2085. PMID: 17573797.
14. Zhao XL, Zhu SF, Xue GJ, Li J, Liu YL, Wan MH, et al. Early oral refeeding based on hunger in moderate and severe acute pancreatitis: a prospective controlled, randomized clinical trial. *Nutrition.* 2015; 31: 171-175. PMID: 25441594.
15. Eckerwall GE, Tingstedt BB, Bergenzaun PE, Andersson RG. Immediate oral feeding in patients with mild acute pancreatitis is safe and may accelerate recovery--a randomized clinical study. *Clin Nutr.* 2007; 26: 758-763. PMID: 17719703.
16. Lariño-Noia J, Lindkvist B, Iglesias-Garcia J, Seijo-Rios S, Iglesias-Canle J, Domínguez-Muñoz JE. Early and/or immediately full caloric diet versus standard refeeding in mild acute pancreatitis: a randomized open-label trial. *Pancreatology.* 2014; 14: 167-173. PMID: 24854611.
17. Whitcomb DC. Clinical practice. Acute pancreatitis. *N Engl J Med.* 2006; 354: 2142-2150. PMID: 16707751.
18. Jacobson BC, Vander Vliet MB, Hughes MD, Maurer R, McManus K, Banks PA. A prospective, randomized trial of clear liquids versus low-fat solid diet as the initial meal in mild acute pancreatitis. *Clin Gastroenterol Hepatol.* 2007; 5: 946-951; quiz 886. PMID: 17613280.
19. Moraes JM, Felga GE, Chebli LA, Franco MB, Gomes CA, Gaburri PD, et al. A full solid diet as the initial meal in mild acute pancreatitis is safe and result in a shorter length of hospitalization: results from a prospective, randomized, controlled, double-blind clinical trial. *J Clin Gastroenterol.* 2010; 44: 517-522. PMID: 20054282.
20. Meng WB, Li X, Li YM, Zhou WC, Zhu XL. Three initial diets for management of mild acute pancreatitis: a meta-analysis. *World J Gastroenterol.* 2011; 17: 4235-4241. PMID: 22072857.
21. Ockenga J, Löser C, Kraft M, Madl C. S3-Leitlinie der Deutschen Gesellschaft für Ernährungsmedizin e. V. Klinische Ernährung in der Gastroenterologie (Teil 3). *Aktuelle Ernährungsmedizin.* 2014; 39: 7143-7156.
22. Migliori M, Pezzilli R, Tomassetti P, Gullo L. Exocrine pancreatic function after alcoholic or biliary acute pancreatitis. *Pancreas.* 2004; 28: 359-363. PMID: 15097850.
23. Glasbrenner B, Büchler M, Uhl W, Malfertheiner P. Exocrine pancreatic function in the early recovery phase of acute oedematous pancreatitis. *J Gastroenterol Hepatol.* 1992; 4: 563-567.

24. Gullo L, Sarles H, Mott CB. Functional investigation of the exocrine pancreas following acute pancreatitis. *Rendiconti di Gastroenterologia.* 1972; 4: 18-21.
25. Buchler M, Hauke A, Malfertheiner A. Follow-up after acute pancreatitis: Morphology and function. In: HG Beger, MW Buchler, eds. *Acute Pancreatits.* Berlin: Springer Verlag; 1987: 367-374.
26. Kahl S, Schutte K, Glasbrenner B, Mayerle J, Simon P, Henniges F, et al. The effect of oral pancreatic enzyme supplementation on the course and outcome of acute pancreatitis: a randomized, double-blind parallel-group study. *JOP.* 2014; 15: 165-174. PMID: 24618443.
27. Airey MC, McMahon MJ. *Pancreatic Enzymes in Health and Disease*. Berlin: Springer Verlag; 1991.

Chronic Pancreatitis

Section Editors: Julia Mayerle and Pramod K. Garg

Chapter 35

Epidemiology of chronic pancreatitis

Jorge D Machicado[1], Vinciane Rebours[2], and Dhiraj Yadav[1]*

[1]*Division of Gastroenterology & Hepatology, University of Pittsburgh Medical Center, Pittsburgh, PA;*
[2]*Pancreatology Unit, Beaujon Hospital, University Paris 7, Clichy, France.*

Introduction

Epidemiologic descriptions of chronic pancreatitis (CP) have changed over time. The focus of reports from the 1950s through 1990s was to describe the clinical profile and natural history in series of patients. Many landmark studies performed during this period are crucial to our understanding of the disease. In the past 25 years, researchers have also focused on describing population distributions of CP, its risk based on the presence of environmental and genetic risk factors, impact of CP on quality of life (QOL), and frequency and factors that affect the evolution of acute and recurrent acute pancreatitis (RAP) to CP. In this chapter, we will review the current epidemiology of CP, changes that have been observed over the past half-century, and their potential explanations. For detailed descriptions of the role of environmental risk factors in CP, natural history of disease, and medical and surgical management, the reader is encouraged to refer to chapters of this book dedicated to these topics.

Changing role of imaging tests in CP diagnosis

A diagnosis of CP can be made by the presence of definitive morphology or histology changes. Although tissue diagnosis remains the gold standard, pancreatic tissue sampling has been historically difficult.[1] Therefore, in clinical practice, the diagnosis relies mainly on the presence of typical clinical presentation and morphologic changes on imaging studies. In the first half of the 20th century, the presence of epigastric calcifications on plain radiography was the mainstay for CP diagnosis.[2] In the 1970s, abdominal ultrasound, endoscopic retrograde cholangiopancreatography (ERCP), and computed tomography (CT) emerged as diagnostic tests for CP.[3-5] In 1983, a group of experts met in Cambridge and developed a grading system using these diagnostic modalities to define CP.[6] CT quickly became the modality of choice for diagnosis because it was noninvasive and widely available. With continuing advances in technology over the past 30 years, high-resolution CT, magnetic resonance imaging (MRI), and endoscopic ultrasound (EUS) have evolved as important tools for evaluation of CP[7-11] and have replaced the use of ERCP for diagnosis.[12-16]

Due to poor sensitivity of abdominal x-ray, ultrasound, and earlier generation CT scanners, it is likely that many patients in earlier studies received a CP diagnosis only in the presence of advanced changes (e.g., large calcifications). With advances in technology, it is conceivable that high-resolution CT, MRI/MRCP, and EUS would diagnose CP at an earlier stage by detecting subtle morphologic changes in the pancreas (e.g., smaller calcifications, duct irregularities, etc.). However, the impact of improvement in imaging techniques on CP epidemiology has not been empirically studied.

Incidence and prevalence

The number of studies examining the population distributions of CP is scarce, and it is important to note that these data are not available from large areas of the world. This is probably related to difficulties in conducting such studies due to low disease prevalence, establishing an accurate diagnosis, and the focus of earlier studies to describe the clinical profile and natural history of the disease. In the past two decades, there has been an interest in documenting population distributions for pancreatic disease. The results of the most representative studies on CP incidence are presented in **Table 1**, and incidence data from Olmsted County, Minnesota are shown in **Figure 1**.[17] The overall incidence ranges from 2-14/100,000 population and shows some variability based on study design and country. In the United States, the incidence of CP has increased modestly from 3.3 during 1940-1969 to 4.3 per 100,000 in 1997-2006.[17,18] In Europe, the incidence of CP appears to be higher than in the U.S.[19-25] In Asia, seven separate surveys from Japan conducted in the past 42 years show a trend toward a much

*Corresponding author. Email: yadavd@upmc.edu

Table 1. CP incidence in selected population-based studies

Country	Year(s) studied	Incidence of CP (all causes)[a]		
		All	Male	Female
Denmark (Andersen)[19]	1970-1976	6.9	NA	NA
	1975-1979	10.0	NA	NA
U.S. (O'Sullivan, Yadav)[17,18]	1940-1969	3.3	NA	NA
	1977-2006	4.0	4.2	2.6
Poland (Dzieniszewski)[20]	1982-1987	5.0	NA	NA
Germany (Lankisch)[21]	1988-1995	6.4	8.2	1.9
Czech Republic (Dite)[22]	1999	7.9	NA	NA
Japan (Lin, Hirota, Hirota)[27-29]	1994	5.4	8.4	2.7
	2007	11.9	NA	NA
	2011	14.0	NA	NA
Netherlands (Spanier)[23]	2000-2005	1.8	2.2	1.4
France (Levy)[24]	2003	7.7	12.9	2.6
Spain (Dominguez)[25]	2011	5.5	NA	NA

[a] Incidence rate per 100,000 of the population.

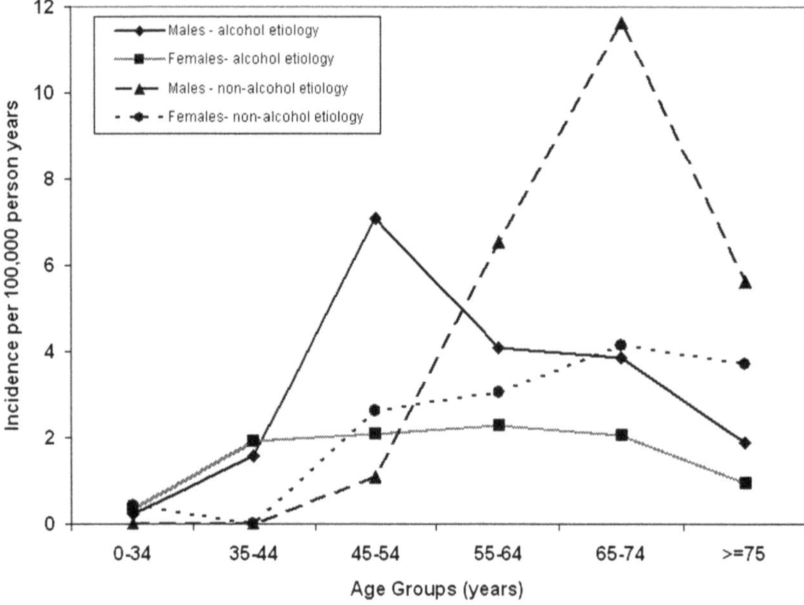

Figure 1. Incidence of CP by age and sex in 2006 in Olmsted County, Minnesota. Data derived from Yadav et al.[17]

greater increase in CP incidence (from 2 to 14/100,000).[26-29] It is likely that wide availability of better imaging technology may have contributed to this increase. The contribution of changing trends for environmental exposures may also be of importance, especially in developing countries where alcohol consumption is on the rise with increasing affluence and data on population distributions are lacking.

Prevalence estimates for CP are limited to only a few populations and are presented in **Table 2**. The overall prevalence of CP shows high variability. In recent studies, the prevalence ranges around 40-50 per 100,000 population. Prevalence data from Olmsted County, Minnesota are shown in **Figure 2**.[17] Prevalence is low below age 35 and reaches 100-120 in middle-aged and older males.[17] A Chinese study showed increasing prevalence of CP from 3.1/100,000 in 1996 to 13.5/100,000 population in 2003.[30] The 7 nationwide epidemiological surveys conducted in Japan, have demonstrated increasing prevalence of CP from 28.5/100,000 in 1994 to 52.4/100,000 in 2011.[27,29] A much higher prevalence of idiopathic CP termed "tropical pancreatitis" was reported from southern India in up to 126 per 100,000 population in 1994.[31] Environmental risk factors (e.g., diet) were suspected to be the main etiologic factors, but recent studies have highlighted an important role of genetic mutations (*SPINK1*, *CFTR*, *CTRC*) in this condition and suggested that the term tropical pancreatitis was a misnomer.[32,33]

Table 2. CP prevalence in selected population-based studies

Country	Year(s) studied	Prevalence of CP (all causes)[a]		
		All	Male	Female
Poland (Dzieniszewski)[20]	1987	17	NA	NA
India (Balaji)[31]	1994	126.1	NA	NA
France (Levy)[24]	2003	26.4	43.8	9.0
China (Wang)[30]	2003	13.5	NA	NA
U.S. (Yadav)[17]	2006	41.8	51.5	33.9
Japan				
Lin[27]	1994	28.5	45.4	12.4
Otsuki[63]	1999	32.9	43.9	22.4
Hirota[28]	2007	36.9	53.2	21.2
Hirota[29]	2011	52.4	NA	NA
Spain (Dominguez)[25]	2011	49.3	NA	NA

[a] Prevalence rate per 100,000 of the population.

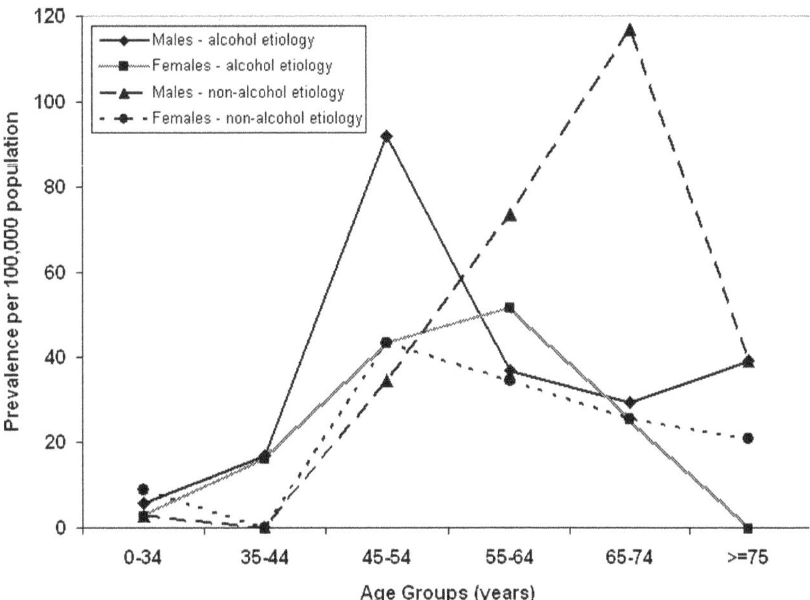

Figure 2. Prevalence of CP by age group, sex, and etiology in 2006 in Olmsted County, Minnesota. Data derived from Yadav et al.[17]

Demographics

The mean or median age at time of study enrollment or diagnosis in most published studies shows little variation over time and geographical area (**Table 3**). The mean age in European studies was 40 years in the 1970s to 1990s[34,35] and more recently between 50 and 55 years.[24,36] In Japan, the mean age in the 1960s was 48 years,[37] and most recently 59 years in 2007.[28] In two populations studies from Olmsted County, Minnesota, the median age at CP diagnosis was 51 in the 1940s to 1960s[18] and 58 in the 1970s to 2006.[17] In the large multicenter North American Pancreatitis study (NAPS2, 2000-2013), the mean age at diagnosis was 47.[51] From these studies, we can conclude that CP mainly affects middle-aged individuals.

In most studies, 60%-80% of CP patients are male (**Table 3**), and population studies have revealed higher incidence and prevalence of CP in males compared with females (**Tables 1** and **2**). In the recently conducted cross-sectional NAPS2 studies, as well as a population-based study in the U.S., there was only a marginal overrepresentation of males (52%-55%).[17,38,51] The reason for a lower than expected prevalence of males in these cohorts is unclear; at least in the NAPS2 studies, accrual of patients from secondary and tertiary referral centers may have accounted for this observation.

Differences in sex and age distribution are primarily related to CP etiology (**Figures 1** and **2**). Alcohol is the most common cause of CP in the 35-54-year-old age group.[17,21] A greater risk of alcoholic pancreatitis in males

Table 3. Age, sex, and CP etiology in selected studies

Country	Year(s) studied	N	Male (%)	Age (mean or median)	EtOH etiology (%)
Switzerland (Ammann)[76]	1963-1986	245	88%	46	71%
Brazil (Dani)[116]	1963-1987	797	91%	38	90%
Italy (Cavallini)[34]	1971-1995	715	88%	41	74%
Mexico (Robles-Diaz)[117]	1975-1987	150	82%	NA	67%
U.S. (Layer)[48]	1976-1982	448	65%	NA	56%
Denmark (Nøjgaard)[93]	1977-1982	249	72%	51	45%
Japan (Lin)[27]	1994	2,523	77%		56%
Italy (Frulloni)[36]	2000-2005	893	74%	54	34%
U.S. (Wilcox)[51]	2000-2014	1,159	55%	47	49%
France (Levy)[24]	2003	1,748	83%	51	84%
India (Balakrishnan)[53]	2007	1,033	71%	40	39%
Netherlands (Ahmed)[54]	2010-2013	1,218	67%	48	53%
Japan (Hirota)[29]	2011	1,734	82%	62	68%
Spain (Dominguez-Munoz)[25]	2011	937	NA	NA	75%

is primarily attributed to the higher prevalence of heavy drinking.[39,40] However, results of recent studies suggest that genetic factors also play an important role in this difference.[41-43] Nonalcoholic etiologies are more evenly distributed between the sexes. Genetic causes are more common in patients diagnosed earlier in life (<35 years of age),[32,44-47] whereas idiopathic CP has a bimodal age distribution.[48]

Few groups have evaluated racial differences in CP. A multicenter study reported that half of all CP patients discharged from three hospitals in Portugal and the U.S. during a 16-year period were black.[49] In comparison to white patients, black patients were 2-3 times more likely to be hospitalized for CP than for cirrhosis.[49] A population study using the National Inpatient Sample in the U.S. revealed that the discharges for alcoholic CP between 1988 and 2004 was higher in blacks (11.3/100,000) compared with whites (5.1/100,000), Hispanics (3.7/100,000), Asians (1.4/100,000), and American Indians (2.3/100,000).[50] In a recent study from the NAPS2 cohort, patient level data was compared between black and white CP patients. The ages at symptom onset and diagnosis were similar based on race, but blacks were more likely to be male compared with white CP patients (61 vs. 53%, $P<0.05$), a difference attributed to differences in CP etiology (see below).[51]

Etiology

Alcohol is the most frequent cause of CP worldwide (**Table 1**). The proportions of cases attributed to alcohol were as high as 80%-90% in earlier studies. In some recent analyses, alcohol as the primary cause of CP was less frequently identified by physicians. In the multicenter NAPS2 studies from the U.S., alcohol was assigned as the etiology in 49% of 1,158 white and black CP patients[51] "Blacks were more likely to have alcohol etiology (77 vs. 42%), and physicians were 4.3 times more likely to identify alcohol as their etiology compared with white CP patients".[51] Similarly, a large multicenter survey of 893 CP patients from Italy evaluated from 2000-2005 attributed alcohol as the the etiology in only 34% (36), which is much lower than the value of 74%-79% reported in other Italian series from 1971-1995.[34,52] Other recent studies also identified a similar pattern.[53,54] A growing recognition of the importance of genetic factors in causing pancreatitis, wide availability of cross-sectional imaging studies such as MRCP that can identify anatomic abnormalities (e.g., pancreas divisum), acceptance of the relationship with smoking, and that autoimmune and other factors could explain a patient's disease are some of the likely explanations for physicians to entertain the possibility of factors other than alcohol as the potential cause of CP in an individual patient. This has led to the proposal of the TIGAR-O classification system, which recognizes the contribution of different factors to pancreatitis development.[1] While smoking is an independent and dose-dependent risk factor, its association with pancreatitis is stronger in the presence of alcohol.[55,56]

In the past 20 years, several genetic susceptibility factors for pancreatitis have been identified, of which mutations in four genes (*PRSS1*, *SPINK1*, *CFTR*, *CTRC*) are now routinely used in clinical practice, especially in patients with idiopathic CP.[57] In contrast to alcoholic pancreatitis, which is more frequent in middle-aged males, genetic factors are more common in early onset disease, and are equally distributed among males and females. Other well-recognized causes of CP include hypercalcemia, hyperlipidemia, autoimmune, postnecrotic, and duct obstruction (e.g., tumor, inflammatory stricture),[1] while the role of pancreas divisum and sphincter of Oddi dysfunction remains uncertain.[58-61]

Nonalcoholic etiologies are identified more frequently among females and can account for up to 70% of cases.[62]

After alcohol, the largest subgroup among CP patients is those in whom no specific cause has been identified. These patients are labeled to have idiopathic CP. The fraction of patients with idiopathic disease varies from 10%-30% in most studies from 1970-2006,[21,24,27,34,36,63,64] but can be up to 60% in India and China.[53,65] Due to differences in clinical symptoms and course, these subjects have been subdivided into early onset (i.e., <35 years of age) and late-onset (>35 years) disease.[48]

Clinical features

The most common clinical features of CP are abdominal pain and one or more attacks of acute pancreatitis; either of these are seen in approximately 90% of patients at some time during the clinical course. These are also the presenting symptoms in the majority of patients. Presence, type, and severity of pain and the number of episodes of AP during the clinical course can be highly variable.[34,48,66-68] Exocrine or endocrine insufficiency are uncommon at initial presentation,[48] but their probability increases over time, and during the clinical course up to 80% and 87% develop diabetes and exocrine insufficiency respectively.[48,66,67,69] Clinical steatorrhea occurs only in the presence of severe exocrine insufficiency.[70] However, consequences of fat malabsorption such as vitamin deficiencies or metabolic bone disease are observed more frequently and occur even with moderate insufficiency.[71-75] Other features include local complications such as pseudocysts, abnormal liver function tests or jaundice from common bile duct stricture, vascular complications, or gastric outlet obstruction.[48,66,67]

Differences in the initial presentation and natural course of CP have been observed based on etiology and age at presentation (see chapter on natural course of disease). In general, patients with alcoholic CP have more aggressive disease with evolution from initial presentation to advanced disease occurring over 5 to 10 years. Patients with early onset idiopathic CP have a prolonged clinical course with a long period of symptomatic disease, development of morphological features, and functional impairment over two to three decades. Patients with late-onset idiopathic CP have less symptomatic disease and are often diagnosed with obvious morphological changes and functional impairment at initial presentation.[48,76]

In CP patients who present with AP or pain as the initial manifestation, a subset may have morphologic features and/or functional abnormalities at initial presentation, while in the remaining patients these develop over a variable period of time. Many recent studies have evaluated the probability of disease progression among patients who present with their first attack of AP without coexistent CP. In a recent meta-analysis of 14 studies, 10% of patients with first attack AP and 36% with RAP progress to CP.[77] The risk of progression was higher among smokers, alcoholics, and males.[78]

QOL

The impact of CP on the patient's overall wellbeing and functioning has become a topic of growing interest in clinical research and practice. This subjective patient's perception has been assessed using different validated health-related QOL instruments, such as the SF-36, SF-12, and EORTC QL-C30.[79-81] More recently, a disease specific instrument has been developed to evaluate QOL in CP (PANQOLI).[82,83] This includes unique features not found in generic instruments (economic factors, stigma, and spiritual factors).

A uniform finding on these studies has been that QOL in CP patients is significantly affected compared with historical controls.[79-81,84-88] Moreover, the QOL in CP is noted to be worse than many other chronic disorders or malignancies.[89] In the NAPS2 study, the independent effect of CP was also evaluated after controlling for demographics, etiology, risk factors, and comorbidities using the SF-12 questionnaire.[89] These data showed that CP has a profound independent effect on physical QOL (~10 points lower) and a clinically significant effect on mental QOL (~4 points lower) compared with control subjects without pancreatitis. Few studies have assessed the factors that determine impaired QOL in CP patients. Among the factors assessed, pancreatic pain seems to be the predominant factor, especially if it is constant.[68,79,80,84,85] The effects of interventions, smoking, alcohol consumption, diabetes, exocrine pancreatic insufficiency, and disease duration are still not well known.

Pancreatic cancer, comorbidities, and mortality

The risk of pancreatic cancer is increased in subjects with CP. In a landmark multicenter cohort study, the risk of pancreatic cancer in CP patients from six different countries was 2.8% during a mean follow-up of 7 years.[90] Other studies have reported similar incidence of pancreatic cancer that ranges from 1.2%-3.8%.[91-93] A meta-analysis showed that compared with controls, there is a 13-fold greater lifetime risk of pancreatic cancer in CP.[94] In subsets of CP patients, this risk is even more pronounced; the risk of pancreatic cancer in patients with hereditary pancreatitis is 69-fold,[44,95,96] and in those with tropical pancreatitis it is 100-fold greater.[97]

Recently, a nationwide Danish study reported the overall risk of having any type of cancer in CP patients to be 20% greater than general population controls.[98] The risks of liver cancer (hazard ratio [HR], 2), small intestinal cancer (HR, 3), and lung cancer (HR, 1.5) were found to be significantly increased in subjects with CP. This risk was not different between alcoholic and nonalcoholic CP.[98] The same study also revealed higher risks of cerebrovascular disease (HR, 1.3), chronic pulmonary disease (HR, 1.9), ulcer disease (HR, 3.6), diabetes (HR, 5.2), and chronic renal disease (HR, 1.7) among CP patients.

In a large multicenter study that enrolled 2,015 CP patients from 1946-1992 in six countries (Switzerland, Germany, U.S., Italy, Sweden, Denmark), the overall mortality rates at 10 and 20 years from diagnosis were 30% and 55%, respectively.[99] Other studies have reported similar findings.[92,100] Based on this data, it is believed that the overall median survival of patients with CP is between 15 and 20 years from onset. Patients with early-onset idiopathic CP may live longer. A study from India reported 17% mortality among patients with idiopathic CP at 35 years after disease onset.[32] Well-designed studies have also compared the mortality rates of CP patients with the general population. In a retrospective study from 30 years ago, Levy et al reported a higher mortality rate in CP patients compared with a matched French population.[101] These data have been replicated in more recent studies. In a study from Olmsted, Minnesota (1977-2006), CP patients had twofold higher mortality compared with an age- and sex-matched Minnesota white population.[17] Likewise, two Danish studies (1977-1982 and 1995-2010) found mortality among CP patients to be four- to fivefold higher compared with a background population.[93,98] This effect was independent of comorbidities and socioeconomic status. Even though mortality rates increased with age in both CP patients and controls, CP patients died at a younger age than controls (8 years earlier) and had a higher adjusted relative risk of death for younger than older patients.[98]

Almost three-quarters of deaths are unrelated to pancreatitis.[17] The most common causes of death in CP patients include malignancy (22%-23%), and diseases of the alimentary tract (15%-23%) and circulatory system (12%-21%).[17,98,99] Pancreatic cancer is the most frequent cancer-related cause of death (1/3 of malignancies), followed by lung cancer.[98] While age at diagnosis, smoking, and alcohol use were major predictors of mortality in the study of Lowenfels et al,[99] a more recent study by Nøjgaard et al reported that smoking, alcohol, CP etiology, exocrine pancreatic insufficiency, and diabetes had no impact on survival.[93] Interestingly, unemployment was associated with higher mortality in their study.

Healthcare utilization and cost of care

Hospitalization in patients with CP could be due to AP flares, pain, maldigestion, and local complications. More than 90% of patients are hospitalized on at least one occasion in their lifetime for pain related to CP.[68] In several European studies, there has been a steady increase in the rates of admission for CP. In a UK study that compared annual hospital admissions between 1960-1965 and 1980-1984, the hospitalization admissions increased from 8.3 to 32 per million population.[102] In another study, the incident hospitalization rate increased from 4.3/100,000 in 1988 to 8.6/100,000 in 2000.[103] This trend has also been seen in two studies from the Netherlands (from 5.2/100,000 in 1992 to 8.5/100,000 in 2004)[104] and Finland (10.4/100,000 in 1977 to 13.4/100,000 in 1989).[105] In contrast, two U.S. population studies (study periods 1988-2004 and 1996-2005) found hospital admissions for CP to be stable over time (8 per 100,000).[50,106] Hospital admissions are disproportionately higher in blacks, alcoholics, and in those with constant pain.[68,106] The median length of stay ranges from 4 to 6 days and is not different between alcoholic and nonalcoholic pancreatitis.[106,107]

CP patients often undergo interventions, mainly for treatment of pain or local complications; this used to be surgery (resection or drainage procedures),[48,66] but endoscopic therapy, if feasible, is being performed more frequently.[108,109] There is paucity of population-level data on the use of endoscopic therapy for CP. A recent study found the trends for pancreatic surgeries performed for CP to be stable in the U.S. population from 1998-2011.[110] The number of drainage operations decreased significantly, which is likely a reflection of more frequent endoscopic drainage. In the NAPS2 cohort, up to 61% of CP patients underwent at least one pancreatic endoscopic intervention.[111] This high rate is likely an overestimation due to referral bias.

There are limited data on the direct and indirect costs related to CP management. Direct costs include the value of services used in CP treatment and care. Indirect costs are related to the personal or family economic loss secondary to the illness. The estimated direct annual cost related to CP in the U.S. is approximately $638 million.[112] Based on prescription data, the cost related to AP and CP was $88 million, of which the cost of pancreatic enzymes was $75 million and that of narcotics and anti-emetics was approximately $13 million.[113] In a recent study from the UK, the estimated direct annual cost was $460 million.[114] The annual costs of hospital admissions and diabetes treatment were $90 million and $145 million respectively.[114] The costs related to interventions are unknown.

Regarding indirect costs, more than a third of CP patients are unemployed, more than a quarter are on disability benefits, and the majority report missing significant time from work due to their illness.[68,115] Loss of productivity among CP patients is comparable to other chronic diseases, such as Crohn's disease, chronic obstructive pulmonary disease, and urologic dysfunction.[115]

Future directions

Studies in the past few decades have informed different aspects of CP epidemiology. However, much of these data are limited to Europe, North America, and some parts of Asia. Future studies should focus on the population distributions of

CP in other parts of the world; the impact of imaging studies, environmental, and other factors on disease estimates and trends between and within populations; and determinants of healthcare utilization and health care cost from CP.

References

1. Etemad B, Whitcomb DC. Chronic pancreatitis: diagnosis, classification, and new genetic developments. *Gastroenterology*. 2001; 120: 682-707. PMID: 11179244.
2. Wirts CW Jr, Snape WJ. Disseminated calcification of the pancreas; subacute and chronic pancreatitis. *Am J Med Sci*. 1947; 213: 290-299. PMID: 20288155.
3. Filly RA, Freimanis AK. Echographic diagnosis of pancreatic lesions. Ultrasound scanning techniques and diagnostic findings. *Radiology*. 1970; 96: 575-582. PMID: 5468845.
4. Zimmon DS, Falkenstein DB, Abrams RM, Seliger G, Kessler RE. Endoscopic retrograde cholangiopancreatography (ERCP) in the diagnosis of pancreatic inflammatory disease. *Radiology*. 1974; 113: 287-292. PMID: 4424116.
5. Haaga JR, Alfidi RJ, Zelch MG, Meany TF, Boller M, Gonzalez L, et al. Computed tomography of the pancreas. *Radiology*. 1976; 120: 589-595. PMID: 781727.
6. Sarner M, Cotton PB. Classification of pancreatitis. *Gut*. 1984; 25: 756-759. PMID: 6735257.
7. Haaga JR. Magnetic resonance imaging of the pancreas. *Radiol Clin North Am*. 1984; 22: 869-877. PMID: 6393210.
8. Semelka RC, Shoenut JP, Kroeker MA, Micflikier AB. Chronic pancreatitis: MR imaging features before and after administration of gadopentetate dimeglumine. *J Magn Reson Imaging*. 1993; 3: 79-82. PMID: 8428105.
9. Sica GT, Braver J, Cooney MJ, Miller FH, Chai JL, Adams DF. Comparison of endoscopic retrograde cholangiopancreatography with MR cholangiopancreatography in patients with pancreatitis. *Radiology*. 1999; 210: 605-610. PMID: 10207456.
10. Lees WR. Endoscopic ultrasonography of chronic pancreatitis and pancreatic pseudocysts. *Scand J Gastroenterol Suppl*. 1986; 123: 123-129. PMID: 3535028.
11. Wiersema MJ, Hawes RH, Lehman GA, Kochman ML, Sherman S, Kopecky KK. Prospective evaluation of endoscopic ultrasonography and endoscopic retrograde cholangiopancreatography in patients with chronic abdominal pain of suspected pancreatic origin. *Endoscopy*. 1993; 25: 555-564. PMID: 8119204.
12. Kahl S, Glasbrenner B, Leodolter A, Pross M, Schulz HU, Malfertheiner P. EUS in the diagnosis of early chronic pancreatitis: a prospective follow-up study. *Gastrointest Endosc*. 2002; 55: 507-511. PMID: 11923762.
13. Pungpapong S, Wallace MB, Woodward TA, Noh KW, Raimondo M. Accuracy of endoscopic ultrasonography and magnetic resonance cholangiopancreatography for the diagnosis of chronic pancreatitis: a prospective comparison study. *J Clin Gastroenterol*. 2007; 41: 88-93. PMID: 17198070.
14. Hansen TM, Nilsson M, Gram M, Frokjaer JB. Morphological and functional evaluation of chronic pancreatitis with magnetic resonance imaging. *World J Gastroenterol*. 2013; 19: 7241-7246. PMID: 24259954.
15. Buscail L, Escourrou J, Moreau J, Delvaux M, Louvel D, Lapeyre F, et al. Endoscopic ultrasonography in chronic pancreatitis: a comparative prospective study with conventional ultrasonography, computed tomography, and ERCP. *Pancreas*. 1995; 10: 251-257. PMID: 7624302.
16. Sherman S, Freeman ML, Tarnasky PR, Wilcox CM, Kulkarni A, Aisen AM, et al. Administration of secretin (RG1068) increases the sensitivity of detection of duct abnormalities by magnetic resonance cholangiopancreatography in patients with pancreatitis. *Gastroenterology*. 2014; 147: 646-654. PMID: 24906040.
17. Yadav D, Timmons L, Benson JT, Dierkhising RA, Chari ST. Incidence, prevalence, and survival of chronic pancreatitis: a population-based study. *Am J Gastroenterol*. 2011; 106: 2192-2199. PMID: 21946280.
18. O'Sullivan JN, Nobrega FT, Morlock CG, Brown AL Jr, Bartholomew LG. Acute and chronic pancreatitis in Rochester, Minnesota, 1940 to 1969. *Gastroenterology*. 1972; 62: 373-379. PMID: 5011528.
19. Andersen BN, Pedersen NT, Scheel J, Worning H. Incidence of alcoholic chronic pancreatitis in Copenhagen. *Scand J Gastroenterol*. 1982; 17: 247-252. PMID: 7134849.
20. Dzieniszewski J, Jarosz M, Ciok J. Chronic pancreatitis in Warsaw. *Mater Med Pol*. 1990; 22: 202-204. PMID: 2132427.
21. Lankisch PG, Assmus C, Maisonneuve P, Lowenfels AB. Epidemiology of pancreatic diseases in Luneburg County. A study in a defined german population. *Pancreatology*. 2002; 2: 469-477. PMID: 12378115.
22. Dite P, Stary K, Novotny I, Precechtelova M, Dolina J, Lata J, et al. Incidence of chronic pancreatitis in the Czech Republic. *Eur J Gastroenterol Hepatol*. 2001; 13: 749-750. PMID: 11434607.
23. Spanier B, Bruno MJ, Dijkgraaf MG. Incidence and mortality of acute and chronic pancreatitis in the Netherlands: a nationwide record-linked cohort study for the years 1995-2005. *World J Gastroenterol*. 2013; 19: 3018-302. PMID: 23716981.
24. Lévy P, Barthet M, Mollard BR, Amouretti M, Marion-Audibert AM, Dyard F. Estimation of the prevalence and incidence of chronic pancreatitis and its complications. *Gastroenterol Clin Biol*. 2006; 30: 838-844. PMID: 16885867.
25. Dominguez-Muñoz JE, Lucendo A, Carballo LF, Iglesias-García J, Tenías JM. A Spanish multicenter study to estimate the prevalence and incidence of chronic pancreatitis and its complications. *Rev Esp Enferm Dig*. 2014; 106: 239-245. PMID: 25075654.
26. Ishii K, Nakamura K, Takeuchi T, Hirayama T. Chronic calcifying pancreatitis and pancreatic carcinoma in Japan. *Digestion*. 1973; 9: 429-437. PMID: 4784704.
27. Lin Y, Tamakoshi A, Matsuno S, Takeda K, Hayakawa T, Kitagawa M, et al. Nationwide epidemiological survey of chronic pancreatitis in Japan. *J Gastroenterol*. 2000; 35: 136-141. PMID: 10680669.
28. Hirota M, Shimosegawa T, Masamune A, Kikuta K, Kume K, Hamada S, et al. The sixth nationwide epidemiological survey of chronic pancreatitis in Japan. *Pancreatology*. 2012; 12: 79-84. PMID: 22487515.

29. Hirota M, Shimosegawa T, Masamune A, Kikuta K, Kume K, Hamada S, et al. The seventh nationwide epidemiological survey for chronic pancreatitis in Japan: clinical significance of smoking habit in Japanese patients. *Pancreatology*. 2014; 14: 490-496. PMID: 25224249.
30. Wang LW, Li ZS, Li SD, Jin ZD, Zou DW, Chen F. Prevalence and clinical features of chronic pancreatitis in China: a retrospective multicenter analysis over 10 years. *Pancreas*. 2009; 38: 248-254. PMID: 19034057.
31. Balaji LN, Tandon RK, Tandon BN, Banks PA. Prevalence and clinical features of chronic pancreatitis in southern India. *Int J Pancreatol*. 1994; 15: 29-34. PMID: 8195640.
32. Midha S, Khajuria R, Shastri S, Kabra M, Garg PK. Idiopathic chronic pancreatitis in India: phenotypic characterisation and strong genetic susceptibility due to SPINK1 and CFTR gene mutations. *Gut*. 2010; 59: 800-807. PMID: 20551465.
33. Paliwal S, Bhaskar S, Mani KR, Reddy DN, Rao GV, Singh SP, et al. Comprehensive screening of chymotrypsin C (CTRC) gene in tropical calcific pancreatitis identifies novel variants. *Gut*. 2013; 62: 1602-1606. PMID: 22580415.
34. Cavallini G, Frulloni L, Pederzoli P, Talamini G, Bovo P, Bassi C, et al. Long-term follow-up of patients with chronic pancreatitis in Italy. *Scand J Gastroenterol*. 1998; 33: 880-889. PMID: 9754738.
35. Talamini G, Bassi C, Falconi M, Frulloni L, Di Francesco V, Vaona B, et al. Cigarette smoking: an independent risk factor in alcoholic pancreatitis. *Pancreas*. 1996; 12: 131-137. PMID: 8720658.
36. Frulloni L, Gabbrielli A, Pezzilli R, Zerbi A, Cavestro GM, Marotta F, et al. Chronic pancreatitis: report from a multicenter Italian survey (PanCroInfAISP) on 893 patients. *Dig Liver Dis*. 2009; 41: 311-317. PMID: 19097829.
37. Oomi K, Amano M. The epidemiology of pancreatic diseases in Japan. *Pancreas*. 1998; 16: 233-237. PMID: 9548660.
38. Whitcomb DC, Yadav D, Adam S, Hawes RH, Brand RE, Anderson MA, et al. Multicenter approach to recurrent acute and chronic pancreatitis in the United States: the North American Pancreatitis Study 2 (NAPS2). *Pancreatology*. 2008; 8: 520-531. PMID: 18765957.
39. Yadav D, Hawes RH, Brand RE, Anderson MA, Money ME, Banks PA, et al. Alcohol consumption, cigarette smoking, and the risk of recurrent acute and chronic pancreatitis. *Arch Intern Med*. 2009; 169: 1035-1045. PMID: 19506173.
40. Kristiansen L, Gronbaek M, Becker U, Tolstrup JS. Risk of pancreatitis according to alcohol drinking habits: a population-based cohort study. *Am J Epidemiol*. 2008; 168: 932-937. PMID: 18779386.
41. Whitcomb DC, LaRusch J, Krasinskas AM, Klei L, Smith JP, Brand RE, et al. Common genetic variants in the CLDN2 and PRSS1-PRSS2 loci alter risk for alcohol-related and sporadic pancreatitis. *Nat Genet*. 2012; 44: 1349-1354. PMID: 23143602.
42. Derikx MH, Kovacs P, Scholz M, Masson E, Chen JM, Ruffert C, et al. Polymorphisms at PRSS1-PRSS2 and CLDN2-MORC4 loci associate with alcoholic and non-alcoholic chronic pancreatitis in a European replication study. *Gut*. 2015; 64: 1426-1433. PMID: 25253127.
43. Aghdassi AA, Weiss FU, Mayerle J, Lerch MM, Simon P. Genetic susceptibility factors for alcohol-induced chronic pancreatitis. *Pancreatology*. 2015; 15 4 Suppl: S23-S31. PMID: 26149858.
44. Howes N, Lerch MM, Greenhalf W, Stocken DD, Ellis I, Simon P, et al. Clinical and genetic characteristics of hereditary pancreatitis in Europe. *Clin Gastroenterol Hepatol*. 2004; 2: 252-261. PMID: 15017610.
45. Rebours V, Boutron-Ruault MC, Schnee M, Ferec C, Le Marechal C, Hentic O, et al. The natural history of hereditary pancreatitis: a national series. *Gut*. 2009; 58: 97-103. PMID: 18755888.
46. Joergensen MT, Brusgaard K, Crüger DG, Gerdes AM, de Muckadell OB. Genetic, epidemiological, and clinical aspects of hereditary pancreatitis: a population-based cohort study in Denmark. *Am J Gastroenterol*. 2010; 105: 1876-1883. PMID: 20502448.
47. Weiss FU, Simon P, Witt H, Mayerle J, Hlouschek V, Zimmer KP, et al. SPINK1 mutations and phenotypic expression in patients with pancreatitis associated with trypsinogen mutations. *J Med Genet*. 2003; 40: e40. PMID: 12676913.
48. Layer P, Yamamoto H, Kalthoff L, Clain JE, Bakken LJ, DiMagno EP. The different courses of early- and late-onset idiopathic and alcoholic chronic pancreatitis. *Gastroenterology*. 1994; 107: 1481-1487. PMID: 7926511.
49. Lowenfels AB, Maisonneuve P, Grover H, Gerber E, Korsten MA, Antunes MT, et al. Racial factors and the risk of chronic pancreatitis. *Am J Gastroenterol*. 1999; 94: 790-794. PMID: 10086667.
50. Yang AL, Vadhavkar S, Singh G, Omary MB. Epidemiology of alcohol-related liver and pancreatic disease in the United States. *Arch Intern Med*. 2008; 168: 649-656. PMID: 18362258.
51. Wilcox CM, Sandhu BS, Singh V, Gelrud A, Abberbock JN, Sherman S, et al. Racial differences in the clinical profile, causes and outcome of chronic pancreatitis. *Am J Gastroenterol*. 2016. In press.
52. Talamini G, Bassi C, Falconi M, Sartori N, Salvia R, Rigo L, et al. Alcohol and smoking as risk factors in chronic pancreatitis and pancreatic cancer. *Dig Dis Sci*. 1999; 44: 1303-1311. PMID: 10489910.
53. Balakrishnan V, Unnikrishnan AG, Thomas V, Choudhuri G, Veeraraju P, Singh SP, et al. Chronic pancreatitis. A prospective nationwide study of 1,086 subjects from India. *JOP*. 2008; 9: 593-600. PMID: 18762690.
54. Ahmed Ali U, Issa Y, van Goor H, van Eijck CH, Nieuwenhuijs VB, Keulemans Y, et al. Dutch Chronic Pancreatitis Registry (CARE): design and rationale of a nationwide prospective evaluation and follow-up. *Pancreatology*. 2015; 15: 46-52. PMID: 25511908.
55. Greer JB, Thrower E, Yadav D. Epidemiologic and Mechanistic Associations Between Smoking and Pancreatitis. *Curr Treat Options Gastroenterol*. 2015; 13: 332-346. PMID: 26109145.
56. Andriulli A, Botteri E, Almasio PL, Vantini I, Uomo G, Maisonneuve P, et al. Smoking as a cofactor for causation of chronic pancreatitis: a meta-analysis. *Pancreas*. 2010; 39: 1205-1210. PMID: 20622705.

57. Whitcomb DC. Genetic risk factors for pancreatic disorders. *Gastroenterology*. 2013; 144: 1292-1302. PMID: 23622139.
58. Cotton PB. Congenital anomaly of pancreas divisum as cause of obstructive pain and pancreatitis. *Gut*. 1980; 21: 105-114. PMID: 7380331.
59. Fogel EL, Toth TG, Lehman GA, DiMagno MJ, DiMagno EP. Does endoscopic therapy favorably affect the outcome of patients who have recurrent acute pancreatitis and pancreas divisum? *Pancreas*. 2007; 34: 21-45. PMID: 17198181.
60. Tarnasky PR. Division of the sphincter of Oddi for treatment of dysfunction associated with recurrent pancreatitis. *Gastrointest Endosc*. 1997; 45: 444-446. PMID: 9165338.
61. Cote GA, Imperiale TF, Schmidt SE, Fogel E, Lehman G, McHenry L, et al. Similar efficacies of biliary, with or without pancreatic, sphincterotomy in treatment of idiopathic recurrent acute pancreatitis. *Gastroenterology*. 2012; 143: 1502-1509. PMID: 22982183.
62. Romagnuolo J, Talluri J, Kennard E, Sandhu BS, Sherman S, Cote GA, et al. Clinical Profile, Etiology, and Treatment of Chronic Pancreatitis in North American Women: Analysis of a Large Multicenter Cohort. *Pancreas*. 2016; 45: 934-940. PMID: 26967451.
63. Otsuki M. Chronic pancreatitis in Japan: epidemiology, prognosis, diagnostic criteria, and future problems. *J Gastroenterol*. 2003; 38: 315-326. PMID: 12743770.
64. Cote GA, Yadav D, Slivka A, Hawes RH, Anderson MA, Burton FR, et al. Alcohol and smoking as risk factors in an epidemiology study of patients with chronic pancreatitis. *Clin Gastroenterol Hepatol*. 2011; 9: 266-273; quiz e227. PMID: 21029787.
65. Garg PK, Tandon RK. Survey on chronic pancreatitis in the Asia-Pacific region. *J Gastroenterol Hepatol*. 2004; 19: 998-1004. PMID: 15304116.
66. Ammann RW, Akovbiantz A, Largiader F, Schueler G. Course and outcome of chronic pancreatitis. Longitudinal study of a mixed medical-surgical series of 245 patients. *Gastroenterology*. 1984; 86: 820-828. PMID: 6706066.
67. Lankisch PG, Lohr-Happe A, Otto J, Creutzfeldt W. Natural course in chronic pancreatitis. Pain, exocrine and endocrine pancreatic insufficiency and prognosis of the disease. *Digestion*. 1993; 54: 148-155. PMID: 8359556.
68. Mullady DK, Yadav D, Amann ST, O'Connell MR, Barmada MM, Elta GH, et al. Type of pain, pain-associated complications, quality of life, disability and resource utilisation in chronic pancreatitis: a prospective cohort study. *Gut*. 2011; 60: 77-84. PMID: 21148579.
69. Malka D, Hammel P, Sauvanet A, Rufat P, O'Toole D, Bardet P, et al. Risk factors for diabetes mellitus in chronic pancreatitis. *Gastroenterology*. 2000; 119: 1324-1332. PMID: 11054391.
70. DiMagno EP, Go VL, Summerskill WH. Relations between pancreatic enzyme ouputs and malabsorption in severe pancreatic insufficiency. *N Engl J Med*. 1973; 288: 813-815. PMID: 4693931.
71. Dutta SK, Bustin MP, Russell RM, Costa BS. Deficiency of fat-soluble vitamins in treated patients with pancreatic insufficiency. *Ann Intern Med*. 1982; 97: 549-552. PMID: 6922690.
72. Sikkens EC, Cahen DL, Koch AD, Braat H, Poley JW, Kuipers EJ, et al. The prevalence of fat-soluble vitamin deficiencies and a decreased bone mass in patients with chronic pancreatitis. *Pancreatology*. 2013; 13: 238-242. PMID: 23719594.
73. Duggan SN, Smyth ND, Murphy A, Macnaughton D, O'Keefe SJ, Conlon KC. High prevalence of osteoporosis in patients with chronic pancreatitis: a systematic review and meta-analysis. *Clin Gastroenterol Hepatol*. 2014; 12: 219-228. PMID: 23856359.
74. Duggan SN, Purcell C, Kilbane M, O'Keane M, McKenna M, Gaffney P, et al. An association between abnormal bone turnover, systemic inflammation, and osteoporosis in patients with chronic pancreatitis: a case-matched study. *Am J Gastroenterol*. 2015; 110: 336-345. PMID: 25623657.
75. Munigala S, Agarwal B, Gelrud A, Conwell DL. Chronic Pancreatitis and Fracture: A Retrospective, Population-Based Veterans Administration Study. *Pancreas*. 2016; 45: 355-361. PMID: 26199986.
76. Ammann RW, Buehler H, Muench R, Freiburghaus AW, Siegenthaler W. Differences in the natural history of idiopathic (nonalcoholic) and alcoholic chronic pancreatitis. A comparative long-term study of 287 patients. *Pancreas*. 1987; 2: 368-377. PMID: 3628234.
77. Sankaran SJ, Xiao AY, Wu LM, Windsor JA, Forsmark CE, Petrov MS. Frequency of progression from acute to chronic pancreatitis and risk factors: a meta-analysis. *Gastroenterology*. 2015; 149: 1490-1500. PMID: 26299411.
78. Lankisch PG, Breuer N, Bruns A, Weber-Dany B, Lowenfels AB, Maisonneuve P. Natural history of acute pancreatitis: a long-term population-based study. *Am J Gastroenterol*. 2009; 104: 2797-2805; quiz 2806. PMID: 19603011.
79. Fitzsimmons D, Kahl S, Butturini G, van Wyk M, Bornman P, Bassi C, et al. Symptoms and quality of life in chronic pancreatitis assessed by structured interview and the EORTC QLQ-C30 and QLQ-PAN26. *Am J Gastroenterol*. 2005; 100: 918-926. PMID: 15784041.
80. Pezzilli R, Morselli-Labate AM, Frulloni L, Cavestro GM, Ferri B, Comparato G, et al. The quality of life in patients with chronic pancreatitis evaluated using the SF-12 questionnaire: a comparative study with the SF-36 questionnaire. *Dig Liver Dis*. 2006; 38: 109-115. PMID: 16243011.
81. Pezzilli R, Morselli-Labate AM, Fantini L, Campana D, Corinaldesi R. Assessment of the quality of life in chronic pancreatitis using Sf-12 and EORTC Qlq-C30 questionnaires. *Dig Liver Dis*. 2007; 39: 1077-1086. PMID: 17692582.
82. Wassef W, DeWitt J, McGreevy K, Wilcox M, Whitcomb D, Yadav D, et al. Pancreatitis Quality of Life Instrument: A Psychometric Evaluation. *Am J Gastroenterol*. 2016. In press. PMID: 27296943.
83. Wassef W, Bova C, Barton B, Hartigan C. Pancreatitis Quality of Life Instrument: Development of a new instrument. *SAGE Open Med*. 2014; 2: 2050312114520856. PMID: 26770703.
84. Wehler M, Reulbach U, Nichterlein R, Lange K, Fischer B, Farnbacher M, et al. Health-related quality of life in chronic pancreatitis: a psychometric assessment. *Scand J Gastroenterol*. 2003; 38: 1083-1089. PMID: 14621285.

85. Mokrowiecka A, Pinkowski D, Malecka-Panas E, Johnson CD. Clinical, emotional and social factors associated with quality of life in chronic pancreatitis. *Pancreatology*. 2010; 10: 39-46. PMID: 20332660.
86. Pezzilli R, Bini L, Fantini L, Baroni E, Campana D, Tomassetti P, et al. Quality of life in chronic pancreatitis. *World J Gastroenterol*. 2006; 12: 6249-6251. PMID: 17072944.
87. Pezzilli R, Fantini L, Calculli L, Casadei R, Corinaldesi R. The quality of life in chronic pancreatitis: the clinical point of view. *JOP*. 2006; 7: 113-116. PMID: 16407631.
88. Pezzilli R, Morselli Labate AM, Fantini L, Gullo L and Corinaldesi R. Quality of life and clinical indicators for chronic pancreatitis patients in a 2-year follow-up study. *Pancreas*. 2007; 34: 191-196. PMID: 17312457.
89. Amann ST, Yadav D, Barmada MM, O'Connell M, Kennard ED, Anderson M, et al. Physical and mental quality of life in chronic pancreatitis: a case-control study from the North American Pancreatitis Study 2 cohort. *Pancreas*. 2013; 42: 293-300. PMID: 23357924.
90. Lowenfels AB, Maisonneuve P, Cavallini G, Ammann RW, Lankisch PG, Andersen JR, et al. Pancreatitis and the risk of pancreatic cancer. International Pancreatitis Study Group. *N Engl J Med*. 1993; 328: 1433-1437. PMID: 8479461.
91. Talamini G, Falconi M, Bassi C, Sartori N, Salvia R, Caldiron E, et al. Incidence of cancer in the course of chronic pancreatitis. *Am J Gastroenterol*. 1999; 94: 1253-1260. PMID: 10235203.
92. Pedrazzoli S, Pasquali C, Guzzinati S, Berselli M, Sperti C. Survival rates and cause of death in 174 patients with chronic pancreatitis. *J Gastrointest Surg*. 2008; 12: 1930-1937. PMID: 18766421.
93. Nøjgaard C, Bendtsen F, Becker U, Andersen JR, Holst C, Matzen P. Danish patients with chronic pancreatitis have a four-fold higher mortality rate than the Danish population. *Clin Gastroenterol Hepatol*. 2010; 8: 384-390. PMID: 20036762.
94. Raimondi S, Lowenfels AB, Morselli-Labate AM, Maisonneuve P, Pezzilli R. Pancreatic cancer in chronic pancreatitis; aetiology, incidence, and early detection. *Best Pract Res Clin Gastroenterol*. 2010; 24: 349-358. PMID: 20510834.
95. Lowenfels AB, Maisonneuve P, DiMagno EP, Elitsur Y, Gates LK Jr, Perrault J, et al. Hereditary pancreatitis and the risk of pancreatic cancer. International Hereditary Pancreatitis Study Group. *J Natl Cancer Inst*. 1997; 89: 442-446. PMID: 9091646.
96. Rebours V, Boutron-Ruault MC, Schnee M, Ferec C, Maire F, Hammel P, et al. Risk of pancreatic adenocarcinoma in patients with hereditary pancreatitis: a national exhaustive series. *Am J Gastroenterol*. 2008; 103: 111-119. PMID: 18184119.
97. Chari ST, Mohan V, Pitchumoni CS, Viswanathan M, Madanagopalan N, Lowenfels AB. Risk of pancreatic carcinoma in tropical calcifying pancreatitis: an epidemiologic study. *Pancreas*. 1994; 9: 62-66. PMID: 8108373.
98. Bang UC, Benfield T, Hyldstrup L, Bendtsen F, Beck Jensen JE. Mortality, cancer, and comorbidities associated with chronic pancreatitis: a Danish nationwide matched-cohort study. *Gastroenterology*. 2014; 146: 989-994. PMID: 24389306.
99. Lowenfels AB, Maisonneuve P, Cavallini G, Ammann RW, Lankisch PG, Andersen JR, et al. Prognosis of chronic pancreatitis: an international multicenter study. International Pancreatitis Study Group. *Am J Gastroenterol*. 1994; 89: 1467-1471. PMID: 8079921.
100. Thuluvath PJ, Imperio D, Nair S, Cameron JL. Chronic pancreatitis. Long-term pain relief with or without surgery, cancer risk, and mortality. *J Clin Gastroenterol*. 2003; 36: 159-165. PMID: 12544201.
101. Levy P, Milan C, Pignon JP, Baetz A, Bernades P. Mortality factors associated with chronic pancreatitis. Unidimensional and multidimensional analysis of a medical-surgical series of 240 patients. *Gastroenterology*. 1989; 96: 1165-1172. PMID: 2925060.
102. Johnson CD, Hosking S. National statistics for diet, alcohol consumption, and chronic pancreatitis in England and Wales, 1960-88. *Gut*. 1991; 32: 1401-1405. PMID: 1752477.
103. Tinto A, Lloyd DA, Kang JY, Majeed A, Ellis C, Williamson RC, et al. Acute and chronic pancreatitis-diseases on the rise: a study of hospital admissions in England 1989/90-1999/2000. *Aliment Pharmacol Ther*. 2002; 16: 2097-2105. PMID: 12452943.
104. Spanier BW, Dijkgraaf MG, Bruno MJ. Trends and forecasts of hospital admissions for acute and chronic pancreatitis in the Netherlands. *Eur J Gastroenterol Hepatol*. 2008; 20: 653-658. PMID: 18679068.
105. Jaakkola M, Nordback I. Pancreatitis in Finland between 1970 and 1989. *Gut*. 1993; 34: 1255-1260. PMID: 8406164.
106. Yadav D, Muddana V, O'Connell M. Hospitalizations for chronic pancreatitis in Allegheny County, Pennsylvania, USA. *Pancreatology*. 2011; 11: 546-552. PMID: 22205468.
107. Jupp J, Fine D, Johnson CD. The epidemiology and socioeconomic impact of chronic pancreatitis. *Best Pract Res Clin Gastroenterol*. 2010; 24 219-231. PMID: 20510824.
108. Clarke B, Slivka A, Tomizawa Y, Sanders M, Papachristou GI, Whitcomb DC, et al. Endoscopic therapy is effective for patients with chronic pancreatitis. *Clin Gastroenterol Hepatol*. 2012; 10: 795-802. PMID: 22245964.
109. Dumonceau JM, Delhaye M, Tringali A, Dominguez-Munoz JE, Poley JW, Arvanitaki M, et al. Endoscopic treatment of chronic pancreatitis: European Society of Gastrointestinal Endoscopy (ESGE) Clinical Guideline. *Endoscopy*. 2012; 44: 784-800. PMID: 22752888.
110. Dudekula A, Munigala S, Zureikat AH, Yadav D. Operative Trends for Pancreatic Diseases in the USA: Analysis of the Nationwide Inpatient Sample from 1998-2011. *J Gastrointest Surg*. 2016; 20: 803-811. PMID: 26791389.
111. Glass LM, Whitcomb DC, Yadav D, Romagnuolo J, Kennard E, Slivka AA, et al. Spectrum of use and effectiveness of endoscopic and surgical therapies for chronic pancreatitis in the United States. *Pancreas*. 2014; 43: 539-543. PMID: 24717802.
112. Garcea G, Pollard CA, Illouz S, Webb M, Metcalfe MS, Dennison AR. Patient satisfaction and cost-effectiveness following total pancreatectomy with islet cell transplantation for chronic pancreatitis. *Pancreas*. 2013; 42: 322-328. PMID: 23407482.

113. Everhart JE, Ruhl CE. Burden of digestive diseases in the United States Part III: Liver, biliary tract, and pancreas. *Gastroenterology*. 2009; 136: 1134-1144. PMID: 19245868.
114. Hall TC, Garcea G, Webb MA, Al-Leswas D, Metcalfe MS, Dennison AR. The socio-economic impact of chronic pancreatitis: a systematic review. *J Eval Clin Pract*. 2014; 20: 203-207. PMID: 24661411.
115. Gardner TB, Kennedy AT, Gelrud A, Banks PA, Vege SS, Gordon SR, et al. Chronic pancreatitis and its effect on employment and health care experience: results of a prospective American multicenter study. *Pancreas*. 2010; 39: 498-501. PMID: 20118821.
116. Dani R, Mott CB, Guarita DR, Nogueira CE. Epidemiology and etiology of chronic pancreatitis in Brazil: a tale of two cities. *Pancreas*. 1990; 5: 474-478. PMID: 2381901.
117. Robles-Diaz G, Vargas F, Uscanga L, Fernandez-del Castillo C. Chronic pancreatitis in Mexico City. *Pancreas*. 1990; 5: 479-483. PMID: 2381902.

Chapter 36

Pathogenesis of chronic pancreatitis

Ali A. Aghdassi*

Department of Medicine A, University Medicine Greifswald, Greifswald, Germany.

Introduction

Chronic pancreatitis is a progressive inflammatory disorder characterized by loss of functional pancreatic tissue, fibrous tissue conversion and ultimately loss of endocrine and exocrine function. Although its morphologic and clinical features have been well described, the pathogenesis of chronic pancreatitis is incompletely understood. There is no single etiology that inevitably leads to chronic pancreatitis, and it is rather considered as a complex disease with several contributing factors.[1,2] Currently, development of chronic pancreatitis is considered to be the result of a pathology involving pancreatic acinar, ductal, and stellate cells. Our current understanding of the pathogenesis arises from experimental animal models as well as epidemiological and genetic studies in humans. This section addresses both pathophysiological mechanisms, including results from established animal models and known genetic and etiological factors that are associated with chronic pancreatitis.

Pancreatic cells and cellular components that promote fibrosis

Histologically, the pancreas consists of 3 main cell lineages: acinar, ductal, and endocrine. In addition, terminal end ductal cells that interface with acini are called centroacinar cells.[3] Adjacent to the basolateral part of acinar cells, and to a minor extent around small pancreatic ducts and blood vessels, are pancreatic stellate cells, which account for around 4% to 7% of all parenchymal cells.[4,5]

Each cell type found in the pancreas–acinar, ductal, or stellate cells–is suspected to contribute to chronic pancreatitis. The extra-pancreatic environment, including inflammatory cells, also contributes to the progress of both acute and chronic inflammatory pancreatic diseases.

There is strong evidence that pancreatic proteases, and their premature intracellular activation, are responsible for the pathogenesis of *acute* pancreatitis. Therefore, these enzymes also might be of interest in *chronic* pancreatitis, not least because findings of genetic studies in humans underline their critical role. Six major genes that target either acinar cells through a trypsin-dependent pathway (PRSS1, PRSS2, CTRC, CASR, SPINK) or duct cells (CFTR) have been identified. These cellular constituents are comprehensively discussed below. Both (extra-) pancreatic cell types and frequently cited genes and their aberrations are depicted in **Figure 1**.

Acinar cells

Cationic and anionic trypsinogen (PRSS1/PRSS2)

The smallest functional units of the exocrine pancreas are acinar cells whose primary function is the synthesis, storage and secretion of digestive enzymes (zymogens). One of them is trypsin, a serine proteinase that is stored as its inactive precursor, trypsinogen, in zymogen granules. Under physiologic conditions these enzymes remain inactive during intracellular transport, secretion, and passage through the pancreatic duct. When they reach the duodenum, trypsinogen is activated by the brush border enzyme enterokinase. This activation leads to a cascade-like activation of the other pancreatic protease precursors.[6] There are 3 isoforms of trypsinogen in the human pancreas, and they differ in charge. They are cationic trypsinogen (PRSS1), anionic trypsinogen (PRSS2), and mesotrypsinogen (PRSS3). Cationic and anionic trypsinogen comprise the overwhelming majority of trypsinogen content whereas mesotrypsinogen makes up only about 5%.[1,7]

One of the key events in acute pancreatitis is the intracellular and premature activation of pancreatic digestive enzymes that ultimately leads to organ injury and autolysis.[8] Trypsinogen plays a pivotal role in the beginning of acute pancreatitis as it activates other zymogens intracellularly, such as chymotrypsin, elastase, carboxypeptidase A2 or phospholipase.[9-11] Since enterokinase is absent inside the pancreas, other activators for trypsinogen must exist. According to the co-localization hypothesis, this activation occurs by the action of lysosomal protease

*Corresponding author. Email: aghdassi@uni-greifswald.de

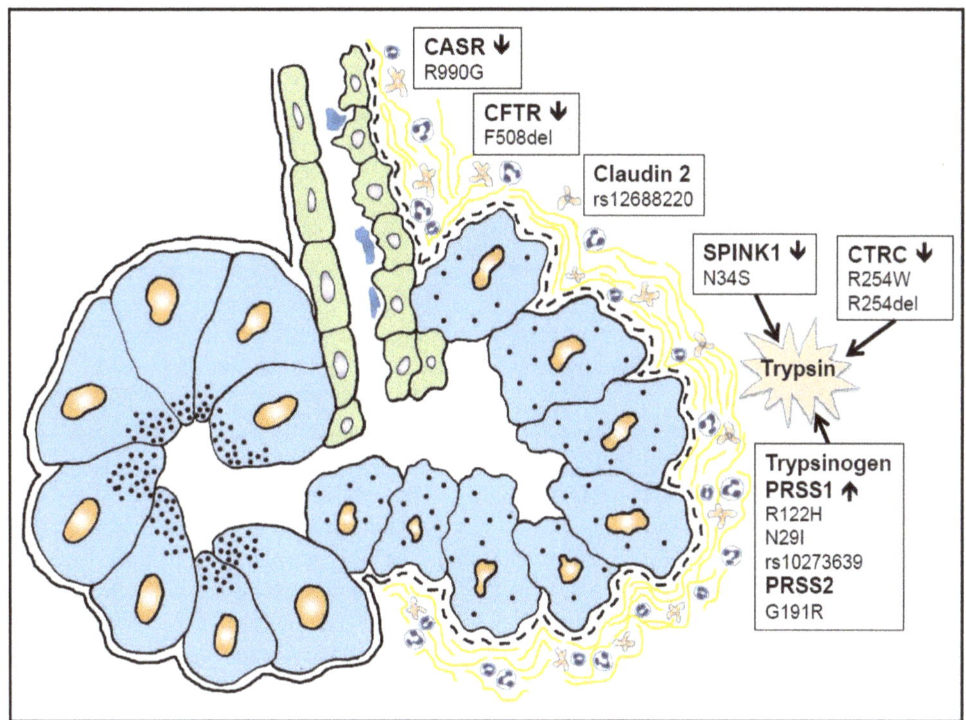

Figure 1. The pathogenesis of chronic pancreatitis. Acinar, ductal, and profibrotic cells all contribute to pathogenesis. In addition, an invasion of immune cells occurs. Some very frequently cited proteins and their genomic aberrations are listed here.

cathepsin B. Lysosomal hydrolases and digestive zymogens co-localize during experimental pancreatitis, with accumulation of cathepsin B in a zymogen enriched subcellular fraction.[12,13] *In-vitro* experiments have shown that cathepsin B directly activates trypsinogen by proteolytic cleavage,[14] and deficiency of cathepsin B markedly reduced trypsinogen activation in a mouse model.[15]

There is strong evidence from genetic studies in humans that trypsinogen is an important pathogenetic factor for chronic pancreatitis as well. In 1996 Whitcomb and coworkers identified a gain-of-function mutation of the cationic trypsinogen (*p.R122H*) gene in patients with hereditary pancreatitis associated with inappropriate trypsin activation because of increased resistance to hydrolysis of this mutated form of trypsin.[16] A second mutation (*p.N29I*) of cationic trypsinogen was found in the same exon in patients with recurrent acute and chronic pancreatitis just 1 year later.[17] Meanwhile other PRSS1 mutations have been identified in association with hereditary pancreatitis.[18-21] A complete loss-of-function mutation was found by Witt et al. in the anionic trypsinogen gene (*PRSS2*) that was significantly underrepresented in patients with chronic pancreatitis compared to healthy control subjects (*G191R* in exon 4).[22] These results indicate that not only are *PRSS1* mutations associated with idiopathic or hereditary chronic pancreatitis, but inactivating mutations of trypsinogen can also modify susceptibility to chronic pancreatitis.

Taken together these observations support the critical role of the protease/antiprotease system, especially trypsin, in the pathogenesis of pancreatitis. However, it should be mentioned that fewer than 60% of patients with hereditary chronic pancreatitis and fewer than 20% of patients with idiopathic chronic pancreatitis harbor mutations in the *PRSS1* gene so that an inappropriate trypsinogen cannot be the only causative factor for chronic pancreatitis.[23-25]

In an attempt to mimic the role of trypsinogen deduced from the human genetics findings, mouse strains carrying over expressed forms of mutated trypsinogen (R122H and N29I) as well as wildtype human PRSS1 were created.[26] All 3 strains not only developed more severe acute pancreatitis upon cerulein treatment but also spontaneously displayed characteristics of chronic pancreatitis including vacuolization, inflammatory infiltrates, and fibrosis, as was expected from human genetics data. Interestingly the phenotypes of the transgenic strains did not differ significantly. One underlying reason might be that human trypsinogen has a higher propensity for auto activation compared with trypsinogens from other species.[27]

Recent experimental animal models questioned the detrimental effects of trypsinogen in chronic pancreatitis. Mice lacking trypsinogen 7 (T-/-) did not show pathologic intracellular trypsinogen activation during caerulein-induced acute pancreatitis but surprisingly still developed chronic pancreatitis showing indistinguishable histomorphologic features like wild types. Previous works indicated that a genetic deletion of trypsinogen isoform 7 in mice led to a 60% reduction of pancreatic trypsinogen content.[28] Similar to these observations cathepsin B deficient mice - that fail to activate trypsinogen by limited proteolysis - developed chronic pancreatitis.[29] Both knockout and wildtype mice showed comparable intracellular transcriptional activation as demonstrated by activation of nuclear factor (NF)-κB and similar COX-2 overexpression. Both COX-2 and NF-κB are key mediators of chronic inflammation.[30] More studies and most likely the application of alternative mouse models will be necessary to further investigate the trypsin-centered theory of chronic pancreatitis.

Interactions between genetic and environmental factors in patients with recurrent acute and chronic pancreatitis have recently been investigated in the North American Pancreatitis Study 2 (NAPS2) using genome wide association studies.[31] A single nucleotide polymorphism (SNP) was detected in the *PRSS1–PRSS2* locus in the 5'-promoter region of *PRSS1* and might affect expression of the trypsinogen gene. Another SNP was found at the *CLDN2* locus. CLDN2 encodes Claudin-2, a tight-junction protein physiologically expressed between duct cells and endocrine islets but also found in an atypical localization along the basolateral membrane of acinar cells in chronic pancreatitis.[32] The findings of the PRSS1-PRSS2 and CLDN2 variants were replicated in a large European cohort with alcoholic and nonalcoholic chronic pancreatitis, and a strong association was found in subjects with alcohol pancreatitis.[33] When compared with patients with alcoholic liver cirrhosis there was no significant association, suggesting that those variants are not susceptibility factors for alcoholism per se or for fibrosing disorders associated with alcohol abuse in general. More studies will be necessary for complete understanding the underlying cellular events.

Serine protease inhibitor Kazal type 1 (SPINK1)

As trace amounts of trypsinogen normally become activated within the pancreas, there are protective mechanisms that prevent the digestive enzyme activation cascade.[34] One of them is the serine protease inhibitor Kazal type 1 SPINK1 (or pancreatic secretory trypsin inhibitor, PSTI; OMIM 167790), which acts as an intracellular inhibitor for intrapancreatic active trypsin.[35] SPINK1 is synthesized inside the acinar cells and stored in zymogen granules, the same compartment as trypsinogen. It is also secreted into the pancreatic juice where it protects against trypsinogen activation inside the pancreatic ducts. It presumably has other activities in addition to its physiological function in the pancreas because this protein is also detected in sera and various malignant tissues.[36] The active site of SPINK1 binds covalently to the catalytic serine residue of trypsin and is considered to inhibit approximately 20% of total trypsin activity inside the acinar cell.[37]

Because SPINK1 maintains a balance of active and inhibited trypsin inside the pancreas, its inactivation is considered to be an important factor for the development of inflammatory pancreatic disorders, including chronic pancreatitis. In accordance with its biological role, several studies have described the association of *SPINK1* gene mutations and pancreatitis. The most commonly observed mutation leads to an exchange of asparagine for serine of codon 34 (p.N34S) and has been reported in idiopathic and hereditary chronic pancreatitis as well as in alcoholic chronic and tropical pancreatitis.[38-40] However, it is worth mentioning that the incidence of this mutation is around 0.5% to 2.5% in the general population, indicating that it cannot be the only causative factor for chronic pancreatitis and probably acts instead as a disease modifier.[37,41] Novel polymorphisms were identified in patients with chronic pancreatitis such as the D50E mutation and a variety of intronic polymorphisms, but their frequency is extremely low and some were found in single patients.[23]

Functional analysis of N34S recombinant SPINK1 did not show any reduced trypsin inhibitor capacity in-vitro so that the exact pathophysiologic action of this mutation has not been clarified so far. Maybe the impaired function of SPINK1 is based on an intronic mutation rather than the N34S itself as N34S is usually associated with intronic sequence variants.[35,38,42] Further research on the exact function of SPINK1 exonic and intronic mutations is inevitable to gain deeper knowledge on its pathophysiologic role in chronic pancreatitis.

Chymotrypsin C (CTRC)

Chymotrypsin C appeared to be identical to Rinderknecht's enzyme Y that he initially found in the pancreatic juice[43] and has seemingly ambivalent functions on trypsinogen. The prevailing Ca^{2+} concentration regulates the balance between activation and degradation of cationic trypsinogen. At high Ca^{2+} concentrations, it facilitates autoactivation by limited proteolysis of trypsinogen activation peptide.[44,45] On the other hand, in a milieu with low Ca^{2+} concentration it selectively cleaves a peptide bond in the calcium-binding loop of trypsinogen, which results in its degradation.[46] Since higher Ca^{2+} concentrations (>1 mM) occur in the upper small intestine, trypsinogen is activated more easily as it is also designated for digestion of proteins. In the lower small intestine, along with falling Ca^{2+} levels, trypsinogen degradation predominates.[46] Intracellular Ca^{2+} signaling is important for acinar cell physiology and also regulates secretion of enzymes. In pathological conditions release of Ca^{2+} from intracellular stores into the cytosol, especially in the apical cell pole and for a prolonged time (>100 sec), is thought to account for premature intracellular protease activation.[47,48]

Mutations of the cationic trypsinogen gene interfere with the cleaving effects of CTRC that can be shown in in-vitro studies.[49-51] Absence of chymotrypsin C increased the autoactivation of R122H mutated trypsinogen only slightly, whereas addition of CTRC drastically increased activation leading to high trypsin levels.[49] In contrast to the situation in humans the R122H mutation did not have a relevant effect on autoactivation of T8 trypsinogen by CTRC in mice.[52] Again, introduction of known human mutations into mouse trypsinogen isoforms can have different effects than in humans. Therefore, mutagenesis techniques might have limitations when investigating chronic pancreatitis in animal models.

Several genetic variations have been found in the chymotrypsin C gene that have been associated with chronic pancreatitis. Variants of the CTRC gene have been found in 3.3% of individuals with idiopathic or hereditary chronic pancreatitis. The most frequent variants were the c.760C>T (p.R254W) mutation and a deletion on exon 7 (p.K247_R254del).[53] These CTRC variants were associated with reduced enzymatic activity, and were secreted to a lesser extent. They thus are considered to be loss-of-function mutations. In a Chinese population, additional CTRC variations were detected in chronic pancreatitis patients, however the overall frequency was 2.3% and thus much lower than in the German study.[54] Taken together these data support the importance of the protease/antiprotease system for pathogenesis of chronic pancreatitis as shown above for cationic/anionic trypsinogen and SPINK1. In this context CTRC variants may represent an extra risk factor.

Calcium-sensing receptor (CASR)

Besides digestive proteases millimolar quantities of calcium ions are released from the zymogen granules that, when precipitated, cause intraductal pancreatic stones. The Ca^{2+} sensing receptor (CASR) is capable of monitoring changes of extracellular calcium concentrations. Besides its expression in the parathyroid gland, kidney and small intestine this molecule was found on the luminal side of ductal cells and more diffusely distributed inside acinar cells.[55] Functional studies showed that CASR regulates hydrogencarbonate (HCO_3^-) efflux into the ducts and thus ensuring a milieu with sufficient fluid secretion to prevent calcium stone precipitation.

Mutations in the CASR gene have been associated with chronic pancreatitis. Recent studies reported that CASR gene mutations in combination of SPINK1 N34S mutation increased the risk of chronic pancreatitis.[1,56] Furthermore the CASR exon 7 polymorphism R990G was associated with chronic pancreatitis and this association was stronger in individuals who reported moderate or heavy alcohol consumption.[57] Presumably subjects with considerable alcohol abuse represent a risk group in which the addition of another risk factor (CASR mutation) enhances the overall risk for development of chronic pancreatitis.[57]

Ductal cells

Cystic fibrosis transmembrane conductance regulator (CFTR)

The CFTR gene encodes for an ABC (acronym for ATP-binding cassette) transporter protein that is expressed on epithelial cells and thus also on pancreatic ductal epithelium. It functions as a Cl^- selective channel and permits chloride-anions and water to enter the ductal lumen, which finally allows highly concentrated pancreatic secretory proteins (including trypsinogen) secreted by the acinar cells to remain in a soluble state.[58,59] Cystic fibrosis is quite common in people of Northern European descent, affects approximately one in 2500 births among whites and is characterized by a heterogeneous clinical course. The exocrine pancreas is invariably affected in cystic fibrosis, with signs of chronic pancreatitis and exocrine insufficiency.[60] In 1989 the CFTR gene was found to be located at chromosome 7 (7q31).[61] More than 1000 different mutations have been reported in cystic fibrosis patients. The most common aberration is a deletion found at position 508 (p.F508del), which results in a deletion of phenylalanine.[62] In 1998 an association of CFTR mutations and chronic pancreatitis was discovered in patients with idiopathic chronic pancreatitis and alcoholic chronic pancreatitis.[63,64] In a comprehensive genetic analysis of the CFTR gene including all 27 exons and the flanking intronic regions, abnormal CFTR alleles were found to be twice as frequent in patients with idiopathic chronic pancreatitis than in healthy controls (18.6% vs. 9.2%, $p < 0.05$).[62]

Recent functional studies underlined the role of CFTR in pancreatitis, as high levels of alcohol consumption impair the function of CFTR in pancreatic duct cells, there by disturbing exocrine pancreatic secretion and sensitizing the organ to pathological stimuli.[65]

Pancreatic stellate cells (PSCs)

Although not activated in an uninjured pancreas, stellate cells fulfill important functions for tissue architecture as they control synthesis and degradation of extracellular matrix.[66] In particular, tissue homeostasis results from secretion of matrix metalloproteinases (MMP) and their inhibitors (tissue inhibitors of matrix metalloproteinases, TIMPs),[67] and secondarily by phagocytosis of necrotic acinar cells.[68] During pancreatic injury, stellate cells are activated and secrete a high amount of extracellular matrix proteins.[66] These extracellular matrix (ECM) proteins consist of collagens, fibronectin and laminin. Furthermore, there is an increase of MMP2 production. In addition, activated PSCs show an increased capacity of cell proliferation and migration. Several activators of PSCs have been identified, including a variety of chemokines, alcohol and its metabolites, fatty acid ethyl esters, oxidative stress or endotoxins.[4]

Theories of pathogenesis of chronic pancreatitis

In the past decades multiple theories to explain the pathogenesis of chronic pancreatitis have emerged. Some well-known concepts are outlined briefly in the following. The traditional and more recent theories are described in more detail in a review by Stevens et al., including arguments for and against these hypotheses.[69]

Oxidative stress theory: Chronic exposure to oxidative stress leads to fibrosis. Because of an aberrant function of hepatic mixed-function, oxidases, byproducts of hepatic detoxification such as lipid peroxidation products, free radicals and other toxic compounds, are excreted in the bile and reach the pancreas through reflux in the pancreatic duct.[70] Reactive oxygen species further damage cellular membranes, intracellular proteins and DNA. Ethanol is a well-known inducer of oxidative stress and one of the mediators is cytochrome P450 2E1 (CYP2E1). Ethanol thereby serves both as a substrate and an enhancer of the enzymatic activity of CYP2E1 that is found overexpressed in the pancreas after chronic abuse.[71]

Toxic–metabolic theory: Alcohol and its metabolites have a direct toxic effect on acinar cells, leading to cellular necrosis, fatty degeneration, and eventually fibrosis.[72] Alcohol is mainly metabolized by the oxidative pathway including alcohol- and aldehyde-dehydrogenases, or to lesser extent, enzymes of the microsomal oxidizing system. In an alternative pathway, the nonoxidative pathway, ethanol is esterified with fatty esters that result in the synthesis of fatty acid ethyl esters.[73] Although the primary site of alcohol metabolism is in the liver, the pancreas is also capable of both oxidative and nonoxidative metabolism, causing local damage.[74,75.]

Stone and ductal obstruction theory: This hypothesis was evoked by the fact that after a variable time, most patients with chronic pancreatitis develop calcifications and intraductal pancreatic stones.[76] Chronic obstruction leads to local damage and stasis that further enhance stone formation and finally fibrosis. Besides, formation of protein plugs and pancreatic stones are increased by alcohol itself. Experimental animal models show that partial or complete pancreatic duct obstruction in combination with ethanol feeding[77] or repetitive secretagogue stimulation,[78] markedly increased severity of acute pancreatitis and induced chronic disease as well.

Necrosis–Fibrosis Theory: Chronic pancreatitis is considered to be a result of recurrent bouts of acute pancreatitis if they are sufficiently severe.[79]Acute inflammation leads to periductal injury and fibrosis that eventually compress the ductal lumen. This obstruction favors acinar cell atrophy, calculi precipitation because stasis, and further fibrous tissue formation.[69] Further support for this theory is provided by data from genetic studies and animal experiments: Activating trypsinogen (PRSS1) mutations lead to a gain-of-function associated with unregulated protease activation, acute pancreatitis, and lastly, chronic pancreatitis. Animal models mimicking chronic pancreatitis use induction of recurrent bouts of acute pancreatitis by repeated injections of cholecystokinin analogues such as caerulein. When animals develop acute pancreatitis, they either recover completely, once the pathogenic stimuli have been stopped, or they develop atrophy of the organ and fibrosis, especially if the pathogenic stimulus was given during the recovery period, during which animals are extremely susceptible to any harmful event.[80,81]

Primary duct hypothesis: An autoimmune mechanism has been considered to be causative for chronic pancreatitis. Resembling primary sclerosing cholangitis to a certain extent, the pancreatic duct is affected by an autoimmune reaction ending up in obliteration of the main and secondary pancreatic ducts.[82] Coincidence of chronic pancreatitis and autoimmune disorders of the gastrointestinal tract has been observed, and autoimmune pancreatitis is a form of chronic pancreatitis that is a pancreatic manifestation of IgG4-related disease.[83] This process can be triggered by alcohol consumption, extending beyond its direct toxic effects on ductal cells.

Sentinel acute pancreatitis event (SAPE) hypothesis: In order to create a unifying theory for development of chronic pancreatitis and to include recent advances in pancreatitis and the immunological contributions, a new hypothesis was introduced in 1999.[34,84] The new features of this hypothesis are on the one hand that an initiating event (sentinel event) is necessary for causing acute pancreatitis and acinar cell injury first, and that subsequent anti-inflammatory and pro-fibrotic events enable the progression to chronic pancreatitis.[84] It should be noted that even before the sentinel event occurs, the pancreas can be exposed to toxic agents such as alcohol, nicotine, lipids, or other compounds that induce chronic metabolic or oxidative stress. During acute pancreatitis, unrestrained trypsinogen activation occurs as described above. Simultaneous with early protease activation, there is a proinflammatory reaction, with invasion of inflammatory cells into the pancreas, that perpetuate protease activation and cellular damage. This event is mediated by tumor necrosis factor (TNF)-α in a cathepsin B- and calcium-dependent manner.[85] In the late phase of acute pancreatitis, an anti-inflammatory reaction is observed that usually limits the inflammatory reaction and initiates the healing process. During this phase, there is an activation of profibrotic cells, including stellate cells. However, a sustained anti-inflammatory reaction drives pancreatic fibrosis. This occurs when causative factors such as oxidative stress, alcohol, or its metabolites are not removed and thus continuously stimulate PSCs to synthesize components of extracellular matrix, causing fibrosis.[69,84]

One of the challenges of the SAPE hypothesis is its intention to combine divergent etiologies for chronic pancreatitis through a common pathway leading to the same endpoint, i.e. chronic pancreatitis. This hypothesis also explains why some individuals with mutations in the trypsin-dependent pathway such as PRSS1, SPINK1 or CTRC, as well as the majority of alcoholics, do not eventually develop acute or chronic pancreatitis because they lack the sentinel event, a *sine qua non* for initiation of chronic pancreatitis.

Conclusions

Recent knowledge on the pathogenesis of chronic pancreatitis has been gained from both genetic linkage analyses and experimental in-vitro and animal studies. There are multiple genetic susceptibility factors, which primarily involve the protease/antiprotease system of the exocrine pancreas. Recent genome wide association studies have identified genetic variants affecting proteins seemingly unrelated to the "trypsin-centered pathway" whose underlying cellular mechanisms are still unclear. From animal models, we have learned that at least 2 principal mechanisms seem to predispose to the development of chronic pancreatitis. These are recurrent pathologic stimuli on the pancreas or a single severe event such as an obstruction of the bile or pancreatic duct.[86] Furthermore new theories postulate that a sequence of 2 events is essential for the pathogenesis of chronic pancreatitis.

It can be assumed that not a single, but rather a combination of different pathologic stimuli, including immune-mediated processes, are necessary to develop chronic pancreatitis. The pathogenesis of this disease is too complex to be reduced to one single event.

References

1. Whitcomb DC. Genetic risk factors for pancreatic disorders. *Gastroenterology.* 2013; 144: 1292-1302. PMID: 23622139.
2. Muniraj T, Aslanian HR, Farrell J, and Jamidar PA. Chronic pancreatitis, a comprehensive review and update. Part I: epidemiology, etiology, risk factors, genetics, pathophysiology, and clinical features. *Dis Mon.* 2014; 60: 530-550. PMID: 25510320.
3. Reichert M and Rustgi AK. Pancreatic ductal cells in development, regeneration, and neoplasia. *J Clin Invest.* 2011; 121: 4572-4578. PMID: 22133881.
4. Apte MV, Pirola RC, and Wilson JS. Pancreatic stellate cells: a starring role in normal and diseased pancreas. *Front Physiol.* 2012; 3: 344. PMID: 22973234.
5. Bachem MG, Schneider E, Gross H, Weidenbach H, Schmid RM, Menke A, et al. Identification, culture, and characterization of pancreatic stellate cells in rats and humans. *Gastroenterology.* 1998; 115: 421-432. PMID: 9679048.
6. Halangk W and Lerch MM. Early events in acute pancreatitis. *Clin Lab Med.* 2005; 25: 1-15. PMID: 15749229.
7. Scheele G, Bartelt D, and Bieger W. Characterization of human exocrine pancreatic proteins by two-dimensional isoelectric focusing/sodium dodecyl sulfate gel electrophoresis. *Gastroenterology.* 1981; 80: 461473. PMID: 6969677.
8. Chiari H. Über die Selbstverdauung des menschlichen Pankreas. *Z. Heilkunde.* 1896; 17: 69-96.
9. Lerch MM, Saluja AK, Dawra R, Ramarao P, Saluja M, and Steer ML. Acute necrotizing pancreatitis in the opossum: earliest morphological changes involve acinar cells. *Gastroenterology.* 1992; 103: 205-213. PMID: 1612327.
10. Lerch MM and Gorelick FS. Early trypsinogen activation in acute pancreatitis. *Med Clin North Am.* 2000; 84: 549-563. PMID: 10872413.
11. Hofbauer B, Saluja AK, Lerch MM, Bhagat L, Bhatia M, Lee HS, et al. Intra-acinar cell activation of trypsinogen during caerulein-induced pancreatitis in rats. *Am J Physiol Gastrointest Liver Physiol.* 1998; 275: G352-G362. PMID: 9688663.
12. Watanabe O, Baccino FM, Steer ML, and Meldolesi J. Supramaximal caerulein stimulation and ultrastructure of rat pancreatic acinar cell: early morphological changes during development of experimental pancreatitis. *Am J PhysiolGastrointest Liver Physiol.* 1984; 246: G457-G467. PMID: 6720895.
13. Saluja A, Hashimoto S, Saluja M, Powers RE, Meldolesi J, and Steer ML. Subcellular redistribution of lysosomal enzymes during caerulein-induced pancreatitis. *Am J Physiol Gastrointest Liver Physiol.* 1987; 253: G508-G516. PMID: 2821825.
14. Figarella C, Miszczuk-Jamska B, and Barrett AJ. Possible lysosomal activation of pancreatic zymogens. Activation of both human trypsinogens by cathepsin B and spontaneous acid. Activation of human trypsinogen 1. *Biol Chem Hoppe Seyler.* 1988; 369 Suppl: 293-298. PMID: 3202969.
15. Halangk W, Lerch MM, Brandt-Nedelev B, Roth W, Ruthenbuerger M, Reinheckel T, et al. Role of cathepsin B in intracellular trypsinogen activation and the onset of acute pancreatitis. *J Clin Invest.* 2000; 106: 773-781. PMID: 10995788.
16. Whitcomb DC, Gorry MC, Preston RA, Furey W, Sossenheimer MJ, Ulrich CD, et al. Hereditary pancreatitis is caused by a mutation in the cationic trypsinogen gene. *Nat Genet.* 1996; 14: 141-145. PMID: 8841182.
17. Gorry MC, Gabbaizedeh D, Furey W, Gates LK, Jr., Preston RA, Aston CE, et al. Mutations in the cationic trypsinogen gene are associated with recurrent acute and chronic pancreatitis. *Gastroenterology.* 1997; 113: 1063-1068. PMID: 9322498.
18. Teich N, Ockenga J, Hoffmeister A, Manns M, Mossner J, and Keim V. Chronic pancreatitis associated with an activation peptide mutation that facilitates trypsin activation. *Gastroenterology.* 2000; 119: 461-465. PMID: 10930381.
19. Witt H, Luck W and Becker M. A signal peptide cleavage site mutation in the cationic trypsinogen gene is strongly associated with chronic pancreatitis. *Gastroenterology.* 1999; 117: 7-10. PMID: 10381903.
20. Ferec C, Raguenes O, Salomon R, Roche C, Bernard JP, Guillot M, et al. Mutations in the cationic trypsinogen gene and evidence for genetic heterogeneity in hereditary pancreatitis. *J Med Genet.* 1999; 36: 228-232. PMID: 10204851.
21. Simon P, Weiss FU, Sahin-Toth M, Parry M, Nayler O, Lenfers B, et al. Hereditary pancreatitis caused by a novel PRSS1 mutation (Arg-122 --> Cys) that alters autoactivation

and autodegradation of cationic trypsinogen. *J Biol Chem.* 2002; 277: 5404-5410. PMID: 11719509.
22. Witt H, Sahin-Toth M, Landt O, Chen JM, Kahne T, Drenth JP, et al. A degradation-sensitive anionic trypsinogen (PRSS2) variant protects against chronic pancreatitis. *Nat Genet.* 2006; 38: 668-673. PMID: 16699518.
23. Pfutzer RH, Barmada MM, Brunskill AP, Finch R, Hart PS, Neoptolemos J, et al. SPINK1/PSTI polymorphisms act as disease modifiers in familial and idiopathic chronic pancreatitis. *Gastroenterology.* 2000; 119: 615-623. PMID: 10982753.
24. Dasouki MJ, Cogan J, Summar ML, Neblitt W, 3rd, Foroud T, Koller D, et al. Heterogeneity in hereditary pancreatitis. *Am J Med Genet.* 1998; 77: 47-53. PMID: 9557894.
25. Creighton J, Lyall R, Wilson DI, Curtis A, and Charnley R. Mutations of the cationic trypsinogen gene in patients with chronic pancreatitis. *Lancet.* 1999; 354: 42-43. PMID: 10406366.
26. Athwal T, Huang W, Mukherjee R, Latawiec D, Chvanov M, Clarke R, et al. Expression of human cationic trypsinogen (PRSS1) in murine acinar cells promotes pancreatitis and apoptotic cell death. *Cell Death Dis.* 5: e1165. PMID: 24722290.
27. Kereszturi E and Sahin-Toth M. Intracellular autoactivation of human cationic trypsinogen mutants causes reduced trypsinogen secretion and acinar cell death. *J Biol Chem.* 2009; 284: 33392-33399. PMID: 19801634.
28. Dawra R, Sah RP, Dudeja V, Rishi L, Talukdar R, Garg P, et al. Intra-acinar trypsinogen activation mediates early stages of pancreatic injury but not inflammation in mice with acute pancreatitis. *Gastroenterology.* 2011; 141: 2210-2217 e2212. PMID: 21875495.
29. Sah RP, Dudeja V, Dawra RK, and Saluja AK. Cerulein-induced chronic pancreatitis does not require intra-acinar activation of trypsinogen in mice. *Gastroenterology* 144(5): 1076-1085 e1072, 2013. PMID: 23354015.
30. Sah RP, Dawra RK, and Saluja AK. New insights into the pathogenesis of pancreatitis. *Curr Opin Gastroenterol.* 2013; 29: 523-530. PMID: 23892538.
31. Whitcomb DC, Yadav D, Adam S, Hawes RH, Brand RE, Anderson MA, et al. Multicenter approach to recurrent acute and chronic pancreatitis in the United States: the North American Pancreatitis Study 2 (NAPS2). *Pancreatology.* 2008; 8: 520-531. PMID: 18765957.
32. Whitcomb DC, LaRusch J, Krasinskas AM, Klei L, Smith JP, Brand RE, et al. Common genetic variants in the CLDN2 and PRSS1-PRSS2 loci alter risk for alcohol-related and sporadic pancreatitis. *Nat Genet.* 2008; 44(12): 1349-1354. PMID: 23143602.
33. Derikx MH, Kovacs P, Scholz M, Masson E, Chen JM, Ruffert C, et al. Polymorphisms at PRSS1-PRSS2 and CLDN2-MORC4 loci associate with alcoholic and non-alcoholic chronic pancreatitis in a European replication study. *Gut.* 2015; 64: 1426-1433.PMID: 25253127.
34. Whitcomb DC. Hereditary pancreatitis: new insights into acute and chronic pancreatitis. *Gut.* 1999; 45: 317-322. PMID: 10446089.
35. Witt H, Apte MV, Keim V, and Wilson JS. Chronic pancreatitis: challenges and advances in pathogenesis, genetics, diagnosis, and therapy. *Gastroenterology.* 2007; 132: 1557-1573. PMID: 17466744.
36. Horii A, Kobayashi T, Tomita N, Yamamoto T, Fukushige S, Murotsu T, et al. Primary structure of human pancreatic secretory trypsin inhibitor (PSTI) gene. *Biochem Biophys Res Commun.* 1987; 149: 635-641. PMID: 3501289.
37. Ohmuraya M and Yamamura K. Roles of serine protease inhibitor Kazal type 1 (SPINK1) in pancreatic diseases. *Exp Anim.* 2011; 60: 433-444. PMID: 22041280.
38. Witt H, Luck W, Hennies HC, Classen M, Kage A, Lass U, et al. Mutations in the gene encoding the serine protease inhibitor, Kazal type 1 are associated with chronic pancreatitis. *Nat Genet.* 2000; 25: 213-216. PMID: 10835640.
39. Witt H, Luck W, Becker M, Bohmig M, Kage A, Truninger K, et al. Mutation in the SPINK1 trypsin inhibitor gene, alcohol use, and chronic pancreatitis. *JAMA.* 2001; 285: 2716-2717. PMID: 11386926.
40. Chandak GR, Idris MM, Reddy DN, Bhaskar S, Sriram PV, and Singh L. Mutations in the pancreatic secretory trypsin inhibitor gene (PSTI/SPINK1) rather than the cationic trypsinogen gene (PRSS1) are significantly associated with tropical calcific pancreatitis. *J Med Genet.* 2002; 39: 347-351. PMID: 12011155.
41. Schneider A. Serine protease inhibitor kazal type 1 mutations and pancreatitis. *Clin Lab Med.* 2005; 25: 61-78. PMID: 15749232.
42. Kuwata K, Hirota M, Shimizu H, Nakae M, Nishihara S, Takimoto A, et al. Functional analysis of recombinant pancreatic secretory trypsin inhibitor protein with amino-acid substitution. *J Gastroenterol.* 2002; 37: 928-934. PMID: 12483248.
43. Rinderknecht H, Adham NF, Renner IG, and Carmack C. A possible zymogen self-destruct mechanism preventing pancreatic autodigestion. *Int J Pancreatol.* 1988; 3: 33-44. PMID: 3162506.
44. Szabo A and Sahin-Toth M. Determinants of chymotrypsin C cleavage specificity in the calcium-binding loop of human cationic trypsinogen. *FEBS J.* 2012; 279: 4283-4292. PMID: 23035638.
45. Nemoda Z and Sahin-Toth M. Chymotrypsin C (caldecrin) stimulates autoactivation of human cationic trypsinogen. *J Biol Chem.* 2006; 281: 11879-11886. PMID: 16505482.
46. Szmola R and Sahin-Toth M. Chymotrypsin C (caldecrin) promotes degradation of human cationic trypsin: identity with Rinderknecht's enzyme Y. *Proc Natl Acad Sci U S A.* 2007; 104: 11227-11232. PMID: 17592142.
47. Ward JB, Petersen OH, Jenkins SA, and Sutton R. Is an elevated concentration of acinar cytosolic free ionised calcium the trigger for acute pancreatitis? *Lancet.* 1995; 346: 1016-1019. PMID: 7475553.
48. Kruger B, Albrecht E, and Lerch MM. The role of intracellular calcium signaling in premature protease activation and the onset of pancreatitis. *Am J Pathol.* 2000; 157: 43-50. PMID: 10880374.
49. Geisz A, Hegyi P, and Sahin-Toth M. Robust autoactivation, chymotrypsin C independence and diminished secretion define a subset of hereditary pancreatitis-associated cationic trypsinogen mutants. *FEBS J.* 2013; 280: 2888-2899. PMID: 23601753.

50. Szabo A and Sahin-Toth M. Increased activation of hereditary pancreatitis-associated human cationic trypsinogen mutants in presence of chymotrypsin C. *J Biol Chem.* 2012; 287: 20701-20710. PMID: 22539344.
51. Nemeth BC and Sahin-Toth M. Human cationic trypsinogen (PRSS1) variants and chronic pancreatitis. *Am J Physiol Gastrointest Liver Physiol.* 2014; 306: G466-G473. PMID: 24458023.
52. Nemeth BC, Wartmann T, Halangk W, and Sahin-Toth M. Autoactivation of mouse trypsinogens is regulated by chymotrypsin C via cleavage of the autolysis loop. *J Biol Chem.* 2013; 288: 24049-24062. PMID: 23814066.
53. Rosendahl J, Witt H, Szmola R, Bhatia E, Ozsvari B, Landt O, et al. Chymotrypsin C (CTRC) variants that diminish activity or secretion are associated with chronic pancreatitis. *Nat Genet.* 2008; 40: 78-82. PMID: 18059268.
54. Chang MC, Chang YT, Wei SC, Liang PC, Jan IS, Su YN, et al. Association of novel chymotrypsin C gene variations and haplotypes in patients with chronic pancreatitis in Chinese in Taiwan. *Pancreatology.* 2009; 9: 287-292. PMID: 19407484.
55. Bruce JI, Yang X, Ferguson CJ, Elliott AC, Steward MC, Case RM, et al. Molecular and functional identification of a Ca^{2+} (polyvalent cation)-sensing receptor in rat pancreas. *J Biol Chem.* 1999; 274: 20561-20568. PMID: 10400686.
56. Felderbauer P, Klein W, Bulut K, Ansorge N, Dekomien G, Werner I, et al. Mutations in the calcium-sensing receptor: a new genetic risk factor for chronic pancreatitis? *Scand J Gastroenterol.* 2006; 41: 343-348. PMID: 16497624.
57. Muddana V, Lamb J, Greer JB, Elinoff B, Hawes RH, Cotton PB, et al. Association between calcium sensing receptor gene polymorphisms and chronic pancreatitis in a US population: role of serine protease inhibitor Kazal 1 type and alcohol. *World J Gastroenterol.* 2008; 14: 4486-4491. PMID: 18680227.
58. Wang Y, Wrennall JA, Cai Z, Li H, and Sheppard DN. Understanding how cystic fibrosis mutations disrupt CFTR function: from single molecules to animal models. *Int J Biochem Cell Biol.* 2014; 52: 47-57. PMID: 24727426.
59. Wilschanski M and Novak I. The cystic fibrosis of exocrine pancreas. *Cold Spring Harb Perspect Med.* 2008; 3: a009746. PMID: 23637307.
60. Lebenthal E, Lerner A and Rolston DDK. The pancreas in cystic fibrosis. In: The pancreas: biology, pathobiology, and disease. Go VLW, DiMagno EP, Gardner JD, Lebenthal E, Reber HA, and Scheele GA, eds. New York, Raven Press. 1993: 1041-1081.
61. Riordan JR, Rommens JM, Kerem B, Alon N, Rozmahel R, Grzelczak Z, et al. Identification of the cystic fibrosis gene: cloning and characterization of complementary DNA. *Science.* 1989; 245: 1066-1073. PMID: 2475911.
62. Weiss FU, Simon P, Bogdanova N, Mayerle J, Dworniczak B, Horst J, et al. Complete cystic fibrosis transmembrane conductance regulator gene sequencing in patients with idiopathic chronic pancreatitis and controls. *Gut.* 2005; 54: 1456-1460. PMID: 15987793.
63. Cohn JA, Friedman KJ, Noone PG, Knowles MR, Silverman LM, and Jowell PS. Relation between mutations of the cystic fibrosis gene and idiopathic pancreatitis. *N Engl J Med.* 1998; 339(10): 653-658. PMID: 9725922.
64. Sharer N, Schwarz M, Malone G, Howarth A, Painter J, Super M, et al. Mutations of the cystic fibrosis gene in patients with chronic pancreatitis. *N Engl J Med.* 1998; 339: 645-652. PMID: 9725921.
65. Maleth J, Balazs A, Pallagi P, Balla Z, Kui B, Katona M, et al. Alcohol disrupts levels and function of the cystic fibrosis transmembrane conductance regulator to promote development of pancreatitis. *Gastroenterology.* 2015; 148: 427-439 e416. PMID: 25447846.
66. Apte M, Pirola R, and Wilson J. The fibrosis of chronic pancreatitis: new insights into the role of pancreatic stellate cells. *Antioxid Redox Signal.* 2011; 15: 2711-2722. PMID: 21728885.
67. Phillips PA, McCarroll JA, Park S, Wu MJ, Pirola R, Korsten M, et al. Rat pancreatic stellate cells secrete matrix metalloproteinases: implications for extracellular matrix turnover. *Gut.* 2003; 52: 275-282. PMID: 12524413.
68. Shimizu K, Kobayashi M, Tahara J, and Shiratori K. Cytokines and peroxisome proliferator-activated receptor gamma ligand regulate phagocytosis by pancreatic stellate cells. *Gastroenterology.* 2005; 128: 2105-2118. PMID: 15940641.
69. Stevens T, Conwell DL, and Zuccaro G. Pathogenesis of chronic pancreatitis: an evidence-based review of past theories and recent developments. *Am J Gastroenterol* 99(11): 2256-2270, 2004. PMID: 15555009.
70. Braganza JM. Pancreatic disease: a casualty of hepatic "detoxification"? *Lancet.* 1983; 2: 1000-1003. PMID: 6138545.
71. Norton ID, Apte MV, Haber PS, McCaughan GW, Pirola RC, and Wilson JS. Cytochrome P4502E1 is present in rat pancreas and is induced by chronic ethanol administration. *Gut.* 1998; 42: 426-430. PMID: 9577353.
72. Bordalo O, Goncalves D, Noronha M, Cristina ML, Salgadinho A, and Dreiling DA. Newer concept for the pathogenesis of chronic alcoholic pancreatitis. *Am J Gastroenterol.* 1977; 68: 278-285. PMID: 596358.
73. Wilson JS and Apte MV. Role of alcohol metabolism in alcoholic pancreatitis. *Pancreas.* 27: 311-315. PMID: 14576493.
74. Edenberg HJ. The genetics of alcohol metabolism: role of alcohol dehydrogenase and aldehyde dehydrogenase variants. *Alcohol Res Health.* 2007; 30: 5-13. PMID: 17718394.
75. Fjeld K, Weiss FU, Lasher D, Rosendahl J, Chen JM, Johansson BB, et al. A recombined allele of the lipase gene CEL and its pseudogene CELP confers susceptibility to chronic pancreatitis. *Nat Genet.* 2015; 47: 518-522. PMID: 25774637.
76. Sarles H, Bernard JP, and Gullo L. Pathogenesis of chronic pancreatitis. *Gut.* 1990; 31: 629-632. PMID: 2199345.
77. Tanaka T, Miura Y, Matsugu Y, Ichiba Y, Ito H, and Dohi K. Pancreatic duct obstruction is an aggravating factor in the canine model of chronic alcoholic pancreatitis. *Gastroenterology.* 1998; 115: 1248-1253. PMID: 9797381.
78. Yamasaki M, Takeyama Y, Shinkai M, and Ohyanagi H. Pancreatic and bile duct obstruction exacerbates rat caerulein-induced pancreatitis: a new experimental model of acute hemorrhagic pancreatitis. *J Gastroenterol.* 2006; 41: 352-360. PMID: 16741615.
79. Kloppel G and Maillet B. Chronic pancreatitis: evolution of the disease. *Hepatogastroenterology.* 1991; 38: 408-412. PMID: 1765357.

80. Adler G, Hupp T, and Kern HF. Course and spontaneous regression of acute pancreatitis in the rat. *Virchows Arch A Pathol Anat Histol.* 1979; 382: 31-47. PMID: 157597.
81. Neuschwander-Tetri BA, Burton FR, Presti ME, Britton RS, Janney CG, Garvin PR, et al. Repetitive self-limited acute pancreatitis induces pancreatic fibrogenesis in the mouse. *Dig Dis Sci.* 2000; 45: 665-674. PMID: 10759232.
82. Cavallini G and Frulloni L. Autoimmunity and chronic pancreatitis: a concealed relationship. *JOP.* 2001; 2: 61-68. PMID: 11867865.
83. Hart PA, Zen Y, and Chari ST. Recent Advances in Autoimmune Pancreatitis. *Gastroenterology*, 2015. PMID: 25770706.
84. Schneider A and Whitcomb DC. Hereditary pancreatitis: a model for inflammatory diseases of the pancreas. *Best Pract Res Clin Gastroenterol.* 2002; 16: 347-363. PMID: 12079262.
85. Sendler M, Dummer A, Weiss FU, Kruger B, Wartmann T, Scharffetter-Kochanek K, et al. Tumour necrosis factor alpha secretion induces protease activation and acinar cell necrosis in acute experimental pancreatitis in mice. *Gut.* 2013; 62: 430-439. PMID: 22490516.
86. Lerch MM and Gorelick FS. Models of acute and chronic pancreatitis. *Gastroenterology.* 2013; 144: 1180-1193. PMID: 23622127.

Chapter 37

Pancreatic fibrosis

Shin Hamada*, Atsushi Masamune, and Tooru Shimosegawa

Division of Gastroenterology, Tohoku University Graduate School of Medicine.

Abstract

Pancreatic fibrosis develops as a result of abnormal activation of stromal cells and deposition of extracellular matrix (ECM) proteins and is characteristic of chronic pancreatitis. Fibrosis impairs both exocrine and endocrine functions of the pancreas, leading to severe impairment of a patient's quality of life. Identification of key regulators of pancreatic fibrosis, especially pancreatic stellate cells (PSCs), has greatly contributed to the understanding of its cellular and molecular pathogenesis. Various external stimuli activate PSCs, and promote cell proliferation and migration, production of ECM proteins and cytokine secretion. Recruitment of other inflammatory cells exacerbates pancreatic inflammation, leading to destruction of acinar and islet cells, which are replaced by extensive fibrosis. Dissection of the signaling pathways involved in pancreatic inflammation has enabled therapeutic intervention with specific inhibitors or antioxidants that contribute to the resolution of symptoms related to chronic pancreatitis. However, recovery of pancreatic tissue damaged by human chronic pancreatitis has not yet been achieved, despite the favorable effects of therapeutic agents evaluated in animal models of chronic pancreatitis. This discrepancy might be attributable to the timing of therapeutic interventions. In animal models, treatments are generally administered at the same time as pancreatic injury. Failure to recognize early stage chronic pancreatitis in humans delays the start of therapy to preserve organ function.

Introduction

Characteristic features of advanced chronic pancreatitis are destruction of acinar and islet cells, increase in the number of stromal cells, and prominent fibrosis. These histological changes result from activation of multiple signaling pathways that lead to the remodeling of pancreatic tissue structure. Ongoing inflammation produces irreversible damage to exocrine and endocrine pancreatic functions, resulting in the severe impairment of quality of life due to the malabsorption of nutrients and pancreatic diabetes. Even though pancreatic enzyme supplementation and insulin therapy are now available, treating end-stage pancreatic insufficiency is still problematic. Therefore, therapeutic intervention should begin before reversible fibrosis has been established. Unfortunately, this has not yet been achieved in clinical practice.

Numerous studies have described the complex mechanisms of pancreatic fibrosis and their dependence on cellular function or molecular regulation. Identification of the cell types that contribute to fibrosis has led to clarification of the fibrosis-promoting mechanisms, which consist of a multicellular inflammatory response. Recent research has revealed essential inflammatory signaling pathways and their downstream targets. Experimental approaches to attenuate fibrosis-promoting processes using inhibitors of specific signaling pathways and oxidative stress have shown promise, but their clinical application needs further validation.

This chapter reviews the basic characteristics of pancreatic fibrosis, including the cellular origin of fibrosis, The signaling pathways that promote fibrosis or cell-to-cell interactions, and the available therapeutic interventions against fibrosis. Current knowledge of the mechanisms of fibrogenesis, fibrosis-promoting cell types and their functions. The signaling pathways involved, and effects of their inhibition, are also discussed.

Pancreatic Fibrosis and Symptoms of Chronic Pancreatitis

Exocrine pancreas insufficiency is a typical symptom of advanced chronic pancreatitis. Destruction of acinar cells leads to reduced secretion of digestive enzymes, which causes maldigestion. Deposition of type I collagen is a characteristic feature of advanced chronic pancreatitis. Stromal cells are sparsely distributed around acinar cells in

*Corresponding author. Email: hamadas@med.tohoku.ac.jp

the normal pancreas, but in chronic pancreatitis, the ECM is prominent and stromal cells surround acinar cells Along with extensive fibrosis, there is evidence of damage to pancreatic acinar tissue. This was confirmed, by immunohistochemical demonstration of 4-hydroxynonenal–protein, an adduct derived by lipid peroxidation[1] and suggestive of increased oxidative stress within the inflamed pancreas. In addition to this tissue injury marker, the study also confirmed expression of transforming growth factor (TGF)-β1 a wound healing and fibrosis-related cytokine. Based on these findings, pancreatic fibrosis is seen as an active inflammatory process, accompanied by dynamic signaling and cell-to-cell interactions. Pancreatic fibrosis also involves the macroscopic ductal structure of the pancreas, typically with dilatation of the main pancreatic duct or formation of pancreatic stones that develop in response to inadequate drainage of pancreatic juice.[2] Obstruction of the main pancreatic duct can cause acute exacerbation of chronic pancreatitis, which further promotes the necrosis-fibrosis sequence.

In addition to the exocrine pancreas, islet cells are also affected by pancreatic fibrosis. However, pancreatic diabetes only becomes evident at later stages of the disease,[3] which reflects the difference in vulnerability and reserve function. Assessment of pancreatic volume, apoptosis of acinar cells and islet cells in chronic pancreatitis patients and controls showed a decrease of beta-cell content by 29% in chronic pancreatitis, but apoptosis of islet cells was not significantly different from controls. In contrast, acinar cell apoptosis in chronic pancreatitis increased by 10-fold compared with controls, suggesting acinar cells are more vulnerable to inflammatory insults.[4] A recent report described that β-cell dysfunction in chronic pancreatitis correlates with the decreased expression of pancreatic duodenal homeobox protein 1 (PDX-1),[5] an essential transcriptional factor for the maintenance of normal islet function.[6] Isolated islets revealed impaired glucose-stimulated insulin secretion, indicating pancreatic diabetes in chronic pancreatitis might result from both quantitative and qualitative changes of endocrine pancreas along with fibrosis.

Pancreatic fibrosis is also related to the abdominal pain of chronic pancreatitis. Stricture of main pancreatic duct or pancreatic stones can increase the pressure in the pancreatic duct, leading to the abdominal pain.[7] Treatment of ductal mechanical obstruction in chronic pancreatitis can follow several strategies, including drainage surgery (Frey's or Berger's procedure), endoscopic stent placement, or extracorporeal shock wave lithotripsy.[8,9] These treatments are generally effective for pain reduction, but some patients experience persisting abdominal pain. In addition to pain from mechanical obstruction, pancreatic fibrosis also causes abdominal pain by affecting nerves in the pancreas. Friess et al. reported that the number of nerves and the area of neural tissue increased in chronic pancreatitis following surgical treatment compared with the normal pancreas, and was accompanied by neuronal alterations.[10] These morphological changes did not differ with the etiology of pancreatitis, suggesting that they are a universal phenomenon. The increase in tissue enervation was accompanied by inflammatory cell infiltration, possibly causing neuronal pain. The detailed mechanisms of neuronal damage have been revealed. Immunohistochemical analysis of nerve fibers within the pancreas to distinguish sympathetic (tyrosine hydroxylase positive) and parasympathetic (choline acetyltransferase positive) innervation confirmed a marked decrease of sympathetic innervation.[11] As reduction in sympathetic nerve fibers has been correlated with the severity of abdominal pain, this neural remodeling is assumed to be an additional cause of pain in chronic pancreatitis. Expression of growth factors and chemokines affecting neuronal function and inflammation is also altered in chronic pancreatitis tissue, and the change in expression varies with the degree of pancreatic fibrosis. For example, fractalkine, a chemokine that induces migration and extravasation of immune cells, is highly expressed in chronic pancreatitis tissues. Its expression level is correlated with the degree of pancreatic fibrosis and severity of pain.[12] The therapeutic effect of anti-nerve growth factor antibody administration in has been demonstrated a rat model of chronic pancreatitis.[13] Elevated expression of both nerve growth factor and its receptor tyrosine kinase receptor A in human chronic pancreatitis has been previously described.[14] and thus might become alternative targets of pain therapy in chronic pancreatitis.

In summary, pancreatic fibrosis has a fundamental role in the pathogenesis of chronic pancreatitis and might be an attractive therapeutic target for the improvement of clinical outcome and maintenance of pancreatic function. **Figure 1** shows the relationships of pancreatic fibrosis with the symptoms of chronic pancreatitis. The cellular and molecular mechanisms of pancreatic fibrosis are being extensively studied with the aim of developing novel therapies of chronic pancreatitis.

Pancreatic Stellate Cells and Fibrogenesis

The star shaped hepatic stellate cells (HSCs) located within the space of Disse[15] are in close contact with hepatocytes and endothelial cells, and contribute to the development of liver fibrosis due to a variety of liver injuries. HSCs contain lipid droplets and stay in a quiescent state in normal liver tissue. Activation of HSCs leads to morphological and functional changes that cause tissue remodeling such as extracellular matrix (ECM) deposition. Similar star-shaped cells located in the pancreatic periacinar space were reported in 1998 by Apte et al and Bachem et al,[16,17] Those cells were named pancreatic stellate cells (PSCs). Quiescent PSCs contain lipid droplets rich in vitamin A,

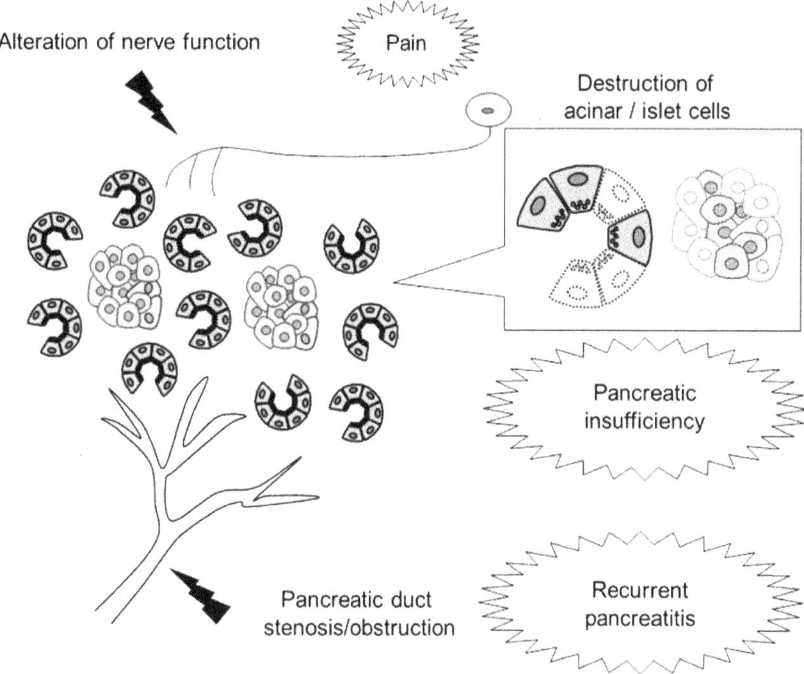

Figure 1. Relationships of pancreatic fibrosis and symptoms of chronic pancreatitis.

a feature that allows isolation of these cells by density-gradient centrifugation. Inflammation within the pancreas activates PSCs, causing loss of lipid droplets, increased cellular proliferation, and production of cytokines and ECM proteins. *In vitro* culture also activates PSCs, resulting in the expression of several specific markers such as desmin, glial fibrillary acidic protein (GFAP) and α-smooth muscle actin (α-SMA) (18). These PSC markers have been used to identify the cellular components of pancreatic fibrosis, and have confirmed that PSCs play a key role in fibrogenesis.[19]

Increased production of ECM proteins is essential for the formation of fibrosis. Activated PSCs secrete ECM proteins, such as type I collagen, fibronectin and periostin.[20] Deposition of ECM proteins alters the cellular microenvironment, and is one of the steps in the pathogenesis of chronic pancreatitis. As in other fibrotic diseases, pancreatic fibrosis is a result of an imbalance in fibrogenesis and fibrosis resolution in response to persisting inflammation or abnormal stimuli.[21] PSCs express several enzymes that degrade ECM proteins including members of the matrix metalloproteinase (MMP) family and tissue inhibitors of metalloproteinases (TIMPs).[22] This finding suggested a role for PSCs in fibrosis resolution, which is inhibited during the progression of chronic pancreatitis. A recent study confirmed that an acute phase protein, pancreatitis-associated protein (PAP), reduced the expression of MMP-1, MMP-S, TIMP-1 and TIMP-2 in PSCs, as well as their concentrations in culture supernatants.[23] This partially explains how pathogenic alteration of PSC function by inflammation might lead to pancreatic fibrosis. In addition, production of ECM-degrading enzymes by PSCs suggests the possibility of fibrosis resolution by specific attenuation of the fibrogenic activity of PSCs. To investigate this mechanism, upstream regulators of PSC activation have been examined.

A wide variety of growth factors, cytokines, small molecules, and environmental changes activate stellate cells. TGF-β1 and platelet derived growth factor (PDGF) are well-known growth factors that activate PSCs.[24,25] Other inflammatory cytokines, tumor necrosis factor-α (TNF-α) and interleukins also increase α-SMA expression in PSCs, a hallmark of activation.[26] These factors are released from various kinds of cells including damaged acinar cells, neutrophils, macrophages and PSCs themselves.[27] Therefore, these growth factors and cytokines form a feed-forward loop of fibrogenic processes during the progression of pancreatitis. In addition to the endogenous factors, exogenous molecules also activate PSCs. Necroinflammatory processes following tissue injury, ethanol, and its acetaldehyde metabolite directly activate PSCs.[28] This activation involves increased oxidative stress within the PSCs, which is also caused by the respiratory burst of neutrophils in acute inflammation.[29] Gram-negative bacteria-derived lipopolysaccharide (LPS) also activates PSCs, which was shown to facilitate ethanol-induced pancreatic fibrosis in a rat model.[30] As a result of excess ECM deposition, interstitial pressure increases, resulting in poor blood perfusion. Environmental factors such as external pressure and

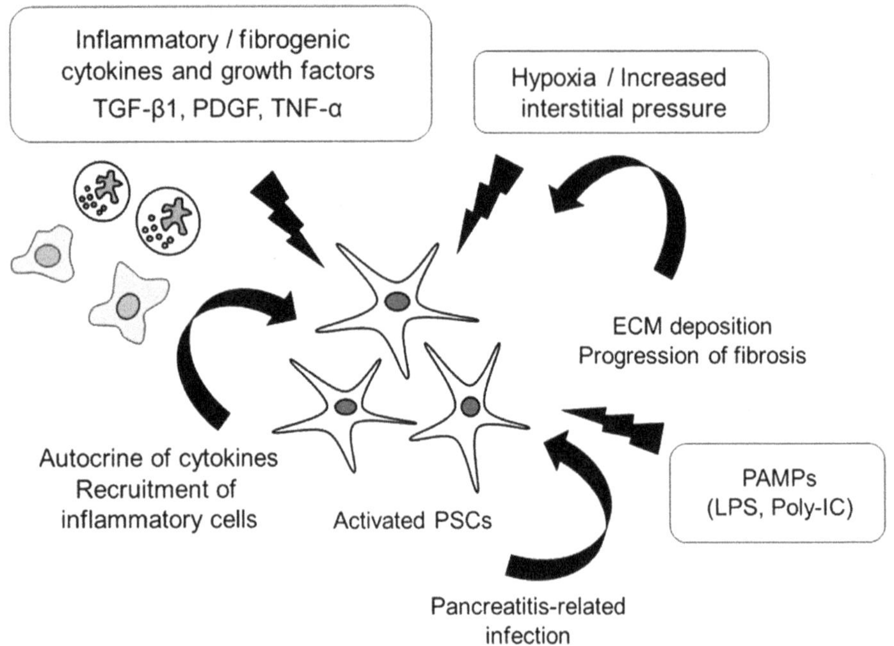

Figure 2. Activators of PSCs and the feed-forward loop of PSC activation.

hypoxia also cause PSC activation. Mechanical compression of cultured rat PSCs by helium gas increased production of intracellular reactive oxygen species (ROS), leading to the increased expression of α-SMA, α1(I)-procollagen, and TGF-β1.[31] Hypoxia also increases the production of ECM proteins, periostin, and type I collagen by cultured human PSCs.[32] **Figure 2** illustrates how these PSC-activation factors interact with each other, to perpetuate inflammation and fibrosis. Following the identification of PSC-activating factors, their downstream signaling pathways and specific inhibitors were identified.

Pancreatic Fibrogenesis-Related Signaling Pathways

Numerous signaling pathways are involved in pancreatic fibrosis. The signaling pathways that activate PSCs have been well studied. Activation of the mitogen-activated protein kinase (MAPK) pathway activation is indispensable for PSC activation, cellular proliferation, migration, cytokine and ECM production.[33] Three kinds of MAPK pathways, extracellular signal regulated kinase (ERK), p38 MAPK, c-jun N-terminal kinase (JNK) have been described and they are activated by various PSC-activating stimuli. For example, ethanol and acetaldehyde activate ERK, p38 and JNK in rat PSCs. McCaroll et al studied the inhibition of each pathway using specific inhibitors (U0126 for ERK pathway inhibition, SB203580 for p38 MAPK pathway inhibition, and SP600125 for JNK pathway inhibition); only inhibition of the p38 MAPK pathway could attenuate the ethanol or acetaldehyde-induced α-SMA expression of PSCs.[34] Another report confirmed activation of all three MAPK pathways and activator protein-1 by an ethanol metabolite, palmitic acid ethyl ester, in PSCs.[35] TGF-β1 also activates the ERK pathway, whose inhibition was shown to lead to the attenuation of the TGF-β1 autocrine loop in PSCs.[36] PDGF-induced cellular migration is mediated by the phosphatidylinositol 3-kinase (PI3-kinase) pathway, which also activates ERK pathway, suggesting signaling cross-talk.[37]

Other signaling pathways are involved in PSC activation in addition to the small molecule-activated or growth factor-activated MAPK pathways. PSCs express Toll-like receptors (TLRs), which recognize pathogen-associated molecular pattern molecules (PAMPs).[38] PSCs express TLR2, 3, 4, 5, and the associated molecules CD14 and MD2. These TLRs recognize various molecules derived from pathogens. The TLR ligands, lipoteichoic acid, polyinosinic–polycytidylic acid, LPS and flagellin, increase production of monocyte chemoattractant protein-1 (MCP-1) and cytokine-induced neutrophil chemoattractant-1 (CINC-1) by PSCs. The nuclear factor-κB (NF-κB) pathway, a typical inflammatory signaling pathway may also be activated,[38] but the MAPK inhibitors failed to show uniform inhibition of MCP-1 and CINC-1 production, as the NF-κB inhibitor did, suggesting a central role of NF-κB in TLR-mediated chemokine production. This observation suggests that PSCs are not only activated by inflammatory signals, but also act to amplify the inflammatory response within the pancreas. Another extracellular ligand affecting the function of PSCs is Indian hedgehog (Ihh), a member of the hedgehog peptide

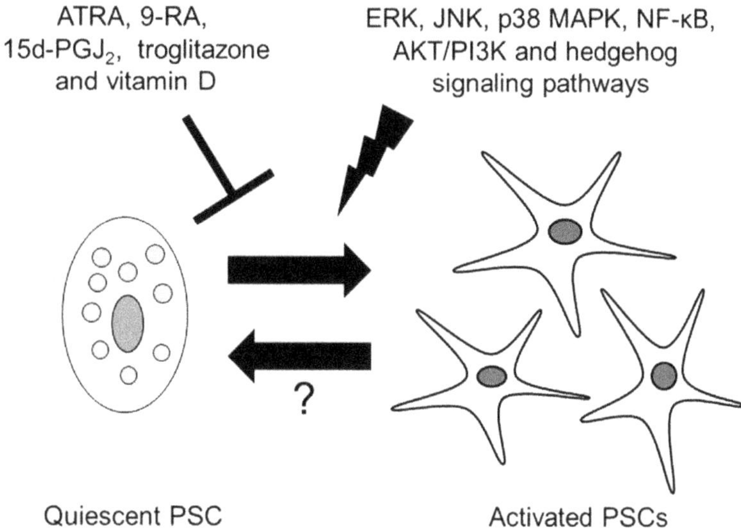

Figure 3. PSC-activating signals and quiescence-maintaining factors.

family, which are involved in the developmental processes and tissue patterning.[39] PSCs were found to express hedgehog receptor components, patched (Ptc-1) and smoothened (Smo),[40] and binding of hedgehog ligand to Ptc-1 abrogates its inhibitory effect on Smo, leading to downstream signal activation as indicated by the nuclear accumulation of Gli transcriptional factor.[41] Ihh-treatment of PSCs increased cellular migration, without alteration of proliferation or ECM protein production. Ihh increased the amount of membrane-type I MMP in the PSCs, which was attenuated by TIMP-2, a metalloproteinase inhibitor. This observation indicates that ECM-degrading enzymes are regulated by external stimuli affect the cellular function of PSCs.

The quiescent state of PSCs is maintained by several signaling pathways. Quiescent PSCs have intracellular lipid droplets containing Vitamin A. Vitamin A and its metabolites bind to nuclear receptors, leading to the alteration of gene expression through retinoic acid responsive elements.[42] Vitamin A and its metabolites all-trans retinoic acid (ATRA) and 9-cis retinoic acid (9-RA) were found to suppress cell proliferation, α-SMA expression, ECM protein production, and MAPK activation.[43] Cultured PSCs retained the expression of retinol-converting enzyme and nuclear receptors for ATRA and 9-RA, which may contribute to the attenuation of activated PSC functions. This suggests that the morphological changes in PSCs reflect the functional alterations in activated PSCs, possibly causing the loss of endogenous factors for quiescence. Similarly, another nuclear receptor, peroxisome proliferator-activated receptor-γ (PPAR-γ) was also found to regulate PSC activation. Oxidative metabolites of poly-unsaturated fatty acids and prostaglandins bind to this ligand-activated transcriptional factor, regulating inflammatory responses.[44] Cultured PSCs expressed PPAR-γ, and its ligands (15d-PGJ_2 and troglitazone) inhibited PDGF-induced proliferation of PSCs.[45] Expression of α-SMA and production of type I collagen or MCP-1 were suppressed by 15d-PGJ_2 and troglitazone treatments, indicating PPAR-γ-mediated signalling contributes to the inhibition of PSC activation. In addition to these ligands of nuclear receptors, vitamin D also has antifibrogenic properties. A recent report identified the expression of vitamin D receptor in PSCs, and the potent vitamin D analogue, calcipotriol induced reprogramming of activated PSCs into the quiescent state.[46]

According to these studies, signaling pathways promoting pancreatic fibrosis are mainly activated by extracellular stimuli of PSCs, which harbor endogenous quiescence-maintaining machinery in the normal pancreas. **Figure 3** illustrates pro- and antifibrogenic signaling pathways in PSCs.

Cell-To-Cell Interactions in Pancreatic Fibrosis

Pancreatic fibrosis also involves other cell types in addition to PSCs. Activated PSCs secrete a wide variety of inflammatory cytokines such as IL-1β, IL-6, MCP-1 and TNF-α that contribute to the recruitment of inflammatory cells to the pancreas. RelA/p65, a component of the NF-κB pathway in myeloid cells, was found essential for the establishment of pancreatic fibrosis in a mouse model (47). This suggests that production of TNF-α and TGF-β1 by macrophages infiltrating the pancreas is regulated by NF-κB. A similar study has confirmed the contribution of alternatively activated macrophages (AAMs, M2) in the pancreatic fibrosis.[48] Unlike classical macrophages (M1, induced by interferon gamma (IFNγ), or LPS), AAMs are induced by IL-4 or IL-13, and play an important role in fibrosis and tumorigenesis.[49] The AAM-inducing factors are secreted by PSCs when IFNγ production is low.[48] Suppression of IL-4 and IL-13 improved established chronic pancreatitis in a mouse model, suggesting that they might be a candidate therapeutic target.

Similar cell-to-cell interactions have been reported in mast cells, an immediate mediator of allergic reactions. The presence of mast cells in chronic pancreatitis tissue was reported by Esposito et al, where there was a correlation of the extent of fibrosis with the intensity of inflammation.[50] Mast cell infiltration was observed in chronic pancreatitis regardless of the etiology. Zimnoch et al noted an increase in the number of degranulated mast cells in chronic pancreatitis that occurred in parallel to increase in the degree of fibrosis, suggesting that mast cell-derived factors are involved in PSC activation.[51] Finally, a recent study found that the mutual activation of PSCs and mast cells plays a pivotal role in progression of pancreatic cancer. Mast cell-derived IL-13 and tryptase were found to stimulate PSC proliferation, and PSCs were also found to facilitate cytokine and tryptase release from human mast cell lines.[52] T-cell function is also affected by chronic pancreatitis. Comparison of patient-derived T cells from chronic pancreatitis, pancreatic cancer and healthy individuals revealed that regulatory T cells recognizing pancreatitis-associated antigens were expanded in chronic pancreatitis, leading to a regulatory cytokine profile characterized by IL-10 production.[53] Taken together, these cell-to-cell interactions alter local and systemic inflammatory responses in chronic pancreatitis, resulting in the fibrotic tissue remodeling.

Cell-to-cell interactions in chronic pancreatitis affect additional cell types in a variety of ways. As mentioned earlier, pancreatic endocrine functions are impaired in chronic pancreatitis, and the mechanisms are partially understood. Coculture with PSCs reduced insulin production and induced apoptosis in a the RIN-5F pancreatic β-cell line.[54] The study also confirmed the existence of α-SMA-positive activated PSCs within the islets in chronic pancreatitis, indicating that cell-to-cell interaction between PSCs and islet cells contributes to the impairment of pancreatic endocrine function. An ECM protein, secreted protein acidic and rich in cysteine (SPARC), has been reported to attenuate growth factor-stimulated signaling, cellular growth and cell survival in INS-1 β-cell line and primary mouse islet cells.[55] SPARC inhibited hepatocyte growth factor- and IGF-1-induced activation of ERK and Akt, leading to reduced cellular growth and cell survival. Since SPARC is predominantly produced by PSCs,[56] these results partially explain how PSCs inhibit islet function. Hgh glucose also affects PSC function. Treatment of PSCs by high concentrations of glucose (30 mM) caused increased production of reactive oxygen species (ROS), as detected by dichlorodihydrofluorescein diacetate (DCF) fluorescence. This treatment led to the increased production of α-SMA, IL-6, and collagen, accompanied by proliferation of PSCs.[57] This observation means if a diabetic state has been established, activation of PSCs would be further promoted, by a feed-forward loop. This was confirmed in a diabetic rat model rat where transplantation of PSCs isolated from 8-week-old Wistar rats into Goto-Kakizaki rats resulted in the exacerbation of impaired glucose tolerance, while Wistar rats with transplanted PSCs were not affected. The islets of PSC-transplanted Goto-Kakizaki rats showed increased fibrosis compared with PSC-transplanted Wistar rats, suggesting that increased blood glucose concentration enhanced PSC function.[58] PSC-conditioned culture medium (PSC-CM) and high glucose additively increased C/EBP Homologous Protein (CHOP) expression, a hallmark of ER stress, in the INS-1 cells used in that study.

Based on these observations, cell-to-cell-interactions, especially with PSCs, have important roles in the tissue remodeling during chronic pancreatitis. **Figure 4** illustrates these interactions and their mediators. Profibrogenic signaling pathways and fibrosis-related interactions have been investigated as candidate anti-fibrosis therapy.

Therapeutic Intervention Targeting Fibrogenesis

As activation of PSCs and their interaction with other cell types contribute to the pathogenesis of chronic pancreatitis, therapeutic interventions against these interactions have been evaluated. A variety of growth factors and extracellular stimuli activate multiple signaling pathways including MAPK, Akt and NF-κB. Effective inhibition of these pathways by single inhibitor presumably has limited therapeutic potential, and selection of a specific target on which these stimuli converge would be ideal. One such candidate is increased oxidative stress in PSCs. There is evidence of a substantial contribution of NADPH oxidase in PSCs.[59] A number of cytokines and growth factors such as PDGF, IL-1 and angiotensin II increase ROS production in PSCs. Their activity is effectively suppressed by treatment with the NADPH oxidase inhibitors, diphenylene iodonium and apocynin, which results in decreased proliferation of PSCs and cytokine production. Other antioxidants such as curcumin or ellagic acid have similar effects,[60,61] suggesting antioxidants might be a promising therapeutic strategy against chronic pancreatitis. Two recent meta-analyses of antioxidant therapy for pain reduction in chronic pancreatitis concluded that antioxidant therapy is safe and has a beneficial role in pain reduction.[62,63] As described earlier, pancreatic fibrosis mechanistically and functionally affects pancreatic nerve fibers, and attenuation of inflammatory processes might contribute to improvement of clinical outcomes. Other food-derived compounds also have inhibitory effects on PSC function. Tocotrienol and tocopherol are vitamin E compounds, and have been reported to inhibit

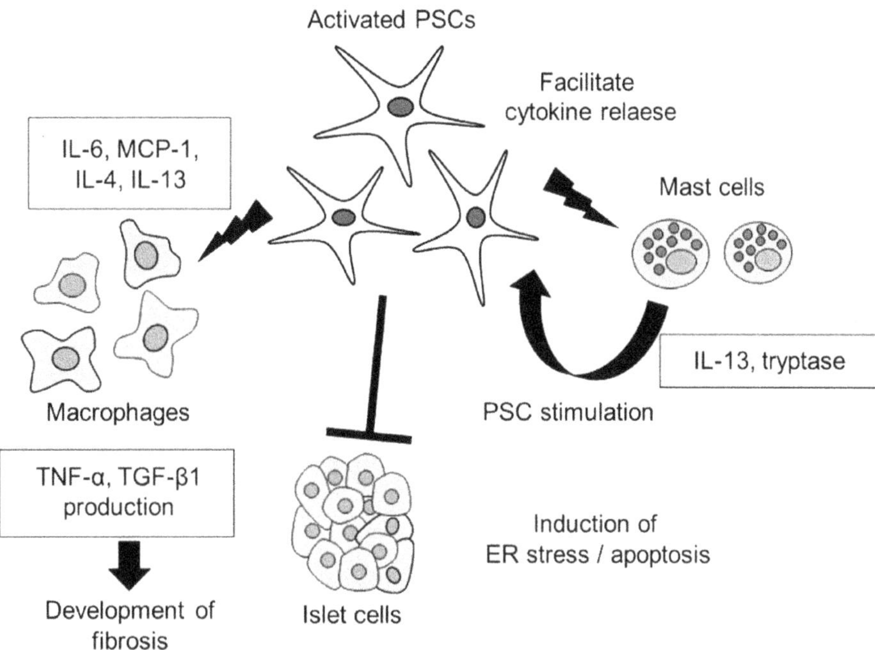

Figure 4. Cell-to-cell interactions and their mediators involved in pancreatic fibrosis.

PSC activation.[64,65] Tocotrienol but not tocopherol caused apoptosis of PSCs *in vitro*[64] accompanied by development of autophagy and sustained mitochondrial permeability transition, resulting in the cell death of activated PSCs. Interestingly, tocotrienol did not affect the viability of acinar cells or quiescent PSCs, showing a safety favorable profile as a therapeutic agent.

In addition to antioxidants and NADPH oxidase inhibitors, other fibrogenic signaling pathways have been targeted in PSCs. Administration of halofuginone, a plant alkaloid analog, inhibited TGF-β1 signaling, ECM production, and activation of MAPK signals.[66] Similarly, transgenic expression of Smad7, an inhibitory Smad against TGF-β1 signaling, protected against caerulein-induced pancreatic fibrosis in a mouse model.[67] A recent report described an effective antifibrosis therapy using the novel prostacyclin analog ONO-1301 in a rat pancreatitis model.[68] ONO-1301 improved experimental pancreatic fibrosis in dibutyltin dichloride-induced pancreatitis, with reduced expression of TGF-β1, TNF-α, IL-1β, and MCP-1. These effects were mediated by the induction of hepatocyte growth factor, which inhibited cytokine and chemokine production by monocytes. Production of connective tissue growth factor (CTGF) by injured acinar cells plays a pivotal role in the production of inflammatory cytokines such as IL-1β and CCL3 in ethanol and caerulein-induced chronic pancreatitis in mice. An inhibitor of chemokine receptor, BX471, attenuated the chemotaxis of macrophage cells toward cultured AR42J acinar cells.[69] Administration of camostat mesilate, an oral protease inhibitor, also reduced the severity of pancreatic fibrosis in dibutyltin dichloride-induced chronic pancreatitis.[70] Camostat mesilate reduced MCP-1 and TNF-α production from LPS-stimulated monocytes and inhibited of proliferation and MCP-1 production by PSCs.[70] These results indicate that inflammation-triggering signaling pathways and their mediators are attractive targets for antifibrosis therapy.

However, these therapeutic interventions have limited benefit for patients with advanced chronic pancreatitis, whose pancreatic parenchyma has already lost functional acinar and islet cells. Since these therapeutic interventions were applied in animal models at the same time as pancreatic injury, their efficacy in human disease is unclear. Lack of a diagnostic method for subclinical chronic pancreatitis hampers early intervention, such as alcohol abstinence or smoking cessation.[71] Japanese clinical diagnostic criteria for chronic pancreatitis were revised in 2009 to define a new disease entity, early chronic pancreatitis.[72] Diagnosis of early chronic pancreatitis is based on abdominal symptoms, laboratory data, and imaging findings characteristic of chronic pancreatitis, with the intent to classify patients with early stage disease. The effectiveness of antifibrosis therapy for these patients needs to be clarified. Similar validation could be performed in patients with hereditary pancreatitis, in whom effective prophylactic therapies are not yet available.[73] In summary, accurate identification of patients with early stage disease must be available for the establishment of an effective anti-fibrosis therapy.

Conclusion

Recent research progress in the field of pancreatic fibrosis has identified intriguing cellular components, signaling pathways, and upstream regulators. Inhibition of fibrogenic processes has shown therapeutic efficacy in animal models, but the clinical applications have not yet resulted For this goal, identification of patients with early stage chronic pancreatitis using novel diagnostic strategies is necessary.

References

1. Casini A, Galli A, Pignalosa P, Frulloni L, Grappone C, Milani S, et al. Collagen type I synthesized by pancreatic periacinar stellate cells (PSC) co-localizes with lipid peroxidation-derived aldehydes in chronic alcoholic pancreatitis. *J Pathol*. 2000; 192: 81-89. PMID: 10951404.
2. Braganza JM, Lee SH, McCloy RF, McMahon MJ. Chronic pancreatitis. *Lancet*. 2011; 377: 1184-1197. PMID: 21397320.
3. Lankisch PG. Natural course of chronic pancreatitis. *Pancreatology*. 2001; 1: 3-14. PMID: 12120264.
4. Schrader H, Menge BA, Schneider S, Belyaev O, Tannapfel A, Uhl W, et al. Reduced pancreatic volume and beta-cell area in patients with chronic pancreatitis. *Gastroenterology*. 2009; 136: 513-522. PMID: 19041312.
5. Mitnala S, Pondugala PK, Guduru VR, Rabella P, Thiyyari J, Chivukula S, et al. Reduced expression of PDX-1 is associated with decreased beta cell function in chronic pancreatitis. *Pancreas*. 2010; 39: 856-862. PMID: 20467340.
6. Ashizawa S, Brunicardi FC, Wang XP. PDX-1 and the pancreas. *Pancreas*. 2004; 28: 109-120. PMID: 15028942.
7. Di Sebastiano P, di Mola FF, Buchler MW, Friess H. Pathogenesis of pain in chronic pancreatitis. *Dig Dis*. 2004; 22: 267-272. PMID: 15753609.
8. Dumonceau JM. Endoscopic therapy for chronic pancreatitis. *Gastrointest Endosc Clin N Am*. 2013; 23: 821-832. PMID: 24079792.
9. Ni Q, Yun L, Roy M, Shang D. Advances in surgical treatment of chronic pancreatitis. *World J Surg Oncol*. 2015; 13: 34. PMID: 25845403.
10. Friess H, Shrikhande S, Shrikhande M, Martignoni M, Kulli C, Zimmermann A, et al. Neural alterations in surgical stage chronic pancreatitis are independent of the underlying aetiology. *Gut*. 2002; 50: 682-686. PMID: 11950816.
11. Ceyhan GO, Demir IE, Rauch U, Bergmann F, Muller MW, Buchler MW, et al. Pancreatic neuropathy results in "neural remodeling" and altered pancreatic innervation in chronic pancreatitis and pancreatic cancer. *Am J Gastroenterol*. 2009; 104: 2555-2565. PMID: 19568227.
12. Ceyhan GO, Deucker S, Demir IE, Erkan M, Schmelz M, Bergmann F, et al. Neural fractalkine expression is closely linked to pain and pancreatic neuritis in human chronic pancreatitis. *Lab Invest*. 2009; 89: 347-361. PMID: 19153557.
13. Zhu Y, Mehta K, Li C, Xu GY, Liu L, Colak T, et al. Systemic administration of anti-NGF increases A-type potassium currents and decreases pancreatic nociceptor excitability in a rat model of chronic pancreatitis. *Am J Physiol Gastrointest Liver Physiol*. 2012; 302: G176-181. PMID: 22038828.
14. Friess H, Zhu ZW, di Mola FF, Kulli C, Graber HU, Andren-Sandberg A, et al. Nerve growth factor and its high-affinity receptor in chronic pancreatitis. *Ann Surg*. 1999; 230: 615-624. PMID: 10561084.
15. Lee YA, Wallace MC, Friedman SL. Pathobiology of liver fibrosis: a translational success story. *Gut*. 2015; 64: 830-841. PMID: 25681399.
16. Apte MV, Haber PS, Applegate TL, Norton ID, McCaughan GW, Korsten MA, et al. Periacinar stellate shaped cells in rat pancreas: identification, isolation, and culture. *Gut*. 1998; 43: 128-133. PMID: 9771417.
17. Bachem MG, Schneider E, Gross H, Weidenbach H, Schmid RM, Menke A, et al. Identification, culture, and characterization of pancreatic stellate cells in rats and humans. *Gastroenterology*. 1998; 115: 421-432. PMID: 9679048.
18. Vonlaufen A, Phillips PA, Yang L, Xu Z, Fiala-Beer E, Zhang X, et al. Isolation of quiescent human pancreatic stellate cells: a promising in vitro tool for studies of human pancreatic stellate cell biology. *Pancreatology*. 2010; 10: 434-443. PMID: 20733342.
19. Masamune A, Watanabe T, Kikuta K, Shimosegawa T. Roles of pancreatic stellate cells in pancreatic inflammation and fibrosis. *Clin Gastroenterol Hepatol*. 2009; 7: S48-54. PMID: 19896099.
20. Erkan M, Adler G, Apte MV, Bachem MG, Buchholz M, Detlefsen S, et al. StellaTUM: current consensus and discussion on pancreatic stellate cell research. *Gut*. 2012; 61: 172-178. PMID: 22115911.
21. Hansen NU, Genovese F, Leeming DJ, Karsdal MA. The importance of extracellular matrix for cell function and in vivo likeness. *Exp Mol Pathol*. 2015; 98: 286-294. PMID: 25595916.
22. Phillips PA, McCarroll JA, Park S, Wu MJ, Pirola R, Korsten M, et al. Rat pancreatic stellate cells secrete matrix metalloproteinases: implications for extracellular matrix turnover. *Gut*. 2003; 52: 275-282. PMID: 12524413.
23. Li L, Bachem MG, Zhou S, Sun Z, Chen J, Siech M, et al. Pancreatitis-associated protein inhibits human pancreatic stellate cell MMP-1 and -2, TIMP-1 and -2 secretion and RECK expression. *Pancreatology*. 2009; 9: 99-110. PMID: 19077460.
24. Vogelmann R, Ruf D, Wagner M, Adler G, Menke A. Effects of fibrogenic mediators on the development of pancreatic fibrosis in a TGF-beta1 transgenic mouse model. *Am J Physiol Gastrointest Liver Physiol*. 2001; 280: G164-172. PMID: 11123210.
25. Schneider E, Schmid-Kotsas A, Zhao J, Weidenbach H, Schmid RM, Menke A, et al. Identification of mediators stimulating proliferation and matrix synthesis of rat pancreatic stellate cells. *Am J Physiol Cell Physiol*. 2001; 281: C532-543. PMID: 11443052.
26. Mews P, Phillips P, Fahmy R, Korsten M, Pirola R, Wilson J, et al. Pancreatic stellate cells respond to inflammatory cytokines: potential role in chronic pancreatitis. *Gut*. 2002; 50: 535-541. PMID: 11889076.
27. Vonlaufen A, Apte MV, Imhof BA, Frossard JL. The role of inflammatory and parenchymal cells in acute pancreatitis. *J Pathol*. 2007; 213: 239-248. PMID: 17893879.
28. Apte MV, Pirola RC, Wilson JS. Battle-scarred pancreas: role of alcohol and pancreatic stellate cells in pancreatic

fibrosis. *J Gastroenterol Hepatol*. 2006; 21 Suppl 3: S97-S101. PMID: 16958684.

29. Xue J, Sharma V, Habtezion A. Immune cells and immune-based therapy in pancreatitis. *Immunol Res*. 2014; 58: 378-386. PMID: 24710635.
30. Vonlaufen A, Xu Z, Daniel B, Kumar RK, Pirola R, Wilson J, et al. Bacterial endotoxin: a trigger factor for alcoholic pancreatitis? Evidence from a novel, physiologically relevant animal model. *Gastroenterology*. 2007; 133: 1293-1303. PMID: 17919500.
31. Asaumi H, Watanabe S, Taguchi M, Tashiro M, Otsuki M. Externally applied pressure activates pancreatic stellate cells through the generation of intracellular reactive oxygen species. *Am J Physiol Gastrointest Liver Physiol*. 2007; 293: G972-978. PMID: 17761838.
32. Erkan M, Reiser-Erkan C, Michalski CW, Deucker S, Sauliunaite D, Streit S, et al. Cancer-stellate cell interactions perpetuate the hypoxia-fibrosis cycle in pancreatic ductal adenocarcinoma. *Neoplasia*. 2009; 11: 497-508. PMID: 19412434.
33. Masamune A, Shimosegawa T. Signal transduction in pancreatic stellate cells. *J Gastroenterol*. 2009; 44: 249-260. PMID: 19271115.
34. McCarroll JA, Phillips PA, Park S, Doherty E, Pirola RC, Wilson JS, et al. Pancreatic stellate cell activation by ethanol and acetaldehyde: is it mediated by the mitogen-activated protein kinase signaling pathway? *Pancreas*. 2003; 27: 150-160. PMID: 12883264.
35. Masamune A, Satoh A, Watanabe T, Kikuta K, Satoh M, Suzuki N, et al. Effects of ethanol and its metabolites on human pancreatic stellate cells. *Dig Dis Sci*. 2010; 55: 204-211. PMID: 19165599.
36. Ohnishi H, Miyata T, Yasuda H, Satoh Y, Hanatsuka K, Kita H, et al. Distinct roles of Smad2-, Smad3-, and ERK-dependent pathways in transforming growth factor-beta1 regulation of pancreatic stellate cellular functions. *J Biol Chem*. 2004; 279: 8873-8878. PMID: 14688282.
37. McCarroll JA, Phillips PA, Kumar RK, Park S, Pirola RC, Wilson JS, et al. Pancreatic stellate cell migration: role of the phosphatidylinositol 3-kinase(PI3-kinase) pathway. *Biochem Pharmacol*. 2004; 67: 1215-1225. PMID: 15006556.
38. Masamune A, Kikuta K, Watanabe T, Satoh K, Satoh A, Shimosegawa T. Pancreatic stellate cells express Toll-like receptors. *J Gastroenterol*. 2008; 43: 352-362. PMID: 18592153.
39. Nybakken K, Perrimon N. Hedgehog signal transduction: recent findings. *Curr Opin Genet Dev*. 2002; 12: 503-511. PMID: 12200154.
40. Shinozaki S, Ohnishi H, Hama K, Kita H, Yamamoto H, Osawa H, et al. Indian hedgehog promotes the migration of rat activated pancreatic stellate cells by increasing membrane type-1 matrix metalloproteinase on the plasma membrane. *J Cell Physiol*. 2008; 216: 38-46. PMID: 18286538.
41. Hu L, Lin X, Lu H, Chen B, Bai Y. An overview of hedgehog signaling in fibrosis. *Mol Pharmacol*. 2015; 87: 174-182. PMID: 25395043.
42. Chambon P. A decade of molecular biology of retinoic acid receptors. *FASEB J*. 1996; 10: 940-954. PMID: 8801176.
43. McCarroll JA, Phillips PA, Santucci N, Pirola RC, Wilson JS, Apte MV. Vitamin A inhibits pancreatic stellate cell activation: implications for treatment of pancreatic fibrosis. *Gut*. 2006; 55: 79-89. PMID: 16043492.
44. Jiang C, Ting AT, Seed B. PPAR-gamma agonists inhibit production of monocyte inflammatory cytokines. *Nature*. 1998; 391: 82-86. PMID: 9422509.
45. Masamune A, Kikuta K, Satoh M, Sakai Y, Satoh A, Shimosegawa T. Ligands of peroxisome proliferator-activated receptor-gamma block activation of pancreatic stellate cells. *J Biol Chem*. 2002; 277: 141-147. PMID: 11606585.
46. Sherman MH, Yu RT, Engle DD, Ding N, Atkins AR, Tiriac H, et al. Vitamin D receptor-mediated stromal reprogramming suppresses pancreatitis and enhances pancreatic cancer therapy. *Cell*. 2014; 159: 80-93. PMID: 25259922.
47. Treiber M, Neuhofer P, Anetsberger E, Einwachter H, Lesina M, Rickmann M, et al. Myeloid, but not pancreatic, RelA/p65 is required for fibrosis in a mouse model of chronic pancreatitis. *Gastroenterology*. 2011; 141: 1473-1485, 1485. e1-7. PMID: 21763242.
48. Xue J, Sharma V, Hsieh MH, Chawla A, Murali R, Pandol SJ, et al. Alternatively activated macrophages promote pancreatic fibrosis in chronic pancreatitis. *Nat Commun*. 2015; 6: 7158. PMID: 25981357.
49. Gordon S. Alternative activation of macrophages. *Nat Rev Immunol*. 2003; 3: 23-35. PMID: 12511873.
50. Esposito I, Friess H, Kappeler A, Shrikhande S, Kleeff J, Ramesh H, et al. Mast cell distribution and activation in chronic pancreatitis. *Hum Pathol*. 2001; 32: 1174-1183. PMID: 11727255.
51. Zimnoch L, Szynaka B, Puchalski Z. Mast cells and pancreatic stellate cells in chronic pancreatitis with differently intensified fibrosis. *Hepatogastroenterology*. 2002; 49: 1135-1138. PMID: 12143220.
52. Ma Y, Hwang RF, Logsdon CD, Ullrich SE. Dynamic mast cell-stromal cell interactions promote growth of pancreatic cancer. *Cancer Res*. 2013; 73: 3927-3937. PMID: 23633481.
53. Schmitz-Winnenthal H, Pietsch DH, Schimmack S, Bonertz A, Udonta F, Ge Y, et al. Chronic pancreatitis is associated with disease-specific regulatory T-cell responses. *Gastroenterology*. 2010; 138: 1178-1188. PMID: 19931255.
54. Kikuta K, Masamune A, Hamada S, Takikawa T, Nakano E, Shimosegawa T. Pancreatic stellate cells reduce insulin expression and induce apoptosis in pancreatic beta-cells. *Biochem Biophys Res Commun*. 2013; 433: 292-297. PMID: 23500461.
55. Ryall CL, Viloria K, Lhaf F, Walker AJ, King A, Jones P, et al. Novel role for matricellular proteins in the regulation of islet beta cell survival: the effect of SPARC on survival, proliferation, and signaling. *J Biol Chem*. 2014; 289: 30614-30624. PMID: 25204658.
56. Mantoni TS, Schendel RR, Rodel F, Niedobitek G, Al-Assar O, Masamune A, et al. Stromal SPARC expression and patient survival after chemoradiation for non-resectable pancreatic adenocarcinoma. *Cancer Biol Ther*. 2008; 7: 1806-1815. PMID: 18787407.
57. Ryu GR, Lee E, Chun HJ, Yoon KH, Ko SH, Ahn YB, et al. Oxidative stress plays a role in high glucose-induced activation of pancreatic stellate cells. *Biochem Biophys Res Commun*. 2013; 439: 258-263. PMID: 23973482.

58. Zha M, Xu W, Zhai Q, Li F, Chen B, Sun Z. High glucose aggravates the detrimental effects of pancreatic stellate cells on Beta-cell function. *Int J Endocrinol.* 2014; 165612. PMID: 25097548.
59. Masamune A, Watanabe T, Kikuta K, Satoh K, Shimosegawa T. NADPH oxidase plays a crucial role in the activation of pancreatic stellate cells. *Am J Physiol Gastrointest Liver Physiol.* 2008; 294: G99-G108. PMID: 17962358.
60. Masamune A, Satoh M, Kikuta K, Suzuki N, Satoh K, Shimosegawa T. Ellagic acid blocks activation of pancreatic stellate cells. *Biochem Pharmacol.* 2005; 70: 869-878. PMID: 16023081.
61. Masamune A, Suzuki N, Kikuta K, Satoh M, Satoh K, Shimosegawa T. Curcumin blocks activation of pancreatic stellate cells. *J Cell Biochem.* 2006; 97: 1080-1093. PMID: 16294327.
62. Rustagi T, Njei B. Antioxidant Therapy for Pain Reduction in Patients With Chronic Pancreatitis: A Systematic Review and Meta-analysis. *Pancreas.* 2015; 44: 812-818. PMID: 25882696.
63. Talukdar R, Murthy HV, Reddy DN. Role of methionine containing antioxidant combination in the management of pain in chronic pancreatitis: a systematic review and meta-analysis. *Pancreatology.* 2015; 15: 136-144. PMID: 25648074.
64. Rickmann M, Vaquero EC, Malagelada JR, Molero X. Tocotrienols induce apoptosis and autophagy in rat pancreatic stellate cells through the mitochondrial death pathway. *Gastroenterology.* 2007; 132: 2518-2532. PMID: 17570223.
65. Apte MV, Phillips PA, Fahmy RG, Darby SJ, Rodgers SC, McCaughan GW, et al. Does alcohol directly stimulate pancreatic fibrogenesis? Studies with rat pancreatic stellate cells. *Gastroenterology.* 2000; 118: 780-794. PMID: 10734030.
66. Zion O, Genin O, Kawada N, Yoshizato K, Roffe S, Nagler A, et al. Inhibition of transforming growth factor beta signaling by halofuginone as a modality for pancreas fibrosis prevention. *Pancreas.* 2009; 38: 427-435. PMID: 19188864.
67. He J, Sun X, Qian KQ, Liu X, Wang Z, Chen Y. Protection of cerulein-induced pancreatic fibrosis by pancreas-specific expression of Smad7. *Biochim Biophys Acta.* 2009; 1792: 56-60. PMID: 19015026.
68. Niina Y, Ito T, Oono T, Nakamura T, Fujimori N, Igarashi H, et al. A sustained prostacyclin analog, ONO-1301, attenuates pancreatic fibrosis in experimental chronic pancreatitis induced by dibutyltin dichloride in rats. *Pancreatology.* 2014; 14: 201-210. PMID: 24854616.
69. Charrier A, Chen R, Kemper S, Brigstock DR. Regulation of pancreatic inflammation by connective tissue growth factor (CTGF/CCN2). *Immunology.* 2014; 141: 564-576. PMID: 24754049.
70. Gibo J, Ito T, Kawabe K, Hisano T, Inoue M, Fujimori N, et al. Camostat mesilate attenuates pancreatic fibrosis via inhibition of monocytes and pancreatic stellate cells activity. *Lab Invest.* 2005; 85: 75-89. PMID: 15531908.
71. Braganza JM, Lee SH, McCloy RF, McMahon MJ. Chronic pancreatitis. *Lancet.* 2011; 377: 1184-1197. PMID: 21397320.
72. Shimosegawa T, Kataoka K, Kamisawa T, Miyakawa H, Ohara H, Ito T, et al. The revised Japanese clinical diagnostic criteria for chronic pancreatitis. *J Gastroenterol.* 2010; 45: 584-591, 2010. PMID: 20422433.
73. Rebours V, Levy P, Ruszniewski P. An overview of hereditary pancreatitis. *Dig Liver Dis.* 2012; 44: 8-15. PMID: 21907651.

Chapter 38

Natural course of chronic pancreatitis

Paul Georg Lankisch[1*] and Albert B. Lowenfels[2]

[1]Department of General Internal Medicine and Gastroenterology, Clinical Center of Lüneburg, Lüneburg, Germany;
[2]New York Medical College, Department of Surgery, Department Family and Community Medicine, Valhalla, New York, USA.

Introduction

In the minority of patients (i.e., 5.8% to 20%), chronic pancreatitis takes a primarily painless course with exocrine and endocrine insufficiency the dominating symptoms.[1-7] However, for the majority of patients, pain is the decisive symptom, causing much discomfort in their daily lives. Some studies have correlated the course of pain in chronic pancreatitis with disease duration, progressing exocrine and endocrine pancreatic insufficiency, and morphological changes such as pancreatic calcification and duct abnormalities. The course of chronic pancreatitis-associated pain has also been studied following alcohol abstinence and after surgery in some groups.

This review of the natural course of chronic pancreatitis focuses on pain but also pays attention to the course of exocrine and endocrine pancreatic insufficiency and concludes by describing the socioeconomic situation of patients and disease mortality and prognosis.

Pain decrease and duration of chronic pancreatitis

Whether progressive parenchymal destruction leads to decreased pain has been debated.[8,9] Ammann's group has claimed that pain decreases with increasing disease duration.[3,10,11] In one long-term study, 85% of 145 patients with chronic pancreatitis felt no more pain after 4.5 years (median) than at disease onset.[3] In another series, in which the interval between the onset of alcohol-induced chronic pancreatitis and pain relief was compared in surgically and nonsurgically treated patient groups, the curves were virtually parallel: pain relief was obtained in about 50% within 6 years and in >80% within 10 years of illness onset.[12]

Reports from Zurich are at variance with studies from Japan and Germany. Miyake et al. found that only 48.2% of the patients with chronic pancreatitis became free of pain within 5 years, but this increased to 66%-73% after more than 5 years.[6] This showed that every third or fourth patient still suffered from relapsing pain attacks even after a long observation period. The Göttingen group[†] reported that the incidence of relapsing pain attacks decreased during the observation period, but more than half of the patients (53%) still suffered from relapsing pain attacks even after more than 10 years of observation.[7]

At present, the course of pain in alcoholic and idiopathic chronic pancreatitis remains unclarified. Layer et al. investigated a group of patients with idiopathic chronic pancreatitis who had never consumed alcoholic beverages.[13] They found that patients with early onset pancreatitis (under 35 years of age) have a long course of severe pain from the start of their illness, whereas patients with late-onset pancreatitis (over 35 years) have a mild and often painless course. Both forms differ from alcoholic pancreatitis in having an equal gender distribution and a much slower rate of calcification. In contrast, the Göttingen group found that the course of pain is the same in alcohol- and nonalcohol-induced chronic pancreatitis.[14] Even when we divided the nonalcoholic group into teetotalers and patients with little alcohol consumption and separately compared their course of pain with alcoholics, there were no differences concerning pain relief among the three groups.[15] Further studies are required to clarify this finding.

[†] Under the leadership of Prof. Dr. Werner Creutzfeldt, a group of clinicians at the University of Göttingen, Germany, began to work on the diagnosis and prognosis of pancreatic diseases, in particular chronic pancreatitis, in 1964. From the mid-1970s this group was headed by one of us (P.G.L.). For the sake of simplicity we refer to this group as the "Göttingen group."

*Corresponding author. Email: paulgeorg.lankisch@t-online.de

Pain decrease and progressing exocrine and endocrine pancreatic insufficiency

The Swiss group has repeatedly observed pain decrease when exocrine and endocrine pancreatic function declines.[8-11] Similarly, Girdwood et al. reported from South Africa that pain decreased as exocrine pancreatic function deteriorated.[16]

Conversely, groups from Denmark and Germany have reported the opposite. Thorsgaard Pedersen et al. from Copenhagen found no correlation between pain and exocrine pancreatic function.[17] The Göttingen group used the secretin-pancreozymin test and fecal fat analysis to evaluate exocrine pancreatic insufficiency,[7] whereas the Swiss group used only indirect pancreatic function tests (i.e., chymotrypsin measurements) to evaluate exocrine pancreatic insufficiency.[3] A clear-cut grading of the severity of exocrine pancreatic insufficiency was used: mild impairment was defined as reduced enzyme output, moderate impairment as a decreased bicarbonate concentration along with reduced enzyme output but normal fecal fat excretion, and severe impairment was equated with an abnormal secretin-pancreozymin test plus steatorrhea. At the end of the observation period, 141 (45%) of 311 patients with painful chronic pancreatitis had severe exocrine pancreatic insufficiency. The majority of them (81/144; 57%) still suffered from pain attacks.[7]

Additionally, the course of pain was studied in correlation with endocrine pancreatic insufficiency, which was classified as absent, moderate (diabetes mellitus treated only by diet with or without oral medication), or severe (requiring insulin). At the end of the observation period, 117 (38%) patients were classified as having severe endocrine pancreatic insufficiency. The majority of them (69/117; 59%) still suffered from pain attacks.[7,18]

Thus, according to these results, the progression of exocrine and endocrine pancreatic insufficiency has a limited influence, if any, on the course of pain in chronic pancreatitis.

Pain decrease and development of morphologic changes of the pancreas (pancreatic calcifications and/or duct abnormalities)

The Swiss group showed an increased incidence of pancreatic calcifications, which in turn was associated with pain decrease.[3,10] However, in a later survey the same group reported a regression of pancreatic calcifications in a long-term study of patients with chronic pancreatitis.[19] Thus, the prognostic role of pancreatic calcifications in determining the course of pain is unclear.

Furthermore, the Swiss results are at variance with two other reports. Malfertheiner et al. found that 89% of patients had pain despite pancreatic calcifications observed on computed tomography, of whom 39% had very intense pain.[20] In the Göttingen group study, freedom of pain was significantly higher in the calcification group than in the noncalcification group. However, the majority of patients with pancreatic calcifications (56%) still had relapsing pain attacks.[7]

The correlation between pain and pancreatic duct changes or pressure in the duct system is also not clear. Ebbehøj et al. measured pancreatic tissue fluid pressure percutaneously or intraoperatively and found a significant correlation with pain in patients with chronic pancreatitis but not with the results of endoscopic retrograde cholangiopancreatography (ERCP). That is, regional pressure tended to be highest in the region of the pancreas with the largest but not the smallest duct diameter.[21,22] Jensen et al. found no correlation between pancreatic duct changes and pain.[23] Warshaw et al. found that 2 of 10 patients had no pain relief 1 year after a lateral pancreaticojejunostomy despite a patent anastomosis detected by ERCP.[24]

Two investigations confirmed the nonparallelism between pancreatic duct changes and pain relief. Malfertheiner et al. found severe pain in only 62% of patients who had advanced pancreatic duct changes demonstrated by ERCP.[20] The Göttingen group found no significant correlation between pancreatic duct abnormalities detected by ERCP and pain in 88 patients with chronic pancreatitis.[7] Severe pancreatic duct abnormalities, as defined by the Cambridge classification[25] were present in 42 patients, but only 16 (31%) of these became free of pain. Despite a normal pancreatic duct in 14 patients, 10 (71%) suffered from persisting pain.[7]

Thus, morphological changes such as pancreatic calcifications or pancreatic duct abnormalities are not necessarily helpful in determining the prognosis of chronic pancreatitis or predicting the course of pain.

Smoking has an effect on the natural course of the disease since it increases the risk of pancreatic calcification in late-onset but not early onset idiopathic chronic pancreatitis.[26]

Pain decrease and alcohol abuse

Since alcoholism is the leading etiologic factor in chronic pancreatitis, several studies have investigated whether alcohol abstinence influences pain or progression of the disease. Sarles and Sahel reported that 50% of their patients with chronic pancreatitis experienced pain relief when alcohol abuse was discontinued,[27] whereas Trapnell reported a figure of 75% when alcohol abuse was discontinued.[28]

Two other investigations have confirmed that abstinence can be helpful. Miyake et al. demonstrated pain relief in 60% of their patients who discontinued or reduced alcohol intake, whereas spontaneous pain relief was seen in only 26% of the group who continued drinking.[6] In a study by the Göttingen group, 66 (31%) of 214 patients with alcoholic chronic pancreatitis were motivated to stop drinking.[7] Pain relief was obtained in 52% of these patients, whereas spontaneous relief in alcoholics was seen in 37%. Thus, alcohol abstinence will probably lead to some improvement of pain in every other patient with chronic pancreatitis, but why exactly abstinence helps some cases but not others remains to be investigated.

Pain decrease and interventional procedures

Interventional procedures for pain treatment in chronic pancreatitis include fragmentation of stones by extracorporeal shock wave lithotripsy (ESWL), endoscopic stone extraction, and bridging of pancreatic strictures by stent applications. Reports of the effect of these procedures on pain are controversial, and controlled studies are lacking. A large Japanese study of 555 patients who underwent ESWL for pancreatic stones report a success rate of 92.4% (fragmentation of stones) and a complete stone clearance rate of 72.6% after ESWL alone or in combination with interventional endoscopy.[29] Symptom relief was achieved in 91.1% of the patients, and complications developed in 6.3% of the patients, including acute pancreatitis in 5.4%. A total of 504 patients were followed up for a mean of 44.3 months, during which 122 (22%) suffered stone recurrence (mean time to recurrence, 25.1 months) and 22 (4.1%) required surgery.[29] In another series from Japan, a total of 117 patients with pancreatic stones underwent ESWL and endoscopic treatment. Immediate pain relief was achieved in 97% and complete removal of stones in 56%. During long-term follow-up over 3 years, 70% of the patients continued to be asymptomatic.[30] These results are at variance with a smaller German study in 80 patients with chronic pancreatitis in whom ESWL was always followed by a further endoscopic procedure. Treatment success was defined as complete clearance of the main pancreatic duct or partial clearance that allowed implantation of a pancreatic stent. Successful treatment was more frequent in patients with solitary stones. The mean duration of follow-up was 40 (range 24-92) months. Pain relief and necessity for further analgesia was independent of ESWL results.[31] Thus, in this study, pancreatic drainage by ESWL and endoscopy had almost no effect on pain in chronic pancreatitis in the long term.[31] This finding is in sharp contrast to the results of a new, albeit retrospective study of 636 patients with idiopathic chronic pancreatitis from a high-volume tertiary care center for endoscopy and gastrointestinal diseases in India.[32] The patients were monitored after ESWL and ERCP and divided into an intermediate group (follow-up 24-60 months, n = 364) and a long-term group (follow-up >60 months, n = 272). Absence of pain was seen in 250 (68.7%) patients, mild to moderate pain in 94 (25.4%) patients, and severe pain in 20 (5.5%) patients of the intermediate group. In the long-term group, 164 (60.3%) patients had no pain, 97 (35.7%) patients had mild or moderate episodes of pain, and 11 (4.04%) patients had episodic severe pain. Recurrence of calculi was seen in 51 (14.01%) patients in the intermediate follow-up group and in 62 (22.8%) patients in the long-term group.

The Indian group freely admits that their study was a single-center retrospective analysis and that visual analog scale scores for pain and quality of life were not validated. Nevertheless, they drew several conclusions from their findings. First, patients who have been relieved of pain during the intermediate period (2-5 years) after ESWL are likely to continue to benefit in the long term. It is probable that early intervention with ESWL and endotherapy, especially in young patients with chronic pancreatitis, alters the course of the disease. Furthermore, early ESWL could even obviate surgical intervention, although this needs to be confirmed in a randomized, controlled trial.[32]

The effect of pancreatic stents on pain in chronic pancreatitis is even more controversial. Patients undergoing pancreatic duct stent placement for disrupted ducts, isolated strictures, pancreas divisum, and hypertensive pancreatic sphincters showed subsequent ductal changes consistent with chronic pancreatitis in 36% of the cases, even though 72% of these patients had a normal initial pancreatogram.[33] Furthermore, patients with preoperative endoscopic pancreatic stenting had frequent postoperative complications, mostly septic, and a prolonged hospital stay.[34] A surgical review of the pitfalls and limitations of stenting in chronic pancreatitis reported that the indications for surgery in patients with a pancreatic stent were severe abdominal pain in 100%, relapsing pain attacks in 77%, and necrotizing pancreatitis in 14%. Before being selected for surgery, 4.5 ERCPs and 3.7 stent exchanges were performed per patient. Thus, from the surgical point of view, endoscopic pancreatic duct stenting in chronic pancreatitis seems not to be indicated because of a low success rate and a substantial risk for complications.[35] The same direction was taken by Holm and Matzen.[36] They performed a retrospective study of patients with chronic pancreatitis and large-duct disease who had undergone decompressing treatment with stenting and/or ESWL. Overall, the authors observed only a small increase in weight and a small reduction in the number of opioid users. In their opinion, these changes may not be different from the natural course of the disease.[36]

The latter results are in sharp contrast to a long-term outcome study of pancreatic stenting in severe chronic pancreatitis in 100 patients from Belgium. The majority of patients (70%) who responded to pancreatic stenting remained pain free after definite stent removal. However, a significantly higher restenting rate was observed in patients with chronic pancreatitis and pancreas divisum.[37] Obviously, the results are also different in special subgroups. Endoscopic stenting of biliary strictures in chronic pancreatitis provided excellent short-term but only moderate long-term results in another study from Germany. Patients without calcifications of the pancreatic head benefit from biliary stenting. However, patients with calcifications have a 17-fold increased risk of failure during 12-month follow-up.[38]

Of special interest are three prospective randomized trials that compared endoscopic with surgical treatment of chronic pancreatitis. Endoscopic treatment included pancreatic sphincterotomy in all and additional stenting of the pancreatic duct in 33 (52%) patients. Mean duration of stent treatment was 16 (range 12-27) months, and stents were exchanged six times (range 4-9). Surgical treatment included pancreatic resection in 61 (80%) and drainage procedures in 15 (20%) patients. Although the short-term effects were similar, the results after 5 years' follow-up showed a comparatively low rate of patients with complete absence of abdominal pain. However, the results for surgery were significantly better than for endotherapy.[39] The study has been criticized for the randomization, which was agreed to by only 51.4% of the patients.

A second study was carried out in the Netherlands. The authors investigated patients with chronic pancreatitis and a distal obstruction of the pancreatic duct but without an inflammatory mass. The patients were randomly assigned to undergo endoscopic transampullary drainage (n, = 19, 16 of whom underwent lithotripsy) of the pancreatic duct or operative pancreaticojejunostomy (n = 20). During the 24 months of follow-up, patients who underwent surgery had lower Izbicki pain scores and better physical health summary scores than those treated endoscopically. At the end of follow-up, complete or partial pain relief was achieved in 32% of patients assigned to endoscopic drainage compared with 75% of patients assigned to surgical drainage ($P = 0.007$). Complication rates, lengths of hospital stay, and changes of pancreatic function were similar in the two treatment groups, but patients receiving endoscopic treatment required more procedures than those in the surgery group ($P>0.001$). The authors concluded that surgical drainage of the pancreatic duct was more effective than endoscopic treatment for patients of this category.[40]

The design of the study from the Netherlands was in contrast to the study by Díte et al. in the Czech Republic,[39] in which the surgical arm included various operations with drainage and the endoscopic treatment did not include lithotripsy. The Dutch study thus seems to be the only one to compare two closely defined drainage options. Nevertheless, it was heavily criticized because of its short observation period. However, the authors later published a second analysis (third study).[41] Surgery remained superior in terms of pain relief (80% vs. 38%, $P = 0.042$). A total of 68% of the patients in the endoscopy group required additional drainage, compared with 5% in the surgery group ($P = 0.001$). Moreover, 47% of the patients in the endoscopy group had to undergo surgery at a later date. The collective results suggest that surgical drainage should currently be preferred to endoscopic measures.

Pain decrease and surgery

During the course of the disease, every second to fourth patient needs surgical treatment because of pain and/or organ complications, such as pancreatic pseudocysts.[3,7] The choice of the surgical procedure is dependent on the special circumstances of each patient and the surgeon's expertise.

On the assumption that pain was caused by obstruction of pancreatic secretion into the duodenum due to inflammation or scarring, longitudinal pancreaticojejunostomy according to Partington and Rochelle was once the method of choice for patients with painful chronic pancreatitis in whom conservative treatment had not reduced the pain.[42] It later became clear that the principal source of pain was actually inflammatory swelling of the head of the pancreas. The classic Kausch-Whipple resection, originally the standard intervention for papillary cancer of the pancreas,[43,44] was subsequently the standard operation for chronic pancreatitis with involvement of the pancreatic head over a period of decades, before being gradually replaced by the pylorus-preserving Whipple procedure.[45] Later, various operations and modifications were introduced to resect the head of the pancreas while preserving the duodenum.

The first duodenum-preserving resection of the head of the pancreas was introduced by Beger and coworkers in 1972.[46] The enlarged pancreatic head was resected without sacrificing the gastroduodenal and bilioduodenal passage, and a drainage operation was performed comparable with the Partington-Rochelle procedure. Subtotal resection of the pancreatic head was carried out before gland transection above the portal vein.

A modification of this procedure was introduced by Frey.[47] A limited duodenum-preserving excision of the pancreatic head was accomplished by coring out the head of the pancreas, leaving a small cuff along the duodenal wall. In contrast to the Beger procedure, the pancreas was not divided above the superior mesenteric portal vein, and the main pancreatic duct was open in the body and tail of the organ.[48] Two further modifications of these operations were later proposed. Groups led by Büchler combined the advantages of the Frey and Beger in the Berne procedure.[49] A deep duodenal-preserving resection of the pancreatic head is accomplished according to Beger, and transection of the gland over the superior mesenteric portal vein is avoided.[48]

The Hamburg procedure also combines aspects of the Beger and Frey operations. Subtotal resection of the pancreatic head including the uncinate processes is carried out, but transection of the gland over the superior mesenteric portal vein is again avoided, and the excision is combined with the longitudinal V-shaped excision of the ventral aspect of the body and tail of the pancreas.[50] Only a small number of randomized controlled studies have compared the different surgical procedures for chronic pancreatitis treatment .[48]

To what extent surgical treatment influences the course of pain in different studies cannot be compared for the following reasons:

- The definition of freedom from pain is often vague, and pain symptoms were usually not measured.
- Not all patients received the same surgical treatment for the same indication. In the past, some authors recommended not performing an indicated resection in alcoholics because of problematic postoperative treatment of diabetes mellitus in those patients.[51,52] It is unclear to what extent these recommendations were or are followed, if at all.

Although continued alcohol abuse distinctly worsens the effect of surgical treatment,[53-55] it is still difficult to determine whether postoperative deterioration results from chronic pancreatitis, continued alcohol abuse, or the surgical treatment.

Overall, the postoperative results of a large number of studies over a period of decades show that independent of the surgical procedure freedom of pain will be obtained in up to 90% of the patients over several years of follow-up (**Table 1**).[7,48,56-104]

Only a few trials have compared pancreaticoduodenectomy with the subsequently developed duodenum-preserving resection of the pancreatic head.[48] Farkas et al. compared a modification of duodenum-preserving resection of the pancreatic head with pancreaticoduodenectomy and found that although their modified procedure did not reduce pain compared with the other group, operation time, length of hospital stay, and morbidity were much lower and weight gain was much higher.[92,95] Klempa et al. compared the Beger procedure with pancreaticoduodenectomy without preservation of the pylorus and found a significant benefit of the Beger procedure with regard to the postoperative hormone status.[105] There was no difference in freedom from pain, but all patients in the Whipple group needed enzyme substitution in contrast with only 10% of those treated according to Beger.

Büchler et al. found that the Beger procedure was superior to pylorus-preserving pancreaticoduodenectomy, but this was after a relatively brief follow-up period.[80] Patients treated according to Beger had less pain, a better quality of life, and higher body weight than those who received the "old" operation.[80] Seven and 14 years later, however, these advantages had disappeared; there was no longer any truly relevant difference between the two operations.[94] The authors assumed reason for the loss of the initial advantage of the Beger procedure was that the latter may be able to delay burn-out of the gland but cannot prevent it entirely.

Only the Hamburg group compared the outcome of the Frey procedure with pylorus-preserving pancreaticoduodenectomy.[87] Twenty-four months after surgery, patients treated according to Frey had less pain, better quality of life, and lower perioperative morbidity. Seven years later there were no differences with regard to mortality, frequency of exocrine or endocrine pancreatic insufficiency, or need for reoperation.[106] After a long-term follow-up (15 years), there were still no differences regarding quality of life or pain, but long-term survival was significantly better after the Frey procedure.[97]

The various modifications of pancreatic head resection were compared in two controlled studies. Köninger et al. compared the Beger procedure with the Berne modification and found the latter technically simpler as reflected in significantly shorter operation times and hospital stays.[96] Quality of life was similar after both procedures.

Izbicki et al. compared the Beger and Frey procedures.[82] After 1.5 years, freedom from pain was the same for both interventions, but perioperative morbidity was significantly lower after the Frey procedure. Eight years after surgery there was no difference between the two groups regarding mortality, quality of life, pain, or exocrine and endocrine pancreatic insufficiency.[91] The situation was the same 16 years after operation; quality of life, pain control, mortality, and rates of exocrine and endocrine pancreatic insufficiency were the same in both groups.[48]

A meta-analysis comparing duodenum-preserving resection of the pancreatic head with pancreaticoduodenectomy was published somewhat earlier.[107] There was no difference between the two procedures regarding pain relief or survival. Duodenum-preserving resection was superior to pancreaticoduodenectomy because of better perioperative and early postoperative outcomes and greater quality of life.[107]

Course of exocrine pancreatic insufficiency

Exocrine pancreatic insufficiency does not play a major prognostic role. Occasionally, massive steatorrhea leading to cachexia and susceptibility to infection has prognostic significance. Whether exocrine pancreatic insufficiency becomes worse during the course of the disease is disputed. Ammann et al. found that severe exocrine pancreatic insufficiency developed within 5.65 years (median) in 122 (86.6%) of 145 patients,[3] whereas Thorsgaard Pedersen et al. observed no significant changes in exocrine pancreatic insufficiency in their patients during an observation

Table 1. Pain freedom after different surgical procedures for chronic pancreatitis.

Reference	Surgical procedure	Mean/median observation period, years	n	Pain relief, %
Way et al.[56]	Drainage/resection	~5	37	64
Lankisch et al.[57]	Drainage/resection	2 6/12	40	60
Mangold et al.[58]	Partial duodenopancreatectomy	1 8/12	44	73
	Total duodenopancreatectomy	2 10/12	18	91
	Partial left-sided resection	3 5/12	37	60
	Subtotal left-sided resection	2 10/12	17	83
Proctor et al.[59]	Pancreaticojejunostomy	11/12	22	50
Rosenberger et al.[60]	Resection	6	67	69
	Nonresective procedures	6	40	50
Lankisch et al.[61]	Pancreaticojejunostomy	3 1/12	17	76
	Resection	3 1/12	22	64
Prinz and Greenlee[62]	Pancreaticojejunostomy	6 1/12-7 11/12	91	35
Sato et al.[63]	Pancreaticojejunostomy	6 6/12	38	68
	Left-sided resection	6 6/12	14	79
	Whipple's operation	6 6/12	9	67
Gall et al.[64]	Whipple's operation, pancreatic duct occlusion	>1	67	93
Morrow et al.[65]	Pancreatic duct drainage	4-13	46	46
	40%-80% left-sided resection	4-13	21	33
	80%-95% left sided resection	4-13	8	100
	Drainage	6	46	80
	Subtotal pancreatectomy	7	21	24
Sato et al.[66]	Left-sided resection	>6/12	21	91
	Whipple's operation	>6/12	11	55
	Pancreaticojejunostomy	>6/12	43	91
Bradley[67]	Lateral pancreaticojejunostomy	5 9/12	46	28
	Caudal pancreaticojejunostomy	5 9/12	18	17
Cooper et al.[68]	Total pancreatectomy	1 6/12	83	72
Frick et al.[69,70]	Left-sided resection	6 6/12	74	50
	Partial duodenopancreatectomy	6 6/12	62	45
	Total duodenopancreatectomy	6 6/12	22	55
	Drainage	4 7/12	156	48
Lambert et al.[71]	Duodenum-preserving total pancreatectomy	9 5/12	14	64
Rossi et al.[72]	Whipple's operation	6/12	61	72
		2	44	61
		5	33	61
		10	18	61
		15	6	83
Mannell et al.[73]	Drainage/resection	8 6/12	100	77
Stone et al.[74]	Whipple's operation	6 2/12	15	53
	Total duodenopancreatectomy	9 1/12	15	27
Beger et al.[75]	Duodenum-preserving pancreatic head resection	3 8/12	128	77
Peiper and Köhler[76]	Resection	10	51	79
	Drainage	10	24	65
Beger and Büchler[77]	Duodenum-preserving pancreatic head resection	3 6/12	141	77
Lankisch et al.[7]	Drainage/resection	6	70	57
Adams et al.[78]	Lateral pancreaticojejunostomy	6 4/12	62	42
Frey and Amikura[79]	Local pancreatic head resection with longitudinal pancreaticojejunostomy	6/12	50	34
Hakaim et al.[98]	Different operations: Pancreatic duct drainage 56%, left-sided resection 20%, cyst drainage 24%	5 2/12	50	30
Büchler et al.[80]	Duodenum-preserving pancreatic head resection	6/12	15	40
	Pylorus-preserving Whipple's operation	6/12	16	75

(Continued)

Table 1. Continued

Reference	Surgical procedure	Mean/median observation period, years	n	Pain relief, %
Fleming and Williamson[81]	Total pancreatectomy	3 6/12	40	79
Izbicki et al.[82]	Duodenum-preserving pancreatic head resection			
	- Beger's procedure	1 6/12	20	95
	- Frey's procedure	1 6/12	22	94
Martin et al.[83]	Pylorus-preserving pancreaticoduodenectomy	5 3/12	45	92
Stapleton and Williamson[84]	Proximal pancreaticoduodenectomy: pylorus-preserving (n = 45), Whipple's operation (n = 7)	4 6/12	52	80
Amikura et al.[99]	Pancreaticojejunostomy	≥6/12	69	75
	Pancreaticojejunostomy plus pancreatic head resection	≥6/12	11	90
	Left-sided resection	≥6/12	37	80
	Whipple's operation	≥6/12	13	65
Rumstadt et al.[85]	Whipple's operation	8 4/12	134	66
Traverso and Kozarek[86]	Whipple's operation	3 6/12	47	76
	Total pancreatectomy	3 6/12	10	76
Izbicki et al.[87]	Longitudinal pancreaticojejunostomy combined with local pancreatic head excision	5 1/12	31	Decreased pain scores in both groups
	Pylorus-preserving pancreaticoduodenectomy	5 1/12	30	
Beger et al.[100]	Duodenum-preserving pancreatic head resection	5 8/12	303	88
Berney et al.[88]	Different procedures of pancreatic resection	6 4/12	68	62
Jimenez et al.[101]	Whipple's operation	3 5/12	33	53
	Pylorus-preserving pancreatic head resection	3 5/12	39	40
Sakorafras et al.[89]	Whipple's operation	6 7/12	66	67
White et al.[90]	Total pancreatectomy	6/12	24	82
Nealon and Matin[102]	Pancreaticojejunostomy	6 9/12	124	86
	Left-sided resection	6 9/12	29	67
	Pancreatic head resection (duodenum-preserving or pylorus-preserving pancreatic head resection	6 9/12	46	91
Sakorafas et al.[103]	Left-sided resection	6 8/12	31	49
Hutchins et al.[104]	Left-sided resection	2 10/12	84	48
Strate et al.[91]	Duodenum-preserving pancreatic head resection			No differences between groups
	- Beger's procedure	8 8/12	34	
	- Frey's procedure	8 8/12	33	
Farkas et al.[92]	Duodenum-preserving pancreatic head resection (authors' modification)	1	40	85
	Pylorus-preserving Whipple's operation	1	40	90
Yekebas et al.[93]	"V-shaped excision" of the anterior aspects of the pancreas	11 6/12	37	89
Müller et al.[94]	Duodenum-preserving pancreatic head resection (Beger)	7	19	No differences between groups
	Pylorus-preserving Whipple's operation	14	20	
Farkas et al.[95]	Duodenum-preserving pancreatic head resection (authors' modification)	4	135	89
Köninger et al.[96]	Duodenum-preserving pancreatic head resection			Quality of life equal in both groups
	- Beger's procedure	2	26	
	- Berne modification	2	29	
Bachmann et al.[97]	Pancreaticoduodenectomy	7	32	Pain control equal in both groups; lower mortality after Frey's procedure
	Frey's procedure	7	32	
Bachmann et al.[48]	Duodenum-preserving pancreatic head resection			Quality of life and pain control equal in both groups
	- Beger's procedure	8	38	
	- Frey's procedure	8	36	

Only reports of "total freedom of pain" were included. Further stages of postoperative improvement (e.g., partly freedom of pain, etc.) were not considered. Closure of literature research June 2014.

period of 4 years.[17] The Göttingen group found no change in the degree of severity of exocrine pancreatic insufficiency in 66 (46.2%) patients, but deterioration occurred in 61 (42.6%). Functional improvement was even seen in 16 (11.2%) of their patients, several of whom no longer required pancreatic enzyme substitution.[7]

Several other studies have furnished evidence of functional improvement in cases of exocrine pancreatic insufficiency in chronic pancreatitis.[6,108-110] Improvement was observed in patients who stopped drinking and/or where exocrine pancreatic insufficiency was moderate (not severe) prior to conservative and/or surgical treatment.[7]

Course of endocrine pancreatic insufficiency

Whereas almost all patients with chronic pancreatitis have exocrine pancreatic insufficiency to some degree at the time of diagnosis, this is not the case for endocrine pancreatic insufficiency. The Göttingen group found moderate to severe endocrine pancreatic insufficiency in all 335 patients with chronic pancreatitis, including 24 patients with painless chronic pancreatitis; however, only 260 (78%) suffered from diabetes, and only 133 (40%) needed insulin treatment. After almost 10 years of observation, the incidence of diabetes had increased 10-fold in only 28 (8%) patients. However, even after this long observation period, 75 (22%) patients (i.e., every fifth patient) still had no diabetes.[7]

In a large prospective cohort study, Malka et al. compared patients who had undergone elective pancreatic surgery with those who had never had surgical treatment.[111] The prevalence of diabetes mellitus did not increase in the surgical group overall but was higher 5 years after distal pancreatectomy than after pancreaticoduodenectomy or pancreatic, cystic, biliary, or digestive drainage. There were no differences between the other surgical procedures. Pancreatic drainage did not prevent diabetes mellitus onset. The risk seemed to be largely caused by disease progression because it increased by more than threefold after the onset of pancreatic calcifications. Endocrine complications may play a major prognostic role, especially after surgical treatment of chronic pancreatitis, because of possible hypoglycemia.[112] Hypoglycemia frequently occurs after subtotal left-sided pancreatic resection and may contribute to an unfavorable prognosis.[52]

The frequencies of some complications of diabetes mellitus secondary to chronic pancreatitis have been studied. Earlier investigations showed that diabetic retinopathy is a rare complication of pancreatogenic diabetes, with an occurrence rate of 7.4%-18%.[113-115] Gullo et al. showed that the risk of retinopathy and the characteristics of this complication in patients with chronic pancreatitis and secondary diabetes are the same as for patients with type 1 diabetes.[116] About half of the patients in each group had retinopathy; this was background, minimal, or mild to moderate without visual function impairment. The only significant difference was the longer duration of diabetes in patients with retinopathy than in those without. A longer observation period may explain the higher frequency of diabetic retinopathy in this study[116] compared with the earlier investigations.[113-115] Similarly, Tiengo et al.[117] and Couet et al.[118] found retinopathy in 31% and 41%, respectively, of patients with chronic pancreatitis. In 1995, Levitt et al. showed that microvascular complications (retinopathy, nephropathy) are equally common and severe in pancreatic diabetes and insulin-dependent diabetes mellitus.[119]

Nondiabetic retinal lesions and retinal function abnormalities (increased threshold of dark adaptation, difficulty with night vision) are also common in patients with chronic pancreatitis, even in the absence of steatorrhea, compared with healthy controls.[120] Electrocardiographic evidence of ischemic heart disease was found twice as often in genetic diabetics as in pancreatic diabetes (37% vs 18%).[121] Diabetic neuropathy was reported in about 30% of patients with chronic pancreatitis (no control group).[122]

Finally, lower extremity arterial disease occurred in 25.3% of patients with chronic pancreatitis and had the same prevalence and distribution as in idiopathic pancreatitis.[123] Whether these complications have major prognostic significance has not yet been investigated.

Course of complications of chronic pancreatitis

The list of complications in chronic pancreatitis includes pancreatic pseudocysts and abscesses; stenosis of the common bile duct, duodenum and colon; development of pleural ascites; and gastrointestinal bleeding. All these complications surely have severe implications for disease prognosis. However, since these have not been investigated in larger studies, their exact influence on outcomes is uncertain, and they are therefore not discussed here.

Course of pancreatic and extrapancreatic carcinomas in chronic pancreatitis

In clinical studies, the incidence of pancreatic carcinoma in patients with chronic pancreatitis has been reported as varying from 1.4% to 2.7%.[3,7,17,124,125] A multicenter historical cohort study of 2015 subjects with chronic pancreatitis involved clinical centers in six countries, and patients were followed for at least 2 years.[126] The cumulative risk of pancreatic carcinoma increased noticeably and was 1.8% and 4%, respectively, 10 and 20 years after the diagnosis of chronic pancreatitis (**Fig. 1**).[126] The risk of pancreatic carcinoma was significantly elevated in patients with chronic pancreatitis, so chronic pancreatitis has to be included in the precanceroses.[126]

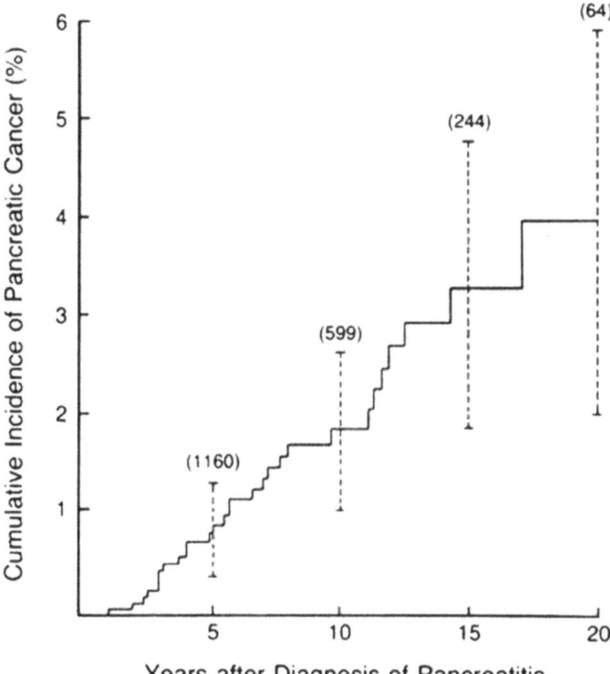

Figure 1. Cumulative incidence of pancreatic cancer in 1,552 subjects with chronic pancreatitis with a minimum of 2 years' follow-up. The vertical lines represent 95% confidence intervals. In parentheses are the numbers of subjects at risk. One additional case of cancer developed after 25 years of follow-up. From Lowenfels et al.[126]

Unfortunately, it is very difficult to diagnose pancreatic carcinoma in chronic pancreatitis. Carcinoma of the pancreas should certainly be suspected in a patient with chronic pancreatitis if there is increasing abdominal discomfort, progressive weight loss, jaundice, and radiologic evidence including nodularity of the duodenal sweep.

Extrapancreatic carcinomas in chronic pancreatitis are not rare events and have been reported with varying incidence, from 3.9% to 12.5%.[6,7,17,125,127] In some of these and other studies,[6,7,125,128] a considerable number of extrapancreatic carcinomas involving the upper respiratory tract (oral cavity, larynx, bronchial tree) have been observed. Since alcohol abuse is the dominating etiology of chronic pancreatitis and because many alcoholics probably smoke, extrapancreatic carcinomas involving the upper respiratory tract may reflect the consequences of another form of substance abuse.

Socioeconomic situation in chronic pancreatitis

Some attention has been paid to the socioeconomic situation of patients with chronic pancreatitis: Gastard et al. found that one out of two male patients continued to work normally, despite pain or diabetes, while one out of three was regarded as unfit for regular work, being totally incapacitated or absent from work for more than 3 months a year.[129] The figures improved after 15 years due to the death of patients with severe disease; at this stage, 68% of the patients were working regularly, and 6% were totally incapacitated. Thorsgaard Pedersen et al. found a decline during an observation period of 5 years (median).[17] Only 15 (40%) of their 38 surviving patients still worked, whereas the remainder were either on prolonged sick-leave or retired. Miyake et al. reported that while 63 (71%) of their 89 patients continued to work, almost all the other patients, who were either retired or who suffered socioeconomically, continued their alcohol abuse.[6] The Göttingen group reported that the incidence of unemployed patients increased from 3% to 15% and the proportion of those retired from 3% to 25% during an observation period of about 11 years. Almost half of the retirements were due to chronic pancreatitis.[7]

Mortality in chronic pancreatitis

The question of whether chronic pancreatitis affects mortality, and if so then how, was addressed by the Copenhagen Pancreatitis Study, a prospective study of patients admitted to the five main hospitals in Copenhagen, Denmark, between 1977 and 1982. Follow-up data in 2008 comprised 249 patients with definite chronic pancreatitis. These patients had a 4-fold higher mortality rate than the background population. Being unemployed or underweight had a significant impact on survival.[130] Data on the mortality rate for chronic pancreatitis are difficult to interpret since etiology and mean observation times vary. Three studies with a similar observation period (median 6.3-9.8 years) revealed a general death rate of 28.8%-35%, but the death rate related to chronic pancreatitis was only 12%-19.8%.[3,6,7] Continued alcohol abuse after conservative treatment and/or surgery has been associated with significantly lower survival rates (**Fig. 2**).[3,6,7,51,52,81]

Prognosis of chronic pancreatitis

The prognosis of chronic pancreatitis is independent of conservative or surgical treatment. A multicenter investigation in seven hospitals of six countries including 2,015 patients with chronic pancreatitis showed that the mortality rate was 3.6 times higher than in patients without pancreatitis. The 10- and 20-year survival rates were 70% and 45%, compared with 93% and 65%, respectively, in patients without pancreatitis.

The following factors were found:

1. Medium or high age at the time of diagnosis: the mortality rates in patients of medium or high age were 2.3- and 6.3-fold, respectively, compared with patients with

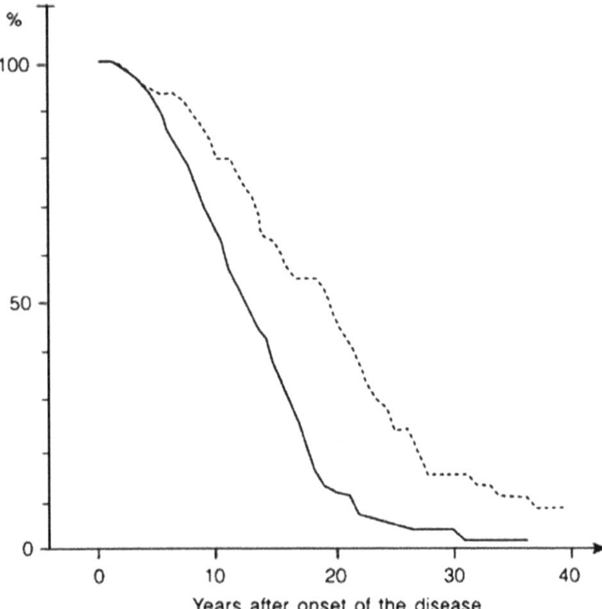

Figure 2. Cumulative survival curve for 230 patients with alcoholic (—) and 105 patients with nonalcoholic (- - -) chronic pancreatitis ($P = 0.0001$). The mean age of onset of the disease (i.e., first pancreatitis-related symptoms) was 37 ± 9 (mean ± SD) years in patients with alcoholic and 39 ± 17 in patients with nonalcoholic chronic pancreatitis. From Lankisch et al.[7] with permission from S. Karger AG, Basel, Switzerland.

chronic pancreatitis in whom the disease was diagnosed before age 40.
2. Consistent alcohol abuse: hazard ratio 1.6.
3. Smoking: hazard ratio 1.4.
4. Liver cirrhosis: hazard ratio 2.5.

Neither sex nor surgical history had any influence on disease prognosis.[131]

Outlook

It will not have escaped the attention of the reader that to date there have been only a few well-performed and valid studies, and even some of these have produced partly diverging results. More controlled studies with larger numbers of patients than any one single center can provide are necessary. This means we have to consider our resources and develop common criteria for diagnosing chronic pancreatitis and following its course. Hence, this review is both an up-to-date survey of studies on the natural course of chronic pancreatitis and an appeal to the readership to take up this task.

References

1. Creutzfeldt W, Fehr H, Schmidt H. [Follow-up and diagnostic procedure in chronically recurrent and chronic pancreatitis]. *Schweiz Med Wochenschr*. 1970; 100: 1180-1189. PMID: 5513763.
2. Ammann RW, Hammer B, Fumagalli I. Chronic pancreatitis in Zurich, 1963-1972. Clinical findings and follow-up studies of 102 cases. *Digestion*. 1973; 9: 404-415. PMID: 4784702.
3. Ammann RW, Akovbiantz A, Largiader F, Schueler G. Course and outcome of chronic pancreatitis. Longitudinal study of a mixed medical-surgical series of 245 patients. *Gastroenterology*. 1984; 86: 820-828. PMID: 6706066.
4. Gullo L, Costa PL, Labò G. Chronic pancreatitis in Italy. Aetiological, clinical and histological observations based on 253 cases. *Rendic Gastroenterol*. 1977; 9: 97-104.
5. Goebell H. [Onset and development of chronic pancreatitis]. *Internist (Berl)*. 1986; 27: 172-174. PMID: 3519503.
6. Miyake H, Harada H, Kunichika K, Ochi K, Kimura I. Clinical course and prognosis of chronic pancreatitis. *Pancreas*. 1987; 2: 378-385. PMID: 3628235.
7. Lankisch PG, Lohr-Happe A, Otto J, Creutzfeldt W. Natural course in chronic pancreatitis. Pain, exocrine and endocrine pancreatic insufficiency and prognosis of the disease. *Digestion*. 1993; 54: 148-155. PMID: 8359556.
8. Ammann RW. Die chronische Pankreatitis. Zur Frage der Operationsindikation und Beitrag zum Spontanverlauf der chronisch-rezidivierenden Pankreatitis. *Dtsch Med Wochenschr*. 1970; 95: 1-7. PMID.
9. Ammann R. [Treatment of chronic pancreatitis]. *Dtsch Med Wochenschr*. 1970; 95: 1234-1235. PMID: 5424968.
10. Ammann RW, Largiader F, Akovbiantz A. Pain relief by surgery in chronic pancreatitis? Relationship between pain relief, pancreatic dysfunction, and alcohol withdrawal. *Scand J Gastroenterol*. 1979; 14: 209-215. PMID: 86198.
11. Ammann R. [Clinical aspects, spontaneous course and therapy of chronic pancreatitis. With special reference to the problem of nomenclature]. *Schweiz Med Wochenschr*. 1989; 119: 696-706. PMID: 2667122.
12. Ammann RW, Muellhaupt B. The natural history of pain in alcoholic chronic pancreatitis. *Gastroenterology*. 1999; 116: 1132-1140. PMID: 10220505.
13. Layer P, Yamamoto H, Kalthoff L, Clain JE, Bakken LJ, DiMagno EP. The different courses of early- and late-onset idiopathic and alcoholic chronic pancreatitis. *Gastroenterology*. 1994; 107: 1481-1487. PMID: 7926511.
14. Lankisch PG, Seidensticker F, Lohr-Happe A, Otto J, Creutzfeldt W. The course of pain is the same in alcohol- and nonalcohol-induced chronic pancreatitis. *Pancreas*. 1995; 10: 338-341. PMID: 7792289.
15. Lankisch PG, Seidensticker F, Löhr-Happe A, Creutzfeldt W. The course of pain is the same in alcoholics, alcohol consumers, and teetotalers (abstr). *Pancreas*. 1996; 13: 446. PMID.
16. Girdwood AH, Marks IN, Bornman PC, Kottler RE, Cohen M. Does progressive pancreatic insufficiency limit pain in calcific pancreatitis with duct stricture or continued alcohol insult? *J Clin Gastroenterol*. 1981; 3: 241-245. PMID: 7288117.
17. Thorsgaard Pedersen N, Nyboe Andersen B, Pedersen G, Worning H. Chronic pancreatitis in Copenhagen. A retrospective

study of 64 consecutive patients. *Scand J Gastroenterol.* 1982; 17: 925-931. PMID: 7156887.

18. Lankisch PG, Andren-Sandberg A. Standards for the diagnosis of chronic pancreatitis and for the evaluation of treatment. *Int J Pancreatol.* 1993; 14: 205-212. PMID: 8113622.
19. Ammann RW, Muench R, Otto R, Buehler H, Freiburghaus AU, Siegenthaler W. Evolution and regression of pancreatic calcification in chronic pancreatitis. A prospective long-term study of 107 patients. *Gastroenterology.* 1988; 95: 1018-1028. PMID: 3410215.
20. Malfertheiner P, Buchler M, Stanescu A, Ditschuneit H. Pancreatic morphology and function in relationship to pain in chronic pancreatitis. *Int J Pancreatol.* 1987; 2: 59-66. PMID: 3681034.
21. Ebbehøj N, Borly L, Bülow J, Rasmussen SG, Madsen P. Evaluation of pancreatic tissue fluid pressure and pain in chronic pancreatitis. A longitudinal study. *Scand J Gastroenterol.* 1990; 25: 462-466. PMID: 2359973.
22. Ebbehøj N, Borly L, Madsen P, Matzen P. Comparison of regional pancreatic tissue fluid pressure and endoscopic retrograde pancreatographic morphology in chronic pancreatitis. *Scand J Gastroenterol.* 1990; 25: 756-760. PMID: 2396092.
23. Jensen AR, Matzen P, Malchow-Moller A, Christoffersen I. Pattern of pain, duct morphology, and pancreatic function in chronic pancreatitis. A comparative study. *Scand J Gastroenterol.* 1984; 19: 334-338. PMID: 6740208.
24. Warshaw AL, Popp JW Jr, Schapiro RH. Long-term patency, pancreatic function, and pain relief after lateral pancreaticojejunostomy for chronic pancreatitis. *Gastroenterology.* 1980; 79: 289-293. PMID: 7399232.
25. Axon AT, Classen M, Cotton PB, Cremer M, Freeny PC, Lees WR. Pancreatography in chronic pancreatitis: international definitions. *Gut.* 1984; 25: 1107-1112. PMID: 6479687.
26. Imoto M, DiMagno EP. Cigarette smoking increases the risk of pancreatic calcification in late-onset but not early-onset idiopathic chronic pancreatitis. *Pancreas.* 2000; 21: 115-119. PMID: 10975703.
27. Sarles H and Sahel J. Die chronische pankreatitis. In Forell M, ed. *Handbuch der Inneren Medizin, vol. 3/6, Pankreas.* Berlin–Heidelberg–New York: Springer; 1976.
28. Trapnell JE. Chronic relapsing pancreatitis: a review of 64 cases. *Br J Surg.* 1979; 66: 471-475. PMID: 466039.
29. Inui K, Tazuma S, Yamaguchi T, Ohara H, Tsuji T, Miyagawa H, et al. Treatment of pancreatic stones with extracorporeal shock wave lithotripsy: results of a multicenter survey. *Pancreas.* 2005; 30: 26-30. PMID: 15632696.
30. Tadenuma H, Ishihara T, Yamaguchi T, Tsuchiya S, Kobayashi A, Nakamura K, et al. Long-term results of extracorporeal shockwave lithotripsy and endoscopic therapy for pancreatic stones. *Clin Gastroenterol Hepatol.* 2005; 3: 1128-1135. PMID: 16271345.
31. Adamek HE, Jakobs R, Buttmann A, Adamek MU, Schneider AR, Riemann JF. Long term follow up of patients with chronic pancreatitis and pancreatic stones treated with extracorporeal shock wave lithotripsy. *Gut.* 1999; 45: 402-405. PMID: 10446109.
32. Tandan M, Reddy DN, Talukdar R, Vinod K, Santosh D, Lakhtakia S, et al. Long-term clinical outcomes of extracorporeal shockwave lithotripsy in painful chronic calcific pancreatitis. *Gastrointest Endosc.* 2013; 78: 726-733. PMID: 23891416.
33. Kozarek RA. Pancreatic stents can induce ductal changes consistent with chronic pancreatitis. *Gastrointest Endosc.* 1990; 36: 93-95. PMID: 2335298.
34. Chaudhary A, Negi SS, Masood S, Thombare M. Complications after Frey's procedure for chronic pancreatitis. *Am J Surg.* 2004; 188: 277-281. PMID: 15450834.
35. Schwarz M, Isenmann R, Beger HG. [Stenting in chronic pancreatitis--the mistakes and limitations]. *Z Gastroenterol.* 2000; 38: 367-374. PMID: 10875146.
36. Holm M, Matzen P. Stenting of extracorporeal shock wave lithotripsy in chronic pancreatitis. *Scand J Gastroenterol.* 2003; 38: 328-331. PMID: 12737450.
37. Eleftherladis N, Dinu F, Delhaye M, Le Moine O, Baize M, Vandermeeren A, et al. Long-term outcome after pancreatic stenting in severe chronic pancreatitis. *Endoscopy.* 2005; 37: 223-230. PMID: 18556820.
38. Kahl S, Zimmermann S, Genz I, Glasbrenner B, Pross M, Schulz HU, et al. Risk factors for failure of endoscopic stenting of biliary strictures in chronic pancreatitis: a prospective follow-up study. *Am J Gastroenterol.* 2003; 98: 2448-2453. PMID: 14638347.
39. Dite P, Ruzicka M, Zboril V, Novotny I. A prospective, randomized trial comparing endoscopic and surgical therapy for chronic pancreatitis. *Endoscopy.* 2003; 35: 553-558. PMID: 12822088.
40. Cahen DL, Gouma DJ, Nio Y, Rauws EA, Boermeester MA, Busch OR, et al. Endoscopic versus surgical drainage of the pancreatic duct in chronic pancreatitis. *N Engl J Med.* 2007; 356: 676-684. PMID: 17301298.
41. Cahen DL, Gouma DJ, Laramee P, Nio Y, Rauws EA, Boermeester MA, et al. Long-term outcomes of endoscopic vs surgical drainage of the pancreatic duct in patients with chronic pancreatitis. *Gastroenterology.* 2011; 141: 1690-1695. PMID: 21843494.
42. Partington PF, Rochelle RE. Modified Puestow procedure for retrograde drainage of the pancreatic duct. *Ann Surg.* 1960; 152: 1037-1043. PMID: 13733040.
43. Kausch W. Das Carcinom der Papilla duodeni und seine radikale Entfernung. *Beitr Klin Chir.* 1912; 78: 439-486. PMID.
44. Whipple AO, Parsons WB, Mullins CR. Treatment of carcinoma of the ampulla of vater. *Ann Surg.* 1935; 102: 763-779. PMID: 17856666.
45. Traverso LW, Longmire WP Jr. Preservation of the pylorus in pancreaticoduodenectomy. *Surg Gynecol Obstet.* 1978; 146: 959-962. PMID: 653575.
46. Beger HG, Witte C, Krautzberger W, Bittner R. [Experiences with duodenum-sparing pancreas head resection in chronic pancreatitis]. *Chirurg.* 1980; 51: 303-307. PMID: 7408575.
47. Frey CF, Smith GJ. Description and rationale of a new operation for chronic pancreatitis. *Pancreas.* 1987; 2: 701-707. PMID: 3438308.
48. Bachmann K, Tomkoetter L, Erbes J, Hofmann B, Reeh M, Perez D, et al. Beger and Frey procedures for treatment of

chronic pancreatitis: comparison of outcomes at 16-year follow-up. *J Am Coll Surg*. 2014; 219: 208-216. PMID: 24880955.

49. Gloor B, Friess H, Uhl W, Buchler MW. A modified technique of the Beger and Frey procedure in patients with chronic pancreatitis. *Dig Surg*. 2001; 18: 21-25. PMID: 11244255.
50. Bachmann K, Kutup A, Mann O, Yekebas E, Izbicki JR. Surgical treatment in chronic pancreatitis timing and type of procedure. *Best Pract Res Clin Gastroenterol*. 2010; 24: 299-310. PMID: 20510830.
51. White TT, Keith RG. Long term follow-up study of fifty patients with pancreaticojejunostomy. *Surg Gynecol Obstet*. 1973; 136: 353-358. PMID: 4688800.
52. Frey CF, Child CG and Fry W. Pancreatectomy for chronic pancreatitis. *Ann Surg*. 1976; 184: 403-413. PMID: 1015887.
53. Leger L, Lenriot JP, Lemaigre G. Five to twenty year followup after surgery for chronic pancreatitis in 148 patients. *Ann Surg*. 1974; 180: 185-191. PMID: 4842980.
54. Holmberg JT, Isaksson G, Ihse I. Long term results of pancreaticojejunostomy in chronic pancreatitis. *Surg Gynecol Obstet*. 1985; 160: 339-346. PMID: 2580360.
55. Capitaine Y, Roche B, Wiesner L, Hahnloser P. [Chronic pancreatitis: natural history and development in relation to alcoholism]. *Schweiz Med Wochenschr*. 1988; 118: 817-820. PMID: 3387981.
56. Way LW, Gadacz T, Goldman L. Surgical treatment of chronic pancreatitis. *Am J Surg*. 1974; 127: 202-209. PMID: 4812121.
57. Lankisch PG, Fuchs K, Schmidt H, Peiper HJ, Creutzfeldt W. [Results of operative treatment of chronic pancreatitis, especially exocrine and endocrine functions (author's transl)]. *Dtsch Med Wochenschr*. 1975; 100: 1048-1050, 1059-1060. PMID: 1126291.
58. Mangold G, Neher M, Oswald B, Wagner G. [Results of resection treatment of chronic pancreatitis (author's transl)]. *Dtsch Med Wochenschr*. 1977; 102: 229-234. PMID: 836384.
59. Proctor HJ, Mendes OC, Thomas CG Jr, Herbst CA. Surgery for chronic pancreatitis. Drainage versus resection. *Ann Surg*. 1979; 189: 664-671. PMID: 443918.
60. Rosenberger J, Stock W, Altmann P, Pichlmaier H. [Late results after surgery in chronic pancreatitis (author's transl)]. *Leber Magen Darm*. 1980; 10: 22-27. PMID: 7374323.
61. Lankisch PG, Fuchs K, Peiper HJ, Creutzfeldt W. Pancreatic function after drainage or resection for chronic pancreatitis. In: Mitchell CJ, Kelleher J, eds. *Pancreatic Disease in Clinical Practice*. London: Pitman Books; 1981.
62. Prinz RA, Greenlee HB. Pancreatic duct drainage in 100 patients with chronic pancreatitis. *Ann Surg*. 1981; 194: 313-320. PMID: 7271348.
63. Sato T, Noto N, Matsuno S, Miyakawa K. Follow-up results of surgical treatment for chronic pancreatitis. Present status in Japan. *Am J Surg*. 1981; 142: 317-323. PMID: 7283020.
64. Gall FP, Gebhardt C, Zirngibl H. Chronic pancreatitis–results in 116 consecutive, partial duodenopancreatectomies combined with pancreatic duct occlusion. *Hepatogastroenterology*. 1982; 29: 115-119. PMID: 7106696.
65. Morrow CE, Cohen JI, Sutherland DE, Najarian JS. Chronic pancreatitis: long-term surgical results of pancreatic duct drainage, pancreatic resection, and near-total pancreatectomy and islet autotransplantation. *Surgery*. 1984; 96: 608-616. PMID: 6435270.
66. Sato T, Miyashita E, Yamauchi H, Matsuno S. The role of surgical treatment for chronic pancreatitis. *Ann Surg*. 1986; 203: 266-271. PMID: 2420294.
67. Bradley EL 3rd. Long-term results of pancreatojejunostomy in patients with chronic pancreatitis. *Am J Surg*. 1987; 153: 207-213. PMID: 3812895.
68. Cooper MJ, Williamson RC, Benjamin IS, Carter DC, Cuschieri A, Linehan IP, et al. Total pancreatectomy for chronic pancreatitis. *Br J Surg*. 1987; 74: 912-915. PMID: 3664222.
69. Frick S, Jung K, Ruckert K. [Surgery of chronic pancreatitis. I. Late results after resection management]. *Dtsch Med Wochenschr*. 1987; 112: 629-635. PMID: 3569054.
70. Frick S, Ebert M, Ruckert K. [Surgery in chronic pancreatitis. II. Late results following non-resection operations]. *Dtsch Med Wochenschr*. 1987; 112: 832-837. PMID: 3107963.
71. Lambert MA, Linehan IP, Russell RC. Duodenum-preserving total pancreatectomy for end stage chronic pancreatitis. *Br J Surg*. 1987; 74: 35-39. PMID: 3828733.
72. Rossi RL, Rothschild J, Braasch JW, Munson JL, ReMine SG. Pancreatoduodenectomy in the management of chronic pancreatitis. *Arch Surg*. 1987; 122: 416-420. PMID: 3566523.
73. Mannell A, Adson MA, McIlrath DC, Ilstrup DM. Surgical management of chronic pancreatitis: long-term results in 141 patients. *Br J Surg*. 1988; 75: 467-472. PMID: 3390681.
74. Stone WM, Sarr MG, Nagorney DM, McIlrath DC. Chronic pancreatitis. Results of Whipple's resection and total pancreatectomy. *Arch Surg*. 1988; 123: 815-819. PMID: 3382346.
75. Beger HG, Buchler M, Bittner RR, Oettinger W, Roscher R. Duodenum-preserving resection of the head of the pancreas in severe chronic pancreatitis. Early and late results. *Ann Surg*. 1989; 209: 273-278. PMID: 2923514.
76. Peiper HJ, Kohler H. [Surgical therapy of chronic pancreatitis]. *Schweiz Med Wochenschr*. 1989; 119: 712-716. PMID: 2667124.
77. Beger HG, Buchler M. Duodenum-preserving resection of the head of the pancreas in chronic pancreatitis with inflammatory mass in the head. *World J Surg*. 1990; 14: 83-87. PMID: 2305590.
78. Adams DB, Ford MC, Anderson MC. Outcome after lateral pancreaticojejunostomy for chronic pancreatitis. *Ann Surg*. 1994; 219: 481-487; discussion 487-489. PMID: 8185399.
79. Frey CF, Amikura K. Local resection of the head of the pancreas combined with longitudinal pancreaticojejunostomy in the management of patients with chronic pancreatitis. *Ann Surg*. 1994; 220: 492-504; discussion 504-497. PMID: 7524454.
80. Buchler MW, Friess H, Muller MW, Wheatley AM, Beger HG. Randomized trial of duodenum-preserving pancreatic head resection versus pylorus-preserving Whipple in chronic pancreatitis. *Am J Surg*. 1995; 169: 65-69; discussion 69-70. PMID: 7818000.
81. Fleming WR, Williamson RC. Role of total pancreatectomy in the treatment of patients with end-stage chronic pancreatitis. *Br J Surg*. 1995; 82: 1409-1412. PMID: 7489180.

82. Izbicki JR, Bloechle C, Knoefel WT, Kuechler T, Binmoeller KF, Broelsch CE. Duodenum-preserving resection of the head of the pancreas in chronic pancreatitis. A prospective, randomized trial. *Ann Surg*. 1995; 221: 350-358. PMID: 7726670.
83. Martin RF, Rossi RL, Leslie KA. Long-term results of pylorus-preserving pancreatoduodenectomy for chronic pancreatitis. *Arch Surg*. 1996; 131: 247-252. PMID: 8611088.
84. Stapleton GN, Williamson RC. Proximal pancreatoduodenectomy for chronic pancreatitis. *Br J Surg*. 1996; 83: 1433-1440. PMID: 8944465.
85. Rumstadt B, Forssmann K, Singer MV, Trede M. The Whipple partial duodenopancreatectomy for the treatment of chronic pancreatitis. *Hepatogastroenterology*. 1997; 44: 1554-1559. PMID: 9427021.
86. Traverso LW, Kozarek RA. Pancreatoduodenectomy for chronic pancreatitis: anatomic selection criteria and subsequent long-term outcome analysis. *Ann Surg*. 1997; 226: 429-435; discussion 435-428. PMID: 9351711.
87. Izbicki JR, Bloechle C, Broering DC, Knoefel WT, Kuechler T, Broelsch CE. Extended drainage versus resection in surgery for chronic pancreatitis: a prospective randomized trial comparing the longitudinal pancreaticojejunostomy combined with local pancreatic head excision with the pylorus-preserving pancreatoduodenectomy. *Ann Surg*. 1998; 228: 771-779. PMID: 9860476.
88. Berney T, Rudisuhli T, Oberholzer J, Caulfield A, Morel P. Long-term metabolic results after pancreatic resection for severe chronic pancreatitis. *Arch Surg*. 2000; 135: 1106-1111. PMID: 10982519.
89. Sakorafas GH, Farnell MB, Nagorney DM, Sarr MG, Rowland CM. Pancreatoduodenectomy for chronic pancreatitis: long-term results in 105 patients. *Arch Surg*. 2000; 135: 517-523; discussion 523-514. PMID: 10807274.
90. White SA, Sutton CD, Weymss-Holden S, Berry DP, Pollard C, Rees Y, et al. The feasibility of spleen-preserving pancreatectomy for end-stage chronic pancreatitis. *Am J Surg*. 2000; 179: 294-297. PMID: 10875989.
91. Strate T, Taherpour Z, Bloechle C, Mann O, Bruhn JP, Schneider C, et al. Long-term follow-up of a randomized trial comparing the beger and frey procedures for patients suffering from chronic pancreatitis. *Ann Surg*. 2005; 241: 591-598. PMID: 15798460.
92. Farkas G, Leindler L, Daroczi M, Farkas G Jr. Prospective randomised comparison of organ-preserving pancreatic head resection with pylorus-preserving pancreaticoduodenectomy. *Langenbecks Arch Surg*. 2006; 391: 338-342. PMID: 16680474.
93. Yekebas EF, Bogoevski D, Honarpisheh H, Cataldegirmen G, Habermann CR, Seewald S, et al. Long-term follow-up in small duct chronic pancreatitis: A plea for extended drainage by "V-shaped excision" of the anterior aspect of the pancreas. *Ann Surg*. 2006; 244: 940-946; discussion 946-948. PMID: 17122619.
94. Muller MW, Friess H, Martin DJ, Hinz U, Dahmen R, Buchler MW. Long-term follow-up of a randomized clinical trial comparing Beger with pylorus-preserving Whipple procedure for chronic pancreatitis. *Br J Surg*. 2008; 95: 350-356. PMID: 17933005.
95. Farkas G, Leindler L, Daroczi M, Farkas G Jr. Long-term follow-up after organ-preserving pancreatic head resection in patients with chronic pancreatitis. *J Gastrointest Surg*. 2008; 12: 308-312. PMID: 17906905.
96. Koninger J, Seiler CM, Sauerland S, Wente MN, Reidel MA, Muller MW, et al. Duodenum-preserving pancreatic head resection--a randomized controlled trial comparing the original Beger procedure with the Berne modification (ISRCTN No. 50638764). *Surgery*. 2008; 143: 490-498. PMID: 18374046.
97. Bachmann K, Tomkoetter L, Kutup A, Erbes J, Vashist Y, Mann O, et al. Is the Whipple procedure harmful for long-term outcome in treatment of chronic pancreatitis? 15-years follow-up comparing the outcome after pylorus-preserving pancreatoduodenectomy and Frey procedure in chronic pancreatitis. *Ann Surg*. 2013; 258: 815-820; discussion 820-811. PMID: 24096767.
98. Hakaim AG, Broughan TA, Vogt DP, Hermann RE. Long-term results of the surgical management of chronic pancreatitis. *Am Surg*. 1994; 60: 306-308. PMID: 8161075.
99. Amikura K, Arai K, Kobari M, Matsuno S. Surgery for chronic pancreatitis--extended pancreaticojejunostomy. *Hepatogastroenterology*. 1997; 44: 1547-1553. PMID: 9427020.
100. Beger HG, Schlosser W, Friess HM, Buchler MW. Duodenum-preserving head resection in chronic pancreatitis changes the natural course of the disease: a single-center 26-year experience. *Ann Surg*. 1999; 230: 512-519; discussion 519-523. PMID: 10522721.
101. Jimenez RE, Fernandez-del Castillo C, Rattner DW, Chang Y, Warshaw AL. Outcome of pancreaticoduodenectomy with pylorus preservation or with antrectomy in the treatment of chronic pancreatitis. *Ann Surg*. 2000; 231: 293-300. PMID: 10714621.
102. Nealon WH, Matin S. Analysis of surgical success in preventing recurrent acute exacerbations in chronic pancreatitis. *Ann Surg*. 2001; 233: 793-800. PMID: 11371738.
103. Sakorafas GH, Sarr MG, Rowland CM, Farnell MB. Postobstructive chronic pancreatitis: results with distal resection. *Arch Surg*. 2001; 136: 643-648. PMID: 11387000.
104. Hutchins RR, Hart RS, Pacifico M, Bradley NJ, Williamson RC. Long-term results of distal pancreatectomy for chronic pancreatitis in 90 patients. *Ann Surg*. 2002; 236: 612-618. PMID: 12409667.
105. Klempa I, Spatny M, Menzel J, Baca I, Nustede R, Stockmann F, et al. [Pancreatic function and quality of life after resection of the head of the pancreas in chronic pancreatitis. A prospective, randomized comparative study after duodenum preserving resection of the head of the pancreas versus Whipple's operation]. *Chirurg*. 1995; 66: 350-359. PMID: 7634946.
106. Strate T, Bachmann K, Busch P, Mann O, Schneider C, Bruhn JP, et al. Resection vs drainage in treatment of chronic pancreatitis: long-term results of a randomized trial. *Gastroenterology*. 2008; 134: 1406-1411. PMID: 18471517.
107. Diener MK, Rahbari NN, Fischer L, Antes G, Buchler MW, Seiler CM. Duodenum-preserving pancreatic head resection versus pancreatoduodenectomy for surgical

treatment of chronic pancreatitis: a systematic review and meta-analysis. *Ann Surg*. 2008; 247: 950-961. PMID: 18520222.

108. Kondo T, Hayakawa T, Noda A, Ito K, Yamazaki Y, Iinuma Y, et al. Follow-up study of chronic pancreatitis. *Gastroenterol Jpn*. 1981; 16: 46-53. PMID: 7227758.
109. Begley CG, Roberts-Thomson IC. Spontaneous improvement in pancreatic function in chronic pancreatitis. *Dig Dis Sci*. 1985; 30: 1117-1120. PMID: 4064863.
110. Garcia-Puges AM, Navarro S, Ros E, Elena M, Ballesta A, Aused R, et al. Reversibility of exocrine pancreatic failure in chronic pancreatitis. *Gastroenterology*. 1986; 91: 17-24. PMID: 3486791.
111. Malka D, Hammel P, Sauvanet A, Rufat P, O'Toole D, Bardet P, et al. Risk factors for diabetes mellitus in chronic pancreatitis. *Gastroenterology*. 2000; 119: 1324-1332. PMID: 11054391.
112. Linde J, Nilsson LH, Barany FR. Diabetes and hypoglycemia in chronic pancreatitis. *Scand J Gastroenterol*. 1977; 12: 369-373. PMID: 867001.
113. Sevel D, Bristow JH, Bank S, Marks I, Jackson P. Diabetic retinopathy in chronic pancreatitis. *Arch Ophthalmol*. 1971; 86: 245-250. PMID: 5095550.
114. Creutzfeldt W, Perings E. Is the infrequency of vascular complications in human secondary diabetes related to nutritional factors? *Acta Diabetol Lat*. 1972; 9: 432-445.
115. Verdonk CA, Palumbo PJ, Gharib H, Bartholomew LG. Diabetic microangiopathy in patients with pancreatitic diabetes mellitus. *Diabetologia*. 1975; 11: 394-400. PMID: 1181665.
116. Gullo L, Parenti M, Monti L, Pezzilli R, Barbara L. Diabetic retinopathy in chronic pancreatitis. *Gastroenterology*. 1990; 98: 1577-1581. PMID: 2338195.
117. Tiengo A, Segato T, Briani G, Setti A, Del Prato S, Devide A, et al. The presence of retinopathy in patients with secondary diabetes following pancreatectomy or chronic pancreatitis. *Diabetes Care*. 1983; 6: 570-574. PMID: 6653314.
118. Couet C, Genton P, Pointel JP, Louis J, Gross P, Saudax E, et al. The prevalence of retinopathy is similar in diabetes mellitus secondary to chronic pancreatitis with or without pancreatectomy and in idiopathic diabetes mellitus. *Diabetes Care*. 1985; 8: 323-328. PMID: 4042797.
119. Levitt NS, Adams G, Salmon J, Marks IN, Musson G, Swanepoel C, et al. The prevalence and severity of microvascular complications in pancreatic diabetes and IDDM. *Diabetes Care*. 1995; 18: 971-974. PMID: 7555558.
120. Toskes PP, Dawson W, Curington C, Levy NS, Fitzgerald C. Non-diabetic retinal abnormalities in chronic pancreatitis. *N Engl J Med*. 1979; 300: 942-946. PMID: 431561.
121. Joffe BI, Novis B, Seftel HC, Krut L, Bank S. Ischaemic heart-disease and pancreatic diabetes. *Lancet*. 1971; 2: 269. PMID: 4104810.
122. Bank S, Marks IN, Vinik AI. Clinical and hormonal aspects of pancreatic diabetes. *Am J Gastroenterol*. 1975; 64: 13-22. PMID: 808121.
123. Ziegler O, Candiloros H, Guerci B, Got I, Crea T, Drouin P. Lower-extremity arterial disease in diabetes mellitus due to chronic pancreatitis. *Diabete Metab*. 1994; 20: 540-545. PMID: 7713277.
124. Mohr P, Ammann R, Largiader F, Knoblauch M, Schmid M and Akovbiantz A. [Pancreatic carcinoma in chronic pancreatitis]. *Schweiz Med Wochenschr*. 1975; 105: 590-592. PMID: 1145157.
125. Ammann RW, Knoblauch M, Mohr P, Deyhle P, Largiader F, Akovbiantz A, et al. High incidence of extrapancreatic carcinoma in chronic pancreatitis. *Scand J Gastroenterol*. 1980; 15: 395-399. PMID: 7433900.
126. Lowenfels AB, Maisonneuve P, Cavallini G, Ammann RW, Lankisch PG, Andersen JR, et al. Pancreatitis and the risk of pancreatic cancer. International Pancreatitis Study Group. *N Engl J Med*. 1993; 328: 1433-1437. PMID: 8479461.
127. Rocca G, Gaia E, Iuliano R, Caselle MT, Rocca N, Calcamuggi G, et al. Increased incidence of cancer in chronic pancreatitis. *J Clin Gastroenterol*. 1987; 9: 175-179. PMID: 3571892.
128. Marks IN, Girdwood AH, Bank S, Louw JH. The prognosis of alcohol-induced calcific pancreatitis. *S Afr Med J*. 1980; 57: 640-643. PMID: 7376029.
129. Gastard J, Joubaud F, Farbos T, Loussouarn J, Marion J, Pannier M, et al. Etiology and course of primary chronic pancreatitis in Western France. *Digestion*. 1973; 9: 416-428. PMID: 4784703.
130. Nojgaard C, Bendtsen F, Becker U, Andersen JR, Holst C, Matzen P. Danish patients with chronic pancreatitis have a four-fold higher mortality rate than the Danish population. *Clin Gastroenterol Hepatol*. 2010; 8: 384-390. PMID: 20036762.
131. Lowenfels AB, Maisonneuve P, Cavallini G, Ammann RW, Lankisch PG, Andersen JR, et al. Prognosis of chronic pancreatitis: an international multicenter study. International Pancreatitis Study Group. *Am J Gastroenterol*. 1994; 89: 1467-1471. PMID: 8079921.

Chapter 39

Recurrent acute pancreatitis and progression to chronic pancreatitis

Nalini M. Guda* and Camilla Nøjgaard*

Aurora St. Luke's Medical Center, Milwaukee WI and Hvidovre University Hospital, Copenhagen, Denmark.

Introduction

Acute pancreatitis (AP) is a common clinical condition with significant morbidity and mortality. AP has many causes and can be multifactorial. The role of genetic factors appears to be complex, and is expanding as genetic mutations and their interactions with environmental influences undergo further investigation. If not corrected, any causative factor is capable of producing relapsing pancreatitis, hence it is important to carefully evaluate the patient and address the underlying issue.

The problem is compounded because multiple etiologies are present in at least 7% of patients, especially genetic predispositions plus another factor (toxic or obstructive). Establishment of the etiology of acute pancreatitis often requires expensive and sometimes invasive evaluation that may present risk of significant complications, including further pancreatitis.

From AP to CP

Increasingly, it is understood that a continuum exists between recurrent AP and chronic pancreatitis (CP). When thoroughly evaluated using newer, sensitive techniques such as secretin-enhanced magnetic retrograde cholangiopancreatography (S-MRCP), endoscopic ultrasound (EUS), and pancreatic function tests, many patients presenting with isolated recurrent acute episodes of pancreatitis, and a minority of those presenting with their first acute attack, are found to have morphologic evidence of CP, ranging from subtle "minimal change" disease to obvious disease with calcifications. Over time, some patients with AP and apparently normal morphology progress to obvious CP with calcifications and loss of endocrine and exocrine function.[1-4] The exact mechanism by which acute pancreatitis progresses to chronic pancreatitis is not well understood.

It is not clear whether a sentinel event starts an inflammatory process that does not resolve (sentinel AP event = SAPE hypothesis) or the pathology simply represents accumulated damage from prior attacks that has not fully healed. It remains to be established why, after either a single or a few attacks of AP, some patients have an aggressive disabling course leading to CP with permanent structural changes of the gland, chronic abdominal pain and exocrine and endocrine dysfunction. Others have a harmless course without development of fibrosis or dysfunction. The etiology of AP is thought to have an influence on the course of the disease, as previous studies indicate that a majority of alcohol-induced AP seems to progress to CP, whereas this is only rarely occurs in biliary-induced AP. Necrotizing AP, however, can lead to pancreatic insufficiency and permanent ductal lesions.[5] Impairment of exocrine and endocrine function has been described even after mild non-alcoholic AP.[6] In patients with acute recurrent pancreatitis and CP, a disconnect between symptoms and morphology is often seen, such that patients with obvious CP by morphology may have minimal chronic symptoms between attacks of AP. Patients with a normal-appearing pancreas between attacks of acute relapsing pancreatitis may suffer intractable chronic pain. In these patients, it is not clear whether the pain is from low-level chronic inflammation or has a functional cause unrelated to the pancreatitis. Data are limited on the natural history of acute pancreatitis. In one study evaluating the natural history after the first attack of AP, recurrent pancreatitis was seen in up to 16.5% of the patients at a mean follow-up of 7.8 years.[7]

The annual relapse rates were higher for those with alcohol and gallstones as an etiology and about 1% per year or less for other etiologies, including those termed "idiopathic". In other studies the recurrence rate of pancreatitis over 2 to 3 years of follow-up were up to 3 or 4 times this rate. Genetic mutations are thought to play a significant role in recurrence or disease progression and may serve as a cofactor (multi-hit hypothesis). Various genetic mutations have been recognized as a cause. The interplay between genetics and environmental risk factors is not well

*Corresponding authors. Email: nguda@wisc.edu, mille@dadlnet.dk

Table 1. Etiology of acute relapsing pancreatitis (Based on TIGAR-O Classification).

Toxic–metabolic
Alcoholic—continued consumption
Smoking—possible risk factor/important cofactor*
Hypercalcemia/hyperparathyroidism
Hypertriglyceridemia
Medications
Toxins
Organotin compounds [e.g., di-n-butyltindichloride (DBTC)]
Idiopathic
Early onset
Late onset
Tropical
Genetic**
Anionic trypsinogen PRSS2 (rare)
Autosomal recessive/modifier genes
CFTR mutations
SPINK1 mutations
Cationic trypsinogen (codon 16, 22, 23 mutations)
α1-antitrypsin deficiency (possible)
Monocyte chemoprotectant protein (MCP-1)
Autoimmune
Isolated/associated with other autoimmune disorders
Obstructive
Pancreatic divisum (controversial/often in conjunction with genetic causes)
Sphincter of Oddi disorders (controversial—no added benefit of pancreatic sphincterotomy)
Duct obstruction (e.g., tumor including periampullary lesions, parasite)
Choledochal cysts and abnormal pancreatobiliary unions
Inflammatory bowel disease/celiac sprue (rare)

Adapted from the TIGAR-O classification system[1].
*Compounding effect in association with alcohol.
**Routine genetic testing not done in clinical practice.

understood, and the utility of routine clinical testing for genetic mutations is unclear (8).

Several interventions are offered for the management of acute recurrent pancreatitis. Data to support the role of minor papillotomy for those with pancreas divisum and recurrent acute pancreatitis are limited, and long-term data are lacking. Similarly, the role of sphincter of Oddi dysfunction as a cause of recurrent acute pancreatitis is very controversial. Evaluation by manometry and endosphincterotomy has not shown that addition of pancreatic sphincterotomy to biliary sphincterotomy provides any additional benefit.[9]

One should be careful when offering endoscopic therapies for these entities, and when they are performed, they should be done in the setting of a carefully planned research study. Measurement of treatment success in a disease where multiple factors play a role is difficult, and defining the end-points is also difficult. There is also a concern of further, intervention-related damage, such as post ERCP pancreatitis. Stents can induce strictures in the pancreatic duct even when they are placed for a short time to prevent post-ERCP pancreatitis.[10] When endoscopic procedures, such as ERCP for possible sphincter of Oddi dysfunction or pancreas divisum are done, one should carefully weigh the risk of complications. The procedures are best done in the setting of clinical research. In a disease with a natural history and significant interaction with other cofactors, determining the end points of therapy and measurement of outcomes are difficult.[11]

Mortality and Risk Factors for Progression to CP

In a Danish prospective study of 352 patients with AP and a full 30-year follow-up in the Danish registries, 24.1% of the patients progressed to CP after the first attack of AP (progressive AP).[2] CP was diagnosed a mean of 3.5 years after first admission for AP. The mortality in patients with progressive acute pancreatitis was 2.7 times higher than the mortality in patients who did not progress to chronic pancreatitis. Compared with the background population, mortality was 5.3 to 6.5 times higher in patients with progressive PA. The risk of progression decreased with increasing age, and in a Cox regression analysis with age as a cofactor, smoking was the most important variable associated with progression from AP to CP, and gallstone-induced AP showed

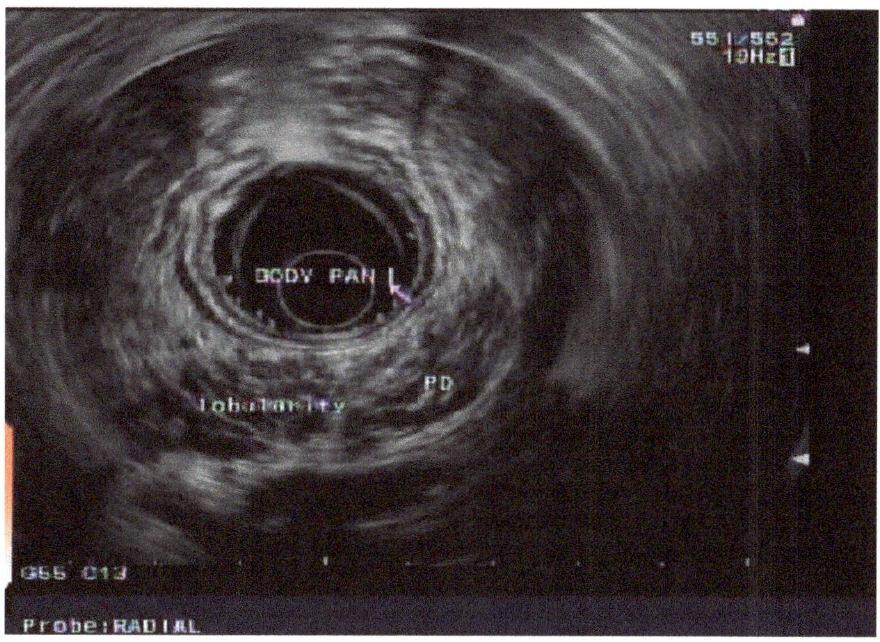

Figure 1. EUS image of a patient with idiopathic acute recurrent pancreatitis. No calcifications are seen but the gland shows lobularity and honeycomb structures suggestive of, but not definitive for, chronic pancreatitis.

a trend towards significance. Gender and employment showed nonproportionality. Alcohol had no significant influence on progression.[2,12]

Conclusions

Recurrent AP is a common clinical condition. After confirming that the attacks are truly pancreatitis, the etiology is easily determined in at least 70 to 80% of cases. Another 10 to 15% of the etiologies can be found with more advanced testing, and up to 10% are idiopathic. However, certain etiologies identified by these tests are not universally agreed upon as being important or relevant. The role of empiric cholecystectomy is unclear. Genetic predisposition is a common cofactor, but the role of routine testing is still unclear, except in those with a family history and suspected PRSS1 mutation (which identifies a higher cancer risk). Evolving research in medical therapy of patients with CFTR mutation may change this, and expand the role of genetic testing. The natural history of the disease and the treatment effects are poorly understood. Recurrent AP is thus a syndrome of various causes, symptoms and outcomes. Long term follow-up and well-designed, preferably randomized, studies with adequate sample size are needed. Invasive procedures, especially ERCP, performed solely for diagnosis (without manometry or divisum-targeted therapy) should be avoided. MRCP and EUS are recommended after a complete history and physical evaluation, routine laboratory tests including evaluation of triglycerides, and imaging studies, especially in recurrent disease. EUS is preferred in older patients and in those with a gallbladder, because of its superior performance for detecting small tumors and subtle gallbladder lithiasis (small stones or sludge in the gallbladder).

Efforts to find subtle evidence of CP may be worthwhile in patients with intractable pain between attacks, and the role of aggressive resection in recurrent AP without CP is evolving. One should not rely on morphological features alone to diagnose chronic pancreatitis. A classification based on a combination of morphological features, tests of pancreatic exocrine function tests, and imaging procedures is recommended.[7]

AP can progress to CP (**Figure 1**), and smoking is the strongest risk factor associated with progression. The mortality is 5 to 6 times higher compared with the background population, indicating that patients with AP and risk factors for CP should be followed. As the disease is multifaceted, treatment for smoking dependency, alcohol dependency, and nutritional support is encouraged. Endoscopic investigations and therapy should be carefully weighed against the risks and should preferably done in expert centers. There are no definitive guidelines and no consensus regarding clinical follow-up for patients with recurrent AP. There is consensus that such patients should avoid smoking to reduce the risk of progression of the disease. Any other triggering risk factors should be carefully avoided including alcohol and any suspected medicine. Triglycerides should be checked. Clinical follow-up and further evaluation of clinical symptoms is appropriate. There are no data to support routine periodic surveillance with invasive procedures such as EUS or to carry out routine CT scans as radiation exposure is a significant risk. There are currently no biomarkers available to monitor disease progression. If a patient develops a recurrent episode once the acute episode resolves,

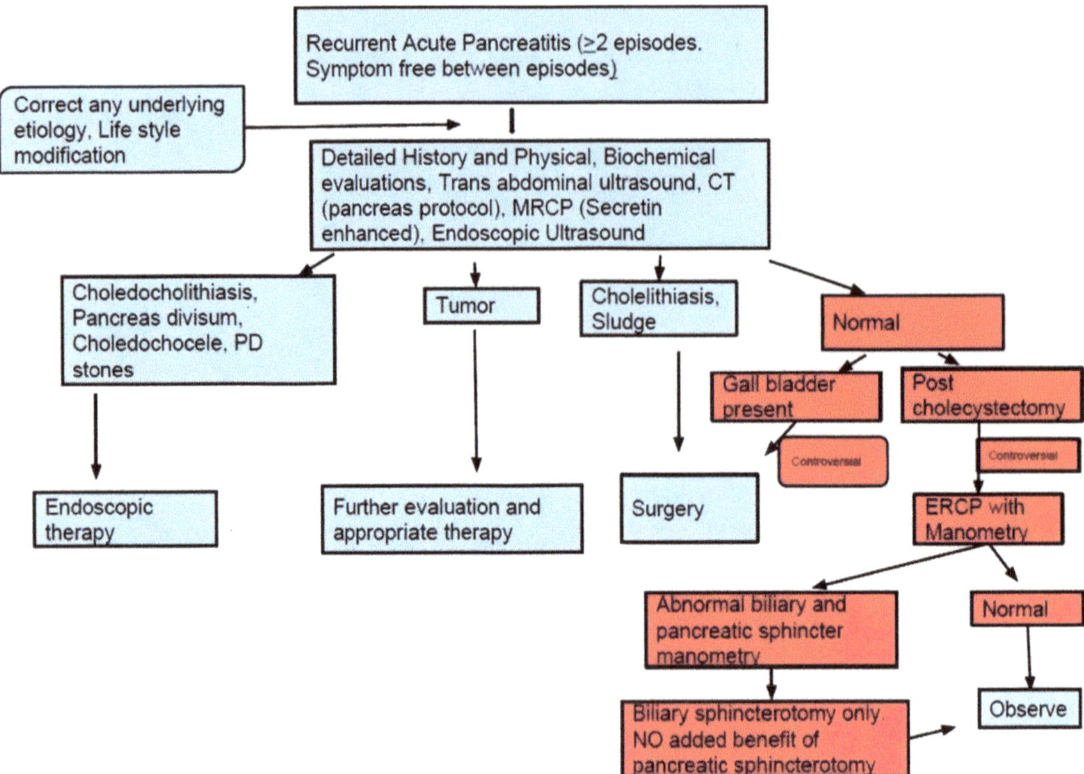

Figure 2. Algorithm for management of patients with recurrent acute pancreatitis. The work-up on the left (blue boxes) with less risky interventions has more proven benefits of its interventions than those on the right (red boxes). Adapted from Guda et al.[13]

further evaluation, as appropriate, should be performed. It might not be unreasonable to repeat endoscopic ultrasound or in appropriate circumstances offer other endoscopic/surgical interventions (**Figure 2**).

References

1. Etemad B, Whitcomb DC. Chronic pancreatitis: diagnosis, classification, and new genetic developments. *Gastroenterology*. 2001; 120(3): 682-707. PMID: 11179244.
2. Nøjgaard C, Becker U, Matzen P, Andersen JR, Holst C, Bendtsen F. Progression from acute to chronic pancreatitis: prognostic factors, mortality, and natural course. *Pancreas*. 2011; 40(8): 1195-1200. PMID: 21926938.
3. Yadav D, O'Connell M, Papachristou GI. Natural history following the first attack of acute pancreatitis. *Am J Gastroenterol*. 2012; 107(7): 1096-1103. PMID: 22613906.
4. Umapathy C, Raina A, Saligram S, Papachristou GI, Rabinovitz M, Chennat J, et al. 591b Natural History After Acute Necrotizing Pancreatitis (NP): A Large U.S. Tertiary Care Experience. *Gastroenterology*. 2015; 148(4): S-113-S-114.
5. Tsiotos GG, Luque-de Leon E, Sarr MG. Long-term outcome of necrotizing pancreatitis treated by necrosectomy. *Br J Surg*. 1998; 85(12): 1650-1653. PMID: 9876068.
6. Symersky T, van Hoorn B, Masclee AA. The outcome of a long-term follow-up of pancreatic function after recovery from acute pancreatitis. *JOP*. 2006; 7(5): 447-453. PMID: 16998241.
7. Lankisch PG, Breuer N, Bruns A, Weber-Dany B, Lowenfels AB, Maisonneuve P. Natural history of acute pancreatitis: a long-term population-based study. *Am J Gastroenterol*. 2009; 104(11): 2797-2805. PMID: 19603011.
8. Shelton CA, Whitcomb DC. Genetics and treatment options for recurrent acute and chronic pancreatitis. *Curr Treat Options Gastroenterol*. 2014; 12(3): 359-371. PMID: 24954874.
9. Cote GA, Imperiale TF, Schmidt SE, Fogel E, Lehman G, McHenry L, et al. Similar efficacies of biliary, with or without pancreatic, sphincterotomy in treatment of idiopathic recurrent acute pancreatitis. *Gastroenterology*. 2012; 143(6): 1502-1509 e1501. PMID: 22982183.
10. Bakman YG, Safdar K, Freeman ML. Significant clinical implications of prophylactic pancreatic stent placement in previously normal pancreatic ducts. *Endoscopy*. 2009; 41(12): 1095-1098. PMID: 19904701.
11. Romagnuolo J, Guda N, Freeman M, Durkalski V. Preferred designs, outcomes, and analysis strategies for treatment trials in idiopathic recurrent acute pancreatitis. *Gastrointest Endosc*. 2008; 68(5): 966-974. PMID: 18725158.
12. Yadav D, Slivka A, Sherman S, Hawes RH, Anderson MA, Burton FR, et al. Smoking is under recognized as a risk factor for chronic pancreatitis. *Pancreatology*. 2010; 10(6): 713-719. PMID: 21242712.
13. Guda NM, Romagnuolo J, Freeman ML. Recurrent and relapsing pancreatitis. *Curr Gastroenterol Rep*. 2011; 13(2): 140-149. PMID: 21286872.

Chapter 40

Clinical and laboratory diagnosis of chronic pancreatitis

J.-Matthias Löhr*

Gastrocentrum, Karolinska Institutet & Karolinska University Hospital, Stockholm, Sweden.

Introduction

Chronic pancreatitis (CP) is still far too rarely diagnosed as symptoms are nonspecific and training of physicians in clinical pancreatology is minimal.[1] With an incidence of 3-4/100,000 inhabitants and a prevalence of 10-40/100,000 inhabitants, CP is a relatively common disease in industrialized countries.[2] CP represents the far end of a disease continuum that begins with acute pancreatitis.[3] This chapter aims to cover the essentials of diagnosing CP and, at the same time, point to open issues for clinical research.

Clinical diagnosis

The clinical picture of CP can vary depending on the underlying etiology, the stage of disease, and the age of the patient.[4] The typical clinical picture of CP is that of a patient who, after years of alcohol abuse and smoking, and a history of recurrent abdominal pain, develops steatorrhea and general malnutrition. Together with weight loss and bloating, these are the four cardinal symptoms of CP and pancreatic exocrine insufficiency (**Table 1**). In the late phase, a diagnosis is easy to establish, as morphological changes can be readily seen with any kind of imaging.

The description of the clinical picture and the clinical diagnosis has not changed since the inaugural descriptions of Gülzow[5] and Amman.[6,7] Of the four cardinal symptoms, abdominal pain is the most prevalent, however it is a symptom common to a broad variety of diseases of the abdomen and beyond.[4,8] At later stages, pancreatic pain can become independent of the inflammatory process in the pancreas.[9]

The most important issue for the clinician is to think of the pancreas as a source of these symptoms. Once this connection is made, and appropriate laboratory tests (below) and imaging are done, the diagnosis of CP can be easily established – or disregarded.

In summary, there is no single symptom pathognomonic to CP, i.e., the diagnosis cannot be established solely on the basis of clinical symptoms. However, in the said enigmatic patient, the clinical diagnosis is still very likely.

On physical examination, signs may be subtle. Patients not reporting pain may have a tenderness of the abdomen to palpation. The head/body region of the pancreas can be easily palpated against the vertebrae. A special procedure involving deep palpation of the pancreas with the patient turned to the right side, more towards the spleen, (Mallet-Guy maneuver) may yield the only positive finding.[10] Palpable resistance stemming from pancreatic pseudocysts can be a typical finding (after an acute episode). In the case of (isolated) splenic vein thrombosis, an enlarged spleen (splenomegaly) can be palpated (also best in a position to the right). A rare but typical sign in patients with longstanding CP and pain may be marmorized skin on the abdomen, called *erythema ab igne*, which is the result of repetitive application of hot water bottles to the stomach in an effort to alleviate pain.[11] Other nonspecific indicators supporting the diagnosis include signs of nicotine abuse (coloring of fingers and sometimes the beard) or alcohol abuse (poor oral hygiene, *foetor ex ore*) as well as any sign of malnourishment pointing to malnutrition (e.g., low body mass index, thin skinfold, broken skin/nails, or perioral rhagadae).

Serum markers

Generic markers

The conventional markers of inflammation, i.e., elevated erythrocyte sedimentation rate and elevated leucocytes (WBC) are of no use in establishing the diagnosis of CP. Depending on the character of the respective disease form, stage, and time, these may or may not be elevated. As CP is a smoldering disease with subclinical inflammation progressing in the pancreas, ordinary serum markers of inflammation will not be elevated.

*Corresponding author. Email: matthias.lohr@ki.se

Table 1. Cardinal symptoms of CP

Abdominal pain
Loose stools/steatorrhea
Weight loss
Bloating

Pancreatic enzymes

Seventy-seven years ago, it was stated that "elevated amylase has become a cornerstone in the diagnosis of pancreatitis".[12] Although the specificity of both serum amylase and lipase for CP is acceptable, in the range of 90%–95%, their sensitivity is extremely low, varying around 10%. As a consequence, serum markers cannot be used to establish the diagnosis of CP. There are many possible reasons for elevated serum amylase and lipase levels, thus, elevated levels in patients with abdominal pain have a low specificity for chronic pancreatitis.[13] Serum elastase-1 is useful in acute pancreatitis[14] but has no better performance in CP.[15]

Plasma trypsin-like activity has been claimed to be a sensitive and specific marker for early (mild) CP; however, the only study in this patient population comprised 16 patients and had some methodological ambiguities.[16] Trypsinogen concentrations have also been suggested to be a good indicator for CP.[17] While plasma trypsin-like activity and trypsinogen concentrations are elevated in a quarter of patients with established CP, they seem to remain normal in early CP. While we could not demonstrate significant differences for absolute values of cationic (PRSS1) and anionic trypsinogen (PRSS2)[18] in AIP, CP and healthy controls, we found a change in the PRSS1:PRSS2 ratio. In healthy individuals (ratio 1:3) and in AIP (ratio 1:2) PRSS2 dominates.[18] In non-AIP CP.[17] the ratio is shifted towards PRSS1 (ratio 2:1).

If one reflects on how amylase, like any other digestive enzyme, reaches the circulation (serum),[19] its low specificity and sensitivity are not surprising. After massive damage of exocrine pancreatic tissue, leakage through dead cells causes serum levels to rise significantly; however, this condition is not indicative of CP, but rather acute pancreatitis.

Pancreatic enzymes below the lower level of normal (LLN) are routinely detected in patients with CP. If such LLN amylase is detected, advanced CP with significant, if not severe pancreatic exocrine insufficiency can be expected (20). However, newer studies comparing pancreatic enzyme serum levels with fecal elastase-1 (see below) and other pancreatic function tests are lacking.

Other promising markers such as pancreatic stone protein[21] and procarboxypeptidase B[22] have also not fulfilled their promise as sensitive markers for CP. None of the available evidence supports either a generic marker or use serum levels of pancreatic enzymes to establish the diagnosis of CP.

Table 2. Decreased serum components that can serve as markers of malnutrition

Prealbumin
Hemoglobulin
Retinol binding protein
Vitamin D (25-OH cholecalciferol)
Vitamin E (alpha-tocopherol)
Magnesium
Zinc

Markers of malnutrition

CP cannot be diagnosed with blood tests, but the resulting malnutrition can be diagnosed in cases where the patient with CP has already developed pancreatic exocrine insufficiency (PEI). In the field of malnutrition, a variety of serum parameters are established as markers of malnutrition (**Table 2**). They have proven useful in CP to predict PEI[23] and are correlated with other symptoms of malnutrition such as osteoporosis.[24]

Other markers

For the diagnosis of (chronic) pancreatitis, some other body fluids might be used. One would be pancreatic juice collected during ERCP or in the duodenum after stimulation by secretin injection. We attempted to describe markers in pancreatic juice samples, but could not detect any differences with high-resolution 2D-PAGE.[25] Cytological analysis does not reveal anything diagnostically relevant for establishing the diagnosis of CP, however, it may help in identifying individuals at risk of pancreatic cancer.[26]

Fecal elastase-1 (FE-1), a marker of PEI can also be measured. In itself, however, FE-1 is not specific, i.e., it cannot be used to establish the diagnosis of CP, but represents a screening test.[27] It is a rather crude marker, that if positive (below 200 ug/g), constitutes a diagnosis of PEI, and in so doing would confirm any sort of CP diagnosis. The threshold is under debate,[28] especially in patients not undergoing pancreatic surgery. However, a result of < 100 ug/g can safely be considered indicative of a significant, if not severe PEI according to the latest European guidelines.[29]

Conclusion

There are clinical symptoms indicative of CP, however none of them are specific or even pathognomonic. They should make a physician think of the pancreas as a source of the patient's symptoms. Laboratory tests are also indicative at best, as there is no positive test to confirm the diagnosis of CP. Very low (LLN) pancreatic serum enzymes can be a sign of significant PEI with CP as a major etiology. The same holds true for low fecal elastase as an indicator of PEI and with CP being the most frequent cause.

References

1. Schmid R. Pancreatologists: an endangered species? *Gastroenterology*. 2010; 138: 1236. PMID: 20175967.
2. Levy P, Dominguez-Munoz E, Imrie C, Löhr M, and Maisonneuve P. Epidemiology of chronic pancreatitis: burden of the disease and consequences. *United European Gastroenterol J*. 2014; 2: 345-354, 2014. PMID: 25360312.
3. Klöppel G and Maillet B. The morphological basis for the evolution of acute pancreatitis into chronic pancreatitis. *Virch Arch A*. 1992; 420: 1-4. PMID: 1539444.
4. Di Lorenzo C, Colletti RB, Lehmann HP, Boyle JT, Gerson WT, Hyams JS, et al. Chronic Abdominal Pain In Children: a Technical Report of the American Academy of Pediatrics and the North American Society for Pediatric Gastroenterology, Hepatology and Nutrition. *J Pediatr Gastroenterol Nutr*. 2005; 40: 249-261. PMID: 15735476.
5. Gülzow M. Erkrankungen des exkretorischen Pankreas. In: *Erkrankungen des exkretorischen Pankreas*. Jena, VEB Gustav Fischer; 1975.
6. Ammann RW. Zur Klinik und Differentialdiagnose der chronischen Pankreatitis. *Dtsch Med Wchnschr*. 1980; 110: 1322-1327. PMID: 7003706.
7. Ammann RW, Akovbiantz A, Largiader F, and Schueler G. Course and outcome of chronic pancreatitis. Longitudinal study of a mixed medical-surgical series of 245 patients. *Gastroenterology*. 1984; 86: 820-828. PMID: 6706066.
8. Natesan S, Lee J, Volkamer H, and Thoureen T. Evidence-Based Medicine Approach to Abdominal Pain. *Emerg Med Clin North Am*. 2016; 34: 165-190. PMID: 27133239.
9. Ceyhan GO, Michalski CW, Demir IE, Muller MW, and Friess H. Pancreatic pain. *Best Pract Res Clin Gastroenterol*. 2008; 22: 31-44. PMID: 18206811.
10. Lankisch PG. Klinik und Prognose der chronischen Pankreatitis. In: *Erkrankungen des exkretorischen Pankreas*. Mössner J, Adler G, Fölsch UR, and Singer MV. Jena, Gustav Fischer; 1995: 334-339.
11. Mok DW and Blumgart LH. Erythema ab igne in chronic pancreatic pain: a diagnostic sign. *J R Soc Med*. 1984; 77: 299-301. PMID: 6232383.
12. Elman R, Arneson N, and Graham EA. Value of blood amylase estimations in the diagnosis of pancreatic disease. *Arch Surg*. 1929; 19: 943-967.
13. Frulloni L, Patrizi F, Bernardoni L and Cavallini G. Pancreatic hyperenzymemia: clinical significance and diagnostic approach. *JOP*. 2005; 6: 536-551. PMID: 16286704.
14. Wilson RB, Warusavitarne J, Crameri DM, Alvaro F, Davies DJ, and Merrett N. Serum elastase in the diagnosis of acute pancreatitis: a prospective study. *ANZ J Surg*. 2005; 75: 152-156. PMID: 15777396.
15. Gunkel U, Bitterlich N, and Keim V. Value of combinations of pancreatic function tests to predict mild or moderate chronic pancreatitis. *Z Gastroenterol*. 2001; 39: 207-211. PMID: 11324137.
16. Hernandez CA, Nicolas JC, Fernandez J, and Pizarro P. Determination of plasma trypsin-like activity in healthy subjects, patients with mild to moderate alcoholic chronic pancreatitis, and patients with nonjaundice pancreatic cancer. *Dig Dis Sci*. 2005; 50: 2165-2169. PMID: 16240234.
17. Rinderknecht H, Stace NH, and Renner IG. Effects of chronic alcohol abuse on exocrine pancreatic secretion in man. *Dig Dis Sci*. 1985; 30: 65-71. PMID: 3965275.
18. Löhr JM, Faissner R, Koczan D, Bewerunge P, Bassi C, Brors B, et al. Autoantibodies against the exocrine pancreas in autoimmune pancreatitis: gene and protein expression profiling and immunoassays identify pancreatic enzymes as a major target of the inflammatory process. *Am J Gastroenterol*. 2010; 105: 2060-2071. PMID: 20407433.
19. Rohr G. Entry of pancreatic enzymes into the circulation. In: *Diagnostic procedures in pancreatic disease*. Ditschuneit H. Berlin, Springer; 1986: 63-66.
20. Malferteiner P and Glasbrenner B. Exokrine Pankreasfunktionstests. In: *Erkrankungen des exkretorischen Pankreas*. Mössner J, Adler G, Fölsch R, and Singer MV. Jena/Stuttgart, G. Fischer Verlag; 1995: 147-159.
21. Schmiegel W, Burchert M, Kalthoff H, Roeder C, Butzow G, Grimm H, et al. Immunochemical characterization and quantitative distribution of pancreatic stone protein in sera and pancreatic secretions in pancreatic disorders. *Gastroenterology*. 1990; 99: 1421-1430. PMID: 1698685.
22. Printz H, Siegmund H, Wojte C, Schafer C, Hesse H, Rothmund M, et al. "Human pancreas-specific protein" (procarboxypeptidase B): a valuable marker in pancreatitis? *Pancreas*. 1995; 10: 222-230. PMID: 7624299.
23. Lindkvist B, Dominguez-Munoz JE, Luaces-Regueira M, Castineiras-Alvarino M, Nieto-Garcia L, and Iglesias-Garcia J. Serum nutritional markers for prediction of pancreatic exocrine insufficiency in chronic pancreatitis. *Pancreatology*. 2012; 12: 305-310. PMID: 22898630.
24. Haas SL, Krins S, and Löhr JM. Altered bone metabolism and bone density in patients with chronic pancreatitis and pancreatic exocrine insufficiency. *JOP*. 2015; 16: 58-62. PMID: 25640785.
25. Wandschneider S, Fehring V, Jacobs-Emeis S, Thiesen HJ, and Löhr M. Autoimmune pancreatic disease: preparation of pancreatic juice for proteome analysis. *Electrophoresis*. 2001; 22: 4383-4390. PMID: 11824606.
26. Löhr M, Müller P, Mora J, Brinkmann B, Ostwald C, Farre A, et al. p53 and K-ras mutations in pancreatic juice samples from patients with chronic pancreatitis. *Gastrointest Endosc*. 2001; 53: 734-743. PMID: 11375580.
27. Domingues-Munoz JE, Frulloni L, Hardt P, Lerch MM, Levy P, and Löhr JM. Potential for screening for chronic pancreatitis and pancreatic exocrine insufficiency using the faecal elastase-1 test. *Pancreatology* in press, 2016.
28. Benini L, Amodio A, Campagnola P, Agugiaro F, Cristofori C, Micciolo R, et al. Fecal elastase-1 is useful in the detection of steatorrhea in patients with pancreatic diseases but not after pancreatic resection. *Pancreatology*. 2013; 13: 38-42. PMID: 23395568.
29. HaPanEU. (2016) The UEG Evidence-based guidelines for the diagnosis and therapy of chronic pancreatitis. *United European Gastroenterol J*. in press.

Chapter 41

Imaging in chronic pancreatitis

Raju Sharma* and Devasenathipathy Kandasamy

Department of Radiodiagnosis, All India Institute of Medical Science, New Delhi 110029.

Introduction

Pancreatitis is the most common benign condition affecting the pancreas, and it occurs in two forms—acute and chronic—characterized by different clinical, morphological and histological features.[1] Chronic pancreatitis (CP) is characterized by progressive inflammation and fibrosis of the pancreas leading to irreversible structural changes that cause both endocrine and exocrine dysfunction. The hallmarks of CP include abdominal pain, malabsorption, malnutrition, diabetes, and pancreatic calcification. Currently there is no effective medical treatment, especially when it is first recognized at a late stage. Early detection of this condition may prevent further progression of the disease process. Diagnosis and evaluation of CP can be quite challenging, and usually needs a battery of tests. Endoscopic retrograde cholangio-pancreatography (ERCP) was previously considered as the gold standard for the diagnosis of CP, but today other modalities such as ultrasonography (US), computed tomography (CT), magnetic resonance imaging (MRI) and endoscopic ultrasound (EUS) are used to evaluate the structural changes of the parenchyma and pancreatic duct. Furthermore, many indirect and direct methods are available to evaluate exocrine function. Fecal elastase 1 (FE 1) is a frequently used indirect assay that is easy to perform but has low sensitivity, and its utility in diagnosing CP is controversial.[2-4] The tubed secretin test is a direct method that involves prolonged intubation and serial collection of pancreatic juice after hormonal stimulation. In spite of many issues with this technique, it is considered as a reference standard for the evaluation of pancreatic exocrine function.[5,6] Secretin-enhanced magnetic resonance cholangio-pancreatography (S-MRCP), in which secretin is used to stimulate secretion of pancreatic juice is emerging as a one-stop-shop modality for the evaluation of both structural and functional status in CP.[5] Advances in MRI technique allow using diffusion-weighted imaging (DWI) and apparent diffusion coefficient (ADC) to study the microscopic diffusion of water molecules. This gives a unique insight into the characteristics of pancreas tissue that will be discussed later in this chapter.[7-9]

Etiopathogenesis of CP

Alcohol abuse is a common causes of CP, accounting for up to 90% of cases in western countries.[9] Other factors in addition to alcohol, such as cigarette smoking, genetic predisposition, and a high protein diet are also thought to play an important causative role.[10] Pancreatic or periampullary neoplasms, sphincter of Oddi dysfunction, ampullary stricture, and congenital lesions such as abnormal pancreaticobiliary junction and pancreatic divisum are also important causes of CP. Hereditary pancreatitis is a rare form of CP caused by trypsinogen gene mutation. Other causes of CP include hypercalcemia, hyperparathyroidism and chronic renal failure.

Autoimmune pancreatitis (AIP) is an unusual and distinct form of CP which will be discussed later in the chapter.

Imaging Modalities

Various imaging modalities are available for the diagnosis of CP, each of which has unique advantages and limitations. No single modality provides all the desired information.

Abdominal Radiographs

Decades ago, before the advent of cross sectional modalities, the imaging diagnosis of CP was based on plain radiography. CP is manifested on abdominal radiographs as multifocal calcifications in the epigastric region (**Figure 1a**). These calcifications are typically seen across the spine

*Corresponding author. Email: raju152@yahoo.com

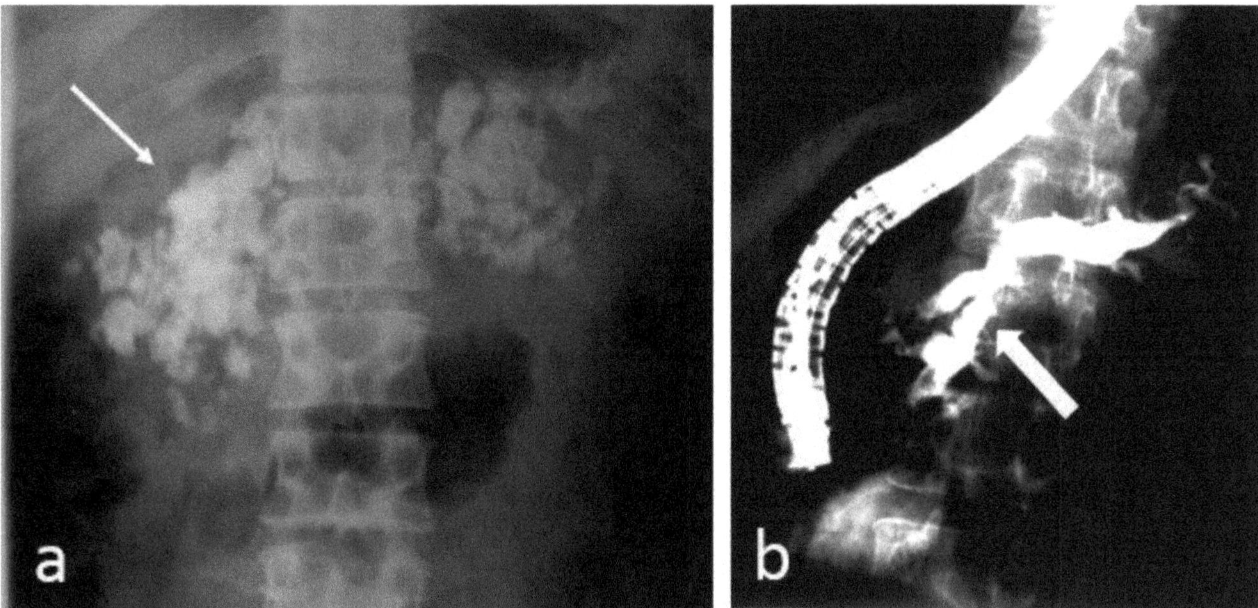

Figure 1. Abdominal radiograph in AP projection showing (a) multiple well defined calcific opacities (thin arrow) seen along the expected course of pancreas on either side of the spine and suggestive of pancreatic calcification. ERCP image of a different patient showing (b) dilated and tortuous MPD and its side branches (thick arrow). These findings are suggestive of chronic pancreatitis.

along the course of pancreas. Since calcifications are usually seen in advanced cases and only in certain types of CP, radiographs have low, sensitivity (30 to 70%).[9] Although the calcifications are specific they have to be differentiated from calcifications due to other causes and in overlying organs. Because of these limitations, abdominal radiographs are not routinely used to evaluate CP. Radiographs are often used in this setting to rule out other causes of abdominal pain.

ERCP

ERCP is considered as the gold standard for the diagnosis of CP because of its superior spatial resolution and its ability to depict side-branch abnormalities in early CP. It has an added advantage of therapeutic intervention whenever needed. Its limitations are the invasive nature of the procedure and procedure-related complications. Since the advent of MRCP, which is a noninvasive technique, the popularity of ERCP for diagnostic evaluation has considerably decreased.[11] However, ERCP has the advantage of showing the ductal system in a distended state, which is very helpful in detecting subtle lesions such as pancreatic divisum. The diameter of the normal main pancreatic duct (MPD) varies with the region of pancreas, from 3 to 4 mm in the head to 2 to 3 mm in the body, and 1 to 2 mm in the tail region.[9] Multiple side branches are seen to join the MPD at right angles in alternating fashion. The earliest features of CP may be seen only on ERCP as irregularity and dilatation of side branches. These changes can become more severe along with dilatation, loss of normal tapering, and irregularity of the MPD as the disease progresses (**Figure 1b**). Alternate dilatation and stenosis of the MPD can give the appearance of a chain of lakes with intraductal calculi seen as filling defects. ERCP is also helpful in diagnosing other obstructive causes of CP such as ampullary lesions, intraductal neoplasms, and congenital anomalies such as pancreatic divisum. The Cambridge Classification of CP is based on ERCP and is used to group patients into equivocal, mild, moderate, or marked types. The status of the MPD and side branches, presence of calculi, and ductal strictures are taken in to account in the Cambridge Classification.[12]

AIP unlike other forms of CP shows focal, segmental, or diffuse narrowing of MPD and nonvisualization of side branches on ERCP.[13] Narrowing can also be seen in the lower end of the common bile duct (CBD) causing biliary dilatation. AIP may be associated with primary sclerosing cholangitis, which is seen as multifocal narrowing in more proximal biliary ducts.

Ultrasonography (US)

Sonography of the pancreas is challenging because of its retroperitoneal location and overlapping bowel loops. It is also dependent on the body habitus of the patient and the skill of the operator. Various maneuvers such as changing the position of patient, distending the stomach with

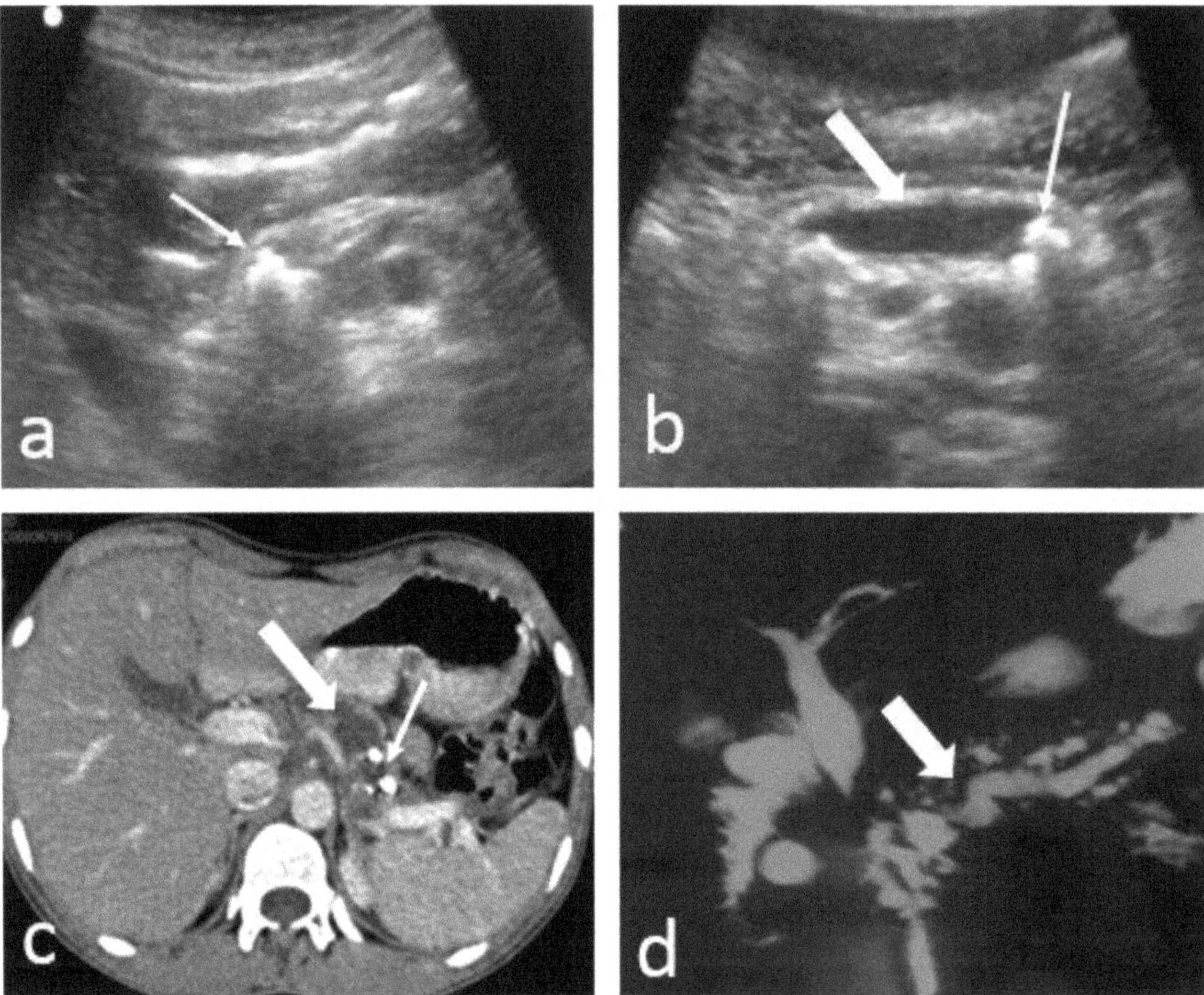

Figure 2. Transabdominal sonography images showing (a,b) calcification (thin arrow) in the head and tail of pancreas with dilated MPD (thick arrow). Axial contrast enhanced CT image showing (c) multiple intraductal calcifications (thin arrow) and dilated MPD (thick arrow). Heavily T2W thick-slab MRCP image showing (d) irregularly dilated MPD and its side branches (thick arrow). A small fluid collection is seen in the region of head of pancreas, and the common bile duct is dilated untill the lower end, with smooth tapering suggestive of benign stricture. The above findings are typical of chronic calcific pancreatitis (CCP).

water and using the spleen as a window to visualize the tail of pancreas may be necessary to image the pancreas in its entirety. In spite of the above limitations, US is still the first-line modality for the evaluation of abdominal pain because of its easy availability, relatively low cost, and lack of ionizing radiation. Pancreatic evaluation is done in the fasting state to avoid bowel gas obscuring the visualization.

The normal pancreas is iso- or hyperechogenic compared with the normal liver, and progressive fatty replacement can occur with age.[14] In the early stage of CP, the pancreas loses its hyperechogenicity and becomes heterogeneous because of focal inflammation. With progression from moderate to severe disease, the changes become more prominent, and they are appreciable in up to 70% of patients.[15,16] In late-stage disease, changes in the form of an irregular, dilated MPD with pancreatic and intraductal calculi and associated atrophy of pancreas are striking, and are characteristic of CP.[16,17] (**Figure 2a,b**). US can also show collections or pseudocysts around the pancreas and occasional focal pancreatic lesions that are responsible for the development of obstructive types of CP.

Elastography is a novel method to evaluate tissue hardness. It can be used to determine the extent of organ involvement in CP and also to evaluate the extent of fibrosis, which can be a prognostic indicator in patients undergoing surgical procedures. Elastography can be used along with transabdominal and endoscopic US. Two types of

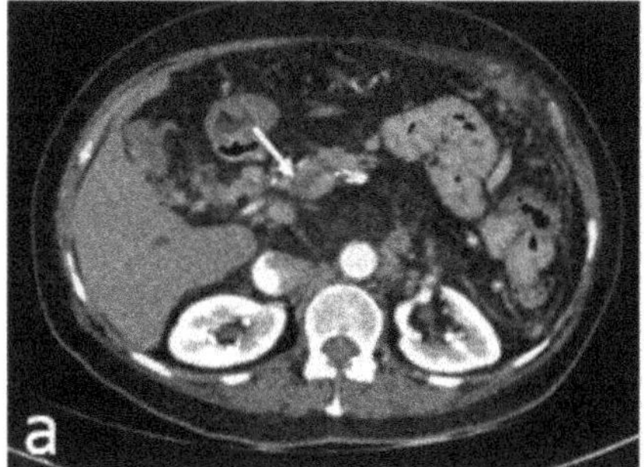

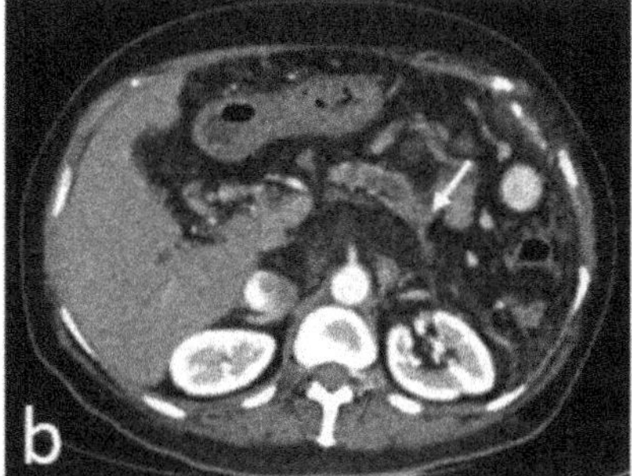

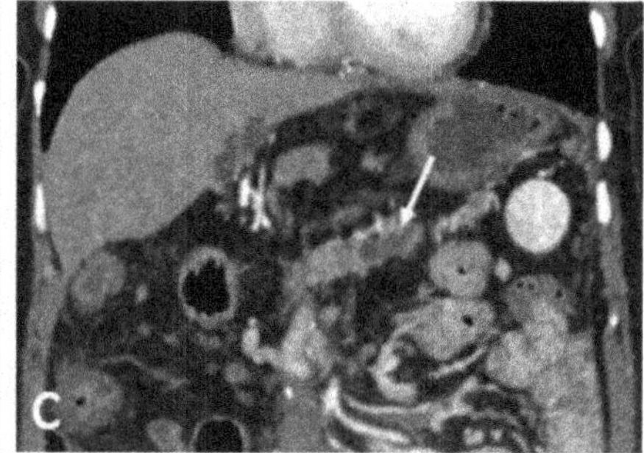

Figure 3. Contrast enhanced CT in axial (a,b) and coronal plane (c) in a patient with chronic pancreatitis show that the pancreatic parenchyma is atrophied and the MPD is dilated (arrow). In this patient, calcifications are conspicuously absent.

elastography are commercially available.[14] The first is strain imaging, which qualitatively evaluates the tissue strain in response to an exogenous acoustic pulse. The second is shearwave elastography, which quantitatively evaluates tissue hardness based on the velocity of shear waves in the tissues. In both methods, an elastogram is represented as a color map superimposed over B-mode images.

Computed Tomography (CT)

Wider availability and technical advances in the past two decades have made CT the imaging modality of choice for the evaluation of CP. The pancreatic calcifications that are crucial for clinching the diagnosis of CP are best seen on CT (**Figure 2c**). CT is sensitive to even small punctate calcifications, which can be missed by other imaging modalities.

However, lack of information on the exocrine function of pancreas, limited contrast resolution, and exposure to radiation are the most important limitations of CT. The complete evaluation of CP on CT is optimally done using a multiphase protocol that includes an unenhanced scan, a pancreatic phase scan, and a venous phase scan.

Pancreatic parenchymal and intraductal calcifications are detected on unenhanced scans. Detection of arterial complications and arterial mapping as a part of surgical planning is done using the pancreatic phase scan. Evaluation of pancreatic parenchyma and ducts, pseudocysts, and focal lesions is done on venous phase scans.

On CT, normal pancreas is seen as a homogeneous structure with smooth, lobulated borders. Any inflammation of the pancreas leads to focal or diffuse hypodensity and stranding of surrounding fat. The characteristic features of CP are atrophy of pancreas (54%), ductal dilatation (up to 68%), and multiple parenchymal and intraductal calcifications (50%).[18] The pancreatic head is the most common location of parenchymal calcifications. Calcifications can vary in size and morphology, and the degree of calcification is directly proportional to the duration of the disease.[9,19] Calcifications are seen earlier in alcoholic CP and some hereditary forms of pancreatitis compared with obstructive CP. Calcification appears in 20 to 40% of patients with alcohol-related CP, usually after 5 to 10 years.[20] The MPD shows segments of stenosis alternating with dilatations containing multiple calculi of varying size and irregular morphology.

In patients with cystic fibrosis having CFTR mutations, calcifications appear late and are smaller than those seen in other genetic mutation-related CP.[21] Stones in genetic mutation-related CP other than cystic fibrosis are usually round or oval in shape and measure more than 2 to 3 cm.[20] On CT they have a typical "bulls-eye" appearance with a hypodense center and hyperdense periphery due to a lack of calcium in the center.[20,22,23] These stones are usually arranged linearly within the dilated MPD.[24] The presence of multiple, large round-to-oval bulls-eye stones should point towards a diagnosis of CP secondary to genetic mutation. Tropical pancreatitis, which is predominantly a disease of developing countries, also presents with parenchymal atrophy (50%), ductal dilatation, and large calculi (80%) that can reach up to 5 cm in size and can extend into side branches.[13,25,26] This finding contrasts with alcoholic CP, in which the calcifications are small and speckled. In this scenario, CT has an edge over MRI in giving a specific diagnosis.

In patients with obstructive CP the MPD is dilated, but parenchymal or intraductal calcifications are usually not seen, differentiating it from other nonobstructive causes.[27] Ductal dilatation is best seen on venous phase after administration of contrast that makes the hypodense MPD stand out against the enhanced parenchyma. In the early stage of CP, changes in the MPD and side branches are not noticeable on CT, and the contrast enhancement is also relatively homogeneous. With disease progression, multifocal fibrotic changes lead to heterogeneity of enhancement. The normal parenchyma enhances earlier in the venous phase whereas the fibrotic areas show delayed enhancement. Progressive fibrosis causes atrophy of the parenchyma and ductal dilatation (**Figure 3**). Another important role of CT is to evaluate the cause of obstructive CP. Focal lesions such as pancreatic adenocarcinoma, periampullary carcinoma, and

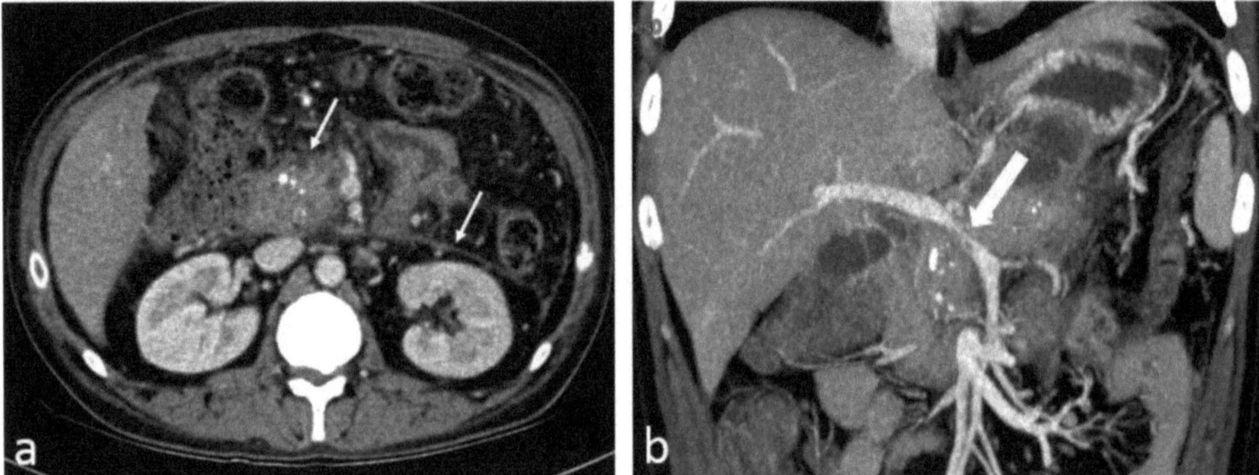

Figure 4. Contrast enhanced CT images in axial plane (a) and thin maximum intensity projection in coronal plane (b) of a patient with CCP who presented with acute abdominal pain showing features of CCP as evidenced by the presence of multiple calcific densities distributed throughout the pancreas. In addition, there is marked fat stranding and fascial thickening (thin arrow) seen around the pancreas. There is pressure effect seen over the main portal vein (thick arrow) caused by the inflamed pancreas. These findings are suggestive of acute exacerbation of CCP.

rarely, nonfunctioning neuroendocrine tumors can lead to MPD obstruction and cause repeated attacks of pancreatitis that eventually present as CP. Cystic tumors of the pancreas, including serous, mucinous, and intraductal tumors, can also cause obstructive forms of CP. CT is very helpful in characterizing these solid tumors and, to some extent, cystic tumors. Pancreatic divisum is a common congenital cause of CP for which the imaging modality of choice is MRI. However, in advanced stages, CT can recognize the changes due to pancreatic divisum. The characteristic inflammatory, fibrotic and ductal changes are limited to the dorsal pancreas, whereas the ventral pancreas appears normal.[28] Rarely, duodenal dystrophy, which is thought to be due to the presence of ectopic pancreatic tissue in the duodenal wall, can be the cause of CP. Recurrent inflammation leads to fibrosis and cyst formation in the duodenal wall, leading to MPD compression and an obstructive type of CP that can be recognized on CT. On contrast enhanced CT (CECT), the fibrotic area enhances late in the delayed phase compared with the rest of the normal pancreas. If the lesion is predominantly solid, then it can mimic pancreatic adenocarcinoma. Since it is primarily a duodenal pathology, the mass effect causes shifting of gastroduodenal artery to the left. A mass in the primary head of pancreas, such as adenocarcinoma, causes the artery to shift to the right. In equivocal cases, sampling will clinch the diagnosis.[29]

CT can be used to evaluate complications related to CP. One of the most important complications is the formation of pseudocysts, which are cystic lesions with a wall and are usually well defined. They occur in up to 25% of cases of CP,[9] and they can be seen in the peripancreatic region, intraperitoneal or retroperitoneal, or even in remote locations such as the chest. In CP, pseudocysts are generally formed during the evolution of peripancreatic fluid that collects after an episode of pancreatitis. Pseudocysts are closely mimicked by retention cysts that occur in the pancreas as a result of MPD or side branch obstruction by calculi, or as a result of fibrosis.[20] The resulting cystic lesions are seen on CT as nonenhancing, well defined lesions, and they are not usually associated with an acute episode of pancreatitis. Pseudocysts, along with peripancreatic inflammation, can involve venous structures in the vicinity, leading to phlebitis and thrombosis. These complications can be seen in the splenic, superior mesenteric, and portal veins on contrast enhanced CT as filling defects or occlusions (**Figure 4**). The resulting portal hypertension, which is usually limited to left side, can lead to the development of multiple collaterals. When the inflammation involves arteries in the vicinity, it can cause pseudoaneurysm. In CP, the gastroduodenal, pancreaticoduodenal, and splenic arteries are the ones most often involved. The affected arteries can rupture and bleed into the peritoneal cavity, bowel, or biliary system, which may present as an acute emergency. Sometimes they are detected on routine imaging, in which case they have to be treated immediately to prevent catastrophic complications. Pseudoaneurysms are best seen on arterial phase CT scan when the concentration of contrast in the arteries is at its peak. They can be missed on routine portal venous scan, which makes the arterial phase acquisition important in this situation. In CP, pancreatic fistula can develop within the peritoneal or even the pleural cavity[30] secondary to rupture of a pseudocyst. On CT they are seen as ascites or pleural effusion, however the actual fistula site may not be demonstrated on CT scans. Biliary complications due to CP can manifest as fistulae or inflammatory strictures that are better evaluated by MRCP. The risk of pancreatic adenocarcinoma, which is a dreaded complication, is increased in CP, especially in hereditary and tropical CP. In patients with CP, pancreatic carcinoma can mimic inflammatory mass-forming CP, focal AIP, or groove pancreatitis. Reliable distinction between these lesions on imaging is quite challenging and is not always possible. Advances in CT techniques in the form of perfusion CT have added another dimension to the diagnostic capability of CT scanners. Perfusion CT is a novel technique in which scans of a particular area are acquired in quick succession. The data collected is post processed and the contrast dynamics of the given area are depicted as color coded maps. Perfusion parameters such as blood flow and blood volume can be quantified. There are promising reports in which researchers have used perfusion CT to differentiate pancreatic carcinoma from mass forming chronic pancreatitis.[31]

Magnetic Resonance Imaging (MRI)

MRI is a noninvasive imaging modality for biliary and pancreatic pathology, and can accurately characterize various pancreatic lesions. MRCP has replaced ERCP for the diagnostic imaging of biliary and pancreatic ducts. It is a specialized MR technique in which heavily T2 weighted sequences are used to image fluid filled structures without a need for contrast agent (**Figure 2d**). MR has the additional advantage of having excellent contrast resolution without using ionizing radiation. Normal pancreas appears hyperintense on T1 weighted sequences with or without fat saturation. It is the most T1 hyperintense structure in the abdomen with the exception of fatty liver.[32] The hyperintensity of the pancreas is due to the presence of proteinaceous secretions within the gland. T1 fat-saturated sequences are very sensitive for the identification of any focal lesions within the pancreas, as many of the focal lesions appear hypointense and are easily recognized. Similarly, any inflammation in the pancreas leads to a drop in signal on T1 weighted sequences. In the early stages of CP, because of the inflammation and onset of fibrosis there is a drop in the T1 signal.[33] The gland may be heterogeneous because of focal areas of inflammation and fibrosis. There is heterogeneous and delayed enhancement in the post contrast images because of fibrosis, and this delayed enhancement, compared with the normal pancreas is considered as an early marker of CP.[34]

Ductal changes are better visualized on MRCP than on CT; however, subtle side branch changes can be missed.[35] The ductal findings of early disease can range from normal looking MPD to mild irregularity of the MPD and side branches. With progression of disease there is progressive glandular atrophy, poor enhancement in portal venous phase, and increased enhancement in delayed phase.

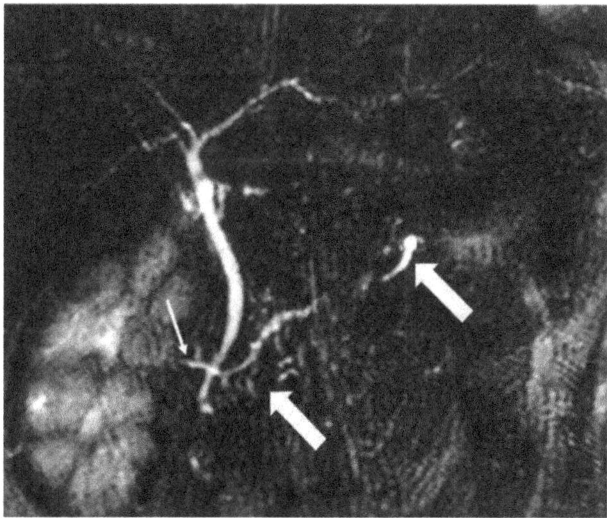

Figure 5. T2W thick-slab MRCP image of a young male patient who presented with multiple episodes of abdominal pain showing the dorsal pancreatic duct draining separately in to the minor papilla (thin arrow). There is no communication with the ventral duct, which is suggestive of pancreatic divisum. In addition, there is mild dilatation of the dorsal duct in the tail region and side branches in the head region (thick arrow). These findings favor the diagnosis of pancreatic divisum with chronic pancreatitis.

Severe ductal changes in the form of irregular dilatation of both the MPD and side branches along with interposed strictures give the appearance of chain of lakes on MRCP. MR is also good at visualizing associated complications such as pseudocysts and fistulae. Intraductal calcifications are seen as filling defects against the hyperintense background of fluid. The sensitivity of MR for small calcifications is limited when compared to CT, but MR can also detect ductal abnormalities such as pancreatic divisum and any solid or cystic focal lesion causing obstructive type CP (**Figure 5**).

MR can also differentiate CP from mimics such as intraductal papillary mucinous neoplasms (IPMN) and variants such as groove pancreatitis and AIP.

Even on MRI, it is challenging to differentiate masses of chronic pancreatitis from pancreatic adenocarcinoma. Duct penetrating sign on MRCP indicating that a normal or smoothly stenotic MPD is seen to penetrate the mass, has been reported to be associated with inflammatory masses rather than carcinoma. It has a reported sensitivity of 85% and specificity of 96%.[36] Recently, diffusion weighted imaging (DWI) has been used to accurately differentiate mass-forming pancreatitis from carcinoma.[37] The role of flurodeoxyglucose-positron emission tomography (FDG-PET) in this scenario is controversial.[38,39]

A major limitation of MRCP in the evaluation of CP is the lack of functional information and inability to image the ductal system when it is distended. This drawback can be overcome by using secretin and acquiring serial MR images, which is known as secretin enhanced MRCP or secretin stimulated MRCP (S-MRCP). Secretin is an amino acid polypeptide normally secreted by the duodenal mucosa. It acts primarily on the pancreas and to some extent on the biliary tree,[7] causing transient increase in the tone of the sphincter of Oddi and increased secretion of bicarbonate-rich fluid. Secretin is a safe drug, and it can be administered easily without any serious side effects. Patients should be fasting for 4 to 6 hours, and are given oral negative contrast 30 minutes before the study to suppress signals from pre-existing fluid in the duodenum. Following baseline imaging, secretin is injected as a slow intravenous injection to prevent side effects. After injection, T2 weighted images are acquired every 30 seconds for 15 minutes. This leads to the dilatation of MPD, which peaks at 2 to 5 minutes, after which the sphincteric tone decreases; the MPD diameter returns to baseline after 10 minutes. The pancreatic secretions can be seen in the duodenum and can be graded quantitatively or semiquatitatively to indicate the exocrine function of the pancreas.[6] The MPD should increase least 1 mm in diameter compared to baseline in patients with a normal sphincter. Absence of increase implies impaired ductal compliance.[7] In normal pancreas the side branches are not visualized after secretin administration, whereas in patients with early CP because of subtle fibrosis the side branches can show dilatation which are not otherwise seen on conventional MRCP.[7] This is an important advantage of S-MRCP, as it distends the MPD, showing even subtle abnormalities better than ERCP can. For the same reason it is superior to conventional MRCP in delineating ductal anomalies such as pancreas divisum. Exocrine function can be graded as follows. Fluid confined to the duodenal bulb is grade 1. Fluid confined to first and second part of duodenum is grade 2, and fluid reaching into the third part is grade 3. Grade 3 is considered normal, grades 1 and 2 are considered to result from impaired exocrine function. This grading is consistently correlated with fecal elastase 1 values.[6] Thus S-MRCP can provide both structural and functional information that is crucial for the management of these patients. The apparent diffusion coefficient (ADC), derived from diffusion weighted imaging (DWI) is also used to evaluate CP. The ADC of the pancreas in patients with CP was found to be lower than that in normal patients. This occurs because decreased exocrine reserve of the pancreas leads to decreased water diffusion and because fibrosis can by itself restrict diffusion. ADC values can potentially be used as an indicator of fibrosis and its extent in patients with CP, and can be used to predict outcomes of patients who undergo surgery. Furthermore, DWI has been combined with S-MRCP to study the increase in ADC following administration of secretin, which increases secretion and hence promotes water diffusion. In normal pancreas, the ADC is expected to increase in the early part of the S-MRCP procedure, but in high-risk patients and in those with CP, the expected ADC peak may either be delayed or not occur at all.[40] This has potential for quantification of pancreatic exocrine function in clinical practice in the future.

Miscellaneous Types of Chronic Pancreatitis

Autoimmune Pancreatitis (AIP)

AIP is an unusual type of CP, also known as lymphoplasmacytic sclerosing pancreatitis or chronic sclerosing pancreatitis, and is thought to reflect pancreatic involvement in IgG4 systemic disease. It is a systemic chronic fibroinflammatory disease that can affect other organs such as the biliary duct (primary sclerosing cholangitis), salivary glands, retroperitoneum (retroperitoneal fibrosis), mesentery (sclerosing mesenteritis), and bowel (inflammatory bowel disease). AIP constitutes around 1.8 to 11% of all cases of chronic pancreatitis.[13] On histology, lymphoplasmacytic infiltration is seen around the veins and ducts, sparing the arterioles.[41,42] It can be differentiated from other types of pancreatitis and focal lesions by immunostaining with IgG4. Because of variations in diagnostic criteria, the diagnosis of AIP is not uniform among different countries. Based on the current understanding, AIP has two distinct subtypes.[43,44] Type 1 is known as lymphoplasmacytic sclerosing pancreatitis (LPSP), which is characterized by elevated serum IgG4 levels, abundant infiltration of IgG4-positive cells, and extrapancreatic involvement. Type 2 is known as idiopathic duct-centric pancreatitis (IDCP), which is characterized by the presence of granulocyte epithelial lesions (GEL). Unlike Type 1, IDCP usually does not have elevated serum levels of IgG4 and infiltration of IgG4-positive cells. In addition, extrapancreatic involvement is not seen in IDCP, except for possible association with inflammatory bowel disease.

Imaging plays a crucial role in the evaluation of AIP and detection of associated extrapancreatic manifestations of IgG4 disease. The Japan Pancreatic Society criteria are often used to diagnose AIP, and are based on imaging features supported by either positive serology or histopathology.[45] The Mayo Clinic HISORt criteria are based on typical imaging features, histology, serology, involvement of other organs, and response to steroid therapy, are also widely accepted.[46] In 2011, the international consensus diagnostic criteria (ICDC) were developed using various existing and commonly applied criteria.[47] The ICDC is considered to be the most sensitive and specific scoring system for diagnosing AIP.[48] It is based on the imaging features of pancreatic parenchyma, ducts, serology, involvement of other organs, histology, and response to steroid therapy. CT scan is the diagnostic modality of choice, three distinct patterns (diffuse, focal, and multifocal) have been described

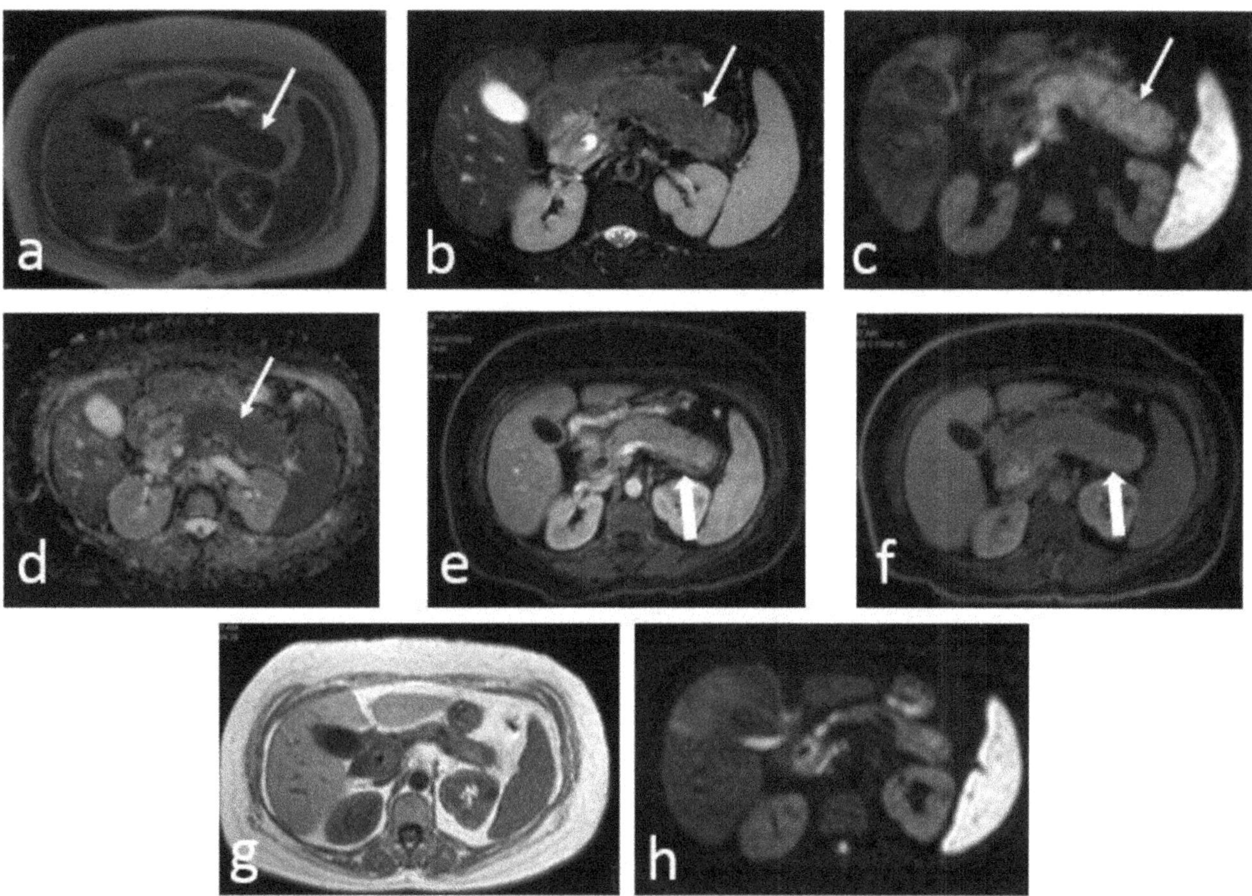

Figure 6. T1W axial MR image showing (a) hypointense and swollen pancreas with loss of normal peripheral lobulations (thin arrow). The tail of the pancreas shows a rounded contour. T2W image with fat suppression showing (b) a swollen pancreas with a hypointense peripheral rim. Intrapancreatic CBD is dilated with a stent in situ. Diffusion weighted image with b value of 800 showing (c) diffuse hyperintensity of pancreas. ADC map (d) at the same level shows hypointensity suggestive of diffusion restriction. Post-contrast image in pancreatic phase (e) shows diffusely hypoenhancing pancreas with a hypointense rim (thick arrow). In the delayed phase image (f) the peripheral rim is retaining contrast, suggesting its fibrous nature. Based on these findings and elevated serum IgG4 levels, a diagnosis of autoimmune pancreatitis was made, and the patient was treated with corticosteroids. The patient's symptoms resolved, and follow-up images after three months (g, h) show both significant reduction in the size of the pancreas and normalization of diffusion.

on imaging; the imaging features vary with the pattern. The diffuse pattern, which is the most common type, is seen as a featureless or sausage-like pancreas because of the loss of lobular architecture. The involved pancreas is homogeneous, and the MPD is either nondilated or diffusely narrowed, which is a characteristic finding in AIP. Calcification is rare, unlike other types of chronic pancreatitis. There can be a hypoattenuating rim with associated fat stranding and involution of the pancreatic tail. The rim shows a characteristic delayed enhancement. On ERCP, the characteristic finding is focal, segmental or diffuse narrowing, and irregularity of the MPD.[13] MRI may show a mildly enlarged pancreas with loss of signal intensity on T1 weighted images and mild hyperintensity on T2 weighted images. After contrast administration, the involved part of the pancreas shows delayed enhancement (**Figure 6**). The rim around the pancreas is hypointense on both T1 and T2 weighted images and shows delayed enhancement.[9] MRCP may show features similar to ERCP as well as associated strictures in the biliary tree that occur in primary sclerosing cholangitis.

The diffuse form of AIP can mimic lymphoma and other diffuse infiltrative disorders. The focal type of AIP can present as a focal mass lesion on all imaging modalities, mimicking carcinoma of the pancreas. Because of this morphological similarity, 2 to 6% of all resections for suspected carcinoma pancreas turn out to be AIP.[49] Focal type AIP can also present with upstream dilatation of the MPD, in which case the dilatation is less severe than in carcinoma of the pancreas.[50] Delayed enhancement in AIP is another feature that differentiates it from carcinoma of the pancreas. Corticosteriods are used to treat AIP, and the response is usually dramatic.

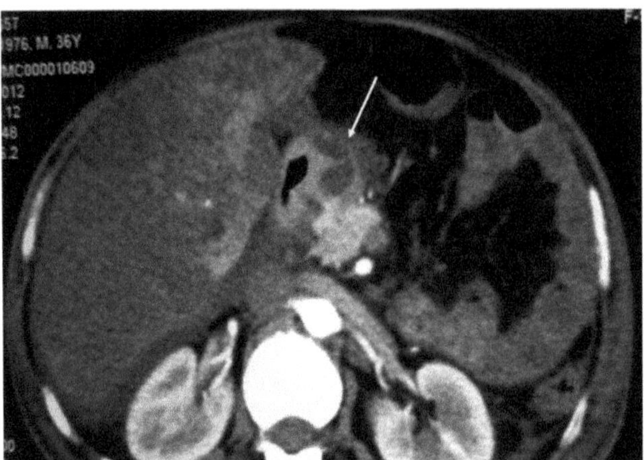

Figure 7. Axial CECT image of a chronic alcoholic patient who presented with abdominal pain showing hypodense plaque-like soft tissue in the pancreatico-duodenal groove (thin arrow) with relative sparing of the uncinate process of pancreas. The rest of the pancreas (not shown here) is also normal. There is mild free fluid in abdomen and abnormal enhancement of liver which became homogeneous on portal venous phase (not shown here) suggestive of transient hepatic attenuation differences. Based on these findings a diagnosis of groove pancreatitis was made.

Groove Pancreatitis

Groove pancreatitis is a rare type of CP which is localized to the pancreaticoduodenal groove, a potential space between the head of pancreas, duodenum, and CBD.[51] The pathogenesis of this entity is not fully understood. Several factors such as penetrating duodenal ulcer post-gastric resection, duodenal wall cysts, pancreatic heterotopia, and obstructed flow of pancreatic secretions have been implicated.[52] It is also unclear whether groove pancreatitis, cystic dystrophy of the duodenum, and paraduodenal wall cysts are different or related entities. These entities have many features in common, hence they are collectively categorized as paraduodenal pancreatitis.[53] There are two forms of groove pancreatitis: pure and segmental. In the pure form, scar tissue is localized to the groove without involving the pancreas. In the segmental form, the head of pancreas is also involved. On CT, groove pancreatitis is characterized by a sheet of relatively hypoenhancing tissue that usually shows delayed enhancement relative to normal pancreas (**Figure 7**). In the segmental form, scar tissue involves the pancreatic head and mimics pancreatic carcinoma. The displacement of the gastroduodenal artery toward the pancreatic head and cystic changes of the duodenal wall that occur in groove pancreatitis and the abrupt cut-off of the MPD that occurs in carcinoma of the pancreas can help in differentiation. On MRI, scar tissue is hypointense on T1, hyperintense on T2 weighted images, and shows delayed enhancement on contrast administration. Cystic lesions and associated thickening in the wall of the duodenum are better visualized on MR. These changes can cause tapering of the MPD and lower CBD.

Chronic Pancreatitis in Cystic Fibrosis

Cystic fibrosis is an autosomal recessive inherited disease that is associated with a mutation of the chloride channel gene. It is a common cause of pancreatic exocrine failure in young patients. The mutation causes inspissation of secretions that obstructs flow and triggers the disease process. Patients presenting with frank acute pancreatitis are rare, and the ongoing low grade inflammation causes progressive fibrosis and calcification.[54] Eventually, the parenchyma is replaced by fat, which is a characteristic feature. This fatty replacement correlates with exocrine dysfunction, and it is seen as hyperechogenicity on US and hypodensity on CT on the background of CP.

Parenchymal and intraductal calcification is unusual unlike other hereditary pancreatitis. Rarely, the entire pancreas is replaced by multiple cysts of varying sizes, which is a condition known as pancreatic cystosis. MRI is more sensitive than CT in detecting this abnormality. Pancreatic signal intensity on T1 weighted images can be variable depending on the extent of fatty replacement. Irregularity and dilatation of the ducts are better visualized on MRI. MRI has an additional advantage of not using ionizing radiation, which is all the more relevant in young patients.

Chronic Pancreatitis and Pancreatic Adenocarcinoma

Focal pancreatitis in the form of mass-forming chronic pancreatitis can closely mimic carcinoma of the pancreas on all imaging modalities, and CP itself predisposes to development of pancreatic carcinoma.

It is of paramount importance to detect the development of carcinoma of the pancreas in the setting of CP and to differentiate mass-forming chronic pancreatitis from carcinoma of the pancreas. Any abnormal contour bulge or change in the morphology in the form of mass effect and alteration or disappearance of pre-existing calcification should raise the suspicion of carcinoma of the pancreas (**Figure 8**). Advances in CT and MR imaging have enhanced the ability to differentiate an inflammatory mass from carcinoma. Smoothly stenotic or nonstenotic MPD on MRI (a duct penetrating sign) should favor the diagnosis of inflammatory mass (**Figure 9**) whereas abrupt cut off of grossly dilated MPD, and peripancreatic vascular invasion should favor the diagnosis of carcinoma of the pancreas. Pancreatic perfusion CT can generate perfusion parameters that help to make this distinction. Although blood flow and blood volume are reduced in both inflammatory masses and carcinoma, the values are much lower in carcinoma than in inflammatory masses (**Figure 10**).[31]

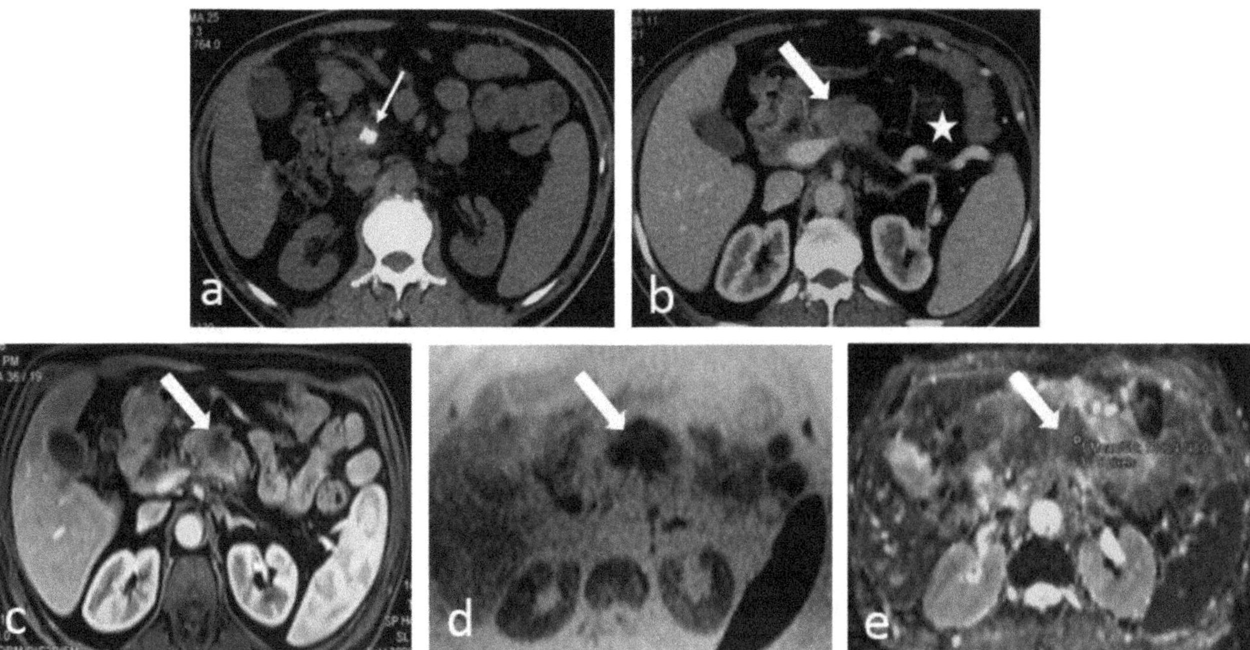

Figure 8. Axial noncontrast CT (a) of a patient with CCP who presented with worsening of pain showing calcification in the head of pancreas (thin arrow) with parenchymal atrophy. Axial CECT (b) showing a hypoenhancing mass lesion in the body of pancreas (thick arrow) causing contour bulge. Multiple peripancreatic collaterals are also seen (asterisk) due to narrowing of the splenic vein. Post-contrast MRI (c) confirmed this hypoenhancing lesion (thick arrow). Diffusion-weighted MRI (d) using b value of 1000 with inverted grey scale showing profound hypointensity; the focal lesion (thick arrow) is hypointense on ADC mapping (e). These imaging features are suggestive of pancreatic carcinoma on a background of CCP, and this was confirmed on cytology.

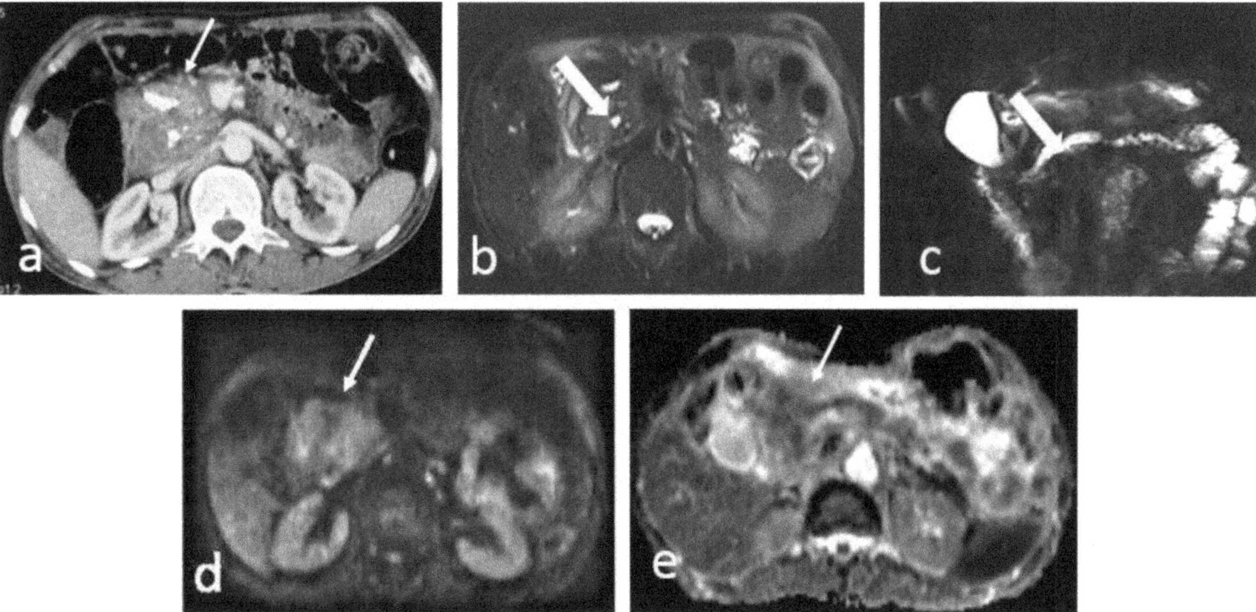

Figure 9. Axial contrast-enhanced CT (a) in a patient with CCP shows a heterogeneous mass lesion in the head of the pancreas (thin arrow) with multiple calcific foci. Heavily T2W MR images (b,c) show the dilated tortuous MPD coursing through the mass lesion (thick arrow). Diffusion-weighted image (d) and ADC map (e) showing that there is no significant diffusion restriction in the mass. Based on the above findings, a diagnosis of mass-forming chronic pancreatitis was made. The patient was later subjected to EUS guided sampling, which confirmed the diagnosis.

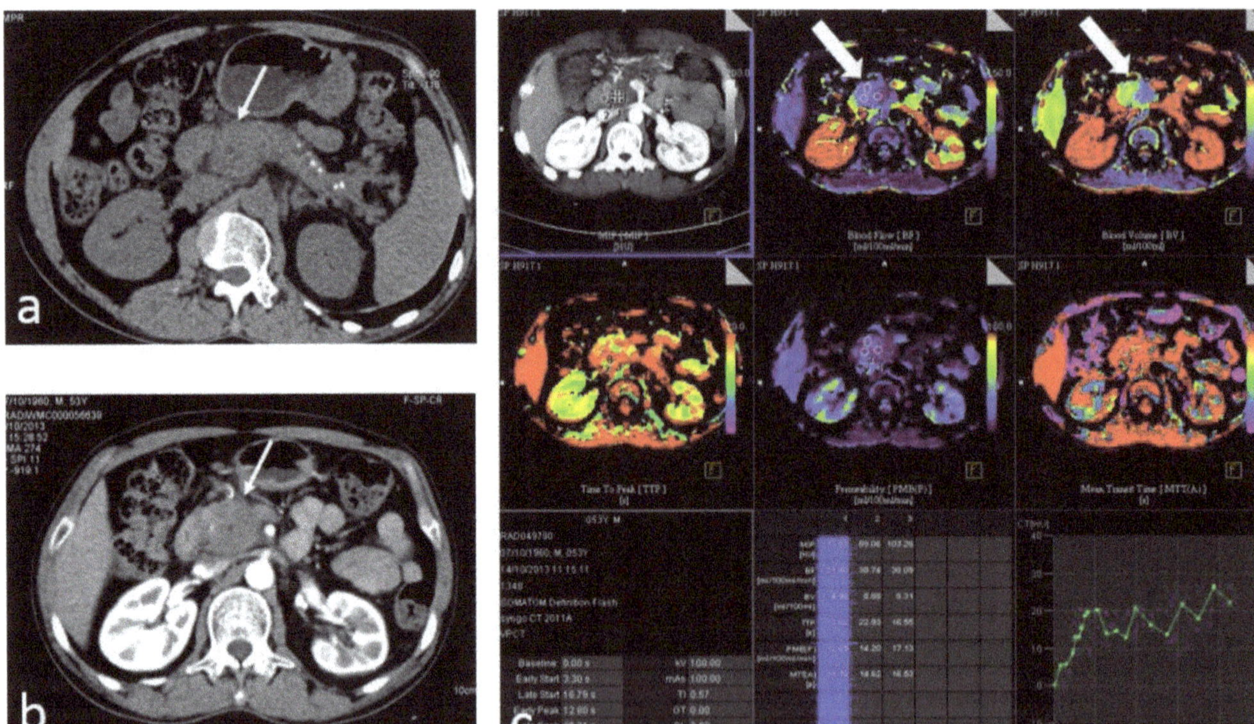

Figure 10. Axial noncontrast CT and contrast-enhanced CT (a,b) of a patient with CCP showing an ill-defined hypoenhancing mass lesion in the head of pancreas (thin arrow). Perfusion CT of the pancreas with color-coded maps depicting various perfusion parameters (c) shows that blood volume and blood flow are decreased (blue color) in the head region comparison with the rest of pancreas (thick arrow), which is shown in green. Decreased perfusion parameters are also seen in pancreatic carcinoma, but the extent of decrease is significantly more in carcinoma. EUS guided sampling revealed only inflammatory cells suggestive of mass-forming chronic pancreatitis.

Diffusion-weighted imaging is emerging as a helpful tool to differentiate inflammatory masses from carcinoma, in which carcinoma is shown to restrict diffusion.[37] FDG-PET CT has also been used for the same purpose with a varying degree of success.[38,39]

References

1. De Backer AI, Mortelé KJ, Ros RR, Vanbeckevoort D, Vanschoubroeck I, De Keulenaer B. Chronic pancreatitis: diagnostic role of computed tomography and magnetic resonance imaging. *JBR-BTR*. 2002; 85(6): 304-310. PMID: 12553661.
2. Brydon WG, Kingstone K, Ghosh S. Limitations of faecal elastase-1 and chymotrypsin as tests of exocrine pancreatic disease in adults. *Ann Clin Biochem*. 2004; 41(1): 78-81. PMID: 14713391.
3. Wali PD, Loveridge-Lenza B, He Z, Horvath K. Comparison of fecal elastase-1 and pancreatic function testing in children. *J Pediatr Gastroenterol Nutr*. 2012; 54(2): 277-280. PMID: 22266489.
4. Glasbrenner B, Kahl S, Malfertheiner P. Modern diagnostics of chronic pancreatitis. *Eur J Gastroenterol Hepatol*. 2002; 14(9): 935-941. PMID: 12352212.
5. Sanyal R, Stevens T, Novak E, Veniero JC. Secretin-enhanced MRCP: review of technique and application with proposal for quantification of exocrine function. *AJR Am J Roentgenol*. 2012; 198(1): 124-132. PMID: 22194487.
6. Bian Y, Wang L, Chen C, Lu J-P, Fan J-B, Chen S-Y, et al. Quantification of pancreatic exocrine function of chronic pancreatitis with secretin-enhanced MRCP. *World J Gastroenterol*. 2013; 19(41): 7177-7182. PMID: 24222963.
7. Balcı C. MRI assessment of chronic pancreatitis. *Diagn Interv Radiol Ank Turk*. 2011; 17(3): 249-25. PMID: 20945291.
8. Hansen TM, Nilsson M, Gram M, Frøkjær JB. Morphological and functional evaluation of chronic pancreatitis with magnetic resonance imaging. *World J Gastroenterol*. 2013; 19(42): 7241-7246. PMID: 24259954.
9. Perez-Johnston R, Sainani NI, Sahani DV. Imaging of chronic pancreatitis (including groove and autoimmune pancreatitis). *Radiol Clin North Am*. 2012; 50(3): 447-466. PMID: 22560691.
10. Lévy P, Mathurin P, Roqueplo A, Rueff B, Bernades P. A multidimensional case-control study of dietary, alcohol, and tobacco habits in alcoholic men with chronic pancreatitis. *Pancreas*. 1995; 10(3): 231-238. PMID: 7624300.

11. Mitchell RMS, Byrne MF, Baillie J. Pancreatitis. *The Lancet.* 2003; 361(9367): 1447-1455. PMID: 12727412.
12. Sarner M, Cotton PB. Classification of pancreatitis. *Gut.* 1984; 25(7): 756-759. PMID: 6735257.
13. Shanbhogue AKP, Fasih N, Surabhi VR, Doherty GP, Shanbhogue DKP, Sethi SK. A clinical and radiologic review of uncommon types and causes of pancreatitis. *Radiogr Rev Publ Radiol Soc N Am Inc.* 2009; 29(4): 1003-1026. PMID: 19605653.
14. Dimcevski G, Erchinger FG, Havre R, Gilja OH. Ultrasonography in diagnosing chronic pancreatitis: new aspects. *World J Gastroenterol.* 2013; 19(42): 7247-7257. PMID: 24259955.
15. Jones SN, Lees WR, Frost RA. Diagnosis and grading of chronic pancreatitis by morphological criteria derived by ultrasound and pancreatography. *Clin Radiol.* 1988; 39(1): 43-8. PMID: 3276430.
16. Bolondi L, Priori P, Gullo L, Santi V, Bassi SL, Barbara L, et al. Relationship between morphological changes detected by ultrasonography and pancreatic exocrine function in chronic pancreatitis. *Pancreas.* 1987; 2(2): 222-229. PMID: 3306660.
17. Homma T, Harada H, Koizumi M. Diagnostic criteria for chronic pancreatitis by the Japan Pancreas Society. *Pancreas.* 1997; 15(1): 14-15. PMID: 9211487.
18. Luetmer PH, Stephens DH, Ward EM. Chronic pancreatitis: reassessment with current CT. *Radiology.* 1989; 171(2): 353-357. PMID: 2704799.
19. DiMagno MJ, DiMagno EP. Chronic pancreatitis. *Curr Opin Gastroenterol.* 2005; 21(5): 544-554. PMID: 16093768.
20. Graziani R, Tapparelli M, Malagò R, Girardi V, Frulloni L, Cavallini G, et al. The various imaging aspects of chronic pancreatitis. *JOP.* 2005; 6(1 Suppl): 73-88. PMID: 15650290.
21. Frulloni L, Castellani C, Bovo P, Vaona B, Calore B, Liani C, et al. Natural history of pancreatitis associated with cystic fibrosis gene mutations. *Dig Liver Dis.* 2003; 35(3): 179-185. PMID: 12779072.
22. Hoshina K, Kimura W, Ishiguro T, Tominaga O, Futakawa N, Bin Z, et al. Three generations of hereditary chronic pancreatitis. *Hepatogastroenterology.* 2003; 46(26): 1192-1198. PMID: 10370690.
23. Rohrmann CA, Surawicz CM, Hutchinson D, Silverstein FE, White TT, Marchioro TL. The diagnosis of hereditary pancreatitis by pancreatography. *Gastrointest Endosc.* 1981; 27(3): 168-173. PMID: 7297825.
24. Kattwinkel J, Lapey A, di Sant'Agnese PA, Edwards WA, Hufty MP. Hereditary pancreatitis: three new kindreds and a critical review of the literature. *Pediatrics.* 1973; 51(1): 55-69. PMID: 4567584.
25. Barman KK, Premalatha G, Mohan V. Tropical chronic pancreatitis. *Postgrad Med J.* 2003; 79(937): 606-615. PMID: 146545.
26. Moorthy TR, Nalini N, Narendranathan M. Ultrasound imaging in tropical pancreatitis. *J Clin Ultrasound.* 1992; 20(6): 389-393. PMID: 1328310.
27. Suda K, Mogaki M, Oyama T, Matsumoto Y. Histopathologic and immunohistochemical studies on alcoholic pancreatitis and chronic obstructive pancreatitis: special emphasis on ductal obstruction and genesis of pancreatitis. *Am J Gastroenterol.* 1990; 85(3): 271-276. PMID: 2178399.
28. Procacci C, Graziani R, Vasori S, Venturini S. Diagnostica per immagini della pancreatite cronica. *Gastroenterol Clin.* 2001; 5: 195-205.
29. Procacci C, Graziani R, Zamboni G, Cavallini G, Pederzoli P, Guarise A, et al. Cystic dystrophy of the duodenal wall: radiologic findings. *Radiology.* 1997; 205(3): 741-747. PMID: 9393530.
30. Bedingfield JA, Anderson MC. Pancreatopleural fistula. *Pancreas.* 1986; 1(3): 283-290. PMID: 3575310.
31. Lu N, Feng X-Y, Hao S-J, Liang Z-H, Jin C, Qiang J-W, et al. 64-slice CT perfusion imaging of pancreatic adenocarcinoma and mass-forming chronic pancreatitis. *Acad Radiol.* 2011; 18(1): 81-88. PMID: 20951612.
32. Winston CB, Mitchell DG, Outwater EK, Ehrlich SM. Pancreatic signal intensity on T1-weighted fat saturation MR images: clinical correlation. *J Magn Reson Imaging.* 1995; 5(3): 267-271. PMID: 7633102.
33. Miller FH, Keppke AL, Wadhwa A, Ly JN, Dalal K, Kamler V-A. MRI of pancreatitis and its complications: part 2, chronic pancreatitis. *AJR Am J Roentgenol.* 2004; 183(6): 1645-52. PMID: 15547204.
34. Zhang X-M, Shi H, Parker L, Dohke M, Holland GA, Mitchell DG. Suspected early or mild chronic pancreatitis: enhancement patterns on gadolinium chelate dynamic MRI. Magnetic resonance imaging. *J Magn Reson Imaging.* 2003; 17(1): 86-94. PMID: 12500277.
35. Takehara Y, Ichijo K, Tooyama N, Kodaira N, Yamamoto H, Tatami M, et al. Breath-hold MR cholangiopancreatography with a long-echo-train fast spin-echo sequence and a surface coil in chronic pancreatitis. *Radiology.* 1994; 192(1): 73-78. PMID: 8208969.
36. Ichikawa T, Sou H, Araki T, Arbab AS, Yoshikawa T, Ishigame K, et al. Duct-penetrating sign at MRCP: usefulness for differentiating inflammatory pancreatic mass from pancreatic carcinomas. *Radiology* 2001; 221(1): 107-116. PMID: 11568327.
37. Niu X, Das SK, Bhetuwal A, Xiao Y, Sun F, Zeng L, et al. Value of diffusion-weighted imaging in distinguishing pancreatic carcinoma from mass-forming chronic pancreatitis: a meta-analysis. *Chin Med J (Engl).* 2014; 127(19): 3477-3482. PMID: 25269917.
38. Santhosh S, Mittal BR, Bhasin D, Srinivasan R, Rana S, Das A, et al. Role of (18)F-fluorodeoxyglucose positron emission tomography/computed tomography in the characterization of pancreatic masses: experience from tropics. *J Gastroenterol Hepatol.* 2013; 28(2): 255-261. PMID: 23278193.
39. Kato K, Nihashi T, Ikeda M, Abe S, Iwano S, Itoh S, et al. Limited efficacy of (18)F-FDG PET/CT for differentiation between metastasis-free pancreatic cancer and mass-forming pancreatitis. *Clin Nucl Med.* 2013; 38(6): 417-421. PMID: 23486318.
40. Erturk SM, Ichikawa T, Motosugi U, Sou H, Araki T. Diffusion-weighted MR imaging in the evaluation of pancreatic exocrine function before and after secretin stimulation. *Am J Gastroenterol.* 2006; 101(1): 133-136. PMID: 16405545.

41. Weber SM, Cubukcu-Dimopulo O, Palesty JA, Suriawinata A, Klimstra D, Brennan MF, et al. Lymphoplasmacytic sclerosing pancreatitis: inflammatory mimic of pancreatic carcinoma. *J Gastrointest Surg*. 2003; 7(1): 129-139 PMID: 12559194.
42. Notohara K, Burgart LJ, Yadav D, Chari S, Smyrk TC. Idiopathic chronic pancreatitis with periductal lymphoplasmacytic infiltration: clinicopathologic features of 35 cases. *Am J Surg Pathol*. 2003; 27(8): 1119-1127. PMID: 12883244.
43. Matsubayashi H, Kakushima N, Takizawa K, Tanaka M, Imai K, Hotta K, et al. Diagnosis of autoimmune pancreatitis. *World J Gastroenterol*. 2014; 20(44): 16559-16569. PMID: 25469024.
44. Crosara S, D'Onofrio M, De Robertis R, Demozzi E, Canestrini S, Zamboni G, et al. Autoimmune pancreatitis: Multimodality non-invasive imaging diagnosis. *World J Gastroenterol*. 2014; 20(45): 16881-16890. PMID: 25493001.
45. Okazaki K, Kawa S, Kamisawa T, Naruse S, Tanaka S, Nishimori I, et al. Clinical diagnostic criteria of autoimmune pancreatitis: revised proposal. *J Gastroenterol*. 2006; 41(7): 626-631. PMID: 16932998.
46. Chari ST, Smyrk TC, Levy MJ, Topazian MD, Takahashi N, Zhang L, et al. Diagnosis of autoimmune pancreatitis: the Mayo Clinic experience. *Clin Gastroenterol Hepatol*. 2006; 4(8): 1010-1016. PMID: 16843735.
47. Shimosegawa T, Chari ST, Frulloni L, Kamisawa T, Kawa S, Mino-Kenudson M, et al. International consensus diagnostic criteria for autoimmune pancreatitis: guidelines of the International Association of Pancreatology. *Pancreas*. 2011; 40(3): 352-358. PMID: 21412117.
48. Naitoh I, Nakazawa T, Hayashi K, Miyabe K, Shimizu S, Kondo H, et al. Clinical evaluation of international consensus diagnostic criteria for type 1 autoimmune pancreatitis in comparison with Japanese diagnostic criteria 2011. *Pancreas*. 2013; 42(8): 1238-1244. PMID: 24152949.
49. Yadav D, Notahara K, Smyrk TC, Clain JE, Pearson RK, Farnell MB, et al. Idiopathic tumefactive chronic pancreatitis: clinical profile, histology, and natural history after resection. *Clin Gastroenterol Hepatol*. 2003; 1(2): 129-135. PMID: 15017505.
50. Kamisawa T, Egawa N, Nakajima H, Tsuruta K, Okamoto A, Kamata N. Clinical difficulties in the differentiation of autoimmune pancreatitis and pancreatic carcinoma. *Am J Gastroenterol*. 2003; 98(12): 2694-2699. PMID: 14687819.
51. Stolte M, Weiss W, Volkholz H, Rösch W. A special form of segmental pancreatitis: "groove pancreatitis". *Hepatogastroenterology*. 1982; 29(5): 198-208. PMID: 7173808.
52. Irie H, Honda H, Kuroiwa T, Hanada K, Yoshimitsu K, Tajima T, et al. MRI of groove pancreatitis. *J Comput Assist Tomogr*. 1998; 22(4): 651-5. PMID: 9676462.
53. Adsay NV, Zamboni G. Paraduodenal pancreatitis: a clinico-pathologically distinct entity unifying "cystic dystrophy of heterotopic pancreas", "para-duodenal wall cyst", and "groove pancreatitis". *Semin Diagn Pathol*. 2004; 21(4): 247-254. PMID: 16273943.
54. De Boeck K, Weren M, Proesmans M, Kerem E. Pancreatitis among patients with cystic fibrosis: correlation with pancreatic status and genotype. *Pediatrics*. 2005; 115(4): e463-469. PMID: 15772171.

Chapter 42

Endoscopic ultrasound for the diagnosis of chronic pancreatitis

Jintao Guo and Siyu Sun*

Endoscopy Center, Shengjing Hospital of China Medical University, Shenyang, China.

Chronic pancreatitis (CP) is a consequence of various disorders—primarily chronic alcoholism, biliary disease, and trauma—and is signaled by specific risk factors, known signs and symptoms, and distinct abnormalities on imaging and laboratory diagnostics. Pancreatic calcification and dilatation of the pancreatic duct are characteristics findings of CP on noninvasive imaging studies, such as computed tomography (CT) and magnetic resonance imaging (MRI).[1] Although the latter are considered the modalities of choice, endoscopic ultrasound (EUS) is now also viewed as one of the most sensitive methods for detecting pancreatic lesions, given the close proximity of the transducer to the pancreas.[2-5] Since 1986, numerous studies have reported on the use of EUS for the diagnosis of CP and compared it with noninvasive cross-sectional imaging and endoscopic retrograde cholangiopancreatography (ERCP)[6-12] for accurate diagnosis of CP (**Table 1**). EUS is able to demonstrate subtle alterations in pancreatic structure that escape traditional imaging and laboratory tests of pancreatic function. The sensitivity of EUS may be further heightened by limiting the core criteria required to diagnose CP.

In EUS studies of the pancreas, nonhomogenous changes of parenchyma, particularly hyperechoic foci or strands, lobulation, calcifications, and cysts; ductal alterations, including a hyperechoic wall, dilatation and/or tortuosity of the main duct, intraductal hyperechoic foci, and ectatic side branches are grounds for a diagnosis of CP.[2-5] The severity of CP (mild, moderate, severe) may also be estimated by EUS,[2] but standardized diagnostic guidelines have yet to be adopted.

The most frequently used classification, described by Wiersema et al. in 1993, includes 9 pancreatic criteria: hyperechoic foci, hyperechoic strands, lobularity, cyst, calcification, main pancreatic duct dilatation, side branch dilatation, pancreatic duct irregularity, and hyperechoic duct margins.[13] A new classification was proposed as part of an international consensus meeting in Rosemont, Illinois In April 2007. The new criteria assigns different values to different features and establishes major and minor criteria depending on the features found.[14,15] The Rosemont major criteria are hyperechoic foci with shadowing and main pancreatic duct calculi (Major A) and lobularity with honeycombing (Major B). Minor criteria include cysts, dilated ducts ≥3.5 mm, irregular pancreatic duct contour, dilated side branches ≥1 mm, hyperechoic duct wall, strands, nonshadowing hyperechoic foci, and lobularity with noncontiguous lobules. These criteria define 4 patient groups: normal pancreas, indeterminate, suggestive, and consistent with CP.[14] The EUS diagnosis of CP based on Rosemont criteria is shown in **Table 2**. Jimeno-Ayllón et al.,[16] used both the Wiersema criteria and the Rosemont classification for diagnosis of CP. They concluded that the new classification was useful in patients with high suspicion of chronic pancreatitis and with <4 of the standard criteria, but with more significance such as parenchymal lithiasis, lobularity, or ductal calcifications.

EUS provides high-resolution imaging of the entire pancreas, enabling detailed parenchymal and ductal assessment. Normally, the parenchyma is homogeneous, with a finely reticular pattern, and the main duct has a smooth wall that is not dilated or hyperechoic. As a rule, the diameter of pancreatic duct is <3 mm at the head, <2 mm at the neck, and <1 mm at the tail; and side branches are not visible.[2,3] Allowing for anatomic variation, the ventral pancreas may be more hypoechoic and heterogeneous than the dorsal pancreas (**Figure 1-3**).

It is difficult to determine whether hypoechoic and cystic lesions are inflammatory or neoplastic via conventional B-mode EUS imaging,[17] but interpretation is aided significantly by fine needle aspiration (FNA).[18] Pancreatic neoplasms may coexist as complications of chronic

*Corresponding author. Email: sun-siyu@163.com

Table 1. Published studies comparing EUS with other modalities in diagnosing chronic pancreatitis.

Study	Comparison modality	Criterion standard	No. of patients	Results
Uskudar, 2009 (6)	ERCP	Fecal elastase	24	EUS and ERCP comparable severity scores were 1 in 0-2 patients, 2 in 6-8 patients, and 3 in 18-14 patients.
Pungpapong, 2009 (7)	MRCP	MRCP	99	Compared with MRCP, EUS was more sensitive but was equally specific, but only to diagnose CP. The combination of EUS and MRCP resulted in 98% sensitivity for either EUS or MRCP and 100% specificity for both EUS and MRCP.
Chong, 2007 (8)	Pathology	Pathology	71	Three or more EUS criteria provided the best balance of sensitivity (83.3%) and specificity (80.0%) for predicting abnormal histology.
Varadarajulu, 2007 (9)	Pathology	Pathology	42	EUS features associated with histopathologic noncalcific CP were as follows: hyperechoic foci, stranding, and lobulations of parenchyma; dilated or irregular main pancreatic duct, ectatic side branches, and hyperechoic duct margins.
Kahl, 2002 (10)	ERCP	ERCP	38	Of patients with EUS findings of CP and normal initial ERCP, 69% had CP confirmed by repeat ERCP (median follow-up time, 18 months).
Iglesias et al, 2012 (11)	EUS, CT, MRI	Pathology		EUS, CT, and MRI may all provide valuable and complementary information for differentiating mass-forming chronic pancreatitis, autoimmune pancreatitis, and pancreatic adenocarcinoma. There is the unique opportunity to obtain specimens via EUS for histopathologic diagnosis, thus playing a pivotal role in patients with inconclusive findings on initial examinations. EUS-guided elastography and use of contrast agents with harmonic echo are also helpful in this setting.

Table 2. EUS diagnosis of CP on the basis of Rosemont criteria.

I. Consistent with chronic pancreatitis	1 major A feature plus 3 or more minor features
	1 major A feature plus 1 major B feature
	2 major A features
II. Suggestive of CP	1 major A feature plus 3 minor features
	1 major B feature with or without plus 3 minor features
	5 or more minor features (any)
III. Indeterminate for CP	3 to 4 minor features, no major features
	Major B feature alone or with <3 minor features
IV. Normal	Less than 2 minor features, no major features

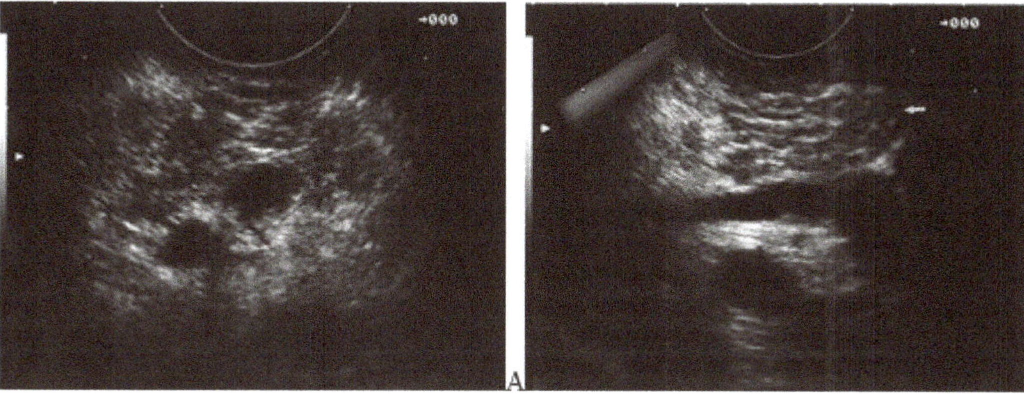

Figure 1. Chronic pancreatitis (Case 1). A 45-year-old man presented with chronic pancreatitis of 5 years duration. EUS showed a heterogeneous echo pattern in the body (A) and neck (B) of the pancreas: hyperechoic foci (dots); hyperechoic strands (linear); lobulation (pancreatic parenchyma is lobulated by linear hyperechos); irregular hypoechoic areas. Multiple FNA results were negative (with no signs of malignancy).

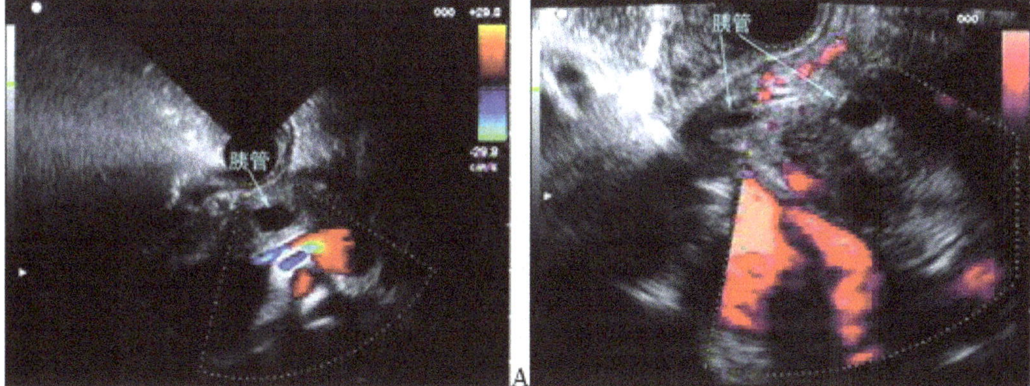

Figure 2. Chronic pancreatitis (Case 2). A 37-year-old man presented with cholecystolithiasis and recurrent pancreatitis of 5 years duration. (A) Radial EUS showed that the main pancreatic duct in the neck of pancreas was dilated (6 mm). (B) EUS showed that the main pancreatic duct in the head of pancreas was dilated, while the main pancreatic duct near the ampulla was not dilated. No tumor was found in the pancreatic head, and combined with other clinical data, the lesion was finally diagnosed as chronic pancreatitis.

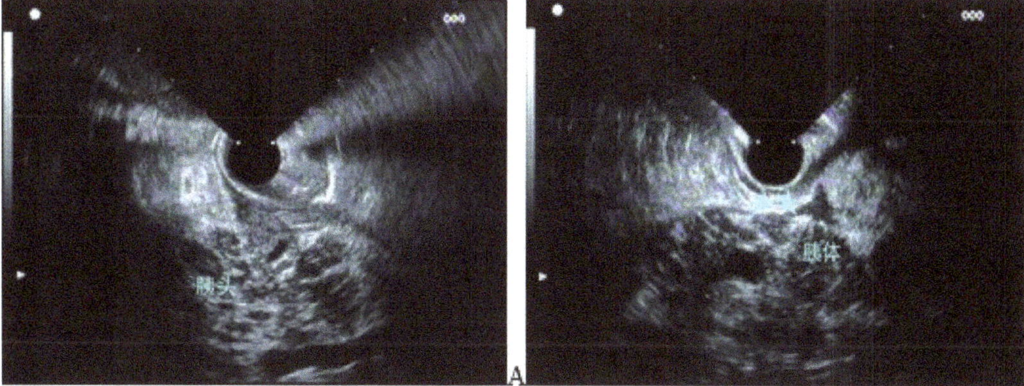

Figure 3. Chronic pancreatitis (Case 3). A 42-year-old man presented with cholecystolithiasis and chronic pancreatitis of 3 years duration. EUS showed heterogeneous, hyperechoic parenchyma in the head (A) and body (B) of pancreas, representing fibrosis.

pancreatitis,[19] and cysts or inflammation may result from neoplastic obstruction of the pancreatic duct.

In that context, the accuracy of EUS-guided FNA is quite high, and has a sensitivity of 80-85% and a specificity near 100%.[20,21] However, this technique is technically demanding, and often requires multiple passes to obtain enough tissue for a diagnosis.[22,23] Furthermore, despite repeated sampling, cytohistologic preparations may be falsely negative in patients with advanced chronic pancreatitis who develop solid masses.[24]

Differentiating ductal adenocarcinoma from mass lesions of pancreatitis may be improved by spectral Doppler analysis owing to the curious absence of venules in adenocarcinomas (only arterioles are present). Venules are generally not a prominent component of tumors, possibly due to the accompanying desmoplasia. On the other hand, both arterioles and venules of inflammatory lesions are usually detectable by Doppler.[25,26]

New techniques have emerged to address this issue, namely contrast-enhanced EUS (CE-EUS) and EUS elastography.[27-37] CE-EUS is a novel approach where the normal high-resolution of ultrasound is intensified by contrast agents.[27] CE-EUS may help to recognize and delineate necrotizing foci of acute pancreatitis, which ordinarily are not enhanced at a very early stage.[28] The lack of nephrotoxicity shown by these agents is of particular importance, because most patients who are severely ill with pancreatitis also develop renal failure. In such instances, CT contrast enhancement is contraindicated. Interestingly, focal uptake of contrast in pancreatitis.[29] or diffuse uptake in autoimmune pancreatitis.[30] is often similar to or better than that seen in normal pancreatic parenchyma. This feature may be useful in differentiating ductal adenocarcinoma.

Elastography is a method for assessing tissue rigidity in real time. Currently, elastographic evaluations of the gastrointestinal tract are done in conjunction with conventional EUS. The EUS probe is equipped with a processor and software that generate real-time elastographic data. Unlike first-generation technology, which is limited to qualitative estimates, the second generation tools now available allow quantitative analysis of tissue rigidity.[31-37]

In qualitative elastography, compression-induced structural deformation is quantified in B-mode images using the degree of deformation as an index of tissue rigidity.[31,32] As shown by Iglesias-Garcia et al,[34] qualitative elastography of patients with CP were irregularly colored, exhibiting green areas with predominantly blue heterogeneous strands. Analogous findings in control subjects without pancreatic disease were were predominantly green and yellow homogeneous patterns.

Quantitative elastography offers two alternatives, the hue histogram and the calculated strain ratio. A hue histogram is a graphic representation of color distribution (hues) in a selected image field and is derived from qualitative EUS elastography data for a manually selected ROI within a standard elastographic image. The calculated strain ratio attempts to offset the comparative nature of qualitative elastographic patterns by analyzing the elastographic image of a target lesion relative to surrounding tissues.[33-37] Similar to a hue histogram, the strain ratio is

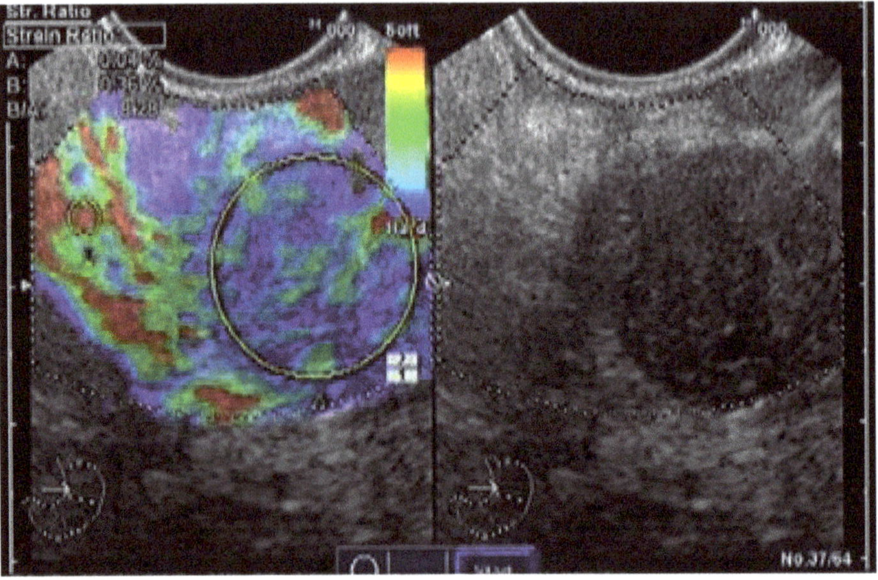

Figure 4. Quantitative EUS elastography based on strain ratio analysis of a solid pancreatic mass (pancreatic adenocarcinoma). Area A shows pancreatic parenchyma, and area B shows a soft area of the gut wall. The B/A ratio is displayed at the bottom of the image.

calculated from standard qualitative EUS elastographic data, selecting two differing areas (A and B) for quantitative analysis. Area A encompasses as much of the target lesion as possible and excludes adjacent tissues. Area B is within a soft (red) reference area extraneous to the target lesion and preferably in the gut wall. The strain ratio is the quotient of B/A.[34] The strain ratios of Rosemont categories significantly different, 1.80 (95% CI: 1.73-1.80) for normal pancreas, 2.40 (95% CI: 2.21-2.56) for indeterminate of CP, 2.85 (95% CI: 2.69-3.02) for suggestive of CP; and 3.62 (95% CI: 3.24-3.99) for consistent with CP ($P < 0.001$) (**Figure 4**). Dominguez-Muñoz' et al,[37] used the strain ratio to predict pancreatic exocrine insufficiency (PEI) in patients with chronic pancreatitis. They found that the degree of pancreatic fibrosis as measured by EUS-guided elastography allowed estimation of the probability of PEI in patients with CP.

References

1. Gleeson FC, Topazian M. Endoscopic retrograde cholangiopancreatography and endoscopic ultrasound for diagnosis of chronic pancreatitis. *Curr Gastroenterol Rep.* 2007; 9: 123-129. PMID: 17418057.
2. Irisawa A, Katakura K, Ohira H, Sato A, Bhutani MS, Hernandez LV, et al. Usefulness of endoscopic ultrasound to diagnose the severity of chronic pancreatitis. *J Gastroenterol.* 2007; 42 Suppl 17: 90-94. PMID: 17238035.
3. Noh KW, Pungpapong S, Raimondo M. Role of endosonography in non-malignant pancreatic diseases. World J Gastroenterol. 2007; 13(2): 165-169. PMID: 17226895.
4. Catalano MF. Diagnosing early-stage chronic pancreatitis: is endoscopic ultrasound a reliable modality? *J Gastroenterol.* 2007; 42 Suppl 17: 78-84. PMID: 17238033.
5. LeBlanc JK, Chen JH, Al-Haddad M, Juan M, Okumu W, McHenry L et al. Endoscopic ultrasound and histology in chronic pancreatitis: how are they associated? Pancreas. 2014; 43(3): 440-444. PMID: 24622076.
6. Uskudar O, Oguz D, Akdogan M, Altiparmak E, Sahin B. Comparison of endoscopic retrograde cholangiopancreatography, endoscopic ultrasonography, and fecal elastase 1 in chronic pancreatitis and clinical correlation. Pancreas. 2009; 38: 503-506. PMID: 19287334.
7. Pungpapong S, Wallace MB, Woodward TA, Noh KW, Raimondo M. Accuracy of endoscopic ultrasonography and magnetic resonance cholangiopancreatography for the diagnosis of chronic pancreatitis: a prospective comparison study. *J Clin Gastroenterol.* 2007; 41: 88-93. PMID: 17198070.
8. Chong AK, Hawes RH, Hoffman BJ, Adams DB, Lewin DN, Romagnuolo J. Diagnostic performance of EUS for chronic pancreatitis: a comparison with histopathology. *Gastrointest Endosc.* 2007; 65: 808-814. PMID: 17466199.
9. Varadarajulu S, Eltoum I, Tamhane A, Eloubeidi MA. Histopathologic correlates of noncalcific chronic pancreatitis by EUS: a prospective tissue characterization study. *Gastrointest Endosc.* 2007; 66: 501-509. PMID: 17640639.
10. Kahl S, Glasbrenner B, Leodolter A, Pross M, Schulz HU, Malfertheiner P. EUS in the diagnosis of early chronic pancreatitis: a prospective follow-up study. *Gastrointest Endosc.* 2002; 55: 507-511. PMID: 11923762.
11. Iglesias-García J, Lindkvist B, Lariño-Noia J, Domínguez-Muñoz JE. The role of EUS in relation to other imaging modalities in the differential diagnosis between mass forming chronic pancreatitis, autoimmune pancreatitis and ductal pancreatic adenocarcinoma. *Rev Esp Enferm Dig.* 2012; 104(6): 315-321. PMID: 22738702.
12. Gardner TB, Michael J. Levy. EUS diagnosis of chronic pancreatitis. *Gastrointest Endosc.* 2010; 71(5): 1280-1289. PMID: 20598255.
13. Wiersema MJ, Hawes RH, Lehman GA, Kochman ML, Sherman S, Kopecky KK. Prospective evaluation of endoscopic ultrasonography and endoscopic retrograde cholangiopancreatography in patients with chronic abdominal pain of suspected pancreatic origin. *Endoscopy.* 1993; 25(9): 555-564. PMID: 8119204.
14. Catalano MF, Sahai A, Levy M, Romagnuolo J, Wiersema M, Brugge W, et al. EUS-based criteria for the diagnosis of chronic pancreatitis: the Rosemont classification. Gastrointest *Endoscopy.* 2009; 69(7): 1251-1261. PMID: 19243769.
15. Petrone MC, Terracciano F, Perri F, Carrara S, Cavestro GM, Mariani A, et al. Pancreatic abnormalities detected by endoscopic ultrasound (EUS) in patients without clinical signs of pancreatic disease: any difference between standard and Rosemont classification scoring? *Pancreatology.* 2014; 14(3): 227-230. PMID: 24854620.
16. Jimeno-Ayllón C, Pérez-García JI, Gómez-Ruiz CJ, García-Cano-Lizcano J, Morillas-Ariño J, Martínez-Fernández R, et al. Standard criteria versus Rosemont classification for EUS-diagnosis of chronic pancreatitis. *Rev Esp Enferm Dig.* 2011; 103(12): 626-631. PMID: 22217346.
17. Jenssen C, Dietrich CF. Endoscopic ultrasound in chronic pancreatitis. *Z Gastroenterol.* 2005; 43(8): 737-749. PMID: 16088771.
18. Ardengh JC, Lopes CV, Campos AD, Pereira de Lima LF, Venco F, Módena JL. Endoscopic ultrasound and fine needle aspiration in chronic pancreatitis: differential diagnosis between pseudotumoral masses and pancreatic cancer. *JOP.* 2007; 8(4): 413-421. PMID: 17625292.
19. Barthet M, Portal I, Boujaoude J, Bernard JP, Sahel J. Endoscopic ultrasonographic diagnosis of pancreatic cancer complicating chronic pancreatitis. *Endoscopy.* 1996; 28(6): 487-491. PMID: 8886634.
20. Dumonceau JM, Polkowski M, Larghi A, Vilmann P, Giovannini M, Frossard JL, et al. Indications, results, and clinical impact of endoscopic ultrasound (EUS)-guided sampling in gastroenterology: European Society of Gastrointestinal Endoscopy (ESGE) Clinical Guideline. *Endoscopy.* 2011; 43: 897-912. PMID: 21842456.
21. Turner BG, Cizinger S, Agarwal D, Yang J, Pitman MB, Brugge WR. Diagnosis of pancreatic neoplasia with EUS-FNA: a report of accuracy. *Gastrointest Endosc.* 2010; 71: 91-98. PMID: 19846087.
22. Erickson RA, Sayage-Rabie L, Beisner RS. Factors' predicting the number of EUS-guided fine-needle passes for diagnosis of pancreatic malignancies. *Gastrointest Endosc.* 2000; 51: 184-190. PMID: 10650262.

23. Binmoeller KF, Rathod VD. Difficult pancreatic mass FNA: tips for success. *Gastrointest Endosc.* 2002; 56: S86-S93. PMID: 12297756.
24. Varadarajulu S, Tamhane A, Eloubeidi MA. Yield of EUS-guided FNA of pancreatic masses in the presence or the absence of chronic pancreatitis. *Gastrointest Endosc.* 2005; 62: 728-736. PMID: 16246688.
25. Hocke M, Schulze E, Gottschalk P, Topalidis T, Dietrich CF. Contrast-enhanced endoscopic ultrasound in discrimination between focal pancreatitis and pancreatic cancer. *World J Gastroenterol.* 2006; 12: 246-250. PMID: 16482625.
26. Saftoiu A, Iordache SA, Gheonea DI, Popescu C, Maloş A, Gorunescu F, et al. Combined contrast-enhanced power Doppler and real-time sonoelastography performed during EUS, used in the differential diagnosis of focal pancreatic masses (with videos). *Gastrointest Endosc.* 2010; 72: 739-747. PMID: 20674916.
27. Dietrich CF, Ignee A, Frey H. Contrast-enhanced endoscopic ultrasound with low mechanical index: a new technique. *Z Gastroenterol.* 2005; 43: 1219-1223. PMID: 16267707,
28. Ripolles T, Martinez MJ, Lopez E, Castelló I, Delgado F. Contrast-enhanced ultrasound in the staging of acute pancreatitis. *Eur Radiol.* 2010; 20: 2518-2523. PMID: 20532782.
29. D'Onofrio M, Zamboni G, Tognolini A, Malago R, Faccioli N, Frulloni L, et al. Mass-forming pancreatitis: value of contrast-enhanced ultrasonography. *World J Gastroenterol.* 2006; 12: 4181-4184. PMID: 16830370.
30. Hocke M, Ignee A, Dietrich CF. Contrast-enhanced endoscopic ultrasound in the diagnosis of autoimmune pancreatitis. *Endoscopy.* 2011; 43: 163-165. PMID: 21165827.
31. Giovannini M. Contrast-enhanced endoscopic ultrasound and elastosonoendoscopy. *Best Prac Res Clin Gastroenterol.* 2009; 23: 767-779. PMID: 19744639.
32. Giovannini M. Endoscopic Ultrasound Elastography. *Pancreatology.* 2011; 11: 34-39. PMID: 21464585.
33. Hirooka Y, Itoh A, Kawashima H, Ohno E, Ishikawa T, Matsubara H, et al. Diagnosis of pancreatic disorders using contrast-enhanced endoscopic ultrasonography and endoscopic elastography. *Clin Gastroenterol Hepatol.* 2009; 7: S63-S67. PMID: 19896102.
34. Iglesias-Garcia J, Lindkvist B, Lariño-Noia J, Domínguez-Muñoz JE. Endoscopic ultrasound elastography. *Endosc Ultrasound.* 2012; 1(1): 8-16. PMID: 24949330.
35. Itoh Y, Itoh A, Kawashima H, Ohno E, Nakamura Y, Hiramatsu T, et al. Quantitative analysis of diagnosing pancreatic fibrosis using EUS-elastography (comparison with surgical specimens). *J Gastroenterol.* 2014; 49(7): 1183-1192. PMID: 24026103.
36. Iglesias-Garcia J, Domínguez-Muñoz JE, Castiñeira-Alvariño M, Luaces-Regueira M, Lariño-Noia J. Quantitative elastography associated with endoscopic ultrasound for the diagnosis of chronic pancreatitis. *Endoscopy.* 2013; 45(10): 781-788. PMID: 24019131.
37. Dominguez-Muñoz JE, Iglesias-Garcia J, Castiñeira Alvariño M, Luaces Regueira M, Lariño-Noia J. EUS elastography to predict pancreatic exocrine insufficiency in patients with chronic pancreatitis. *Gastrointest Endosc.* 2015; 81(1): 136-142. PMID: 25088920.

Chapter 43

Diagnosis of pancreatic exocrine insufficiency in chronic pancreatitis

Jutta Keller* and Peter Layer

Department of Medicine, Israelitisches Krankenhaus, Hamburg, Germany.

Introduction

Pancreatic exocrine insufficiency (PEI) is defined as partial or complete loss of digestive enzyme and bicarbonate secretion. In chronic pancreatitis this is caused by a progressive destruction of functioning pancreatic tissue. The overt clinical symptoms of PEI are steatorrhea, weight loss and abdominal discomfort due to maldigestion. Due to the large reserve capacity of the pancreas symptoms frequently become apparent in only advanced stages. However, patients with mild to moderate PEI also have an increased risk of nutritional deficiencies. Several direct and indirect function tests are available for assessment of pancreatic exocrine function, but until today diagnosis of PEI remains difficult because the available tests have either limited availability due to invasiveness and/or high cost or have limited sensitivity and specificity, particularly in patients with mildly impaired pancreatic exocrine function.

Pathophysiology

Progressive inflammatory destruction of pancreatic tissue in chronic pancreatitis leads to reduced synthesis and secretion of pancreatic enzymes in response to food intake. With rare exceptions, clinically overt malabsorption only occurs when enzyme secretion is reduced by more than 90%.[1,2] In alcoholic chronic pancreatitis, this usually takes 10 to 20 years. Steatorrhea usually occurs earlier, and is more severe than malabsorption of other nutrients. This is explained by an earlier decrease in lipase secretion compared with amylase and proteases,[3] higher susceptibility of lipase to acidic pH caused by concomitant impairment of bicarbonate secretion, increased susceptibility of lipase to proteolytic destruction during small intestinal transit, additional acidic denaturation of bile acids, and marked inhibition of bile acid secretion in states of malabsorption.[4] Moreover, only gastric lipase can serve as an extrapancreatic source of lipolytic activity in humans, and this enzyme does not compensate for pancreatic lipase deficiency, although it may be elevated in patients with chronic pancreatitis compared with healthy individuals.[5] By contrast, more than 80% of carbohydrates can be digested and absorbed in the absence of pancreatic amylase activity,[6] and the colonic flora can further metabolize malabsorbed carbohydrates.

Different natural courses suggest that pancreatic exocrine function is preserved longer, and consequently exocrine insufficiency may generally be milder, in "early onset" idiopathic chronic pancreatitis than in alcoholic and "late onset" idiopathic chronic pancreatitis.[7] However, direct comparisons of pancreatic exocrine function in patients with varying etiologies of chronic pancreatitis have so far been few.[8]

In an unselected group of patients with chronic pancreatitis, mean pancreatic exocrine function is reduced by around 50 to 80% compared with healthy controls, and 80 to 90% show some degree of PEI.[4] In about 65 to 75% of patients, morphologic alterations and functional impairment develop in parallel. PEI without morphologic alterations is rare (<5% of patients) yet possible.

In severe PEI with less than 5% of normal enzyme output, about 40% of nutrients from a readily digestible low-calorie meal are malabsorbed and enter the colon.[9] Maldigestion can be decreased by oral enzyme supplementation. However, even with clinically established doses of pancreatic lipase, duodenal enzyme delivery remains far below physiologic levels and lipid malabsorption is rarely normalized.[10,11]

Clinical Symptoms of PEI

Typical symptoms of PEI are abdominal discomfort, weight loss, steatorrhea, malnutrition and signs of vitamin deficiency.[12] Steatorrhea and azotorrhoea, an excessive discharge of nitrogenous substances in the feces, occur when secretion of lipase and trypsin fall below 5 to 10% of

*Corresponding author. Email: j.keller@ik-h.de

normal levels. Typical features of steatorrhea are voluminous, fatty ("shiny" and "sticky") stools. However, while it is important to evaluate these parameters, stool characteristics are neither sensitive nor specific for detection of steatorrhea.[13,14]

Steatorrhea is conventionally diagnosed when daily stool fat excretion exceeds 7 g during ingestion of a diet containing 100 g fat per day.[1] Often steatorrhea is accompanied by diarrhea. This is caused in part by accelerated gastric emptying and intestinal transit in patients with exocrine insufficiency that can be reversed by enzyme supplementation.[9]

As a consequence of fat malabsorption, fat-soluble vitamins are insufficiently absorbed so that patients may exhibit low vitamin D levels and develop osteopathy, i.e., osteopenia, osteoporosis and osteomalacia. Reduced fecal elastase is observed in significantly more individuals suffering from osteoporotic bone fractures than in healthy controls (a 65% reduction). This study excluded patients with overt steatorrhea, suggesting that mild to moderate PEI is a risk factor for development of osteoporosis.[15-18] Moreover, there are reports of vitamin A deficiency causing night-blindness, visual impairment, and other ocular afflictions. Neurologic symptoms or coagulopathy can occur as a consequence of vitamin E and K deficiency.[12]

Pancreatic Function Tests

Exocrine function tests are either based on the measurement of secreted enzymes and bicarbonate (direct tests) or they investigate secondary effects which are the result of lack of enzymes (indirect tests).[19-21]

Direct Tests

Stool Tests

The fecal excretion of pancreatic enzymes correlates with duodenal enzyme secretion.[22] However, pancreatic enzymes are inactivated to different degrees during gastrointestinal transit. Chymotrypsin and elastase-1 are relatively more stable enzymes and are therefore suitable for stool testing.

The activity of chymotrypsin in stool can be tested photometrically. To improve the sensitivity of the test, three different stool samples are necessary, and this partially explains why chymotrypsin measurements have been largely replaced by measurement of fecal elastase-1, which only requires a single stool sample (compare below). Moreover, since the test does not differentiate human and substituted chymotrypsin, the test results are influenced by pancreatin supplementation. Thus, it is important that these enzyme supplements are discontinued at least 5 days before the examination. On the other hand, the chymotrypsin test can also be used to monitor compliance with enzyme supplementation in refractory cases. The main drawbacks of this test are its low sensitivity and specificity in patients with mild or moderate PEI.[23]

Currently, measurement of fecal elastase-1 concentration in a single stool sample is the preferred and most widely available pancreatic function test. The concentration of elastase-1 is by an enzyme-linked immunosorbent assay (ELISA) using a specific antibody against the human enzyme, so that pancreatin supplements have no influence on the results and there is no need to discontinue them. Normal stool-concentration of elastase-1 exceeds 200 µg/g stool, depending on the method, and a concentration less than 100 µg/g stool usually means severe PEI. Measurement of fecal elastase-1 is more sensitive and specific than chymotrypsin testing.[24] However, as a stand alone test in early chronic pancreatitis, the lack of sensitivity (50 to 93%) and specificity (62 to 93%) limit its diagnostic value.[24,25] Moreover, in the differential diagnosis of diarrhea, specificity of the test is rather low since increased stool-water content leads to false positive results.[26]

Secretin Test

The secretin (or secretin-pancreozymin) test is an invasive test that requires placement of a duodenal tube. It is regarded as the reference method for evaluation of pancreatic exocrine function. It can also detect mild and moderate PEI but has several disadvantages including invasiveness, high cost, need of special equipment and trained personnel,[26] and lack of standardization among different centers.

In order to achieve reliable test results, pancreatin preparations have to be discontinued several days in advance. Nicotine and drugs with sedative or anticholinergic effects have to be discontinued at least 24 hours before the secretin-test is performed, and the patient has to fast for at least 12 hours. The test is contraindicated in patients with acute pancreatitis for the first 8 to 12 weeks after the acute episode.

A commonly applied test protocol requires that the tip of a double-lumen nasoduodenal tube be placed near the ligament of Treitz. One lumen is placed in the gastric antrum for continuous aspiration of gastric secretions, which are discarded. Duodenal contents are aspirated via the second lumen of the tube for 30 min under basal conditions followed by a 60 min collection period with intravenous application of secretin. Subsequently, secretion volume, bicarbonate concentration, and activity of pancreatic enzymes (trypsin, chymotrypsin, lipase and amylase) are determined in duodenal juice samples. Secretin stimulation leads to maximal bicarbonate output but induces only moderate stimulation of pancreatic enzyme secretion. This is why a second stimulation period using a combination of secretin and cholecystokinin (CCK) or the CCK-analog cerulein is usually performed. However, these substances are currently not available in many countries. To compensate for incomplete aspiration of duodenal contents, a dilution marker can be added but this further complicates the procedure.

Endoscopy based modifications are used by some specialized centers.[27,28] The endoscopic secretin test includes aspiration of duodenal juice through the suction channel of the endoscope at 15, 30, 45, and 60 min after secretin stimulation. A bicarbonate concentration greater than 80 mmol/L in any of the samples is considered normal. The endoscopic secretin test has demonstrated good sensitivity and specificity compared with conventional tube based stimulation tests; however, a considerable limitation is that it takes approximately 1 h to perform. Reducing the length to 45 minutes with fluid collections at 30 and 45 minutes provides 94% accuracy compared with the 1 hour test but further abbreviations appear to lead to inaccurate results, although it is feasible to inject secretin prior to endoscopy so that the duration of intubation can be limited.[28,29] CCK alone or CCK in combination with secretin has also been used in endoscopic function tests.[28]

Lundh Test

The Lundh test[30] also requires intestinal intubation for direct measurement of enzyme output in duodenal juice. However, in contrast to the secretin test, pancreatic exocrine secretion is stimulated by a standardized test meal. This consists of 300 ml of liquid composed of dried milk, vegetable oil and dextrose (67% fat, 5% protein, 15% carbohydrate). Accordingly, release of regulatory mediators from the intestinal mucosa is needed for stimulation of pancreatic secretion, and false positive results may occur in intestinal diseases such as celiac sprue or altered gastroduodenal anatomy. Usually only trypsin activity is measured.

Indirect Tests

Fluorecein Dilaurate and NBT PABA Tests

The fluorescein dilaurate (pancreolauryl test=PLT) and the NBT-PABA test (N-benzoyl-L-tyrosyl-p-aminobenzoic acid test) are no longer commercially available in many countries. Briefly, for both tests, the patient ingests a substrate that is metabolized into two or more products by pancreatic enzymes. At least one of the metabolites (fluorescein or PABA) is absorbed from the gut, conjugated, and excreted in urine, where it can be measured. Increased fecal excretion of the unsplit molecule, and decreased absorption, blood levels, and urinary excretion of the metabolite will occur in patients with PEI. To account for inter-individual variability of intestinal absorption and renal function, the fluorescein dilaurate test includes application of the absorbable metabolite (fluorescein) on a second day and the results of the test are expressed as the ratio of excreted fluorescein on the test and the control day in percent. A ratio of less than 20% is clearly abnormal. A modified serum test eliminates the need for a second test day but does not increase sensitivity and specificity.[24]

^{13}C-Breath Tests

Several breath tests using ^{13}C-labeled substrates for measurement of pancreatic function have been developed recently.[26] Of these, tests using ^{13}C-labeled lipids are the most promising because, in chronic pancreatitis, lipase synthesis and secretion tend to be impaired earlier than those of other pancreatic enzymes (compare above). The labeled lipids are ingested orally together with a test meal and need to be digested to monoglycerides and free fatty acids by pancreatic lipase prior to absorption. Hepatic metabolism of the absorbed lipids leads to production of $^{13}CO_2$ which is transported to the lungs and exhaled. Thus, the ratio of $^{13}CO_2/^{12}CO_2$ in the breath over time reflects intestinal lipolysis by pancreatic lipase as the rate-limiting step of lipid absorption. Available substrates include 1,3 distearyl-2[^{13}C]-octanoate, called ^{13}C-mixed triglyceride, which has several advantages over other lipid markers and is the most commonly used. Other potential lipid markers are uniformly labeled Hiolein® (a mixture of long chain triglycerides) and cholesteryl-^{13}C-octanoate.[26] Sensitivity and specificity of certain test modifications have been reported to exceed 90%.[31] Moreover, a modified version of the ^{13}C-mixed triglyceride breath test has been shown to also detect mild to moderate PEI.[32] A major disadvantage of the test is the need for prolonged breath sampling. Retrospective comparison of test results in a large group of patients has shown that an abbreviated version requiring breath sampling for 4 hours still provides a high accuracy, but that shorter tests lack specificity.[33] Apart from diagnosis of PEI ^{13}C-breath tests can also be used to monitor the effect of enzyme replacement therapy.[34]

Fecal Fat Analysis

Quantitative measurement of fecal fat excretion over 72 h during ingestion of a diet containing 100 g fat per day is the reference method for diagnosis of steatorrhea. Under these circumstances, fecal fat excretion of more than 7 g/day is abnormal.[35] The levels of steatorrhea seen in CP tend to be much higher (often > 20 g/day). Due to its numerous disadvantages including nonspecificity for pancreatic disease, need for prolonged abstinence from pancreatic enzyme preparations, and unpleasant sampling, storage and mixing of stool, it is no longer performed in most centers for clinical reasons. Instead, Sudan staining of a random stool sample for fecal fat can be used but is relatively insensitive for fat malabsorption.[36]

Combined Morphological and Functional Investigations

Secretin-enhanced magnetic resonance cholangiopancreatography (S-MRCP) reveals ductal morphological alterations and simultaneously gives semiquantitative information on functional changes by evaluation of the degree of duodenal filling.[37] However, the number of relevant studies is limited and the sensitivity of this technique for exocrine insufficiency is only about 70%. Thus, normal duodenal filling does not rule out its existence.[38] Endoscopic ultrasonography has recently also been combined with secretin-stimulation. With that method, fluid filling in the descending part of duodenum was a predictor of pancreatic insufficiency.[39]

Clinical Role of Pancreatic Function Tests in Chronic Pancreatitis

Most experts agree that diagnosis of CP depends on a combination of clinical, histological, imaging and functional criteria.[38,40-42] Proof of impaired exocrine function by function testing is particularly important for diagnosis of CP in patients with inconclusive morphological findings. Moreover, staging of disease according to various classifications requires assessment of exocrine function. Function testing is generally recommended to screen patients with a new diagnosis of chronic pancreatitis for exocrine insufficiency. Some national guidelines recommend repetitive testing at annual intervals in patients with previously normal results.[40] When symptoms of exocrine insufficiency persist in spite of adequate enyzme tretament, function tests (^{13}C-breath test, measurement of fecal fat) are to be considered for evaluation of treatment efficacy. From a practical point of view, verification of PEI by a pathological pancreatic function test is a prerequisite for reimbursement of enzyme treatment in some countries.

References

1. DiMagno EP, Go VL, Summerskill WH. Relations between pancreatic enzyme ouputs and malabsorption in severe pancreatic insufficiency. *N Engl J Med.* 1973; 288(16): 813-815. PMID: 4693931.
2. DiMagno EP, Go VL, Summerskill HJ. Intraluminal and postabsorptive effects of amino acids on pancreatic enzyme secretion. *J Lab Clin Med.* 1973; 82(2): 241-248. PMID: 4721379.
3. DiMagno EP, Malagelada JR, Go VL. Relationship between alcoholism and pancreatic insufficiency. *Ann N Y Acad Sci.* 1975; 252: 200-207. PMID: 1056723.
4. Keller J and Layer P. Human pancreatic exocrine response to nutrients in health and disease. *Gut.* 2005; 54 Suppl 6: vi1-28. PMID: 15951527.
5. Carriere F, Laugier R, Barrowman JA, Douchet I, Priymenko N, Verger R. Gastric and pancreatic lipase levels during a test meal in dogs. *Scand J Gastroenterol.* 1993; 28(5): 443-454. PMID: 8511506.
6. Layer P, Go VL and DiMagno EP. Fate of pancreatic enzymes during small intestinal aboral transit in humans. *Am J Physiol Gastrointest Liver Physiol.* 1986; 251: G475-480. PMID: 2429560.
7. Layer P, Yamamoto H, Kalthoff L, Clain JE, Bakken LJ, DiMagno EP. The different courses of early- and late-onset idiopathic and alcoholic chronic pancreatitis. *Gastroenterology.* 1994; 107(5): 1481-1487. PMID: 7926511.
8. Sarles H, Augustine P, Laugier R, Mathew S, Dupuy P. Pancreatic lesions and modifications of pancreatic juice in tropical chronic pancreatitis (tropical calcific diabetes). *Dig Dis Sci.* 1994; 39(6): 1337-1344. PMID: 8200268.
9. Layer P, von der Ohe MR, Holst JJ, Jansen JB, Grandt D, Holtmann G, et al. Altered postprandial motility in chronic pancreatitis: role of malabsorption. *Gastroenterology.* 1997; 112(5): 1624-1634. PMID: 9136842.
10. Keller J, Holst JJ, Layer P. Inhibition of human pancreatic and biliary output but not intestinal motility by physiological intraileal lipid loads. *Am J Physiol Gastrointest Liver Physiol.* 2006; 290(4): G704-709. PMID: 16322090.
11. Regan PT, Malagelada JR, DiMagno EP, Glanzman SL, Go VL. Comparative effects of antacids, cimetidine and enteric coating on the therapeutic response to oral enzymes in severe pancreatic insufficiency. *N Engl J Med.* 1977; 297(16): 854-858. PMID: 20572.
12. Andersen DK. Mechanisms and emerging treatments of the metabolic complications of chronic pancreatitis. *Pancreas.* 2007; 35(1): 1-15. PMID: 17575539.
13. Lankisch PG, Droge M, Hofses S, Konig H, Lembcke B. Steatorrhoea: you cannot trust your eyes when it comes to diagnosis [letter] [see comments]. *Lancet.* 1996; 347(9015): 1620-1621. PMID: 8667884.
14. Dumasy V, Delhaye M, Cotton F, Deviere J. Fat malabsorption screening in chronic pancreatitis. *Am J Gastroenterol.* 2004; 99(7): 1350-1354. PMID: 15233677.
15. Moran CE, Sosa EG, Martinez SM, Geldern P, Messina D, Russo A, et al. Bone mineral density in patients with pancreatic insufficiency and steatorrhea. *Am J Gastroenterol .* 1997; 92(5): 867-871. PMID: 9149203.
16. Dujsikova H, Dite P, Tomandl J, Sevcikova A, Precechtelova M. Occurrence of metabolic osteopathy in patients with chronic pancreatitis. *Pancreatology.* 2008; 8(6): 583-586. PMID: 18824882.
17. Mann ST, Mann V, Stracke H, Lange U, Klor HU, Hardt P, et al. Fecal elastase 1 and vitamin D3 in patients with osteoporotic bone fractures. *Eur J Med Res.* 2008; 13(2): 68-72. PMID: 18424365.
18. Haas S, Krins S, Knauerhase A, Lohr M. Altered bone metabolism and bone density in patients with chronic pancreatitis and pancreatic exocrine insufficiency. *JOP.* 2015; 16(1): 58-62. PMID: 25640785.
19. Chowdhury RS, Forsmark CE. Review article: Pancreatic function testing. *Aliment Pharmacol Ther.* 2003; 17(6): 733-750. PMID: 12641496.
20. Niederau C, Grendell JH. Diagnosis of chronic pancreatitis. *Gastroenterology.* 1985; 88(6): 1973-1995. PMID: 3888772.

21. Ochi K, Mizushima T, Harada H, Matsumoto S, Matsumura N, Seno T. Chronic pancreatitis: functional testing. *Pancreas.* 1998; 16(3): 343-348. PMID: 9548677.
22. Katschinski M, Schirra J, Bross A, Goke B, Arnold R. Duodenal secretion and fecal excretion of pancreatic elastase-1 in healthy humans and patients with chronic pancreatitis. *Pancreas.* 1997; 15(2): 191-200. PMID: 9260205.
23. Lankisch PG, Schreiber A, Otto J. Pancreolauryl test. Evaluation of a tubeless pancreatic function test in comparison with other indirect and direct tests for exocrine pancreatic function. *Dig Dis Sci.* 1983; 28(6): 490-493. PMID: 6602697.
24. Siegmund E, Lohr JM, Schuff-Werner P. [The diagnostic validity of non-invasive pancreatic function tests-a meta-analysis]. *Z Gastroenterol.* 2004; 42(10): 1117-1128. PMID: 15508057.
25. Stein J, Jung M, Sziegoleit A, Zeuzem S, Caspary WF, Lembcke B. Immunoreactive elastase I: clinical evaluation of a new noninvasive test of pancreatic function. *Clin Chem.* 1996; 42(2): 222-226. PMID: 8595714.
26. Keller J, Aghdassi AA, Lerch MM, Mayerle JV, Layer P. Tests of pancreatic exocrine function-clinical significance in pancreatic and non-pancreatic disorders. *Best Pract Res Clin Gastroenterol.* 2009; 23(3): 425-439. PMID: 19505669.
27. Stevens T, Conwell DL, Zuccaro G, Jr., Van Lente F, Lopez R, Purich E, et al. A prospective crossover study comparing secretin-stimulated endoscopic and Dreiling tube pancreatic function testing in patients evaluated for chronic pancreatitis. *Gastrointest Endosc.* 2008; 67(3): 458-466. PMID: 18294508.
28. Stevens T and Parsi MA. Update on endoscopic pancreatic function testing. *World J Gastroenterol.* 2011; 17(35): 3957-3961. PMID: 22046082.
29. Erchinger F, Engjom T, Tjora E, Hoem D, Hausken T, Gilja OH, et al. Quantification of pancreatic function using a clinically feasible short endoscopic secretin test. *Pancreas.* 2013; 42(7): 1101-1106. PMID: 23921960.
30. James O. The Lundh test. *Gut.* 1973; 14(7): 582-591. PMID: 4581004.
31. Iglesias-Garcia J, Vilarino-Insua M, Iglesias-Rey M, Lourido V and Dominguez-Munoz E. Accuracy of the optimized ^{13}C-mixed triglyceride breath test for the diagnosis of steatorrhea in clinical practice. *Gastroenterology.* 2003; 124(4): Suppl1: A631.
32. Keller J, Bruckel S, Jahr C, Layer P. A modified ^{13}C-mixed triglyceride breath test detects moderate pancreatic exocrine insufficiency. *Pancreas.* 2011; 40(8): 1201-1205. PMID: 21705945.
33. Keller J, Meier V, Wolfram KU, Rosien U, Layer P. Sensitivity and specificity of an abbreviated (13)C-mixed triglyceride breath test for measurement of pancreatic exocrine function. *United European Gastroenterol J.* 2014; 2(4): 288-294. PMID: 25083286.
34. Dominguez-Munoz JE, Iglesias-Garcia J, Vilarino-Insua M, Iglesias-Rey M. ^{13}C-mixed triglyceride breath test to assess oral enzyme substitution therapy in patients with chronic pancreatitis. *Clin Gastroenterol Hepatol.* 2007; 5(4): 484-488. PMID: 17445754.
35. Safdi M, Bekal PK, Martin S, Saeed ZA, Burton F, Toskes PP. The effects of oral pancreatic enzymes (Creon 10 capsule) on steatorrhea: a multicenter, placebo-controlled, parallel group trial in subjects with chronic pancreatitis. *Pancreas.* 2006; 33(2): 156-162. PMID: 16868481.
36. Lieb JG II, Draganov PV. Pancreatic function testing: here to stay for the 21st century. *World J Gastroenterol.* 2008; 14(20): 3149-3158. PMID: 18506918.
37. Balci NC, Smith A, Momtahen AJ, Alkaade S, Fattahi R, Tariq S, et al. MRI and S-MRCP findings in patients with suspected chronic pancreatitis: correlation with endoscopic pancreatic function testing (ePFT). *J Magn Reson Imaging.* 2010; 31(3): 601-606. PMID: 20187202.
38. Martinez J, Abad-Gonzalez A, Aparicio JR, Aparisi L, Boadas J, Boix E, et al. The Spanish Pancreatic Club recommendations for the diagnosis and treatment of chronic pancreatitis: part 1 (diagnosis). *Pancreatology.* 2013; 13(1): 8-17. PMID: 23395564.
39. Engjom T, Erchinger F, Tjora E, Laerum BN, Georg D, Gilja OH. Diagnostic accuracy of secretin-stimulated ultrasonography of the pancreas assessing exocrine pancreatic failure in cystic fibrosis and chronic pancreatitis. *Scand J Gastroenterol.* 2015; 50(5): 601-610. PMID: 25623422.
40. Hoffmeister A, Mayerle J, Beglinger C, Buchler MW, Bufler P, Dathe K, et al. [S3-Consensus guidelines on definition, etiology, diagnosis and medical, endoscopic and surgical management of chronic pancreatitis German Society of Digestive and Metabolic Diseases (DGVS)]. *Z Gastroenterol.* 2012; 50(11): 1176-1224. PMID: 23150111.
41. Delhaye M, Van Steenbergen W, Cesmeli E, Pelckmans P, Putzeys V, Roeyen G, et al. Belgian consensus on chronic pancreatitis in adults and children: statements on diagnosis and nutritional, medical, and surgical treatment. *Acta Gastroenterol Belg.* 2014; 77(1): 47-65. PMID: 24761691.
42. Frulloni L, Falconi M, Gabbrielli A, Gaia E, Graziani R, Pezzilli R, et al. Italian consensus guidelines for chronic pancreatitis. *Dig Liver Dis.* 2010; 42 Suppl 6: S381-406. PMID: 21078490.

Chapter 44

Hereditary pancreatitis

Celeste A. Shelton[1,2] and David C. Whitcomb[1-4*]

[1]*Department of Medicine, University of Pittsburgh;*
[2]*Department of Human Genetics, University of Pittsburgh;*
[3]*Department of Cell Biology and Physiology, University of Pittsburgh;*
[4]*UPMC Medical Center, Pittsburgh, PA 15213.*

Introduction

Hereditary pancreatitis (HP) is a rare genetic disorder characterized by recurrent acute pancreatitis (RAP) and chronic pancreatitis (CP) that runs in families.[1-4] HP typically presents in childhood with attacks of acute pancreatitis (AP) that become more frequent, leading to the morphologic changes of chronic pancreatitis. Over time, patients may develop the common complications of CP, including pancreatic fibrosis, pancreatic exocrine insufficiency (PEI), diabetes mellitus (Type 3c; T3cDM),[5] chronic pain syndromes and pancreatic ductal adenocarcinoma (PDAC). However, the age of onset, clinical course, and types of complications vary markedly between individuals and families, suggesting that modifier genes and environmental factors play an important role in individual patients.[6,7]

Historically, HP has functioned as a model to understand the progression of AP to RAP and CP. The disease originates primarily from gain-of-function mutations in the cationic trypsinogen gene (protease, serine, 1; PRSS1; OMIM *276000), i.e., *PRSS1* N29I and R122H.[8-10] Specifically, the identification of gain-of-function mutations in the trypsinogen gene brought new insights into the field of pancreatology by indicating that (1) trypsin activity is the proximal cause of AP, (2) CP develops as a result of RAP, and (3) genetic and environmental factors modify the phenotype of RAP and CP.

Following the insights from HP and related advances, the concept of CP has been changed from diagnosing CP by end-stage features, to a new paradigm based on a progression model beginning with asymptomatic risk stage, and proceeding to inflammation (typically AP and RAP) and variable dysfunction of the relevant cell types that contribute to fibrosis, PEI, diabetes mellitus and pancreatic cancer. The new mechanistic definition highlights the essence of the disorder (mechanistic pathophysiology), as well as the characteristic features.[11]

> **CP definition (essence):** "Chronic pancreatitis is a pathologic fibro-inflammatory syndrome of the pancreas in individuals with genetic, environmental and/or other risk factors who develop persistent pathologic responses to parenchymal injury or stress".
> **CP definition (characteristics):** "Common features of established and advanced CP include pancreatic atrophy, fibrosis, pain syndromes, duct distortion and strictures, calcifications, pancreatic exocrine dysfunction, pancreatic endocrine dysfunction and dysplasia".

This new approach to defining and identifying CP should facilitate a rational approach to early diagnosis, classification, and prognosis for HP and other inflammatory disorders of the pancreas.

Diagnosis and classification

The term "hereditary pancreatitis" is used with both broad and narrow definitions. Online Mendelian Inheritance in Man (OMIM) #167800 defines 'PANCREATITIS, HEREDITARY; PCTT' broadly to include multiple genes associated with RAP and CP including *PRSS1, PRSS2, SPINK1, CFTR* and *CTRC*. Clinical researchers and geneticists generally define HP as autosomal dominant pancreatitis, and use the term "familial pancreatitis" to describe recessive or complex phenotypes in the absence of a recessive syndrome such as cystic fibrosis

*Corresponding author. Email: whitcomb@pitt.edu, whitcomb@pancreas.org

(CF) or a cystic fibrosis transmembrane conductance regulator gene (*CFTR*)-related disorder.[12] In this chapter, we define HP as 2 or more individuals with RAP or CP in 2 or more generations of a family (i.e., an autosomal dominant pattern of inheritance) or pancreatitis associated with a known, gain-of-function germline variant in *PRSS1*.[13,14]

Familial pancreatitis

Familial pancreatitis is a broader term to describe families in which the incidence of pancreatitis is higher than expected compared with the frequency of pancreatitis in the general population. Since pancreatitis, especially CP, is rare, 2 first- or second-degree relatives with pancreatitis are sufficient for classification as a familial pancreatitis kindred. However, other causes of pancreatitis, including gallstones, and trauma, must be excluded. Furthermore, episodic abdominal pain from AP may not be diagnosed in stoic patients, and older members of the family with diabetes mellitus or PDAC may represent late stages of undiagnosed CP. Thus, collecting an accurate family history and identifying familial pancreatitis may be challenging.

The contribution of genetics to familial pancreatitis is often broad and complex. Known genetic contributors to familial pancreatitis include recessive inheritance of mild variable or borderline *CFTR* mutations, pathogenic variants in *SPINK1*, and variants in other genes with small but interacting or additive effects. Whitcomb *et al.* demonstrated the complexity of gene-environment interactions that contribute to familial pancreatitis with a genome-wide association study (GWAS) carried out with next-generation sequencing.[15] In this HP kindred, 2 key affected family members were found to have completely different complex combinations of genetic and environmental risk factors.[15] The classification of hereditary pancreatitis and familial pancreatitis and examples of genotype-phenotype correlations are given in **Table 1**.

Clinical presentation

The penetrance for *PRSS1* hereditary pancreatitis has been estimated at 80%.[6,16-18] However, penetrance may vary by the presence of modifying risk factors and type of mutation. For example, one study reported a *PRSS1* R122H kindred in Venezuela with low penetrance, as demonstrated by the presence of only 2 affected individuals in a large family.[19]

The complications of HP are similar to those of CP. Early on it was recognized that some patients had severe AP with portal vein thrombosis,[4] but this does not appear to be the most common characteristic. The primary distinguishing features of HP from other forms of pancreatitis are an early age of onset and a family history in the absence of environmental risk factors (e.g., alcohol, tobacco). Furthermore, HP patients who progress to CP have higher cumulative risks for diabetes mellitus and exocrine insufficiency, and a higher overall risk for PDAC. This may be attributed to an early age of onset, resulting in longer lifetime exposure of the pancreas to injury and inflammation. As compared to the general population, lifespan is not reduced in HP patients who do not develop pancreatic cancer.[20]

Acute pancreatitis

HP typically presents in childhood at a median age of 10-12 years (**Figure 1**).[16,21] However, age at onset can vary dramatically by family, as demonstrated by one kindred where 58% of *PRSS1* R122H family members developed pancreatitis before the age of 5 years.[18] A number of studies have shown that the age of onset is earlier in R122H *PRSS1* kindreds compared to N29I *PRSS1* and mutation-negative patients.[9,16,18] Severity, length, and frequency of attacks can also vary substantially between families. As with other forms of pancreatitis, epigastric abdominal pain is the most common and disabling symptom, affecting at least 83% of HP patients.[21] Though attacks are typically 7 or less days in length,[16] smoldering pancreatitis and/or persistent pain occur in some cases.[22] Almost 90% of patients report more

Table 1. Genotype-phenotype correlations of hereditary pancreatitis

Genotype (variants)	Phenotype (syndromes)	Comment
PRSS1 GOF e.g., p.N29I, p. R122H, p.R122C	Autosomal dominant hereditary pancreatitis	Unregulated trypsin activity with premature activation Genetic counseling recommended for families and predictive testing
PRSS1 LOF e.g., p.D100H, p.C139F, p.K92N, p.S124F, p.G208A	Sporadic pancreatitis	Unfolded protein stress response. Genetic counseling optional
PRSS1 regulation e.g., rs10273639, rs4726576 A	Protection from trypsin-associated pancreatitis	Focus on non-trypsin-associated causes of pancreatitis

GOF, gain-of-function; LOF, loss-of-function.

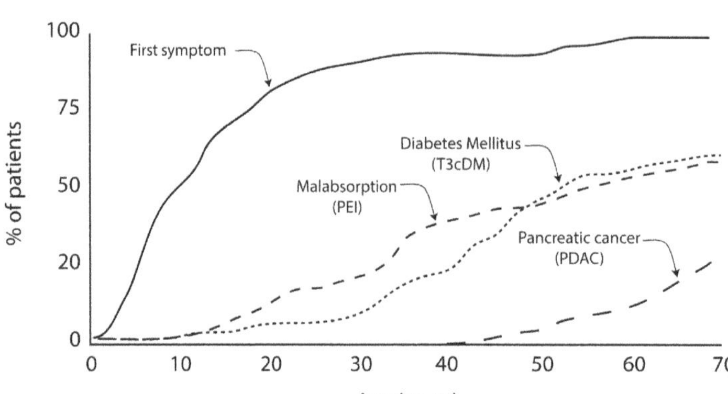

Figure 1. Historic data on the time from birth to detection of first symptoms (e.g. AP), malabsorption (e.g., PEI), Diabetes mellitus (e.g., T3cDM), and pancreatic cancer (i.e., PDAC). Figure based on models by Howes.[16]

than 5 hospitalizations, with a higher reported hospital admission rate for *PRSS1* R122H carriers than for N29I carriers (0.33 and 0.19 per year, respectively) (16). The same study found no significant difference in the number of attacks by type of mutation, suggesting that the R122H mutation may be associated with more severe attacks but not greater susceptibility.[16]

Chronic pancreatitis

The majority of HP patients with RAP progress to CP by the second or third decade of life. The degree of fibrosis is influenced by the number of attacks and other modifying factors. Eventually, progressive inflammation and fibrosis lead to PEI in a significant amount of patients. The cumulative risk for exocrine failure at 50 years of age has been estimated at 37.2%, with a median age of 53 years.[16] Diabetes arising from destruction of the islets of Langerhans by exocrine pancreatic disease is classified as T3cDM. Destruction of insulin-secreting beta cells also leads to glucose intolerance, followed by pancreatic endocrine insufficiency. Furthermore, loss of glucagon-secreting alpha cells reduces counter-regulatory hormones and places patients at risk for hypoglycemia and "brittle" disease. The cumulative risk for endocrine failure is 47.6% at 50 years of age, with a median age of diabetes mellitus onset of 53 years.[16]

Pancreatic cancer

Patients with HP have a >50-fold increased risk for pancreatic adenocarcinoma,[16,20,23] with a cumulative risk of 40-<54% at 70 years of age.[16,21,24] Risk is further increased in the presence of smoking and diabetes mellitus.[24,25] The increased risks of pancreatic cancer appear to result from prolonged pancreatic exposure to chronic inflammation[26-29] particularly in HP patients who develop pancreatitis in adolescence. However, the risk of PDAC does not tightly correlate with the severity of pancreatic inflammation and fibrosis.[23,30] The presence of shared risk and/or protective factors likely modifies the risk for pancreatic cancer among families, as evidenced by extensive variations in pancreatic cancer incidence between HP kindreds.

Epidemiology

HP is rare and is primarily a disease of Caucasians. The majority of identified families originate from the United States and European countries, including Italy,[8,31] England and Wales,[17] Germany,[32] France,[21,33] Turkey,[34] Denmark,[7] Spain,[35] and others.[16] Reports of HP from Asia are rare, though a few kindreds have been reported from Japan and China.[36-39]

In South America, 1 Brazilian family[40] and 1 Venezuelan patient[19] were reported to have HP originating from gain-of-function *PRSS1* mutations. In Mexico, single pancreatitis patients with *PRSS1* V39E or N42S variants were identified, but no *PRSS1*, R122H, or N29I variants were observed.[41]

No reports of HP families or individuals of African ancestry have been published to date. A *SPINK1* c.36G>C (p.L12F) variant has been observed in some African patients with pancreatitis, but functional analysis showed no detrimental effects from this common polymorphism.[42]

One HP family of Aboriginal descent was reported from New Zealand and found to carry the *PRSS1* R122H variant.[43] However, a number of this family's ancestors were European, suggesting that the mutation may have been inherited from European ancestors rather than Aboriginals.

The frequency of HP seen in clinical practice varies widely by geographic region. In the United States for example, there are large numbers of HP families throughout

Appalachia, including Pennsylvania, Ohio, West Virginia, Kentucky, Tennessee, Georgia, Northern Florida, Oklahoma, Minnesota, and California[44] (and personal observation). The elevated concentration of HP kindreds in these regions is believed to originate from early founders of the disease within large families who tended to remain within the previously described geographic regions. An early estimate of the prevalence of HP in the United States was about 1000 cases,[45] although the actual numbers are not known. A sampling of cases from 30 centers in the United States in the North American Pancreatitis Study (NAPS2)[46], and samples used in the first pancreatitis GWAS,[15] found that 19 of 1586 RAP and CP cases (excluding HP families) (1.2%) had *PRSS1* gain-of-function mutations. Overall, among NAPS2 cases the prevalence of *PRSS1* N29I, R122H and R122C was 2.8%, with no gain-of-function mutations in unrelated controls, although referral bias for the cases in this cohort is also possible. The population prevalence in France is estimated to be at least 0.3 per 100,000 according to a national series of HP patients.[21]

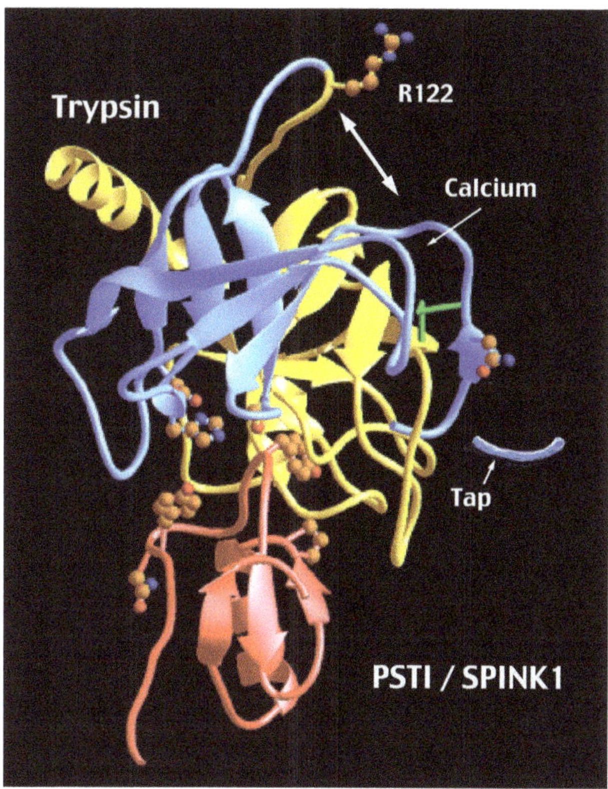

Figure 2. Structural representation of cationic trypsin (PRSS1, blue and yellow) interacting with the suicide inhibitor, pancreatic secretory trypsin inhibitor, SPINK1 (PRSST/SPINK1). The flexible side chain connecting the 2 globular domains illustrates the location of R122 as an autolysis site, which is the amino acid substituted in the R122H gain-of-function variant. The 2 calcium-binding sites are illustrated by the arrows from calcium, with the activation site of calcium binding being lost by activation and release of TAP. Figure constructed by William Furey and David Whitcomb.

Pathogenesis and pathology

Molecular genetics

PRSS1 hereditary pancreatitis

The pathogenesis of HP was discovered by Whitcomb *et al.* to be caused by mutations in the cationic trypsinogen gene (*PRSS1*).[47] Trypsinogen is the zymogen precursor to trypsin, a serine protease that hydrolyzes peptide bonds following an arginine or lysine, preferably in the small intestine. Two gain-of-function mutations were identified, the first being R122H and the second, N29I (initially designated R117H and N21I using the chymotrypsin numbering system).[9] These 2 mutations have been identified in the vast majority of HP kindreds in the United States and Europe, and comprise 90% of *PRSS1*-positive HP cases. A list of known *PRSS1* variants can be found at http://www.pancreasgenetics.org.

Analysis of trypsinogen's crystal structure provides insight into the pathogenic mechanisms of gain-of-function mutations. **Figure 2** is an x-ray crystallography figure of cationic trypsinogen illustrating 2 calcium-binding sites and 2 sites of trypsin-catalyzed hydrolysis. The trypsinogen activation peptide (TAP) at the N-terminus maintains the zymogen in an inactive form. First, trypsin can activate other trypsinogen molecules by cleaving the TAP [at residue K12] in the process of autoactivation.[48] This process is facilitated by calcium binding to the first calcium-binding pocket, which stabilizes the TAP. Once trypsinogen is activated, other trypsin molecules can induce autolysis by hydrolyzing arginine 122 on a flexible side chain (or autolysis loop) that links the 2 globular domains of trypsin.[49,50] The site is flexible, but protected from trypsin by calcium-binding to a second, adjacent pocket. Additional inhibitors of trypsin activity include CTRC, which cleaves the calcium-binding loop, and SPINK1, which binds to the trypsin active site as a suicide inhibitor. It has been observed that in the presence of elevated calcium concentrations (>1 mM Ca^{2+}), the hydrolysis of trypsin by another trypsin or by chymotrypsin C (CTRC) is blocked.[51] From a functional standpoint, the trypsinogen or trypsin molecule is susceptible to hydrolysis in low calcium concentrations, as seen inside the pancreatic acinar cell after synthesis, or in the distal intestine, but is resistant to hydrolysis when the calcium levels are high, as seen in the pancreatic duct duodenum and jejunum.[52] Thus, in high calcium concentrations, trypsin is more easily activated, whereas in lower trypsin concentrations, activation is minimized. The degradation of trypsin is a complex and well-orchestrated process involving both an additional trypsin molecule and CTRC. The interaction of these molecules under various conditions has been defined.[53,54]

Table 2.

Trypsin AA#	16	29	122
PRSS1	A	N	R
PRSS2	A	I	R
PRSS3	V	T	R
T6	A	N	H

Conversion Mutations between trypsinogen genes and pseudogenes. Comparison of amino acid sequences in PRSS1 with PRSS2, PRSS3 and T6. A alanine; H, Histidine; I, isoleucine; N, asparagine; R, arginine; T, threonine.

In the human trypsinogen family, anionic trypsinogen (PRSS2), meso trypsinogen (PRSS3) and 3 pseudogene paralogs exist that contain variants corresponding to the R122H mutation in *PRSS1* (e.g., T6, **Table 2**). Pseudogenes are noncoding relatives of functional genes that have typically acquired mutations rendering them nonfunctional. Generally, pseudogenes are harmless, except in cases where sequence homology with its functional paralog leads to recombination and acquisition of a pathogenic variant in the expressed gene. In the first report of a gene conversion event leading to a pathogenic *PRSS1* allele, 2 patients were identified where recombination events between exon 3 of *PRSS1* and the pseudogene *PRSS3P2* resulted in the accumulation of R122H within *PRSS1*.[55] *PRSS3P2* also contains variants corresponding to the known pathogenic A16V and N29T variants, which may also be acquired by *PRSS1* in a gene conversion event.

In 1 HP family, a novel 9 nucleotide intragenic duplication (c.63_71dup) was identified.[56] Functional studies supported this variant as a gain-of-function mutation, as evidenced by a $\geq$ 10-fold increase in both autoactivation and activation by human cathepsin B.[56]

In addition to gain-of function-mutations, trypsin activity can be markedly increased by copy number variations (CNVs). A variety of CNVs have been identified in HP families, and additional copies of *PRSS1* act as gain-of-function mutations by increasing trypsin expression, which predisposes to recurrent pancreatitis and hereditary pancreatitis.[57,58]

Additional mutations have been identified in the trypsin molecule that are associated with CP, but do not appear to be inherited as highly penetrant autosomal dominant variants. The most common one is the *PRSS1* A16V variant, which appears to act as a secondary or modifier variant to increase risk of pancreatitis.[59] Furthermore, not all trypsinogen mutations found in pancreatitis patients are gain-of-function variants. At least a dozen *PRSS1* variants that are rare and scattered throughout the molecule have been identified in case reports, and functional studies suggest that these variants are associated with misfolding of the mutant trypsinogen protein, triggering acinar cell stress through the unfolded protein response.[60,61] Further genotype-phenotype and therapeutic response studies need to be conducted to fully understand the implications of these findings for affected patients.

Other genes

Additional genes have been associated with recurrent acute and CP, a number of which regulate trypsin activity. Loss-of-function mutations in chymotrypsinogen C (*CTRC*) and the serine protease inhibitor, Kazal-type 1 (*SPINK1*) reduce the protective functions of these trypsin inhibitors in the pancreas.[51,53,62,63] Mutations in the CFTR that impair bicarbonate conductance are associated with RAP, CP and other CFTR-related disorders.[64] Next-generation sequencing suggests that more complex combinations of genes also play a significant role in the development and progression of CP.[65]

Histology

The pathogenicity of the *PRSS1* R122H variant was supported in a transgenic mouse model. Mice expressing the R122H_mPRSS1 transgene presented with early pancreatic acinar cell injury and inflammation, as well as progressive fibrosis and acinar cell dedifferentiation.[66] A later study examined pancreata from 10 *PRSS1*-mutation-positive (R122H, N29I, and IVS4-24 C>T) HP patients following a total pancreatectomy. Inspection of pancreatic tissue revealed progressive lipomatous atrophy and fat replacement, with thin and loosely packed fibrosis in comparison to alcoholic and obstructive CP.[67]

Genetic testing and counseling

The goals of genetic testing differ depending on the circumstances surrounding the patient. In general, asymptomatic subjects are not tested, especially if they are not in an HP family. However, testing may be indicated when a mutation has been previously identified in the family and/or for reproductive decision making. In patients with RAP or early signs of CP, genetic testing is medically indicated to make a diagnosis, and to develop a management plan. In established CP, genetic testing may be useful for anticipating and managing complications of CP. In end-stage disease, genetic testing is most useful for establishing risk to family members and for research purposes.

HP should be suspected in cases of idiopathic pancreatitis, early onset pancreatitis, and in families with multiple affected individuals. At least a 3-generation pedigree should be ascertained and evaluated for pancreatitis, pancreatic cancer, diabetes mellitus, PEI, CF, and exposures to smoking and alcohol to establish a HP kindred.[68] Risk calculation should always be taken in the context of the family history, particularly genotype (if known), inheritance pattern, environmental exposures, penetrance, ages of onset, and severity.

Following careful evaluation of the patient's personal and family history, targeted genetic testing of members of an established HP family may be considered in cases of unexplained RAP and/or CP, an affected individual with a first or second-degree relative with pancreatitis, unexplained pancreatitis in a child requiring hospitalization and/or when there is a known mutation in the family.[69] The patient should be provided with both pre- and post-test counseling to ensure that they understand the benefits, implications, and limitations of testing.[70,71] Insurance discrimination is a major concern for genetic testing in HP patients. Patients in the United States should be informed of the *Genetic Information Nondiscrimination Act of 2008* (GINA, Pub. L, 110–233), which protects against genetic discrimination in health insurance and employment, but affords no protection for life, disability, or long-term care insurance.

Commercial genetic testing is currently available for *PRSS1**, *SPINK1*, *CFTR*, and *CTRC*. As noted above, the trypsinogen gene family is complex, and both genes and pseudogenes are highly homologous. Therefore, specially designed genetic tests are required, and next-generation sequencing approaches such as whole exome sequencing or whole genome sequencing should not be used for *PRSS1* testing because of challenges in sequence alignment.

If a mutation is not identified from sequencing or a targeted mutation analysis, a deletion/duplication analysis can be considered. When a *PRSS1* mutation is identified, patients can be counseled on a 50% or 1 in 2 chance for each child to inherit the deleterious allele from a carrier parent. If the deleterious allele is inherited, the risk to develop HP is about 80%. Notably, these calculations should always be provided in the context of family history, as many HP families demonstrate significant differences in penetrance and severity.

Symptomatic patients

When genetic testing is indicated in a family, testing should always begin in a symptomatic individual. Test results may identify a genetic etiology in a family, thereby accelerating the diagnosis of other affected family members. Results may also have implications for risk to develop other complications, risk to other family members, and family planning. Not all families meeting clinical criteria for HP have an identifiable *PRSS1* mutation. Therefore, negative genetic test results in the affected proband of a family does not preclude the diagnosis of HP.

* Testing for hereditary pancreatitis has been patented (US 6406846 B1) owned by Dr. Whitcomb and licensed initial to Ambry Genetics, but now licensed to Arial Precision Medicine (www.arielmedicine.com).

Asymptomatic patients

In families where a deleterious variant has been identified, predictive genetic testing may be considered in close family members. Single-site testing for this mutation can provide information on risk and risk to descendants. Generally, risk of pancreatitis in an asymptomatic, mutation-positive adult decreases with age.

A family member who tests negative for the familial mutation has a significantly reduced, but not absent, risk for HP. Family members may have other unknown risk factors and are still at risk of pancreatitis of nongenetic etiology.

Genetic testing of asymptomatic family members in a family without an identifiable mutation is uninformative. As always, genetic counseling for risk should be provided in the context of family history.

Children

Genetic testing may be indicated in a child with diagnosed or suspected pancreatitis. Parents or legal guardians are responsible for the decision to pursue genetic testing. However, children 7 years of age and older should provide consent for the testing. Predictive genetic testing for asymptomatic patients less than 16 years of age is not recommended and does not have clear benefits.[69] The lifestyle practices that may be relevant to at risk carriers, such as a healthy low-fat diet and avoidance of alcohol, tobacco, and stress, are recommended for all children.[72]

Management and treatment

HP represents a complex syndrome, and studies on management are limited. Acute pancreatitis episodes are managed identically to AP from other etiologies, with attention to intravascular fluid status, oxygenations and pain control.[73]

Once the diagnosis is established, the focus is on minimizing recurrence and complications. Generally, patients should be counseled to avoid alcohol and tobacco, and referral to special programs for alcohol and/or smoking cessation in active users is advised. Alcohol lowers the threshold for attacks of AP and contributes to progression to CP. Smoking further increases the risk for pancreatic cancer by two-fold.[25] A low-fat diet in the form of multiple small meals a day and good hydration is often recommended but remains unproven. Stress reduction with activities such as running has been reported to be of major benefit in some patients (unpublished communication).

Pain

Pancreatic pain is complex and multifactorial.[74] Analgesics are commonly required to help control pain, ranging from acetaminophen and NSAIDs to narcotics. In some patients, antioxidants may also reduce pain by reducing oxidative stress in acinar cells.[75,76] As with other forms of pancreatitis, endoscopic or surgical interventions may also be indicated to alleviate pain. There is growing use of total pancreatectomy with islet autotransplantation (TP-IAT) in the United States, and this appears to be an effective (and radical) treatment in some patients.[77,78] (see below).

Pancreatic exocrine insufficiency

About a third to a half of the patients with HP will develop PEI in their lifetime.[21,79] PEI is a complex condition of insufficient pancreatic enzymes for digestion and absorption of nutrients. The threshold between sufficiency and insufficiency is vague because it depends on the meal, the diet and the capacity of the intestines in addition to the capacity of the pancreas to deliver enzymes.[80] If PEI is suspected because of symptoms of maldigestion and/or malnutrition, then function testing or a trial of pancreatic enzyme replacement therapy should be initiated.

Pancreatic endocrine insufficiency

Patients with CP should be monitored for development of T3cDM.[81] Diminished insulin secretion resulting from loss of beta islet cells may be further reduced by declines in proximal gut digestion and incretin secretion. Due to loss of glucagon and pancreatic polypeptide secreting alpha and polypeptide producing (gamma) cells, patients are at risk to develop "brittle" diabetes, characterized by difficult to control swings in blood glucose levels.

Total pancreatectomy

Total pancreatectomy with islet autotransplantation may be considered in younger patients for unmanageable pain.[77,82] Older patients with longstanding CP may benefit from total pancreatectomy without islet autotransplantation for pain alleviation and to reduce the risk of pancreatic cancer.[82,83]

Clinical trials

Calcium-channel blockers are being investigated as a therapy to reduce symptoms in individuals with HP. A pilot study demonstrated that amlodipine does not increase risk for an acute attack, cause pain, or significantly reduce quality of life.[84] The small trial also demonstrated a trend toward pain alleviation and reduction in quality of life.[84]

References

1. Comfort MW and Steinberg AG. Pedigree of a family with hereditary chronic relapsing pancreatitis. *Gastroenterology*. 1952; 21: 54-63. PMID: 14926813.
2. Gross JB and Comfort MW. Hereditary pancreatitis: report on two additional families. *Gastroenterology*. 1957; 32: 829-854. PMID: 13438142.
3. Gross JB, Gambill EE, and Ulrich JA. Hereditary pancreatitis. Description of a fifth kindred and summary of clinical features. *Am J Med*. 1962; 33: 358-364. PMID: 13902224.
4. McElroy R and Christiansen PA. Hereditary pancreatitis in a kinship associated with portal vein thrombosis. *Am J Med*. 1972; 52: 228-241. PMID: 5062005.
5. American Diabetes Assoc. Diagnosis and classification of diabetes mellitus. *Diabetes Care*. 2014; 37 Suppl 1: S81-S90. PMID: 24357215.
6. Amann ST, Gates LK, Aston CE, Pandya A and Whitcomb DC. Expression and penetrance of the hereditary pancreatitis phenotype in monozygotic twins. *Gut*. 2001; 48: 542-547. PMID: 11247900.
7. Joergensen MT, Brusgaard K, Cruger DG, Gerdes AM and Schaffalitzky de Muckadell OB. Genetic, epidemiological, and clinical aspects of hereditary pancreatitis: a population-based cohort study in Denmark. *Am J Gastroenterol*. 2010; 105(8): 1876-1883. PMID: 20502448.
8. Whitcomb DC, Gorry MC, Preston RA, Furey W, Sossenheimer MJ, Ulrich CD, et al. Hereditary pancreatitis is caused by a mutation in the cationic trypsinogen gene. *Nature Genetics*. 1996; 14: 141-145. PMID: 8841182.
9. Gorry MC, Gabbaizedeh D, Furey W, Gates LK, Jr., Preston RA, Aston CE, et al. Mutations in the cationic trypsinogen gene are associated with recurrent acute and chronic pancreatitis. *Gastroenterology*. 1997; 113: 1063-1068. PMID: 9322498.
10. Schneider A and Whitcomb DC. Hereditary pancreatitis: a model for inflammatory diseases of the pancreas. *Best Pract Res Clin Gastroenterol*. 2002; 16: 347-363. PMID: 12079262.
11. Whitcomb DC, Frulloni L, Garg P, Greer JB, Schneider A, Yadav D, et al. Chronic pancreatitis: An international draft consensus proposal for a new mechanistic definition. *Pancreatology*. 2016; 16: 218-224. PMID: 26924663.
12. Bombieri C, Claustres M, De Boeck K, Derichs N, Dodge J, Girodon E, et al. Recommendations for the classification of diseases as CFTR-related disorders. *J Cystic Fibrosis*. 2011; 10 Suppl 2: S86-S102. PMID: 21658649.
13. Solomon S, Whitcomb DC, and LaRusch J. PRSS1-Related Hereditary Pancreatitis. *GeneReviews*. RA Pagon, TD Bird, CR Dolan and K Stephens. Seattle, 2012.
14. Whitcomb DC and Lowe ME. Hereditary, Familial and Genetic Disorders of the Pancreas and Pancreatic Disorders in Childhood *Sleisenger and Fordtran's Gastrointestinal and Liver Disease: Pathophysiology / Diagnosis / Management*. M Feldman, LS Friedman and LJ Brandt. Philadelphia, W. B. Saunders Company. 2010; 1: 931-957.
15. Whitcomb DC, LaRusch J, Krasinskas AM, Klei L, Smith JP, Brand RE, et al. Common genetic variants in the CLDN2 and PRSS1-PRSS2 loci alter risk for alcohol-related and sporadic pancreatitis. *Nat Genet*. 2012; 44: 1349-1354. PMID: 23143602.
16. Howes N, Lerch MM, Greenhalf W, Stocken DD, Ellis I,Simon P, et al. Clinical and genetic characteristics of hereditary pancreatitis in Europe. *Clin Gastroenterol Hepatol*. 2004; 2(3): 252-261. PMID: 15017610.

17. Sibert JR. Hereditary pancreatitis in England and Wales. *J Med Genet*. 1978; 15: 189-201. PMID: 671483.
18. Sossenheimer MJ, Aston CE, Preston RA, Gates LK, Jr., Ulrich CD, Martin SP, et al. Clinical characteristics of hereditary pancreatitis in a large family, based on high-risk haplotype. The Midwest Multicenter Pancreatic Study Group (MMPSG). *Am J Gastroenterol*. 1997; 92: 1113-1116. PMID: 9219780.
19. Solomon S, Gelrud A, and Whitcomb DC. Low penetrance pancreatitis phenotype in a Venezuelan kindred with a PRSS1 R122H mutation. *JOP*. 2013; 14: 187-189. PMID: 23474566.
20. Rebours V, Boutron-Ruault MC, Jooste V, Bouvier AM, Hammel P, Ruszniewski P, et al. Mortality rate and risk factors in patients with hereditary pancreatitis: uni- and multidimensional analyses. *Am J Gastroenterol*. 2009; 104: 2312-2317. PMID: 19550412.
21. Rebours V, Boutron-Ruault MC, Schnee M, Ferec C, Le Marechal C, Hentic O, et al. The natural history of hereditary pancreatitis: a national series. *Gut*. 2009; 58: 97-103. PMID: 18755888.
22. Bellin MD, Freeman ML, Schwarzenberg SJ, Dunn TB, Beilman GJ, Vickers SM, et al. Quality of life improves for pediatric patients after total pancreatectomy and islet autotransplant for chronic pancreatitis. *Clin Gastroenterol Hepatol*. 2011; 9: 793-799. PMID: 21683160.
23. Rebours V, Boutron-Ruault MC, Schnee M, Ferec C, Maire F, Hammel P, et al. Risk of pancreatic adenocarcinoma in patients with hereditary pancreatitis: a national exhaustive series. *Am J Gastroenterol*. 2008; 103: 111-119. PMID: 18184119.
24. Lowenfels A, Maisonneuve P, DiMagno E, Elitsur Y, Gates L, Perrault J, et al. Hereditary pancreatitis and the risk of pancreatic cancer. *J Nat Cancer Inst*. 1997; 89: 442-446. PMID: 9091646.
25. Lowenfels AB, Maisonneuve P, Whitcomb DC, Lerch MM, and DiMagno EP. Cigarette smoking as a risk factor for pancreatic cancer in patients with hereditary pancreatitis. *JAMA*. 2001; 286: 169-170. PMID: 11448279.
26. Hengstler JG, Bauer A, Wolf HK, Bulitta CJ, Tanner B, Oesch F, et al. Mutation analysis of the cationic trypsinogen gene in patients with pancreatic cancer. *Anticancer Res*. 2000; 20: 2967-2974. PMID: 11062709.
27. Weiss FU. Pancreatic cancer risk in hereditary pancreatitis. *Front Physiol*. 2014; 5: 70. PMID: 24600409.
28. Whitcomb DC. Inflammation and Cancer V. Chronic pancreatitis and pancreatic cancer. *Am J Physiol Gastrointest Liver Physiol*. 2004; 287: G315-319. PMID: 15246966.
29. Whitcomb DC, Shelton CA, and Brand RE. Genetics and Genetic Testing in Pancreatic Cancer. *Gastroenterology*. 2015; 149: 1252-1264; e1254. PMID: 26255042.
30. Rebours V, Levy P, Mosnier JF, Scoazec JY, Soubeyrand MS, Flejou JF, et al. Pathology analysis reveals that dysplastic pancreatic ductal lesions are frequent in patients with hereditary pancreatitis. *Clin Gastroenterol Hepatol*. 2010; 8: 206-212. PMID: 19765677.
31. Scuro LA, Dobrilla G, Angelini G, Cavaliini G, Vantini I, and Barba A. Hereditary pancreatitis: report of the first kindred in Italy. *Acta Hepato Gastroenterologica*. 1973; 20: 70-76. PMID: 4757781.
32. Teich N, Ockenga J, Manns MP, Mössner J, and Keim V. Evidence for further mutations of the cationic trypsinogen in hereditary pancreatitis (abstract). *Digestion*. 1999; 60: 401.
33. Le Bodic L, Schnee M, Georgelin T, Soulard F, Ferec C, Bignon J, et al. An exceptional genealogy for hereditary chronic pancreatitis. *Dig Dis Sci*. 1996; 41: 1504-1510. PMID: 8689932.
34. Tautermann G, Ruebsamen H, Beck M, Dertinger S, Drexel H and Lohse P. R116C mutation of cationic trypsinogen in a Turkish family with recurrent pancreatitis illustrates genetic microheterogeneity of hereditary pancreatitis. *Digestion*. 2001; 64: 226-232. PMID: 11842279.
35. de las Heras-Castano G, Castro-Senosiain B, Fontalba A, Lopez-Hoyos M, and Sanchez-Juan P. Hereditary pancreatitis: clinical features and inheritance characteristics of the R122C mutation in the cationic trypsinogen gene (PRSS1) in six Spanish families. *JOP*. 2009; 10: 249-255. PMID: 19454815.
36. Nishimori I and Onishi S. Hereditary pancreatitis in Japan: a review of pancreatitis-associated gene mutations. *Pancreatology*. 2001; 1: 444-447. PMID: 12120222.
37. Lee YJ, Cheon CK, Kim K, Oh SH, Park JH, and Yoo HW. The PRSS1 c.623G>C (p.G208A) mutation is the most common PRSS1 mutation in Korean children with hereditary pancreatitis. *Gut*. 2015; 64: 359-360. PMID: 24780743.
38. Sun XT, Hu LH, Xia T, Shi LL, Sun C, Du YQ, et al. Clinical Features and Endoscopic Treatment of Chinese Patients With Hereditary Pancreatitis. *Pancreas*. 2015; 44: 59-63. PMID: 25058887.
39. Nishimori I, Kamakura M, Fujikawa-Adachi K, Morita M, Onishi S, Yokoyama K, et al. Mutations in exon 2 and 3 of the cationic trypsinogen gene in japanese families with hereditary pancreatitis. *Gut*. 1999; 44: 259-263. PMID: 9895387.
40. Dytz MG, Mendes de Melo J, de Castro Santos O, da Silva Santos ID, Rodacki M,Conceicao FL, et al. Hereditary Pancreatitis Associated With the N29T Mutation of the PRSS1 Gene in a Brazilian Family: A Case-Control Study. *Medicine (Baltimore)*. 2015; 94: e1508. PMID: 26376395.
41. Pelaez-Luna M, Robles-Diaz G, Canizales-Quinteros S and Tusie-Luna MT. PRSS1 and SPINK1 mutations in idiopathic chronic and recurrent acute pancreatitis. *World J Gastroenterol*. 2014; 20: 11788-11792. PMID: 25206283.
42. Kiraly O, Boulling A, Witt H, Le Marechal C, Chen JM, Rosendahl J, et al. Signal peptide variants that impair secretion of pancreatic secretory trypsin inhibitor (SPINK1) cause autosomal dominant hereditary pancreatitis. *Hum Mutat*. 2007; 28: 469-476. PMID: 17274009.
43. McGaughran JM, Kimble R, Upton J, and George P. Hereditary pancreatitis in a family of Aboriginal descent. *J Paediatr Child Health*. 2004; 40: 487-489. PMID: 15265195.
44. Applebaum-Shapiro SE, Finch R, Pfützer RH, Hepp LA, Gates L, Amann S, et al. Hereditary Pancreatitis in North America: The Pittsburgh - Midwest Multi-Center Pancreatic Study Group Study. *Pancreatology*. 2001; 1: 439-443. PMID: 12120221.
45. Lowenfels AB and Whitcomb DC. Estimating the number of hereditary panceatitis (HP) patients in the USA. *Pancreas*. 1997; 15: 444.
46. Whitcomb DC, Yadav D, Adam S, Hawes RH, Brand RE, Anderson MA, et al. Multicenter approach to recurrent acute

and chronic pancreatitis in the United States: the North American Pancreatitis Study 2 (NAPS2). *Pancreatology*. 2008; 8: 520-531. PMID: 18765957.

47. Whitcomb DC, Gorry MC, Preston RA, Furey W, Sossenheimer MJ, Ulrich CD, et al. Hereditary pancreatitis is caused by a mutation in the cationic trypsinogen gene. *Nat Genet*. 1996; 14: 141-145. PMID: 8841182.
48. Whitcomb DC and Lowe ME. Human pancreatic digestive enzymes. *Dig Dis Sci*. 2007; 52: 1-17. PMID: 17205399.
49. Varallyay E, Pal G, Patthy A, Szilagyi L, and Graf L. Two mutations in rat trypsin confer resistance against autolysis. *Biochem Biophys Res Commun*. 1998; 243: 56-60. PMID: 9473479.
50. Rovery M. Limited proteolyses in pancreatic chymotrypsinogens and trypsinogens. *Biochimie*. 1988; 70(9): 1131-1135. PMID: 3147704.
51. Szmola R and Sahin-Toth M. Chymotrypsin C (caldecrin) promotes degradation of human cationic trypsin: identity with Rinderknecht's enzyme Y. *Proc Natl Acad Sci U S A*. 2007; 104: 11227-11232. PMID: 17592142.
52. Colomb E, Guy O, Deprez P, Michel R, and Figarella C. The two human trypsinogens: catalytic properties of the corresponding trypsins. *Biochim Biophys Acta*. 1978; 525: 186-193. PMID: 28765.
53. Beer S, Zhou J, Szabo A, Keiles S, Chandak GR, Witt H, et al. Comprehensive functional analysis of chymotrypsin C (CTRC) variants reveals distinct loss-of-function mechanisms associated with pancreatitis risk. *Gut*. 2013; 62: 1616-1624. PMID: 22942235.
54. Szabo A and Sahin-Toth M. Increased activation of hereditary pancreatitis-associated human cationic trypsinogen mutants in presence of chymotrypsin C. *J Biol Chem*. 2012; 287: 20701-20710. PMID: 22539344.
55. Rygiel AM, Beer S, Simon P, Wertheim-Tysarowska K, Oracz G, Kucharzik T, et al. Gene conversion between cationic trypsinogen (PRSS1) and the pseudogene trypsinogen 6 (PRSS3P2) in patients with chronic pancreatitis. *Hum Mutat*. 2015; 36: 350-356. PMID: 25546417.
56. Joergensen MT, Geisz A, Brusgaard K, Schaffalitzky de Muckadell OB, Hegyi P, Gerdes AM, et al. Intragenic duplication: a novel mutational mechanism in hereditary pancreatitis. *Pancreas*. 2011; 40: 540-546. PMID: 21499207.
57. Masson E, Le Marechal C, Delcenserie R, Chen JM, and Ferec C. Hereditary pancreatitis caused by a double gain-of-function trypsinogen mutation. *Hum Genet*. 2008; 123: 521-529. PMID: 18461367.
58. Chen JM, Masson E, Le Marechal C, and Ferec C. Copy number variations in chronic pancreatitis. *Cytogenet Genome Res*. 2008; 123: 102-107. PMID: 19287144.
59. Grocock CJ, Rebours V, Delhaye MN, Andren-Sandberg A, Weiss FU, Mountford R, et al. The variable phenotype of the p.A16V mutation of cationic trypsinogen (PRSS1) in pancreatitis families. *Gut*. 2010; 59: 357-363. PMID: 19951905.
60. Kereszturi E and Sahin-Toth M. Intracellular autoactivation of human cationic trypsinogen mutants causes reduced trypsinogen secretion and acinar cell death. *J Biol Chem*. 2009; 284: 33392-33399. PMID: 19801634.
61. Schnur A, Beer S, Witt H, Hegyi P, and Sahin-Toth M. Functional effects of 13 rare PRSS1 variants presumed to cause chronic pancreatitis. *Gut*. 2014; 63: 337-343. PMID: 23455445.
62. Witt H, Luck W, Hennies HC, Classen M, Kage A, Lass U, et al. Mutations in the gene encoding the serine protease inhibitor, Kazal type 1 are associated with chronic pancreatitis. *Nat Genet*. 2000; 25: 213-216. PMID: 10835640.
63. Rosendahl J, Witt H, Szmola R, Bhatia E, Ozsvari B, Landt O, et al. Chymotrypsin C (CTRC) variants that diminish activity or secretion are associated with chronic pancreatitis. *Nat Genet*. 2008; 40: 78-82. PMID: 18059268.
64. LaRusch J, Jung J, General IJ, Lewis MD, Park HW, Brand RE, et al. Mechanisms of CFTR functional variants that impair regulated bicarbonate permeation and increase risk for pancreatitis but not for cystic fibrosis. *PLoS Genet*. 2014; 10: e1004376. PMID: 25033378.
65. Sofia VM, Da Sacco L, Surace C, Tomaiuolo AC, Genovese S, Grotta S, et al. Extensive molecular analysis suggested the strong genetic heterogeneity of idiopathic chronic pancreatitis. *Mol Med*. 2016; 22. PMID: 27264265.
66. Archer H, Jura N, Keller J, Jacobson M, and Bar-Sagi D. A mouse model of hereditary pancreatitis generated by transgenic expression of R122H trypsinogen. *Gastroenterology*. 2006; 131: 1844-1855. PMID: 17087933.
67. Singhi AD, Pai RK ,Kant JA, Bartholow TL, Zeh HJ, Lee KK, et al. The histopathology of PRSS1 hereditary pancreatitis. *Am J Surg Pathol*. 2014; 38: 346-353. PMID: 24525505.
68. Solomon S and Whitcomb DC. Genetics of pancreatitis: an update for clinicians and genetic counselors. *Curr Gastroenterol Rep*. 2012; 14: 112-117. PMID: 22314809.
69. Ellis I, Lerch MM, Whitcomb DC, and Consensus Committees of the European Registry of Hereditary Pancreatic Diseases MM-CPSGIAoP. Genetic testing for hereditary pancreatitis: guidelines for indications, counselling, consent and privacy issues. *Pancreatology*. 2001; 1: 405-415. PMID: 12120217.
70. Applebaum SE, Kant JA, Whitcomb DC, and Ellis IH. Genetic testing. Counseling, laboratory, and regulatory issues and the EUROPAC protocol for ethical research in multicenter studies of inherited pancreatic diseases. *Med Clin North Am*. 2000; 84: 575-588,viii. PMID: 10872415.
71. Fink EN, Kant JA, and Whitcomb DC. Genetic counseling for nonsyndromic pancreatitis. *Gastroenterol Clin North Am*. 2007; 36: 325-333,ix. PMID: 17533082.
72. Ross LF, Saal HM, David KL, Anderson RR, American Academy of Pediatrics, American College of Medical Genetics and Genomics, et al. Technical report: Ethical and policy issues in genetic testing and screening of children. *Genet Med*. 2013; 15: 234-245. PMID: 23429433.
73. Janisch N and Gardner T. Recent Advances in Managing Acute Pancreatitis. *F1000Res*. 2015; 4. PMID: 26918139.
74. Anderson MA, Akshintala V, Albers KM, Amann ST, Belfer I, Brand R, et al. Mechanism, assessment and management of pain in chronic pancreatitis: Recommendations of a multidisciplinary study group. *Pancreatology*. 2016; 16: 83-94. PMID: 26620965.
75. Burton F, Alkaade S, Collins D, Muddana V, Slivka A, Brand RE, et al. Use and perceived effectiveness of non-analgesic medical therapies for chronic pancreatitis in the United States. *Aliment Pharmacol Ther*. 2011; 33: 149-159. PMID: 21083584.

76. Uomo G, Talamini G and Rabitti PG. Antioxidant treatment in hereditary pancreatitis. A pilot study on three young patients. *Dig Liver Dis*. 2001; 33: 58-62. PMID: 11303976.
77. Chinnakotla S, Radosevich DM, Dunn TB, Bellin MD, Freeman ML, Schwarzenberg SJ, et al. Long-term outcomes of total pancreatectomy and islet auto transplantation for hereditary/genetic pancreatitis. *J Am Coll Surg*. 2014; 218: 530-543. PMID: 24655839.
78. Bellin MD, Freeman ML, Gelrud A, Slivka A, Clavel A, Humar A, et al. Total pancreatectomy and islet autotransplantation in chronic pancreatitis: recommendations from PancreasFest. *Pancreatology*. 2014: 14: 27-35. PMID: 24555976.
79. Howes N, Lerch MM, Greenhalf W, Stocken DD, Ellis I, Simon P, et al. Clinical and genetic characteristics of hereditary pancreatitis in Europe. *Clin Gastroenterol Hepatol*. 2004; 2: 252-261. PMID: 15017610.
80. Keller J and Layer P. Human pancreatic exocrine response to nutrients in health and disease. *Gut*. 2005; 54 Suppl 6: vi1-28. PMID: 15951527.
81. Rickels MR, Bellin M, Toledo FG, Robertson RP, Andersen DK, Chari ST, et al. Detection, evaluation and treatment of diabetes mellitus in chronic pancreatitis: recommendations from PancreasFest 2012. *Pancreatology*. 2013; 13: 336-342. PMID: 23890130.
82. Chinnakotla S, Beilman GJ, Dunn TB, Bellin MD, Freeman ML, Radosevich DM, et al. Factors Predicting Outcomes After a Total Pancreatectomy and Islet Autotransplantation Lessons Learned From Over 500 Cases. *Ann Surg*. 2015; 262: 610-622. PMID: 26366540.
83. Ulrich CD and Consensus Committees of the European Registry of Hereditary Pancreatic Diseases MM-CPSGIAoP. Pancreatic cancer in hereditary pancreatitis: consensus guidelines for prevention, screening and treatment. *Pancreatology*. 2001; 1(5): 416-422. PMID: 12120218.
84. Morinville VD, Lowe ME, Elinoff BD and Whitcomb DC. Hereditary pancreatitis amlodipine trial: a pilot study of a calcium-channel blocker in hereditary pancreatitis. *Pancreas*. 2007; 35(4): 308-312. PMID: 18090235.

Chapter 45

Idiopathic chronic pancreatitis: Genetic predisposition

Pramod Kumar Garg[1*] and Atsushi Masamune[2]

[1]*Department of Gastroenterology, All India Institute of Medical Sciences, New Delhi, India;*
[2]*Division of Gastroenterology, Tohoku University Graduate School of Medicine, Sendai, Japan.*

Introduction

The major causes of chronic pancreatitis (CP) include toxic injury due to alcohol and smoking, hereditary and nonhereditary genetic predisposition, metabolic derangements in the form of hypercalcemia and hypertriglyceridemia, anatomical abnormalities such as pancreas divisum, obstructive pathology such as tumors, and idiopathic. The cause of idiopathic CP has long been unclear. Initial thinking regarding the pathogenesis of idiopathic CP revolved around multiple environmental factors such as diet and toxins, but such hypotheses were never proven in well-designed case-control studies.[1] During the last decade, attention has dramatically shifted toward underlying genetic susceptibility as a risk factor in developing CP. With regard to alcohol as the cause of CP, it is not known why only a minority of patients who abuse alcohol develop CP, again suggesting that genetic predisposition as a significant risk factor. Indeed, intense research has revealed a strong genetic influence in CP pathogenesis and has renewed interest in the study of gene-environment interactions, similar to other common polygenic and poorly understood diseases such as diabetes.

Historical perspective

The role of genetic susceptibility in CP has been considered for over 30 years. Initial efforts were directed toward the association of human leukocyte antigen (HLA) genes with CP. In 1979, Faucet et al. studied 90 patients and 523 controls and showed that HLA B40 was associated with chronic alcoholic pancreatitis ($P<0.01$).[2] In 1981, Homma et al. showed HLA B5 to be associated with idiopathic CP but not alcoholic pancreatitis.[3] Abnormal class I and class II major histocompatibility complex antigen expression was shown in pancreatic ductular epithelial cells in 57% of patients with CP (mainly alcohol-related) along with T lymphocyte infiltration.[4] HLA association study results are summarized in **Table 1**. The limitations of these studies were (i) a lack of consistency among studies with many different loci associated with both idiopathic and alcohol-related CP; (ii) small sample sizes in most studies, although they did show significant differences between cases and controls; and (iii) the basic concept of autoimmunity as an underlying cause for CP was flawed to a large extent. The current concept of autoimmune pancreatitis had not been established when these studies were conducted. Nevertheless, the findings did point toward a possible genetic predisposition for CP development.

We will review various studies dealing with genetic predisposition to different types of CP. There is mounting evidence of strong genetic susceptibility in different types of CP with increasing numbers of identified genetic mutations.

Hereditary pancreatitis

Hereditary pancreatitis (HP) is a type of CP that affects multiple members of a family. It is transmitted as an autosomal dominant disease with penetrance as high as 80% (lower for some of the mutations) and variable expressivity. HP offered itself as a perfect model to identify causal genetic mutations. Indeed, in a landmark study, a mutation in the cationic trypsinogen gene (*PRSS1*) was found in a large kindred of HP with multiple affected members through genetic linkage analysis. Whitcomb et al. reported arginine to histidine substitution at residue 122 (p.R122H, p. designates protein coding; originally named R117H in the chymotrypsin numbering system) in *PRSS1* on the long arm of chromosome 7 (7q35).[5] Subsequent studies confirmed this exciting finding and revealed many more mutations in the *PRSS1* gene. The second-most common *PRSS1* mutation is p.N29I mutation in exon 2 with a change of

*Corresponding author. Email: pkgarg@aiims.ac.in

Table 1. Summary of the studies on the association of HLA with CP

Author	Year	Cases, n	Controls, n	Gene of interest	*P* value
Faucet[2]	1979	90	523	HLA B40	<0.01
Homma[3]	1981	46	120	HLA B5	<0.05
Gullo[73]	1982	64	425	HLA B13	<0.02
Wilson[88]	1984			HLA Bw39	<0.02
Forbes[89]	1987	50		HLA Cw5 (alcoholic CP)	<0.05
				A25, Cw1 (idiopathic CP)	<0.05
Anderson[90]	1988	88	344	HLA B21 (alcoholic CP)	<0.01
				HLA A1 (idiopathic CP)	<.002

isoleucine to asparagine at position 29.[6] HP is covered in another chapter in more detail.

Idiopathic CP

The pathogenesis of idiopathic CP has long been shrouded in mystery. Different hypotheses such as immune-mediated injury and environmental toxins were proposed but subsequently discarded. However, there has been tremendous advancement in the field of genetic mutations in the pathogenesis of idiopathic CP, leading to numerous studies on this subject. It is now generally accepted that genetic mutations are the most important risk factor for idiopathic CP; it is thought to be a polygenic disorder with strong environmental influence. Mutations in two important genes (i.e., *CFTR* and *SPINK1*) have been strongly implicated in idiopathic CP.

CFTR **mutations and idiopathic CP**

In 1998, two groups simultaneously showed that *CFTR* gene mutations were significantly associated with idiopathic CP. Sharer et al. showed that the frequency of minor *CFTR* mutations was increased 2.5 times in patients with idiopathic CP compared with healthy controls in an English population.[7] Similarly, Cohn et al. reported that the frequency of minor *CFTR* mutations was 11 times more common in patients with idiopathic CP compared with controls in an American population of predominantly northern European ancestry.[8] These groups introduced the concept of pancreas sufficiency in such patients with minor *CFTR* mutations who have no overt manifestations of cystic fibrosis (CF) but with isolated pancreatitis, a situation akin to absent vas deferens, which is also associated with some minor *CFTR* mutations. In contrast, patients with classical *CFTR* mutations have pancreatic insufficiency and atrophy but no pancreatitis. A recent study confirmed this concept of pancreas sufficiency and pancreatitis. Of 505 Israeli patients with CF, 139 (27.5%) were found to be pancreas sufficient, and none of them harbored the two mutations associated with severe disease; 20 (14.3%) of the 139 patients developed pancreatitis versus none of the 366 pancreatic insufficient patients.[9] Other groups subsequently confirmed the observations that minor mutations in the gene are common in patients with idiopathic CP compared with the general populations (**Table 2**). A German study revealed that the frequency of minor *CFTR* gene mutations was two times more common in patients with idiopathic CP as compared to controls.[10] In another large study of 381 patients from the USA, 32% (122/381) of patients had 166 mutated *CFTR* alleles, including 12 novel *CFTR* variants: c.4243-20A>G, p.F575Y, p.K598E, p.L1260P, p.G194R, p.F834L, p.S573C, c.2657+17C>T, 621+83 A>G, p.T164S, c.489+25A>G, and c.3368-19G>A.[11] [The CFTR gene mutations in intronic regions are expressed as c. (coding DNA sequence) ### (position of the last nucleotide in the adjacent exon) +/- ## (position of the change in the intron) followed by nucleotide change.][12] In a study of Brazilian patients, *CFTR* gene mutations were found to be common in patients with idiopathic CP.[13] However, in a study of 92 children with CP or recurrent acute pancreatitis from Poland, there was no definite association with *CFTR* gene mutations.[14] The natural history of patients with *CFTR* gene mutation-associated pancreatitis was analyzed in a study, which showed that it is characterized by recurrent attacks of pancreatitis over many years, finally leading to CP development, but endocrine and exocrine insufficiencies are rare or delayed.[15]

Association of CFTR mutations with idiopathic CP in non-Caucasian populations

As CF is generally more common among Caucasians, it is important to find out if *CFTR* mutations/polymorphisms are associated with idiopathic CP in non-Caucasian patients. In a Japanese study of 65 patients with CP, high associations of p.Q1352H (12.3% in CP patients vs. 3.7% in controls) and p.R1453W (6.2% vs. 3.1%) were found, suggesting an association of *CFTR* variants with CP in Japan where CF is

Table 2. Summary of studies on the association of *CFTR* mutations with idiopathic CP

Author	Year	cases, n	Controls	Gene of interest	*P* value*
Sharer[7]	1998	134	600	CFTR (13.4% vs. 5.3%)	<0.001
				5T allele (10.4%)	0.008
Cohn[8]	1998	27		CFTR (37% cases)	<0.001
Truninger[91]	2001	82		CFTR (21.4%, 4.8 times)	<0.05
Audrezet[92]	2002	39		CFTR (20%)	<0.05
Fujiki[16]	2004	65	121	CFTR (12.3% vs. 3.7%)	<0.05
Weiss[10]	2005	67	60	CFTR (25/134 vs. 11/120)	<0.05
Chang[20]	2007	78	200	CFTR 22/156 vs. 19/400)	0.001
Zoller[93]	2008	133		CFTR (12.7% vs. 3.2% controls)	<0.05
Aoyagi[94]	2009	20	110	5T in intron 8 (20% vs. 4.5%)	<0.05

very rare.[16] In this study, none of the common CF-causing mutations found in Caucasian populations were detected. Very recently, Nakano et al. reported a comprehensive analysis of *CFTR* variants in Japanese patients with CP by aid of next-generation sequencing.[17] They found 10 non-synonymous *CFTR* variants (p.R31C, p.R31H, p.I125T, p.K411E, p.V470M, p.I556V, p.L957fs, p.L1156F, p.Q1352H, and p.R1453W) in patients with idiopathic CP. The frequency of the p.L1156F variant was higher in patients with idiopathic CP than that in controls (10/121 vs. 46/1136, $P = 0.033$). A report from South Korea showed that the haplotype containing p.Q1352H showed the strongest association with bronchiectasis and CP ($P = 0.02$ and 0.008, respectively).[18] Another study from Japan showed the association of polythymidine tract 5T splicing variants of the intron 9 acceptor splice site [c.1210-12T(5_9)] with CP.[19] In a study from China, the occurrence of abnormal *CFTR* alleles was found to be thrice as frequent in idiopathic CP patients as in controls (22/156 vs. 19/400, $P<0.0001$).[20] The 5T allele was associated with early onset of idiopathic CP. The haplotype containing c.125G/c.1001+11C, (TG)12 repeats, p.470M, c.2694T, and c.4521G haplotype was associated with an increased risk of idiopathic CP (odds ratio [OR] 11.3; 95% confidence interval [CI] 2.3–54.6, $P = 0.008$) in Chinese patients. In a study of Indian patients with idiopathic CP, we found that minor *CFTR* variants were five times more common when compared with healthy controls, and six novel variants c.2280G>A, c.2988+35A>T, c.3718-41C>G, c.473G>A, c.1680-99C>T, and c.1392+4G>T) were detected.[21]

Mechanism of CFTR gene mutation in pancreatitis

The mechanism(s) involved in pancreatitis in patients with minor *CFTR* mutations is not known. A study showed that ion channel transport measured by sweat chloride and nasal transepithelial potential difference varied in patients with pancreatitis and minor *CFTR* mutations, but ion channel measurements worsened with increasing number and severity of *CFTR* mutations.[22] Another study showed abnormal ion transport in patients with two minor *CFTR* mutations and pancreatitis, which suggested that quantitatively the loss in CFTR function lies between that observed in CF patients and in normal carriers.[23] A recent study has shown that p.M348V minor *CFTR* mutation resulted in decreased chloride and bicarbonate fluxes across the *Xenopus* oocyte, indicating the possibility of similar defects in the pancreas.[24] However, whether such a putative defect in ionic fluxes operates across acinar or ductal cells is not known, and how such an effect leads to the initiation of pancreatitis is also not understood. It could be a result of different ion concentrations in the pancreatic juice within the ducts due to the defect in ductal cells, which leads to protein precipitation and obstruction, or a defect in acinar cells could perturb the internal milieu, resulting in disturbance in enzyme activation or secretion. As CF is a disease associated with overt bacterial infections, studies on the role of intestinal flora in CP progression are also warranted.

In summary, major and minor mutations in the *CFTR* gene are associated with idiopathic CP in both Caucasians and non-Caucasian patients.

Serine Protease Inhibitor Kazal Type 1 (*SPINK1*) gene and idiopathic CP

SPINK1 is an acute phase reactant protein. It is a natural protease inhibitor and inhibits active trypsin within the acinar cells of the pancreas. Thus, it provides protection against prematurely activated trypsin in acinar cells. In 2000, three important studies reported significantly higher frequencies of the p.N34S mutation in exon 3 of the *SPINK1* gene in patients with idiopathic CP.[25–27] Subsequently, many other studies described *SPINK1* gene mutations in patients with idiopathic CP of different ethnic origins. Studies from India showed that *SPINK1* gene mutations were quite common in patients with idiopathic (tropical) CP.[28,29] In addition to

N34S mutation, another mutation p.P55S in the *SPINK1* gene is also common in patients with idiopathic CP.[30] Other rare variants include p.D50E, p.Y54H, p.R65Q, and p.R67C. A meta-analysis in 2007 of all the studies on *SPINK1* mutations in CP found that the P.N34S mutation was detected in 469 of 4,842 patient alleles and in 96 of 9,714 control alleles, yielding a pooled OR of 11.00 (95% CI 7.59–15.93) based on allelic frequency for all CP etiologies.[31] The OR was higher for idiopathic CP compared with that for alcoholic CP [14.97 (95% CI 9.09–24.67) vs. 4.98 (95% CI 3.16–7.85)]. A comprehensive list of the studies included in the meta-analysis is available.[31]

In a more recent study of patients with idiopathic CP from Taiwan, *SPINK1* mutations were found in 32.4% of patients with early-onset and 2.1% of those with late-onset CP.[32] The most common mutation was the intronic variant IVS3+2T>C (c.194+2>C) rather than p.N34S as reported in other studies. The association of the IVS3+2T>C with CP was first reported in Japanese patients with CP.[33] This study showed a clear distinction between early- and late-onset CP with regard to genetic mutation, suggesting that mutation leads to early onset and more severe pancreatitis.

In Korea, *SPINK1* mutations p.N34S and IVS3+2T>C were identified in 3 and 11 out of 37 patients with idiopathic CP, respectively, including one with compound p.N34S/IVS3+2T>C heterozygote. The prevalence of *SPINK1* IVS3+2T>C mutation was 26.8% in patients with idiopathic CP.[34]

In a Japanese study, the frequencies of p.N34S and IVS3+2T>C in the *SPINK1* gene were significantly higher in patients with idiopathic CP (10.6% and 11.6%, respectively) than in controls (0.4% and 0%).[35]

The highest frequency of *SPINK1* p.N34S mutation was found in Indian patients with idiopathic CP. Three studies reported that *SPINK1* p.N34S mutation was present in 42% to 47% of patients with idiopathic (tropical) CP.[21,28,29]

Mechanism of SPINK1 *mutation and pancreatitis*

The mechanism as to how *SPINK1* p.N34S mutation causes CP is not well understood.[36] One study showed that p.N34S mutation was not associated with alternative splicing.[37] Two other studies almost simultaneously showed that the common p.N34S and p.P55S polymorphisms involve amino-acid substitutions with similar physicochemical properties but do not cause any significant reduction in terms of mature SPINK1 peptide expression.[38,39] On the other hand, the IVS3+2T>C mutation caused skipping of the entire exon 3, including the region containing the trypsin binding site. This leads to production of a mutated protein and lowered expression (62% of that observed in healthy controls).[40] The p.R65Q missense mutation involves substitution of a positively charged amino acid by a neutral one and causes a ~60% reduction in protein expression.[38] Other rare polymorphisms p.G48E, p.D50E, p.Y54H, and p.R67C involve charged amino acids and lead to complete or nearly complete loss of SPINK1 expression, possibly due to intracellular retention and degradation.[39]

In summary, *SPINK1* gene mutations, particularly P.N34S and IVS3+2T>C, are associated with idiopathic CP although geographical differences might exist.

Mutations in other genes and idiopathic CP

Since mutations in the cationic trypsinogen gene (*PRSS1*) were significantly associated with hereditary pancreatitis, mutations in anionic trypsinogen (*PRSS2*) were also tested in patients with CP. *PRSS2* p.G191R might actually confer protection against CP in Europeans; however, its protective role has been questioned in other populations.[41,42]

Chymotrypsinogen C (CTRC) degrades trypsinogen, and loss-of-function variants have been found in European patients with CP. In Indian and Japanese patients with idiopathic CP, no significant association with *CTRC* variants was found initially,[43] but a unique loss-of-function p.R29Q variant was identified in Japanese patients, and significant association has been shown for Indian patients with CP as well.[43–45]

A mutation in the calcium-sensing receptor (*CASR*) gene has been suggested to play a role in idiopathic CP in German patients.[46] In a US population, the *CASR* exon 7 p.R990G polymorphism was significantly associated with CP (OR, 2.01, 95% CI, 1.12-3.59, $P = 0.015$).[47] The association between *CASR* p.R990G and CP was stronger in subjects who reported moderate or heavy alcohol consumption (OR, 3.12, 95% CI, 1.14-9.13, $P = 0.018$). An association with the *CASR* gene mutation was also observed in Indian patients with idiopathic CP.[48]

Pancreatic stone protein (PSP) is a stress secretory protein considered to be a major component of pancreatic stones in CP.[49] The human PSP or Reg protein is encoded by the *reg1*a gene (regenerating gene). However, polymorphisms in *reg1*a, including the regulatory variants, were not found to be associated with idiopathic CP.[50]

Angiotensin-converting enzyme (ACE) activity might be related to pancreatic stellate cell activation and pancreatic fibrosis. However, no significant differences were found in the prevalence of the ACE-deletion genotype frequencies when patients with alcoholic (27.5%), nonalcoholic (26.4%), and acute pancreatitis (32.7%) were compared with controls (26.9%) in a recent European study.[51]

The hemochromatosis (*HFE*) gene is a major risk factor for hereditary hemochromatosis, but whether it might increase susceptibility to CP is not known. No significant differences were found in heterozygosities for p.C282Y and p.H63D among patients with alcoholic (8.0, 21.5%), idiopathic (7.3, 24.5%), or familial (9.8, 23.0%) pancreatitis, or pancreatic adenocarcinoma (5.4, 28.6%) or among healthy (6.2, 24.8%) and alcoholic (7.0, 25.0%) controls in a recent study.[52]

In a study from Taiwan, polymorphism of the tumor necrosis factor (TNF)-alpha gene was shown to be a risk factor for CP. The 2863A allele of the TNF-alpha promoter was associated with an increased risk for CP (OR 4.949, 95% CI 2.678–9.035). In multivariate analysis, 2863A and 21031C were independently associated with higher susceptibility to CP (P<0.0001).[53]

Genome-wide association studies

It has been recognized that hypothesis-driven investigations might take a long time and still not produce satisfactory results. In more complex polygenic diseases such as CP, multiple genes contribute to the pathogenesis through quantitative rather than qualitative change. Thus, a hypothesis-independent approach through genome wide association studies (GWAS) was initiated to find genes that influence disease risk.[54] Applying the GWAS approach, Whitcomb et al. identified two loci at *PRSS1-PRSS2* and X-linked *CLDN2* as robustly associated with recurrent acute pancreatitis and alcohol-related CP in subjects of European ancestry.[55] Subsequent studies have confirmed the association of these loci with idiopathic CP in patients of different ancestry (i.e., Chinese, Europeans, Japanese, and Indians).[56–59] Another GWAS recently showed a novel association between alcoholic CP and polymorphisms in the genes encoding fucosyltransferase 2 nonsecretor status (*FUT2* locus rs632111 and rs601338) and blood group B (ABO locus rs8176693).[60]

Is idiopathic CP a genetic disease?

In a study of 381 patients with CP, 32% had 166 mutant *CFTR* alleles, including 12 novel *CFTR* variants: c.4243-20A>G4375-20 A>G, p.F575Y, p.K598E, p.L1260P, p.G194R, p.F834L, p.S573C, c.2657+17C>T2789 + 17 C>T, 621+83 A>G, p.T164S, c.489+25A>G 621+25 A>G, and c.3368-19G>A3500-19 G>A. *SPINK1* mutation was seen in 14.5% (55/381), and *PRSS1* mutation was present in 8.1% (31/381) of patients.[11] Thus, 49% (185/381) of the patients had one or more mutations. In Indian patients with idiopathic CP, up to 51% of patients had *SPINK1* and/or *CFTR* mutations.[21] These observations lend strong support to the concept that the majority of idiopathic CP pattents have an underlying genetic predisposition. In addition, there must be environmental influences modulating the overt presentation and phenotype of the disease. Thus, it seems that the term "idiopathic CP" may no longer be justified, and a more meaningful term such a "CP-G" is proposed, where "G" denotes genetic susceptibility.

Genetic mutations/polymorphisms and alcoholic pancreatitis

The discovery of a variety of gene mutations in idiopathic and hereditary CP led to considerable enthusiasm, and it was thought that the same might hold true for alcohol-related CP. However unlike idiopathic CP, genetic mutations in the usually suspected genes (i.e., *SPINK1*, *PRSS1*, and *CFTR*) are not common in patients with alcoholic CP.

A study in European patients did not find any significant association with any of the three genes (i.e., *CFTR*, *PRSS1*, and *SPINK1*).[61] Neither *CFTR* nor cationic trypsinogen mutations were found to be predisposing risk factors for alcohol-related pancreatitis in a study from the US.[62] *CFTR* mutations did not seem to play an important role in alcoholic CP.[63] Another American study did not find *SPINK1* p.N34S mutation more commonly in alcoholic CP than in controls (6.3%, vs. 1.1% controls; P>0.05).[64] Studies from other parts of the world reported similar results. A Korean group did not find any association of chronic alcoholic pancreatitis with *CFTR* or *SPINK1* gene mutations.[65]

Polymorphisms at the known loci in the TNF-alpha, transforming growth factor (TGF)-beta(1), interleukin (IL)-10, and interferon (IFN)-gamma genes involved in inflammation were not found to be associated with alcoholic CP.[66] It was initially thought that pancreatitis-associated protein (PAP) might be involved in CP pathogenesis. However, there was no evidence for polymorphism of the *PAP* gene in patients with alcoholic pancreatitis.[67]

Polymorphisms of the genes related to the metabolism of the oxidative compounds such as NADPH-quinone oxidoreductase 2 (*NQO2*), multidrug resistance 1 (*MDR1*), and lipoprotein lipase (*LPL*) were analyzed in alcoholic CP. No significant differences were found between patients and controls with regard to these genes.[68] Similarly, polymorphisms in genes encoding other metabolizing enzymes such as glutathione-S-transferase P1 (*GSTP1*) and manganese-superoxide dismutase (*MnSOD*) and detoxifying phase II biotransformation enzymes such as the UDP-glucuronosyltransferases have not been found to be associated with susceptibility to alcoholic CP. [69,70] However, one study did find a significant association between UDP-glucuronosyltransferases and CP with an increased risk with the UGT1A7*3 allele (K129-K131-R208) (OR 1.76, 95% CI 1.26–2.46, P = 0.0009). Moreover, the UGT1A7*3 allele was specifically associated with the subgroup of patients with alcoholic pancreatitis, of whom 89% were smokers (OR 2.24, 95% CI 1.46-3.43, P = 0.0001).[71]

Polymorphisms in the monocyte chemotactic protein-1 (*MCP-1*) and heat-shock protein 70-2 (*HSP70-2*) were not found associated with alcoholic CP.[72]

Since alcohol is considered to cause toxic pancreas injury, polymorphisms in alcohol-metabolizing enzymes have been studied as a basis of individual susceptibility to pancreatitis. In the alcohol dehydrogenase 1B (*ADH1B*) gene, the ADH1B*1 wild-type allele frequency was significantly lower in alcoholic CP compared with alcoholics without CP.[73] No significant difference was found between the patient and control groups for aldehyde dehydrogenase enzyme *ADH2* genotypes, but another study did report a significant difference between the two groups in the acetaldehyde dehydrogenase enzyme *ALDH2* locus.[74] The frequency of the ALDH2*1 wild-type allele was found to be 0.681 and that of the ALDH2*2 allele (p.E504K) was 0.319 in controls, while the corresponding values in patients were 0.935 and 0.065. The ALDH2 isoenzyme exists in two isoforms (1 and 2 code for active and inactive subunits, respectively). It is expressed as ALDH2*1 or ALDH2*2. A person can be homozygous or heterozygous (i.e., ALDH2*1/*1 or ALDH2*1/*2). Most of the patients (27 of 31) were ALDH2*1/*1; only four were ALDH2*1/*2, and none of the patients were ALDH2*2/*2. Thus, genetic polymorphism of the *ALDH2* gene might influence the risk of developing alcoholic pancreatitis.[74] In another study, the frequencies of *ADH3* and *CYP2E1* c1c2 genotypes did not differ among CP patients, alcoholics, and healthy controls.[75] In a Polish study, ADH2*1, ADH3*1 alleles and ADH2*1/*1, ADH3*1/*1 genotypes were statistically more frequent among patients with alcoholic CP compared to controls.[76] In an Australian study, alcoholic cirrhosis but not alcoholic CP was associated with ADH3*2/*2 and perhaps with ADH2*1/*1.[77] Thus, there are contradictory and variable reports, and the data so far do not suggest any definite association with polymorphisms in either alcohol-metabolizing or detoxifying enzymes.

Genetic mutations in other types of CP

Some of the specific causes of CP are related to metabolic derangements or anatomical defects, and it is generally believed that these abnormalities are the sole cause for pancreatitis. However, recent studies have assessed the role of genetic predisposition in such patients.

In a study of patients with primary hyperparathyroidism, 4 (16%) of 25 patients with pancreatitis carried the p.N34S mutation in *SPINK1*, while none of 50 controls (hyperparathyroidism without pancreatitis) had *SPINK1* or *PRSS1* mutations ($P<0.05$ vs. controls, $P<0.001$ vs. general population).[78] In addition, *CFTR* mutations were present in four patients ($P<0.05$ vs. general population), while one patient carried a 5T allele. One patient was transheterozygous (*SPINK1*: p.N34S/*CFTR*: p.R553X). Importantly, the mean serum calcium level in pancreatitis patients did not significantly differ from that of patients without pancreatitis, thus questioning the value of serum calcium levels in pancreatitis causation or initiation. The authors concluded that genetic mutations significantly increase the risk of pancreatitis in patients with hyperparathyroidism.

In hypertriglyceridemia (HTG)-related CP, Chang et al. reported a higher frequency of *CFTR* gene mutations, suggesting that the mechanism of pancreatitis may be related to genetic predisposition.[79] In their study of 126 HTG patients, 13 (10.3%) carried a *CFTR* mutation (all p.I556V), the *CFTR* mutation rate was significantly higher in those with than those without pancreatitis (26.1% [12 of 46] vs. 1.3% [1 of 80]; $P<0.0001$). A multivariate analysis of HTG patients indicated that triglycerides, *CFTR* 470Val, and *TNF* promoter 863A were independent risk markers for HTG-associated pancreatitis.

There is considerable controversy whether or not pancreas divisum causes recurrent pancreatitis.[80] In patients with pancreas divisum presenting with recurrent pancreatitis, a study showed lower nasal transepithelial potential difference, suggesting a functional defect in the *CFTR* gene to account for the risk of pancreatitis in pancreas divisum.[81] Another case report identified minor *CFTR* mutations in two patients with pancreas divisum presenting with recurrent pancreatitis.[82] Another study showed that *SPINK1* gene mutations were present in 38% of patients with pancreas divisum and recurrent pancreatitis compared with 2% in healthy controls, suggesting that pancreas divisum alone is unlikely to cause pancreatitis and that pancreatitis may be a result of both genetic predisposition and anatomical defect, a two-hit theory.[83]

Genetic mutations not associated with CP

Polymorphisms in the *TNF* promoter region and the entire coding region of the corresponding TNF receptor 1 (*TNFR1*) gene were not associated with hereditary, familial, or idiopathic CP.[84]

Functional polymorphisms in the TGF-beta1, IL-10, and IFN-gamma genes were not found to be associated with hereditary, familial, or sporadic pancreatitis.[85]

Mutation in the genes coding for glutathione s-transferases (*MGST1*) and *GSTM3* genes or common deletions in the *GSTT1* and *GSTM1* genes were also not associated with hereditary pancreatitis.[86]

Keratin 8 gene mutation was not found to be associated with either hereditary or idiopathic CP.[87]

Future prospects

Although there have been significant gains in our understanding of genetic predisposition in CP, there are equally significant gaps in our knowledge. Currently known genetic mutations are associated with 50%-60% of cases in idiopathic CP.[11,21] Furthermore, the causative roles of genetic mutation in pancreatitis initiation and progression are not clear. For example, the *SPINK1* p.N34S mutation, which is the commonest mutation reported in patients with CP, does not result in any functional loss of protein activity. How this leads to pancreatitis is unknown. Whether it is just a bystander or modifier and not the causal mutation remains to be determined. In alcohol-related pancreatitis, it is not known why only <5%-10% of alcoholics develop pancreatitis. The genetic predisposition to alcohol-related pancreatitis has so far not yielded much information.

The modest effect of common variations, which is the basis of current GWAS screening technology, on many human diseases and related traits is helping shift interest to studies on rarer variants with larger effects on disease outcome. Thus, stringent selection of clinical phenotypes and prioritization of smaller patient cohorts for direct whole genome sequencing might be the best solution to identify putative causative variants.

References

1. Midha S, Singh N, Sachdev V, Tandon RK, Joshi YK, Garg PK. Cause and effect relationship of malnutrition with idiopathic chronic pancreatitis: prospective case-control study. *J Gastroenterol Hepatol*. 2008; 23: 1378-1383. PMID: 18554234.
2. Fauchet R, Genetet B, Gosselin M, Gastard J. HLA antigens in chronic alcoholic pancreatitis. *Tissue Antigens*. 1979; 13: 163-166. PMID: 442066.
3. Homma T, Aizawa T, Nagata A, Oguchi H. HLA antigens in chronic idiopathic pancreatitis compared with chronic alcoholic pancreatitis. *Dig Dis Sci*. 1981; 26: 449-452. PMID: 7249884.
4. Jalleh RP, Gilbertson JA, Williamson RC, Slater SD, Foster CS. Expression of major histocompatibility antigens in human chronic pancreatitis. *Gut*. 1993; 34: 1452-1457. PMID: 8244120.
5. Whitcomb DC, Gorry MC, Preston RA, Furey W, Sossenheimer MJ, Ulrich CD, et al. Hereditary pancreatitis is caused by a mutation in the cationic trypsinogen gene. *Nat Genet*. 1996; 14: 141-145. PMID: 8841182.
6. Gorry MC, Gabbaizedeh D, Furey W, Gates LK Jr, Preston RA, Aston CE, et al. Mutations in the cationic trypsinogen gene are associated with recurrent acute and chronic pancreatitis. *Gastroenterology*. 1997; 113: 1063-1068. PMID: 9322498.
7. Sharer N, Schwarz M, Malone G, Howarth A, Painter J, Super M, et al. Mutations of the cystic fibrosis gene in patients with chronic pancreatitis. *N Engl J Med*. 1998; 339: 645-652. PMID: 9725921.
8. Cohn JA, Friedman KJ, Noone PG, Knowles MR, Silverman LM, Jowell PS. Relation between mutations of the cystic fibrosis gene and idiopathic pancreatitis. *N Engl J Med*. 1998; 339: 653-658. PMID: 9725922.
9. Augarten A, Ben Tov A, Madgar I, Barak A, Akons H, Laufer J, et al. The changing face of the exocrine pancreas in cystic fibrosis: the correlation between pancreatic status, pancreatitis and cystic fibrosis genotype. *Eur J Gastroenterol Hepatol*. 2008; 20: 164-168. PMID: 18301294.
10. Weiss FU, Simon P, Bogdanova N, Mayerle J, Dworniczak B, Horst J, et al. Complete cystic fibrosis transmembrane conductance regulator gene sequencing in patients with idiopathic chronic pancreatitis and controls. *Gut*. 2005; 54: 1456-1460. PMID: 15987793.
11. Keiles S, Kammesheidt A. Identification of CFTR, PRSS1, and SPINK1 mutations in 381 patients with pancreatitis. *Pancreas*. 2006; 33: 221-227. PMID: 17003641.
12. Ogino S, Gulley ML, den Dunnen JT, Wilson RB, Association for Molecular Pathol Training and Education Committee. Standard mutation nomenclature in molecular diagnostics: practical and educational challenges. *J Mol Diagn*. 2007; 9: 1-6. PMID: 17251329.
13. Bernardino AL, Guarita DR, Mott CB, Pedroso MR, Machado MC, Laudanna AA, et al. CFTR, PRSS1 and SPINK1 mutations in the development of pancreatitis in Brazilian patients. *JOP*. 2003; 4: 169-177. PMID: 14526128.
14. Sobczynska-Tomaszewska A, Bak D, Oralewska B, Oracz G, Norek A, Czerska K, et al. Analysis of CFTR, SPINK1, PRSS1 and AAT mutations in children with acute or chronic pancreatitis. *J Pediatr Gastroenterol Nutr*. 2006; 43: 299-306. PMID: 16954950.
15. Frulloni L, Castellani C, Bovo P, Vaona B, Calore B, Liani C, et al. Natural history of pancreatitis associated with cystic fibrosis gene mutations. *Dig Liver Dis*. 2003; 35: 179-185. PMID: 12779072.
16. Fujiki K, Ishiguro H, Ko SB, Mizuno N, Suzuki Y, Takemura T, et al. Genetic evidence for CFTR dysfunction in Japanese: background for chronic pancreatitis. *J Med Genet*. 2004; 41: e55. PMID: 15121783.
17. Nakano E, Masamune A, Niihori T, Kume K, Hamada S, Aoki Y, et al. Targeted next-generation sequencing effectively analyzed the cystic fibrosis transmembrane conductance regulator gene in pancreatitis. *Dig Dis Sci*. 2015; 60: 1297-1307. PMID: 25492507.
18. Lee JH, Choi JH, Namkung W, Hanrahan JW, Chang J, Song SY, et al. A haplotype-based molecular analysis of CFTR mutations associated with respiratory and pancreatic diseases. *Hum Mol Genet*. 2003; 12: 2321-2332. PMID: 12952861.
19. Kimura S, Okabayashi Y, Inushima K, Yutsudo Y, Kasuga M. Polymorphism of cystic fibrosis gene in Japanese patients with chronic pancreatitis. *Dig Dis Sci*. 2000; 45: 2007-2012. PMID: 11117575.
20. Chang MC, Chang YT, Wei SC, Tien YW, Liang PC, Jan IS, et al. Spectrum of mutations and variants/haplotypes of CFTR and genotype-phenotype correlation in idiopathic chronic pancreatitis and controls in Chinese by complete analysis. *Clin Genet*. 2007; 71: 530-539. PMID: 17539902.

21. Midha S, Khajuria R, Shastri S, Kabra M, Garg PK. Idiopathic chronic pancreatitis in India: phenotypic characterisation and strong genetic susceptibility due to SPINK1 and CFTR gene mutations. *Gut*. 2010; 59: 800-807. PMID: 20551465.
22. Bishop MD, Freedman SD, Zielenski J, Ahmed N, Dupuis A, Martin S, et al. The cystic fibrosis transmembrane conductance regulator gene and ion channel function in patients with idiopathic pancreatitis. *Hum Genet*. 2005; 118: 372-381. PMID: 16193325.
23. Noone PG, Zhou Z, Silverman LM, Jowell PS, Knowles MR, Cohn JA. Cystic fibrosis gene mutations and pancreatitis risk: relation to epithelial ion transport and trypsin inhibitor gene mutations. *Gastroenterology*. 2001; 121: 1310-1319. PMID: 11729110.
24. Weiss FU, Simon P, Bogdanova N, Shcheynikov N, Muallem S, Lerch MM. Functional characterisation of the CFTR mutations M348V and A1087P from patients with pancreatitis suggests functional interaction between CFTR monomers. *Gut*. 2009; 58: 733-734. PMID: 19359437.
25. Chen JM, Mercier B, Audrezet MP, Ferec C. Mutational analysis of the human pancreatic secretory trypsin inhibitor (PSTI) gene in hereditary and sporadic chronic pancreatitis. *J Med Genet*. 2000; 37: 67-69. PMID: 10691414.
26. Pfutzer RH, Barmada MM, Brunskill AP, Finch R, Hart PS, Neoptolemos J, et al. SPINK1/PSTI polymorphisms act as disease modifiers in familial and idiopathic chronic pancreatitis. *Gastroenterology*. 2000; 119: 615-623. PMID: 10982753.
27. Witt H, Luck W, Hennies HC, Classen M, Kage A, Lass U, et al. Mutations in the gene encoding the serine protease inhibitor, Kazal type 1 are associated with chronic pancreatitis. *Nat Genet*. 2000; 25: 213-216. PMID: 10835640.
28. Chandak GR, Idris MM, Reddy DN, Bhaskar S, Sriram PV, Singh L. Mutations in the pancreatic secretory trypsin inhibitor gene (PSTI/SPINK1) rather than the cationic trypsinogen gene (PRSS1) are significantly associated with tropical calcific pancreatitis. *J Med Genet*. 2002; 39: 347-351. PMID: 12011155.
29. Bhatia E, Choudhuri G, Sikora SS, Landt O, Kage A, Becker M, et al. Tropical calcific pancreatitis: strong association with SPINK1 trypsin inhibitor mutations. *Gastroenterology*. 2002; 123: 1020-1025. PMID: 12360463.
30. Drenth JP, te Morsche R, Jansen JB. Mutations in serine protease inhibitor Kazal type 1 are strongly associated with chronic pancreatitis. *Gut*. 2002; 50: 687-692. PMID: 11950817.
31. Aoun E, Chang CC, Greer JB, Papachristou GI, Barmada MM, Whitcomb DC. Pathways to injury in chronic pancreatitis: decoding the role of the high-risk SPINK1 N34S haplotype using meta-analysis. *PLoS One*. 2008; 3: e2003. PMID: 18414673.
32. Chang YT, Wei SC, L PC, Tien YW, Jan IS, Su YN, et al. Association and differential role of PRSS1 and SPINK1 mutation in early-onset and late-onset idiopathic chronic pancreatitis in Chinese subjects. *Gut*. 2009; 58: 885. PMID: 19433603.
33. Kaneko K, Nagasaki Y, Furukawa T, Mizutamari H, Sato A, Masamune A, et al. Analysis of the human pancreatic secretory trypsin inhibitor (PSTI) gene mutations in Japanese patients with chronic pancreatitis. *J Hum Genet*. 2001; 46: 293-297. PMID: 11355022.
34. Oh HC, Kim MH, Choi KS, Moon SH, Park DH, Lee SS, et al. Analysis of PRSS1 and SPINK1 mutations in Korean patients with idiopathic and familial pancreatitis. *Pancreas*. 2009; 38: 180-183. PMID: 18852684.
35. Masamune A. Genetics of pancreatitis: the 2014 update. *Tohoku J Exp Med*. 2014; 232: 69-77. PMID: 24522117.
36. Chen JM, Ferec C. The true culprit within the SPINK1 p.N34S-containing haplotype is still at large. *Gut*. 2009; 58: 478-480. PMID: 19299380.
37. Masamune A, Kume K, Takagi Y, Kikuta K, Satoh K, Satoh A, et al. N34S mutation in the SPINK1 gene is not associated with alternative splicing. *Pancreas*. 2007; 34: 423-428. PMID: 17446841.
38. Boulling A, Le Marechal C, Trouve P, Raguenes O, Chen JM, Ferec C. Functional analysis of pancreatitis-associated missense mutations in the pancreatic secretory trypsin inhibitor (SPINK1) gene. *Eur J Hum Genet*. 2007; 15: 936-942. PMID: 17568390.
39. Kiraly O, Wartmann T, Sahin-Toth M. Missense mutations in pancreatic secretory trypsin inhibitor (SPINK1) cause intracellular retention and degradation. *Gut*. 2007; 56: 1433-1438. PMID: 17525091.
40. Kume K, Masamune A, Kikuta K, Shimosegawa T. [-215G>A; IVS3+2T>C] mutation in the SPINK1 gene causes exon 3 skipping and loss of the trypsin binding site. *Gut*. 2006; 55: 1214. PMID: 16849362.
41. Sundaresan S, Chacko A, Dutta AK, Bhatia E, Witt H, Te Morsche RH, et al. Divergent roles of SPINK1 and PRSS2 variants in tropical calcific pancreatitis. *Pancreatology*. 2009; 9: 145-149. PMID: 19077465.
42. Mahurkar S, Bhaskar S, Reddy DN, Rao GV, Singh SP, Thomas V, et al. The G191R variant in the PRSS2 gene does not play a role in protection against tropical calcific pancreatitis. *Gut*. 2009; 58: 881-882. PMID: 19433599.
43. Derikx MH, Szmola R, te Morsche RH, Sunderasan S, Chacko A, Drenth JP. Tropical calcific pancreatitis and its association with CTRC and SPINK1 (p.N34S) variants. *Eur J Gastroenterol Hepatol*. 2009; 21: 889-894. PMID: 19404200.
44. Paliwal S, Bhaskar S, Mani KR, Reddy DN, Rao GV, Singh SP, et al. Comprehensive screening of chymotrypsin C (CTRC) gene in tropical calcific pancreatitis identifies novel variants. *Gut*. 2013; 62: 1602-1606. PMID: 22580415.
45. Masamune A, Nakano E, Kume K, Kakuta Y, Ariga H, Shimosegawa T. Identification of novel missense CTRC variants in Japanese patients with chronic pancreatitis. *Gut*. 2013; 62: 653-654. PMID: 23135764.
46. Felderbauer P, Klein W, Bulut K, Ansorge N, Dekomien G, Werner I, et al. Mutations in the calcium-sensing receptor: a new genetic risk factor for chronic pancreatitis? *Scand J Gastroenterol*. 2006; 41: 343-348. PMID: 16497624.
47. Muddana V, Lamb J, Greer JB, Elinoff B, Hawes RH, Cotton PB, et al. Association between calcium sensing receptor gene polymorphisms and chronic pancreatitis in a US population: role of serine protease inhibitor Kazal 1type

and alcohol. *World J Gastroenterol*. 2008; 14: 4486-4491. PMID: 18680227.

48. Murugaian EE, Premkumar RM, Radhakrishnan L, Vallath B. Novel mutations in the calcium sensing receptor gene in tropical chronic pancreatitis in India. *Scand J Gastroenterol*. 2008; 43: 117-121. PMID: 18938753.
49. Bimmler D, Schiesser M, Perren A, Scheele G, Angst E, Meili S, et al. Coordinate regulation of PSP/reg and PAP isoforms as a family of secretory stress proteins in an animal model of chronic pancreatitis. *J Surg Res*. 2004; 118: 122-135. PMID: 15100001.
50. Mahurkar S, Bhaskar S, Reddy DN, Rao GV, Chandak GR. Comprehensive screening for reg1alpha gene rules out association with tropical calcific pancreatitis. *World J Gastroenterol*. 2007; 13: 5938-5943. PMID: 17990360.
51. Hucl T, Kylanpaa ML, Kunzli B, Witt H, Lempinen M, Schneider A, et al. Angiotensin-converting enzyme insertion/deletion polymorphism in patients with acute and chronic pancreatitis. *Eur J Gastroenterol Hepatol*. 2009; 21: 1032-1035. PMID: 19307975.
52. Hucl T, Kylanpaa-Back ML, Witt H, Kunzli B, Lempinen M, Schneider A, et al. HFE genotypes in patients with chronic pancreatitis and pancreatic adenocarcinoma. *Genet Med*. 2007; 9: 479-483. PMID: 17666895.
53. Chang MC, Chang YT, Tien YW, Liang PC, Wei SC, Wong JM. Association of tumour necrosis factor alpha promoter haplotype with chronic pancreatitis. *Gut*. 2006; 55: 1674-1676. PMID: 16809418.
54. Hirschhorn JN, Daly MJ. Genome-wide association studies for common diseases and complex traits. *Nat Rev Genet*. 2005; 6: 95-108. PMID: 15716906.
55. Whitcomb DC, LaRusch J, Krasinskas AM, Klei L, Smith JP, Brand RE, et al. Common genetic variants in the CLDN2 and PRSS1-PRSS2 loci alter risk for alcohol-related and sporadic pancreatitis. *Nat Genet*. 2012; 44: 1349-1354. PMID: 23143602.
56. Wang W, Sun XT, Weng XL, Zhou DZ, Sun C, Xia T, et al. Comprehensive screening for PRSS1, SPINK1, CFTR, CTRC and CLDN2 gene mutations in Chinese paediatric patients with idiopathic chronic pancreatitis: a cohort study. *BMJ Open*. 2013; 3: e003150. PMID: 24002981.
57. Derikx MH, Kovacs P, Scholz M, Masson E, Chen JM, Ruffert C, et al. Polymorphisms at PRSS1-PRSS2 and CLDN2-MORC4 loci associate with alcoholic and non-alcoholic chronic pancreatitis in a European replication study. *Gut*. 2015; 64: 1426-1433. PMID: 25253127.
58. Masamune A, Nakano E, Hamada S, Kakuta Y, Kume K, Shimosegawa T. Common variants at PRSS1-PRSS2 and CLDN2-MORC4 loci associate with chronic pancreatitis in Japan. *Gut*. 2015; 64: 1345-1346. PMID: 26002935.
59. Giri AK, Midha S, Banerjee P, Agrawal A, Mehdi SJ, Dhingra R, et al. Common Variants in CLDN2 and MORC4 Genes Confer Disease Susceptibility in Patients with Chronic Pancreatitis. *PLoS One*. 2016; 11: e0147345. PMID: 26820620.
60. Weiss FU, Schurmann C, Teumer A, Mayerle J, Simon P, Volzke H, et al. ABO blood type B and fucosyltransferase 2 non-secretor status as genetic risk factors for chronic pancreatitis. *Gut*. 2016; 65: 353-354. PMID: 26061595.
61. Perri F, Piepoli A, Stanziale P, Merla A, Zelante L, Andriulli A. Mutation analysis of the cystic fibrosis transmembrane conductance regulator (CFTR) gene, the cationic trypsinogen (PRSS1) gene, and the serine protease inhibitor, Kazal type 1 (SPINK1) gene in patients with alcoholic chronic pancreatitis. *Eur J Hum Genet*. 2003; 11: 687-692. PMID: 12939655.
62. Monaghan KG, Jackson CE, KuKuruga DL, Feldman GL. Mutation analysis of the cystic fibrosis and cationic trypsinogen genes in patients with alcohol-related pancreatitis. *Am J Med Genet*. 2000; 94: 120-124. PMID: 10982968.
63. Whitcomb DC. Genetic polymorphisms in alcoholic pancreatitis. *Dig Dis*. 2005; 23: 247-254. PMID: 16508289.
64. Schneider A, Pfutzer RH, Barmada MM, Slivka A, Martin J, Whitcomb DC. Limited contribution of the SPINK1 N34S mutation to the risk and severity of alcoholic chronic pancreatitis: a report from the United States. *Dig Dis Sci*. 2003; 48: 1110-1115. PMID: 12822871.
65. Lee KH, Ryu JK, Yoon WJ, Lee JK, Kim YT, Yoon YB. Mutation analysis of SPINK1 and CFTR gene in Korean patients with alcoholic chronic pancreatitis. *Dig Dis Sci*. 2005; 50: 1852-1856. PMID: 16187186.
66. Schneider A, Barmada MM, Slivka A, Martin JA, Whitcomb DC. Analysis of tumor necrosis factor-alpha, transforming growth factor-beta 1, interleukin-10, and interferon-gamma polymorphisms in patients with alcoholic chronic pancreatitis. *Alcohol*. 2004; 32: 19-24. PMID: 15066699.
67. Keim V, Hoffmeister A, Teich N, Halm U, Scheurlen M, Tannapfel A, et al. The pancreatitis-associated protein in hereditary and chronic alcoholic pancreatitis. *Pancreas*. 1999; 19: 248-254. PMID: 10505755.
68. Maruyama K, Harada S, Yokoyama A, Naruse S, Hirota M, Nishimori I, et al. Association analysis among polymorphisms of the various genes and chronic alcoholic pancreatitis. *J Gastroenterol Hepatol*. 2008; 23 Suppl 1: S69-S72. PMID: 18336668.
69. Verlaan M, Drenth JP, Truninger K, Koudova M, Schulz HU, Bargetzi M, et al. Polymorphisms of UDP-glucuronosyltransferase 1A7 are not involved in pancreatic diseases. *J Med Genet*. 2005; 42: e62. PMID: 16199544.
70. Osterreicher CH, Schultheiss J, Wehler M, Homann N, Hellerbrand C, Kunzli B, et al. Genetic polymorphisms of manganese-superoxide dismutase and glutathione-S-transferase in chronic alcoholic pancreatitis. *Mutagenesis*. 2007; 22: 305-310. PMID: 17548864.
71. Ockenga J, Vogel A, Teich N, Keim V, Manns MP, Strassburg CP. UDP glucuronosyltransferase (UGT1A7) gene polymorphisms increase the risk of chronic pancreatitis and pancreatic cancer. *Gastroenterology*. 2003; 124: 1802-1808. PMID: 12806614.
72. Lee SH, Ryu JK, Jeong JB, Lee KY, Woo SM, Park JK, et al. Polymorphisms of the MCP-1 and HSP70-2 genes in Korean patients with alcoholic chronic pancreatitis. *Dig Dis Sci*. 2008; 53: 1721-1727. PMID: 17940904.
73. Gullo L, Tabacchi PL, Corazza GR, Calanca F, Campione O, Labo G. HLA-B13 and chronic calcific pancreatitis. *Dig Dis Sci*. 1982; 27: 214-216. PMID: 6951694.
74. Kimura S, Okabayashi Y, Inushima K, Kochi T, Yutsudo Y, Kasuga M. Alcohol and aldehyde dehydrogenase

polymorphisms in Japanese patients with alcohol-induced chronic pancreatitis. *Dig Dis Sci.* 2000; 45: 2013-2017. PMID: 11117576.

75. Verlaan M, Te Morsche RH, Roelofs HM, Laheij RJ, Jansen JB, Peters WH, et al. Genetic polymorphisms in alcohol-metabolizing enzymes and chronic pancreatitis. *Alcohol.* 2004; 39: 20-24. PMID: 14691069.
76. Cichoz-Lach H, Celinski K, Slomka M. Alcohol-metabolizing enzyme gene polymorphisms and alcohol chronic pancreatitis among Polish individuals. *HPB (Oxford).* 2008; 10: 138-143. PMID: 18773092.
77. Frenzer A, Butler WJ, Norton ID, Wilson JS, Apte MV, Pirola RC, et al. Polymorphism in alcohol-metabolizing enzymes, glutathione S-transferases and apolipoprotein E and susceptibility to alcohol-induced cirrhosis and chronic pancreatitis. *J Gastroenterol Hepatol.* 2002; 17: 177-182. PMID: 11966948.
78. Felderbauer P, Karakas E, Fendrich V, Bulut K, Horn T, Lebert R, et al. Pancreatitis risk in primary hyperparathyroidism: relation to mutations in the SPINK1 trypsin inhibitor (N34S) and the cystic fibrosis gene. *Am J Gastroenterol.* 2008; 103: 368-374. PMID: 18076731.
79. Chang YT, Chang MC, Su TC, Liang PC, Su YN, Kuo CH, et al. Association of cystic fibrosis transmembrane conductance regulator (CFTR) mutation/variant/haplotype and tumor necrosis factor (TNF) promoter polymorphism in hyperlipidemic pancreatitis. *Clin Chem.* 2008; 54: 131-138. PMID: 17981921.
80. Quest L, Lombard M. Pancreas divisum: opinio divisa. *Gut.* 2000; 47: 317-319. PMID: 10940261.
81. Gelrud A, Sheth S, Banerjee S, Weed D, Shea J, Chuttani R, et al. Analysis of cystic fibrosis gener product (CFTR) function in patients with pancreas divisum and recurrent acute pancreatitis. *Am J Gastroenterol.* 2004; 99: 1557-1562. PMID: 15307877.
82. Dray X, Fajac I, Bienvenu T, Chryssostalis A, Sogni P, Hubert D. Association of pancreas divisum and recurrent acute pancreatitis with the IVS8-5T-12TG allele of the CFTR gene and CFTR dysfunction. *Pancreas.* 2007; 35: 90-93. PMID: 17575549.
83. Garg PK, Khajuria R, Kabra M, Shastri SS. Association of SPINK1 gene mutation and CFTR gene polymorphisms in patients with pancreas divisum presenting with idiopathic pancreatitis. *J Clin Gastroenterol.* 2009; 43: 848-852. PMID: 19593166.
84. Schneider A, Pogue-Geile K, Barmada MM, Myers-Fong E, Thompson BS, Whitcomb DC. Hereditary, familial, and idiopathic chronic pancreatitis are not associated with polymorphisms in the tumor necrosis factor alpha (TNF-alpha) promoter region or the TNF receptor 1 (TNFR1) gene. *Genet Med.* 2003; 5: 120-125. PMID: 12644782.
85. Schneider A, Barmada MM, Slivka A, Martin JA, Whitcomb DC. Transforming growth factor-beta1, interleukin-10 and interferon-gamma cytokine polymorphisms in patients with hereditary, familial and sporadic chronic pancreatitis. *Pancreatology.* 2004; 4: 490-494. PMID: 15316224.
86. Schneider A, Togel S, Barmada MM, Whitcomb DC. Genetic analysis of the glutathione s-transferase genes MGST1, GSTM3, GSTT1, and GSTM1 in patients with hereditary pancreatitis. *J Gastroenterol.* 2004; 39: 783-787. PMID: 15338373.
87. Schneider A, Lamb J, Barmada MM, Cuneo A, Money ME, Whitcomb DC. Keratin 8 mutations are not associated with familial, sporadic and alcoholic pancreatitis in a population from the United States. *Pancreatology.* 2006; 6: 103-108. PMID: 16327287.
88. Wilson JS, Gossat D, Tait A, Rouse S, Juan XJ, Pirola RC. Evidence for an inherited predisposition to alcoholic pancreatitis. A controlled HLA typing study. *Dig Dis Sci.* 1984; 29: 727-730. PMID: 6589150.
89. Forbes A, Schwarz G, Mirakian R, Drummond V, Chan CK, Cotton PB, et al. HLA antigens in chronic pancreatitis. *Tissue Antigens.* 1987; 30: 176-183. PMID: 3686517.
90. Anderson RJ, Dyer PA, Donnai D, Klouda PT, Jennison R, Braganza JM. Chronic pancreatitis, HLA and autoimmunity. *Int J Pancreatol.* 1988; 3: 83-90. PMID: 3162507.
91. Truninger K, Malik N, Ammann RW, Muellhaupt B, Seifert B, Muller HJ, et al. Mutations of the cystic fibrosis gene in patients with chronic pancreatitis. *Am J Gastroenterol.* 2001; 96: 2657-2661. PMID: 11569691.
92. Audrezet MP, Chen JM, Le Marechal C, Ruszniewski P, Robaszkiewicz M, Raguenes O, et al. Determination of the relative contribution of three genes-the cystic fibrosis transmembrane conductance regulator gene, the cationic trypsinogen gene, and the pancreatic secretory trypsin inhibitor gene-to the etiology of idiopathic chronic pancreatitis. *Eur J Hum Genet.* 2002; 10: 100-106. PMID: 11938439.
93. Zoller H, Egg M, Graziadei I, Creus M, Janecke AR, Loffler-Ragg J, et al. CFTR gene mutations in pancreatitis: Frequency and clinical manifestations in an Austrian patient cohort. *Wien Klin Wochenschr.* 2007; 119: 527-533. PMID: 17943404.
94. Aoyagi H, Okada T, Hasatani K, Mibayashi H, Hayashi Y, Tsuji S, et al. Impact of cystic fibrosis transmembrane conductance regulator gene mutation on the occurrence of chronic pancreatitis in Japanese patients. *J Int Med Res.* 2009; 37: 378-384. PMID: 19383231.

Chapter 46

Pathogenesis and treatment of pain in chronic pancreatitis

Søren Schou Olesen[1], Elke Tieftrunk[2], Güralp O. Ceyhan[2], and Asbjørn Mohr Drewes[1*]

[1]*Department of Gastroenterology & Hepatology, Aalborg University Hospital and Denmark;*
[2]*Clinic and Polyclinic for Surgery, Technical University of Munich, Germany.*

Introduction

Chronic pancreatitis (CP) is an inflammatory process of the pancreas characterized by fibrosis and progressive destruction. In most patients, the early phase is dominated by pain or recurrent episodes of pancreatitis and complications. In the advanced phase, symptoms related to exocrine and/or endocrine insufficiency are also seen.[1] Hence, apart from local complications the three major clinical features of CP are pain, maldigestion, and diabetes. Pain can affect the complications of CP. For example, if postprandial pain results in patients refraining from eating, then enzyme treatment may not be very helpful against malnutrition. Eating habits can also influence diabetes regulation, immune system function, and quality of life. Therefore, pain can be regarded as the most severe complication of CP, especially as it is poorly understood and difficult to treat.

Characterization of pain

Abdominal pain is present in most patients and is the primary cause of hospitalization.[2] Pancreatic pain is characteristically described as a constant, severe, dull, epigastric pain that often radiates to the back and typically worsens after meals. However, many different pain patterns have been described. The pain has previously been thought to decrease over time, the so-called "burn-out" hypothesis. However, evidence against this hypothesis was provided by two large prospective studies that found no association between the duration of CP and the quality or frequency of pain.[3] Today the "burn-out" hypothesis is regarded as obsolete, and most patients have a chronisc pain pattern with exacerbations of variable frequency. The economic burden is also of major importance. CP has a profound impact on social life and employment patterns mainly due the complications, pain being the most severe.[4] In the year 2000 in the USA, the disease accounted for 327,000 hospitalizations, 200,000 emergency room visits, and 532,000 physician visits costing $2.5 billion.[5]

Pain pathogenesis

Even though the pain can be caused by a variety of factors, obstruction of the flow from acinar cells and destruction of the nerves are thought to be of major importance. This has led to a dispute between supporters of the so called "plumbing" and "wiring" hypotheses.[2] Advocates of the plumbing hypothesis cite findings that indicate pain is generated by increased pressure in the pancreatic duct or in the pancreatic parenchyma. This mechanistic understanding of pain has been the most widely accepted explanation and it is the theoretical basis of most interventions including surgical and endoscopic drainage procedures. However, endoscopic manometry has not documented ductal hypertension in CP, and no difference in pressure has been observed in patients with or without pain.[6] In a recent study, our group found no association between the degree of pathology–fibrosis, atrophy, and ductal abnormality on magnetic resonance cholangiopancreatography with diffusion weighted imaging and pain.[7] However, pancreatic atrophy and ductal pathology were associated with diabetes and phosphate and hemoglobin levels. Hence, the plumbing hypothesis may not be relevant for pain in pancreatitis in general, although relief of obstruction is undoubtedly helpful in selected cases.

Other potential mechanisms resulting in pain are microstructural changes caused by the histopathological changes during evolution of the disease. There is increasing evidence that pancreatic stellate cells are key mediators of fibrosis, the formation of extracellular matrix in the interstitial space, leading to areas where acinar cells have disappeared or duct cells have been injured. This ultimately leads to progressive loss of the lobular morphology and structure of the pancreas.

*Corresponding author. Email: amd@rn.dk

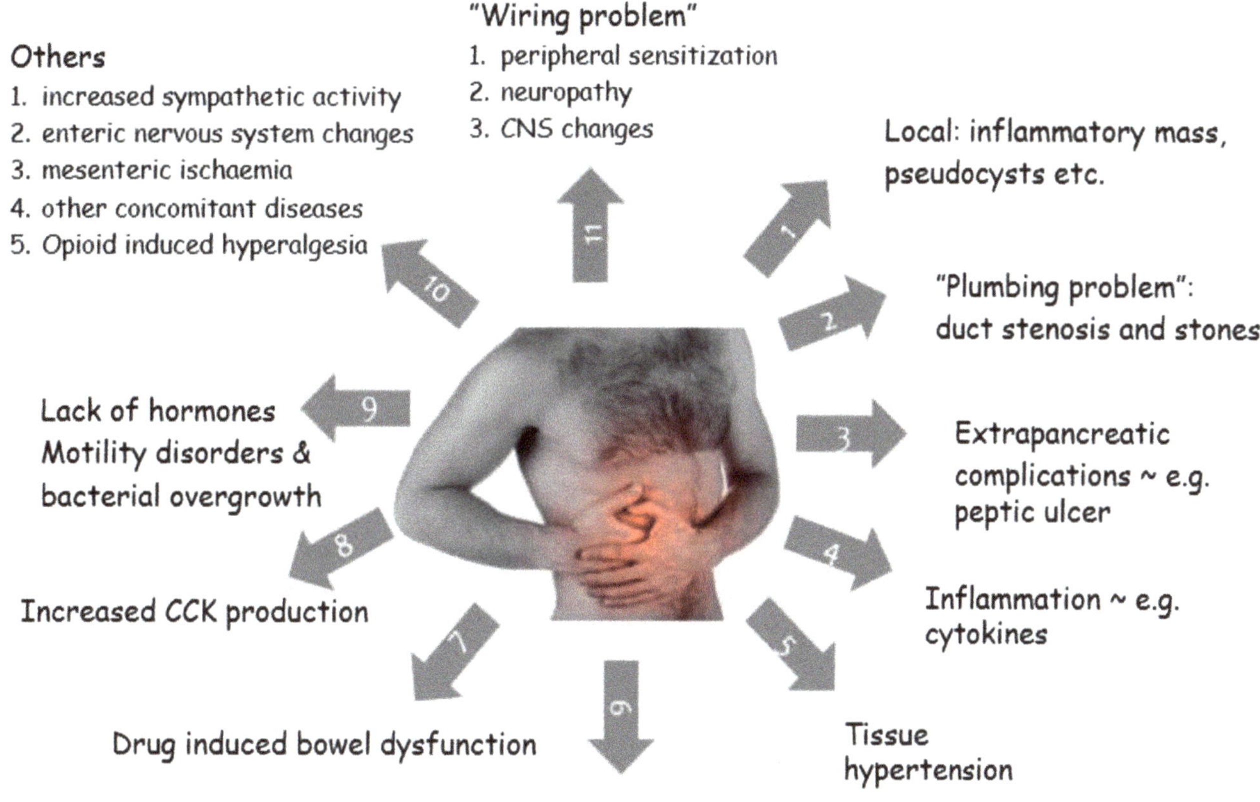

Figure 1: Various factors and mechanisms that may be responsible for pain in patients with CP

The process can lead to ischemia and local changes in the gut, which by themselves can cause pain. There is also destruction of nerves, and the accompanying features of the neuropathic pain that are likely to occur have been reviewed.[8] As discussed later in this chapter, upregulation of signalling molecules involved in inflammation, pronociceptive mediators, and neurotropic factors may occur in the pancreatic parenchyma in patients with CP.[9] Increased neural density and hypertrophy, sprouting, and neuritis of the intrapancreatic nerves, as well as activation of glia and immune cells have also been reported in pancreatic tissue from CP patients.[10] Finally, and also described in detail later, several studies have reported CP findings compatible with central sensitization. In addition to other findings, this was manifested as increase in areas of referred pain, decreased pain threshold, and neuroplastic changes in the brain.[8,10] Malnutrition following the development of exocrine and endocrine insufficiency further aggravates the situation as changes in the immune system and brain-gut axis are likely consequences.[12] Many CP patients are alcoholics with a certain "addiction potential", which complicates treatment, especially the treatment of pain.

It is important not to overlook pain due to the disease complications and to the adverse effects of treatment. These additional sources of pain are often easier to treat on a permanent basis. The many causes of pain are shown in **Figure 1**. Each of these must be thoroughly investigated and treated if possible. The new neurobiological view of pain following CP is somewhat in opposition to the traditional view of pain etiology, where pain was assumed to arise from pathology in, or in close proximity to, the pancreatic gland. However, these theories are not mutually exclusive, and aspects of both may contribute in the generation and perpetuation of pain. In addition, adverse effects and complications of medical and interventional therapies may account for substantial morbidity in many patients and should be considered as additional sources of pain. Therefore, it is important to consider the appropriate mechanisms when evaluating the origin of pain in pancreatitis patients. It is plausible that the "collective" abdominal pain is a result of a complex interplay of several mechanisms.

In conclusion, the novel and improved understanding of pain pathophysiology in CP advocates a paradigm shift in pain management. Hence, modern mechanism-based pain treatment, where the cause of pain is thoroughly investigated, and drug therapy tailored to the findings, may replace the usual "trial and error approach". Furthermore, each individual patient should undergo careful evaluation as shown in **Figure 1** to determine the most likely source(s) of pain.

Notably, invasive therapies (surgery or endotherapy) should be reserved for special, carefully selected cases demonstrating pathology suitable for interventions and with a clear temporal relationship between the appearance of pathology and symptoms. In this chapter, we highlight recent evidence for a neuropathic source of pain in many patients with CP and propose a theoretical framework for treatment.

Peripheral pain mechanisms in CP

Pain sensation in CP includes a complex interaction between the peripheral and central nervous systems.[1] Both arms of the nervous system undergo "neuroplastic" alterations during chronic inflammation of the pancreas, and this neuroplasticity seems to contribute considerably to the chronic and intensive character of the neuropathic pain syndrome in CP.[13] It is widely acknowledged that the central nociceptive circuits involved in chronic neuropathic pain are independent of input from the periphery, However, there is also evidence of amelioration of neuropathic pain following removal of the source of a noxious, painful input from the periphery.[14] A prime example is the significant reduction or even disappearance of pain following pancreatic resection for CP.[15] Therefore, it is reasonable that many of the peripheral neuropathic alterations that occur during CP may be not only be an adaptive mechanism, but also the origin of and reason for severe pain in CP patients. In the following discussion, the peripheral pain mechanisms in CP are divided into *morphological* and *functional* alterations.

Morphological alterations

The characteristic features of pancreatic neuropathy in CP are 1) increased neural density, 2) neural hypertrophy, and 3) pancreatic neuritis.[16] Increased neural density and neural hypertrophy have been recently summarized as "pancreatic neuroplasticity" and "pancreatic hyperinnervation". Systematic analysis of human CP tissues revealed that intrapancreatic nerves are enlarged in the resected inflammatory mass, regardless of the etiology of CP.[17] These neuroplastic alterations during pancreatic neuropathy seem to have an impact on the clinical course of CP because the extent of neuroplasticity is closely correlated to the severity of pain.[9] On the other hand, neuro-inflammation is a characteristic feature of neuropathic pain syndromes.[18] The intrapancreatic equivalent of neuro-inflammation during CP is pancreatic neuritis, which is characterized by targeted peri- or endoneural immune-cell infiltration.[19] Pancreatic neuritis was reported to be independent of the etiology of CP, i.e., having a similar severity in alcoholic, tropical and idiopathic pancreatitis.[17] Recently, immunophenotyping revealed that infiltrating perineural immune cells from CP patients with pancreatic neuritis immune cell infiltrations are mainly composed of macrophages, cytotoxic T lymphocytes, and mast cells. However, only mast cells were specifically enriched around the intrapancreatic nerves of patients who experienced more severe pain.[20] Indeed, mast cells are typically localized in proximity of peptidergic nerve fibers containing substance P (SP) and calcitonin-gene-related peptide (CGRP). Mast cells can secrete numerous neuro-excitatory agents including histamine, serotonin, nerve growth factor (NGF), and proteases including mast cell tryptase. These agents can bind to their corresponding receptors present on neurons [H1-4, 5HT-3, tyrosine kinase receptor (Trk)A, and protease activated receptor (PAR-1)] to trigger pain and neuronal over activation. This recent evidence indicates that CP patients show mast-cell induced hypersensitivity similar to patients with irritable bowel syndrome (IBS), ulcerative colitis, migraine, or interstitial cystitis.[20]

The most likely molecular mediators of pancreatic neuropathy in CP have been considered to be neurotrophic factors and neuronal chemokines. The tissue levels of NGF and glial-cell-line derived neurotrophic factor (GDNF) family members artemin and neurturin in CP tissues are correlated with the extent of neural hypertrophy and the degree of pain sensation in these patients.[9,21] Similarly, overexpression of the neuronal chemokine fractalkine in CP tissues and pancreatic nerves is correlated with pancreatic neuritis and with the severity and duration of the pain syndrome in CP.[22] However, study of the relation of morphological alterations and function is limited by the lack of animal models that exhibit similar neuroplastic-neuropathic alterations. Nonetheless, in recent *in vitro* models, stimulation of dorsal root ganglia neurons with extracts of tissue resected from CP patients mimicked the increased neural density and neuron hypertrophy seen in CP.[23] Blockade of the neurotrophic factor neurturin, similar to the blockade of NGF or TGF-beta-1, suppressed the neurotrophic potential of CP extracts.[24] Studies of neurturin as a potential analgesic target in CP are lacking.

Functional alterations

Understanding pancreatic neuropathy in CP at a functional level is even more likely to provide clues about the actual pathomechanism of the neuropathic pain syndrome in CP. From the perspective of autonomic innervation, CP has been reported to exhibit "neural remodeling", i.e., decreased sympathetic innervation, particularly with increasing degree of pain sensation or pancreatic neuritis.[10,16] Hence, it seems that the generation of pain in CP is coupled with the suppression of pancreatic adrenergic input. This observation also seems to be in line with the clinical ineffectiveness of thoracic splanchnectomy involving transsection of sympathetic and sensory nerves.[16] At the same time, nerves in CP tissues provide indicators of glial activation, as they contain reduced amounts of Sox10-immunoreactive peripheral glia and nestin-expressing cells in their interior.[10] Therefore, at a functional level, both sympathetic suppression and glial activation seem to significantly contribute to the generation of neuropathic pain in CP.

Although human-like neuroplasticity has yet not been demonstrated in animal models of CP, the models do allow study of molecular agents that may trigger pancreatic nociception during CP. Agents such as protons, bradykinin, hydrogen sulfide, serotonin, and calcium are released after acinar cell damage, and can activate nociceptive fibers via the respective receptors.[13] In the pancreas, proteinase-activated receptor 2 (PAR-2) and transient receptor potential vanilloid 1 (TRPV1) are the two leading receptor subtypes that can be directly stimulated by those agents.[25-27] Hoogerwerf et al. showed that infusion of trypsin into the pancreatic duct of rats increased Fos immunoreactivity within sensory dorsal root ganglia (DRG) neurons by binding to PAR-2.[25] In a similar model, infusion of trinitrobenzene sulfonic acid (TNBS) into the pancreatic duct, resulted in more depolarized resting potentials and increased suppression of A-type potassium current density were recorded in pancreas-specific DRG neurons.[26] In a follow-up study in the same rat model, intraperitoneal injection of NGF-blocking antibodies was found to reverse these alterations.[28] Importantly, reactive changes in central glia, particularly microglia, have been studied in the same animal model of CP.[29] In the preclinical animal models, NGF suppresses A-type potassium currents in pancreas-specific DRG neurons and triggers neuronal hyperexcitability. However, studies that target NGF in clinical studies of CP patients are still lacking.

Summary

Peripheral neuropathic-neuroplastic alterations, together with the abundance of nociceptive/noxious agents in pancreatic tissue during CP suggest that pain may be induced and maintained by the interaction of both neuropathic and nociceptive mechanisms. Therefore, as stated in the introduction, pain due to CP should be considered "mixed-type" pain.[13] Understanding the peripheral component of the CP-associated pain syndrome may provide valuable clues to help understand the generation of pancreatic neuroplasticity and mechanisms of visceral pain in several other gastrointestinal disorders.

Central pain mechanisms in chronic pancreatitis

Central sensitization

An increased input of peripheral pain signals to the spinal cord may result in increased responsiveness of central pain-transmitting neurons. This phenomenon is known as *central sensitization* and refers to an increased synaptic activity of sensory neurons in the dorsal horn of the spinal cord following stimulation by intense peripheral noxious stimuli, tissue injury, or nerve damage.[30,31] Ultimately, this results in a state where pain processing is uncoupled from the presence, intensity, or duration of noxious peripheral stimuli. Various mechanisms have been associated with central sensitization, which comprises two temporal phases. 1) The first is an early phosphorylation-dependent and transcription-independent phase that results primarily from rapid changes in the properties of glutamate receptors and ion channels. 2) The second is a later, longer lasting transcription-dependent phase that drives synthesis of new proteins responsible for the longer-lasting form of central sensitization observed in various pathological conditions.[32] One of the best characterized mechanisms in the early phase of central sensitization is activation of the N-methyl-D-aspartic acid (NMDA) receptor, revealing the key involvement of glutamate in this process.[33] In an experimental model, blocking the NMDA receptor by ketamine reversed the hyperalgesia associated with CP.[34]

Central sensitization manifests as hyperalgesia (extreme sensitiveness and prolonged after effects of painful stimuli), allodynia (pain in response to a non-noxious stimulus), and secondary hyperalgesia (a receptive field expansion that enables input from noninjured tissue to produce pain).[30] Several studies have reported findings compatible with central sensitization in CP. In one, increased area of referred pain in response to electrical stimulation of the esophagus, stomach, and duodenum, which share spinal segmental innervations with the pancreas and thus act as proxies of true pancreatic simulation, was reported in CP patients compared with controls.[35] Other studies have reported decreased pain thresholds in CP patients in response to visceral stimulation of the rectosigmoid or somatic stimulation of muscle and bone,[36,37] and the hyperalgesia seemed to be linked to disease severity.[38] Taken together, these findings characterize a generalized hyperalgesia in the pain system that most likely reflects widespread sensitization of the central nervous system, as seen in many other chronic pain disorders.[30]

Cortical reorganization and hyperexcitability

Several experimental and clinical studies have reported that deafferentation, chronic pain, and hyperalgesia in CP patients are associated with a functional reorganization of the cerebral cortex.[39] For example, in people with arm or hand amputations, the mouth to hand representation in the primary somatosensory cortex shifts, with a correlation of the extent of cortical reorganization and subjective pain ratings.[40] In patients with CP, damage to the peripheral nerves in the pancreas may, to some degree, mimic the peripheral nerve pathology seen in patients following amputation.

In this context, experimental pain studies of somatic stimulation of the epigastric skin area, which shares spinal segmental innervation with the pancreas, and visceral stimulation of the upper and lower gut, with concomitant recording of evoked brain potentials and brain source localization, found that chronic pain and hyperalgesia were associated with functional reorganization of the cerebral cortex.[35,41,42] Compared with healthy controls, reorganization of the brain areas involved in visceral pain processing, including the insula, secondary somatosensory cortex, and cingulate cortex parallel to what is seen in phantom pain, occurred in CP patients. In addition to reorganization of brain areas involved in visceral pain processing, the excitability of those neural networks was abnormal, with evidence of impaired habituation to noxious stimuli, possibly reflecting cortical neuronal hyperexcitability (i.e., cortical sensitization.[43] Finally, the thalamus, a key relay site in the pain system, has been implicated in chronic pain. Disturbance of thalamocortical interplay, seen as global changes in the rhythmicity of the cerebral cortex, has been observed in patients with neuropathic pain of mixed origin.[44] Parallel findings were observed in CP patients by spectral analysis of visceral evoked brain potentials and resting state electroencephalography.[45,46]

Structural correlates of functional cortical reorganization and hyperexcitability are shown in studies using advanced magnetic resonance imaging (MRI). Microstructural changes in the insular and frontal brain regions found on diffusion weighted MRI, were associated with clinical pain intensity and function scores.[47] Patients with a constant pain pattern had more severe microstructural abnormalities than patients with an attack-related pain pattern. This translates well to the clinic, where patients with constant pain were recently reported to have the most reduced quality of life.[3] In another MRI study of cortical volumetry, brain areas involved in visceral pain processing were shown to have a reduced thickness.[48] This finding suggests a central neurodegenerative response to severe and chronic pain.

Impaired pain modulation

The pain system has several inherent mechanisms to modulate inflowing pain signals. Among these, descending pathways from the brain stem and higher cortical structures play a key role in modulating endogenous pain and controlling the input of afferent pain signals at the spinal level. This process can lead to either an increase in the spinal transmission of pain impulses (facilitation) or a decrease in transmission (inhibition). The balance between these states ultimately determines the quality and strength of the pain signals perceived by the brain.[49] Alterations in the state of descending modulation from inhibition towards facilitation have been implicated in the transition of acute to chronic and neuropathic pain. Studies in both animals and humans have documented the involvement of brainstem structures in the generation and maintenance of central sensitization and hyperalgesia.[50,51] In the context of pain and CP, impaired descending inhibitory pain modulation has been reported in experimental models of human pain.[37,38] In addition, brainstem facilitation was reported to maintain pancreatic pain in an animal model of CP.[52]

Central pain mechanisms in chronic pancreatitis: chicken or egg?

As can be seen in the above sections, several lines of evidence indicate that central pain processing is abnormal in CP. However, from the current evidence, it is difficult to determine whether these central abnormalities are an epiphenomenon maintained by a sustained nociceptive drive from the pancreas or have become independent of peripheral input.[53] However, as outlined in the following section, there is evidence that generalized hyperalgesia, independent of the initial peripheral nociceptive drive, is the cause of pain in many patients. In that case, treatment should be directed toward the mechanisms involved in neuronal sensitization.

Theoretical framework for treatment

Although not well documented, it seems likely that prevention of recurrent clinical or subclinical pancreatitis attacks by risk-factor modification, translates into a slowing of disease progression, less exocrine and endocrine insufficiency, and most important, decreased abdominal pain. Therefore, pain treatment is a *sine qua non* in the clinical approach to the patient. A comprehensive review of pain treatment deserves some comments on the framework suggested here. As mentioned previously, extrapancreatic causes of pain should always be considered, and any complications that can give rise to pain should be treated as well as possible. For example, peptic ulcers are reported to have an increased prevalence in CP. This could result from a reduction of blood flow to the mucosa following attacks of acute pancreatitis as well as deterioration of pancreatic exocrine function, and an increased prevalence of *H. pylori*.[54] The resulting reduction of bicarbonate concentration contributes to acidification of the milieu. Pseudocysts are also an important source of pain and should be evaluated by an appropriate radiological work-up and treated accordingly. Some patients may have pain as a consequence of obstruction of adjacent viscera (e.g., the duodenum or common bile duct). Other factors that should always be considered and treated are bacterial overgrowth (seen in up to 40% of the patients), mesenteric ischemia, and side-effects of medications such as opioids.[55] As the pain experienced by most patients is multifactorial and neuropathic, that should always be considered. Although the neurobiological view of pain following CP is novel and somewhat in opposition to the traditional view of pain etiology, these theories are not mutually exclusive, and aspects of both may contribute in the generation and perpetuation of pain. Therefore, it is important to consider a number of different mechanisms when evaluating the origin of pain (**Figure 1**). It is plausible that "collective" abdominal pain is a result of a complex interplay of several mechanisms. In addition, establishing a stable doctor-patient relationship as well as collaboration with other professions helps achieve a successful treatment outcome.[56] The reader can also refer to the chapter "Medical therapy for chronic pancreatitis: Diet, enzymes, and analgesics" by Joachim Mössner.

An improved understanding of pain mechanisms in CP will undoubtedly pave the way for new treatments, and future strategies should be based on up-to-date mechanisms and personalized pain treatment. In the clinical setting, many patients with chronic abdominal pain suffer from comorbidities, such as nausea, narcotic addiction, physical and emotional disability, and malnutrition. Therefore, a detailed characterization of pain symptoms is often difficult to obtain, and is often blurred by symptoms of the associated comorbidities and medications. This is particularly problematic when underlying pain mechanisms are investigated. To avoid this problem, experimental pain models based on quantitative sensory testing can be used.[57,58] Quantitative sensory testing provides information on sensory function at the peripheral and central levels of the nervous system by subjective or objective recording of subject responses to various external stimuli of controlled intensity. The primary advantages are that a pain stimulus can be controlled, delivered repeatedly, and modulated, and that the responses can be assessed qualitatively and quantitatively using psychophysical, neurophysiological, or other imaging methods (**Figure 2**). As outlined in the previous sections these methods have proven to be important instruments to characterize basic physiology as well as mechanisms underlying pathological pain disorders in CP. A major problem in pain medicine is the lack of knowledge of the best treatment for a specific patient. We recently investigated the ability of quantitative sensory testing to predict the analgesic effect of pregabalin and placebo in patients with CP.[59] A positive pregabalin effect was associated with pretreatment sensitivity to electric tetanic stimulation of the upper abdominal area, which shares spinal segmental innervation with the pancreas. Hence, patients expressing lower pain thresholds in the "pancreatic viscerotome" were more likely to benefit from pregabalin treatment than were patients with normal sensitivity. These findings suggest sensitization of spinal neurons in the segment innervated by pancreatic visceral afferents are an important predictor of pregabalin efficacy in these patients. This method may be used to tailor pain medication based individual sensory profiles and thus represents a significant step towards personalized pain medicine.

Importantly, surgeons and gastroenterologists often overlook pain mechanisms because they have limited expertise. Hence, they often treat the patient with either surgery or endoscopy, and in case of failure, the patient is left with symptomatic treatment at the general practitioner. This is unsatisfactory, as modern pain treatment is based on a thorough knowledge of pain mechanisms and the variety of available treatment modalities. In many centers, pain is still treated according to the macrostructural appearance of the pancreas as briefly outlined above. However, as the procedures are neither evidence nor mechanistically based, the outcome is variable and often unsatisfactory. Even though studies have compared endoscopy and surgery,[60] no placebo-controlled studies have been performed, and this calls the effectiveness of invasive treatments into question. Surgery has been described as the most effective treatment of pain in CP, and recent studies suggest early surgery for CP may actually increase the likelihood of long-term complete postoperative pain relief.[61] For example, total pancreatectomy with islet cell transplantation is an emerging approach to treat patients with pancreatic pain. However, there has been no documentation that such advanced surgery is better than placebo as no studies have included sham surgery or sham endoscopy of the pancreas. As pain often resolves during the natural course of disease, future studies should try to better characterize pain pathogenesis in order to select the right patients. In patients with pain of neuropathic origin, surgical or endoscopic procedures may do more harm than good and deteriorate several hormonal systems regulating metabolism, gut motility, and related functions.

Surgical procedures to treat phantom pain in amputees have been abandoned by most centers, and here has been a shift towards a more complex neurobiological understanding of pain generation and treatment. The inflammation and fibrosis of CP are invariably linked to damage of the pancreatic nerves along with peripheral and central sensitization of the pain system. An important outcome of such neural-generated pain is that once the disease has advanced and the pathophysiological processes are firmly established, the generation of pain become self-perpetuating and independent of the initial nociceptive drive. This is in line with a small cross-sectional study that found generalized hyperalgesia, as a clinically measurable proxy of central sensitization, was associated with failure of thoracoscopic splanchnic denervation.[62] The authors proposed that in hyperalgesic patients, the generation of pain was independent of the initial peripheral nociceptive drive, consequently denervation of peripheral nerves was ineffective.

Conclusion

The improved understanding of pain mechanisms focusing on neuropathic pain may pave the way for new treatments.

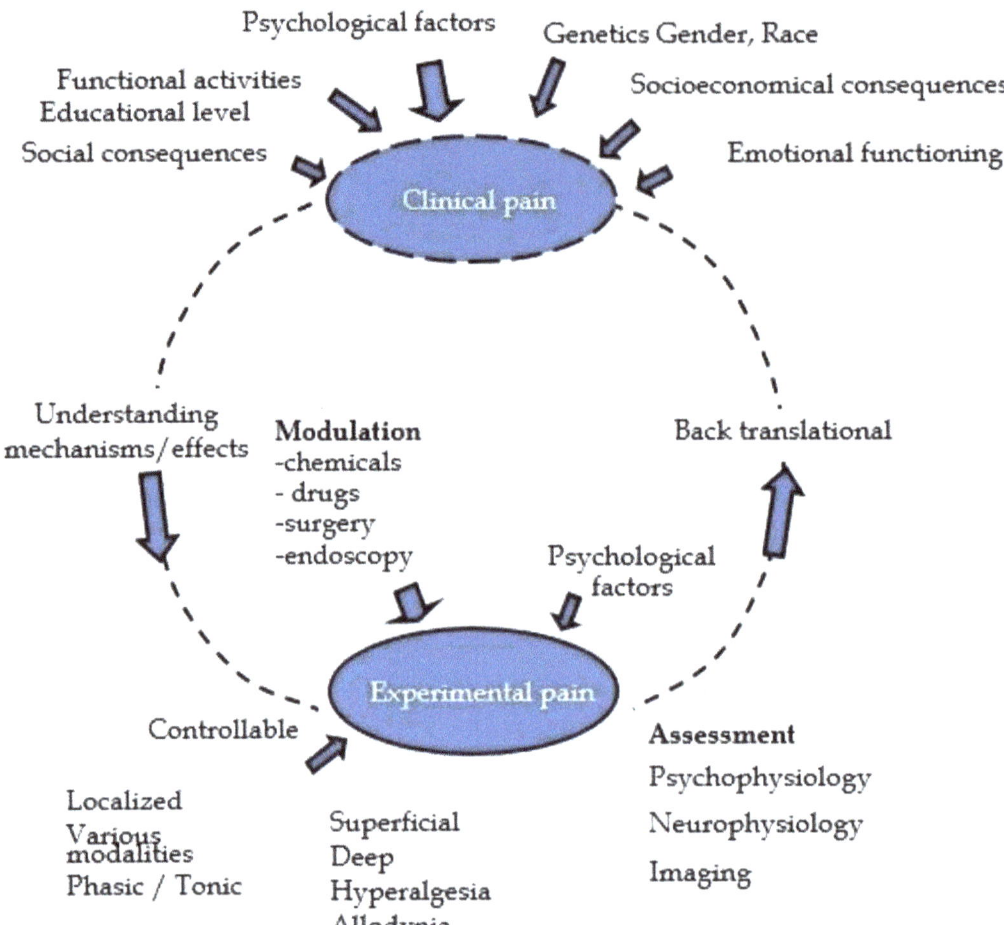

Figure 2. Overview of factors influencing a patient's perception of pain in the clinic (top) and illustration of concepts in experimental assessment of pain (bottom). Experimental pain is better suited to investigate not only pain mechanisms but also the effects of treatment. It is essential that intensity, duration, frequency, and localization of the experimental stimuli are controlled. When a given experimental stimulus results in a stable and reproducible response, it is possible to modulate the stimulus. The evoked pain sensation can be assessed in a subjective manner by use of visual analogue scales (VAS) or questionnaires, but to go beyond this one-dimensional pain assessment, subjective measurements can be combined with objective methods such as electroencephalography or functional MRI To mimic the clinical situation, where many mechanisms come into play, various modalities (e.g., electrical, thermal, mechanical, or chemical), combinations of phasic and tonic models, and models inducing hyperalgesia are often used. Compared to complex clinical conditions, phasic models are short lasting and have limitations, whereas models inducing hyperalgesia can act as proxies for the clinical manifestations (i.e., are back translational) and hence are more clinically relevant than superficial pain models.

Analgesics specifically targeting neural or humoral mediators of pain, such as NGF and TRPV1 antagonists, are currently being tested in clinical trials and hold promise for the future, although these drugs have yet to be tested in patients with pancreatitis. Recently, a NGF antagonist (Tanezumab) was shown to relieve pain in patients with knee pain due to gonarthrosis.[63] As mentioned in the chapter about peripheral pain mechanisms, NGF is upregulated in CP patients, and is known to play a pivotal role in the process of peripheral sensitization. It may prove to be effective for pain relief in patients.

Patients referred for pain treatment should, under ideal circumstances, be offered an extensive work-up of the pain system to avoid failures relating to irreversible central sensitization and phantom-like pain. Unfortunately, such pain assessment can only be done in the most advanced laboratories. Future studies should focus on identification of simple biomarkers to identify effective bedside treatments and ensure a framework for personalized pain medicine in pancreatology.

References

1. Braganza JM, Lee SH, McCloy RF, McMahon MJ. Chronic pancreatitis. *Lancet*. 2011; 377: 1184-1197. PMID: 21397320
2. Pasricha, PJ. Unraveling the mystery of pain in chronic pancreatitis. *Nat Rev Gastroenterol Hepatol*. 2012; 9: 140-151. PMID: 22269952
3. Mullady DK, Yadav D, Amann ST, O'Connell MR, Barmada MM, Elta GH, et al. Type of pain, pain-associated

complications, quality of life, disability and resource utilisation in chronic pancreatitis: a prospective cohort study. *Gut.* 2011; 60: 77-84. PMID: 21148579

4. Gardner TB, Kennedy AT, Gelrud A, Banks PA, Vege SS, Gordon SR, et al. Chronic pancreatitis and Its effect on employment and health care experience. Results of a Prospective American multicenter study. *Pancreas.* 2010; 39: 498-501. PMID: 20118821
5. Lowenfels AB, Sullivan T, Fiorianti J, Maisonneuve P. The epidemiology and impact of pancreatic diseases in the United States. *Curr Gastroenterol Rep.* 2005; 7: 90-95. PMID: 15802095
6. Novis, BH, Bornman, PC, Girdwood, AW, Marks, IN. Endoscopic manometry of the pancreatic duct and sphincter zone in patients with chronic pancreatitis. *Dig Dis Sci.* 1985; 30: 225-228. PMID: 3971834
7. Frokjaer, JB, Drewes, AM, Olesen, SS. Fibrosis, atrophy and ductal pathology in chronic pancreatitis are associated with pancreatic function but independent of symptoms. *Pancreas.* 2013; 42: 1182-1187. PMID: 24048457
8. Drewes AM, Krarupa L, Detlefsen S, Malmstrøm M-L, Dimcevski G, Funch-Jensen P. Pain in chronic pancreatitis: the role of neuropathic pain mechanisms. *Gut.* 2008; 57: 1616-1627. PMID: 18566105
9. Friess, H, Zhu, ZW, Di Mola, FF, Kulli, C, Graber, HU, Andren-Sandberg, A, et al. Nerve growth factor and its high-affinity receptor in chronic pancreatitis. *Ann Surg.* 1999; 230: 615-624. PMID: 10561084
10. Ceyhan GO, Demir IE, Rauch U, Bergmann F, Muller MW, Buchler MW, et al. Pancreatic neuropathy results in "neural remodeling" and altered pancreatic innervation in chronic pancreatitis and pancreatic cancer. *Am J Gastroenterol.* 2009; 104: 2555-2565. PMID: 19568227
11. Poulsen JL, Olesen SS, Frøkjær JB, Malver LP, Drewes AM. Pain and chronic pancreatitis: A Complex Interplay of Multiple Mechanisms. *World J Gastroenterol.* 2013; 19: 7282-7291. PMID: 24259959
12. Brock C, Søfteland E, Gunterberg V, Frøkjær JB, Lelic D, Dimcevski G, et al. Diabetic autonomic neuropathy affects symptom generation and brain-gut axis. *Diabetes Care.* 2013; 36: 3698-3705. PMID: 24026548
13. Demir IE, Tieftrunk E, Maak M, Friess H, Ceyhan GO. Pain mechanisms in chronic pancreatitis: of a master and his fire. *Langenbecks Arch Surg.* 2011; 396: 151-160. PMID: 21153480
14. Devor M. Centralization, central sensitization and neuropathic pain. Focus on "sciatic chronic constriction injury produces cell-type-specific changes in the electrophysiological properties of rat substantia gelatinosa neurons". *J Neurophysiol.* 2006; 96: 522-523. PMID: 16835360
15. Diener MK, Rahbari NN, Fischer L, Antes G, Buchler MW, Seiler CM. Duodenum-preserving pancreatic head resection versus pancreatoduodenectomy for surgical treatment of chronic pancreatitis: a systematic review and meta-analysis. *Ann Surg.* 2008; 247: 950-961. PMID: 18520222
16. Ceyhan GO, Demir IE, Maak M, Friess H. Fate of nerves in chronic pancreatitis: Neural remodeling and pancreatic neuropathy. *Best Pract Res Clin Gastroenterol.* 2010; 24: 311-322.
17. Friess H, Shrikhande S, Shrikhande M, Martignoni M, Kulli C, Zimmermann A, et al. Neural alterations in surgical stage chronic pancreatitis are independent of the underlying aetiology. *Gut.* 2012; 50: 682-686. PMID: 11950816
18. Scholz J, Woolf CJ. The neuropathic pain triad: neurons, immune cells and glia. *Nat Neurosci.* 2007; 10: 1361-1368. PMID: 17965656
19. Di Sebastiano P, Fink T, Weihe E, Friess H, Innocenti P, Beger HG, et al. Immune cell infiltration and growth-associated protein 43 expression correlate with pain in chronic pancreatitis. *Gastroenterology.* 1997; 112: 1648-1655. PMID: 9136844
20. Demir IE, Schorn S, Schremmer–Danninger E, Wang K, Kehl T, et al. Perineural mast cells are specifically enriched in pancreatic neuritis and neuropathic pain in pancreatic cancer and chronic pancreatitis. *PLoS One.* 2013; 8: e60529. PMID: 23555989
21. Ceyhan GO, Bergmann F, Kadihasanoglu M, Erkan M, Park W, Hinz U, et al. The neurotrophic factor artemin influences the extent of neural damage and growth in chronic pancreatitis. *Gut.* 2007; 56: 534-544. PMID: 17047099
22. Ceyhan GO, Deucker S, Demir IE, Erkan M, Schmelz M, Bergmann F, et al. Neural fractalkine expression is closely linked to pain and pancreatic neuritis in human chronic pancreatitis. *Lab Invest.* 2009; 89: 347-361. PMID: 19153557
23. Demir IE, Ceyhan GO, Rauch U, Altintas B, Klotz M, Muller MW, et al. The microenvironment in chronic pancreatitis and pancreatic cancer induces neuronal plasticity. *Neurogastroenterol Motil.* 2010; 22: 480-490, e112-113. PMID: 19912545
24. Demir IE, Wang K, Tieftrunk E, Giese NA, Xing B, Friess H, et al. Neuronal plasticity in chronic pancreatitis is mediated via the neurturin/GFRalpha2 axis. *Am J Physiol Gastrointest Liver Physiol.* 2012; 303: G1017-G1028. PMID: 22961804
25. Hoogerwerf WA, Shenoy M, Winston JH, Xiao SY, He Z, Pasricha PJ. Trypsin mediates nociception via the proteinase-activated receptor 2: a potentially novel role in pancreatic pain. *Gastroenterology.* 2014; 127: 883-891. PMID: 15362043
26. Xu GY, Winston JH, Shenoy M, Yin H, Pasricha PJ. Enhanced excitability and suppression of A-type K^+ current of pancreas-specific afferent neurons in a rat model of chronic pancreatitis. *Am J Physiol Gastrointest Liver Physiol.* 2006; 291: G424-431. PMID: 16645160
27. Xu GY, Winston JH, Shenoy M, Yin H, Pendyala S, Pasricha PJ. Transient receptor potential vanilloid 1 mediates hyperalgesia and is up-regulated in rats with chronic pancreatitis. *Gastroenterology.* 2007; 133: 1282-1292. PMID: 17698068
28. Zhu Y, Mehta K, Li C, Xu GY, Liu L, Colak T, et al. Systemic administration of anti-NGF increases A-type potassium currents and decreases pancreatic nociceptor excitability in a rat model of chronic pancreatitis. *Am J Physiol Gastrointest Liver Physiol.* 2012; 302: G176-G181. PMID: 22038828
29. Liu PY, Lu CL, Wang CC, Lee IH, Hsieh JC, Chen CC, et al. Spinal microglia initiate and maintain hyperalgesia in a rat model of chronic pancreatitis. *Gastroenterology.* 2012; 142: 165-173. PMID: 21963786
30. Woolf CJ. Central sensitisation: implications for the diagnosis and treatment of pain. *Pain.* 2011; 152: S2-S15. PMID: 20961685

31. Latremoliere A, Woolf CJ. Central Sensitisation: A Generator of pain hypersensitivity by central neural plasticity. *J. Pain.* 2009; 10: 895-926. PMID: 19712899
32. Woolf CJ, Salter MW. Neuronal plasticity: increasing the gain in pain. Science 2000; 288: 1765-1769.
33. Willert RP, Woolf CJ, Hobson AR, Delaney C, Thompson DG, Aziz Q. The development and maintenance of human visceral pain hypersensitivity is dependent on the N-methyl-D-aspartate receptor. *Gastroenterology.* 2004; 126: 683-692. PMID: 14988822
34. Bouwense SA, Buscher HC, van Goor H, Wilder-Smith OH. S-ketamine modulates hyperalgesia in patients with chronic pancreatitis pain. *Reg. Anesth. Pain Med.* 2011; 36: 303-307. PMID: 21490522
35. Dimcevski G, Sami S, Funch-Jensen P, Le Pera D, Valeriani M, Arendt-Nielsen L, et al. Pain in chronic pancreatitis: the role of reorganization in the central nervous system. *Gastroenterology.* 2007; 132: 1546-1556. PMID: 17408654
36. Buscher HC, Wilder-Smith OH, van Goor H. Chronic pancreatitis patients show hyperalgesia of central origin: a pilot study. *Eur J Pain.* 2006; 10: 363-370. PMID: 16087373
37. Olesen SS, Brock C, Krarup AL, Funch-Jensen P, Arendt-Nielsen L, Wilder-Smith OH, et al. Descending inhibitory pain modulation is impaired in patients with chronic pancreatitis. *Clin. Gastroenterol Hepatol.* 2010; 8: 724-730. PMID: 20304100
38. Bouwense SA, Olesen SS, Drewes AM, Frokjaer JB, van Goor H, Wilder-Smith OH. Is altered central pain processing related to disease stage in chronic pancreatitis patients with pain? An exploratory study. *PLoS One.* 2013; 8: e55460. PMID: 23405154
39. Flor H, Nikolajsen L, Jensen TS. Phantom limb pain : a case of maladaptive CNS plasticity? *Nat Rev Neurosci.* 2006; 7: 873-881. PMID: 17053811
40. Flor H, Elbert T, Knecht S, Wienbruch C, Pantev C, Birbaumer N, et al. Phantom-limb pain as a perceptual correlate of cortical reorganization following arm amputation. *Nature.* 1995; 375: 482-484. PMID: 7777055
41. Lelic D, Olesen SS, Hansen TM, Valeriani M, Drewes AM. Functional reorganization of brain networks in patients with painful chronic pancreatitis space. *Eur J Pain.* 2014; 18: 968-977. PMID: 24402765
42. Olesen SS, Frøkjær JB, Lelic D, Valeriani M, Drewes AM. Pain-associated adaptive cortical reorganisation in chronic pancreatitis. *Pancreatology.* 2010; 10: 742-751. PMID: 21273802
43. Olesen SS, Hansen TM, Graversen C, Valeriani M, Drewes AM. Cerebral excitability is abnormal in patients with painful chronic pancreatitis. *Eur. J. Pain.* 2013; 17: 46-54. PMID: 22508470
44. Sarnthein J, Stern J, Aufenberg C, Rousson V, Jeanmonod D. Increased EEG power and slowed dominant frequency in patients with neurogenic pain. *Brain.* 2006; 129: 55-64. PMID: 16183660
45. Drewes AM. Is the pain in chronic pancreatitis of neuropathic origin? Support from EEG studies during experimental pain. *World J Gastroenterol.* 2008; 14: 4020-4027. PMID: 18609686
46. Olesen SS, Hansen TM, Graversen C, Steimle K, Wilder-Smith OHG, Drewes AM. Slowed EEG rhythmicity in patients with chronic pancreatitis: evidence of abnormal cerebral pain processing? *Eur J Gastroenterol Hepatol.* 2011; 23: 418-424. PMID: 21399506
47. Frøkjær JB, Olesen SS, Gram M, Yavarian Y, Bouwense SAW, Wilder-Smith OHG, et al. Altered brain microstructure assessed by diffusion tensor imaging in patients with chronic pancreatitis. *Gut* 2011; 60: 1554-1562. PMID: 21610272
48. Frøkjær JB, Bouwense SAW, Olesen SS, Lundager FH, Eskildsen SF, van Goor H van, et al. Reduced cortical thickness of brain areas involved in pain processing in patients with chronic pancreatitis. *Clin Gastroenterol Hepatol.* 2012; 10: 434-438. PMID: 22155560
49. Heinricher MM, Tavares I, Leith JL, Lumb BM. Descending control of nociception: Specificity, recruitment and plasticity. *Brain Res Rev.* 2009; 60: 214-225. PMID: 19146877
50. Gebhart GF. Descending modulation of pain. *Neurosci Biobehav Rev.* 2004; 27: 729-737. PMID: 15019423
51. Zambreanu L, Wise RG, Brooks JCW, Iannetti GD, Tracey I. A role for the brainstem in central sensitisation in humans. Evidence from functional magnetic resonance imaging *Pain.* 2005; 114: 397-407. PMID: 15777865
52. Vera-Portocarrero LP, Xie JY, Yie JX, Kowal J, Ossipov MH, King T, et al. Descending facilitation from the rostral ventromedial medulla maintains visceral pain in rats with experimental pancreatitis. *Gastroenterology.* 2006; 130: 2155-2164. PMID: 16762636
53. Gebhart GF. It's chickens and eggs all over again: is central reorganization the result or cause of persistent visceral pain? *Gastroenterology.* 2007; 132: 1618-1620. PMID: 17418168
54. Chebli, JM, de Souza, AF, Gaburri, PD, Bastos, KV, Ribeiro, TC, Filho, RJ, et al. Prevalence and pathogenesis of duodenal ulcer in chronic alcoholic pancreatitis. *J Clin Gastroenterol* 2002; 35: 71-74. PMID: 12080230
55. Brock C, Olesen SS, Olesen AE, Frøkjær JF, Andresen T, Drewes AM. Opioid-induced bowel dysfunction: pathophysiology and management. *Drugs.* 2012; 14: 1847-1865. PMID: 22950533
56. Forsmark, CE, Liddle, RA. The challenging task of treating painful chronic pancreatitis. *Gastroenterol.* 2012; 143: 533-535. PMID: 22841737
57. Drewes AM, Gregersen H, Arendt-Nielsen L. Experimental pain in gastroenterology: a reappraisal of human studies. *Scand J Gastroenterol.* 2003; 38: 1115-1130. PMID: 14686714
58. Olesen AE, Andresen T, Staahl C, Drewes AM. Human experimental pain models for assessing the therapeutic efficacy of analgesic drugs. *Pharmacol Rev.* 2012; 64(3): 722-779. PMID: 22722894
59. Olesen SS, Graversen C, Bouwense SAW, van Goor H, Wilder-Smith OHG, Drewes AM. Quantitative sensory testing predicts pregabalin efficacy in painful chronic pancreatitis. *PLOS ONE.* 2013; 8: e57963. PMID: 23469256
60. Cahen DL, Gouma DJ, Laramée P, Nio Y, Rauws EA, Boermeester MA, et al. Long-term outcomes of endoscopic vs surgical drainage of the pancreatic duct in patients with chronic pancreatitis. *Gastroenterology.* 2011; 141: 1690-1705. PMID: 21843494
61. Yang CJ, Bliss LA, Schapira EF, Freedman SD, Ng SC, Windsor JA, et al. Systematic review of early surgery for

chronic pancreatitis: impact on pain, pancreatic function, and re-intervention. *J Gastrointest Surg*. 2014; 18: 1863-1869. PMID: 24944153

62. Bouwense SAW, Buscher HCJL, van Goor H, Wilder-Smith OHG. Has central sensitisation become independent of nociceptive input in chronic pancreatitis patients who fail thoracoscopic splanchnicectomy? *Reg. Anesth. Pain Med.* 2011; 36: 531-536. PMID: 22005656

63. Lane, NE, Schnitzer, TJ, Birbara, CA, Mokhtarani, M, Shelton, DL, Smith, MD, et al. Tanezumab for the treatment of pain from osteoarthritis of the knee. *N Engl J Med*. 2010; 363: 1521-1531. PMID: 20942668

Chapter 47

Conservative therapy of chronic pancreatitis

Joachim Mössner*

Division of Gastroenterology and Rheumatology, Department of Medicine, Neurology, and Dermatology University Hospitals of Leipzig, Liebigstrasse 20 D-04103 Leipzig / Germany.

Introduction

Medical treatment of chronic pancreatitis is based on the 3 main characteristics of the disease, pain and exocrine and endocrine insufficiency. Pain is the leading symptom of chronic pancreatitis. Patients may suffer from continuous pain or relapsing pain in parallel with relapses of the chronic inflammatory process or complications. Pain may decrease over time because of what is called "burn out" disease. Treatment of pain should be based on its pathogenesis. However, in many instances the pathogenesis of pain remains unclear. Pain may be caused by an inflammatory mass of the pancreatic head that doesn't resolve with time and is best treated by resection surgery; e.g. duodenum preserving pancreatic head resection. Pain due to obstruction of the main pancreatic duct by calcified protein plaques may be treated by ESWL (extracorporeal shock wave lithotripsy) with or without endoscopic placement of a stent into the pancreatic duct. These options are discussed in other chapters. Complications of chronic pancreatitis such as development of pseudocysts, bleeding of a pseudoaneurysm of the splenic artery, obstruction of the bile duct leading to cholestasis are generally not amenable to conservative, medical treatment. Cholangitis because of obstruction of the bile duct is primarily treated by endoscopic drainage with sphincterotomy and placement of a biliary stent, usually in addition to antibiotics. Development of pancreatic cancer may require surgical resection and chemotherapy. Pain not responding to medical treatment may be treated by endoscopic ultrasound-guided celiac plexus blockade. Again, interventional endoscopic possibilities will not be discussed in this chapter. This review on medical treatment of chronic pancreatitis is based on two recent publications of the author.[1,2] Thus, some degree of overlap is inevitable. However, some new clinical studies on treatment are included as well.

Treatment of a severe, acute inflammatory relapse of chronic pancreatitis is similar to treatment of acute pancreatitis. Thus, medical treatment of SIRS (systemic inflammatory response syndrome), MODS (multiorgan dysfunction syndrome), including treatment of renal insufficiency or sepsis are discussed in the section on "Acute Pancreatitis". The role of enteral nutrition in acute relapses is similar to nutrition in acute pancreatitis as well.

Pain syndrome

Clinical symptoms are often unspecific. Symptoms such as belt-like upper abdominal pain and vomiting, together with a more than 3-fold rise in serum amylase or lipase levels above normal, point the way to the diagnosis of either acute pancreatitis or a relapse of chronic pancreatitis. Initially, it may not be possible to differentiate acute alcohol-induced pancreatitis with the potential for full recovery from an attack of previously unrecognized, yet already established chronic pancreatitis. The pain syndrome – either acute relapses of pain, chronic pain, or relapses of pain with decreasing pain severity during the course of the disease – has been extensively described by Ammann and Melhaupt.[3] According to a long-term study, the course of early-stage chronic pancreatitis is characterized by episodes of relapsing pain. Chronic pain is often associated with local complications such as pseudocysts. According to the Ammann study in advanced chronic pancreatitis, all patients achieved complete pain relief. This observation has not been completely confirmed by others. However, in some patients, pain may remit spontaneously because of the chronic inflammatory destruction of the pancreas (i.e., "burn out").

Pain score

A validated pain score, such as that published by Bloechle et al. in 1995, or the visual analog scale (VAS), should be used as a tool for quantifying pain.[4] Rated on a scale from

*Corresponding author. Email: moej@medizin.uni-leipzig.de

0 to 100 are frequency of pain attacks (0 never, 100 daily), intensity of pain (1 to 100), use of analgesics (100 morphine, 1 acetylsalicyclic acid), and pain-related absence from work (100 permanent, 0 not in the last year). The review of Pezilli et al. describes measurements of quality of life comparing the SF-12 with the SF-36.[5] Both the SF-12 and the SF-36 have been validated, albeit only for the assessment of quality of life. The pain score published in 1995 is therefore the only validated score explicitly for pain in patients with chronic pancreatitis.

Pain medications

Analgesics

Analgesics are indicated to treat patients with pain from chronic pancreatitis in order to achieve pain relief or reduction of pain until spontaneous improvement resulting from cessation of a relapse or definitive treatment (e.g., endoscopy or surgery). Pain management in chronic pancreatitis follows the World Health Organization (WHO) three-step analgesic ladder. However, because of a lack of studies in chronic pancreatitis, the effectiveness of the WHO pain management plan cannot be answered at present.

Adequate pain management is essential. Patients with an acute exacerbation of pancreatitis often suffer from severe visceral pain. Analgesia is therefore one of the most important and often most urgent, aims of treatment. The argument that morphine or its analogs may cause contraction of the duodenal papilla, thus creating an additional obstruction for pancreas secretion, is obsolete. This effect either does not occur with the majority of analgesics of this group, or is so inconsequential that it is not clinically significant.[6-8] Some morphine analogs are successfully used for pain control both in acute and chronic pancreatitis. The question whether oxycodone is a stronger analgesic than morphine has to be proven by a large study.[9] One small study found that transdermal fentanyl is useful, but not the ideal first-choice analgesic.[10] Tramadol is generally not preferred because it often causes nausea and vomiting in patients with acute pancreatitis. However, the use of tramadol is associated with fewer gastrointestinal side effects.[11] Some centers have achieved good results with the use of thoracic epidural analgesia (EPA).[12,13] This does not only lead to rapid analgesia, but also prevents or treats paralytic ileus. A prerequisite for the use of EPA is an alert patient; coagulopathy is a contraindication.

The duration of medical therapy with various combinations of pain relievers can be decided on a case-by-case basis. However, re-evaluation should be made regularly in unsuccessful cases in order to augment the treatment with either an endoscopic or surgical procedure. There are no data to guide the duration of pain therapy using conservative means or when endoscopic or surgical treatment is indicated.

Weaning patients from pain medication again can follow the WHO three-step analgesic ladder in reverse order. Conservative pain management follows the WHO three-step analgesic ladder, although its effectiveness has not been specifically tested in chronic pancreatitis.

Somatostatin

Inhibition of exocrine pancreatic secretion by somatostatin in order to decrease intrapancreatic ductal pressure has not been shown to be successful in decreasing pain. Thus, octreotide should not be used to treat pain associated with chronic pancreatitis. Apart from single case reports and retrospective case series, there are only a double blind crossover study[14] and an unblinded crossover study comparing octreotide with octreotide long-acting release (LAR).[15] In both studies, pain was measured by the VAS. The double blind crossover study comparing octreotide with saline administration was unable to detect reduction in pain or analgesic requirement while effectively blocking pancreatic secretion. The unblinded crossover study showed no difference between octreotide and octreotide LAR for pain reduction. The effects of somatostatin in acute pancreatitis are controversial as well as its claimed effect in reducing the complication rate after pancreatic surgery.

Pancreatic enzymes

Inhibition of exocrine pancreatic secretion by porcine pancreatic extracts (negative feedback inhibition) has not been successful in treatment of pain. Thus, pancreatic enzymes should not be used to treat pain associated with chronic pancreatitis.[16-18] The rationale behind pancreatic enzyme therapy for pain relief is based on the assumption of a negative feedback mechanism for the release of cholecystokinin releasing peptides. This in turn leads to a reduced release of cholecystokinin and, by this mechanism, reduced exocrine pancreas secretion. A systematic review published by the Cochrane Collaboration in 2009, identified 10 randomized controlled trials with a total of 361 patients and evaluated various aspects of the effectiveness of pancreatic enzyme supplements.[18] Six of the studies compared enteric encapsulated preparations with placebo, one compared an unencapsulated preparation with placebo, 2 examined different preparations, and one study examined different dosage regimens. The heterogeneity of the selected dependent variables and the lack of statistical characteristic variables did not allow the data to be pooled. Three of 5 studies using a pain score showed a significant reduction in pain; 2 did not. One of 4 studies that quantified analgesic usage reported a reduction in the consumption of analgesics. No study evaluated long-term effects of the various types of treatment. Thus, one may conclude that the use of pancreatic enzyme supplements has no proven positive effect on pain symptoms. Furthermore, no improvement in the quality of life was detected. Because of different inclusion criteria, which often are not clearly explained in the studies, it was not possible to clarify whether the cause of pancreatitis, the presence of exocrine pancreatic insufficiency, or a particular formulation of the preparations that were used was responsible for the lack of therapeutic success. Finally negative feedback inhibition of exocrine pancreatic secretion may either not exist in humans or not play a role in the pathogenesis of pain.[19]

Antioxidants

Increased levels of free oxygen radicals have been detected in the serum and pancreatic juice of patients with chronic pancreatitis. Thus, treatment with antioxidants could help to prevent and treat pain by reducing cellular damage from pancreatitis. An initial study involving patients with recurrent acute and chronic pancreatitis demonstrated a significant improvement in the number of acute exacerbations as well as in chronic pain. However, only 20 of the initial 28 patients were assessed in the per-protocol analysis.[20] In another study, an improvement of pain was also be demonstrated. However, the number of patients who could be analyzed was much too low to allow any conclusions.[21] In a double blind placebo-controlled study from India, 71 patients were treated with antioxidants and 56 with placebo over a period of 6 months. There was a reduction of the days with pain in the treatment arm,[22] but these results were not confirmed in a recent controlled trial carried out in the U.K.[23] A later study, again from India, found a reduction of serum surrogate markers of fibrosis and a reduction of pain in patients treated with antioxidants.[24] A combination of pregabalin (see below) and antioxidants ameliorated pain recurrence in patients who were still free of narcotics and whose pancreatic duct had been cleared of stones.[25] A recent meta-analysis recommended antioxidant supplements for patients with low blood antioxidant levels.[26] Another meta-analysis concluded "that antioxidants can reduce pain slightly in patients with chronic pancreatitis. The clinical relevance of this small reduction is uncertain, and more evidence is needed".[27] However, "adverse events in 1 of 6 patients may prevent the use of antioxidants. Furthermore, the effects of antioxidants on other outcome measures, such as use of analgesics, exacerbation of pancreatitis, and quality of life remain uncertain because reliable data are not available".[27] The pathogenesis of pain in chronic pancreatitis is rather complex and often not understood in the individual patient to be treated. Pain may be caused by inflammatory infiltration of sensory nerves, ductal hypertension because of ductal scars or protein precipitates, an inflammatory mass, or pseudocysts with compression of adjacent organs. Duration of the disease, concomitant smoking or alcohol abuse, prior therapy such as interventional endoscopy or surgery, need for narcotics for pain medication, and numerous additional factors may have influenced the studies that tested the effect of additional supplementation with antioxidants.[28] In summary, convincing evidence that antioxidants have a role in the treatment of pain from chronic pancreatitis is still lacking. Furthermore, in most of the studies mentioned, antioxidant medication contained beta-carotene. Application of beta-carotene may be associated with the development of bronchial carcinoma in smokers, who comprise the majority of patients with alcoholic chronic pancreatitis.[29,30]

Electro-acupuncture and transcutaneous electrical nerve stimulation

Electro-acupuncture and transcutaneous electrical nerve stimulation (TENS) are not effective for treatment of pain in chronic pancreatitis.[31]

Inhibition of leukotrienes, radiotherapy

Treatment with a leukotriene receptor antagonist was not effective in chronic pancreatitis. A 3-month treatment with montelukast did not result in a significant reduction in pain.[32] Radiotherapy cannot be recommended for treatment of pain. In a pilot study, a significant reduction in pain, and avoidance of acute exacerbations, were achieved with one session of radiotherapy in 12 of 15 patients.[33] However, in view of an increased risk of developing pancreatic cancer in chronic pancreatitis, radiation may have the potential to increase this risk.

Pregabalin

Pregabalin has effects similar to gamma aminobutyric acid (GABA). However, it does not bind to GABA receptors. Rather, pregabalin binds to a subunit of voltage-dependent calcium channels in the central nervous system (CNS). Pain processing by the CNS seems to be abnormal in patients with chronic pancreatitis. The additional role of alcohol in pain processing is only partly understood. In a randomized, double blind, placebo-controlled trial in 64 patients with pain of chronic pancreatitis, pregabalin, as an adjuvant analgesic, was superior to placebo after 3 weeks of treatment.[34] The same group found that these inhibitory effects on central sensitization may have resulted from inhibition of spreading hyperalgesia.[35]

Exocrine and endocrine insufficiency

With ongoing destruction of pancreatic acini and pancreatic ducts, inhibition of outflow of digestive enzymes because of scars or protein plaques and the destruction of the islets of Langerhans, exocrine and endocrine insufficiency will develop. The destruction of exocrine acini and endocrine islets does not always proceed in parallel. Thus, exocrine insufficiency may precede the development of diabetes or vice versa. However, most patients with long lasting chronic pancreatitis develop so-called type 3c diabetes.

Definition of exocrine insufficiency

Exocrine pancreatic insufficiency develops when the decrease of digestive enzyme and bicarbonate secretion no longer allows full digestion of dietary intake. The main causes of exocrine pancreatic insufficiency in adults are chronic pancreatitis, pancreatic carcinoma, and a previous pancreas resection. Cystic fibrosis is the main cause of maldigestion that develops in childhood. A functional impairment of digestion, so called pancreato-cibal asynchrony, may be a consequence of (sub-)total gastrectomy, and some forms of bariatric surgery. as well as in patients with atrophy of the duodenal/jejunal mucosa because of celiac disease. Rare causes include Shwachman-Diamond syndrome, Johanson-Blizzard syndrome, and congenital enzyme deficiencies such as trypsinogen, amylase, lipase, enteropeptidase (enterokinase), or α1-antitrypsin deficiency

Clinical features of exocrine pancreatic insufficiency

Typical symptoms of exocrine insufficiency are abdominal symptoms such as cramps, gas, bloating, flatulence, steatorrhea, and signs of malnutrition. The development of steatorrhea and other symptoms of exocrine pancreatic insufficiency are to be expected once the diagnosis of chronic pancreatitis has been made. In patients with alcoholic chronic pancreatitis, clinically manifest exocrine pancreatic insufficiency usually appears approximately 10 to 15 years after appearance of the first symptoms, such as abdominal pain. In patients with early onset of idiopathic or hereditary chronic pancreatitis, exocrine pancreatic insufficiency may develop after even longer periods. The relatively late manifestation of exocrine insufficiency, well after pancreatic tissue destruction has begun, reflects the large functional reserve capacity of the pancreas. It is widely agreed that decompensation associated with steatorrhea and creatorrhea (abnormal excretion of muscle fibers in the feces) does not occur until secretion of the corresponding enzymes has been reduced by more than 90% to 95%.[36] However, this study has not been reproduced. There is no clinical symptom that either unequivocally confirms or excludes exocrine pancreatic insufficiency. Clinically, steatorrhea cannot be reliably detected. Inspection of stools is also unreliable, even when performed by an experienced practitioner.[37] Exocrine pancreatic insufficiency, even without symptomatic steatorrhea, can have a negative effect on nutrition parameters such as body weight.[38] Further studies substantiate reduced absorption of fat-soluble vitamins in patients with only mild to moderate exocrine insufficiency.[39-41] In patients with osteoporotic fractures. reduced fecal elastase levels have been observed. This finding correlates with low vitamin D_3 levels.[37] In the majority of patients with chronic pancreatitis, there is a correlation between the extent of morphological and functional disturbances.[42]

Therapy of exocrine pancreatic insufficiency

The indication for pancreatic enzyme replacement therapy is weight loss of more than 10% of body weight, steatorrhea with fecal fat excretion of more than 15 g/day, and dyspeptic symptoms with severe gas or diarrhea. Pancreatin should also be supplemented even when the increase in fecal fat excretion is modest (7 to 15 g/day) if there are signs of malassimilation (e.g. weight loss) or the patient presents abdominal symptoms that can be attributed to maldigestion and malabsorption. As the quantitative measurement of fecal fat is often no longer performed, the indication for replacement is also presenting with a pathological pancreatic function test in combination with clinical signs of malabsorption. This includes weight loss and abdominal pain with dyspepsia, severe gas, or diarrhea. Therapy with pancreatin as an empiric trial for up to 4 to 6 weeks may also be beneficial if the source of symptoms is uncertain.[1,2]

The majority of enzyme supplements contain pancreatin, a pulverized extract from porcine pancreas with lipase, amylase, trypsin, and chymotrypsin as the main components. Pancreatin is not absorbed from the gastrointestinal tract, but is inactivated by enteric bacteria and digestive juices and eliminated in the feces.[43-46] Encapsulated microsphere formulations, which protect against gastric acid, clearly improve the effectiveness of pancreas enzyme replacement.[47-50] The measure of treatment success is improvement of the disease symptoms. Pancreatic enzyme replacement therapy improves quality of life.[51] Several studies that compared enteric coated porcine pancreatic extracts with placebo showed their superiority.[52-55]

Complete normalization of digestion and absorption of nutrients is usually not attainable. A rapid release of pancreatic enzymes from encapsulation may be hampered by a low pH in the duodenum because of a decrease of bicarbonate secretion in chronic pancreatitis. The success of pancreatin replacement therapy should be monitored primarily using clinical parameters (weight gain, long-term normalization of vitamin status, and disappearance of abdominal symptoms). If there is any doubt whether persistence of symptoms can be explained by a lack of efficacy of enzyme replacement, then fecal fat excretion or pancreatic function tests to measure nutrient digestion under therapy (e.g., breath tests with ^{13}C-labelled lipids) should be performed. The disappearance of clinical signs of malabsorption is the most important criterion for the success of pancreatic enzyme therapy.

Pancreatin should be taken with meals. The effectiveness of pancreatic enzyme supplements presupposes mixing of pancreatin and chyme. If more than 1 capsule/tablet per meal is to be taken, it may be beneficial to take one part of the dose immediately at the beginning of, and the rest distributed throughout, the meal.[56] Because mixing of chyme and pancreatin is required for optimal effectiveness, preparations that consist of acid-protected particles with a diameter of ≤ 2 mm should be chosen. This critical value is in principle only relevant for patients with a preserved pylorus.[57] However, there are no double blind, prospective randomized trials comparing the efficacy of acid-protected microtablets or microspheres with larger acid-protected tablets/capsules. In a randomized study of patients with chronic pancreatitis and steatorrhea the coefficient of fat absorption was measured after application of either acid-protected minimicrospheres (> 90% diameter < 1.25 mm, range 0.7-1.6 mm) with minispheres (> 70% diameter > 1.25 mm, range 1-2 mm). Both preparations were effective and at least equivalent.[58] The number of patients studied was not large enough to determine whether minimicrospheres were superior to minispheres. The administered pancreatin dose should contain adequate enzymatic activity for the digestion of 1 meal. The dose of pancreatin preparations is based on lipase activity. From 20,000 to 40,000 units (Ph. Eur.) should be administered as an initial dose at each meal, and 10,000 to 20,000) lipase units for the digestion of smaller amounts of food eaten between-meals. The enzyme dose should be doubled, if necessary tripled, if the effect is inadequate. Previous studies showed an improvement of the efficacy of pancreatic enzymes by adding a H2-receptor blocker.[59-61] Adding a PPI (proton pump inhibitor) may be more effective.[61] However, a complete resolution of steatorrhea may not be achieved. Thus, pancreatin powder or granulate should be combined with a PPI if the effect is still inadequate. The clinical efficacy of pancreatin preparations is determined by the administered dose, the time when taken, acid protection and size of the pancreatin particles, specific biochemical properties of the preparation, which depend on its origin, and past and concomitant disorders of the patient to be treated.

Almost all available pancreatic enzyme supplements contain porcine pancreatin. Preparations with fungal (*Rhizopus oryzae*, *Aspergillus oryzae*) enzymes have less favorable biochemical properties (higher acid stability, but rapid deactivation in the presence of low bile acid concentrations) and are therefore of only limited clinical value. Bacterial enzymes and human lipase produced using gene technology are not yet of relevance in the treatment of exocrine pancreatic insufficiency. However, microbial lipase may be efficacious and seems to be safe.[62] As some religions prohibit the consumption of pork, the patient should be told of the origin of the preparations.

Long-term treatment with porcine pancreatic extracts is generally safe.[63,64] Minor side effects such as abdominal symptoms in < 10% of patients (abdominal pain, bowel movement changes, nausea/vomiting) are possible, as well as allergic reactions (in < 1% of patients). Very high doses of enzymes (> 10,000 to 20,000 units of lipase/kg/day) should be avoided if possible. Fibrosing colonopathy, a rare disorder, has been reported to occur after the administration of extremely high doses of pancreatin in children with cystic fibrosis. Causality has not been established and is rather unlikely.[65-69] One may consider that ingredients of the encapsulation itself rather than enzymes are responsible.

In patients with diabetes mellitus and newly initiated or increased pancreatic therapy, blood glucose levels should be monitored more closely than usual for a short time because the improved uptake of carbohydrates can result in hyperglycemia. Patients with chronic pancreatitis and associated diabetes mellitus may encounter more significant problems with controlling their blood sugar levels if pancreatin therapy is initiated or discontinued. This includes emergency situations requiring treatment. In a study by O'Keefe et al. symptomatic hypoglycemia developed during placebo treatment and ketoacidosis after recommencing pancreatic therapy.[70]

Therapy of endocrine insufficiency

Endocrine insufficiency in chronic pancreatitis has been designated diabetes type 3c. Endocrine insufficiency will eventually develop in most cases as the inflammatory processes progress. There is some correlation with the development of exocrine insufficiency. Therapy of this type of diabetes is often more difficult for several reasons. 1) In addition to a lack of insulin because of the inflammatory destruction of islets, there is also a lack of counter regulatory islet hormones such as glucagon and somatostatin. 2) Postprandial serum glucose levels depend on the sufficiency of food digestion, which is dependent on the effectiveness of treatment with porcine pancreatic enzymes. 3) Compliance, especially in alcoholics, may play a major negative role to control metabolism. Thus in patients whose daily food intake varies because of their life style or abdominal pain, treatment with insulin needs cautious supervision. The risk of late complications as a consequence of insufficient treatment of diabetes has to be counterbalanced by the risk of severe hypoglycemia. Intensified insulin therapy by patient measurements of preprandial serum glucose and individual selection of the appropriate dosage of insulin may not be possible in many of these patients. However, in patients with good adherence, as is usually the case in patients with hereditary and idiopathic chronic pancreatitis and patients with a rather stable disease course, may be managed with an intensified diabetic regimen. Unfortunately, there are no evidence-based data regarding treatment of diabetes type 3c in patients with alcohol-induced chronic pancreatitis.

Nutrition in chronic pancreatitis

Nutrition during acute relapses of chronic pancreatitis is discussed under "Acute Pancreatitis". The value of "pancreas diets" or "bland diets" for pancreas patients is unproven. Indeed, a randomized trial led to initial fasting for mild acute pancreatitis no longer being recommended.[71] Thus, a reduction in the length of hospital stay and a more rapid recovery can be achieved with oral refeeding.[72] Malnutrition in patients with chronic pancreatitis may not only be the result of exocrine pancreatic insufficiency, but also result from reduced food intake secondary to pain or continued alcohol consumption. Nutritional treatment should provide an adequate supply of nutrients, vitamins, and trace elements. Usually, patients should receive a normal isocaloric diet together with adequate pancreatic enzyme replacement. To improve the response, food intake should be distributed over appropriately 4 to 6 small meals. There is no established specific pancreas diet. Data from animal studies indicate that diets with a high fat and protein content plus adequate enzyme replacement can improve the effectiveness of fat absorption.[73] A low fat diet cannot be generally recommended. Only when clinical symptoms of fat maldigestion occur with further progression of exocrine pancreatic insufficiency despite adequate oral enzyme replacement, should the amount of oral fat be reduced, depending on tolerability. Fat is important as a central source of energy for avoiding and treating catabolism. If dietary fat must be reduced for reasons of intolerability, despite adequate enzyme replacement therapy, it is necessary to ensure that the compensatory oral supply of other sources of energy (carbohydrates, proteins) are appropriately increased to maintain isocaloric nutrition. Medium-chain triglycerides (MCT) can be absorbed without prior digestion by lipase. MCT may improve fat absorption in patients with exocrine insufficiency and not receiving enzyme replacement therapy. However, MCT should not be recommended in conjunction with enzyme administration. In a small study of patients with severe steatorrhea, MCT alone were not superior to regular fat intake together with pancreatic enzyme administration.[74] Diet counseling is very important and is as efficient in malnourished patients as supplementation with MCT.[75] Alcohol consumption should be avoided in chronic pancreatitis. Alcohol consumption is an important pathogenetic factor for the progression of exocrine pancreatic insufficiency.[76] There are numerous studies demonstrating that continuous smoking accelerates the progression of the disease course.[77] Deficits of vitamins and trace elements should be specifically replaced. Patients with chronic pancreatitis and exocrine pancreatic insufficiency usually have a daily intake of vitamins and trace elements that is less than recommended. Thus deficiencies of the fat-soluble vitamins A, D, E, and K, as well as calcium, magnesium, zinc, thiamine, and folic acid are often detected.[78] A reduced intake has also been reported for riboflavin, choline, copper, manganese, and sulfur. The indication to replace vitamins and trace elements should be established in adults, primarily according to clinical symptoms of deficiency.

References

1. Mössner J, Hoffmeister A, and Mayerle J. Chronic Pancreatitis. In: Podolsky DK, Camilleri M, Fitz JG, B. KA, Shanahan F, and Wang TC, editors. *Yamada's Textbook of Gastroenterology, 6th edition.* Hoboken, NJ: John Wiley & Sons; 2015: 1702-1731.
2. Hoffmeister A, Mayerle J, Beglinger C, Buchler MW, Bufler P, Dathe K, et al. English language version of the S3-consensus guidelines on chronic pancreatitis: Definition, aetiology, diagnostic examinations, medical, endoscopic and surgical management of chronic pancreatitis. *Z Gastroenterol.* 2015; 53: 1447-1495. PMID: 26666283.
3. Ammann RW and Muellhaupt B. The natural history of pain in alcoholic chronic pancreatitis. *Gastroenterology.* 1999; 116: 1132-1140. PMID: 10220505.
4. Bloechle C, Izbicki JR, Knoefel WT, Kuechler T, and Broelsch CE. Quality of life in chronic pancreatitis–results after duodenum-preserving resection of the head of the pancreas. *Pancreas.* 1995; 11: 77-85. PMID: 7667246.
5. Pezzilli R, Fantini L, Calculli L, Casadei R, and Corinaldesi R. The quality of life in chronic pancreatitis: the clinical point of view. *JOP.* 2006; 7: 113-116. PMID: 16407631.
6. Staritz M. Pharmacology of the sphincter of Oddi. *Endoscopy.* 1988; 20(Suppl1): 171-174. PMID: 3049055.
7. Thompson DR. Narcotic analgesic effects on the sphincter of Oddi: a review of the data and therapeutic implications in treating pancreatitis. *Am J Gastroenterol.* 2001; 96: 1266-1272. PMID: 11316181.
8. Jakobs R, Adamek MU, von Bubnoff AC, and Riemann JF. Buprenorphine or procaine for pain relief in acute pancreatitis. A prospective randomized study. *Scand J Gastroenterol.* 2000; 35: 1319-1323. PMID: 11199374.
9. Staahl C, Dimcevski G, Andersen SD, Thorsgaard N, Christrup LL, Arendt-Nielsen L, et al. Differential effect of opioids in patients with chronic pancreatitis: an experimental pain study. *Scand J Gastroenterol.* 2007; 42: 383-390. PMID: 17354119.
10. Niemann T, Madsen LG, Larsen S, and Thorsgaard N. Opioid treatment of painful chronic pancreatitis. *Int J Pancreatol.* 2000; 27: 235-240. PMID: 10952406.
11. Wilder-Smith CH, Hill L, Osler W, and O'Keefe S. Effect of tramadol and morphine on pain and gastrointestinal motor

function in patients with chronic pancreatitis. *Dig Dis Sci.* 1999; 44: 1107-1116. PMID: 10389680.

12. Niesel HC, Klimpel L, Kaiser H, Bernhardt A, al-Rafai S, and Lang U. [Epidural blockade for analgesia and treatment of acute pancreatitis]. *Reg Anaesth.* 1991; 14: 97-100. PMID: 1780489.
13. Bernhardt A, Kortgen A, Niesel H, and Goertz A. [Using epidural anesthesia in patients with acute pancreatitis–prospective study of 121 patients]. *Anaesthesiol Reanim.* 2002; 27: 16-22. PMID: 11908096.
14. Malfertheiner P, Mayer D, Buchler M, Dominguez-Munoz JE, Schiefer B, and Ditschuneit H. Treatment of pain in chronic pancreatitis by inhibition of pancreatic secretion with octreotide. *Gut.* 1995; 36: 450-454. PMID: 7698708.
15. Lieb JG, 2nd, Shuster JJ, Theriaque D, Curington C, Cintron M, and Toskes PP. A pilot study of Octreotide LAR vs. octreotide tid for pain and quality of life in chronic pancreatitis. *JOP.* 2009; 10: 518-522. PMID: 19734628.
16. Mossner J, Secknus R, Meyer J, Niederau C, and Adler G. Treatment of pain with pancreatic extracts in chronic pancreatitis: results of a prospective placebo-controlled multicenter trial. *Digestion.* 1992; 53: 54-66. PMID: 1289173.
17. Malesci A, Gaia E, Fioretta A, Bocchia P, Ciravegna G, Cantor P, et al. No effect of long-term treatment with pancreatic extract on recurrent abdominal pain in patients with chronic pancreatitis. *Scand J Gastroenterol.* 1995; 30: 392-398. PMID: 7610357.
18. Shafiq N, Rana S, Bhasin D, Pandhi P, Srivastava P, Sehmby SS, et al. Pancreatic enzymes for chronic pancreatitis. *Cochrane Database Syst Rev* 2009; (4): CD006302. PMID: 19821359.
19. Mossner J, Wresky HP, Kestel W, Zeeh J, Regner U, and Fischbach W. Influence of treatment with pancreatic extracts on pancreatic enzyme secretion. *Gut.* 1989; 30: 1143-1149. PMID: 2767512.
20. Uden S, Bilton D, Nathan L, Hunt LP, Main C, and Braganza JM. Antioxidant therapy for recurrent pancreatitis: placebo-controlled trial. *Aliment Pharmacol Ther.* 1990; 4: 357-371. PMID: 2103755.
21. Kirk GR, White JS, McKie L, Stevenson M, Young I, Clements WD, et al. Combined antioxidant therapy reduces pain and improves quality of life in chronic pancreatitis. *J Gastrointest Surg.* 2006; 10: 499-503. PMID: 16627214.
22. Bhardwaj P, Garg PK, Maulik SK, Saraya A, Tandon RK, and Acharya SK. A randomized controlled trial of antioxidant supplementation for pain relief in patients with chronic pancreatitis. *Gastroenterology.* 2009; 136: 149-159 e142. PMID: 18952082.
23. Siriwardena AK, Mason JM, Sheen AJ, Makin AJ, and Shah NS. Antioxidant therapy does not reduce pain in patients with chronic pancreatitis: the ANTICIPATE study. *Gastroenterology.* 2012; 143: 655-663 e651. PMID: 22683257.
24. Dhingra R, Singh N, Sachdev V, Upadhyay AD, and Saraya A. Effect of antioxidant supplementation on surrogate markers of fibrosis in chronic pancreatitis: a randomized, placebo-controlled trial. *Pancreas.* 2013; 42: 589-595. PMID: 23531998.
25. Talukdar R, Lakhtakia S, Reddy DN, Rao GV, Pradeep R, Banerjee R, et al. Antioxidant cocktail and pregabalin combination ameliorates pain recurrence after ductal clearance in chronic pancreatitis: results of a randomized, double blind, placebo-controlled trial. *J Gastroenterol Hepatol*, 2016. doi: 10.1111/jgh.13332. PMID: 26945817.
26. Zhou D, Wang W, Cheng X, Wie J, and Zheng S. Antioxidant therapy for patients with chronic pancreatitis: A systematic review and meta-analysis. *Clin Nutr.* 2015; 34: 627-634. PMID: 25035087.
27. Ahmed Ali U, Jens S, Busch OR, Keus F, van Goor H, Gooszen HG, et al. Antioxidants for pain in chronic pancreatitis. *Cochrane Database Syst Rev* 2014;(8): CD008945. PMID: 25144441.
28. Garg PK. Antioxidants for chronic pancreatitis: reasons for disappointing results despite sound principles. *Gastroenterology.* 2013; 144: e19-20. PMID: 23352593.
29. Omenn GS, Goodman GE, Thornquist MD, Balmes J, Cullen MR, Glass A, et al. Effects of a combination of beta carotene and vitamin A on lung cancer and cardiovascular disease. *N Engl J Med.* 1996; 334: 1150-1155. PMID: 8602180.
30. The effect of vitamin E and beta carotene on the incidence of lung cancer and other cancers in male smokers. The Alpha-Tocopherol, Beta Carotene Cancer Prevention Study Group. *N Engl J Med.* 1994; 330: 1029-1035. PMID: 8127329.
31. Ballegaard S, Christophersen SJ, Dawids SG, Hesse J, and Olsen NV. Acupuncture and transcutaneous electric nerve stimulation in the treatment of pain associated with chronic pancreatitis. A randomized study. *Scand J Gastroenterol.* 1985; 20: 1249-1254. PMID: 3912961.
32. Cartmell MT, O'Reilly DA, Porter C, and Kingsnorth AN. A double-blind placebo-controlled trial of a leukotriene receptor antagonist in chronic pancreatitis in humans. *J Hepatobiliary Pancreat Surg.* 2004; 11: 255-259. PMID: 15368110.
33. Guarner L, Navalpotro B, Molero X, Giralt J, and Malagelada JR. Management of painful chronic pancreatitis with single-dose radiotherapy. *Am J Gastroenterol.* 2009; 104: 349-355. PMID: 19190609.
34. Olesen SS, Bouwense SA, Wilder-Smith OH, van Goor H, and Drewes AM. Pregabalin reduces pain in patients with chronic pancreatitis in a randomized, controlled trial. *Gastroenterology.* 2011; 141: 536-543. PMID: 21683078.
35. Bouwense SA, Olesen SS, Drewes AM, Poley JW, van Goor H, and Wilder-Smith OH. Effects of pregabalin on central sensitization in patients with chronic pancreatitis in a randomized, controlled trial. *PLoS One.* 2012; 7: e42096. PMID: 22879908.
36. DiMagno EP, Malagelada JR, Go VL, and Moertel CG. Fate of orally ingested enzymes in pancreatic insufficiency. Comparison of two dosage schedules. *N Engl J Med.* 1977; 296: 1318-1322. PMID: 16213.
37. Lankisch PG, Droge M, Hofses S, Konig H and Lembcke B. Steatorrhoea: you cannot trust your eyes when it comes to diagnosis. *Lancet* 1996; 347(9015): 1620-1621. PMID: 8667884.

38. Haaber AB, Rosenfalck AM, Hansen B, Hilsted J, and Larsen S. Bone mineral metabolism, bone mineral density, and body composition in patients with chronic pancreatitis and pancreatic exocrine insufficiency. *Int J Pancreatol.* 2000; 27: 21-27. PMID: 10811020.
39. Kalvaria I, Labadarios D, Shephard GS, Visser L, and Marks IN. Biochemical vitamin E deficiency in chronic pancreatitis. *Int J Pancreatol.* 1986; 1: 119-128. PMID: 3693979.
40. Mann ST, Stracke H, Lange U, Klor HU, and Teichmann J. Vitamin D3 in patients with various grades of chronic pancreatitis, according to morphological and functional criteria of the pancreas. *Dig Dis Sci.* 2003; 48: 533-538. PMID: 12757166.
41. Mann ST, Mann V, Stracke H, Lange U, Klor HU, Hardt P, et al. Fecal elastase 1 and vitamin D3 in patients with osteoporotic bone fractures. *Eur J Med Res.* 2008; 13: 68-72. PMID: 18424365.
42. Bozkurt T, Braun U, Leferink S, Gilly G, and Lux G. Comparison of pancreatic morphology and exocrine functional impairment in patients with chronic pancreatitis. *Gut.* 1994; 35: 1132-1136. PMID: 7523260.
43. Heizer WD, Cleaveland CR, and Iber FL. Gastric Inactivation of Pancreatic Supplements. *Bull Johns Hopkins Hosp.* 1965; 116: 261-270. PMID: 14272432.
44. Pap A and Varro V. Proteolytic inactivation of lipase as a possible cause of the uneven results obtained with enzyme substitution in pancreatic insufficiency. *Hepatogastroenterology.* 1984; 31: 47-50. PMID: 6199274.
45. Marotta F, O'Keefe SJ, Marks IN, Girdwood A, and Young G. Pancreatic enzyme replacement therapy. Importance of gastric acid secretion, H2-antagonists, and enteric coating. *Dig Dis Sci.* 1989; 34: 456-461. PMID: 2563963.
46. Delchier JC, Vidon N, Saint-Marc Girardin MF, Soule JC, Moulin C, Huchet B, et al. Fate of orally ingested enzymes in pancreatic insufficiency: comparison of two pancreatic enzyme preparations. *Aliment Pharmacol Ther.* 1991; 5: 365-378. PMID: 1777547.
47. Bruno MJ, Borm JJ, Hoek FJ, Delzenne B, Hofmann AF, de Goeij JJ, et al. Comparative effects of enteric-coated pancreatin microsphere therapy after conventional and pylorus-preserving pancreatoduodenectomy. *Br J Surg.* 1997; 84: 952-956. PMID: 9240133.
48. Borowitz D, Goss CH, Limauro S, Konstan MW, Blake K, Casey S, et al. Study of a novel pancreatic enzyme replacement therapy in pancreatic insufficient subjects with cystic fibrosis. *J Pediatr.* 2006; 149: 658-662. PMID: 17095338.
49. Wooldridge JL, Heubi JE, Amaro-Galvez R, Boas SR, Blake KV, Nasr SZ, et al. EUR-1008 pancreatic enzyme replacement is safe and effective in patients with cystic fibrosis and pancreatic insufficiency. *J Cyst Fibros.* 2009; 8: 405-417. PMID: 19683970.
50. Dominguez-Munoz JE, and Iglesias-Garcia J. Oral pancreatic enzyme substitution therapy in chronic pancreatitis: is clinical response an appropriate marker for evaluation of therapeutic efficacy? *JOP.* 2010; 11: 158-162. PMID: 20208327.
51. Czako L, Takacs T, Hegyi P, Pronai L, Tulassay Z, Lakner L, et al. Quality of life assessment after pancreatic enzyme replacement therapy in chronic pancreatitis. *Can J Gastroenterol.* 2003; 17: 597-603. PMID: 14571298.
52. Safdi M, Bekal PK, Martin S, Saeed ZA, Burton F, and Toskes PP. The effects of oral pancreatic enzymes (Creon 10 capsule) on steatorrhea: a multicenter, placebo-controlled, parallel group trial in subjects with chronic pancreatitis. *Pancreas.* 2006; 33: 156-162. PMID: 16868481.
53. Whitcomb DC, Lehman GA, Vasileva G, Malecka-Panas E, Gubergrits N, Shen Y, et al. Pancrelipase delayed-release capsules (CREON) for exocrine pancreatic insufficiency due to chronic pancreatitis or pancreatic surgery: A double-blind randomized trial. *Am J Gastroenterol.* 2010; 105: 2276-2286. PMID: 20502447.
54. Toskes PP, Secci A, Thieroff-Ekerdt R, and Group ZS. Efficacy of a novel pancreatic enzyme product, EUR-1008 (Zenpep), in patients with exocrine pancreatic insufficiency due to chronic pancreatitis. *Pancreas.* 2011; 40: 376-382. PMID: 21343835.
55. Thorat V, Reddy N, Bhatia S, Bapaye A, Rajkumar JS, Kini DD, et al. Randomised clinical trial: the efficacy and safety of pancreatin enteric-coated minimicrospheres (Creon 40000 MMS) in patients with pancreatic exocrine insufficiency due to chronic pancreatitis–a double-blind, placebo-controlled study. *Aliment Pharmacol Ther.* 2012; 36: 426-436. PMID: 22762290.
56. Dominguez-Munoz JE, Iglesias-Garcia J, Iglesias-Rey M, Figueiras A, and Vilarino-Insua M. Effect of the administration schedule on the therapeutic efficacy of oral pancreatic enzyme supplements in patients with exocrine pancreatic insufficiency: a randomized, three-way crossover study. *Aliment Pharmacol Ther.* 2005; 21: 993-1000. PMID: 15813835.
57. Meyer JH, Elashoff J, Porter-Fink V, Dressman J, and Amidon GL. Human postprandial gastric emptying of 1-3-millimeter spheres. *Gastroenterology.* 1988; 94: 1315-1325. PMID: 3360258.
58. Halm U, Loser C, Lohr M, Katschinski M, and Mossner J. A double-blind, randomized, multicentre, crossover study to prove equivalence of pancreatin minimicrospheres versus microspheres in exocrine pancreatic insufficiency. *Aliment Pharmacol Ther.* 1999; 13: 951-957. PMID: 10383531.
59. Durie PR, Bell L, Linton W, Corey ML, and Forstner GG. Effect of cimetidine and sodium bicarbonate on pancreatic replacement therapy in cystic fibrosis. *Gut.* 1980; 21: 778-786. PMID: 7429342.
60. Carroccio A, Pardo F, Montalto G, Iapichino L, Soresi M, Averna MR, et al. Use of famotidine in severe exocrine pancreatic insufficiency with persistent maldigestion on enzymatic replacement therapy. A long-term study in cystic fibrosis. *Dig Dis Sci.* 1992; 37: 1441-1446. PMID: 1505293.
61. Bruno MJ, Rauws EA, Hoek FJ, and Tytgat GN. Comparative effects of adjuvant cimetidine and omeprazole during pancreatic enzyme replacement therapy. *Dig Dis Sci.* 1994; 39: 988-992. PMID: 8174440.
62. Heubi JE, Schaeffer D, Ahrens RC, Sollo N, Strausbaugh S, Graff G, et al. Safety and Efficacy of a Novel Microbial Lipase in Patients with Exocrine Pancreatic Insufficiency

due to Cystic Fibrosis: A Randomized Controlled Clinical Trial. *J Pediatr*. 2016. PMID: 27297209.

63. Gubergrits N, Malecka-Panas E, Lehman GA, Vasileva G, Shen Y, Sander-Struckmeier S, et al. A 6-month, open-label clinical trial of pancrelipase delayed-release capsules (Creon) in patients with exocrine pancreatic insufficiency due to chronic pancreatitis or pancreatic surgery. *Aliment Pharmacol Ther.* 2011; 33: 1152-1161. PMID: 21418260.
64. Ramesh H, Reddy N, Bhatia S, Rajkumar JS, Bapaye A, Kini D, et al. A 51-week, open-label clinical trial in India to assess the efficacy and safety of pancreatin 40000 enteric-coated minimicrospheres in patients with pancreatic exocrine insufficiency due to chronic pancreatitis. *Pancreatology.* 2013; 13: 133-139. PMID: 23561971.
65. Smyth RL, Ashby D, O'Hea U, Burrows E, Lewis P, van Velzen D, et al. Fibrosing colonopathy in cystic fibrosis: results of a case-control study. *Lancet.* 1995; 346: 1247-1251. PMID: 7475715.
66. Waters BL. Cystic fibrosis with fibrosing colonopathy in the absence of pancreatic enzymes. *Pediatr Dev Pathol.* 1998; 1: 74-78. PMID: 10463274.
67. Connett GJ, Lucas JS, Atchley JT, Fairhurst JJ, and Rolles CJ. Colonic wall thickening is related to age and not dose of high strength pancreatin microspheres in children with cystic fibrosis. *Eur J Gastroenterol Hepatol.* 1999; 11: 181-183. PMID: 10102230.
68. Serban DE, Florescu P, and Miu N. Fibrosing colonopathy revealing cystic fibrosis in a neonate before any pancreatic enzyme supplementation. *J Pediatr Gastroenterol Nutr.* 2002; 35: 356-359. PMID: 12352527.
69. Taylor CJ. Fibrosing colonopathy unrelated to pancreatic enzyme supplementation. *J Pediatr Gastroenterol Nutr.* 2001; 35: 268-269. PMID: 12352511.
70. O'Keefe SJ, Cariem, and Levy M. The exacerbation of pancreatic endocrine dysfunction by potent pancreatic exocrine supplements in patients with chronic pancreatitis. *J Clin Gastroenterol.* 2001; 32: 319-323. PMID: 11276275.
71. Eckerwall GE, Tingstedt BB, Bergenzaun PE, and Andersson RG. Immediate oral feeding in patients with mild acute pancreatitis is safe and may accelerate recovery–a randomized clinical study. *Clin Nutr.* 2007; 26: 758-763. PMID: 17719703.
72. Teich N, Aghdassi A, Fischer J, Walz B, Caca K, Wallochny T, et al. Optimal timing of oral refeeding in mild acute pancreatitis: results of an open randomized multicenter trial. *Pancreas.* 2010; 39: 1088-1092. PMID: 20357692.
73. Suzuki A, Mizumoto A, Sarr MG, and DiMagno EP. Bacterial lipase and high-fat diets in canine exocrine pancreatic insufficiency: a new therapy of steatorrhea? *Gastroenterology.* 1997; 112: 2048-2055. PMID: 9178698.
74. Caliari S, Benini L, Sembenini C, Gregori B, Carnielli V, and Vantini I. Medium-chain triglyceride absorption in patients with pancreatic insufficiency. *Scand J Gastroenterol.* 1996; 31: 90-94. PMID: 8927947.
75. Singh S, Midha S, Singh N, Joshi YK, and Garg PK. Dietary counseling versus dietary supplements for malnutrition in chronic pancreatitis: a randomized controlled trial. *Clin Gastroenterol Hepatol.* 2008; 6: 353-359. PMID: 18328440.
76. Gullo L, Barbara L, and Labo G. Effect of cessation of alcohol use on the course of pancreatic dysfunction in alcoholic pancreatitis. *Gastroenterology.* 1988; 95: 1063-1068. PMID: 3410221.
77. Rebours V, Vullierme MP, Hentic O, Maire F, Hammel P, Ruszniewski P, et al. Smoking and the course of recurrent acute and chronic alcoholic pancreatitis: a dose-dependent relationship. *Pancreas.* 2012; 41: 1219-1224. PMID: 23086245.
78. Marotta F, Labadarios D, Frazer L, Girdwood A, and Marks IN. Fat-soluble vitamin concentration in chronic alcohol-induced pancreatitis. Relationship with steatorrhea. *Dig Dis Sci.* 1994; 39: 993-998. PMID: 8174441.

Chapter 48

Micronutrient ('antioxidant') therapy for chronic pancreatitis: Basis and clinical experience

Joan M. Braganza* DSc, FRCP, FRCPath

Emeritus Reader, Manchester University c/o Mrs J Parr 3rd Floor, Core Technology Facility, 46 Grafton Street, Manchester M13 9NT, UK

Introduction

Chronic pancreatitis is an ongoing fibro-inflammatory process that causes patchy loss of acinar cells while at the same time favoring the formation of intraductal calcium carbonate stones. It often presents as an attack that is indistinguishable from acute pancreatitis, representing paralysis of apical exocytosis in acinar cells, "pancreastasis",[1-3] which in animal experiments is tied in with a burst of electron transfer reactions (loosely called free radical activity, FRA).[2,4] Until all secretory parenchyma is obliterated, agonizing pain is usually the predominant symptom, whether accompanying recurrent attacks, or constant and disabling. Its treatment is largely empirical, such that addiction to narcotic analgesics is a compounding menace, because there is no consensus on disease pathogenesis.[3] The concept that electrophilic stress is the detonator and inflammatory motor[5,6] offers the opportunity for corrective micronutrient therapy,[7-12] and thereby, pain control.[13] This usage of micronutrients exploits more than "antioxidant" properties.

Stresses and stressors

Electrophilic stress

The phrase indicates the threat realized when electrophilic compounds (i.e., with a relative electron deficit) steal electrons from nucleophiles, which most biological macromolecules are. Xenobiotics (i.e., exogenous lipophilic substrates) are the major pathological source of electrophiles, by way of reactive xenobiotic species (RXS) that are inadvertently generated upon processing by cytochrome P450 monooxygenases (CYP). Highly reactive carbonyl products derived from oxidation of polyunsaturated fatty acids in cell membranes are the most relevant endogenous source.[14]

Oxidative stress

This descriptor points to the threat from an unusually high concentration of reactive oxygen species (ROS), of which many are free radicals (i.e., having an unpaired electron).[15] The best known—leaving aside products of interaction with nitric oxide—are superoxide ($O_2^{-\bullet}$), which is quenched by superoxide dismutase; hydrogen peroxide (H_2O_2), which is removed by catalase and glutathione (GSH) peroxidase; and the highly reactive hydroxyl radical ($OH^\bullet$).[16,17] About 10% of molecular oxygen undergoes ROS-yielding stepwise reduction during such physiological processes as mitochondrial respiration, CYP-mediated processing of endogenous lipophilic compounds, phagocytosis, and synthesis of disulfide (S-S) bonds from cysteine that are needed for proper protein folding in the endoplasmic reticulum (ER).[18] Evidently, cells can tolerate the burden, deliberately allowing low-grade oxidative stress for the cited and many other vital roles including signal transduction, calcium homeostasis, membrane turnover, redox control and genomic stability. A pathological excess of ROS, as is associated with CYP induction,[19] ultraviolet irradiation, xanthine oxidase activity under conditions of ischemia-reperfusion, and the like, threatens cell viability by jettisoning just those homeostatic mechanisms that physiological oxidative stress secures.[14] Transition metals, iron in particular, promote electron transfer reactions.[20] Insofar that ROS are integral to CYP function, the degree of electrophilic stress might be thought to mirror oxidative stress, but studies in the context of ageing show that the level of electrophilic stress can be disproportionately greater than that of its oxidative drive.[21]

Reductive stress

This idiom describes abnormally high electron (reducing) pressure behind a blockade of an enzymic step in the ATP energy production staircase. The blockade may be due to

*Corresponding author. Email: jenny.parr@manchester.ac.uk

absence of an enzyme or to its malfunction. When electron pressure is sufficiently high, some of the electrons may react with O_2 directly to generate ROS. Swings in electron pressure (redox potential) mimic, and are reciprocally linked to, swings in pH (proton pressure).[9,22,23] In fact, just as alkalosis is rarely if ever a problem unless deliberately induced, because all metabolic processes tend to be acid-generating, reducing pressure/reducing stress seems to be the main route to oxidative stress, at least in the long term. The problem is epitomized by alcoholism, hypoxia, redox cycling compounds such as doxorubicin that cause electron dislocation, and uncouplers of electron flow, such as NSAIDs, cyclosporine, and cytokines.

ER stress

If not quickly rectified, any of the above stresses activates ER stress. The unfolded protein response (UPR) is an ER stress response that exacerbates oxidative stress and elicits inflammation by activating stress response genes such as NF-κB.[24,25] The exocrine pancreas, with its huge rate of protein synthesis, is particularly vulnerable when subjected to congestion in the busy protein-trafficking lanes. That is an inevitable consequence of pancreastasis episodes despite the acinar cell's best efforts to compensate by endocrine rerouting of newly synthesized enzymes; removal of zymogen granules via the three-pronged strategy of centripetal dissolution, crinophagy and basolateral redirection; and down-regulation of enzyme synthesis.[2,3,9,26] The close integration of oxidative, electrophilic, ER, and inflammation stress is now regarded as the basis for many chronic diseases[27] and, increasingly, for chronic pancreatitis.[28-30]

Electrophilic stress template

Component clauses

Since it was first mooted in 1983,[31] this disease model has evolved in line with new observations.[5,32] The 1998 version[6] views the acinar cell as the site of mounting electrophilic stress that steadily erodes methyl (CH_3) and thiol (SH)—principally glutathione (GSH)—moieties, as a result of CYP induction, concurrent exposure to a toxicant that yields RXS, and insufficiency of refurbishing micronutrients (**Figure 1**). A fourth factor must now be built into the equation, namely gene mutations that might favor the cytoplasmic presence of trypsin.[28] This enzyme, as also chymotrysin, is readily inhibited by GSH via SH–SS exchange[6] should it break loose of constraint by SPINK1 (serine protease inhibitor Kazal type 1).[33] Less GSH is then available for control of electrophilic / oxidative stress and other vital roles.[6,9,34]

The qualifying clauses help to explain why patients on CYP-inducing anticonvulsant drugs rarely develop chronic pancreatitis, or why profound electrophilic/oxidative stress but with low CYP activity in children with kwashiorkor results in painless loss of acini, not chronic pancreatitis.[35] The concept does allow for a steady buildup of ROS alone, as in elderly people[36] and patients with hereditary pancreatitis.[34,37,38]

Within this framework, each burst of electron transfer reactions hinders apical exocytosis to trigger an attack of pancreatitis by interfering with the methionine-to-GSH metabolic pathway, which interacts closely with ascorbate and selenium. The diversion of free radical oxidation products (FROP) into the interstitium causes mast cells to degranulate (**Figure 1**),[3,39] thereby provoking inflammation, the activation of nociceptive mechanisms that promote a chronic pain syndrome,[13] and profibrotic interactions. It is worth noting here that RXS (including those from opiates), bile salts and radiocontrast media evoke a non-IgE anaphylactoid response.[39] Meanwhile, the acinar cell generates its own proinflammatory mediators under the influence of redox-sensitive signaling cascades,[17] but pancreatitis is said not to ensue when basolateral exocytosis is prevented.[26]

Cystic fibrosis, usually due to severe mutation in both alleles of the *cystic fibrosis transmembrane conductance regulator* (*CFTR*) gene, causes an accelerated noncalcific form of chronic pancreatitis that begins *in utero*: oxidative stress and inflammation are now regarded as integral features of the disease, driven by unfolded CFTR via the ER stress-UPR system.[27,40] This is not the position depicted in **Figure 1**, which instead seeks to understand the increased frequency of *CFTR* mutation(s), with or without mutation in *SPINK1*, among patients with idiopathic chronic pancreatitis,[28] especially the tropical variant.[41]

Thus, neonatal hypertrypsinogenemia in *CFTR* carriers, and the enhanced susceptibility to experimental pancreatitis so conveyed, suggests hindrance to CFTR-facilitated apical exocytosis in the acinar cell under conditions of excessive FRA.[9] Moreover, as predicted,[6] CFTR is easily inactivated by oxidants,[9] which would have the same impact as pancreas-selective mutations in *CFTR*,[42] compromising the delivery, via ductal cells, of bicarbonate into pancreatic juice, and thereby contributing to lithogenicity.[3,43] The ability of the antioxidant curcumin to rescue DF508-CFTR localization in cell lines[44] suggests that oxidants might be responsible for the cytoplasmic mislocalization of CFTR observed in alcoholic, idiopathic, and autoimmune pancreatitis.[43] Of interest, the CFTR channel also transports the antioxidants GSH[9,40] and thiocyanate.[45]

The framework shown in **Figure 1** envisages permutations and combinations among the aforesaid factors plus oxidant attack on CFTR in ductal epithelium as determining outcome of recurrent acute pancreatitis, small-duct chronic pancreatitis or large-duct disease with or without calculi; regardless of age at onset and rate of progression. The worst combination appears to be in patients with

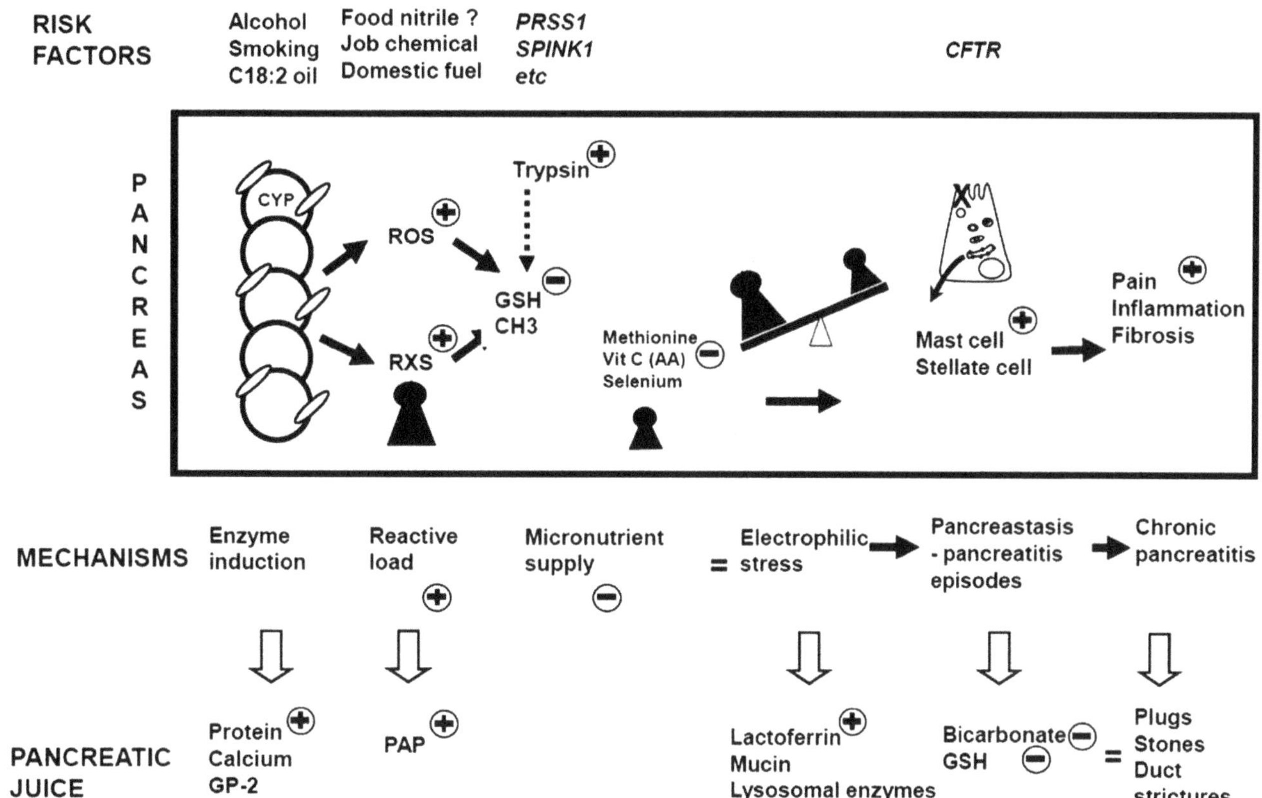

Figure 1. A framework for the pathogenesis of chronic pancreatitis, showing how risk factors interact to generate electrophilic/oxidative stress while also promoting lithiasis. Note that the supply of critical micronutrients might be subnormal in absolute terms due to unaffordability of source foodstuffs (e.g., in Soweto), problems associated with senility,[36] hostile culinary practices (e.g., as in India, resulting in destruction of ascorbic acid),or relative to increased oxidant load. Abbreviations: C18:2, oils rich in bi-unsaturated fatty acids; CYP, cytochrome P450 monooxygenases; *PRSS1, SPINK1, CFTR,* mutation(s) in genes for cationic trypsinogen, the serine protease inhibitor Kazal type 1, and the cystic fibrosis transmembrane conductance regulator; ROS reactive oxygen species; RXS reactive xenobiotic species; GSH, glutathione in bioactive form; CH_3, activated methyl groups; Vit C (AA), the bioactive ascorbic acid form of vitamin C; GP-2, secreted component of zymogen granule membranes analogous to the renal cast protein;[3] PAP, pancreatitis associated protein activated by electrophilic stress.[3] Circled plus and minus symbols represent increases and decreases.

tropical pancreatitis.[9,41,46] The popular notion of pancreatic autodigestion by prematurely activated trypsin in acinar cells has no part in the philosophy,[1,33,39,47] and is increasingly challenged by its former proponents.[48] Although not in the schema, it is conceivable that RXS via CYP might be involved in the genesis of autoimmune pancreatitis, as it is in autoimmune hepatitis.[49] This becomes plausible with the finding from studies in hepatocytes that newly synthesized CYP enters the secretory pathway to arrive at the outer surface of the plasma membrane.[50] As for a connection with ER stress, many xenobiotics have been shown to influence the UPR signaling route, with either prosurvival or prodeath features, which is not surprising given that resident CYP straddles ER membranes.[51]

CYP induction/concurrent toxicants

Although the liver is the primary site of xenobiotic processing by CYP, since around 1986 it has become increasingly evident that many organs including the pancreas possess this archaic, dormant, but inducible machinery.[14,32] The detoxification of xenobiotics and excretion of hydrophilic metabolites is brought about by an initial oxidative step that utilizes ROS followed by conjugation of the intermediate metabolite with glucuronic acid, inorganic sulfur, acetyl groups, or GSH via GSH transferases (GST).[12,52] The phenomenon of "enzyme induction" ensures increased availability of the particular CYP isoform that is appropriate for the substrate in question. This is accomplished by increased synthesis of heme for incorporation into CYP and heme oxygenase.[53] The latter degrades excess toxic heme with release of ferritin, bilirubin (via biliverdin), and carbon monoxide. Heme oxygenase is upregulated by numerous other stressors that share a capacity to decrease tissue GSH. The enzyme is carried in blood and is a potent antioxidant, as are the catalytic end-products. Moreover, it strongly inhibits mast cells.[54] Membrane lipids are integral to proper CYP function.[14] So too is the trace element selenium,

Table 1.

	Hepatocyte	Acinar cell
Compatible with CYP induction	↑ Cell size	↑ Cell size
	Ground glass hepatocytes	
	↑ SER mass	↑ RER mass
	↑ Phospholipids in bile	↑ Protein in pancreatic juice
		↑ Calcium in pancreatic juice
	↑ Drug metabolism	
	BSP-$_{K1}$ [= ↑ ligandin]	
	Antipyrine clearance [= ↑ CYP overall]	? Pancreatic contribution
	Theophylline clearance [= ↑ CYP1A	
	Urinary D-glucaric acid [= ↑ phase-2]	
	↑ CYP by immunochemistry	↑ CYP by immunochemistry
Compatible with electrophilic / oxidative stress	Microvesicular steatosis	Microvesiculation
		Pancreastasis episodes
		Tubular complexes
	Dilated SER	Dilated RER
	↑ Lipofuscin in tissue [= ↑ lipid peroxidation]	↑ Lipofuscin in tissue
	↑ FROP in bile	↑ FROP in pancreatic juice
		↑ Lysosomal enzymes in pancreatic juice
	↑ Bilirubin in bile [= ↑ haem oxygenase in liver]	↑ Mucin and PAP/*reg111* in pancreatic juice
	↑ Copper in bile	↑ Lactoferrin in pancreatic juice
		↑ Albumin in pancreatic juice
	↑ serum caerulopalmin [= ↑ ferroxidase 1]	↑ serum PAP
	↑ serum ferritin	
	Sclerosing cholangitis-like lesions	Sclerosing ductal lesions

Abbreviations: SER = smooth endoplasmic reticulum; RER = rough endoplasmic reticulum; BSP-$_{K1}$ = first-phase corrected disappearance curve after injection of sulphobromophthalein; CYP = cytochrome P450; CYP1A = the isoform inducible by polycyclic and other hydrocarbons; FROP = free radical oxidation products; PAP/*reg111* = secretory stress, pancreatitis- associated protein subtype. Upward arrows indicate increases.

a deficit of which causes hepatic heme to be wasted down the bilirubin route.[55]

The information in **Table 1** is a distillate of many studies in patients with chronic pancreatitis that were itemized in earlier reviews,[3,5,32,56] plus more recent observations in patients mainly with alcoholic disease.[57,58] The findings are readily rationalized by the electrophilic stress concept (**Figure 1**), but not by any other theory on pathogenesis.[3] The information reveals that induction of the xenobiotic processing machinery in liver and pancreas is not innocuous despite mobilization of several natural antioxants.[15,20] Studies on surgically resected specimens afford direct evidence of CYP induction,[59-61] and also on-going oxidative stress: structural aberrations by microscopy (**Table 1**),[6] FRA signals,[62] increased FROP with decreased GSH,[58,63] increased concentrations of pro-oxidant metals (copper, iron) but decreased levels of antioxidant metals (zinc, selenium);[58] and markers of the ER stress-UPR.[30] The last finding might be expected to involve disrupted calcium homeostasis,[27] but studies in isolated rat acini indicate that this is not a factor in toxicity from induced CYP.[64] As to whether oxidative stress contributes to the sclerosing ductal lesions, its involvement in primary sclerosing cholangitis is worth noting,[65] in that similar lesions are not infrequently present in patients with ordinary chronic pancreatitis.[56] Moreover, pancreatic juice,[66] bile,[67] and duodenal aspirates[68,69] from patients with chronic pancreatitis have high concentrations of irritant lipid oxidation products.

The key point is that the pancreas falls clinical victim while liver injury is generally silent—but why? The best explanation is that xenobiotics hit the gland directly via the arterial route, whereas ingested toxicants first encounter the liver which is best equipped to deal with RXS, via its huge complement of both GSH and GST.[14,70] This is illustrated by experimental studies in the 1950s using a subcutaneous dose of carbon tetrachloride, which is processed by CYP, to yield RXS-mediated damage in advance of liver injury. These lesions could be "produced at will" by varying the dose, ranging from patchy lesions of early chronic pancreatitis, with or without concretions, to "pancreatic cirrhosis" or a cystic fibrosis-like appearance.[71] The theme is reinforced by more recent studies with nitriles akin to those in dietary cassava (manioc, tapioca), and the occupational chemical dibutyltin.[70] Prior induction of CYP2E1 by a small dose of ethanol augments dibutyltin injury,[72] as is also true for hepatotoxicity from volatile hydrocarbons.[73,74] As for chronic exposure to ethanol, laboratory studies show that increased FRA precedes pancreatic injury.[75] In the drug metabolism studies from Manchester, UK (**Table 1**), heightened theophylline clearance was the predominant finding in patients with idiopathic or alcoholic disease,[56] indicating induction of CYP1A[52]—as by C18:2 fatty acids (e.g., in corn, peanut, or linseed oil), polycyclic aromatic hydrocarbons, and halogenated hydrocarbons.[76]

Since a proportion of arterial blood first enters islets cells, it is likely that RXS generated in CYP-induced islets are delivered to some acini by the insulo-portal conduit, thus adding to their RXS burden, and potentially explaining the patchy distribution of lesions.[6,60,71] The abundance of GST in islet cells affords insurance against injury in the short term, whereas a dearth of GST in acinar cells,whether absolute,[77] or relative to increased need from CYP induction,[59-61] renders them vulnerable.[9] Moreover, relatively long-lived FROP and RXS generated in the CYP-induced liver (**Table 1**) could aggravate pancreatic injury if they find their way there via refluxed bile[78] or the bloodstream.[56]

Of all the findings in **Table 1**, the increase in bilirubin is most revealing because it indicates induction of heme oxygenase to combat severe oxidative stress. A further surge accompanies a pancreatitis relapse,[56] mimicking the abrupt enzyme rise when phenobarbitone-treated rats are exposed to RXS from halothane gas.[79] The combination of induced CYP1A, increased copper, and induced heme oxygenase is a unique exposé of environmental toxicology in humans.[80,81] The 3 findings cannot be dismissed as a consequence of impaired pancreatic function because there was no correlation with its degree as measured by secretin-pancreozymin tests.[56] However, the normalization of copper and bilirubin data by long-term treatment with pancreatic extracts[56] is of the utmost interest now that a paper documenting the antioxidant potential of such extracts has been found (see below). Both bile and pancreatic juice inhibit copper absorption in experimental models, but studies using radioisotopes did not show any difference in copper absorption by healthy volunteers, patients with untreated chronic pancreatitis, or those taking pancreatic extracts (unpublished data).

Reports from the UK (Manchester),[82,83] southern India (Madras),[84] and South Africa (Soweto),[57,85] have revealed repetitive exposure to volatile hydrocarbons among patients with chronic pancreatitis, whether in a occupational environmental or domestic settings (e.g. kerosene or paraffin lamps and/or cookers in confined spaces). In the first UK study, patients noted freedom from attacks when away from the workplace.[82] The 6-fold decline between 1962 and 1987 in annual hospital admissions with the disease in Kerala province, southern India, coincides with the introduction of electricity, which removed the dependence on traditional lighting.[3] An investigation in Soweto concluded that exposure to occupational chemicals distinguished patients labelled as having "alcoholic chronic pancreatitis" from alcoholic controls with similar cigarette usage and an equally poor diet.[57] These observations add weight to case reports cited in previous reviews.[14,86,87] Although the direct pancreatic toxicity of petrochemicals is documented in lower species,[14] and hepatotoxicicity from kerosene was reported some time ago,[88] the field of inhalation toxicology to the pancreas has been neglected until recent evidence of injury from cigarette smoke in rodents.[3]

This should soon be rectified, scepticism notwithstanding,[89] because the health risk from volatile petrochemicals is currently under intense scrutiny.[90-92]

Methyl/thiol insufficiency

In theory, there are many ways in which a burst of electron transfer reactions can impede apical exocytosis in acinar cells,[14] but the evidence in patients with chronic pancreatitis points to a breakdown in the delivery of CH_3 and SH moieties (**Figure 2**).[5,14,39] The concept of methionine-dependent exocytosis was enunciated in the 1950s.[71,93,94] and is now known to depend on methylation of membrane components, probably of a prenylated cysteine residue.[95]

The supply of CH_3 moieties depends on *de novo* synthesis from S-adenosylmethionine (SAM) via a folate-dependent enzyme which catalyzes the production of S-adenosyl homocysteine (SAH), or by remethylation of the next metabolite, homocysteine, via choline-betaine and vitamin B_{12}-folate cycles that need ATP and are facilitated by ascorbic acid, the bioactive from of vitamin C.[9] Hence lack of folic acid also inhibits secretion.[96] GSH derived from homocysteine by the transsulfuration pathway is another absolute requirement for apical exocytosis, not least by protecting participating enzymes in the methionine metabolic route[6] while also sparing critical protein thiols.[97] Furthermore, *in vitro* studies identified the need of CFTR for exocytosis,[98] while *in vivo* experiments showed that a surfeit of magnesium stabilizes the exocytosis machinery by antagonizing calcium.[99]

Both steps in the onward route from homocysteine to cysteine are powered by vitamin B_6 (pyridoxine)-dependent enzymes. Pyridoxal-5'-phosphate is also a cofactor for 2 other enzymes involved in the synthesis of the gaseous mediator hydrogen sulfide (H_2S) from homocysteine and cysteine,[100] seemingly provoked when the progression to GSH is impeded. Cysteine is pluripotent – the rate-limiting component in GSH synthesis, source of taurine and inorganic sulfate that facilitate the removal of RXS (**Figure 2**), key to proper protein folding in the ER,[18] and seemingly even more important than GSH for redox control.[101] The same is true for GSH, which not only facilitates exocytosis and inhibits proteases, but also helps in redox control, serves as a reservoir for cysteine, mops up hydrogen and lipid peroxides, detoxifies RXS, and contributes to the extracellular antioxidant shield. Whereas its utilization in peroxide control is soon made good via interlocking GSH

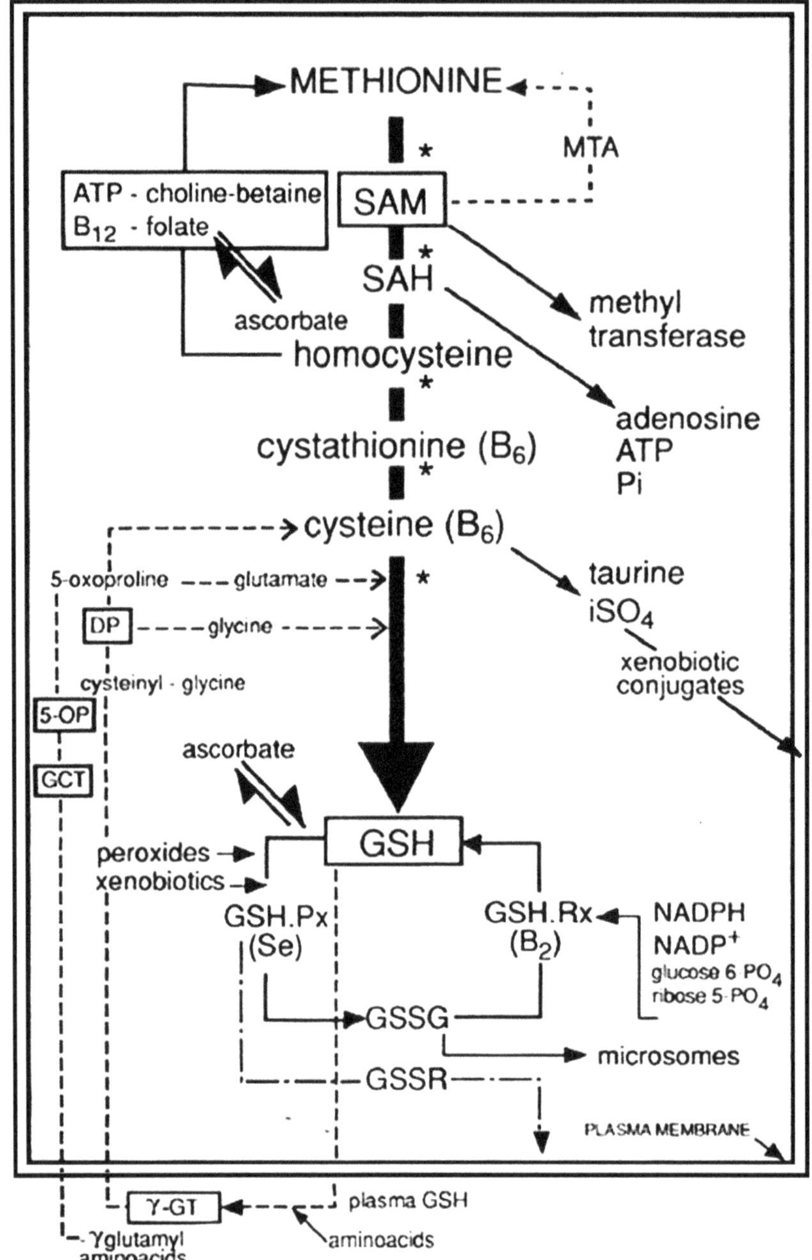

Figure 2. The pathway of methionine metabolism. Key metabolites are SAM, sulfadeosnsyl methionine; SAH, sulfadenosyl homocysteine; and GSH, glutathionine. Other abbreviations: MTA, methylthioadenosine; ATP, adenosyl triosephosphate; Pi, activated phosphate; iSO_4, inorganic sulfate; B_2, B_6, B_{12}, riboflavin, pyridoxine and cobalamin; GSH. Px, glutathione peroxidase; GSH. Rx, glutathione reductase; Se, selenium; GSSG, oxidized glutathione on engaging with peroxides; GSSR, conjugates of glutathione with electrophiles from xenobiotics; NADPH and NADP, the reduced and oxidized forms of nicotinamide adenosine phosphatase; DP, 5-OP and GCT, enzymes involved in the synthesis of glutathione.[70] Asterisks indicate enzymes that are known to be vulnerable to electrophilic/oxidative stress. Reproduced from Braganza[39], with kind permission from S. Karger AG, Basel, Germany.

peroxidase-GSH reductase, NADPH-NADP, and glucose 6 phosphate-ribose 5 phosphate shuttles, it is permanently excreted from cells in conjugates with RXS (**Figure 2**).[14,70] In these circumstances, the ability of ascorbic acid to substitute for GSH by redox and nonredox pathways is invaluable,[9] as is heightened activity of gamma glutamyl transpeptidase (γGT) in the plasma membrane that enables the uptake of reconstituting amino acids from the plasma GSH pool.[57,70] However, these resources are finite.

The pathway of methionine metabolism also impacts on the correction of reductive stress by biomolecules with electrophilic methyl groups. These include SAM, phosphatidylcholine, betaine and carnitine.[22] They appear to act by binding to positively charged nitrogen or sulfur moieties, a poising mechanism that is demonstrable *in vitro* when the reaction mix includes catalytically active iron, H_2O_2 and ascorbic acid. Carbon dioxide and carbon monoxide are formed from the ascorbate molecule in parallel with generation of methane gas. It is now recognized that albumin acts as a sacrificial antireductive protein that emits a signal for proteolytic degradation and elimination when modified by $OH^•$ radicals.[102]

In patients with chronic pancreatitis, there is clear evidence of oxidant-associated breakdown in methionine metabolism. Thus, during a relapse, neutrophils show low GSH but an increase in the oxidized form,[103] while urine and/or blood analysis point to a metabolic block in the transsulfuration pathway distal to cysteine, leading to surges in cysteine and more proximate metabolites,[103,104] and a fall in inorganic sulfur. By the third day, subnormal methionine and a further decline in sulfur levels hint at poor premorbid intake of sulfur amino acids.[9] These twin problems, of hindrance to methionine metabolism within an oxidative environment and methionine insufficiency, are evident in studies of patients with quiescent disease, whether alcoholic or idiopathic. (a) Peripheral blood displays a strong tendency to produce ROS.[105-107] (b) Plasma/serum contains excessive amounts of both protein carbonyls[107] and lipid-based FROP as reported in papers that are too numerous to cite individually. (c) Erythrocytes have subnormal levels of certain antioxidant enzymes, and GSH.[108-110] (d) Transmethylation and transsulfuration pathways remain fractured.[111] (e) ^{11}C methionine scanning demonstrates good pancreatic uptake of the amino acid but then its regurgitation coupled with impaired enzyme secretion into the duodenum.[112,113] (f) Subnormal plasma concentrations are reported of sulphur amino acids[114] and thiols derived via the transsulfuration route,[107, 115] including GSH.[57, 107] Plasma homocysteine level may remain normal[107] or increase in conjunction with subnormal folic acid,[111] vitamin B_6,[116] or vitamin B_{12}.[57] (g) H_2S appears in exhaled air.[117] It is not known whether any of these aberrations has a bearing on displacement of Munc18c into the cytosol of intact acinar cells as noted in a resected specimen of a patient with stable disease: this "SM protein" is involved in pathological basolateral exocytosis.[26]

Toward treatment

Clues for a prescription

Nonenzymic endogenous defenses against electrophilic/oxidative stress are already upregulated in patients with chronic pancreattis (**Table 1**), and it is known that the acinar cell has little copper-superoxide dismutase.[9] The inference is that micronutrient antioxidants fall short in the face of the persisting assault from RXS/ROS.[55,118] Many trace elements, the sulfur amino acids, and several, perhaps all, vitamins contribute in 1 or more ways to the antioxidant repertoire of tissues.[35] Analysis of habitual diets is the only way to glean which items might be crucially lacking in the face of an increased oxidant load, not merely less than in healthy controls. The axiom – which extends to blood levels – cannot be overstated, while appreciating the difficulty in estimating that load.[14-15] Low blood levels reflect the net result of intake, absorption, tissue sequestration and excretion.

Studies in Manchester, UK, identified lower habitual intakes of selenium, vitamin C, riboflavin and vitamin E in patients with idiopathic chronic pancreatitis than in age and gender-matched controls. Selenium was the best discriminator on stepwise analysis, and when examined in relation to theophylline clearance as a marker of CYP1A-related oxidant load,[52] effectively distinguished between patients and controls.[119] When the studies were extended to a control group with a similar, high theophylline clearance—patients with epilepsy on anticonvulsant CYP inducers—a second discriminant function emerged that was equally weighted on lower methionine and vitamin C in the chronic pancreatitis group.[120] This is in line with *in vitro* studies showing heterosynergism between ascorbic acid and sulfur antioxidants.[121] Moreover, whereas the epilepsy group was in a care center insulated from environmental toxicants, regular exposure to volatile hydrocarbons was noted in 4 others who were employed and developed chronic pancreatitis.[120] There are no comparable studies of habitual diets in patients with chronic pancreatitis.

The antioxidant role of selenium is generally linked to its presence at the active site of enzymes that are redox catalysts. The best known are GSH peroxidase which removes H_2O_2 and lipid peroxides, and thioredoxin reductase which is homologous to GSH reductase and is critical for redox regulation of protein function and signaling.[122] However, there is evidence that the element serves other important roles in the detoxification of xenobiotics.[118] Ascorbic acid is pluripotent in combating electrophilic/oxidative stress. It can substitute for GSH, facilitates the homocysteine remethylation cycle (**Figure 2**), scavenges electrophiles, acts as a "Michael donor" in reactions with acrolein and genotoxic FROP,[9] protects against $OH^•$ in plasma,[20] and quenches mast cell histamine,[123] which generates H_2O_2.[124] Not only does the last factor rationalize the virtual absence of ascorbic acid in plasma samples from patients admitted with a pancreatitis attack,[125,126] but it also underlines the involvement of mast cells.[39,47,54]

Lower concentrations of selenium have been noted in the serum/plasma of groups with chronic pancreatitis compared with control groups in diverse geographic regions,[57,58,118,127-131] with subnormal GSH peroxidase activity when selenium level is very low.[129] In Manchester the lowest selenium values accompanied painful disease, and levels fell progressively over 4 days upon repeated exposure to CYP substrates used for drug kinetics studies.[118] There is debate as to whether[128] or not[131,132] malabsorption contributes to the decrease. However, treatment with pancreatic extracts is expected to augment the intake of selenium, zinc, magnesium, and methionine because the gland is a repository of those metals that should, and sulfur amino acids that might, survive the purification procedure. However, the vitamins could be lost. This deduction is supported by a hitherto undiscovered study in patients with cystic fibrosis, in whom increases in plasma selenium and erythrocyte GSH peroxidase activity were attributed to substantial amounts of selenium in commercial preparations.[132] The finding has obvious repercussions on the usage of pancreatic extracts to ease pancreatic pain in patients with small-duct chronic pancreatitis, and indicating micronutrient antioxidant therapy by proxy.[133]

Spectrophotometric assays of vitamin C do not indicate the percentage present in the bioactive ascorbic acid form, but it is revealed when an HPLC assay is run in parallel. Thus, the control levels of plasma vitamin C reported from Madras,[134] Delhi,[108] and Cochin[109] in India are misleading if the Madras results can be generalized. Here the samples contained very little ascorbic acid, the discrepancy likely due to hostile culinary practices that might also destroy β-carotene. By contrast, among controls in Soweto the low level of ascorbic acid in plasma was proportionate to that of vitamin C, reflecting unaffordability of fresh fruit and vegetables, and fell further in the oxidizing milieu of chronic pancreatitis.[57] In Manchester, ascorbic acid values were negligible in patients with calcific disease or cysts/pseudocysts.[8] Against this background, the good value for ascorbic acid reported in French patients seems anomalous,[128] and begs the question as to what fraction of total vitamin C this represented.

The triple whammy in the genesis of pancreatic electrophilic stress—CYP induction, concurrent exposure to volatile toxicants, and insufficiency of particular micronutrients—was highlighted by a report from Manchester on patients with idiopathic disease.[78] Low protein intake, as in Madras and Soweto, impairs CYP induction. Consequently the rate of theophylline clearance in Madras controls was lower than in Manchester controls, yet significantly increased in local non-alcoholic patients,[135] alongside regular close exposure to kerosene fumes and little ascorbic acid.[46,134] At the time the studies were conducted in Soweto, it was not known that chlorzoxazone is a probe of CYP2E1 induction, as by ethanol.[136] In those patients, predominantly with alcoholic disease, theophylline clearance was similar to that in healthy controls, but the impact of RXS was evident from a fall in plasma GSH, increased oxidation of plasma ascorbic acid, decreased urinary inorganic sulfate and increased D-glucaric acid.[57] A subnormal concentration of zinc in serum[57,58] and erythrocytes,[109,128] correlates with reduced exocrine secretory capacity[109] rather than poor intake, and has no bearing on CYP function.

Potential benefit

Treatment with a combination of methionine, vitamin C and selenium should, in theory, help patients with painful chronic pancreatitis by several means. These include protecting the acinar exocytosis machinery, controlling rogue trypsin, removing RXS from halogenated hydrocarbons[94] and petrochemicals,[137] shielding CFTR,[9] curbing NF-κB activation and cytokine production,[138] rectifying reductive stress, as by cyclosporine,[139] inhibiting ER stress and activation of the UPR,[140-142] and reducing the oxidative drive to stellate cells.[143] Moreover, antioxidants stabilize mast cells,[13,47] mediators from which are not only profibrotic, but also implicated in converting peripheral pain sensitization into unrelenting pain from central sensitization.[13]

Insofar as recurrent acute pancreatitis (i.e., with histological restitution 6 or more weeks after the last episode as gauged by normal secretory and imaging studies),[32] and chronic pancreatitis are now regarded as a disease continuum,[3] some areas of overlap and subtle differences are interesting. Genetic studies show an increased frequency of *CFTR* with or without *SPINK1* mutation in patients with pancreas divisum, type-1 hyperlipidemia, or hyperparathyropidism.[9] A pilot study reported regular exposure to volatile hydrocarbons in patients without gallstones,[82] and drug disposal studies indicated induction of CYP and ancillary systems in several of them.[56] Analysis of secretin-stimulated duodenal aspirates identified increased lipid peroxidation, albeit less than in chronic pancreatitis.[69] Dietary inventories showed that data points were on or close to the aforementioned discrimination line based on selenium intake versus theophylline clearance.[144] Oxidative stress has been implicated in the pathogenesis of recurrent pancreatitis due to a deficiency of lipoprotein lipase.[145] Plasma/serum profiles of micronutrients were found to be within normal limits, in contrast to the deficiency profiles seen in chronic pancreatitis.[127] In other words, there seems to be a better match between the availability of micronutrient antioxidants and the degree of electrophilic/oxidative stress in patients with recurrent acute pancreatitis, despite the need to protect a larger mass of functional parenchyma. However, this might not be the only explanation for why recurrent acute pancreatitis does not always progress to chronic pancreatitis.[9,30,127,145,146]

Pilot studies

In the 1980s there was no commercial preparation that could deliver methionine, vitamin C, and selenium simultaneously. Methionine tablets were available from Evans Medical

Ltd, Horsham, UK to treat paracetamol poisoning, which is caused by CYP-derived RXS, A nutraceutical from Wassen International, Leatherhead, UK provided the other 2 micronutrients along with β-carotene and α-tocopherol (vitamin E). The total daily doses that most often reduced attack frequency and/or background pain were identified by trial and error in a group of 23 patients.[8] The group included 5 patients described in case reports of small-duct chronic pancreatitis or large-duct disease without or with huge calculi.[78,120] The doses were 2 gm methionine—although patients exposed to occupational chemicals tended to need twice as much—600 μg organic selenium, 0.54 gm vitamin C, and, invariably with 9000 IU of β-carotene and 270 IU of vitamin E. Side effects were usually minimal (e.g. nausea, or skin discoloration from β-carotene). Schizophrenia has been reported with methionine doses exceeding 10 gm/day, but a patient with a strong family history developed symptoms on 4 gm/day.

A number of exclusion criteria for future placebo-controlled clinical trials were delineated. They include suspected pancreatic cancer; over-the counter vitamins/antioxidants; children; pregnant women; pain that could be explained by concurrent illness such as gallstones, peptic ulcer, or somatic causes that are neither expected to nor respond to micronutrient therapy (unpublished data); large pseudocysts or bile duct stones that need invasive intervention; advanced disease in which oxidants no longer have a target,[105] as evidenced by steatorrhea, secretin tests or, nowadays, assay of fecal elastase;[3,109,133] family history of schizophrenia; chronic renal or liver failure; and addiction to narcotic analgesics—because the associated pain mimics that of chronic pancreatitis and because addicts might have ulterior motives for sickness behavior.[13] Clearly, the earlier that micronutrient therapy is started in patients with relapses, and without gallstones, the greater the chance of success. These exclusion criteria can be relaxed outside of clinical trials when regular clinical and biochemical monitoring is possible.[147]

Assessing outcome

The goal of treatment is to correct electrophilic/oxidative stress and thereby to control pancreatic pain.[13] Hence it stands to reason that there must be evidence of stress before recruitment, or the confident expectation of stress based on numerous published reports, provided that ineligible patients are excluded and that patients do not change their lifestyles for the duration of the trial. Furthermore, any reduction in pain while on active treatment should ideally be shown to occur *pari passu* with correction of such stress, so as to distinguish true improvement from the expected 20% rate of amelioration by placebo.[148] Low plasma/serum levels of 1 or more micronutrients in isolation merely indicates a propensity to oxidative stress. Likewise, increases in plasma levels upon supplementation without reference to oxidant load are not only meaningless, but without benefit in healthy controls,[149] and could be harmful by abolishing low-grade oxidative stress that is so essential physiologically.

In order to assess oxidant load, clinical investigators seek biochemical "fingerprints" of persisting stress. The choice, from the immense library,[15] must be guided by the perceived primary target of attack, and by practicality. If lipids are the all-important target, the best current markers are F_2 isoprostanes[67] and thiobarbituric acid reacting substances (TBARS) the least specific albeit most popular. These are products of the classical lipid peroxidation pathway, but there is another route that accounts for the bulk of so-called "diene conjugates" in biological fluids. This is the isomerization pathway, and it is easily mimicked *in vitro* by irradiating linoleic acid (LA, 9 *cis*, 12 *cis*) in the presence of albumin. Moreover, the route seems to be controlled by a selenium-dependent enzyme, as only 1 isomer (9 *cis*, 11 *trans*) is present in bile, duodenal juice, and serum even though 4 are possible.[150,151] Another reason is that serum selenium when viewed alongside the percent molar ratio of the isomer to the parent fatty acid (%MRLA) allowed distinguishing between data from patients with cystic fibrosis and controls.[152] The isomer's stability under ordinary freezing conditions and ease of batch analysis by automated HPLC makes it an attractive marker, but potential invalidation by food sources and bacterial contamination must be considered.

As argued recently,[13] the triggering attack in pancreatitis is on enzymes and receptors that are protected by ascorbic acid interacting with GSH. Hence, useful measures in plasma/serum might include the percent oxidized ascorbic acid relative to total vitamin C;[57] GSH coupled with γGT activity;[57] protein carbonyls;[107] and allantoin, signifying oxidation of uric acid which, along with albumin, glucose and bilirubin constitute the bulk antioxidants. Convenient tests that measure "total plasma antioxidant activity" by commercial kits, so-called "TRAP" and "FRAP" assays that have been used in clinical trials,[108,153] are misleading when used to monitor micronutrient therapy. They are strongly influenced by ascorbic acid which contributes 20% to the FRAP reading, vitamin E which contributes 5%, β-carotene which contributes very little, and thiols which have no effect.[9] If a nomogram is available to monitor treatment,[104,152] so much the better. Since dysregulated methionine metabolism due to RXS seems to underlie most cases of chronic pancreatitis, an index of its repair by treatment (e.g., by metabolite assay(s)[104,111] and/or ^{11}C methionine scanning[112,113]) would be very helpful. These resources are scarce, but a sustained increase in erythrocyte GSH upon micronutrient therapy appears to be an indirect pointer.[108] It is generally accepted that the identification of oxidative stress and its correction should involve more than a single index of attack on a single target.[14]

As for clinical recording, exclusion criteria as well as criteria for diagnosing chronic pancreatitis should be specified, recognizing that minimal changes on endoscopic pancreatography or endoscopic ultrasonography are insufficient without a test of secretory capacity.[3] The frequency of attacks, pain scores using visual analogue scales for the most common local descriptors of pain, the best available quality-of-life measure that befits pancreatic pain,[154] and analgesic usage are indices of therapeutic efficacy, or lack of it. Questionnaires should be kept to a minimum and administered by the same clinician, given that patients cooperate voluntarily although they may be in much pain. Monitoring of compliance is best achieved by an objective measure, and since the detection of ascorbic acid by urinary dipstick is not quantitative, compliance might only be determined retrospectively when the results of blood analysis become available after completion of active treatment. The wide individual variability in disease pattern favors a switch-over trial design, which is limited by the carry-over effect of today's high potency materials such as Antox (Pharmanord, Morpeth, UK), although the average daily dose of selenium is half that used initially.[155]

Clinical trials

Meta-analyses

The first independent appraisal of antioxidant therapy for pain control in patients with chronic pancreatitis covered reports on randomized controlled trials (RCT) up to 2009, and concluded that the identified micronutrient combination (Section 3) improved outcome in each of 3 placebo-controlled studies,[108,153,156] but that meta-analysis was impossible because different instruments were used to measure pain.[157] In the past 12 months, 3 meta-analyses have appeared that include studies to October 2012[158] December 2012,[159] and February 2014.[160] Despite the indiscriminate inclusion of RCTs judged satisfactory on mechanistic grounds, without considering the basis for treatment or legitimacy, each report concluded that active treatment reduced pain, especially using a micronutrient combination,[159] and that although side effects (e.g., headache, nausea, allergy, constipation, diarrhea) occurred in up to 19% of patients, and were usually mild, they did cause some patients to withdraw from the trials. The first trial, published in 1990,[156] was unique in ticking all the boxes in the report under the Cochrane banner.[158] The questionnaires used to gauge patient quality-of-life were based on studies of chronic backache, which were inappropriate in retrospect but the best tools available at the time. Interestingly, reports that were deemed fit for inclusion were not the same in these meta-analyses. All authors called for further large-scale studies.

Since the *raison d'être* for a micronutrient prescription is to boost the supply of CH_3 and SH moieties (Section 3), the ineffectiveness of the micronutrient curcumin (despite curbing lipid peroxidation and being a potent inhibitor of mast cells) and allopurinol (an inhibitor of xanthine oxidase) in clinical trials indicates that these substances did not achieve the desired goal, notably that curcumin did not increase GSH in erythrocytes. Yet, the curcumin trial[161] was included in each meta-analysis, and the allopurinol trial[162] was included in 2.[158,159] The Cochrane report[158] correctly separated a study showing the benefit of allopurinol or another antioxidant, dimethylsulfoxide, in patients with a pancreatitis relapse,[163] wherein many other factors such as pancreatic ischemia come into play,[5,39] but was included in the other 2 appraisals.[159,160] However, that analysis included 2 studies published only as abstracts[158] and a Polish-language report of vitamin C/E treatment versus no treatment, i.e., not the full micronutrient package,[164] which was also included in another meta-analysis.[160]

Subjective assessments during this period concluded that micronutrient antioxidant therapy was convincing,[7,12] had potential[10,11] could be useful as adjuvant therapy,[165] was poor and based on very limited experience,[166] or useless.[167]

Micronutrient combination

Table 2 summarizes information on studies of the micronutrient combination, whether[104,108,153,156,168,169] or not[34,170] placebo-controlled and excluding studies reported only as abstracts. In the original cross-over trial, clinical improvement was accompanied by migration of data points toward the control zone in the nomogram relating serum levels of a lipid oxidation marker and selenium (**Figure 3**).[104] Amelioration of oxidative stress concurrently with clinical improvement was shown in 2 other trials,[108,168] one of which also noted reduction in markers of fibrosis.[168] Clear benefit from active treatment accrued in all but 1 trial,[169] although its authors argued strongly in favor just 2 years earlier (**Table 2**), in a cross-sectional study, of patients already on micronutrient supplements versus no supplements under a later policy (see below).[154] Unfortunately, serious flaws render the second report invalid,[13] while diluting the value of micronutrient therapy in each meta-analysis.

Of special note in **Table 2** is the observation that the combination of SAM (instead of methionine) (**Figure 2**), plus vitamins A, C, E, and magnesium was beneficial in 3 children with hereditary pancreatitis.[34] Combination therapy was also highly successful in abolishing attacks in patients with lipoprotein lipase deficiency,[145] which is interesting because in this instance xanthine oxidase rather

Table 2.

Author	Clinical	Trial type/Active treatment	Outcome	Biochemistry
Uden[104, 156] Manchester 1990 / 1992	n=20 ACP 7, ICP 8 RAP 5 opiates none Steatorrhoea none	20 week switchover double-dummy double-blind Rx: 6/day Se-=βcar-C-E (WaSSen, UK) 8/day methionine (Evans, UK) Dose/day : Se 600μg, βcar 9000 IU (= 5.4 mg), C 540 mg, E 270 IU (= 270 mg) methionine 2g	Attacks ↓ 11 pain words VAS ↓ Pain diaries 2nd 5-wk ↓ Pain psychology ↔ Placebo effect	Baseline Se, βcar < controls; E, A ↔ ; post-Rx all ↑↑ Baseline SAM < controls; downward drift post-Rx Baseline MRLA > controls; post-Rx ↓ Baseline pGSH. Px, uSO_4 = conlrols; post-Rx ↔ pSAM in attack ↑; Se vs MRLA nomogram useful No carry-over at 10 week
De las Heras Castano[170] Santander 2000	n=19 ACP 11, ICP 5, RAP3 Opiates? Steatorrhoea?	Open trial for 12 months Rx: 4/day (hospital preparation) Dose/day : Se 300μg, βcar 12 mg, C 600 mg, E 188 mg, methionine 1.6g	Admissions vs previous year ↓ Pain word VAS vs previous year ↓ Pancreatic function vs previous year ↔	Not done
Uomo[34] Naples 2001	n=3 children with HP	2 year open in 4 blocks of 6 months, Rx 2nd & 4th Rx: 2/day SAM, 3/day multivitamin (sources?) Dose/day : Se 75μg, A 2.4g, C 180 mg, Mg 300 mg, E 30 mg, SAM 800 mg	Painful days ↓ Analgesics ↓	Not done
Kirk[153] Belfast 2006	n=19 all ACP? Opiates? Steatorrhoea?	Trial type: as Manchester 1990 Rx: 4/day Antox (Pharmanord, UK) Dose/day : Se 300μg, βcar 12 mg, C 600 mg, * E 152 mg, methionine 1.6g	SF-36 Quality of life ↑ Pain ↓ PhySical/social well-being ↑ (Nausea)	No control data; post-Rx Se, βcar, C & E > placebo Post-Rx A,αcar & TAC ↔ Post-Rx Fox1 , MDA, & pGSH ↔ Carry-over at 10 week
Bhardwaj[108] Delhi 2009	n=127 study power 80% ACP 35. ICP 92 Calculi? Opiates? Steatorrhoea 20%	6 month parallel placebo or active Rx: ?/day Belamore G (Osper, India) Dose/day : as Manchester 1990 Plus all on pancreatic enzyme supplements	Admissions ↓ Pain free: active > placebo Pain days/month ↓ Analgesics ↓, man-days lost ↓ Improvement by 3 months (Headache, constipation)	Baseline A, E < controls, C = controls Baseline FRAP, E-TGSH & E-SOD < controls, Post-Rx all these ↑, vitamins by 1 month Baseline S-SOD & TBARS > controls, post-Rx ↓ 3-month data not given
Shah[154] Manchester 2010	n=137 ACP 84 Antox 68, non 69 28 disease-duration matched pairs	Prospective cross - sectional study of concecutive patients already on Antox (Pharmanord, UK) versus standard Rx. Antox dose not stated, likely variable	VAS: Antox vs Non (P= 0.01) EORTC QLC C-30 &QLQ PAN-28 Quality of life: Antox group better on all counts (p<0.001-<0.0001) Opiates Antox vs Non (p<0.01)	Not done
Siriwardena[169] Manchester 2012	n =70 study power 80% ACP 51, ICP 19 CT calculi 66 Opiates? mean 88 mg/d Marked EPI in many Prior intervention 54%	6 month parallel placebo or active Intended 4-block design ie +/− intervention Rx: 6/day Antox v1.2 (Pharmanord, UK) Dose/day : Se 300 μg, C 720 mg *E 228 mg, methionine 2.88g *βcar from coating 2.5 mg	Clinic & Diary numeric pain score ↔ Brief pain inventory ↔ 4 Quality of life scores ↔ In-patient days ↔ Out-patient visits↔ 4-block data not given (Bad taste, heartburn, diarrhea, nausea)	No baseline data; no raw data post-active or placebo All data as change from baseline No evidence of micronutrient lack at baseline No evidence of oxidative stress by MRLA at baseline GSH and MRLA Change post-active =post-placebo Post-active Se, βcar, E, C >> post-placebo Increments post-active suggest major reporting errors
Dhingra[168] Delhi 2013	n=61 ACP 21, ICP 40 strict exclusion criteria Steatorrhoea 15	3 month parallei placebo or active Rx 8/day Belamore G (Osper, India) Dose/day : as Manchester 1990, Dehli 2000	Pain days/month Pain diary, Analgesic use Pain less on active, data sparse	Baseline TBARS > controls, FRAP < controls Baseline TGF- β1 & PDGF-AA > controls (p 0.07) Post-active ↓ drift in TBARS & ↑ FRAP Post-active PDGF-AA ↓, TGF- β1↔

Abbreviations alphabetically. Clinical ACP: alcoholic; HP: hereditary; ICP: idiopathic; RAP: recurrent acute; EPI: exocrine pancreatic insufficiency by faecal elastase assay. Trialtype βcar: β carotene; C, E: vitamins C & E; Mg: magnesium: Rx: active treatment; SAM; sulphadenosylmethionine; Se: selenium. Outcome EORTC QLC-30: European Organization for Research and Treatment of Cancer Quality of Life Questionnaire Core questions 30, and Pancreatic Modification questions 28; VAS: visual analogue score; vs: versus. Biochemistry A: retinol; AA: ascorbic acid: αcar: α carotene; E-TGSH, E-SOD: erythrocyte total glutathione and superoxide dismutase respectively; FRAP: free radical trapping ability of plasma: Fox1: ferrous oxidation; MDA: malondialdehyde; MRLA molar ratio of linoleic acid isomer to parent acid: pGSH: plasma glutathionine; ROS: reactive oxygen species; S-SOD: serum superoxide dismutase; TAC total antioxidant capacity; TSARS thiobarbituric acid reacting products of lipid peroxidation; TGF-β1: transforming growth factor-beta1; PDGF-AA: platelet-derived growth factor-AA. Arrows signify direction & degree of change. *doses from senior technical officer at Pharmanord, Denmark.

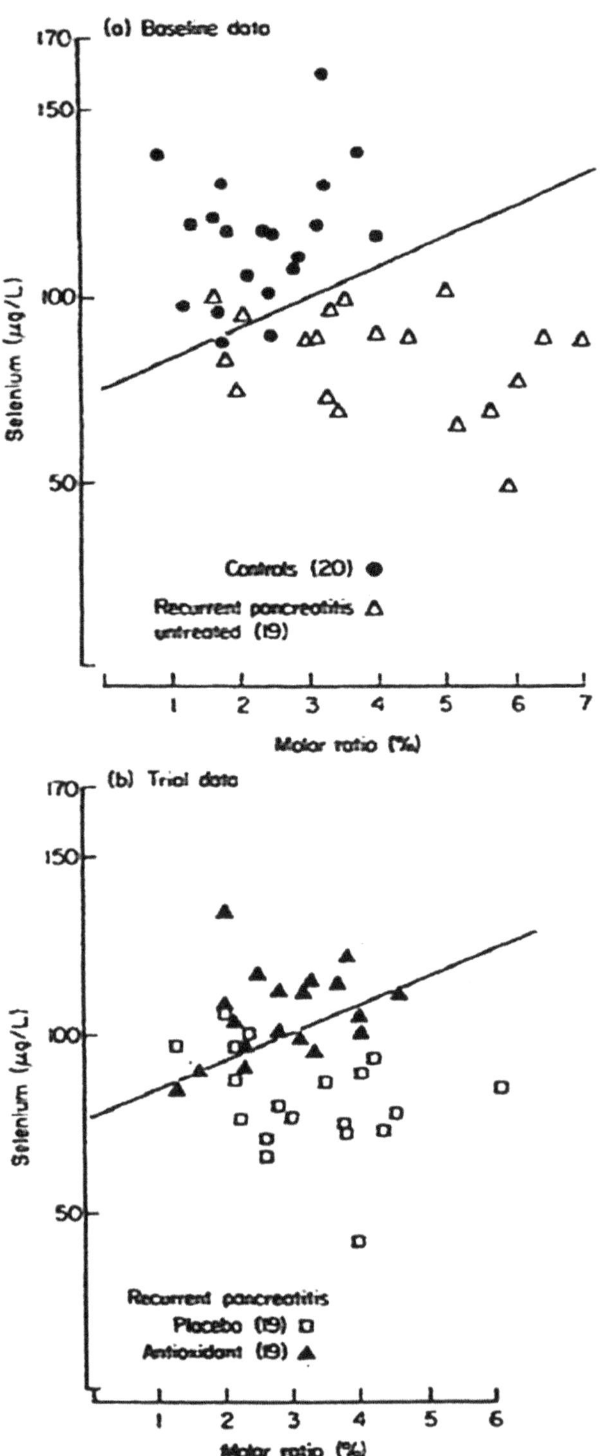

Figure 3. Discriminant analysis of serum selenium and the %molar ratio of the 9 *cis* 11 *trans* isomer of linoleic acid to the parent compound in controls and patients with recurrent pancreatitis. Discriminant function: selenium=8.76 x %MR + 75.74. Note that this function also applies to data from placebo-treated patients but fails to distinguish between controls and antioxidant-treated patients. Moreover, the discriminant function is not dissimilar to that recorded in patients with cystic fibrosis.[152] Reproduced with kind permission from Uden et al.[104]

than induced CYP is the likely source of increased FRA.[5] Intravenous treatment with N-acetylcysteine in lieu of methionine, as a more immediate precursor of GSH (**Figure 2**), plus the other micronutrients by appropriate routes, resulted in rapid pain relief and contraction of the inflammatory calcific head mass in an emaciated patient with impedance to gastric outflow and silent hemochromatosis.[171]

Two RCTs are currently in progress, NCT01528540 testing the micronutrient cocktail plus pregabalin (a presynaptic voltage-gated blocker of the calcium channel) or placebo in all-comers, and EUROPAC-2 a 3-armed trial involving a potent commercial preparation of the antioxidant combination (Antox version 1.2; Pharmanord, UK), versus magnesium, versus placebo in patients with hereditary or idiopathic disease.

Other observations

(a) SAM alone, or with selenium and vitamin E, was ineffective in double-blind placebo-controlled RCTs from the UK.[172] (b) This was also true for selenium and vitamin C in a single-blind RCT from India, which reported no diagnostic criteria, stated gall stones/common bile duct stones as the most frequent etiological factor, did not specify if these problems were on-going, and administered proton pump inhibitors plus pancreatic extracts—both with antioxidant potential—to treatment and no treatment groups.[173] (c) By contrast, in an open, observational study from the Czech Republic, vitamin C (0.5 gm/day) plus vitamin E (100 mg/day) for 12 months resulted in substantial pain reduction, to the point of abolition in 44% of 70 patients mainly with alcoholic disease. This was largely attributable to vitamin C, in that vitamin E levels were inexplicably unchanged by treatment, and with the greatest decrements in ROS generation and lipid peroxides among patients with the most functional parenchyma, judging by pancreatogram abnormality grade.[105] (d) A study reported in Polish[164] is cited in 2 meta-analyses.[158,160] The prescription (vitamin C 0.4 gm/day, vitamin E 300 mg/day) or no treatment was administered in an open RCT for 6 months in 91 patients with alcoholic disease, while blood antioxidant levels were monitored. The English-language abstract reports that 68% of the group of 46 on active treatment became pain free versus 31% of 45 untreated (p=0.002). The treated group also had fewer pancreatitis relapses (p=0.03) and their weight improved (p=0.001), as did pancreatic exocrine (p=0.001) and endocrine function (p=0.015). (e) An anecdotal account from the USA showed impressive improvement in 3 patients treated with a grape-seed extract.[174]

Clinical improvement in the latter 3 studies suggests that methionine intake in those patients was adequate, such that ascorbic acid or potent antioxidants in the grape-seed extract protected enzymes in the methionine metabolic route (**Figure 2**). Moreover, the Czech study shows that it is illogical to expect relief from oxidative stress-induced inflammatory pain in patients whose exocrine pancreatic function is severely compromised.

Long-term treatment

The long-term value of combination micronutrient therapy has been documented in reports from Delhi[41] and Manchester.[147,175] However, the importance of correcting reductive stress is illustrated by the finding that in 3 Manchester patients with recurrent acute pancreatitis, who were referred after the trial, standard treatment failed. The addition of folate to provide more methyl groups did not help, but a choline supplement did (unpublished data). This is in tune with the experimental observation that polyenylphosphatidyl choline protects against pancreatic oxidative stress in alcohol-treated rats.[176] When choline intake falls short, this phospholipid can be synthesized from phosphatidyl ethanolamine, but incurs severe pressure on SAM, "the universal methyl donor"[177] (**Figure 2**). There is now a convergence of thought on mechanisms of liver and pancreatic damage from a protracted excess of alcohol. The combination of 3 methyl donors—SAM, folate, and betaine—(**Figure 2**) alleviated alcoholic liver injury, while at the same time lowering the elevated SAM/SAH ratio and homocysteine level,[178] but the aforesaid evidence also points to the critical importance of ascorbic acid in protecting the exocrine pancreas, as shown by its ameliorating effect in animal models of mild and severe pancreatitis.[9] The inescapable conclusion is that the choline-deficient ethionine-supplemented dietary model of acute pancreatitis, which is easily modified to cause inflammatory fibrosis, is highly relevant to clinical pancreatitis.

A surgical audit was conducted in 1992 of 94 patients attending the Manchester Pancreato-Biliary Unit, with a mean follow-up of 30 months on micronutrient therapy, and more than 5 years in 22% of cases.[147] Imaging studies revealed that 85% had "large-duct disease", i.e., moderate or advanced change pancreatitis by endoscopic pancreatography, with or without calculi, and 15% had "small-duct disease", usually identified by secretin-pancreozymin tests. No patient needed duct decompression or resective pancreatic surgery during 248 patient-years of follow-up. The total number of days spent in hospital while on treatment was significantly lower than in the preceding year; 78% of patients became pain free, and a further 7% had a substantial reduction in pain (although several continued to take simple analgesics as fearful of an attack). Only 2 patients had continuous pain compared with 29 before micronutrient therapy. Of the 76 patients previously unemployed, 88% were back at work, and 80% were doing the same job. Of the 42 patients who drank alcohol excessively, a third continued to drink as previously, half had abstained altogether, and the others had reduced their intake to "safe" limits.[147]

This excellent result, which was continued through to 1998, such that surgery to treat the pain of chronic pancreatitis was virtually obsolete, accrued through strict guidelines. Patient-controlled devices to deliver morphine were forbidden. Routine endoscopic sphincterotomy, pancreatic duct stents, or attempts at clearance of pancreatic calculi were firmly rejected. Psychiatric help was sought early when dependence on narcotic analgesics or despair at social upheaval loomed. Input of primary care practitioners was solicited, and nutritionists, social workers, and pharmacists were engaged from the outset. The prescription of opiates in patients who were already dependent at referral was devolved to the pain team. A weekly medical-surgical clinic was preceded by an interdisciplinary discussion on patients to be seen that day and coordinated by a medical registrar, nurse specialist, and biochemist. Each doctor had a printout of previous antioxidant and %MRLA data, so that selenium dosage could be adjusted with reference to the nomogram (**Figure 3**). Whole blood GSH helped to assess methionine adequacy and adequacy of vitamin C was assessed by reference to the percentage oxidation of ascorbic acid (unpublished data).

The full prescription was usually needed for 6 months, during which dietary advice was given on antioxidant-rich foodstuffs.[147] Negotiation with executives from Pharmanord, UK, resulted in a combination tablet, Antox, that reduced the number to an average of 4 per day compared with 14 per day in the original trial. Further improvements were made by the company so as with Antox version 1.2 to increase the daily dose of methionine, while limiting β-carotene to the shell, because of cosmetic distress from a yellow hue. Treatment failure occurred in approximately 10% of about 300 patients, and was associated with large cysts/pseudocysts, noncompliance in unreformed alcoholics, undiagnosed neoplasia in 2 (adenocarcinoma, papillary mucinous) and in the previously described patients with recurrent acute pancreatitis (unpublished data).

After 1998, new physicians brought their previous experience to bear such that patient-controlled pumps to deliver morphine were introduced, morphine prescriptions soared, invasive intervention increased, and the micronutrient prescription ceased. The change in practice was linked to an increased daily dose of morphine and a 54% prior intervention rate reported in the recent negative trial of combination micronutrient therapy (**Table 2**),[169] compared to none on either count in the 1990 report.[156]

Conclusion

Chronic pancreatitis seems to represent "hepatization" of the gland—a reversion to its ancestral roots—as a result of chronic exposure to xenobiotics that strike parenterally.[32, 71]

Choline intake and status in patients consuming their habitual diet were unfortunately not assessed in the Manchester studies, but are urgently needed. In the meantime, the addition of a choline supplement to the successful micronutrient cocktail is judicious, and probably should take precedence over calls to prescribe zinc, folate, or magnesium. The perception of electrophilic/oxidative stress in acinar cells as the "obligate intermediate phenotype" in the pathogenesis of chronic pancreatitis (**Figure 1**) fulfils a set of postulates derived from Koch's classical work on tuberculosis, as modified for a polygenic disease.[5,6] Hence, it is difficult to see the need for "a new framework for 21st century medicine".[179]

Addendum

The result of NCT01528540 has recently been published on-line. "Narcotic-naive" patients with chronic pancreatitis, and pain despite clearance of ductal calculi, received either a combination of pregabalin plus the Manchester antioxidant prescription or placebos for 2 months; wherepon pregabalin was stopped and all patients had open micronutrient antioxidant therapy for 4 months. Not only did active treatment lower pain compared to placebo when assessed in several ways at 2 months, but also pain was further lowered by 6 months in the first set. Moreover, the mitigating effect of micronutrient therapy was evident at this stage in the set that initially received placebo [Taludkar R et al. J Gastroenterol Hepatol. 2016. DOI: 10.1111/jgh.13332].

References

1. Braganza JM. Free Radicals and Pancreatitis. In: Rice-Evans C, Dormandy TL,eds. Free radicals: chemistry, pathology and medicine. London: Richelieu Press; 1988: 357-381.
2. Braganza JM. Experimental acute pancreatitis. *Curr Opin Gastroenterol*. 1990; 6: 763-768.
3. Braganza JM, Lee S, McCloy RF, McMahon MJ. Seminar. Chronic pancreatitis. *Lancet*. 2011; 377: 1184-1197. PMID: 21397320.
4. Sanfey H, Buckley GB, Cameron JL. The role of oxygen-derived free radicals in the pathogenesis of acute pancreatitis. *Ann Surg*. 1984; 200: 405-412. PMID: 6207783.
5. Braganza JM. The pathogenesis of chronic pancreatitis. *QJM*. 1996; 89: 243-250. PMID: 8733510.
6. Braganza JM. A framework for the aetiogenesis of chronic pancreatitis. *Digestion*. 1998; 59 (suppl 4): 1-12. PMID: 9832631.
7. Bhardwaj P, Yadav RK. Chronic pancreatitis: role of oxidative stress and antioxidants. *Free Radic Res*. 2013; 47: 941-949. PMID: 23668832.
8. Braganza JM. Antioxidant therapy for pancreatitis: clinical experience. In: Braganza JM, ed. The pathogenesis of pancreatitis. Manchester: Manchester University Press; 1991: 178-197.
9. Braganza JM, Dormandy TL. Micronutrient therapy for chronic pancreatitis: Rationale and impact. *JOP*. 2010; 11: 99-112. PMID: 20208316.
10. Grisby B, Dodriguez-Rilo H, Khan K. Antioxidants and chronic pancreatitis: theory of oxidative stress and trials of antioxidant therapy. *Dig Dis Sci*. 2012; 57: 835-841. PMID: 22302241.
11. Shahedi K, Pandol SJ, Hu R. Oxidative stress and alcoholic pancreatitis. *J Gastroenterol Hepatol Res*. 2013; 2: 335-342.
12. Tandon RK, Garg PK. Oxidative stress in chronic pancreatitis: pathophysiological relevance and management. *Antiox Redox Signal*. 2011; 15: 2757-2766. PMID: 21902596.
13. Braganza JM. Micronutrient therapy for chronic pancreatitis: Premises and pitfalls. *JOP*. 2013; 14: 304-308. PMID: 23846913.
14. Braganza JM. Toxicology of the pancreas. In: Braganza JM ed. The pathogenesis of pancreatitis. Manchester: Manchester University Press. 1991: 66-85.
15. Palmieri B, Sblendorio V. Oxidative stress tests: overview on reliability and use. Part 1. *Eur Rev Med Pharmacol Sci*. 2007; 11: 309-342. PMID: 18074940.
16. Chvanov M, Petersen OH, Tepkin A. Free radicals and the pancreatic acinar cells: role in physiology and pathology. *Philos Trans R Soc Lond B Biol Sci*. 2005; 360: 2273-2284. PMID: 16321797.
17. Leung PS, Chan YC. Role of oxidative stress in pancreatic inflammation. *Antiox Redox Signal*. 2009; 11: 135-165. PMID: 18837654.
18. Shimizu Y, Handershot LM. Oxidative folding: cellular strategies for dealing with the resultant equimolar production of reactive oxygen species. *Antiox Redox Signal*. 2009; 11: 2317-2331. PMID: 19243234.
19. Gonzalez FJ. Role of cytochromes P450 in chemical toxicity and oxidative stress: studies with CYP2E1. *Mutat Res*. 2005; 569: 101-110.
20. Gutteridge JMC. Lipid peroxidation and antioxidants as biomarkers of tissue damage. *Clin Chem*. 1995; 41: 1819-1828. PMID: 7497639.
21. Zimniak P. Relationship of electrophilic stress to aging. *Free Radic Biol Med*. 2011; 51: 1087-1105. PMID: 21708248.
22. Ghyczy M, Boros M. Electrophilic methyl groups present in the diet ameliorate pathological states induced by reductive and oxidative stress: a hypothesis. *Br J Nutr*. 2001; 85: 409-414. PMID: 11348555.
23. Ghyczy M, Torday C, Boros M. Simultaneous generation of methane, carbon dioxide, and carbon monoxide from choline and ascorbic acid: a defensive mechanism against reductive stress? *FASEB J*. 2003; 17: 1124-1126. PMID: 12692080.
24. Bhandary D, Marahatta A, Kim H-R, Chae H-J. An involvement of oxidative stress in endoplasmic stress and its associated diseases. *Int J Mol Sci*. 2013; 14: 434-456. PMID: 23263672.
25. Rutkowski DT, Kaufman RJ. A trip to the ER: coping with stress. *Trends Cell Biol*. 2004; 14: 20-28. PMID: 14729177.
26. Dolai S, Liang T, Cosen-Binker LI, Lam PPL, Gaisano H. Regulation of physiologic and pathologic exocytosis in pancreatic acinar cells. *The Pancreapedia: Exocrine Pancreas Knowledge Base*, 2012. DOI: 10.3998/panc.2012.12.
27. Zhang K. Integration of ER stress, oxidative stress and the inflammatory response in health and disease. *Int J Clin Exp Med*. 2010; 3: 33-40. PMID: 20369038.
28. Masamune A. Genetics of pancreatitis: the 2014 update. *Tohoku J Exp Med*. 2014; 232: 69-77. PMID: 24522117.

29. Pandol SJ, Gorelick FS, Gerloff A, Lugea A. Alcohol abuse, endoplasmic reticulum stress and pancreatitis. *Dig Dis.* 2010; 28: 776-782. PMID: 21525762.
30. Sah RP, Garg SK, Dixit AK, Dudeja V, Dawra RK, Saluja AK. Endoplasmic stress is chronically activated in chronic pancreatitis. *J Biol Chem.* 2014; 289: 27551-27561. PMID: 25077966.
31. Braganza JM. Pancreatic disease: a casualty of hepatic 'detoxification'? *Lancet*: 1983; 1000-1003. PMID: 6138545
32. Braganza JM. The pancreas. In: Pounder RE, ed. Recent Adv Gastroenterol. London: Churchill Livingstone; 1986: 251-280.
33. Rinderknecht H. Pancreatic secretory enzymes. In: Go VLW, Gardner JD, Brooks FP, Lebenthal E, DiMagno EP, Scheele GA, eds. The exocrine pancreas: biology, pathobiology and diseases, 2nd edition. New York, NY: Raven Press; 1993: 219-252.
34. Uomo G, Talamini G, Rabitti PG. Antioxidant treatment in hereditary pancreatitis. A pilot study on three young patients. *Dig Liver Dis.* 2001; 33: 58-62. PMID: 11303976.
35. Golden MHN. The exocrine pancreas in severe malnutrition. In: Braganza JM, ed. The pathogenesis of pancreatitis. Manchester: Manchester University Press; 1991: 139-155.
36. Braganza JM. The pancreas. In: Brocklehurst JC, Tallis R, Fillit J, eds. Textbook of geriatric medicine and gerontology, 4th edition. London: Churchill Livingstone; 1991: 527-535.
37. Georgelin T, Schnee M, Sagniez M, Bailly F, Naudot I, Soulard FM, et al. Antioxidant status in patients with hereditary chronic pancreatitis (HCP) and alcoholics. *Gastroenterology.* 1998; 114: A461.
38. Mathew P, Wyllie R, Van Lente F, Steffen RM, Kay MH. Antioxidants in hereditary pancreatitis. *Am J Gastroenterol.* 1996; 91: 1558-1562. PMID: 8759661.
39. Braganza JM. Towards a novel treatment strategy for acute pancreatitis. 1. Reappraisal of the evidence on aetiogenesis. *Digestion.* 2001; 63: 69-91. PMID: 11244246.
40. Rottner M, Freyssinet J-M, Martinez MC. Mechanisms of the noxious inflammatory cycle in cystic fibrosis. *Respiratory Research.* 2009; 10: 23. PMID: 19284656.
41. Midha S, Khaguria R, Shastri S, Kabra M, Garg PK. Idiopathic chronic pancreatitis in India: phenotypic characterisation and strong genetic susceptibility due to *SPINK1* and *CFTR* mutations. *Gut.* 2010; 59: 800-807. PMID: 20551465.
42. LaRusch J, Jung J, General IJ, Lewis MD, Park HW, Brand RE, et al. Mechanisms of *CFTR* functional variants that impair regulated bicarbonate permeation and increase risk for pancreatitis but not for cystic fibrosis. *PLOS Genetics.* 2014; 10: 1-15. PMID: 25033378.
43. Ko SB, Azuma S, Yoshikawa T, Yamamoto A, Kyokane K, Ko MS, et al. Molecular mechanisms of pancreatic stone formation in chronic pancreatitis. *Front Physiol* 2012; 3: 415: 2012. PMID: 23133422.
44. Lipecka J, Norez C, Bensalem N, Baudouin-Legros M, Planelles G, Becq F, et al. Rescue of Delta508-CFTR (cystic fibrosis transmembrane conductance regulator) by curcumin: involvement of the keratin 18 network. *J Pharmacol Exp Ther.* 2006; 317: 500-505. PMID: 16424149.
45. Xu Y, Szép S, Lu Z. The antioxidant role of thiocyanate in the pathogenesis of cystic fibrosis and other inflammation-related diseases. *PNAS.* 2009; 106: 20515-20519. PMID: 19918082.
46. Mohan V, Braganza JM. Xenobiotics in tropical pancreatitis. In: Braganza JM, ed. The pathogenesisis of pancreatitis. Manchester: Manchester University Press.1991: 115-128.
47. Braganza JM. Towards a novel treatment strategy for acute pancreatitis. 2. Principles and potential practice. *Digestion.* 2001; 63: 143-162. PMID: 1351142.
48. Sah RP, Saluja AK. Trypsinogen activation in acute and chronic pancreatitis: is it a prerequisite? *Gut* 2011; 60: 1305-1307. PMID: 21672938.
49. Gilbert KM. Xenobiotic exposure and autoimmune hepatitis. *Hepatitis Research and Treatment* 2010; Article ID 248157. http://dx.doi.org/10.1155/2010/248157.
50. Robin MA, Descatoire V, Le Roy M, Berson A, Lebreton F-R, Maratrat M. Vesicular transport of newly synthesised cytochromes P4501A to the outside of rat hepatocyte plasma membranes. *JPET.* 2000; 294; 1063-1069. PMID: 10945860.
51. Lafleur MA, Stevens JL, Lawrence JW. Xenobiotic perturbation of ER stress and the unfolded protein response. *Toxicol Pathol.* 2013; 41: 235-262. PMID: 23334697.
52. Houston JB. Cytochromes P450 in chronic pancreatitis. In: Braganza JM, ed. The pathogenesis of pancreatitis. Manchester: Manchester University Press; 1991: 103-114.
53. Liu LG, Yan H, Zhang W, Yao P, Zhang XP, Sun XF, et al. Induction of heme oxygenase-1 in human hepatocytes to protect from ethanol-induced cytotoxicity. *Biomed Environ Sci.* 2004; 17: 315-326. PMID: 15602829.
54. Braganza JM. Mast cell control: likely modus operandi of panhaematin in experimental pancreatitis. *Gut.* 2012; 61: 632. PMID: 21757450.
55. Correia MA, Burk RF. Defective utilization of haem in selenium-deficient rat liver. *Biochem J.* 1983; 214: 53-58. PMID: 6615473.
56. Braganza JM. The role of the liver in exocrine pancreatic disease. *Int J Pancreatol.* 1988; 3: S19-S42. PMID: 3062099.
57. Segal I, Ally R, Hunt LP, Sandle LN, Ubbink JB, Braganza JM. Insights into the development of alcoholic chronic pancreatitis at Soweto, south Africa. *Pancreas.* 2011; 40: 508-516. PMID: 21499204.
58. Arumugam G, Padmanaban M, Krishnan D, Panneerselvam S, Rajagopal S. Influence of copper, iron, zinc and Fe_3^+ haemoglobin levels on the etiopathogenesis of chronic calcific pancreatitis - a study in patients with pancreatitis. *Biol Trace Elem Res.* 2011; 142: 424-434. PMID: 20809271.
59. Foster JR, Idle JR, Hardwick JP, Bars R, Scott P, Braganza JM. Induction of drug-metabolizing enzymes in human pancreatic cancer and chronic pancreatitis. *J* Pathol. 1993; 169: 457-463. PMID: 8501544.
60. Standop L, Schneider M, Ulrich A, Büchler MW, Pour PM. Differences in immunohistochemical expression of xenobiotic-metabolizing enzymes between normal pancreas, chronic pancreatitis and pancreatic cancer. *Toxicol Pathol.* 2003; 31: 500-513. PMID: 14692619.
61. Wacke R, Kirchner A, Prall F, Nizze H, Schmidt W, Fischer U, et al. Up-regulaton of cytochrome P4501A2 2C9 and 2E1

in chronic pancreatitis. *Pancreas*. 1998; 16: 521-528. PMID: 9598815.

62. Telek G, Regõly-Mérei J, Kovács GC, Simon L, Hamar J, Jakab F. The first histological demonstration of pancreatic oxidative stress in human acute pancreatitis. *Hepatogastroenterology*. 2001; 48: 1252-1258. PMID: 11677940.
63. Schoenberg MH, Büchler M, Pietrzyk C, Uhl W, Birk D, Eisele S. Lipid peroxidation and glutathione metabolism in chronic pancreatitis. *Pancreas*. 1995; 10: 36-43. PMID: 7899458.
64. Bruce JIE, Elliott AC. Pharmacological evaluation of the role of cytochrome P450 in intracellular calcium signalling in pancreatic acinar cells. *Br J Pharmacol*. 2000; 131: 761-771. PMID: 11030726.
65. Cecere A, Tancredi L, Gattoni A. Primary sclerosing cholangitis. *Panminerva Med*. 2002; 44: 313-323. PMID: 12434113.
66. Santini SA, Spada C, Bononi F, Foschia F, Mutignani M, Perri V, et al. Enhanced lipoperoxidation products in pure pancreatic juice: evidence for organ-specific oxidative stress in chronic pancreatitis. *Dig Liver Dis*. 2003; 35: 888-892. PMID: 14703885.
67. Leo MA, Aleynik SI, Siegel JH, Kasmin FE, Aleynik MK, Leiber CS. F_2-isoprostanes and 4-hydroxynonenal excretion in human bile of patients with biliary tract and pancreatic disorders. *Am J Gastroenterol*. 1997; 92: 2069-2072. PMID: 9362195.
68. Ganesh Pai C, Sreejayan, Rao MN. Evidence for oxidative stress in chronic pancreatitis. *Indian J Gastroenterol*. 1999; 18: 156-157. PMID: 10531717.
69. Guyan PM, Uden S, Braganza JM. Heightened free radical activity in pancreatitis. *Free Radic Biol Med*. 1990; 8: 347-354. PMID: 2379863.
70. Wallig M. Xenobiotic metabolism, oxidant stress and chronic pancreatitis. *Digestion*. 1998; 59 (suppl 4): 13-24. PMID: 9832632.
71. Veghelyi PV, Kemeny TT, Pozsonyi J, Sos J. Toxic lesions of the pancreas. *Am J Dis Child*. 1950; 80: 390-403. PMID: 14770454.
72. Merkord J, Weber H, Jonas L, Nizze H, Heninghausen G. The influence of ethanol on long-term effects of dibutylytin dichloride (DBTC) in pancreas and liver of rats. *Hum Exp Toxicol*. 1998; 17: 144-150. PMID: 9587782.
73. Sato A, Nakajima T, Koyama Y. Effects of chronic ethanol consumption on hepatic metabolism of aromatic and chlorinated hydrocarbons in rats. *Br J Ind Med*. 1980; 37: 382-386. PMID: 7192567.
74. Strubelt O. Interactions between ethanol and other hepatotoxic agents. *Biochem Pharmacol*. 1980; 29: 1445-1449. PMID: 6994745.
75. Iimuro Y, Bradford BU, Gao W, Kadiska M, Mason RP, Stefanovic B, et al. Detection of α-hydroxyethyl free radical adducts in the pancreas after chronic exposure to alcohol in the rat. *Mol Pharmacol*. 1996; 50: 656-661. PMID: 8794907.
76. Ma Q, Lu AYH. Cyp1A induction and human risk assessment: an evolving tale of in vitro and in vivo studies. *Drug Metab Dispos*. 2007; 35: 1009-1016. PMID: 17431034.
77. Ulrich AB, Schmeid BM, Matsuzaki H, Lawson TA, Freiss HY, Andrén-Sandberg A, et al. Increased expression of glutathione S-transferase-π in the islets of patients with primary chronic pancreatitis but not secondary chronic pancreatitis. *Pancreas*. 2001; 22: 388-394. PMID: 11345140.
78. Sandilands D, Jeffrey IJM, Haboubi NY, MacLennan IAM, Braganza JM. Abnormal drug metabolism in chronic pancreatitis. Treatment with antioxidants. *Gastroenterology*. 1990; 98: 766-772. PMID: 2298375.
79. Takahashi T, Akagi R, Shimizu H, Hirakawa M, Sassa S. Heme oxygenase-1. A major player in the defence against the oxidative tissue injury. In: Abraham NG, Alam J, Nath K, eds. Heme oxygenase in biology and medicine. New York, NY: Kluwer Academic/Plenum Publishers; 2002: 387-396.
80. Korashy HM, El-Kadi AO. Modulation of TCCD-mediated induction of cytochrome P-4501A1 by mercury, lead, and copper in human HepG2 cell line. *Toxicol In Vitro*. 2008; 22: 154-158. PMID: 17889500.
81. Ossola JO, Groppa MD, Tomaro MI. Relationship between oxidative stress and heme oxygenase induction by copper sulphate. *Arch Biocem Biophys*. 1997; 227: 332-337. PMID: 9016830.
82. Braganza JM, Jolley JE, Lee WR. Occupational chemicals and pancreatitis: a link? *Int J Pancreatol*. 1986; 1: 9-19. PMID: 3320224.
83. McNamee R, Braganza JM, Hogg J, Leck I, Rose P, Cherry NM. Occupational exposure to hydrocarbons and chronic pancreatitis: a case-referent study. *Occup Environ Med*. 1994; 51: 631-637. PMID: 7951796.
84. Braganza JM, John S, Padmayalam I, Mohan V, Chari S, Madanagopalan M. Xenobiotics and tropical chronic pancreatitis. *Int J Pancreatol*. 1990; 7: 231-245.
85. Jeppe CY, Smith MD. Transverse descriptive study of xenobiotic exposures in patients with chronic pancreatitis and pancreatic cancer. *JOP*. 2008; 9: 235-239. PMID: 18326937.
86. Khurana V, Barkin JS. Pancreatitis induced by environmental toxins. *Pancreas*. 2001; 22: 102-195. PMID: 11138962.
87. Longnecker DS. Environmental factors and diseases of the pancreas. *Environ Health Perspect*. 1977; 20: 105-112. PMID: 598342.
88. Starek K, Kaminski M. [Polish] Toxicity of certain petrochemical derivatives used as dielectrics in electromachining. V. Morphological, cytoenzymic, and biochemical changes in the liver of rats chronically exposed to kerosene hydrocarbons. *Med Pr*. 1982; 33: 9-53.
89. Siriwardena AK. Reappraisal of xenobiotic-induced, oxidative stress-mediated cellular injury in chronic pancreatitis: a systematic review. *World J Gastroenterol*. 2014; 20: 3033-3043. PMID: 24659895.
90. Odewabi AO, Ogundahunsi OA, Oyalowo M. Effect of exposure to petrochemical fumes on plasma antioxidant defense system in petrol attendants. *Br J Pharmacol Toxicol*. 2014; 5: 83-87.
91. Rekhadevi PV, Rahman MF, Mahboob M, Grover P. Genotoxicity in filling station attendants exposed to petroleum hydrocarbons. *Ann Occup Hyg*. 2010; 54: 944-954. PMID: 20956619.
92. Uboh FE, Akpanabiatu MI, Eyong EU, Ebong PE, Eka OO. Evaluation of toxicological implications of inhalation

exposure to kerosene fumes and petrol fumes in rats. *Acta Biol Szeged*. 2005; 49: 19-22.

93. Kahn DR, Carlson AB. On the mechanism of experimentally induced ethionine pancreatitis. *Ann Surg*. 1959; 150: 42-49. PMID: 13661828.
94. Veghelyi PV, Kemeny TT, Pozsonyi J, Sos J. Dietary lesions of the pancreas. *Am J Dis Child*. 1950; 79: 658-665.
95. Capdevila A, Decha-Umphai W, Song KH, Borchardt RT, Wagner C. Pancreatic enzyme secretion is blocked by inhibitors of methylation. *Arch Biochem Biophys*. 1997; 345: 47-55. PMID: 9281310.
96. Balaghi M, Wagner C. Folate deficiency inhibits pancreatic amylase secretion in rats. *Am J Clin Nutr*. 1995; 61: 90-96. PMID: 7529961.
97. Luthen RE, Grendell JH. Thiol metabolism and acute pancreatitis: trying to make the pieces fit. *Gastroenterology*. 1994; 107: 888-892. PMID: 8076778.
98. Quesnel LB, Jaran AS, Braganza JM. Antibiotic accumulation and membrane trafficking in cystic fibrosis cells. *J Antimicrob Chemother*. 1998; 41: 215-221. PMID: 9533463.
99. Schick V, Scheiber JA, Mooren FC, Turi S, Ceyhan GO, Schnekenburger J, et al. Effect of magnesium supplementation and depletion on the onset and course of acute experimental pancreatitis. *Gut*. 2014; 63: 1469-1480. PMID: 24277728.
100. Whiteman M, Le Trionnaire S, Chopra M, Fox B, Whatmore J. Emerging role of hydrogen sulphide in health and disease: critical appraisal of biomarkers and pharmacological tools. *Clin Sci (Lond)*. 2011; 121: 459-488. PMID: 21843150.
101. Moreno ML, Escobar J, Izquierdo-Âlvarez A, Gil A, Pérez S, Pereda J, et al. Disulfide stress : a novel type of oxidative stress in acute pancreatitis. *Free Radic Biol Med*. 2014; 70: 265-277. PMID: 24456905.
102. Lipinski B. Evidence in support of a concept of reductive stress. *Br J Nutr*. 2002; 87: 93-94. PMID: 11895317.
103. Martensson J, Bolin T. Sulfur amino acid metabolism in chronic relapsing pancreatitis. *Am J Gastroenterol*. 1986; 81: 1179-1184. PMID: 3788926.
104. Uden S, Schofield D, Miller PF, Bottiglieri T, Braganza JM. Antioxidant therapy for recurrent pancreatitis: biochemical profiles in a placebo-controlled trial. *Aliment Pharmacol Ther*. 1992; 6: 229-240. PMID: 160043.
105. Ditě P, Prĕcehtelová M, Novooytmny L, Soska V, Źaková A, Lata J. Changes of reactive substance in patients with morphologically different degrees of chronic pancreatitis and effects of long-term therapy with natural antioxidants. *Gastroenterologia Polska*. 2003; 10: 379-383.
106. Szuster-Ciesielska A, Daniluk J, Kandefer-Szerszeńn M. Oxidative stress in blood of patients with alcohol related pancreatitis. *Pancreas*. 2001; 22: 261-266. PMID: 11291927.
107. Verlaan R, Roelofs HM, van-Schaik A, Wanten GJ, Jansen JB, Peters WH, et al. Assessment of oxidative stress in chronic pancreatitis patients. *World J Gastroenterol*. 2006; 12: 5705-5710. PMID: 17007026.
108. Bhardwaj P, Garg PK, Maulik SK, Saraya A, Tandon RK, Acharya SK. A randomized controlled trial of antioxidant supplementation for pain relief in patients with chronic pancreatitis. *Gastroenterology*. 2009; 138: 149-159. PMID: 18952082.
109. Girish BN, Vaidyanathan K, Rajesh G, Balakrishnan V. Effects of micronutrient status on oxidative stress and exocrine pancreatic function in patients with chronic pancreatitis. *Indian J Biochem Biophys*. 2012; 49: 386-391. PMID: 23259326.
110. Kodydkova J, Vavrova L, Stankova B, Macasek J, Krechler T, Zak A. Antioxidant status and oxidative stress markers in pancreatic cancer and chronic pancreatitis. *Pancreas*. 2013; 42: 614-621. PMID: 23558240.
111. Girish BN, Vaidyanathan K, Rao NA, Rajesh G, Reshmi S, Balakrishnan V. Chronic pancreatitis is associated with hyperhomocysteinaemia and derangements in transsulfuration and transmethylation pathways. *Pancreas*. 2010; 39: e11-16. PMID: 20050230.
112. Syrota A, Dop-Ngassa M, Cerf M, Paraf A. ^{11}C-L-methionine for evaluation of pancreatic exocrine function. *Gut*. 1981; 22: 907-915. PMID: 6171485.
113. Takasu A, Shimosegawa E, Hatazawa J, Nagasaki Y, Kimura K, Fujita M, et al. [^{11}C] Methionine positron emission tomography for the evaluation of pancreatic exocrine function in chronic pancreatitis. *Pancreas*. 2001; 22: 203-209. PMID: 11249078.
114. Girish BN, Rajesh G, Vaidyanathan K, Balakrishnan V. Alterations in plasma amino acid levels in chronic pancreatitis. *JOP*. 2011; 12: 11-18. PMID: 21206095.
115. Sajewicz W, Milnerowicz S, Nabzdyk S. Blood plasma antioxidant defense in patients with pancreatitis. *Pancreas*. 2006; 32: 139-144. PMID: 16552332.
116. Braganza JM, Odom N, McCloy RF, Ubbink JB. Homocysteine and chronic pancreatitis. *Pancreas*. 2010; 39: 1303-1304. PMID: 20944492.
117. Morselli-Labate A, Fantini L, Pezzilli R. Hydrogen sulphide, nitric oxide and a molecular mass 66 u substance in the exhaled air of chronic pancreatitis patients. *Pancreatology*. 2007; 7: 497-504. PMID: 17912017.
118. Braganza JM, Hewitt CD, Day JP. Serum selenium in patients with chronic pancreatitis: lowest values during painful exacerbations. *Trace Elements Med*. 1988; 5: 79-84.
119. Rose P, Fraine E, Hunt LP, Acheson DWK, Braganza JM. Dietary antioxidants and chronic pancreatitis. *Hum Nutr Clin Nutr* 1986; 40: 151-164. PMID: 3957720.
120. Uden S, Acheson DWK, Reeves J, Worthington HV, Hunt LP, Brown S, et al. Antioxidants, enzyme induction, and chronic pancreatitis, A reappraisal following studies in patients on anticonvulsants. *Eur J Clin Nutr*. 1988; 42; 561-569. PMID: 3224602.
121. Scott G. Antioxidants *in vitro* and *in vivo*. In: Braganza JM, ed. The pathogenesis of pancreatitis. Manchester: Manchester University Press; 1991: 159-177.
122. Arnĕr ESJ, Holmgren A. Physiological functions of thioredoxin and thioredoxin reductase. *Eur J Biochem*. 2000; 267: 6102-6109. PMID: 11012661.
123. Johnston CS. The antihistamine action of ascorbic acid. *Subcell Biochem*. 1998; 25: 189-213. PMID: 8821975.
124. Nakos G, Gossrau R. Visualization of hydrogen peroxide (H_2O_2)-production from histamine. *Ann Anat*. 1995; 177: 431-438. PMID: 7645739.

125. Bonham MJ, Abu-Zidan FM, Simovic MO, Sluis KB, Wilkinson A, Winterbourne CC, et al. Early ascorbic acid depletion is related to the severity of acute pancreatitis. *Br J Surg*. 1999; 86: 1296-1301. PMID: 10540137.
126. Scott P, Bruce C, Schofield D, Shiel N, Braganza JM, McCloy RF. Vitamin C status in patients with acute pancreatitis. *Br J Surg*. 1993; 80: 750-754. PMID: 8330166.
127. Morris-Stiff GJ, Bowrey DJ, Oleesky D, Davies M, Clark GW, Puntis MC. The antioxidant profiles of patients with recurrent acute and chronic pancreatitis. *Am J Gastroenterol*. 1999; 94: 2135-2140. PMID: 10445540.
128. Quillot D, Walters E, Bonte J-P, Fruchart J-C, Duriez P, Ziegler O. Diabetes mellitus worsens antioxidant status in patients with chronic pancreatitis. *Am J Clin Nutr*. 2005; 81: 1117-1125. PMID: 15883437.
129. Van Gossum A, Closset P, Noel E, Cremer M, Neve J. Deficiency in antioxidant factors in patients with alcohol-related chronic pancreatitis. *Dig Dis Sci*. 1996; 41: 1225-1231. PMID: 8654156.
130. Vaona B, Stanzial AM, Talamini G, Bovo P, Corrocher R, Cavallini G. Serum selenium concentrations in chronic pancreatitis and controls. *DIg Liver Dis*. 2005; 37: 522-525. PMID: 15975540.
131. Yadav S, Day JP, Mohan V, Snehalatha C, Braganza JM. Selenium and diabetes in the tropics. *Pancreas*. 1991; 5: 528-533. PMID: 1946309.
132. Winklhofer-Roob B, Tiran B, Tuchschmid PE, Van't Hof MA, Shmerling DH. Effects of pancreatic enzyme preparations on erythrocyte glutathione peroxidase activities and plasma selenium concentrations in cystic fibrosis. *Free Radic Biol Med*. 1998; 25: 242-249. PMID: 9667502.
133. Braganza JM. Pancreatic extracts for painful chronic pancreatitis: Micronutrient antioxidant therapy by proxy. *JOP*. 2014; 15: 541-543. PMID: 25435568.
134. Braganza JM, Schofield D, Snehalatha C, Mohan V. Micronutrient antioxidant status in tropical compared with temperate-zone chronic pancreatitis. *Scand J Gastroenterol*. 1993; 28: 1098-1104. PMID: 8303214.
135. Chaloner C, Sandle LN, Mohan V, Snehalatha C, Viswanathan M, Braganza JM. Evidence for induction of cytochrome P4501 in patients with tropical pancreatitis. *Int J Pharmacol Ther Toxicol*. 1990; 28: 235-240. PMID: 2376424.
136. Lucas D, Ferrara R, Gonzalez E, Bodenez P, Albores A, Manno M, et al. Chlorzoxazone, a selective probe for phenotyping CYP2E1 in humans. *Pharmacogenetics*. 1999; 9: 377-388. PMID: 10471070.
137. Uboh FE, Ebong PE, Akpan HD, Usoh IF. Hepatoprotective effect of vitamins C and E against gasoline vapour-induced liver injury in male rats. *Turk J Biol*. 2012; 36: 217-223.
138. Blanchard JA, Barve S, Joshi-Barve S, Talwalker R, Gates LK. Antioxidants inhibit cytokine production and suppress NF-kappa B activation in CAPAN-1 and CAPAN-2 cell lines. *Dig Dis Sci*. 2001; 46; 2768-2772. PMID: 11768272.
139. Scott P, Knoop M, McMahon RFT, Braganza JM, Hutchinson IV. *S*-adenosyl-L-methionine protects against haemorrhagic pancreatitis in partially immunosuppressed panreaticoduodenal transplant recipients. *Drug Investigation*. 1992; 4 (suppl 4): 69-77.
140. Ji Y-L, Wang Z, Wang H, Zhang C, Zhang Y, Zhao M, et al. Ascorbic acid protects against cadmium-induced reticulum stress and germ cell apoptosis in testes. *Reproductive Toxicology*. 2012; 34: 357-363. PMID: 22569276.
141. Ji Y-L, Wang H, Zhang C, Zhang Y, Zhao M, Chen Y-H, et al. N-acetylcysteine protects against cadmium-induced germ cell apoptosis by inhibiting endoplasmic reticulum stress in testes. *Asian J Androl*. 2013; 15: 290-296. PMID: 23353715.
142. Malhotra JD, Miao H, Zhang K, Wolfson A, Pennathur S, Pipe SW, Kaufman RL. Antioxidants reduce endoplasmic stress and improve protein secretion. *PNAS*. 2008; 105: 18525-18530. PMID: 19011102.
143. De Las Heras-Castaño G, García-Unzueta T, Dominguez-Diez A, Fernández-Gonzáles MD, García de la Paz AM, Mayorga-Fernández M, et al. Pancreatic fibrosis in rats and its response to antioxidant treatment. *JOP*. 2005; 6: 316-324. PMID: 16006681.
144. Foster JR. Toxicology of the exocrine pancreas. In: Ballantyne B, Marrs TC, Syverson J, eds. General and Applied Toxicology 3rd edition. John Wiley & Sons: UK; 2009: 1411-1456.
145. Heaney AP, Sharer N, Rameh B, Braganza JM, Durrington PN. Prevention of recurrent pancreatitis in familial lipoprotein lipase deficiency with high-dose antioxidant therapy. *J Clin Endocrin Metab*. 1999; 84: 1203-1205. PMID: 10199753.
146. Yadav D, O'Connell M, Papachristou GI. Natural history following the first attack of acute pancreatitis. *Am J Gastroenterol*. 2012; 107: 1096-1103. PMID: 22613906.
147. McCloy RF. Chronic pancreatitis at Manchester, UK. Focus on antioxidant therapy. *Digestion*. 1998; 59 (suppl 4): 36-48. PMID: 9832634.
148. Capurso G, Cocomello L, Benedetto U, Camma C, Delle Fave G. Meta-analysis: the placebo rate of abdominal pain remission in clinical trials of chronic pancreatitis. *Pancreas*. 2012; 41: 125-131. PMID: 22513290.
149. Anderson D, Phillips BJ, Yu TW, Edwards AJ, Ayesh ER, Butterworth KR. The effects of vitamin C supplementation on bilomarkers of oxygen radical generated damage in human volunteers with 'low' or 'high' cholesterol levels. *Environ Mol Mutag*. 1997; 30: 161-174. PMID: 9329641.
150. Cawood P, Wickens DG, Iversen SA, Braganza JM, Dormandy TL. The nature of diene conjugation in human serum, bile and duodenal juice. *FEBS Lett*. 1983; 62: 239-243. PMID: 6628668.
151. Smith GN, Taj M, Braganza JM. On the identification of a conjugated diene component of duodenal bile as 9Z, 11E–octadecanoic acid. *Free Radic Biol Med*. 1991; 10: 13-21. PMID: 20250295.
152. Salh B, Webb K, Guyan PM, Day JP, Wickens J, Griffin J, et al. Aberrant free radical activity in cystic fibrosis. *Clin Chim Acta*. 1989; 181: 65-74. PMID: 2721006.
153. Kirk GR, White JS, McKie L, Stevenson M, Young I, Clements WD, et al. Combined antioxidant therapy reduces pain and improves quality of life in chronic pancreatitis. *J Gastrointest Surg*. 2006; 10: 499-503. PMID: 16627214.
154. Shah NS, Makin AJ, Sheen AJ, Siriwardena AK. Quality of life assessment in patients with chronic pancreatitis receiving antioxidant therapy. *World J Gastroenterol*. 2012; 16: 4066-4071. PMID: 20731021.
155. Schofield D, Rameh B, Leach FN, Braganza JM. Antioxidant profiles after antioxidant regimens for ten weeks: implications for clinical trial design. *Digestion*. 1997; 58 (suppl 2): 26.

156. Uden S, Bilton D, Nathan L. Hunt LP, Main C, Braganza JM. Antioxidant therapy for recurrent pancreatitis: placebo–controlled trial. *Aliment Pharmacol Ther*. 1990; 4: 357-371. PMID: 2103755.
157. Monfared SSMS, Vahidi H, Abdolghaffari AH, Nikfar S, Abdollahl M. Antioxidant therapy in the management of acute, chronic and post ERCP pancreatitis: A systematic review. *World J Gastroenterol*. 2009; 15: 4481-4490. PMID: 19777606.
158. Ahmed Ali U, Jens S, Busch ORC, Keus F, van Goor H, Gooszen HG, et al. Antioxidants for pain in chronic pancreatitis. *Cochrane Database Syst Rev*. 2014; 8: CD008945. PMID: 25144441.
159. Cai GH, Huang J, Chen J, Wu HH, Dong YL, Smith HS, et al. Antioxidant therapy for pain relief in patients with chronic pancreatitis: systematic review and meta-analysis. *Pain Physician*. 2013; 16: 521-532. PMID: 24284838.
160. Zhou D, Wang W, Cheng X, Wei J, Zheng S. Antioxidant therapy for patients with chronic pancreatitis: A systematic review and meta-analysis. *Clin Nutr*. 2015; 34: 627-634. PMID: 25035087.
161. Durgaprasad S, Ganesh Pai C, Vasanthkumar, Alvres JF, Namitha SA. A pilot study of the antioxidant effect of curcumin in tropical pancreatitis. *Indian J Med Res*. 2005; 122: 315-318. PMID: 16394323.
162. Banks PA, Hughes M, Ferrante M, Noordhoek EC, Ramagopal V, Slivka A. Does allopurinol reduce pain of chroniuc pancreatituis? *Int J Pancreatol*. 1997; 22: 171-176. PMID: 9444547.
163. Salim AS. Role of oxygen–derived free radical scavengers in the treatment of recurrent pain produced by chronic pancreatitis. *Arch Surg*. 1991; 126: 1109-1114. PMID: 1929842.
164. Jarosz M, Orzeszko M, Rychlik E, Kozuch M. [Polish] Antioxidants in the treatment of chronic pancreatitis *Gastroenterologia Polska*. 2010; 17: 41-46.
165. Chauhan SS, Pannu DS, Forsmark CE. Antioxidants as adjuvant therapy for pain in chronic pancreatitis. *Practical Gastroenterology: Nutrition issues in Gastroenterology* series #103 2012; Available at https://med.virginia.edu/ginutrition/wp-content/uploads/sites/199/2015/10/Parrish_March_12.pdf.
166. Burton F. Alkaade S, Collins D, Muddana V, Slivka A, Brand RE, et al. Use and perceived effectiveness of non-analgesic medical therapies for chronic pancreatitis in the United States. *Aliment Pharmacol Ther*. 2011; 33: 149-159. PMID: 21083584.
167. Pezzilli R. Antioxidants are not useful in reducing both pain and inflammation in chronic pancreatitis. *Recent Pat Inflamm Allergy Drug Discov*. 2014; 8: 19-23. PMID: 24397820.
168. Dhingra R, Singh N, Sachdev V, Upadhya AD, Saraya A. Effect of antioxidant supplementation on surrogate markers of fibrosis in chronic pancreatitis. A randomized placebo–controlled trial. *Pancreas*. 2013; 42: 589-595. PMID: 23531998.
169. Siriwardena AK, Mason JM, Sheen AJ, Makin AJ, Shah NS. Antioxidant therapy does not reduce pain in patients with chronic pancreatitis. The ANTICIPATE study. *Gastroenterology*. 2012; 143: 655-673. PMID: 22683257.
170. De las Heras Castaño G, Garcia de la Paz A, Fernández MD, Fernández Forcelledo JL. Use of antioxidants to treat pain in chronic pancreatitis. *Rev Esp Enferm Dig*. 2000; 92: 831-835. PMID: 10985097.
171. Sharer NM, Taylor PM, Linaker BD, Gutteridge JMC, Braganza JM. Safe and successful use of vitamin C to treat painful calcific chronic pancreatitis despite iron overload from primary haemochromatosis. *Clin Drug Invest*. 1995; 10: 310-315.
172. Bilton D, Schofield D, Mei G, Kay PM, Bottiglieri T, Braganza JM. Placebo-controlled trials of antioxidant therapy including *S*-adenosylmethionine in patients with recurrent non-gallstone pancreatitis. *Drug Invest*. 1994; 8: 10-20.
173. Khariong PDS, Hajong R, Kundu D, Tongper D, Mibang N, Picardo PJ. A comparative study into pain treatment in chronic pancreatitis between non operative conventional treatment and those treated with antioxidants. *IOSR-JDMS*. 2013; 6: 91-99.
174. Banerjee B, Bagchi D. Beneficial effects of a novel IH636 grape seed proanthocyanidin extract in the treatment of chronic pancreatitis. *Digestion*. 2001; 63: 203-206. PMID: 11351148.
175. Sharer NM, Schwarz M, Malone G, Howarth A, Painter J, Super M, et al. Mutations of the cystic fibrosis gene in patients with chronic pancreatitis *N Engl J Med*. 1998; 339: 645-652. PMID: 9725921.
176. Aleynik S, Leo MA, Aleynik MK, Lieber CS. Alcohol-induced pancreatic oxidative stress: protection by phospholipid repletion. *Free Radic Biol Med*. 1999; 26: 609-619. PMID: 10218649.
177. Wagner C. Some more comments on 'folate deficiency in chronic pancreatitis'. *JOP*. 2010; 11: 646-647.
178. Purohit V, Abdelmalek MF, Barve S, Benevenga NJ, Halsted CH, Kaplowitz N, et al. Role of S-adenosylmethionine, folate, and betaine in the treatment of alcoholic liver disease: summary of a symposium. *Am J Clin Nutr*. 2007; 86: 14-24. PMID: 17616758.
179. Whitcomb DC. Framework for interpretation of genetic variations in pancreatitis patients. *Front Physiol*. 2012; 3: 440.

Chapter 49

Management of endocrine failure in chronic pancreatitis

Dana K. Andersen*

Division of Digestive Diseases and Nutrition
National Institute of Diabetes and Digestive and Kidney Diseases, National Institutes of Health, Bethesda, Maryland.

Introduction

The natural history of chronic pancreatitis (CP) includes progressive loss of exocrine and endocrine function. Endocrine failure occurs because of progressive destruction of the gland by the ongoing inflammatory events of CP, and results in diabetes which is termed pancreatogenic or type 3c diabetes (T3cDM). The pathophysiology of T3cDM includes loss of secretion of the principal glucoregulatory hormones produced by the islets (insulin, glucagon, and pancreatic polypeptide), and is contributed to by abnormal secretion of the incretin hormones glucagon-like peptide 1 (GLP-1) and glucose-dependent insulinotropic polypeptide (GIP), which are adversely affected by the loss of exocrine function. T3cDM is therefore a complex form of secondary diabetes, and it requires careful assessment and management.

Pathophysiology of T3cDM

Definition and Classification of Pancreatogenic or T3cDM

Diabetes caused by agenesis, destruction, or loss of the exocrine pancreas has been termed pancreatogenic diabetes. In 1979, the National Diabetes Data Group of the National Institutes of Health formulated a classification system that defined secondary diabetes caused by pancreatic disease as a third type of diabetes, after type 1 and type 2.[1] The classification was subsequently endorsed by the American Diabetes Association (ADA) and other groups. In 1997, the ADA published a table of diabetes classifications in which pancreatogenic diabetes was listed as T3cDM.[2] The ADA classification table was subsequently republished as an annual supplement from 2002[3] to 2014.[4] In 2015, the classification table included pancreatogenic diabetes as a form of "diabetes due to other causes" without further description or guidelines for diagnosis or therapy.[5] The term T3cDM has been used repeatedly by investigators and clinicians to refer to the diabetes that results from, or is associated with, pancreatitis, trauma/pancreatectomy, neoplasia, cystic fibrosis, hemochromatosis, or fibrocalcific pancreatopathy.

It is uncertain whether pancreatogenic diabetes due to CP is identical to other forms of T3cDM having other causes such as pancreatectomy, pancreatic cancer, or cystic fibrosis, or whether these various causes of T3cDM have similar etiologies. T3cDM caused by CP most closely resembles the form of diabetes associated with pancreatic resection, in that beta cell mass is reduced according to the extent of the resection or disease. A deficiency of pancreatic polypeptide (PP), a regulator of the expression and availability of hepatic insulin receptors, is a consequence of both advanced CP and proximal (or total) pancreatectomy.[6] In diabetes that is a consequence, and frequently a harbinger, of pancreatic ductal adenocarcinoma (PDAC), impaired insulin secretion is believed to be a para-neoplastic phenomenon,[7] and insulin sensitivity is impaired.[8] The impairment in (hepatic) insulin sensitivity may be a consequence of the loss of PP secretion associated with PDAC localized to the pancreatic head.[9] In diabetes associated with cystic fibrosis, the progressive destruction of the pancreas due to impairment in bicarbonate secretion caused by mutations in the cystic fibrosis transmembrane receptor, is associated with insulin deficiency as well as a loss of hepatic insulin sensitivity,[10] which may also be a consequence of impaired PP secretion.[11]

Prevalence of T3cDM

The prevalence of pancreatogenic or T3cDM was believed to be quite low until recent studies by Hardt et al[12] and Ewald et al[13] showed that T3cDM accounted for 8% to

*Corresponding author. Email: dana.andersen@nih.gov

9% of the total population of over 1900 diabetic patients referred to an academic center in Germany (**Figure 1**). No such prevalence study has been published for North America or elsewhere because of uncertainly of the criteria for the designation of T3cDM and its differentiation from type 1 (T1DM) and type 2 diabetes (T2DM). In the German series, half of the patients with probable or definite T3cDM had been previously misdiagnosed as having either T1DM or T2DM. The largest percentage of patients classified as having T3cDM (76%) had antecedent CP.

Natural History of CP-associated T3cDM

The prevalence of diabetes in patients with CP has been reported to range from 20% to 70%.[14,15] Longitudinal studies of 500 patients with (alcohol-induced) CP showed that after 25 years, 83% of patients had developed diabetes, and most required insulin treatment.[16] The morbidity of the diabetes due to small vessel disease (retinopathy and nephropathy) has been shown to be similar for T3cDM as for other types[17], and the mortality of T3cDM from hypoglycemia and other diabetic complications appears comparable to that of diabetes of other causes.

Pathophysiology of T3cDM

Severe T3cDM secondary to complete loss of islet hormone secretion is associated with a form of disease termed "brittle diabetes" because of a loss of both insulin and glucagon secretion. Insulin deficiency results in an increase in peripheral insulin sensitivity and the potential for overmedication despite small doses of insulin. Glucagon deficiency results in a loss of hypoglycemia awareness and responsiveness with resulting neuroglycopenia. A 1981 series of 117 patients treated with partial and total pancreatectomy for CP revealed that half the late deaths after surgery were due to hypoglycemia.[18]

Hyperglycemia in T3cDM results from insulin deficiency, and persistent endogenous glucose production due to the loss of hepatic insulin sensitivity.[6] In laboratory and clinical studies, persistent hepatic glucose production was seen to be associated with the loss of PP secretion,[19,20] and was reversed by PP administration in PP-deficient patients with CP.[21]

Progressive exocrine dysfunction results in lipase deficiency and a failure to digest fats. This results in impaired absorption of the fat-soluble vitamins A, D, E, and K,[22] and is associated with a high prevalence of metabolic bone disease and fractures in CP.[23] The loss of fat digestion also results in impaired incretin-mediated insulin release because of altered GLP-1 and GIP secretion from the proximal and distal small bowel. Pancreatic enzyme replacement therapy (PERT) has been shown to restore incretin secretion and improve nutrient-induced insulin release.[24,25] The clinical and laboratory characteristics that differentiate T1DM, T2DM and T3cDM are compared in **Table 1**.

Differentiation of T3cDM from T1DM and T2DM

The diagnosis of T3cDM due to CP was addressed in a consensus conference held at the annual meeting of PancreasFest in 2012.[26] A definition of the major and minor criteria for diagnosis of T3cDM was described, and included the documentation of antecedent pancreatic exocrine disease established by radiology and exocrine

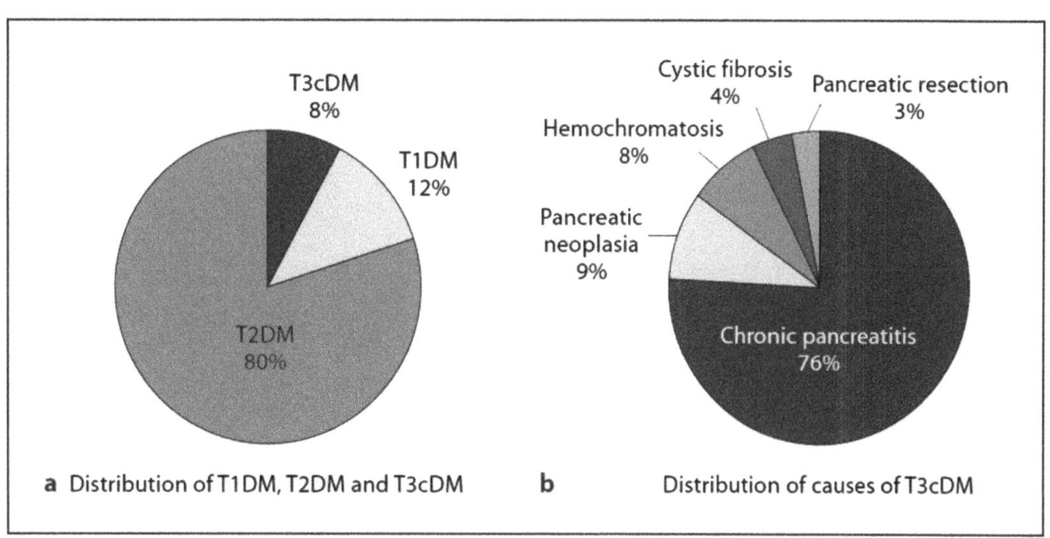

Figure 1. Distribution of types of diabetes (a) and causes of type 3c (pancreatogenic) diabetes (b) based on studies of 1,922 diabetic patients referred to an academic medical center.[6] Used with permission.[12]

Table 1. Clinical and laboratory findings in types of diabetes mellitus.

Parameter	T1DM (IDDM)	T2DM (NIDDM)	T3cDM (Pancreatogenic)
Ketoacidosis	Common	Rare	Rare
Hyperglycemia	Severe	Usually Mild	Mild
Hypoglycemia	Common	Rare	Common
Peripheral insulin sensitivity	Normal or increased	Decreased	Increased
Hepatic insulin sensitivity	Normal	Normal or decreased	Decreased
Insulin levels	Low	High	Low
Glucagon levels	Normal or High	Normal or high	Low
PP levels	Normal or low (late)	High	Low
GIP levels	Normal or low	Variable	Low
GLP-1 levels	Normal	Variable	Variable
Typical age of onset	Childhood or adolescence	Adulthood	Any
Typical etiology	Auto-immune	Obesity or Aging	CP, Post-op, PDAC

T1DM, type 1 diabetes mellitus; T2DM, type 2 diabetes mellitus; T3cDM, type 3c diabetes mellitus; IDDM, insulin dependent diabetes mellitus; NIDDK, non-insulin dependent diabetes mellitus; PP, pancreatic polypeptide; GIP, glucose-dependent insulinotropic polypeptide; GLP-1, glucagon-like peptide-1; CP, chronic pancreatitis; PDAC, pancreatic ductal adenocarcinoma.
Modified, and used with permission.[6]

secretory testing. In addition, the absence of anti-islet antibodies (to rule out T1DM) and PP deficiency (to rule out T2DM) were included as criteria. These criteria have also been used by Ewald et al. in their studies of T3cDM.[27] As the majority of patients with CP will develop diabetes later in their disease course, the most common misdiagnosis is that of T2DM. A proposed set of criteria for the diagnosis of T3cDM is shown in **Table 2**.

PP secretion is increased in obesity associated with diabetes,[28] normal aging, and age-related diabetes.[29] PP secretion is increased in these diabetes groups, presumably as a compensatory response to a progressive decline in insulin sensitivity. However, PP secretion is impaired in T3cDM caused by CP, pancreatic resection, pancreatic carcinoma, and cystic fibrosis[6] (**Table 1**). Therefore, a failure of PP secretion in response to oral nutrients is a useful test to discriminate T3cDM from the more prevalent T2DM. PP secretion is stimulated by glucose, protein, and fat; but glucose alone is a relatively weak stimulant of PP release. This is probably a consequence of the normal enteric stimulation of PP release by cholecystokinin (CCK)[30] and GIP.[29,31] Because oral glucose is a weak stimulant of PP, it is recommended that a mixed meal test be used to document PP levels.[26] Eight ounces of a liquid nutritional supplement such as Boost or Ensure serve as suitable nutrient stimuli for PP release and are usually well tolerated. PP levels normally increase 3- to 5-fold within 30–60 minutes after ingestion of the liquid meal. Plasma levels obtained

Table 2. Proposed criteria for the diagnosis of type 3c diabetes in CP.

Major Criteria (All must be present)
Pancreatic exocrine deficiency (based on FE1 level < 200 ug/g or direct exocrine testing)
Abnormal pancreatic imaging (EUS, MRI, or CT)
Absence of anti-islet antibodies (to rule out T1DM)
Deficient PP response to oral nutrient challenge (to rule out T2DM)
Minor Criteria (Suggestive but non-specific)
Impaired beta cell function (by oral or intravenous GTT, HOMA-B*, or C-peptide/glucose ratio[51])
No excessive insulin resistance (by HOMA-IR[52])
Impaired Incretin secretion (e.g., GIP levels)
Low serum levels of lipid-soluble vitamins (e.g., A, D. E, K)

CP, chronic pancreatitis; FE1, fecal elastase-1; EUS, endoscopic ultrasound; MRI, magnetic resonance imaging; CT, computer-assisted tomography; T1DM, type 1 diabetes mellitus; T2DM, type 2 diabetes mellitus; GTT, glucose tolerance testing; HOMA-B, homeostasis model of assessment for beta cell function; HOMA-IR, homeostasis model of assessment for insulin resistance; GIP, glucose-dependent insulinotropic polypeptide.
Modified, and used with permission.[27]

Table 3. Diabetes surveillance of CP.

Hemoglobin A_{1C} level (HbA_{1C}) (normal < 5. 7%; impaired 5.7-6.5%)
Fasting plasma glucose (FPG) (normal < 100 mg/dL or 5.6 mmol/L; impaired 100-126 mg/dL or 5.6-7.0 mmol/L)
Oral glucose tolerance test* (OGTT) (normal 2 h plasma glucose level < 140 mg/dL or 7.8 mmol/L; impaired 140-200 mg/dL or 7.8-11.1 mmol/L)
Random plasma glucose** (normal <200 mg/dL or 11.1 mmol/L)

*75 g glucose ingested within 5 minutes.
Impaired values for HbA_{1C} or FPG indicate the need for OGTT testing.
Impaired values for OGTT indicate the need for repeat testing in 6 months.
Normal values indicate repeat testing in 3 years.
**Abnormal value sufficient for diagnosis of diabetes when accompanied by classic symptoms.
Used with permission.[26]

before (fasting) and at 30 and 60 minutes after ingestion are sufficient to detect a failure (less than 2-fold increase) in PP secretion.

Practical Importance of Differentiating T3cDM from T2DM

T3cDM differs from T2DM in having a high prevalence of metabolic bone disease and nutritional deficiencies, and an increased risk of pancreatic cancer. Pancreatic exocrine insufficiency is present in most patients with T3cDM, and frequently exists despite the absence of the classic symptom of steatorrhea. When T3cDM is diagnosed or suspected, it is appropriate to assess exocrine function in all patients. The most commonly used test is the fecal elastase 1 (FE1) level.[27] Levels of FE1 above 200 µg/g are considered normal, whereas levels below 100 µg/g indicate significant exocrine impairment.[32] Low FE1 levels or a history suggestive of exocrine insufficiency are indications for PERT.

Metabolic bone disease because of a loss of vitamin D absorption is common in patients with CP and T3cDM. Vitamin D supplements along with PERT are believed to be useful to reduce the risk of osteopenia and bone fractures,[22] and should be considered in all patients.

CP associated with diabetes carries a 12- to 33-fold increased risk of pancreatic cancer.[33–35] Therefore, all patients with T3cDM due to CP should be regularly evaluated for the presence of this malignancy. Indications of the presence of PDAC include unexplained weight loss or a sudden worsening of glycemic control in a patient with known diabetes. Surveillance studies might include CA19-9 levels, although this has not been shown to be a useful marker of early-stage (resectable) PDAC. No published criteria have yet been formalized for the screening of CP patients other than periodic pancreatic imaging. Although CT scanning is the most widely imaging technique, endoscopic ultrasound is more useful for the detection of early-stage disease. Patients with stable CP who suddenly develop diabetes are candidates for pancreatic imaging studies to rule out the possibility of PDAC.

Management of T3cDM

Screening for Diabetes

All patients with CP should be periodically evaluated for the presence or development of T3cDM.[26] Surveillance should include hemoglobin A_{1C} (Hgb A_{1C}) levels or fasting glucose levels as recommended by the ADA (**Table 3**). Values that are suspicious or nondiagnostic for diabetes should be followed by oral glucose tolerance testing (OGTT) to confirm the presence of diabetes. Repeat testing should be performed every 6 months if equivocal or nondiagnostic, or every 3 years if normal.[5] Differentiation of T3cDM from T2DM should include the criteria shown in Table 2 with the measurement of PP responsiveness to a liquid test meal, as described above.

PP deficiency may be the earliest indication of endocrine dysfunction in CP. Because PP-secreting cells are localized predominantly in the pancreatic head and uncinate process, inflammation localized to the pancreatic head may affect PP secretion before global beta cell failure results in hyperglycemia. PP deficiency is associated with impaired hepatic insulin sensitivity, but may not result in diabetes if sufficient residual islet function is present.[20]

Algorithm for Management of Hyperglycemia

The goal of therapy is to lower the HbA_{1C} level to less than 7%. No evidence-based recommendations are available to guide treatment specific to T3cDM. Therefore guidelines that pertain to the management of T2DM are usually followed.[36] Oral therapy beginning with metformin is recommended, although use of this drug may be problematic in patients with CP because of gastrointestinal irritability. A schedule of graduated increases in metformin dose has been recommended to lessen side effects (**Table 4**).

Table 4. Metformin graduated dose schedule.

1. Begin with low dose (500 mg) metformin taken once or twice a day (before breakfast and/or dinner) or 850 mg once a day (before breakfast).
2. After 5-7 days, if gastrointestinal side effects have not occurred, advance dose to 850-1,000 mg twice a day.
3. If gastrointestinal side effects appear as dose is increased, drop back to previous dose and wait an additional 2-4 weeks before increasing dose again.
4. Maximum effective dose is 1,000 mg twice a day, although dose increase to 2,500 mg/day may have greater effectiveness if gastrointestinal side effects do not intervene.
5. Generic metfomin is preferred because of cost considerations, but a longer-acting formulation available in some countries may allow once-a-day dosing. Metformin is contraindicated in patients with renal failure or when glomerular filtration rate falls to < 30 ml/min.

Modified, and used with permission.[36]

Periodic HbA_{1C} testing may be used to assess the effectiveness of therapy.

If metformin is not tolerated or is ineffective, additional or alternative medications include alpha glucosidase inhibitors (αGIs),[37] thiazolidinediones (TZDs),[38] and sodium-glucose cotransporter-2 inhibitors (SGLT2Is).[39] TZDs have been shown in one study to be effective in reversing the hepatic insulin resistance of T3cDM due to CP,[40] but SGLT2Is have been associated with euglycemic acidosis in insulin deficient patients[41] so they should be used with caution.

Insulin secretagogues and incretin-based therapy should be avoided or delayed when possible, because of the increased incidence of hypoglycemia associated with sulfonylurea therapy, and the suspected (but unconfirmed) risk of pancreatitis and pancreatic malignancy associated with incretin-based therapy. It is recommended that until studies of incretin-based therapy are found safe in patients with T3cDM, that these agents be avoided.[26] In CP patients with impaired glucagon secretion, the risk of hypoglycemia is increased. Metformin, TZDs, and αGIs have not been shown to increase the risk of hypoglycemia compared with other therapies.[42] Patients with a history of hypoglycemia might better be managed with a therapeutic goal of maintaining an HbA_{1C} level less than 8%.

When hyperglycemic crises occur, or when HbA_{1C} levels are persistently above 7%, insulin treatment is indicated for the management of T3cDM.[6] Patients with T3cDM frequently require low doses of insulin because of increased peripheral insulin sensitivity. A usual approach is to begin with 10 units of Lantus insulin once per day with subsequent assessment of HbA_{1C} levels and surveillance of hypoglycemia. Additional doses of insulin may be necessary; twice daily administration or greater. Patients with brittle diabetes may be better managed with a programmable insulin pump coupled with a continuous glucose monitor.

Importance of PERT

Pancreatic exocrine insufficiency is present in virtually all patients with T3cDM, and may not be accompanied by the classic symptom of steatorrhea[43], so PERT is recommended for consideration in all cases. Oral enzyme supplements vary in formulation and dosage, and their availability is affected by healthcare coverage and distribution issues. Therefore, multiple formulations of pancreatic enzyme supplements are potentially useful, with selection based on availability (**Table 5**).

In general, 90,000 USP units of enzyme are required for complete digestion and absorption of a normal meal. The amount of enzymes required by an individual patient will depend on residual endogenous exocrine function, and may be limited by side effects. It is recommended that therapy begin with a dose of 50,000-60,000 USP units, or 1,000 USP units of lipase/kg, per meal, taken in divided

Table 5. Pancreatic enzyme formulations.

Product formulation		Manufacturer	Lipase content (USP)/pill or capsule
Zenpep	Enteric-coated porcine capsule	Aptalis	3000, 5000, 10,000, 15,000, 20,000
Creon	Enteric-coated porcine capsule	Abbott/AbVie	3,000, 6,000, 12,000, 24,000
Pancreaze	Enteric-coated porcine capsule	Ortho-McNeil-Janssen	4,200, 10,500, 16,800, 21,000
Pertzye	Enteric-coated porcine plus bicarbonate capsule	Digestive Care	8,000, 16,000
Ultresa	Enteric-coated porcine capsule	Aptalis	13,800, 20,700, 23,000
Viokase	Non-enteric coated tablet	Aptalis	10,440, 20,880

Modified, and used with permission.[44]

doses before and after eating, with subsequent assessment of effectiveness and symptoms.[22] Pancreatic enzyme bioavailability is affected by acid inactivation of lipase, so an antacid medication is usually prescribed to improve efficacy.[44] Multivitamins or vitamin D supplements are also appropriate to consider in patients with T3cDM because of the high prevalence of metabolic bone disease in CP.

Role of Early Intervention in Delaying or Preventing Progressive Endocrine Failure

Progressive endocrine dysfunction is a sign of progressive pancreatic destruction caused by CP. Therefore, therapeutic interventions that halt or delay the continued inflammation may prevent or delay the development of T3cDM. These interventions may include therapeutic endoscopy or surgery to prevent persistent inflammation, in addition to abstinence from toxic agents (e.g., alcohol and nicotine) that are associated with recurrent attacks. The relief of obstructive pancreatopathy by surgical decompression has been shown to prevent or delay the progression of CP by more than 24 months.[45] However, the development and progression of subsequent T3cDM in the 5 years after resectional and hybrid surgical procedures have been found to be similar.[46] The risk of T3cDM after surgical procedures is less in the near-term post-operative period with hybrid procedures (e.g., Beger or Frey procedures) than with proximal pancreatectomy.[47]

Role of Total Pancreatectomy With Islet Auto-transplantation (TPIAT) in Preserving Endocrine Function in CP

The principal symptom that usually prompts treatment of CP is pain. Most patients with recurrent or chronic pain because of CP can be successfully managed with therapeutic endoscopic or surgical resection and/or decompressive approaches. A significant number of patients have persistent symptoms despite prior treatment, and/or are not considered appropriate candidates for decompressive or hybrid procedures. Many of these patients are disabled by their symptoms, and are usually dependent on opioid treatment for relief. For this subset of CP patients who still have endocrine function, an alternative consideration for management is TPIAT.

Total pancreatectomy (alone) is a potentially devastating procedure because of the risk of complete exocrine and endocrine insufficiency. Although such patients can be managed with meticulous attention to nutritional and glycemic homestasis, the requirements of this care are very high. In some patients with disabling symptoms, total pancreatectomy may be a feasible option if endocrine function can be preserved by autologous islet transplantation. TPIAT has been performed since 1977, when it was developed at the University of Minnesota.[48] Currently, there are 15 centers in the United States that offer TPIAT, with 150-200 procedures being performed each year. About 30% of TPIAT patients are insulin-independent 3 years after their procedure, 32% have partial islet function, and more than 85% report significant pain relief and an improved quality of life after recovery.[49] In recent years, TPIAT has been carried out in an increasing number of pediatric patients with hereditary or idiopathic CP, whose disease is often completely disabling. In children 5–12 years of age who have received TPIAT, 56% are insulin-independent and virtually all have returned to normal activities 1 year after the procedure.[50] In adolescent patients 13–19 years of age, 41% of patients are insulin-independent and 90% report relief of symptoms and a return to normal activities 3 years after the procedure.

Summary

Endocrine failure is a common complication of CP, and indicates severe or worsening disease. The development of T3cDM may be hastened by pancreatic resection or preexisting diminished pancreatic reserve. T3cDM is a result of the combined deficiency of insulin, glucagon, and PP, and is worsened by an impaired incretin effect, due to exocrine deficiency-related deficits in the secretion of GLP-1 and GIP. T3cDM is virtually always accompanied by exocrine insufficiency, which results in vitamin D deficiency and metabolic bone disease. Pancreatic enzyme replacement is therefore indicated in almost all cases. The management of T3cDM requires careful attention to the risks of hypoglycemia, and should begin with a trial of therapy with metformin. New onset T3cDM is an indication to consider the possible presence of pancreatic cancer as a cause. Reducing the risk of T3cDM through interventions which delay or prevent its occurrence are important considerations in the treatment of CP.

References

1. National Diabetes Data Group. Classification and diagnosis of diabetes mellitus and other categories of glucose intolerance. *Diabetes*. 1979; 28: 1039-1057. PMID: 510803.
2. Report of the Expert Committee on the Diagnosis and Classification of Diabetes Mellitus. *Diabetes Care*. 1997; 20: 1183-1197. PMID: 9203460.
3. Expert Committee on the Diagonsis and Classification of Diabetes Mellitus. Report of the expert committee on the diagnosis and classification of diabetes mellitus. *Diabetes Care*. 2003; 26(Suppl 1): S5-20. PMID: 12502614.
4. American Diabetes Association. Diagnosis and classification of diabetes mellitus. *Diabetes Care*. 2014; 37(Suppl 1): S81-90. PMID: 24357215.

5. American Diabetes Association. (2) Classification and diagnosis of diabetes. *Diabetes Care*. 2015; 38(Suppl1): S8-S16. PMID: 25537714.
6. Cui Y and Andersen DK. Pancreatogenic diabetes: special considerations for management. *Pancreatology*. 2011; 11: 279-294. PMID: 21757968.
7. Javeed N, Sagar G, Dutta SK, Smyrk TC, Lau JS, Bhattacharya S, et al. Pancreatic cancer-derived exosomes cause paraneoplastic beta-cell dysfunction. *Clin Cancer Res*. 2015; 21: 1722-1733. PMID: 25355928.
8. Cersosimo E, Pisters PW, Pesola G, McDermott K, Bajorunas D, and Brennan MF. Insulin secretion and action in patients with pancreatic cancer. *Cancer*. 1991; 67: 486-493. PMID: 1985741.
9. Hart PA, Baichoo E, Bi Y, Hinton A, Kudva YC, and Chari ST. Pancreatic polypeptide response to a mixed meal is blunted in pancreatic head cancer associated with diabetes mellitus. *Pancreatology*. 2015; 15: 162-166. PMID: 25766398.
10. Kien CL, Horswill CA, Zipf WB, McCoy KS, and O'Dorisio T. Elevated hepatic glucose production in children with cystic fibrosis. *Pediatr Res*. 1995; 37: 600-605. PMID: 7603777.
11. Adrian TE, McKiernan J, Johnstone DI, Hiller EJ, Vyas H, Sarson DL, et al. Hormonal abnormalities of the pancreas and gut in cystic fibrosis. *Gastroenterology*. 1980; 79: 460-465. PMID: 7000612.
12. Hardt PD, Brendel MD, Kloer HU, and Bretzel RG. Is pancreatic diabetes (type 3c diabetes) underdiagnosed and misdiagnosed? *Diabetes Care*. 2008; 31(Suppl 2): S165-169. PMID: 18227480.
13. Ewald N, Kaufmann C, Raspe A, Kloer HU, Bretzel RG, and Hardt PD. Prevalence of diabetes mellitus secondary to pancreatic diseases (type 3c). *Diabetes Metab Res Rev*. 2012; 28: 338-342. PMID: 22121010.
14. Nyboe Andersen B, Krarup T, Thorsgaard Pedersen NT, Faber OK, Hagen C, and Worning H. B cell function in patients with chronic pancreatitis and its relation to exocrine pancreatic function. *Diabetologia*. 1982; 23: 86-89. PMID: 6182047.
15. Bank S. Chronic pancreatitis: clinical features and medical management. *Am J Gastroenterol*. 1986; 81: 153-167. PMID: 3513542.
16. Malka D, Hammel P, Sauvanet A, Rufat P, O'Toole D, Bardet P, et al. Risk factors for diabetes mellitus in chronic pancreatitis. *Gastroenterology*. 2000; 119: 1324-1332. PMID: 11054391.
17. Couet C, Genton P, Pointel JP, Louis J, Gross P, Saudax E, et al. The prevalence of retinopathy is similar in diabetes mellitus secondary to chronic pancreatitis with or without pancreatectomy and in idiopathic diabetes mellitus. *Diabetes Care*. 1985; 8: 323-328. PMID: 4042797.
18. Gall FP, Muhe E, and Gebhardt C. Results of partial and total pancreaticoduodenectomy in 117 patients with chronic pancreatitis. *World J Surg*. 1981; 5: 269-275. PMID: 7245796.
19. Sun YS, Brunicardi FC, Druck P, Walfisch S, Berlin SA, Chance RE, et al. Reversal of abnormal glucose metabolism in chronic pancreatitis by administration of pancreatic polypeptide. *Am J Surg*. 1986; 151: 130-140. PMID: 3946744.
20. Seymour NE, Brunicardi FC, Chaiken RL, Lebovitz HE, Chance RE, Gingerich RL, et al. Reversal of abnormal glucose production after pancreatic resection by pancreatic polypeptide administration in man. *Surgery*. 1988; 104: 119-129. PMID: 3041640.
21. Brunicardi FC, Chaiken RL, Ryan AS, Seymour NE, Hoffmann JA, Lebovitz HE, et al. Pancreatic polypeptide administration improves abnormal glucose metabolism in patients with chronic pancreatitis. *J Clin Endocrinol Metab*. 1996; 81: 3566-3572. PMID: 8855802.
22. Afghani E, Sinha A, and Singh VK. An overview of the diagnosis and management of nutrition in chronic pancreatitis. *Nutr Clin Pract*. 2014; 29: 295-311. PMID: 24743046.
23. Tignor AS, Wu BU, Whitlock TL, Lopez R, Repas K, Banks PA, et al. High prevalence of low-trauma fracture in chronic pancreatitis. *Am J Gastroenterol*. 2010; 105: 2680-2686. PMID: 20736937.
24. Ebert R and Creutzfeldt W. Reversal of impaired GIP and insulin secretion in patients with pancreatogenic steatorrhea following enzyme substitution. *Diabetologia*. 1980; 19: 198-204. PMID: 6997121.
25. Knop FK, Vilsboll T, Larsen S, Hojberg PV, Volund A, Madsbad S, et al. Increased postprandial responses of GLP-1 and GIP in patients with chronic pancreatitis and steatorrhea following pancreatic enzyme substitution. *Am J Physiol Endocrinol Metab*. 2007; 292: E324-330. PMID: 16954337.
26. Rickels MR, Bellin M, Toledo FG, Robertson RP, Andersen DK, Chari ST, et al. Detection, evaluation and treatment of diabetes mellitus in chronic pancreatitis: recommendations from PancreasFest 2012. *Pancreatology*. 2013; 13: 336-342. PMID: 23890130.
27. Ewald N and Bretzel RG. Diabetes mellitus secondary to pancreatic diseases (Type 3c)–are we neglecting an important disease? *Eur J Intern Med*. 2013; 24: 203-206. PMID: 23375619.
28. Glaser B, Zoghlin G, Pienta K, and Vinik AI. Pancreatic polypeptide response to secretin in obesity: effects of glucose intolerance. *Horm Metab Res*. 1988; 20: 288-292. PMID: 3042579.
29. Chia CW, Odetunde JO, Kim W, Carlson OD, Ferrucci L, and Egan JM. GIP contributes to islet trihormonal abnormalities in type 2 diabetes. *J Clin Endocrinol Metab*. 2014; 99: 2477-2485. PMID: 24712564.
30. Lonovics J, Guzman S, Devitt P, Hejtmancik KE, Suddith RL, Rayford PL, et al. Release of pancreatic polypeptide in humans by infusion of cholecystokinin. *Gastroenterology*. 1980; 79: 817-822. PMID: 7419006.
31. Amland PF, Jorde R, Aanderud S, Burhol PG, and Giercksky KE. Effects of intravenously infused porcine GIP on serum insulin, plasma C-peptide, and pancreatic polypeptide in non-insulin-dependent diabetes in the fasting state. *Scand J Gastroenterol*. 1985; 20: 315-320. PMID: 3890139.
32. Loser C, Mollgaard A, and Folsch UR. Faecal elastase 1: a novel, highly sensitive, and specific tubeless pancreatic function test. *Gut*. 1996; 39: 580-586. PMID: 8944569.
33. Maisonneuve P, Lowenfels AB, Bueno-de-Mesquita HB, Ghadirian P, Baghurst PA, Zatonski WA, et al. Past medical history and pancreatic cancer risk: Results from a multicenter

case-control study. *Ann Epidemiol.* 2010; 20: 92-98. PMID: 20123159.

34. Liao KF, Lai SW, Li CI, and Chen WC. Diabetes mellitus correlates with increased risk of pancreatic cancer: a population-based cohort study in Taiwan. *J Gastroenterol Hepatol.* 2012; 27: 709-713. PMID: 21929650.
35. Brodovicz KG, Kou TD, Alexander CM, O'Neill EA, Engel SS, Girman CJ, et al. Impact of diabetes duration and chronic pancreatitis on the association between type 2 diabetes and pancreatic cancer risk. *Diabetes Obes Metab.* 2012; 14: 1123-1128. PMID: 22831166.
36. Nathan DM, Buse JB, Davidson MB, Ferrannini E, Holman RR, Sherwin R, et al. Medical management of hyperglycemia in type 2 diabetes: a consensus algorithm for the initiation and adjustment of therapy: a consensus statement of the American Diabetes Association and the European Association for the Study of Diabetes. *Diabetes Care.* 2009; 32: 193-203. PMID: 18945920.
37. Riccardi G, Giacco R, Parillo M, Turco S, Rivellese AA, Ventura MR, et al. Efficacy and safety of acarbose in the treatment of Type 1 diabetes mellitus: a placebo-controlled, double-blind, multicentre study. *Diabet Med.* 1999; 16: 228-232. PMID: 10227568.
38. Garber AJ, Abrahamson MJ, Barzilay JI, Blonde L, Bloomgarden ZT, Bush MA, et al. AACE comprehensive diabetes management algorithm 2013. *Endocr Pract.* 2013; 19: 327-336. PMID: 23598536.
39. Nair S and Wilding JP. Sodium glucose cotransporter 2 inhibitors as a new treatment for diabetes mellitus. *J Clin Endocrinol Metab.* 2010; 95: 34-42. PMID: 19892839.
40. Zhou X and You S. Rosiglitazone inhibits hepatic insulin resistance induced by chronic pancreatitis and IKK-beta/NF-kappaB expression in liver. *Pancreas* 2014; 43(8): 1291-1298. PMID: 25036911.
41. Hine J, Paterson H, Abrol E, Russell-Jones D, and Herring R. SGLT inhibition and euglycaemic diabetic ketoacidosis. *Lancet Diabetes Endocrinol.* 2015; 3: 503-504. PMID: 26025388.
42. Anderson M, Powell J, Campbell KM, and Taylor JR. Optimal management of type 2 diabetes in patients with increased risk of hypoglycemia. *Diabetes Metab Syndr Obes.* 2014; 7: 85-94. PMID: 24623984.
43. Hardt PD, Hauenschild A, Nalop J, Marzeion AM, Jaeger C, Teichmann J, et al. High prevalence of exocrine pancreatic insufficiency in diabetes mellitus. A multicenter study screening fecal elastase 1 concentrations in 1,021 diabetic patients. *Pancreatology.* 2003; 3: 395-402. PMID: 14526149.
44. Forsmark CE. Management of chronic pancreatitis. *Gastroenterology.* 2013; 144: 1282-1291 e1283. PMID: 23622138.
45. Nealon WH and Thompson JC. Progressive loss of pancreatic function in chronic pancreatitis is delayed by main pancreatic duct decompression. A longitudinal prospective analysis of the modified puestow procedure. *Ann Surg.* 1993; 217: 458-466; discussion 466-458. PMID: 8489308.
46. Strate T, Bachmann K, Busch P, Mann O, Schneider C, Bruhn JP, et al. Resection vs drainage in treatment of chronic pancreatitis: long-term results of a randomized trial. *Gastroenterology.* 2008; 134: 1406-1411. PMID: 18471517.
47. Andersen DK and Frey CF. The evolution of the surgical treatment of chronic pancreatitis. *Ann Surg.* 2010; 251: 18-32. PMID: 20009754.
48. Najarian JS, Sutherland DE, Baumgartner D, Burke B, Rynasiewicz JJ, Matas AJ, et al. Total or near total pancreatectomy and islet autotransplantation for treatment of chronic pancreatitis. *Ann Surg.* 1980; 192: 526-542. PMID: 6775603.
49. Sutherland DE, Radosevich DM, Bellin MD, Hering BJ, Beilman GJ, Dunn TB, et al. Total pancreatectomy and islet autotransplantation for chronic pancreatitis. *J Am Coll Surg.* 2012; 214: 409-424; discussion 424-406. PMID: 22397977.
50. Chinnakotla S, Bellin MD, Schwarzenberg SJ, Radosevich DM, Cook M, Dunn TB, et al. Total pancreatectomy and islet autotransplantation in children for chronic pancreatitis: indication, surgical techniques, postoperative management, and long-term outcomes. *Ann Surg.* 2014; 260: 56-64. PMID: 24509206.
51. Matthews DR, Hosker JP, Rudenski AS, Naylor BA, Treacher DF, and Turner RC. Homeostasis model assessment: insulin resistance and beta-cell function from fasting plasma glucose and insulin concentrations in man. *Diabetologia.* 1985; 28: 412-419. PMID: 3899825.
52. Meier JJ, Menge BA, Breuer TG, Muller CA, Tannapfel A, Uhl W, et al. Functional assessment of pancreatic beta-cell area in humans. *Diabetes.* 2009; 58: 1595-1603. PMID: 19509022.

Chapter 50

Interventional and endoscopic therapy of chronic pancreatitis

Julia Mayerle[1*], Rupjyoti Talukdar[2,3], Georg Beyer[1], and D. Nageshwar Reddy[2]

[1]*Department of Medicine A, University Medicine, Ernst-Moritz-Arndt University, Greifswald, Germany;*
[2]*Asian Institute of Gastroenterology;*
[3]*Asian Healthcare Foundation, Hyderabad, India.*

Introduction

Chronic pancreatitis is a debilitating disease with high socio-economic relevance; it accounts for an increasing number of hospital admissions, on average 16 to 20 days in hospital per year, with 34% of patients constantly taking pain medication, 57% requiring enzyme supplementation, and 29% with diabetes mellitus. One-third of all patients suffering from chronic pancreatitis can no longer work in their original profession. The number of unemployed patients with chronic pancreatitis due to prolonged stays in hospital or continued alcohol abuse is as high as 40%. Continued alcohol abuse, smoking, and liver cirrhosis carry hazard ratios of 1.6, 1.4, and 2.5, respectively, and negatively affect chronic pancreatitis prognosis. Belt-like upper abdominal pain is regarded as a cardinal symptom of chronic pancreatitis, together with weight loss, steatorrhea, and diabetes mellitus. An estimated 30%-60% of patients develop disease complications such as strictures of the common bile duct (CBD), inflammatory space-occupying masses, pancreatic pseudocysts, or pancreatic ductal stones, which require interventional or surgical treatment. In the absence of causal therapeutic options, treatment is restricted to symptom control by means of pain therapy, enzyme replacement, treatment of jaundice, strictures, fluid collection, and optimal control of endocrine insufficiency. We will discuss the indications and options for treatment. The evidence presented is graded according to the Oxford grading system (www.cebm.net) as displayed in **Table 1**.

Indication for endoscopic therapy

Interventional or surgical treatment should be undertaken for long-lasting severe pain requiring analgesics [Evidence 2b]. Severe pain can be effectively treated by both endoscopic as well as surgical procedures [Evidence 2b/3b], depending on the pathogenic cause.[1] Surgical procedures (drainage) are superior to endoscopic procedures with regard to long-term pain reduction; they are, however, associated with higher mortality but lower morbidity. There are several level of evidence grade 2b or 3a studies dealing with the treatment of chronic pancreatitis pain by endoscopy, extracorporeal shockwave lithotripsy (ESWL), thoracoscopic splanchnicectomy, surgical resection, and draining procedures. A direct comparison between surgery and endoscopy was carried out in only two level of evidence grade 1b studies.[2-4] Both demonstrated a long-term advantage for the surgical procedure.

If a resectable pancreatic carcinoma is suspected, then surgery should be performed. [Evidence 2b]. If a space-occupying lesion of the pancreas is present and suspected (resectable) pancreatic carcinoma cannot be excluded, then surgical resection should be performed. Without surgery, life expectancy for patients with pancreatic carcinoma is less than 1 year; after successful resection it may be more than 5 years in 20%-25%. [Evidence 1a].[5-7]

Surgical or interventional treatment should be carried out for persistent clinical symptoms of gastric outlet obstruction or duodenal stenosis secondary to chronic pancreatitis. Unfortunately, there are no comparative studies available to answer whether resection surgery, bypass surgery, and/or endoscopic insertion of self-expanding metal stents are superior.[8] The natural course of chronic pancreatitis predicts that between 30% and 60% of all patients will require intervention. In at least 30% of cases, conservative management supplemented by endoscopic therapeutic interventions appears to be sufficient for an adequate quality of life. CBD stenosis will develop in 10%-40% of cases, requiring intervention. In the presence of an inflammatory tumor of the pancreatic head, primary endoscopy for bile duct obstruction with stent insertion into the bile duct should be performed followed by duct dilatation. However, if symptoms or cholestasis persist after temporary endoscopic therapy, surgical resection should be performed [Evidence 2b]. A retrospective analysis of all

*Corresponding author current address is Department of Medicine 2, University of Munich. Email: julia.mayerle@med.uni-muenchen.de

Table 1. Oxford grading system for level of evidence

Level of evidence grade	Description
1a	"Evidence" from a systematic review of randomized controlled trials (RCTs)
1b	"Evidence" from suitably planned RCTs
1c	All-or-none principle studies
2a	"Evidence" from a systematic review of well-planned cohort studies
2b	"Evidence" from a well-planned cohort study/low-quality RCT [e.g., <80% follow-up)
2c	"Evidence" from outcome research studies
3a	"Evidence" from a systematic review of well-planned case-control studies
3b	"Evidence" from an individual case-control study
4	"Evidence" from case series/poor-quality cohort and moderate case-control studies
5	Expert opinion without explicit critical appraisal, or based on physiology, bench research, or "first principles"

patients treated with an average observation period of 45 months revealed that stent therapy for bile duct obstruction due to chronic pancreatitis does not produce effects beyond 1 year.[9] A prospective study showed a clearly poorer long-term effect of stent management of distal bile duct obstruction if calcifications were associated with chronic pancreatitis.[10,11] A clinical example of a patient with calcifying chronic pancreatitis in the head of the pancreas and subsequent bile duct obstruction that was managed by temporary stent insertion is shown in **Figure 1 A-C**.

A further complication is the development of stenosis of the pancreatic duct **(Figure 1 D-F)**. The indication for the insertion of an endoprosthesis (stent) has not been fully clarified. Just one prospective controlled study has demonstrated a positive effect of stent drainage of a dominant stenosis in the duct of Wirsung. Some studies suggest that the insertion of a stent into the pancreatic duct can induce secondary changes due to the stent with subsequent fibrosis and stricture.[12,13] However, removal of the main pancreatic duct (MPD) obstruction is often effective for pain management in shorter terms, with reported success rates between 37% and 94%.[14] Metabolic side effects of stenting the pancreatic duct over a longer period have not been reported.

A further endoscopic/interventional procedure for treating chronic pancreatitis is extracorporeal shock wave lithotripsy (ESWL) for pancreatic duct stones. Before its introduction in 1989, surgery was often the only option for removing pancreatic duct stones that could not be removed endoscopically. Several retrospective studies have addressed the question of the clinical benefit of ESWL for pancreatic duct stones.

In the following sections, we will discuss the benefits and drawbacks of interventional endoscopic options in more detail. For further reading see Lee & Conwell.[15]

Endoscopic therapy for pseudocysts

The prevalence of pancreatic pseudocysts in chronic pancreatitis is between 20% and 40%.[16] They occur most often in patients with alcoholic chronic pancreatitis (70%-78%).[17] The second most common cause is idiopathic chronic pancreatitis (6%-16%), followed by biliary pancreatitis (6%-8%).[16] Within the first 6 weeks after an acute bout of pancreatitis, 40% of the pseudocysts resolve spontaneously, while in 20% complications such as infection, obstruction of adjacent organs, cystic rupture, or persistent pancreatitis necessitate intervention. Spontaneous remission of pseudocysts after 12 weeks is very rare, and complications are observed in up to two-thirds of such cases. The increase in pseudocyst size to >5 cm in diameter is associated with an increased risk of complications. Patients with pseudocysts that have resulted in complications such as gastric outlet obstruction, hemorrhage, pain, cholestasis, or vascular stenosis should undergo endoscopic or surgical treatment regardless of size [Evidence 2a]. The surgical procedures to treat pseudocysts tend to have higher success rates but a somewhat higher mortality rate than endoscopic pseudocyst drainage into either the duodenum or more usually the stomach. The decisions regarding on whom, when, and by which procedure pancreatic pseudocysts should be treated has been very controversial. Either surgery or percutaneous or endoscopic drainage can be performed for symptomatic pseudocysts.

The literature on interventional therapy of pancreatic pseudocysts as a form of pain management is very limited. Most data are based on retrospective case series,[18-23] but there are three systematic reviews.[24-28] Pain relief will be achieved in a large number of patients either by surgical, endoscopic, or percutaneous drainage techniques. Given that a high rate of pain relief was achieved in these retrospective series (about 80%), all three systematic reviews conclude that although conservative management of chronic pancreatitis also results in pain relief, percutaneous, endoscopic, or surgical drainage is still the more effective form of pain management in a certain percentage of patients. It is not possible to identify significant differences in the comparison of the three procedures from the

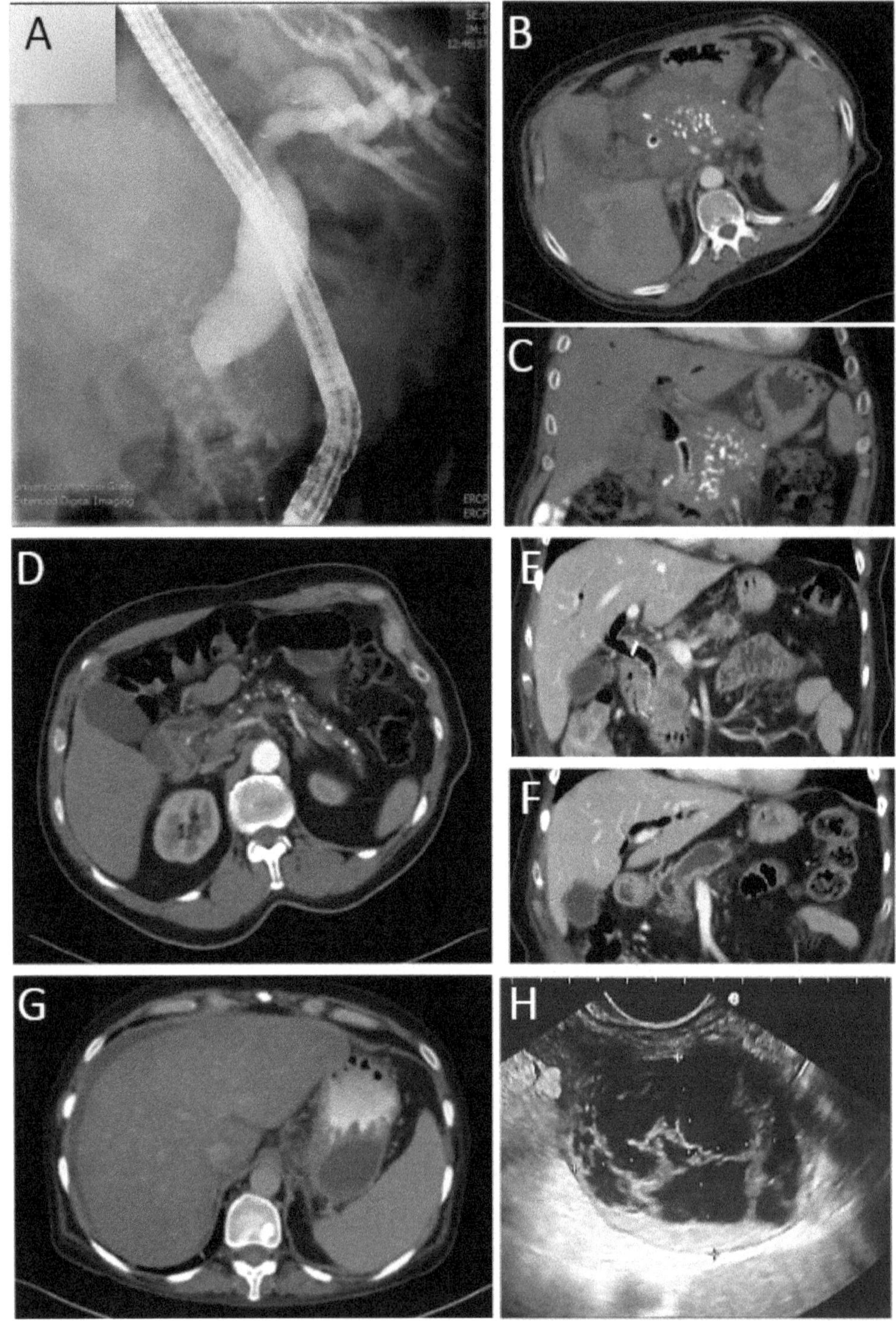

Figure 1. Complications of chronic pancreatitis that could warrant endotherapy are stenosis of the CBD, stricture and subsequent upstream dilatation of the pancreatic duct, and pancreatic pseudocysts. A) ERC image of a patient with alcoholic calcifying groove pancreatitis and initial endoscopic therapy for cholangitis and jaundice. The patient was known to be a heavy smoker **B)** Unenhanced computed tomography (CT) scan showing an enlarged pancreatic head and calcifications. **C)** Sagittal view with a fully covered self-expandable metal stent (FCSEM) in the same patient **D)** Atrophic pancreas in a patient with alcoholic chronic pancreatitis and dilated pancreatic duct, as well as calcifications. **E and F**) Patient with idiopathic chronic pancreatitis due to a chymotrypsin C mutation, jaundice, FCSEM and grossly dilated and atrophic pancreatic duct, no calcification. **G)** CT scan with oral contrast media of a 45-year-old female patient depicting a cystic lesion in the tail of the pancreas. **H)** EUS picture of the same patient illustrating the differential diagnosis between a mucinous cystic neoplasm and pancreatic pseudocyst in the absence of EUS-guided FNA for cyst fluid analysis. EUS FNA revealed grossly elevated lipase levels, while carcinoembryonic antigen level was normal, suggesting the lesion to be pancreatic pseudocyst.

published data. In cases of obstruction of the bile or pancreatic duct by pancreatic pseudocysts, they should be treated. When cholestasis does not improve after pseudocyst drainage alone, stent placement into the bile duct or resection may be indicated.

Further complications that render endoscopic or surgical treatment of the pseudocyst necessary include compression of large abdominal vessels, clinically relevant gastric outlet obstruction or duodenal stenosis, infection of the pseudocyst, and pancreatico-pleural fistula formation. Nausea and vomiting are common symptoms of pancreatic pseudocysts. Endoscopic interventional therapy of a hemorrhagic pseudocyst is associated with a high risk of bleeding. Thus, these pseudocysts should be treated surgically.

Initial therapy for symptomatic pancreatic pseudocysts can be endoscopic drainage of the pseudocyst followed by surgery should the pseudocyst recur [Evidence 3a]. The choice between endoscopic and operative pseudocyst drainage should be decided based on the cyst location and type of additional pathomorphological changes [Evidence 3b]. Endoscopic procedures for draining a pancreatic pseudocyst are less prone to complications than surgical procedures. However, not all pseudocysts are successfully treated by endoscopic drainage alone in the long term. Studies comparing endoscopy with surgery are not available. An interdisciplinary therapeutic concept is intended (**Table 2**).[29]

Asymptomatic pancreatic pseudocysts that have reached a size >5 cm in diameter and do not resolve within 6 weeks can be treated [Evidence 2a]. Pancreatic pseudocysts that show a fibrous wall >5 mm on imaging are particularly suited for endoscopic or surgical drainage. In a multivariate analysis a pseudocyst size <4 cm in diameter was the only favorable factor for spontaneous resolution.[30] Untreated cysts >5 cm may have a higher risk of complications such as rupture, infection, jaundice, or hemorrhage.[31]

Drainage of pseudocysts can be carried out by transgastric, transduodenal, or transpapillary approaches.[29,32] Percutaneous drainage is also possible but is associated with the risk of external fistula formation [Evidence 4].

Table 2. Summary of endoscopic pseudocyst/walled-off pancreatic necrosis drainage

	Number of patients	Success rate	Complete cyst drainage	Recurrence rate	Complications
Kozarek et al., 1985[75]	4	2 (50%)	2 (50%)	0 (0%)	1 (25%) dead
Cremer et al., 1989[76]	33	28 (85%)	30 (91%)	4 (12%)	3 (9%)
Sahel et al., 1991[77]	37	31 (86%)	36 (97%)	2 (5%)	5 (14%)
Kozarek et al., 1991[46]	14	11 (79%)	n.a.	2 (14%)	3 (21%)
Bejanin et al., 1993[78]	26	19 (73%)	n.a.	4 (15%)	4 (15%)
Funnel et al., 1994[79]	5	5 (100%)	5 (100%)	0 (0%)	0 (0%)
Deviere et al., 1995[80]	12	10 (87%)	10 (87%)	0 (0%)	0 (0%)
Vitale et al., 1999[81]	36	31 (86%)	31 (86%)	5 (14%)	1 (3%)
White et al., 2000[82]	20	20 (100%)	20 (100%)	0 (0%)	2 (10%)
Giovannini et al., 2001[83]	15	15 (100%)	15 (100%)	0 (0%)	1 (6.6%)
Libera et al., 2000[84]	25	21 (84%)	20 (80%)	1 (4%)	6 (28%)
Norton et al., 2001[85]	17	14 (82.4%)	13 (76.5%)	1 (7.1%)	3 (17.6%)
Sharma et al., 2002[86]	38	37 (97%)	37 (97%)	7 (16%)	5 (13%)
Binmoeller et al., 1995[47,87,88]	53	43 (81%)	47 (89%)	11 (23%)	6 (11%)
Smits et al., 1995[89]	37	24 (65%)	24 (65%)	3 (12.5%)	6 (16%)
Barthet et al., 1995[37]	30	23 (77%)	26 (87%)	3 (11.5%)	4 (13%)
Baron et al., 2002[90]	64	52 (81%)	59 (92%)	7 (12%)	11 (17%)
Catalano et al., 1995[91]	21	16 (76%)	17 (81%)	1 (6%)	1 (5%)
Antillon et al., 2006[92]	33	31 (94%)	24 (82%)	1 (3%)	2 (6%)
Hookey et al., 2006[93]	116	102 (87.9%)	108 (93.1%)	19 (16.4%)	13 (11%) 6 (5.2%) dead
Kruger et al., 2006[94]	35	33 (94%)	30 (88%)	4 (12%)	0 (0%)
Weckman et al., 2006[95]	165	142 (86.1%)	142 (86.1%)	8 (5.3%)	16 (10%)
Kahaleh et al., 2006[96]	99	93 (94%)	n.a.	n.a.	19 (19%)
Cahen et al., 2005[97]	92	89 (97%)	79 (86%)	4 (5%)	31 (35%) 1 (1%) dead
Varadarajul et al., 2011[98]	154	154 (100%)	144 (93.5%)	1 (1.5%)	8 (5.2%)
Will et al., 2012[99]	32	31 (97%)	k.A.	5 (15.4%)	3 (9.6%)
Total	**1,213**	**1,077 (88.8%)**	**919 (70%)**	**93 (7.7%)**	**161 (13.3%)**

One should select the access route for endoscopic transmural drainage of pseudocysts by endoscopic ultrasound (EUS) assessment. It depends on the size, vessels in the vicinity, and location of the pseudocyst. There are no comparative studies showing superiority of the endoscopic access route, either through the stomach or duodenal wall. Transcutaneous drainage carries the risk of persistent cutaneous fistula formation. Furthermore, an existing transcutaneous drain can adversely affect patient quality of life. Thus, endoscopic transmural drainage is preferred.[29]

Transmural drainage should be done under EUS guidance [Evidence 3]. This procedure can best assess the appearance of the pseudocyst wall, content, location and relationship to adjacent blood vessels. EUS guidance will possibly reduce the rate of failed puncture attempts and complications.[29,32] A direct comparison of the complication rate for transmural needle drainage without ultrasound guidance is not available. The success rate in 1,213 published patients with transmural drainage of a pancreatic pseudocyst was 82.2% (**Table 2**), with more recent studies reporting success rates significantly over 85%. These results are comparable with surgery. The mortality rate in larger case series involving over 30 patients was 0.2%. The recurrence and complication rates are reported to be around 8.5% and 14.4%, respectively.[33] **Figure 2** illustrates a case of a pancreatic pseudocyst in the tail of the pancreas due to pancreatic duct leak, which was managed by using a modern fully covered self-expandable metal stent (FCSEM)

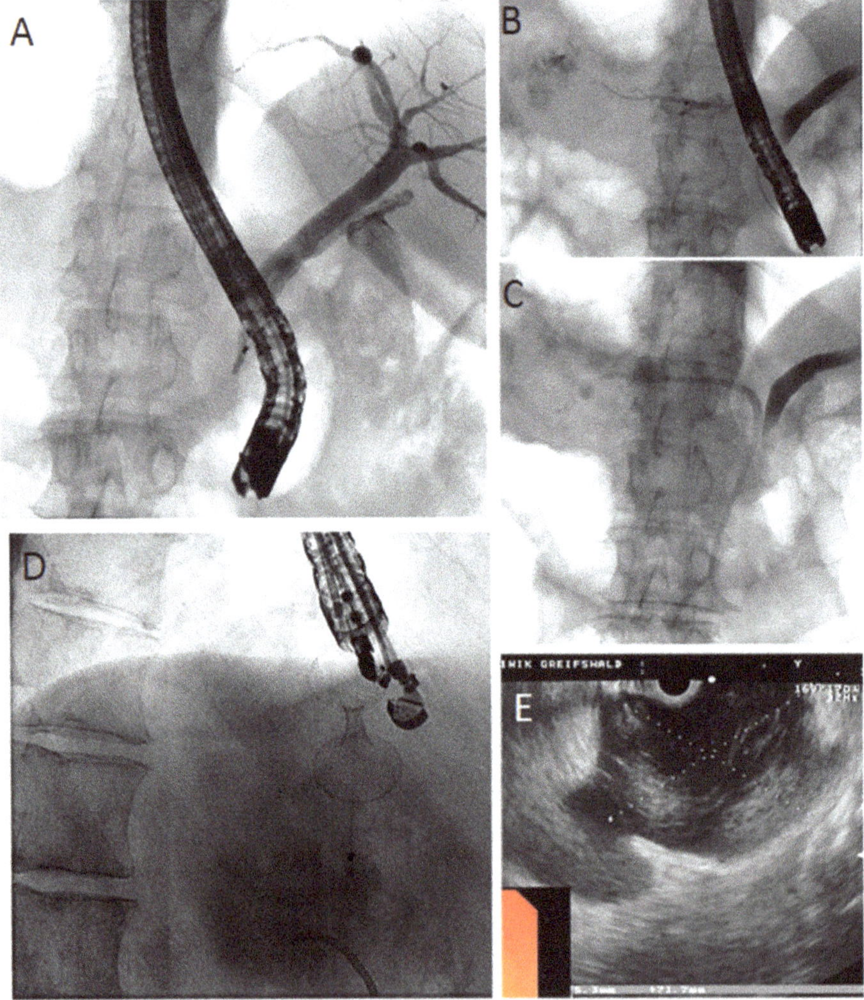

Figure 2. Endoscopic management of pancreatic fluid collection by a combined approach. A) ERC picture of a patient with recurrent acute pancreatitis due to alcohol abuse and a walled-off pancreatic necrosis (WOPN) in the tail of the pancreas. ERC shows a normal cholangiogram and tailored distal CBD in the absence of cholestasis. **B)** ERP with distal leak of the MPD classified as Cambridge IV. **C)** Treatment with a 15-cm 8.5-Fr stent reaching the leak. **D)** Radiograph of the subsequent EUS-guided drainage of the collection in the tail employing a hot AXIOS stent. **E)** EUS picture of the WOPN in the tail of the pancreas before drainage with a lumen opposing stent (hot AXIOS, Boston Scientific®).

system mounted on an electrocautery-enhanced delivery system in addition to conventional pancreatic duct stenting.

Diagnostic needle aspiration of the cyst may be performed for suspected infection or neoplasm [Evidence 4]. If diagnostic needle aspiration of the cyst confirms an infection of the content, then drainage is indicated. Surgical treatment should be carried out if malignancy is suspected. Diagnostic needle aspiration of a pseudocyst with the aid of EUS helps differentiate between mucinous cystic tumors and pseudocysts, as those entities might be difficult to distinguish on modes of imaging alone (**Figure 1 G, H**). When EUS-guided needle aspiration of a cyst reveals a carcinoembryonic antigen level >400 ng/mL, variably increased or low amylase or lipase, high viscosity, mucin, or epithelial cells in the cyst contents, then the presence of a mucinous neoplasm must be assumed.[34-36] If a connection to the pancreatic duct is excluded, the final diagnosis of a mucinous cystic neoplasm can be made.

Visualization of the pancreatic ducts can be performed before endoscopic or surgical drainage of a pseudocyst [Evidence 3b]. Whether endoscopic retrograde cholangiopancreatography (ERCP) with the attempt of draining the pseudocyst via the papilla should be performed instead of a primarily transgastric or transduodenal drainage is still a matter of controversy. On one hand, drainage of the pseudocyst via a stent in the pancreatic duct is the "most physiological" form of drainage. According to one study, 22%-57% of pancreatic pseudocysts have a connection with the pancreatic ductal system.[21] Thus, an ERP can precede endoscopic transmural drainage to detect a connection with the duct or exclude a rupture of pancreatic ducts (8% after acute necrotizing pancreatitis). Transmural drainage in the presence of an undetected rupture of the pancreatic duct or a connection of the pancreatic pseudocyst with an obstructed pancreatic duct is less promising with regard to long-term therapeutic outcome. On the other hand, the success rate of an attempted transpapillary drainage is usually <60%. Furthermore, these attempts impose a risk of ERCP-induced pancreatitis. Direct transgastric or transduodenal cyst drainage is very effective and usually associated with few complications.[29] The procedure-related incidence of infection of a pseudocyst and the risk of development of a pancreatic abscess increase without antibiotic prophylaxis.[37] In patients with advanced pancreatic duct changes, especially pancreatolithiasis, any pseudocyst treatment should be part of a general therapeutic concept [Evidence 2b]. A relative indication to treat pseudocysts is the presence of chronic pancreatitis with respective pancreatic duct anomalies or pancreatic ductal stones because in these cases, the rate of spontaneous regressions, even of small cysts, is at most 10%-26% due to constant inflammatory irritation.[30] Treatment of pancreatic duct obstruction can be undertaken in patients with a pancreatic pseudocyst, prestenotic duct dilatation, or fistula formation [Evidence 4]. Pancreatic pseudocysts are maintained by pancreatic duct obstruction in the presence of prestenotic duct dilatations or fistulae if these stenoses are responsible for a blockade of drainage. Removal of the pancreatic duct obstruction is recommended in these cases.

Therapy of pancreatic duct stenosis and ductal stones

In patients with chronic pancreatitis, the pressure in the pancreatic duct is initially increased, regardless of the etiology or whether dilation of the duct of Wirsung is seen.[38] An important role in the pathogenesis of pain is ascribed to ductal and interstitial hypertension and possible relative pancreatic ischemia. The aim of endoscopic and surgical decompression therapy in patients with chronic pancreatitis and pain and/or clinical episodes of acute pancreatitis is to remove the obstruction preventing outflow of exocrine pancreatic juices. Techniques such as sphincterotomy, dilatation, ESWL, and stent insertion have been modified for the pancreatic duct. Endoscopic decompression of the duct can precede a surgical procedure to predict whether surgical decompression of the pancreatic duct might alleviate pain or reduce acute bouts of chronic pancreatitis. Endoscopy represents an alternative to surgery and is associated with low morbidity and mortality. Endoscopic interventions do not interfere with surgery that might still be necessary later in the disease course. Furthermore, clinical success after endoscopic reduction of the intraductal pressure does provide some indication of the ultimate result of surgical drainage or a resection procedure.

Pancreatic ductal stones may cause pain by obstructing pancreatic juice outflow, inducing recurrent exacerbations, maintaining a pseudocyst or fistula, or causing other complications. Stones can be treated by endoscopic or surgical means [Evidence 4]. Pancreatic ductal stones are the result not the cause of chronic pancreatitis; however, they can lead to consecutive obstruction of the outflow of pancreatic secretions in the duct and duodenum and thus cause pseudocyst or fistula development. They can also cause recurrent exacerbations or contribute to the pathogenesis of pain. Under these conditions, treatment of pancreatic ductal stones appears appropriate, but no available studies have compared the treatment of pancreatic ductal stones with a sham intervention. Case series and one meta-analysis show pain improvement after treatment of pancreatic ductal stones; however, comparative studies involving the spontaneous course or randomized studies have not been published. Endoscopic treatment appears particularly suitable for treating solitary stones and obstructions near the papilla, while surgical drainage procedures are superior for distal obstructions. There are no comparative studies for either endoscopic or surgical procedures with untreated cohorts or directly comparing the natural course of the disorder. In two studies in which endoscopic treatment was compared with surgery (i.e., drainage operation), the results after surgery were significantly better with respect to long-term pain reduction.[2-4]

Pancreatic duct strictures, which may be responsible for pain, recurrent exacerbations, maintenance of a pseudocyst, fistula, or other complications, can be treated by endoscopic dilatation and stent placement [Evidence 4]. In a prospective non-randomized study, rapid improvement of symptoms was achieved by insertion of a pancreatic stent in non-operable patients, although further interventions were frequently necessary.[39] Some studies report that the insertion of a stent into the pancreatic duct can induce secondary changes due to the stent with subsequent fibrosis and strictures.[12-14] Removal of the obstruction of the pancreatic duct is effective for the treatment of pain in the short term. Success rates between 37 and 94% have been reported. In the largest hitherto examined cohort of 1,021 patients, a long-term reduction of pancreas-related pain was achieved in 84% of cases.[40] However, in 79% of the patients stent therapy for control of pain had to be repeated within one year and in 97% within two years. Long-term metabolic side effects have not been examined. The only randomized study recruited 41 consecutive patients with chronic pancreatitis with a dominant stricture of the main pancreatic duct to either receive pancreatic duct stenting or serve as control. Recurrences of pain and pancreatic function were recorded as outcome measures over 3 years. During a mean follow-up period of 62.5 months, pain recurred in 15% of patients with pancreatic duct stenting (3/20) and 50.0% of control patients (11/22) ($p<0.05$). Progression of exocrine insufficiency in the stent group was significantly slower than in the control group ($p<0.05$), while endocrine function was not different between groups.[41]

The endoscopic placement of a stent into the pancreatic duct may be performed if pancreatic ductal stones or stenosis of the pancreatic duct near the papilla obstructs flow. No general recommendations can be made about the necessary duration of stent therapy [Evidence 4]. Benign strictures of the duct of Wirsung can develop as a complication of an impacted stone or due to acute inflammatory parenchymal changes with compression or stricture of the duct;[42] examples of different etiologies are displayed in **Figure 1, D-F**. The success rate of stent insertion was examined considering the rise in pressure due to the stone as a cause of pain development and of chronic pancreatitis exacerbations.[43-51] Pancreatic stent placement is technically successful in about 70% of patients, especially those in whom a pancreatic fistula or a pseudocyst are maintained by an obstruction. Endoscopic drainage with stone extraction and stent therapy is an effective measure to control pain in some patients with a dilated duct of Wirsung.[23] Better pain management, however, was achieved by pancreaticojejunostomy in two randomized controlled studies.[2-4] Endoscopic therapy led to pain reduction or complete pain relief in 32%[4] and 65%,[2,3] respectively, whereas pancreaticojejunostomy led to pain reduction or relief in 75%[4] and 86%,[2,3] respectively. The different success rates of endoscopic therapy in both studies are possibly due to the longer duration of stent therapy in the study by Díte et al.[4]

There are currently no reliable data available regarding the necessary duration of stent therapy. Some authors recommend treatment over 1 year with stent exchange at least every 3 months.

When surgery is not possible, a FCSEMS can be inserted into the duct of Wirsung for pain control [Evidence 4]. Some case reports and series suggest that covered self-expandable metallic stents may be inserted into the pancreatic duct to treat pain. Their potential advantage versus plastic stents is their longer period of patency. Long-term results of their benefit are not available. Uncovered self-expandable metallic stents are not recommended due to the rapid proliferation of duct epithelium as a reaction to the metal mesh.[52,53]

Pancreatic ductal stones, which cause pain by obstruction may be treated by ESWL. There is some evidence that the subsequent endoscopic removal of the pancreatic ductal stones or their fragments is not a prerequisite for procedure effectiveness.[54] ESWL treatment of pain in patients with diffuse calcifications has not been substantiated in any studies [Evidence 2b]. A meta-analysis demonstrated a significant effect on pain reduction, but there was remarkable result heterogeneity.[55] The publications included in the meta-analysis were case studies without untreated or sham-operated control groups. To date, only one randomized controlled study has compared ESWL with and without subsequent ERP to remove fragments from the MPD. In this study, the subsequent endoscopic stone extraction had no influence on pain relief after 2 years.[54]

Endoscopic therapy for biliary stricture

In 10% to 44.6% of cases, obstruction of the CBD will develop in patients with chronic pancreatitis and require intervention. Indications for endoscopic intervention include significant cholestasis, exacerbations of cholangitis, prevention of secondary biliary cirrhosis, and for differentiation of the cause of pain (obstruction of the CBD vs. chronic pancreatitis). Several studies have assessed the efficacy and cost-effectiveness of endoscopic drainage of the CBD. A long-term success rate was achieved in only one-third of patients, so endoscopic therapy is usually only indicated as an interim procedure until definitive surgery (e.g., as an acute intervention in septic patients, in non-operable patients, or in those unwilling to undergo surgery). In principle, there is a risk of developing cholangitis after endoscopic drain placement. The administration of prophylactic antibiotics together with ursodeoxycholic acid has not proven effective in various clinical studies.[56-61]

Commonly occurring complications include stent occlusion by cellular detritus, microcolonies of bacteria, or extracellular fibrillar material.

If chronic pancreatitis causes bile duct obstruction and there are clinical signs of cholangitis, immediate endoscopic drainage of the obstruction should be carried out. There are no published studies comparing endoscopic therapy of cholangitis secondary to mechanical cholestasis to observation without therapy. Treatment of mechanical cholestasis as part of cholangitis therapy is important and well substantiated by clinical experience. If chronic pancreatitis causes distal obstruction of the bile duct with cholestasis or jaundice, then either surgical treatment or endoscopic stent therapy should be performed; the later is illustrated in **Figure 1**. If calcifications are present in the pancreas, surgical treatment should be favored [Evidence 4]. Cholestasis due to obstruction may be treated by either endoscopic or surgical means, although endoscopic stent therapy has lasting success beyond 12 months in only one-third of patients. A prospective study showed an even worse long-term effect of stent management of distal bile duct obstruction in patients with calcifying pancreatitis (long-term effect 9%).[10,11] Therefore, surgical treatment is clearly preferred in these cases. A retrospective analysis of all patients treated with an average observation period of 45 months demonstrated that stent therapy for CBD obstruction in patients with chronic pancreatitis has no additional effect beyond 1 year.[9] Surgical treatment should therefore be pursued for recurrence of CBD obstruction after 1 year of stent therapy.

Treatment by insertion of several plastic stents for distal bile duct obstruction can be recommended [Evidence 3b]. The placement of multiple plastic stents to treat bile duct obstruction in patients with chronic pancreatitis is superior to both insertion of solitary plastic stents and uncovered metal stents. In a prospective, nonrandomized single-center study the long-term success rate after insertion of four to five stents into the CBD was higher than after a single stent.[62] The insertion of FCSEMS can be undertaken for distal bile duct obstruction [Evidence 4]. The insertion of covered metal stents has demonstrated good results in case series. A recent nonrandomized study at 13 centers in 11 countries treated 187 patients with benign biliary strictures by FCSEMS. Removal was scheduled at 10 to 12 months. The rate of stricture recurrence was 14.8% (95% confidence interval, 8.2%-20.9%). In a large prospective multinational study, successful removal of FCSEMS after extended indwell and stricture resolution were achieved for approximately 75% of patients. While FCSEMS might be an attractive option to treat CBD stenosis in patients less fit for surgery, what remains unsolved is the role of calcifications on the long-term treatment effect, as well as a randomized head-to-head comparison between plastic stents versus FCSEMS in benign strictures.[63-66]

There are no randomized studies comparing FCSEMS with single or multiple plastic stents.[67-69] Endoscopic treatment for distal CBD obstruction should not be pursued longer than 12 months. Stent exchange should be undertaken at least every 3 months [Evidence 4] because stent occlusion may cause cholangitis. The exchange interval is less critical with the insertion of multiple stents and is unnecessary if fully coated metal stents are used as they are patent for up to 9 months.[70]

Management of chronic bile duct obstruction after unsuccessful endoscopic treatment attempts should be surgical [Evidence 1b]. Resecting surgical procedures to treat bile duct obstruction in patients with chronic pancreatitis are effective and have lasting success. The long-term results of the various surgical procedures such as "Beger," "Büchler," "Kausch-Whipple," and "Frey" do not differ from each other with regard to quality of life, exocrine pancreatic insufficiency, endocrine pancreatic insufficiency, pain, or recurrence rate.[71-74] If there is an indication to treat cholestasis by surgery, a preoperative endoscopic insertion of a stent into the bile duct should only be undertaken if 1) surgery cannot be done promptly or 2) cholangitis is present [Evidence 2a]. A multicenter prospective randomized study examined the effect of preoperative endoscopic stent insertion into the CBD for mechanical cholestasis secondary to carcinoma of the head of the pancreas before pancreas resection. Preoperative drainage significantly increased the complication rate.[74] A short individual life expectancy; high comorbidity; and difficult, foreseeable technical feasibility of an operation (e.g., marked collateral circulation secondary to portal hypertension) all favor endoscopic treatment of bile duct obstruction.

Conclusion

In a patient cohort burdened with a high comorbidity load, endoscopic therapy can provide short-term symptom relief. In many instances, the benefit of endoscopy therapy is transient, and repeated interventions are necessary. Endotherapy is the first-line management in chronic pancreatitis with symptomatic pancreatobiliary ductal obstruction. Further studies are required in key areas such as the use of FCSEMs for pancreatic ductal and biliary strictures and EUS-guided pancreatobiliary drainage after failed ERCP. However, as endoscopic therapy puts the patient at minimal risk for long-term morbidity or mortality, it plays a major role in an interdisciplinary treatment context.

Funding

This work was supported by the Deutsche Krebshilfe/ Dr. Mildred-Scheel-Stiftung (109102), the Deutsche Forschungsgemeinschaft (DFG GRK840-D2/E3/E4, MA

4115/1-2/3), and the European Union (eU-FP-7: EPC-TM and EU-FP7-REGPOT-2010-1).

References

1. Chauhan S, Forsmark CE. Pain management in chronic pancreatitis: A treatment algorithm. *Best Pract Res Clin Gastroenterol*. 2010; 24: 323-335. PMID: 20510832.
2. Cahen DL, Gouma DJ, Laramee P, Nio Y, Rauws EA, Boermeester MA, et al. Long-term outcomes of endoscopic vs surgical drainage of the pancreatic duct in patients with chronic pancreatitis. *Gastroenterology*. 2011; 141: 1690-1695. PMID: 21843494.
3. Cahen DL, Gouma DJ, Nio Y, Rauws EA, Boermeester MA, Busch OR, et al. Endoscopic versus surgical drainage of the pancreatic duct in chronic pancreatitis. *N Engl J Med*. 2007; 356: 676-684. PMID: 17301298.
4. Díte P, Ruzicka M, Zboril V, Novotný I. A prospective, randomized trial comparing endoscopic and surgical therapy for chronic pancreatitis. *Endoscopy*. 2003; 35: 553-558. PMID: 12822088.
5. Burris HA 3rd, Moore MJ, Andersen J, Green MR, Rothenberg ML, Modiano MR, et al. Improvements in survival and clinical benefit with gemcitabine as first-line therapy for patients with advanced pancreas cancer: a randomized trial. *J Clin Oncol*. 1997; 15: 2403-2413. PMID: 9196156.
6. Neoptolemos JP, Dunn JA, Stocken DD, Almond J, Link K, Beger H, et al. Adjuvant chemoradiotherapy and chemotherapy in resectable pancreatic cancer: a randomised controlled trial. *Lancet*. 2001; 358: 1576-1585. PMID: 11716884.
7. Neoptolemos JP, Stocken DD, Bassi C, Ghaneh P, Cunningham D, Goldstein D, et al. Adjuvant chemotherapy with fluorouracil plus folinic acid vs gemcitabine following pancreatic cancer resection: a randomized controlled trial. *JAMA*. 2010; 304: 1073-1081. PMID: 20823433.
8. Vijungco JD, Prinz RA. Management of biliary and duodenal complications of chronic pancreatitis. *World J Surg*. 2003; 27: 1258-1270. PMID: 14534824.
9. Cahen DL, van Berkel AM, Oskam D, Rauws EA, Weverling GJ, Huibregtse K, et al. Long-term results of endoscopic drainage of common bile duct strictures in chronic pancreatitis. *Eur J Gastroenterol Hepatol*. 2005; 17: 103-108. PMID: 15647649.
10. Kahl S, Zimmermann S, Genz I, Glasbrenner B, Pross M, Schulz HU, et al. Risk factors for failure of endoscopic stenting of biliary strictures in chronic pancreatitis: a prospective follow-up study. *Am J Gastroenterol*. 2003; 98: 2448-2453. PMID: 14638347.
11. Kahl S, Zimmermann S, Glasbrenner B, Pross M, Schulz HU, McNamara D, et al. Treatment of benign biliary strictures in chronic pancreatitis by self-expandable metal stents. *Dig Dis*. 2002; 20: 199-203. PMID: 12566623.
12. Smith MT, Sherman S, Ikenberry SO, Hawes RH, Lehman GA. Alterations in pancreatic ductal morphology following polyethylene pancreatic stent therapy. *Gastrointest Endosc*. 1996; 44: 268-275. PMID: 8885345.
13. Kozarek RA. Pancreatic stents can induce ductal changes consistent with chronic pancreatitis. *Gastrointest Endosc*. 1990; 36: 93-95. PMID: 2335298.
14. Nguyen-Tang T, Dumonceau JM. Endoscopic treatment in chronic pancreatitis, timing, duration and type of intervention. *Best Pract Res Clin Gastroenterol*. 2010; 24: 281-298. PMID: 20510829.
15. Lee LS, Conwell DL. Update on advanced endoscopic techniques for the pancreas: endoscopic retrograde cholangiopancreatography, drainage and biopsy, and endoscopic ultrasound. *Radiol Clin North Am*. 2012; 50: 547-561. PMID: 22560697.
16. Barthet M, Bugallo M, Moreira LS, Bastid C, Sastre B, Sahel J. Management of cysts and pseudocysts complicating chronic pancreatitis. A retrospective study of 143 patients. *Gastroenterol Clin Biol*. 1993; 17: 270-276. PMID: 8339886.
17. Ammann RW, Akovbiantz A, Largiader F, Schueler G. Course and outcome of chronic pancreatitis. Longitudinal study of a mixed medical-surgical series of 245 patients. *Gastroenterology*. 1984; 86: 820-828. PMID: 6706066.
18. Andrén-Sandberg A, Dervenis C. Surgical treatment of pancreatic pseudocysts in the 2000's--laparoscopic approach. *Acta Chir Iugosl*. 2003; 50: 21-26. PMID: 15307493.
19. Traverso LW, Tompkins RK, Urrea PT, Longmire WP Jr. Surgical treatment of chronic pancreatitis. Twenty-two years' experience. *Ann Surg*. 1979; 190: 312-319. PMID: 485605.
20. Usatoff V, Brancatisano R, Williamson RC. Operative treatment of pseudocysts in patients with chronic pancreatitis. *Br J Surg*. 2000; 87: 1494-1499. PMID: 11091235.
21. Nealon WH, Walser E. Duct drainage alone is sufficient in the operative management of pancreatic pseudocyst in patients with chronic pancreatitis. *Ann Surg*. 2003; 237: 614-620; discussion 620-612. PMID: 12724627.
22. Cheruvu CV, Clarke MG, Prentice M, Eyre-Brook IA. Conservative treatment as an option in the management of pancreatic pseudocyst. *Ann R Coll Surg Engl*. 2003; 85: 313-316. PMID: 14594534.
23. Bartoli E, Delcenserie R, Yzet T, Brazier F, Geslin G, Regimbeau JM, et al. Endoscopic treatment of chronic pancreatitis. *Gastroenterol Clin Biol* 2005; 29: 515-521. PMID: 15980744.
24. Balthazar EJ, Freeny PC, vanSonnenberg E. Imaging and intervention in acute pancreatitis. *Radiology*. 1994; 193: 297-306. PMID.
25. Johnson MD, Walsh RM, Henderson JM, Brown N, Ponsky J, Dumot J, et al. Surgical versus nonsurgical management of pancreatic pseudocysts. *J Clin Gastroenterol*. 2009; 43: 586-590. PMID: 19077728.
26. Aghdassi A, Mayerle J, Kraft M, Sielenkamper AW, Heidecke CD, Lerch MM. Diagnosis and treatment of pancreatic pseudocysts in chronic pancreatitis. *Pancreas*. 2008; 36: 105-112. PMID: 18376299.
27. Mayerle J, Hoffmeister A, Werner J, Witt H, Lerch MM, Mossner J. Chronic pancreatitis--definition, etiology, investigation and treatment. *Dtsch Arztebl Int*. 2013; 110: 387-393. PMID: 23826027.
28. Hoffmeister A, Mayerle J, Beglinger C, Buchler MW, Bufler P, Dathe K, et al. English language version of the

S3-consensus guidelines on chronic pancreatitis: Definition, aetiology, diagnostic examinations, medical, endoscopic and surgical management of chronic pancreatitis. *Z Gastroenterol*. 2015; 53: 1447-1495. PMID: 26666283.

29. Barthet M, Lamblin G, Gasmi M, Vitton V, Desjeux A, Grimaud JC. Clinical usefulness of a treatment algorithm for pancreatic pseudocysts. *Gastrointest Endosc*. 2008; 67: 245-252. PMID: 18226686.
30. Gouyon B, Levy P, Ruszniewski P, Zins M, Hammel P, Vilgrain V, et al. Predictive factors in the outcome of pseudocysts complicating alcoholic chronic pancreatitis. *Gut*. 1997; 41: 821-825. PMID.
31. Bradley EL, Clements JL Jr, and Gonzalez AC. The natural history of pancreatic pseudocysts: a unified concept of management. *Am J Surg*. 1979; 137: 135-141. PMID: 758840.
32. Varadarajulu S, Christein JD, Tamhane A, Drelichman ER, Wilcox CM. Prospective randomized trial comparing EUS and EGD for transmural drainage of pancreatic pseudocysts (with videos). *Gastrointest Endosc*. 2008; 68: 1102-1111. PMID: 18640677.
33. Patrzyk M, Maier S, Busemann A, Glitsch A, Heidecke CD. [Therapy of pancreatic pseudocysts: endoscopy versus surgery]. *Chirurg*. 2013; 84: 117-124. PMID: 23371027.
34. Tanaka M, Fernandez-del Castillo C, Adsay V, Chari S, Falconi M, Jang JY, et al. International consensus guidelines 2012 for the management of IPMN and MCN of the pancreas. *Pancreatology*. 2012; 12: 183-197. PMID: 22687371.
35. Brugge WR, Lewandrowski K, Lee-Lewandrowski E, Centeno BA, Szydlo T, Regan S, et al. Diagnosis of pancreatic cystic neoplasms: a report of the cooperative pancreatic cyst study. *Gastroenterology*. 2004; 126: 1330-1336. PMID: 15131794.
36. Spinelli KS, Fromwiller TE, Daniel RA, Kiely JM, Nakeeb A, Komorowski RA, et al. Cystic pancreatic neoplasms: observe or operate. *Ann Surg*. 2004; 239: 651-657; discussion 657-659. PMID: 15082969.
37. Barthet M, Sahel J, Bodiou-Bertei C, Bernard JP. Endoscopic transpapillary drainage of pancreatic pseudocysts. *Gastrointest Endosc*. 1995; 42: 208-213. PMID: 7498684.
38. Widdison AL, Alvarez C, Karanjia ND, Reber HA. Experimental Evidence of Beneficial Effects of Ductal Decompression in Chronic Pancreatitis. *Endoscopy*. 1991; 23: 151-154. PMID.
39. Treacy PJ, Worthley CS. Pancreatic stents in the management of chronic pancreatitis. *Aust N Z J Surg*. 1996; 66: 210-213. PMID: 8611126.
40. Rosch T, Daniel S, Scholz M, Huibregtse K, Smits M, Schneider T, et al. Endoscopic treatment of chronic pancreatitis: a multicenter study of 1000 patients with long-term follow-up. *Endoscopy*. 2002; 34: 765-771. PMID: 12244496.
41. Seza K, Yamaguchi T, Ishihara T, Tadenema H, Tawada K, Saisho H, et al. A long-term controlled trial of endoscopic pancreatic stenting for treatment of main pancreatic duct stricture in chronic pancreatitis. *Hepatogastroenterology*. 2011; 58: 2128-2131. PMID: 22234084.
42. Cremer M, Devière J, Delhaye M, Baize M, Vandermeeren A. Stenting in severe chronic pancreatitis: results of medium-term follow-up in seventy-six patients. *Endoscopy*. 1991; 23: 171-176. PMID.
43. McCarthy J, Geenen JE, Hogan WJ. Preliminary experience with endoscopic stent placement in benign pancreatic diseases. *Gastrointest Endosc*. 1988; 34: 16-18. PMID: 3350298.
44. Huibregtse K, Schneider B, Vrij AA, Tytgat GN. Endoscopic pancreatic drainage in chronic pancreatitis. *Gastrointest Endosc*. 1988; 34: 9-15. PMID: 3350319.
45. Kozarek RA, Patterson DJ, Ball TJ, Traverso LW. Endoscopic placement of pancreatic stents and drains in the management of pancreatitis. *Ann Surg*. 1989; 209: 261-266. PMID: 2923512.
46. Kozarek RA, Ball TJ, Patterson DJ, Freeny PC, Ryan JA, Traverso LW. Endoscopic transpapillary therapy for disrupted pancreatic duct and peripancreatic fluid collections. *Gastroenterology*. 1991; 100: 1362-1370. PMID: 2013381.
47. Binmoeller KF, Jue P, Seifert H, Nam WC, Izbicki J, Soehendra N. Endoscopic pancreatic stent drainage in chronic pancreatitis and a dominant stricture: long-term results. *Endoscopy*. 1995; 27: 638-644. PMID: 8903975.
48. Ponchon T, Bory RM, Hedelius F, Roubein LD, Paliard P, Napoleon B, et al. Endoscopic stenting for pain relief in chronic pancreatitis: results of a standardized protocol. *Gastrointest Endosc*. 1995; 42: 452-456. PMID: 8566637.
49. Kozarek RA, Traverso LW. Endotherapy for chronic pancreatitis. *Int J Pancreatol*. 1996; 19: 93-102. PMID: 8723551.
50. Smits ME, Rauws EA, Tytgat GN, Huibregtse K. Endoscopic treatment of pancreatic stones in patients with chronic pancreatitis. *Gastrointest Endosc*. 1996; 43: 556-560. PMID: 8781932.
51. Smits ME, Rauws EA, van Gulik TM, Gouma DJ, Tytgat GN, Huibregtse K. Long-term results of endoscopic stenting and surgical drainage for biliary stricture due to chronic pancreatitis. *Br J Surg*. 1996; 83: 764-768. PMID: 8696734.
52. Boerma D, van Gulik TM, Rauws EA, Obertop H, Gouma DJ. Outcome of pancreaticojejunostomy after previous endoscopic stenting in patients with chronic pancreatitis. *Eur J Surg*. 2002; 168: 223-228. PMID: 12440760.
53. Sauer B, Talreja J, Ellen K, Ku J, Shami VM, Kahaleh M. Temporary placement of a fully covered self-expandable metal stent in the pancreatic duct for management of symptomatic refractory chronic pancreatitis: preliminary data (with videos). *Gastrointest Endosc*. 2008; 68: 1173-1178. PMID: 19028226.
54. Dumonceau JM, Costamagna G, Tringali A, Vahedi K, Delhaye M, Hittelet A, et al. Treatment for painful calcified chronic pancreatitis: extracorporeal shock wave lithotripsy versus endoscopic treatment: a randomised controlled trial. *Gut*. 2007; 56: 545-552. PMID.
55. Guda NM, Partington S, Freeman ML. Extracorporeal shock wave lithotripsy in the management of chronic calcific pancreatitis: a meta-analysis. *JOP*. 2005; 6: 6-12. PMID: 15650279.
56. Groen AK, Out T, Huibregtse K, Delzenne B, Hoek FJ, Tytgat GN. Characterization of the content of occluded biliary endoprostheses. *Endoscopy*. 1987; 19: 57-59. PMID.
57. Smit JM, Out MM, Groen AK, Huibregtse K, Jansen PL, van Marle J, et al. A placebo-controlled study on the efficacy

of aspirin and doxycycline in preventing clogging of biliary endoprostheses. *Gastrointest Endosc*. 1989; 35: 485-489. PMID: 2689261.

58. Ghosh S, Palmer KR. Prevention of biliary stent occlusion using cyclical antibiotics and ursodeoxycholic acid. *Gut*. 1994; 35: 1757-1759. PMID.
59. Ghosh S, Palmer KR. Preventing biliary stent occlusion. *Lancet*. 1994; 344: 1087-1088; author reply 1088-10894. PMID: 7934468.
60. Barrioz T, Ingrand P, Besson I, de Ledinghen V, Silvain C, Beauchant M. Randomised trial of prevention of biliary stent occlusion by ursodeoxycholic acid plus norfloxacin. *Lancet*. 1994; 344: 581-582. PMID: 7914962.
61. Halm U, Schiefke, Fleig WE, Mössner J, Keim V. Ofloxacin and ursodeoxycholic acid versus ursodeoxycholic acid alone to prevent occlusion of biliary stents: a prospective, randomized trial. *Endoscopy*. 2001; 33: 491-494. PMID: 11437041.
62. Catalano MF, Linder JD, George S, Alcocer E, Geenen JE. Treatment of symptomatic distal common bile duct stenosis secondary to chronic pancreatitis: comparison of single vs. multiple simultaneous stents. *Gastrointest Endosc*. 2004; 60: 945-952. PMID: 15605010.
63. Devière J, Nageshwar Reddy D, Püspök A, Ponchon T, Bruno MJ, Bourke MJ, et al. Successful management of benign biliary strictures with fully covered self-expanding metal stents. *Gastroenterology*. 2014; 147(2): 385-395. PMID: 24801350.
64. Perri V, Boskoski I, Tringali A, Familiari P, Marchese M, Lee DK, et al. Prospective evaluation of the partially covered nitinol "ComVi" stent for malignant non hilar biliary obstruction. *Dig Liver Dis*. 2013; 45: 305-309. PMID: 23218991.
65. Perri V, Boskoski I, Tringali A, Familiari P, Mutignani M, Marmo R, et al. Fully covered self-expandable metal stents in biliary strictures caused by chronic pancreatitis not responding to plastic stenting: a prospective study with 2 years of follow-up. *Gastrointest Endosc*. 2012; 75: 1271-1277. PMID: 22464813.
66. Poley JW, Cahen DL, Metselaar HJ, van Buuren HR, Kazemier G, van Eijck CH, et al. A prospective group sequential study evaluating a new type of fully covered self-expandable metal stent for the treatment of benign biliary strictures (with video). *Gastrointest Endosc*. 2012; 75: 783-789. PMID: 22325806.
67. van Boeckel PG, Vleggaar FP, Siersema PD. Plastic or metal stents for benign extrahepatic biliary strictures: a systematic review. *BMC Gastroenterol*. 2009; 9: 96. PMID: 20017920.
68. Behm B, Brock A, Clarke BW, Ellen K, Northup PG, Dumonceau JM, et al. Partially covered self-expandable metallic stents for benign biliary strictures due to chronic pancreatitis. *Endoscopy*. 2009; 41: 547-551. PMID: 19533560.
69. Kahaleh M, Behm B, Clarke BW, Brock A, Shami VM, De La Rue SA, et al. Temporary placement of covered self-expandable metal stents in benign biliary strictures: a new paradigm? (with video). *Gastrointest Endosc*. 2008; 67: 446-454. PMID: 18294506.
70. Lawrence C, Romagnuolo J, Payne KM, Hawes RH, Cotton PB. Low symptomatic premature stent occlusion of multiple plastic stents for benign biliary strictures: comparing standard and prolonged stent change intervals. *Gastrointest Endosc*. 2010; 72: 558-563. PMID: 20638060.
71. McClaine RJ, Lowy AM, Matthews JB, Schmulewitz N, Sussman JJ, Ingraham AM, et al. A comparison of pancreaticoduodenectomy and duodenum-preserving head resection for the treatment of chronic pancreatitis. *HPB (Oxford)*. 2009; 11: 677-683. PMID: 20495636.
72. Muller MW, Friess H, Martin DJ, Hinz U, Dahmen R, Buchler MW. Long-term follow-up of a randomized clinical trial comparing Beger with pylorus-preserving Whipple procedure for chronic pancreatitis. *Br J Surg*. 2008; 95: 350-356. PMID: 17933005.
73. Riediger H, Adam U, Fischer E, Keck T, Pfeffer F, Hopt UT, et al. Long-term outcome after resection for chronic pancreatitis in 224 patients. *J Gastrointest Surg*. 2007; 11: 949-959; discussion 959-960. PMID: 17534689.
74. van der Gaag NA, Rauws EA, van Eijck CH, Bruno MJ, van der Harst E, Kubben FJ, et al. Preoperative biliary drainage for cancer of the head of the pancreas. *N Engl J Med*. 2010; 362: 129-137. PMID: 20071702.
75. Kozarek RA, Brayko CM, Harlan J, Sanowski RA, Cintora I, Kovac A. Endoscopic drainage of pancreatic pseudocysts. *Gastrointest Endosc*. 1985; 31: 322-327. PMID: 4043685.
76. Cremer M, Deviere J, Engelholm L. Endoscopic management of cysts and pseudocysts in chronic pancreatitis: long-term follow-up after 7 years of experience. *Gastrointest Endosc*. 1989; 35: 1-9. PMID: 2920879.
77. Sahel J. Endoscopic drainage of pancreatic cysts. *Endoscopy*. 1991; 23: 181-184. PMID.
78. Bejanin H, Liguory C, Ink O, Fritsch J, Choury AD, Lefebvre JF, et al. [Endoscopic drainage of pseudocysts of the pancreas. Study of 26 cases]. *Gastroenterol Clin Biol*. 1993; 17: 804-810. PMID: 8143945.
79. Funnell IC, Bornman PC, Krige JE, Beningfield SJ, Terblanche J. Endoscopic drainage of traumatic pancreatic pseudocyst. *Br J Surg*. 1994; 81: 879-881. PMID: 8044609.
80. Deviere J, Bueso H, Baize M, Azar C, Love J, Moreno E, et al. Complete disruption of the main pancreatic duct: endoscopic management. *Gastrointest Endosc*. 1995; 42: 445-451. PMID: 8566636.
81. Vitale GC, Lawhon JC, Larson GM, Harrell DJ, Reed DN Jr, MacLeod S. Endoscopic drainage of the pancreatic pseudocyst. *Surgery*. 1999; 126: 616-621; discussion 621-613. PMID: 10520906.
82. White SA, Sutton CD, Berry DP, Chillistone D, Rees Y, Dennison AR. Experience of combined endoscopic percutaneous stenting with ultrasound guidance for drainage of pancreatic pseudocycts. *Ann R Coll Surg Engl*. 2000; 82: 11-15. PMID: 10700759.
83. Giovannini M, Pesenti C, Rolland AL, Moutardier V, Delpero JR. Endoscopic ultrasound-guided drainage of pancreatic pseudocysts or pancreatic abscesses using a therapeutic echo endoscope. *Endoscopy*. 2001; 33: 473-477. PMID.
84. Libera ED, Siqueira ES, Morais M, Rohr MR, Brant CQ, Ardengh JC, et al. Pancreatic pseudocysts transpapillary and transmural drainage. *HPB Surg*. 2000; 11: 333-338. PMID: 10674749.

85. Norton ID, Clain JE, Wiersema MJ, DiMagno EP, Petersen BT, Gostout CJ. Utility of endoscopic ultrasonography in endoscopic drainage of pancreatic pseudocysts in selected patients. *Mayo Clin Proc*. 2001; 76: 794-798. PMID: 11499818.
86. Sharma SS, Bhargawa N, Govil A. Endoscopic management of pancreatic pseudocyst: a long-term follow-up. *Endoscopy*. 2002; 34: 203-207. PMID: 11870570.
87. Binmoeller KF, Seifert H, Walter A, Soehendra N. Transpapillary and transmural drainage of pancreatic pseudocysts. *Gastrointest Endosc*. 1995; 42: 219-224. PMID: 7498686.
88. Binmoeller KF, Soehendra N. Endoscopic ultrasonography in the diagnosis and treatment of pancreatic pseudocysts. *Gastrointest Endosc Clin N Am*. 1995; 5: 805-816. PMID: 8535629.
89. Smits ME, Rauws EA, Tytgat GN, Huibregtse K. The efficacy of endoscopic treatment of pancreatic pseudocysts. *Gastrointest Endosc*. 1995; 42: 202-207. PMID: 7498683.
90. Baron TH, Harewood GC, Morgan DE, Yates MR. Outcome differences after endoscopic drainage of pancreatic necrosis, acute pancreatic pseudocysts, and chronic pancreatic pseudocysts. *Gastrointest Endosc*. 2002; 56: 7-17. PMID: 12085029.
91. Catalano MF, Geenen JE, Schmalz MJ, Johnson GK, Dean RS, Hogan WJ. Treatment of pancreatic pseudocysts with ductal communication by transpapillary pancreatic duct endoprosthesis. *Gastrointest Endosc*. 1995; 42: 214-218. PMID: 7498685.
92. Antillon MR, Shah RJ, Stiegmann G, Chen YK. Single-step EUS-guided transmural drainage of simple and complicated pancreatic pseudocysts. *Gastrointest Endosc*. 2006; 63: 797-803. PMID: 16650541.
93. Hookey LC, Debroux S, Delhaye M, Arvanitakis M, Le Moine O, Deviere J. Endoscopic drainage of pancreatic-fluid collections in 116 patients: a comparison of etiologies, drainage techniques, and outcomes. *Gastrointest Endosc*. 2006; 63: 635-643. PMID: 16564865.
94. Kruger M, Schneider AS, Manns MP, Meier PN. Endoscopic management of pancreatic pseudocysts or abscesses after an EUS-guided 1-step procedure for initial access. *Gastrointest Endosc*. 2006; 63: 409-416. PMID: 16500388.
95. Weckman L, Kylanpaa ML, Puolakkainen P, Halttunen J. Endoscopic treatment of pancreatic pseudocysts. *Surg Endosc*. 2006; 20: 603-607. PMID: 16424988.
96. Kahaleh M, Shami VM, Conaway MR, Tokar J, Rockoff T, De La Rue SA, et al. Endoscopic ultrasound drainage of pancreatic pseudocyst: a prospective comparison with conventional endoscopic drainage. *Endoscopy*. 2006; 38: 355-359. PMID: 16680634.
97. Cahen D, Rauws E, Fockens P, Weverling G, Huibregtse K, Bruno M. Endoscopic drainage of pancreatic pseudocysts: long-term outcome and procedural factors associated with safe and successful treatment. *Endoscopy*. 2005; 37: 977-983. PMID.
98. Varadarajulu S, Bang JY, Phadnis MA, Christein JD, Wilcox CM. Endoscopic transmural drainage of peripancreatic fluid collections: outcomes and predictors of treatment success in 211 consecutive patients. *J Gastrointest Surg*. 2011; 15: 2080-2088. PMID: 21786063.
99. Will U, Wanzar I, Meyer F. Endoscopic necrosectomy--a feasible and safe alternative treatment option for infected pancreatic necroses in severe Acute pancreatitis: preliminary results of 18 patients in an ongoing single-center prospective observational study. *Pancreas*. 2012; 41: 652-655. PMID: 22504384.

Chapter 51

Current surgical treatment options in chronic pancreatitis

Jan G. D'Haese[1], Djuna L. Cahen[2], and Jens Werner[1*]

[1]*Department of General, Visceral, Transplantation, Vascular and Thoracic Surgery, Campus Grosshadern, Ludwig Maximilians-University, Munich, Germany;*

[2]*Department of Gastroenterology and Hepatology, Erasmus University Medical Center, Rotterdam, the Netherlands.*

Introduction

Chronic pancreatitis (CP) is a benign inflammatory disease that leads to progressive and irreparable destruction of the pancreatic parenchyma, resulting in fibrosis and consequent loss of exocrine and endocrine function.[1,2] This may cause steatorrhea, malabsorption, diabetes, and unbearable pain.[3] Pain – often in combination with obstruction (duodenum, bile duct, pancreatic duct, portal vein) –is the main indication for surgical intervention.

The incidence of CP varies among countries. European studies commonly have incidence rates around 7 per 100,000,[4-6] whereas higher incidence rates of 14.4 per 100,000 have been reported in Japan.[7] The leading cause of CP in Western industrialized countries is alcohol overconsumption (between 65% and 90%) followed by idiopathic (20% to 25%) and other, rare etiologies (5%).[5-7]

Patients typically present with deeply penetrating and dull epigastric pain, which classically radiates to the back.[8] The pathophysiological mechanisms for pain in CP are incompletely understood. An increasingly discussed hypothesis is that neural inflammatory cell infiltration leads to pancreatic neuritis with enlarged nerves, changes in neural plasticity, and formation of a dense intrapancreatic neural network. These neural alterations are thought to cause the characteristic pancreatic neuropathy and consequent neuropathic pain.[9-13] Since the underlying pain mechanisms are just beginning to be understood, treatment of chronic unbearable CP pain is often empirical and insufficient, with surgery remaining the treatment of choice.

Indication for surgery: wait, operate or scope?

Making the correct diagnosis is the initial challenge in the treatment of painful CP, which can be difficult, especially in patients with early forms of CP, lacking the structural changes frequently seen in advanced disease. Most patients require long-term analgesic medications for pain control once the diagnosis is confirmed. Moreover, patients should be advised to maintain strict abstinence from alcohol and tobacco. Pain medication should be employed according to the step up approach of the WHO analgesic ladder. Despite a low level of evidence for efficacy in pancreatic pain, non-narcotic adjunctive medications such as selective serotonin reuptake inhibitors (SSRIs) or pregabalin have become increasingly popular in CP treatment since they were proven effective in other chronic pain states.[14,15] Pancreatic enzyme supplementation is also used, although evidence concerning pain reduction is conflicting.[16-21] If medical therapy proves insufficient, and there is no sign of pancreatic or biliary duct obstruction, more invasive nonoperative strategies like coeliac nerve block may be considered. In this context, endoscopic ultrasound-guided techniques have proven safer, more effective, and longer lasting than fluoroscopy-guided or CT-guided techniques.[22-24] However, coeliac nerve block usually has a transient effect, with only 10% of patients still experiencing pain relief after 24 weeks.[25] Therefore, this option seems more reasonable in patients with malignant disease and an anticipated short life span.

In patients with CP and pancreatic duct obstruction, endoscopic treatment for ductal decompression including papillotomy, stone removal, and/or stent implantation is another widely used treatment option. Classical indications for surgery in CP are pancreatic duct obstruction, vascular obstruction, suspicion of neoplasm, and abdominal pain with failure of conservative treatment options. So far, only two prospective randomized clinical trials have compared endoscopic with surgical drainage to treat symptomatic pancreatic duct obstruction. Dite and colleagues were the first to address this controversial issue in a randomized controlled trial that randomized 72 patients to surgery vs. endoscopy.[26] Resection was the most common surgical procedure (80%) whereas surgical drainage was

*Corresponding author. Email: jens.werner@med.uni-muenchen.de

performed in 20% of patients. On the other hand, sphincterotomy and stenting in 52% and/or stone removal in 23% of patients were the most commonly performed intervention in the endoscopy arm. While the initial success rates for pain relief were similarly high (> 90% of patients with at least a partial pain relief after 1 year follow-up) for both groups, these clinical outcomes changed noticeably after 3 and 5 years follow-up. In the surgical treatment group, 42% of patients had persisting, complete pain relief after 1 year, which only slightly decreased to 41% after 3 and to 37% after 5 years. Initially, an equally good clinical outcome was seen in patients in the endoscopic treatment arm, where 52% of patients showed a complete pain relief after 1 year. But this effect substantially decreased to 11% after 3, and to 14% after 5 years. Accordingly, the percentage of nonresponders was disappointingly high, with 33% to 35% in the endoscopy arm versus only 12% to 14% in the surgical treatment arm after 3 and 5 years. Results were similar for the patients' body weight. Therefore, Dite and colleagues concluded that surgery seems to be superior to endoscopic treatment for long-term pain relief and body weight gain in CP patients. It should be noted however, that endoscopic drainage techniques in this study did not meet current standards as they did not include extracorporeal shockwave lithotripsy, and for some patients only consisted of a sphincterotomy.

In 2007, Cahen et al. published the second randomized trial on this subject,[27] which was updated with long-term outcomes in 2011.[28] In this trial, 39 patients were randomized to either endoscopic (n=19) or surgical drainage by a pancreaticojejunostomy (n=20). The study was terminated early following an unscheduled interim analysis at a median of 24 months that found a significant difference in the mean Izbicki pain score (11 vs. 34) favoring the surgical treatment arm ($p<0.001$). Even more striking were the vast differences in percentage of patients with complete or partial pain relief at the end of the first follow-up. Only 32% of patients in the endoscopic treatment group, but 75% in the surgical treatment group had at least partial pain relief. Furthermore, at long-term follow-up of up to 7 years, these numbers did not change considerably (38% vs. 80%). Additionally, endoscopically treated patients underwent significantly more re-interventions than surgically treated patients (8 vs. 3 at first follow-up and 12 vs. 4 at the second follow-up). Based on these results, the authors concluded that surgical drainage is superior to endoscopic treatment and should be regarded as the preferred treatment option in patients with advanced disease.

Based on these two randomized trials, it can be concluded that surgical therapy is more effective and longer lasting than endoscopic treatment. There may be a role for endoscopic drainage early in the disease course. However, surgical treatment for pain in CP should also be considered early in disease history especially in patients with pancreatic calcifications. Current data on the optimal timing of surgical intervention are not sufficient to make final recommendations. Nealon and colleagues suggested that early operative duct decompression may delay progressive functional destruction of the pancreas.[29] While similar conclusions were drawn by Ihse et al.,[30] others have described progressive functional impairment despite surgery,[31] meaning that to date, the question of optimal timing of surgery remains unclear. From the study by Cahen et al., we know that the large group of patients with surgery following endoscopic failure (47%) also did not do well after surgery (27). This suggests that early intervention may to be a key factor for success in the treatment of CP regardless of the type of intervention. Current guidelines suggest that if endoscopic therapy is insufficiently effective after 1 year, the patient should be referred for surgery.

Surgical options: how to operate – drain or resect?

Two main forms of surgical intervention are currently performed for CP patients with the aim of improved drainage of the pancreatic duct: drainage and resection procedures. Any surgical intervention should aim to relieve pain, while at the same time preserve as much of the pancreatic parenchyma and be as safe as possible. In the early 19th century, the first surgical attempts to relieve pancreatic pain in CP attempted to drain the pancreatic duct by pancreatostomy[32] or pancreatic left resection.[33] Surgical procedures for the treatment of chronic pancreatitis have continuously evolved since then. Puestow and Gillesby were the first to perform a modification with combined pancreatic left resection, longitudinal opening of the pancreatic duct, and an anastomosis to the small intestine (pancreaticojejunostomy).[34] In 1960, Partington and Rochelle published what they called the modified Puestrow-Gilles procedure, a spleen-preserving longitudinal pancreaticojejunostomy, where they preserved the tail of the pancreas and extended the opening of the pancreatic duct.[35] This surgical technique is currently known as the Partington-Rochelle procedure and has been the favored surgical drainage procedure for treatment of CP for many years. These draining procedures preserve a maximum of pancreatic tissue, however the major disadvantage of these procedures is that the frequently associated inflammatory mass in the pancreatic head, and therefore the underlying cause of the disease, is not addressed. Nowadays the only suitable indication for a simple drainage procedure and for longitudinal pancreaticojejunostomy is in patients with isolated pancreatic duct pathology (a dilated duct of > 7 mm; "chain of lakes"), without an inflammatory mass in the pancreatic head. For a select group of patients, the long-term pain relief of this drainage operation has been shown to be around 60% to 70%, and up to 98%, with low mortality and morbidity (approximately 3% and 20%, respectively).[36,37]

Pain in patients without pancreatic duct dilation is thought to evolve from neuropathic changes within the pancreatic head, as described earlier. The pancreatic head has been identified as the derivation of the disease, long before the underlying neural alterations were discovered.[38] Therefore, within the last century, several surgical techniques have been developed for the resection of the pancreatic head. The first resection of the pancreatic head was performed 1909 in Berlin by Walther Carl Eduard Kausch on a patient with periampullary cancer. It was the introduction of a technique, nowadays known as the standard Kausch-Whipple procedure, which encompasses the radical resection of the pancreatic head, the duodenum, the gastric antrum with the pylorus and the gallbladder. While it was initially developed for the treatment of malignancies, it subsequently became used for the resection of inflammatory pancreatic head masses. Because of relatively high rates of gastrointestinal complications and diabetes mellitus, the classic Kausch-Whipple procedure has been replaced by the pylorus preserving Whipple procedure, introduced by Traverso and Longmire in 1978.[39,40] The Traverso-Longmire procedure has been shown to result in long-term pain relief in around 90% of patients with painful CP.[40,41]

In the early 1970s, Beger introduced the duodenum-preserving pancreatic head resection (DPPHR), with the rationale that resection of the gastric antrum, duodenum and common bile duct seemed overtreatment in benign pancreatic disease.[42] For the Beger procedure, a subtotal resection of the pancreatic head prior to a transection of the gland above the portal vein is performed, sparing the duodenum and the intrapancreatic bile duct. The drainage of the remaining pancreatic tail is then achieved by an end-to-end or end-to-side pancreaticojejunostomy using a Roux-en-Y loop.

Frey et al. modified the established procedures to a more limited and organ-preserving resection, which is performed by coring out the head of the pancreas and leaving a small remnant along the duodenal wall.[43] Frey et al. then combined this procedure with a longitudinal incision of the left-sided main pancreatic duct for optimal drainage, comparable to the earlier mentioned Partington-Rochelle drainage procedure. For reconstruction, a longitudinal pancreaticojejunostomy using a Roux-en-Y loop is used for drainage of the pancreatic head cavity and the left-sided main duct. The Frey procedure is commonly regarded as technically easier than the Beger operation, as the head resection is more limited, dissection of the pancreas above the portal vein is not required, and the reconstruction is less complex.

The Beger technique of DPPHR has also been further modified and described by Gloor et al. in 2001, often referred to as the Bern procedure.[44] The idea was to combine the advantages of both the Beger and the Frey procedures. For the Bern procedure, a deep duodenum-preserving resection of the pancreatic head for optimal decompression is performed, without transection of the pancreas above the portal vein. In contrast to the Frey procedure and the Hamburg procedure, no drainage of the main pancreatic duct in the body and tail of the organ is performed. Drainage of the resection cavity of the pancreatic head is achieved as in the Beger procedure, by creating a pancreaticojejunostomy using a Roux-en-Y loop.

When it comes to the question as to which of these procedures one should choose, evidence is limited to some monocentric trials (**Table 1**). Klempa et al. compared the

Table 1. Randomized controlled trials comparing surgical techniques in the treatment of CP

Techniques compared	Publication	No. of patients	Outcome
Classic Whipple vs. Beger	Klempa et al. (45)	43	Beger procedure: less pain, greater weight gain, shorter hospital stay
Pylorus preserving Whipple vs. Beger	Büchler et al. (46)	40	Beger procedure: less pain, greater weight gain, a better glucose tolerance, and a higher insulin secretion capacity
Pylorus preserving Whipple vs. Frey	Izbicki et al. (47)	61	Equally effective for pain relief and definitive control of complications; Frey procedure provides a better quality of life
Pylorus preserving Whipple vs. modification of Frey	Farkas et al. (48)	40	Equally effective for pain relief; Frey superior in morbidity, hospital stay, and weight gain
Beger vs. Frey	Strate et al. (49)	74	Both procedures provide adequate pain relief and quality of life after long-term follow-up with no differences of exocrine and endocrine function
Beger vs. Bern	Köninger et al. (50)	65	No differences in quality of life, significantly shorter operation times and hospital stay for the Büchler procedure
Pylorus preserving Whipple vs. DPPHR (Beger or Frey or Bern)	Diener et al. (51)	recruiting aim=200	Expected 2016

classic Whipple procedure (n=21) with the Beger procedure (n=22) in the first randomized controlled trial on the type of surgical treatment for painful CP in 1995. Here, patients with a Beger procedure had less pain, a better gain in body weight, and a shorter hospital stay.[45] A similar study was published by Büchler et al., comparing the DPPHR (n=20) with the pylorus preserving Whipple procedure (n=20). Again, the duodenum-sparing resection had better pain, weight gain, glucose tolerance, and insulin secretion capacity outcomes.[46] Two randomized trials compared the pylorus preserving Whipple procedure with the Frey procedure, and both showed that these procedures were equally efficient for pain relief, but that the Frey procedure provided better quality of life.[47,48] Strate et al. could not show any difference regarding mortality, quality of life, pain, or exocrine and endocrine function when comparing the Beger procedure (n= 38) with the Frey procedure (n=36).[49] The most recent randomized trial, by Köninger et al., was published in 2008, and shows that the Bern procedure can be performed significantly faster and leads to a shorter hospital stay than the Beger procedure.[50] In 2010, Diener and colleagues published the protocol for the ChroPac Trial, which is the first large randomized controlled multicenter trial comparing DPPHR versus pancreatoduodenectomy, with the primary outcome being patient quality of life 24 months after surgery.[51] The first results of this trial are expected in late 2016. The current evidence is best summarized in a recently published meta-analysis, where DPPHRs (including the Beger, Frey, and Büchler procedures) and pancreatoduodenectomy were shown to be equally effective for pain relief, overall morbidity, and incidence of postoperative endocrine insufficiency.[52] However, the DPPHRs seems to be superior in terms of postoperative weight gain and long-term quality of life. Similar results were obtained for the Beger and Frey procedures. Therefore, despite the lack of clear, multicenter randomized controlled trial evidence, it seems that any of these duodenum-preserving resection techniques is appropriate for the surgical treatment of painful CP, and that to date, these should be preferably performed over pancreatoduodenectomy (Whipple procedure).

Conclusion

Long-term pain relief, resolving complications in organs near the pancreas, and improvements in patient pain and quality of life are the primary goals in treating CP. This should be approached by an interdisciplinary team of radiologists, pain specialists, gastroenterologists, and surgeons. Endoscopic drainage may have a role in early disease. However, if persisting pain reduction and consequent improvement in patient's quality of life cannot be achieved by conservative therapy within 1 year, surgery is the treatment of choice. Surgery is superior to endoscopic treatment in the long-term. Pancreatic resections for CP have low morbidity and mortality rates in high-volume centers and promise long-term pain relief for the vast majority of patients with painful chronic pancreatitis. When it comes to surgical techniques, drainage operations are safe and efficient for short-term pain relief, especially in patients without an enlarged pancreatic head, but often fail in the long-term. The Kausch-Whipple operation has been the standard of care for decades, but was steadily replaced by the pylorus-preserving modification of Longmire and Traverso. Consistently high morbidity and insufficient long-term effects after these extensive resections have led to the development of tissue preserving techniques. Currently, the duodenum-preserving resection techniques offer the best outcomes for patients with painful CP and an inflammatory mass in the pancreatic head and should therefore be considered as the current standard of care. The different variants of this technique seem to achieve similar results.[29-31]

References

1. DiMagno EP. A short, eclectic history of exocrine pancreatic insufficiency and chronic pancreatitis. *Gastroenterology.* 1993; 104: 1255-1262. PMID: 8482439.
2. Sarles H, Bernard JP, and Johnson C. Pathogenesis and epidemiology of chronic pancreatitis. *Annu Rev Med.* 1989; 40: 453-468. PMID: 2658760.
3. Witt H, Apte MV, Keim V, and Wilson JS. Chronic pancreatitis: challenges and advances in pathogenesis, genetics, diagnosis, and therapy. *Gastroenterology* 132(4): 1557-1573, 2007. PMID: 17466744.
4. Pedersen NT and Worning H. Chronic pancreatitis. *Scand J Gastroenterol Suppl.* 1996; 216: 52-58. PMID: 8726279.
5. Dite P, Stary K, Novotny I, Precechtelova M, Dolina J, Lata J, et al. Incidence of chronic pancreatitis in the Czech Republic. *Eur J Gastroenterol Hepatol* 2001; 13: 749-750. PMID: 11434607.
6. Levy P, Barthet M, Mollard BR, Amouretti M, Marion-Audibert AM, and Dyard F. Estimation of the prevalence and incidence of chronic pancreatitis and its complications. *Gastroenterol Clin Biol* 2006; 30: 838-844. PMID: 16885867.
7. Otsuki M and Tashiro M. Chronic pancreatitis and pancreatic cancer, lifestyle-related diseases. *Intern Med.* 2007; 46: 109-113. PMID: 17220612.
8. Lankisch PG. Chronic pancreatitis. *Curr Opin Gastroenterol.* 2007; 23: 502-507. PMID: 17762555.
9. Ceyhan GO, Bergmann F, Kadihasanoglu M, Altintas B, Demir IE, Hinz U, et al. Pancreatic neuropathy and neuropathic pain–a comprehensive pathomorphological study of 546 cases. *Gastroenterology.* 2009; 136: 177-186 e171. PMID: 18992743.
10. Ceyhan GO, Bergmann F, Kadihasanoglu M, Erkan M, Park W, Hinz U, et al. The neurotrophic factor artemin influences the extent of neural damage and growth in chronic pancreatitis. *Gut.* 2007; 56: 534-544. PMID: 17047099.

11. Ceyhan GO, Demir IE, Maak M, and Friess H. Fate of nerves in chronic pancreatitis: Neural remodeling and pancreatic neuropathy. *Best Pract Res Clin Gastroenterol.* 2010; 24: 311-322. PMID: 20510831.
12. Ceyhan GO, Demir IE, Rauch U, Bergmann F, Muller MW, Buchler MW, et al. Pancreatic neuropathy results in "neural remodeling" and altered pancreatic innervation in chronic pancreatitis and pancreatic cancer. *Am J Gastroenterol.* 2009; 104: 2555-2565. PMID: 19568227.
13. Ceyhan GO, Michalski CW, Demir IE, Muller MW, and Friess H. Pancreatic pain. *Best Pract Res Clin Gastroenterol.* 2008; 22: 31-44. PMID: 18206811.
14. Matsuzawa-Yanagida K, Narita M, Nakajima M, Kuzumaki N, Niikura K, Nozaki H, et al. Usefulness of antidepressants for improving the neuropathic pain-like state and pain-induced anxiety through actions at different brain sites. *Neuropsychopharmacology.* 2008; 33: 1952-1965. PMID: 17957217.
15. Giannopoulos S, Kosmidou M, Sarmas I, Markoula S, Pelidou SH, Lagos G, et al. Patient compliance with SSRIs and gabapentin in painful diabetic neuropathy. *Clin J Pain.* 2007; 23: 267-269. PMID: 17314587.
16. Malesci A, Gaia E, Fioretta A, Bocchia P, Ciravegna G, Cantor P, et al. No effect of long-term treatment with pancreatic extract on recurrent abdominal pain in patients with chronic pancreatitis. *Scand J Gastroenterol.* 1995; 30: 392-398. PMID: 7610357.
17. Halgreen H, Pedersen NT, and Worning H. Symptomatic effect of pancreatic enzyme therapy in patients with chronic pancreatitis. *Scand J Gastroenterol.* 1986; 21: 104-108. PMID: 3633631.
18. Mossner J, Secknus R, Meyer J, Niederau C, and Adler G. Treatment of pain with pancreatic extracts in chronic pancreatitis: results of a prospective placebo-controlled multicenter trial. *Digestion.* 1992; 53: 54-66. PMID: 1289173.
19. Vecht J, Symersky T, Lamers CB, and Masclee AA. Efficacy of lower than standard doses of pancreatic enzyme supplementation therapy during acid inhibition in patients with pancreatic exocrine insufficiency. *J Clin Gastroenterol.* 2006; 40: 721-725. PMID: 16940886.
20. Brown A, Hughes M, Tenner S, and Banks PA. Does pancreatic enzyme supplementation reduce pain in patients with chronic pancreatitis: a meta-analysis. *Am J Gastroenterol.* 1997; 92: 2032-2035. PMID: 9362186.
21. Winstead NS and Wilcox CM. Clinical trials of pancreatic enzyme replacement for painful chronic pancreatitis–a review. *Pancreatology.* 2009; 9: 344-350. PMID: 19451744.
22. Puli SR, Reddy JB, Bechtold ML, Antillon MR, and Brugge WR. EUS-guided celiac plexus neurolysis for pain due to chronic pancreatitis or pancreatic cancer pain: a meta-analysis and systematic review. *Dig Dis Sci.* 2009; 54: 2330-2337. PMID: 19137428.
23. Kaufman M, Singh G, Das S, Concha-Parra R, Erber J, Micames C, et al. Efficacy of endoscopic ultrasound-guided celiac plexus block and celiac plexus neurolysis for managing abdominal pain associated with chronic pancreatitis and pancreatic cancer. *J Clin Gastroenterol.* 2010; 44: 127-134. PMID: 19826273.
24. Santosh D, Lakhtakia S, Gupta R, Reddy DN, Rao GV, Tandan M, et al. Clinical trial: a randomized trial comparing fluoroscopy guided percutaneous technique vs. endoscopic ultrasound guided technique of coeliac plexus block for treatment of pain in chronic pancreatitis. *Aliment Pharmacol Ther.* 2009; 29: 979-984. PMID: 19222416.
25. Gress F, Schmitt C, Sherman S, Ciaccia D, Ikenberry S, and Lehman G. Endoscopic ultrasound-guided celiac plexus block for managing abdominal pain associated with chronic pancreatitis: a prospective single center experience. *Am J Gastroenterol.* 2001; 96: 409-416. PMID: 11232683.
26. Dite P, Ruzicka M, Zboril V, and Novotny I. A prospective, randomized trial comparing endoscopic and surgical therapy for chronic pancreatitis. *Endoscopy.* 2003; 35: 553-558. PMID: 12822088.
27. Cahen DL, Gouma DJ, Nio Y, Rauws EA, Boermeester MA, Busch OR, et al. Endoscopic versus surgical drainage of the pancreatic duct in chronic pancreatitis. *N Engl J Med.* 2007; 356: 676-684. PMID: 17301298.
28. Cahen DL, Gouma DJ, Laramee P, Nio Y, Rauws EA, Boermeester MA, et al. Long-term Outcomes of Endoscopic Versus Surgical Drainage of the Pancreatic Duct in Patients With Chronic Pancreatitis. *Gastroenterology.* 2011; 141: 1690-1695. PMID: 21843494.
29. Nealon WH and Thompson JC. Progressive loss of pancreatic function in chronic pancreatitis is delayed by main pancreatic duct decompression. A longitudinal prospective analysis of the modified puestow procedure. *Ann Surg.* 1993; 217: 458-466. PMID: 8489308.
30. Ihse I, Borch K, and Larsson J. Chronic pancreatitis: results of operations for relief of pain. *World J Surg.* 1990; 14: 53-58. PMID: 2407038.
31. Warshaw AL, Popp JW, Jr., and Schapiro RH. Long-term patency, pancreatic function, and pain relief after lateral pancreaticojejunostomy for chronic pancreatitis. *Gastroenterology.* 1980; 79: 289-293. PMID: 7399232.
32. Link G. The Treatment of Chronic Pancreatitis by Pancreatostomy: A New Operation. *Ann Surg.* 1911; 53: 768-782. PMID: 17862691.
33. Duval MK, Jr. Caudal pancreatico-jejunostomy for chronic relapsing pancreatitis. *Ann Surg.* 1954; 140: 775-785. PMID: 13208131.
34. Puestow CB and Gillesby WJ. Retrograde surgical drainage of pancreas for chronic relapsing pancreatitis. *AMA Arch Surg.* 1958; 76: 898-907. PMID: 13532132.
35. Partington PF and Rochelle RE. Modified Puestow procedure for retrograde drainage of the pancreatic duct. *Ann Surg.* 1960; 152: 1037-1043. PMID: 13733040.
36. Greenlee HB, Prinz RA, and Aranha GV. Long-term results of side-to-side pancreaticojejunostomy. *World J Surg.* 1990; 14: 70-76. PMID: 2407040.
37. Gonzalez M, Herrera MF, Laguna M, Gamino R, Uscanga L, Robles-Diaz G, et al. Pain relief in chronic pancreatitis by pancreatico-jejunostomy. An institutional experience. *Arch Med Res.* 1997; 28: 387-390. PMID: 9291636.
38. Beger HG, Büchler M, and Bittner R. The duodenum preserving resection of the head of the pancreas (DPRHP) in patients with chronic pancreatitis and an inflammatory mass in the

head. An alternative surgical technique to the Whipple operation. *Acta Chir Scand.* 1990; 156: 309-315. PMID: 2349851.

39. Traverso LW and Longmire WP, Jr. Preservation of the pylorus in pancreaticoduodenectomy. *Surg Gynecol Obstet.* 1978; 146: 959-962. PMID: 653575.
40. Friess H, Berberat PO, Wirtz M, and Buchler MW. Surgical treatment and long-term follow-up in chronic pancreatitis. *Eur J Gastroenterol Hepatol.* 2002; 14: 971-977. PMID: 12352216.
41. Muller MW, Friess H, Beger HG, Kleeff J, Lauterburg B, Glasbrenner B, et al. Gastric emptying following pylorus-preserving Whipple and duodenum-preserving pancreatic head resection in patients with chronic pancreatitis. *Am J Surg.* 1997; 173: 257-263. PMID: 9136776.
42. Beger HG, Buchler M, and Bittner R. The duodenum preserving resection of the head of the pancreas (DPRHP) in patients with chronic pancreatitis and an inflammatory mass in the head. An alternative surgical technique to the Whipple operation. *Acta Chir Scand.* 1990; 156: 309-315. PMID: 2349851.
43. Fry WJ and Child CG, 3rd. Ninety-five per cent distal pancreatectomy for chronic pancreatitis. *Ann Surg.* 1965; 162: 543-549. PMID: 5833584.
44. Gloor B, Friess H, Uhl W, and Buchler MW. A modified technique of the Beger and Frey procedure in patients with chronic pancreatitis. *Dig Surg.* 2001; 18: 21-25. PMID: 11244255.
45. Klempa I, Spatny M, Menzel J, Baca I, Nustede R, Stockmann F, et al. [Pancreatic function and quality of life after resection of the head of the pancreas in chronic pancreatitis. A prospective, randomized comparative study after duodenum preserving resection of the head of the pancreas versus Whipple's operation]. *Chirurg.* 1995; 66: 350-359. PMID: 7634946.
46. Büchler MW, Friess H, Müller MW, Wheatley AM, and Beger HG. Randomized trial of duodenum-preserving pancreatic head resection versus pylorus-preserving Whipple in chronic pancreatitis. *Am J Surg.* 1995; 169: 65-69. PMID: 7818000.
47. Izbicki JR, Bloechle C, Broering DC, Knoefel WT, Kuechler T, and Broelsch CE. Extended drainage versus resection in surgery for chronic pancreatitis: a prospective randomized trial comparing the longitudinal pancreaticojejunostomy combined with local pancreatic head excision with the pylorus-preserving pancreatoduodenectomy. *Ann Surg.* 1998; 228: 771-779. PMID: 9860476.
48. Farkas G, Leindler L, Daroczi M, and Farkas G, Jr. Prospective randomised comparison of organ-preserving pancreatic head resection with pylorus-preserving pancreaticoduodenectomy. *Langenbecks Arch Surg.* 2006; 391: 338-342. PMID: 16680474.
49. Strate T, Taherpour Z, Bloechle C, Mann O, Bruhn JP, Schneider C, et al. Long-term follow-up of a randomized trial comparing the beger and frey procedures for patients suffering from chronic pancreatitis. *Ann Surg.* 2005; 241: 591-598. PMID: 15798460.
50. Köninger J, Seiler CM, Sauerland S, Wente MN, Reidel MA, Muller MW, et al. Duodenum-preserving pancreatic head resection–a randomized controlled trial comparing the original Beger procedure with the Berne modification (ISRCTN No. 50638764). *Surgery.* 2008; 143: 490-498. PMID: 18374046.
51. Diener MK, Bruckner T, Contin P, Halloran C, Glanemann M, Schlitt HJ, et al. ChroPac-trial: duodenum-preserving pancreatic head resection versus pancreatoduodenectomy for chronic pancreatitis. Trial protocol of a randomised controlled multicentre trial. *Trials.* 2010; 11: 47. PMID: 20429912.
52. Diener MK, Rahbari NN, Fischer L, Antes G, Buchler MW, and Seiler CM. Duodenum-preserving pancreatic head resection versus pancreatoduodenectomy for surgical treatment of chronic pancreatitis: a systematic review and meta-analysis. *Ann Surg.* 2008; 247(6): 950-961. PMID: 18520222.

Chapter 52

Total pancreatectomy and islet auto transplantation for chronic pancreatitis

Sydne Muratore, Martin Freeman*, and Greg Beilman*

Departments of Surgery and Medicine, University of Minnesota, Minneapolis, MN, USA.

Introduction

Surgical management of chronic pancreatitis is in a constant state of evolution. The trials of management reflect the inherent complexity of the organ's function and closeness to neighboring organs. As the irreversible process of chronic pancreatitis progresses, patients are subjected to varying degrees of endocrine and exocrine loss, as well as pain. Management of this process is multifaceted. Endoscopic and surgical drainage procedures can be used to attempt decompression of dilated ducts. Celiac ganglion blocks, narcotic analgesics, and enteral or parenteral nutrition are therapies directed at the recurring or continuous pain of recurrent acute pancreatitis (RAP) or chronic pancreatitis (CP). Patients refractory to these therapies frequently find themselves on escalating doses of narcotics due to intractable pain, and can be faced with countless days of lost time at school or work, depression, and financial burden.

History

Total pancreatectomy was first proposed to relieve pain in patients where other therapies had failed.[1] Islet autotransplantation was added to this procedure to preserve beta-cell mass in an effort to prevent development of brittle diabetes.[1,2] Mirkovitch and Campiche were the first investigators to successfully transplant autologous islets in large animals by injection into the spleens of pancreatectomized dogs.[3,4] The first human total pancreatectomy with islet autotransplantation (TPIAT) in the world was performed at the University of Minnesota in 1977. The patient was insulin-independent and pain-free until her death 6 years later from unrelated causes.[5,6] This success helped to shed light on the etiology of antecedent allograft efforts; failure likely resulting from low viability, poor preservation of deceased donor pancreases, or rejection.[1,6] A small number of other centers began utilizing IAT after TP with variable initial success in the 1980s and modest program expansion occurring in the 1990s-2000s.[4] Complications initially occurred at some centers not using anticoagulation.[7-9] As of 2014, the published literature included reports of over 900 IATs worldwide as several centers developed their programs.[10-23] Advancements in surgical technique, islet isolation, patient selection, and perioperative care are steadily improving the outcomes of this therapy.

Patient Selection

Patient selection for TPIAT is difficult. The primary focus for surgery is to alleviate pain, however, the pathogenesis of pain in chronic pancreatitis is incompletely understood. There are multiple theories based on observational studies that attempt to explain the multifactorial features of this prominent symptom. In the presence of strictures, stones, or disrupted ducts; increased intraductal pressure, interstitial hypertension, and ischemia are thought to be the culprits of pain. The neuropathic theory is based on observation of abnormal intrapancreatic nerves and increased numbers of perineural inflammatory cells.[24-26]

Additionally, pain levels do not correlate well with severity of fibrosis or impairment of organ function.[27] These inconsistencies contribute to the complexity of patient selection for TPIAT. Individualized evaluation is critical for optimal pairing of appropriate therapy. Patients with dilated large ducts or expanded head may be candidates for endoscopic or surgical drainage procedures. Those with a focal stricture, disrupted duct, or tail-only disease may find relief when treated with distal pancreatectomy.[28] However, there are a growing number of patients who are not candidates for classical surgical therapy or endoscopic drainage, including those with small duct pancreatitis and minimal change disease. Additionally, adults and children with genetic causes of chronic or recurrent pancreatitis should be given special consideration for TPIAT given the likelihood of persistent disease, and increased risk of pancreatic malignancy in some patients.[27]

*Corresponding authors. Email: beilm001@umn.edu, freem020@umn.edu

Preoperative Evaluation Criteria

Given the gravity of removing the entire pancreas, the correct diagnosis of CP is paramount to the success of this operation. Criteria for patient selection has evolved over the years as outcomes and better understanding of the disease process help match patients to the appropriate surgical management. Patients should be evaluated at a well-established center with a multidisciplinary approach including surgeons, gastroenterologists, endocrinologists, pain management physicians, and nurse coordinators. Patients should have abdominal pain >6 months duration with impaired quality of life such as inability to attend work, school, or ordinary activities; repeated hospitalizations; and a constant need for narcotics. Their symptoms must have failed to respond to medical or endoscopic therapies.

The criteria for the diagnosis of chronic pancreatitis developed at the University of Minnesota are shown in **Table 1**. They include 1) pancreas calcifications on CT scan, or obviously abnormal ERCP including pancreatic stones, strictures and/or main duct/sidebranch abnormalities, or greater than or equal to 6 of 9 criteria on endoscopic ultrasound (EUS). 2) Two of the 3 following criteria—ductal or parenchymal abnormalities on secretin-stimulated magnetic resonance cholangiopancreatography (MRCP), EUS with 4 of the 9 criteria positive, abnormal endoscopic pancreatic function tests with peak bicarbonate <80 mmol/L)—are present. 3) They have a histopathologically confirmed diagnosis of CP from previous operations or biopsy. 4) They have hereditary pancreatitis (PRSS1, SPINK1, or CFTR gene mutation) with a compatible clinical history; or 5) a history of recurrent acute pancreatitis with >3 episodes of pain associated with imaging diagnostic of AP and/or elevated serum amylase or 3 times normal lipase.[19,29] EUS evaluation features include the "Rosemount Criteria": hyperechoic parenchymal foci, strands, hypoechoic lobules, cysts, main-duct irregularity, ductal dilation, hyperechoic duct walls, visible side branches, and calcifications or stones.[30]

Contraindications include active alcoholism, pancreatic cancer, use of illegal drugs, poorly controlled psychiatric

Table 1. University of Minnesota Criteria[20] To be considered for TPIAT, patients must meet criteria in sections I and II and have no contraindications.

I. Definitions (must have one of the following: a, b, or c)

a. CP (must have one of i, ii, or iii) Patients with chronic abdominal pain, lasting > 6 months, features consistent with that of pancreatitis, and evidence of CP as evidenced by at least one of the following:
   i. Morphologic/functional evidence of CP [CT of abdomen with evidence of CP (calcifications), or ERCP evidence of pancreatitis]
      or
   ii. EUS of ≥ 6/9 criteria positive of CP
      or
   iii. At least 2 of the following 3 findings:
      1. Secretin MRCP or ERCP, with findings suggestive of CP (abnormal duct/side branch) or MRI T2 evidence of fibrosis
      2. EUS with ≥ 4/9 criteria positive for pancreatitis
      3. Abnormal exocrine pancreatic function tests (peak bicarbonate < 80)
      or

b. Relapsing AP (must have both 1 and 2)
   i. Three or more episodes of documented AP with ongoing episodes over > 6 months.
   ii. No evidence of current gallstone disease or other correctable etiology such as autoimmune pancreatitis
      or

c. Documented hereditary pancreatitis with compatible clinical history.

II. Indications for TPIAT (must have each of the following: 1-5)

a. Documented CP or relapsing AP with chronic or severe abdominal pain, directly resulting in at least one of the following:
   i. Chronic narcotic dependence (patient requires narcotics on a daily or nearly daily basis for > 3 months)
   ii. Impaired quality of life, defined by at least one of the following:
      1. Loss of job
      2. Inability or significantly reduced ability to work or attend school
      3. Frequent absences from school
      4. Frequent hospitalizations
      5. Loss of ability to participate in usual age-appropriate activities
   iii. Complete evaluation, with no reversible cause of CP or relapsing AP present or untreated
   iv. Unresponsive to maximal medical therapy and endoscopic therapy, with ongoing abdominal pain requiring routine narcotics for CP or relapsing AP
   v. Adequate islet cell function (non-diabetic, or non-insulin-requiring diabetes with C-peptide positive)

illness, predictable inability to comply with the postoperative regimen, or end-stage cardiopulmonary disease.[19,27] Patients with C-peptide-negative diabetes do not benefit from the IAT portion of the procedure. Therefore it is not recommended at this time.[1] Additionally, preoperative assessment for liver disease; including portal hypertension, portal vein thrombosis, or cirrhosis is important as these are relative contraindications to any major pancreatic resection or islet embolization into the portal vein.[27]

Metabolic Testing

After determining that RAP or CP is the primary diagnosis, and the pain is of pancreatic origin, evaluation of metabolic function should be undertaken prior to surgery. This may include fasting and postprandial blood glucose and HbA1c, glucose tolerance test, and baseline and stimulated C-peptide levels. Studies have demonstrated that fasting and mixed meal test glucose and HbA1c were inversely correlated with IEQ/kg, and that the other factors also have modest correlation with islet isolation outcomes.[31-33]

Other Testing

Immunization status should be assessed and updated to include encapsulated organisms due to the high likelihood of splenectomy associated with removal of the pancreas. Additionally, assessing nutritional status and identifying comorbidities that may impact postoperative management, such as gastroparesis, is important. Exocrine dysfunction is common in preoperative CP patients, however, no routine quantitative preoperative testing is performed at this time. In patients with cystic fibrosis mutations, a pulmonary consult for evaluation and preoperative optimization is appropriate.

Technique

TPIAT is most commonly performed via open laparotomy, although reports of laparoscopic and robotic assisted resection are increasing.[34-39] Surgery involves resection of the entire pancreas, duodenum, distal common bile duct, and typically the spleen. Pylorus preservation is surgeon dependent. During mobilization of the pancreas, preserving the blood supply as long as possible is an important consideration to minimize the duration of warm ischemia of the islet cells. For this, the gastroduodenal artery and the origin of the splenic artery and splenic vein are ligated only after full pancreatic mobilization. The distal pancreas should not be separated from the splenic vessels.[1] In cases of difficult mobilization, the body and tail can be resected and sent separately to the islet processing lab, while the head is removed and sent later.[19,40] After resection, the specimen is placed in cold preservation solution and prepared for processing by removing nonpancreatic tissue before being sent to the lab.[41]

Biliary and enteric reconstruction occur while the islets are being processed. Choledochojejunostomy is typically performed in the end-to-side fashion. Gastrojejunostomy or duodenojejunostomy can be performed in the antecolic or retrocolic fashion. Variations of reconstruction have been described when the patient's anatomy or sequela of chronic pancreatitis necessitate alternative resections.[20]

Spleen resection rates are variable across centers, but is necessary the majority of the time due to disruption of the blood supply.[19,21] After the hilar vessels are taken, the spleen can at times survive off collateral circulation. However, leaving the spleen has risks, including variceal formation, splenomegaly, and both early and late GI bleeding.[1,13]

After processing the pancreas for islet isolation, the islets are returned to the operating room for infusion. The majority of centers perform this infusion through the portal vein with embolization of islets to the liver. There are multiple options for the endovascular access site to the portal vein, such as a recanalized umbilical vein,[42] mesenteric vein,[21,43,44] or splenic vein.[45] Islets are typically infused intraoperatively, or less commonly by interventional radiology after surgery. This is done via percutaneous transhepatic access to the portal vein.[20,45] Heparin is administered at 70 U/kg prior to infusion to minimize thrombotic complications from tissue thromboplastin present in the islet preparation.[1,7] Most centers also measure portal pressures before and during infusion. If there is a persistent increase in portal pressure >25cm H_20 with islet infusion, it is advisable to consider an alternative site such as intraperitoneal, beneath the renal capsule, or the submucosal layer of the stomach.[1]

Preoperative Care

Continuous insulin infusion is initiated immediately after resection of the pancreas to maintain euglycemia and prevent glucose toxicity to the islets as they engraft.[31,40] This is continued postoperatively until the patient has initiated enteral nutrition and can be transitioned to an outpatient regimen. A gastric or jejunal feeding tube may be placed at the discretion of the surgeon at the time of operation. Exocrine supplementation may be administered upon initiation of enteral feeding as well by either route. At the discretion of the surgeon, prophylactic heparin/lovenox should be initiated in the postoperative period when bleeding risk allows. It is the practice of the author's institution to perform a screening right upper quadrant ultrasound at 1 week postoperatively to evaluate portal vein thrombosis. If positive, patients are kept on Coumadin for three months.

Islet Isolation

Islet isolation and purification must be performed at a facility that meets good medical practice standards and has expertise in islet isolation. The basic method of islet preparation will be reviewed, however, enzyme type varies across institutions. First, intraductal infusion of enzyme is performed either manually or via automated pump perfusion. Interstitial perfusion is performed in cases of severe fibrosis or incomplete enzyme dispersion. Next, semi-automated digestion at 34 to 37°C in a Ricordi chamber facilitates tissue dissociation. From 1994 to 2007, Liberase HI was universally used for enzyme digestion, but then it became clinically unavailable and centers now utilize a range of enzyme protocols.[46,47]

After digestion, purification is performed to minimize exocrine cell contamination without compromising islet numbers. Islet purification is performed using isopycnic density gradient centrifugation.[46,47] The islets can also be partially purified or transplanted as an unpurified preparation. The decision to purify is multifactorial, balancing the benefit of avoiding islet exposure to harsh solutions and additional mechanical stress and the desire to minimize increases in portal pressure during islet embolization to the liver. Currently, the author's institution allows up to 0.25 ml/kg for intraportal infusion. Quantities above this are considered for purification.[47,48]

The extent of fibrosis plays a large role in enzymatic digestion of the extracted pancreas. Additionally, age, pancreas weight, and fat infiltration can lead to discrepancies in islet release. Variations in length of enzyme exposure, enzyme dose, digestion chamber size, temperature, circulation speed, and level of mechanical shaking are needed in order to accommodate the discrepancies found in each organ.[47]

Outcomes

The majority of TPIATs reported to date have been performed at the University of Minnesota, encompassing over 500 patients.[20] Other reports of current or past TPIAT programs include centers at the University Hospitals of Leicester, University of Cincinnati, University of Arizona, University of Alabama, Medical University of South Carolina, Digestive Disease Institute Cleveland, and Baylor Research Institute.[12-14,18,21-23] TPIAT for small numbers of patients with benign and malignant tumors are being performed at San Raffaele Scientific Institute in Italy,[10,11] and benign tumors in Korea[15-17] and Geneva.[49]

Examining the demographics (**Table 2**) in the largest series with comprehensive data of TPIAT for CP, patients undergo surgery at a mean 35 to 44 years of age after suffering symptoms of pancreatitis for a range of 5.4 to 9.2 years.[13,19,21] The most common etiology prior to surgery is idiopathic, followed by alcoholic pancreatitis. Anywhere from 12 to 80% of study populations have undergone prior pancreatic resections before TPIAT. This has been shown in multiple studies—particularly for lateral pancreaticojejunostomy or distal pancreatectomy—to have deleterious effects on islet cell harvest, which in turn may confer decreased success of the transplanted beta cell mass.[19,41,45] Starting with the earliest reports of TPIAT done in the late 1970s, centers such as the University of Minnesota are amassing follow-up data on patients spanning decades, which helps to continually improve treatment of this patient population.

The predominant goal of surgery is mitigation of intractable pain. The overall clinical experience of pancreas centers (**Table 3**) has demonstrated that TPIAT can successfully alleviate pain in the majority of CP patients.[12-14,18,19,21-23] Nearly all patients undergoing TPIAT are narcotic dependent at the time of surgery, and studies show rates of narcotic independence at 1 year postop of 55 to 71%.[13,14,19,23] This success shows continued improvement over time, likely due to the effect of tapering long-term narcotic users. Additionally, these same studies demonstrated significant improvement in pain scores postoperatively when compared to the preoperative state.

The addition of islet autotransplantation to attenuate the otherwise complete insulin and glucagon deficiency is also proving positive. Insulin independence rates range from 10 to 47% across studies, though the attrition rate increases over time (**Table 3**). The patients who become insulin dependent but retain partial islet function demonstrated by C-peptide positivity gain a benefit by ameliorating the potentially severe glycemic swings seen in pancreatogenic diabetes, thus improving diabetes management.[31] The centers at Minnesota and Leicester report C-peptide positivity rates of 90% and 100% respectively, demonstrating high success rates in islet autotransplantation.[13,19] Additionally, studies have shown that postoperative insulin use did not negatively impact quality of life scores.[50]

Postoperative Management

It is important to maintain postoperative follow-up of TPIAT patients, as aspects of their anatomy and physiology may be foreign to centers and practitioners not experienced with this treatment. Avoidance of corticosteroids is paramount to avoid harm to the islets.[51] In addition, TPIAT patients with infusion of islets into the liver may have abnormal imaging findings. After infusion, the islets engraft into the hepatic sinusoids. Subsequent blockage of terminal portal vein branches and local insulin release may result in hepatic structural changes.[52] This in turn may lead to an increase in echogenicity with a nodular appearance on ultrasound. A UK study showed 25% of patients had these characteristics, and were stable on imaging at 6 and 12 month follow-up. There was no associated significant loss of liver function or increase in insulin requirements.[52] These changes have also been reported as seen on MRI and are thought to be associated with periportal steatosis.[53]

Table 2. Study Demographics

FACTORS	Minnesota[20]	Leicester[13]	Cincinnati[23]	Cleveland[22]	Arizona^[14]	Alabama^[12]	Baylor *[21]	S. Carolina^[18]
STUDY DATES	1977-2011	1996-2006	2000-2013	2007-2010	2009-2013	2005-2012	2006-2009	2009-2010
NUMBER OF PATIENTS	409	50	112	20	61 (52 TP, 8 CP, 1 partial)	91 (57 TP, 4 CP, 8 DP, 22 whipple)	17	33 (21 TP, 11 CP, 1 DP)
MEAN AGE	35.3	43	37.3	43	42.2	44	40.1	42
BMI	24.5	21	24.2	NR	26.6	23.8	26.1	27
SEX	74% F (303)	52% F (26)	67% F (75)	40% F (8)	63.9% F (39)	54% F (49)	75% F (13)	76% F (25)
FOLLOWUP (median)	NR	8 yrs	74 mo	25 mo	NR (1-24 mo)	19 mo	7.3 mo	9 mo
DURATION of preop narc	3.6 yrs	NR	NR	NR	NR	NR	NR	NR
YEARS of pain symptoms	9.2	5.4	NR	NR	NR	NR	7	NR
DIABETIC preop	8% (33)	0%	12.5% (14)	NR	0%	NR	5.8% (1)	21% (7)
ETIOLOGY								
Idopathic	41% (168)	48% (24)	75% (84)	55% (11)	73% (45)	NR	53% (9)	24% (8)
Alcohol	7% (29)	36% (18)	2.7% (3)	25% (5)	11% (7)	23% (21)	NR	12% (4)
Divisum	17% (70)	0%	8.9% (10)	10% (2)	0%	NR	NR	9% (3)
Biliary	9% (37)	10% (5)	0%	0%	0%	NR	NR	42% (14)
Genetic	14% (57)	0%	13.4% (15)	10% (2)	16% (10)	NR	NR	9% (3)
Other	12% (49)	6% (3)	0%	0%	0%	0%	47% (8)	3% (1)
PRIOR SURG	21% (86)	12% (6)	38% (43)	25% (5)	80% (49)	25% (23)	17% (3)	54% (18)
Whipple/Beger	6% (25)	6% (3)	20.5% (23)	NR	NR	NR	NR	15% (5)
DP/Duval	8% (33)	6% (3)	7.1% (8)	NR	NR	NR	NR	12 % (4)
Puestow/Frey	9% (37)	0%	7.1% (8)	NR	NR	NR	NR	6% (2)
Other	8% (33)	NR	NR	NR	NR	NR	NR	6% (2)

*extrapolated data; ^studies including partial and total pancreatectomies; *DP,* distal pancreatectomy; *TP,* total pancreatectomy; *CP:* completion pancreatectomy; *NR,* data not reported.

Table 3. Comparison of study results across centers

FACTORS	Minnesota[20]	Leicester[13]	Cincinnati[23]	Cleveland[22]	Arizona^[14]	Alabama^[12]	Baylor *[21]	S. Carolina^[18]
STUDY DATES	1977-2011	1996-2006	2000-2013	2007-2010	2009-2013	2005-2012	2006-2009	2009-2010
IEQ/kg	3,050	2,245	6,027	3,846	3,048	1,955	5,278	NR
INSULIN	1yr/3yr	5yr	1yr/5yr	at follow-up	1-24 months	at follow-up	at follow-up	1 yr
independent	28%, 30%	10%	38%, 27%	20%	19%	15%	47%	24%
partial	49%, 33%	NR	38%, 35% <20U/d	NR	27% <10U/d	NR	53%	15% <10U/d
dependent	23%, 37%	NR	24%, 38%	80%	54%	NR	0	NR
INSULIN/DAY preop	NR	0	1	NR	0	NR	NR	NR
INSULIN U/d postop	NR	5 yr: 16*	5 yr: 18.1	11.6	NR	NR	NR	NR
HbA1c preop	NR	NR	NR	6.04	NR	NR	NR	NR
HbA1c postop	82% <7.0	NR	5 yr: 6.9	7.72	NR	NR	NR	NR
NARCOTIC INDEPENDENCE	2 yr: 59%	1 yr: 60%, 5 yr: 84%	1 yr: 55%; 5 yr: 73%	30%	1 yr: 71%	NR	35%	23%
PAIN SCORE	SF-36 integrated pain score	VAS	SF-36 BODLY PAIN SCORE.	VAS %mild/mod/ sev	SF-36 pain score.	SF McGill Pain	VAS	0-10 scale
preop	54	10 for both	9.3	0% mild, 45% mod, 55% severe	25.2	AP: 25.2, NAP: 23.2	7.8	7
postop	1 yr: 31, 2 yr: 30	3 for severity, 2 for frequency	1 yr: 53.2, 5 yr: 59.4	80% mild, 15% mod, 5% severe	1 yr: 57.4	AP: 1yr 20.1, 2yr 15.2; NAP: 1yr 17.5, 2yr 12.8	NR	6 mo: 5, 6+ mo: 4
NARCOTIC USE								
preop (ME/d)	NR	120	118.9	89.2	NR	NR	293	357
post (ME/d)	NR	62	5 yr: 21.1	78	1 mo: 191	NR	76	128
QOL SCORES	SF-36		SF-36	DASS/PDI		SF-36		SF-12
preop	29 PCS, 38 MCS	NR	NR	see study	NR	30.4 PCS 37.1 MCS	NR	25 PCS, 32 MCS
postop	1 yr: 39 PCS, 47 MCS; 2yr: 38 PCS, 49 MCS	NR	1 yr: 92% improved from baseline	79-90% improved across all domains	NR	1 yr: 37.6 PCS, 37.9 MCS; 2yr: 44.4 PCS, 45.5 MCS	NR	1 yr: 36 PCS, 44 MCS
SURVIVAL	1yr: 97%, 5 yr: 90%, 20yr: 62%	NR	5yr: 94.6%	NR	NR	NR	NR	NR
MORBIDITY	15%	15%	NR	45%	NR	NR	NR	48%
MORTALITY	1.2%	2%	0%	0%	0%	NR	NR	0
LOS (days)	NR	20	14	12	12.4		NR	NR
OR time (hrs)	NR	8	9.1	NR	NR	5.9	NR	4.1
EBL (mL)	NR	NR	549	NR	NR	413	NR	679
BLOOD TRANSFUSION	NR	NR	33.9%	NR	NR	NR	NR	24%
ISLET HAREVEST TME (hrs)	4.5	2-4	NR	NR+	NR	NR	NR	4.6
SPLENIC PRESERVATION	30%	96%	routine splenectomy	NR	routine splenectomy	NR	NR	NR

*extrapolated data; ^studies including partial and total pancreatectomies; *DP,* distal pancreatectomy; *TP,* total pancreatectomy; *CP:* completion pancreatectomy; *NR,* data not reported; *QOL:* quality of life; *AP:* alcoholic pancreatitis; *NAP:* non-alcoholoic pancreatitis; *VAS:* visual analogue scale; *DASS/PDI:* depression anxiety stress scale/pain disability index; *SF-36/12:* short form health survey; *PCS/MCS:* physical component score/mental component score; results without time label specified were reported in original study at "time of follow-up".

Conclusion

Thirty-seven years after the first procedure was performed for CP, TPIAT is proving to be a safe and effective treatment strategy for this difficult and complex disease process. Growing experience is allowing earlier and improved selection of patients for TPIAT, which may improve their postoperative endocrine function, pain relief, and quality of life. Ongoing research in islet processing, preoperative patient assessment and selection, as well as islet engraftment will likely contribute to refining outcomes in future patients.

References

1. Blondet JJ, Carlson AM, Kobayashi T, Jie T, Bellin M, Hering BJ, et al. The role of total pancreatectomy and islet autotransplantation for chronic pancreatitis. *Surg Clin North Am*. 2007; 87(6): 1477-1501. PMID: 18053843
2. Najarian JS, Sutherland DE, Baumgartner D, Burke B, Rynasiewicz JJ, Matas AJ, et al. Total or near total pancreatectomy and islet autotransplantation for treatment of chronic pancreatitis. *Ann Surg*. 1980; 192(4): 526-542. PMID: 6775603
3. Mirkovitch V, Campiche M. Successful intrasplenic autotransplantation of pancreatic tissue in totally pancreatectomised dogs. *Transplantation*. 1976; 21(3): 265-269. PMID: 781926
4. Sutton JM, Schmulewitz N, Sussman JJ, Smith M, Kurland JE, Brunner JE, et al. Total pancreatectomy and islet cell autotransplantation as a means of treating patients with genetically linked pancreatitis. *Surgery*. 2010; 148(4): 676-685. PMID: 20846557
5. Farney AC, Najarian JS, Nakhleh RE, Lloveras G, Field MJ, Gores PF, et al. Autotransplantation of dispersed pancreatic islet tissue combined with total or near-total pancreatectomy for treatment of chronic pancreatitis. *Surgery*. 1991; 110(2): 427-437. PMID: 1858051
6. Najarian JS, Sutherland DE, Matas AJ, Goetz FC. Human islet autotransplantation following pancreatectomy. *Transplant Proc*. 1979; 11(1): 336-340. PMID: 109963
7. Mehigan DG, Bell WR, Zuidema GD, Eggleston JC, Cameron JL. Disseminated intravascular coagulation and portal hypertension following pancreatic islet autotransplantation. *Ann Surg*. 1980; 191(3): 287-293. PMID: 6767451
8. Memsic L, Busuttil RW, Traverso LW. Bleeding esophageal varices and portal vein thrombosis after pancreatic mixed-cell autotransplantation. *Surgery*. 1984; 95(2): 238-242. PMID: 6420919
9. Toledo-Pereyra LH, Rowlett AL, Cain W, Rosenberg JC, Gordon DA, MacKenzie GH. Hepatic infarction following intraportal islet cell autotransplantation after near-total pancreatectomy. *Transplantation*. 1984; 38(1): 88-89. PMID: 6429912
10. Balzano G, Maffi P, Nano R, Zerbi A, Venturini M, Melzi R, et al. Extending indications for islet autotransplantation in pancreatic surgery. *Ann Surg*. 2013; 258(2): 210-218. PMID: 23751451
11. Balzano G, Piemonti L. Autologous islet transplantation in patients requiring pancreatectomy for neoplasm. *Curr Diab Rep*. 2014; 14(8): 512. PMID: 24915889
12. Dunderdale J, McAuliffe JC, McNeal SF, Bryant SM, Yancey BD, Flowers G, et al. Should pancreatectomy with islet cell autotransplantation in patients with chronic alcoholic pancreatitis be abandoned? *J Am Coll Surg*. 2013; 216(4): 591-596. PMID: 23521936
13. Garcea G, Weaver J, Phillips J, Pollard CA, Ilouz SC, Webb MA, et al. Total pancreatectomy with and without islet cell transplantation for chronic pancreatitis: A series of 85 consecutive patients. *Pancreas*. 2009; 38(1): 1-7. PMID: 18665009
14. Gruessner RW, Cercone R, Galvani C, Rana A, Porubsky M, Gruessner AC, et al. Results of open and robot-assisted pancreatectomies with autologous islet transplantations: Treating chronic pancreatitis and preventing surgically induced diabetes. *Transplant Proc*. 2014; 46(6): 1978-1979. PMID: 25131087
15. Jin SM, Oh SH, Kim SK, Jung HS, Choi SH, Jang KT, et al. Diabetes-free survival in patients who underwent islet autotransplantation after 50% to 60% distal partial pancreatectomy for benign pancreatic tumors. *Transplantation*. 2013; 95(11): 1396-1403. PMID: 23558506
16. Jung HS, Choi SH, Kim SJ, Choi DW, Heo JS, Lee KT, et al. Delayed improvement of insulin secretion after autologous islet transplantation in partially pancreatectomized patients. *Metabolism*. 2009; 58(11): 1629-1635. PMID: 19604519
17. Lee BW, Jee JH, Heo JS, Choi SH, Jang KT, Noh JH, et al. The favorable outcome of human islet transplantation in korea: Experiences of 10 autologous transplantations. *Transplantation*. 2005; 79(11): 1568-1574. PMID: 15940047
18. Morgan K, Owczarski SM, Borckardt J, Madan A, Nishimura M, Adams DB. Pain control and quality of life after pancreatectomy with islet autotransplantation for chronic pancreatitis. *J Gastrointest Surg*. 2012; 16(1): 129-133. PMID: 22042566
19. Sutherland DE, Radosevich DM, Bellin MD, Hering BJ, Beilman GJ, Dunn TB, et al. Total pancreatectomy and islet autotransplantation for chronic pancreatitis. *J Am Coll Surg*. 2012; 214(4): 409-424; discussion 424-426. PMID: 22397977
20. Sutherland DE, Bellin MD, Blondet JJ, Beilman GJ, Dunn TB, Chinnakotla S, et al. (2012). Total pancreatectomy and islet autotransplantation for chronic pancreatitis. *Chronic Pancreatitis*. ISBN: 978-953-51-0011-9, InTech, http://www.intechopen.com/books/chronic-pancreatitis/total-pancreatectomy-and-islet-autotransplantation-for-chronic-pancreatitis
21. Takita M, Naziruddin B, Matsumoto S, Noguchi H, Shimoda M, Chujo D, et al. Variables associated with islet yield in autologous islet cell transplantation for chronic pancreatitis. *Proc (Bayl Univ Med Cent)*. 2010; 23(2): 115-120. PMID: 20396418
22. Walsh RM, Saavedra JR, Lentz G, Guerron AD, Scheman J, Stevens T, et al. Improved quality of life following total pancreatectomy and auto-islet transplantation for chronic pancreatitis. *J Gastrointest Surg*. 2012; 16(8): 1469-1477. PMID: 22673773
23. Wilson GC, Ahmad SA, Schauer DP, Eckman MH, Abbott DE. Cost-effectiveness of total pancreatectomy and islet

cell autotransplantation for the treatment of minimal change chronic pancreatitis. *J Gastrointest Surg*. 2014; 19(1): 46-55. PMID: 25095749

24. Navaneethan U, Venkataraman J. Recent advancements in the pathogenesis of pain in chronic pancreatitis: The argument continues. *Minerva Gastroenterol Dietol*. 2010; 56(1): 55-63. PMID: 20190725
25. Keith RG, Keshavjee SH, Kerenyi NR. Neuropathology of chronic pancreatitis in humans. *Can J Surg*. 1985; 28(3): 207-211. PMID: 3995416
26. Vardanyan M, Rilo HL. Pathogenesis of chronic pancreatitis-induced pain. *Discov Med*. 1985; 9(47): 304-310. PMID: 20423674
27. Bellin MD, Freeman ML, Gelrud A, Slivka A, Clavel A, Humar A, et al. Total pancreatectomy and islet autotransplantation in chronic pancreatitis: Recommendations from PancreasFest. *Pancreatology*. 2014; 14(1): 27-35. PMID: 24555976
28. Neal CP, Dennison AR, Garcea G. Surgical therapy in chronic pancreatitis. *Minerva Gastroenterol Dietol*. 2012; 58(4): 377-400. PMID: 23207614
29. Bellin MD, Freeman ML, Schwarzenberg SJ, Dunn TB, Beilman GJ, Vickers SM, et al. Quality of life improves for pediatric patients after total pancreatectomy and islet autotransplant for chronic pancreatitis. *Clin Gastroenterol Hepatol*. 2011; 9(9): 793-799. PMID: 21683160
30. Catalano MF, Sahai A, Levy M, Romagnuolo J, Wiersema M, Brugge W, et al. EUS-based criteria for the diagnosis of chronic pancreatitis: The rosemont classification. *Gastrointest Endosc*. 2011; 69(7): 1251-1261. PMID: 19243769
31. Bellin MD, Balamurugan AN, Pruett TL, Sutherland DE. No islets left behind: Islet autotransplantation for surgery-induced diabetes. *Curr Diab Rep*. 2011; 12(5): 580-586. PMID: 22777430
32. Bellin MD, Blondet JJ, Beilman GJ, Dunn TB, Balamurugan AN, Thomas W, et al. Predicting islet yield in pediatric patients undergoing pancreatectomy and autoislet transplantation for chronic pancreatitis. *Pediatr Diabetes*. 2010; 11(4): 227-234. PMID: 19708905
33. Lundberg R, Beilman GJ, Dunn TB, Pruett TL, Chinnakotla SC, Radosevich DM, et al. Metabolic assessment prior to total pancreatectomy and islet autotransplant: Utility, limitations and potential. *Am J Transplant*. 2013; 13(10): 2664-2671. PMID: 23924045
34. Giulianotti PC, Kuechle J, Salehi P, Gorodner V, Galvani C, Benedetti E, et al. Robotic-assisted laparoscopic distal pancreatectomy of a redo case combined with autologous islet transplantation for chronic pancreatitis. *Pancreas*. 2009; 38(1): 105-107. PMID: 19106750
35. Marquez S, Marquez TT, Ikramuddin S, Kandaswamy R, Antanavicius G, Freeman ML, et al. Laparoscopic and da vinci robot-assisted total pancreaticoduodenectomy and intraportal islet autotransplantation: Case report of a definitive minimally invasive treatment of chronic pancreatitis. *Pancreas*. 2010; 39(7): 1109-1111. PMID: 2086169
36. Gustavson SM, Rajotte RV, Hunkeler D, Lakey JR, Edgerton DS, Neal DW, et al. Islet auto-transplantation into an omental or splenic site results in a normal beta cell but abnormal alpha cell response to mild non-insulin-induced hypoglycemia. *Am J Transplant*. 2005; 5(10): 2368-2377. PMID: 16162184
37. Galvani CA, Rodriguez Rilo H, Samame J, Porubsky M, Rana A, Gruessner RW. Fully robotic-assisted technique for total pancreatectomy with an autologous islet transplant in chronic pancreatitis patients: Results of a first series. *J Am Coll Surg*. 2014; 218(3): e73-78. PMID: 24559970
38. Galvani CA, Rilo HR, Samame J, Gruessner RW. First fully robotic-assisted total pancreatectomy combined with islet autotransplant for the treatment of chronic pancreatitis: A case report. *Pancreas*. 2013; 42(7): 1188-1189. PMID: 24048458
39. Zureikat AH, Nguyen T, Boone BA, Wijkstrom M, Hogg ME, Humar A, et al. Robotic total pancreatectomy with or without autologous islet cell transplantation: Replication of an open technique through a minimal access approach. *Surg Endosc*. 2014; 29(1): 176-183. PMID: 25005012
40. Wilson GC, Sutton JM, Abbott DE, Smith MT, Lowy AM, Matthews JB, et al. Long-term outcomes after total pancreatectomy and islet cell autotransplantation: Is it a durable operation? *Ann Surg*. 2014; 260(4): 659-667. PMID: 25203883
41. Bellin MD, Beilman GJ, Dunn TB, Pruett TL, Chinnakotla S, Wilhelm JJ, et al. Islet autotransplantation to preserve beta cell mass in selected patients with chronic pancreatitis and diabetes mellitus undergoing total pancreatectomy. *Pancreas*. 2013; 42(2): 317-321. PMID: 23146918
42. Pollard C, Gravante G, Webb M, Chung WY, Illouz S, Ong SL, et al. Use of the recanalised umbilical vein for islet autotransplantation following total pancreatectomy. *Pancreatology*. 2011; 11(2): 233-239. PMID: 21577042
43. Ali NS, Walsh RM. Total pancreatectomy with islet cell auto-transplantation: Update and outcomes from major centers. *Curr Treat Options Gastroenterol*. 2014; 12(3): 350-358. PMID: 25053231
44. Wang H, Desai KD, Dong H, Owzarski S, Romagnuolo J, Morgan KA, et al. Prior surgery determines islet yield and insulin requirement in patients with chronic pancreatitis. *Transplantation*. 2013; 95(8): 1051-1057. PMID: 23411743
45. Morgan KA, Theruvath T, Owczarski S, Adams DB. Total pancreatectomy with islet autotransplantation for chronic pancreatitis: Do patients with prior pancreatic surgery have different outcomes? *Am Surg*. 2012; 78(8): 893-896. PMID: 22856498
46. Anazawa T, Balamurugan AN, Bellin M, Zhang HJ, Matsumoto S, Yonekawa Y, et al. Human islet isolation for autologous transplantation: Comparison of yield and function using SERVA/Nordmark versus Roche enzymes. *Am J Transplant*. 2009; 9(10): 2383-2391. PMID:
47. Balamurugan AN, Loganathan G, Bellin MD, Wilhelm JJ, Harmon J, Anazawa T, et al. A new enzyme mixture to increase the yield and transplant rate of autologous and allogeneic human islet products. *Transplantation*. 2012; 93(7): 693-702. PMID: 22318245
48. Wilhelm JJ, Bellin MD, Dunn TB, Balamurugan AN, Pruett TL, Radosevich DM, et al. Proposed thresholds for pancreatic tissue volume for safe intraportal islet autotransplantation

after total pancreatectomy. *Am J Transplant*. 2013; 13(12): 3183-3191. PMID: 24148548

49. Berney T, Mathe Z, Bucher P, Demuylder-Mischler S, Andres A, Bosco D, et al. Islet autotransplantation for the prevention of surgical diabetes after extended pancreatectomy for the resection of benign tumors of the pancreas. *Transplant Proc*. 2004; 36(4): 1123-1124. PMID: 15194391
50. Dorlon M, Owczarski S, Wang H, Adams D, Morgan K. Increase in postoperative insulin requirements does not lead to decreased quality of life after total pancreatectomy with islet cell autotransplantation for chronic pancreatitis. *Am Surg*. 2013; 79(7): 676-680. PMID: 23815999
51. Ngo A, Sutherland DE, Beilman GJ, Bellin MD. Deterioration of glycemic control after corticosteroid administration in islet autotransplant recipients: A cautionary tale. *Acta Diabetol*. 2014; 51(1): 141-145. PMID: 21822910
52. Ong SL, Pollard C, Rees Y, Garcea G, Webb M, Illouz S, et al. Ultrasound changes within the liver after total pancreatectomy and intrahepatic islet cell autotransplantation. *Transplantation*. 2008; 85(12): 1773-1777. PMID: 18580470
53. Bhargava R, Senior PA, Ackerman TE, Ryan EA, Paty BW, Lakey JR, et al. Prevalence of hepatic steatosis after islet transplantation and its relation to graft function. *Diabetes*. 2004; 53(5): 1311-1317. PMID: 15111501

Chapter 53

Pharmaceutical developments for chronic pancreatitis: Pipelines and future options

Rajarshi Mukherjee and Robert Sutton*

NIHR Liverpool Pancreas Biomedical Research Unit, Royal Liverpool and Broadgreen University Hospitals NHS Trust and Institute of Translational Medicine, University of Liverpool, Liverpool, UK.

Introduction

Chronic pancreatitis (CP) is a disease that remains without specific treatment and carries with it substantial morbidity. The disease is a chronic inflammatory disease of the pancreas with the key hallmark of progressive fibrotic destruction of the pancreatic secretory parenchyma resulting in loss of acinar and islet cells and subsequent exocrine and endocrine insufficiency.[1,2] There has been significant variation in CP epidemiology among worldwide studies over the last 40 years, mainly concentrated in the western world, indicating a range in incidence from 2.1-13.4/100,000,[3] with a 20-year mortality rate of 35.8%-62%.[4,5] Numerous etiological factors have been identified: alcohol, nicotine, nutrition, hereditary/genetic, efferent duct/obstructive, and autoimmune.[1] Autoimmune pancreatitis, while recognized as a form of CP, is characterized by infiltration of lymphocytes and immunoglobulin G4-positive plasma cells within the pancreatic parenchyma. Unlike other forms of CP, it responds significantly to steroid treatment and so will not be considered further in this review; nor will the management of pancreatic exocrine and/or endocrine insufficiency. While alcohol remains the most common etiological factor in most studies,[6] only a small proportion of alcoholics develop CP,[5] suggesting a multifactorial etiology. Our understanding of the interplay and contribution of risk factors has been greatly enhanced by genetic discovery, starting with the discovery nearly 20 years ago of mutations in the cationic trypsinogen gene (*PRSS1*) causing hereditary pancreatitis,[7] to the recent identification of common genetic variants in *CLDN2* conferring an increased risk of alcohol-related CP, particularly in men.[8]

The demand for novel treatments for CP has never been greater and this is based upon a number of factors. **[1]** The variation in epidemiology may be attributable to problems with long-term follow-up, especially in chronic alcoholics, as well as common delays in obtaining a formal and standardized diagnosis. As a result, the disease burden is likely to be higher than previously reported.[3] **[2]** No treatments are available to halt disease progression, and current treatment options for CP are limited to supportive and palliative care; patients with advanced disease can be managed with endoscopic and/or surgical pancreatic decompression, denervation, resection, bypass, or transplantation.[9,10] **[3]** The patient impact of CP is significant both directly, with recurrent severe pain, which is the primary clinical complaint,[11] and repeated hospital admissions leading to a poor quality of life, as well as indirectly, through the complications of malnutrition and diabetes mellitus that result from exocrine and endocrine insufficiency. **[4]** The health resource burden as a result of the disease is sizeable, with estimated costs for both acute and chronic pancreatitis in the U.S. in 2004 amounting to $3.8 billion.[12] **[5]** A considerable number of patients presenting with acute pancreatitis (AP) may progress on to CP and risk factor control, be it from a hereditary etiology to a predominant alcoholic etiology, remains difficult. Population-based studies report that 20%-45% of patients have a recurrence of AP, with the highest rates among those with alcohol-related AP.[13] Progression to CP after recurring AP has been reported in 4%-24% of patients, again more commonly amongst those with alcoholic recurrent AP.[14] Interestingly, a long-term prospective study (1976-1992) of patients with recurring AP who continued to consume alcohol reported progression to CP in as many as 78%,[15] with a 30-year Danish follow-up study finding that AP (alcohol-related and idiopathic) progressed to CP with a mean interval of 3.5 years.[16] **[6]** CP carries a substantial risk of progression to pancreatic ductal adenocarcinoma (PDA). Patients with CP have a higher incidence of PDA,[17] and individuals with hereditary pancreatitis have a 40% cumulative risk of developing PDA in their lifetime.[18]

These crucial clinical characteristics of CP highlight the need for targeted novel treatment strategies to halt disease progression and thus improve patient outcomes.

*Corresponding author. Email: R.Sutton@liverpool.ac.uk

If novel drugs are combined with better standardized early diagnosis, a potentially significant impact on disease outcome may result. The identification of such putative treatment pipelines rests on a clear understanding of disease pathogenesis and mechanisms so that appropriate targets can be identified for drug discovery programs, as well as open options for drug repositioning.

Pathogenesis of CP and potential treatment strategies

The sentinel acute pancreatitis event (SAPE) hypothesis, first described by Whitcomb in 1999, provides a unified model for CP pathogenesis.[19] After studying cases of hereditary pancreatitis, Whitcomb et al. found that 50% of patients with gain-of-function trypsinogen mutations experienced repeated episodes of AP that later developed into CP.[20] Regardless of the cause of the sentinel event of AP, recurrent episodes of AP can progress to CP. This complex multifactorial disease requires the interaction of various environmental factors (e.g., alcohol consumption), recurrent injury (e.g., trypsin activation and autodigestion) and the immune response.[21] AP is characterized by acinar and ductal cell injury, premature acinar zymogen activation, recruitment of inflammatory cells, autodigestion and necrosis of acinar and ductal cells, and subsequent reparative and anti-inflammatory responses; repetitive episodes drive pancreatic stellate cell (PSC) activation and PSC-dependent fibrosis.[22] Recurrent and/or sustained pancreatic parenchymal injury and inflammation lead to progressive irreversible fibrosis,[22] the pathological hallmark of CP. Pain, however, does not correlate well with morphological features of CP,[23] and the extent to which primary parenchymal injury contributes to the progression of established CP is unclear. Nevertheless, any strategy to modulate outcomes in CP must be based on a detailed understanding of the pathological process of destruction of the pancreatic parenchyma and resultant fibrogenesis.

Our understanding of fibrogenesis in the pancreas of patients with CP improved with the finding that PSCs regulate the synthesis and degradation of the extracellular matrix (ECM) proteins (particularly fibronectin and fibrillary collagen types) that comprise fibrous tissue.[24] Under normal homeostatic conditions, PSCs remain in their quiescent form, but they can be activated by a variety of toxic factors such as ethanol and its metabolites or inflammatory cytokines and chemokines, which are upregulated in pancreatic tissues of patients with CP. Such factors induce PSCs to proliferate and transform into myofibroblast-like cells.[25] Thus, novel therapeutic strategies could target one of three potential areas in the disease process: treatments to reduce primary parenchymal injury, immunomodulation or PSC inhibition (**Figure 1**).

Immunology of CP

How immune factors contribute to disease pathogenesis and specifically PSC activation is an area of pivotal understanding that may produce numerous potential treatment pipelines. Immune cells play a key role in CP pathogenesis with a variety of changes observed in the condition (**Table 1**). Infiltrating myeloid cells have previously been demonstrated to play a crucial role in PSC activation with activated macrophages previously shown to stimulate collagen and fibronectin synthesis by cultured PSCs,[26] and furthermore by the requirement of myeloid (rather than acinar cell) nuclear factor-κB p65 subunit to promote fibrosis in experimental CP.[27]

An increasing number of studies have focused on the role of T cells in CP. An early study demonstrated pancreas samples to have significant increases in CD4+ and CD8+ T-cell infiltrates and *perforin* messenger RNA–expressing cells in CP lesions compared with healthy pancreatic tissue, indicating cell-mediated cytotoxicity.[28] Another study demonstrated no differences in total leukocyte or T-cell populations; however, samples from patients with CP had increased numbers of CD4+ and CD8+ central memory T-cell subsets (CCR7+) compared with controls.[29]

A more recent study investigated pancreas-specific T cell responses to antigens from lysates of human CP lesions obtained during surgical resection.[31] T cells from CP patients had higher levels of interleukin (IL)-10-based responses to pancreatitis-associated antigens compared to normal controls and patients with pancreatic ductal adenocarcinoma, supporting the association between CP and changes in tissue- and disease-specific memory and regulatory T-cell responses.[31] The tragedy remains, however, that even in the light of these significant advances in our understanding of the pathoimmunology of CP, there remains no immune-based therapies for the disease, but this could change in the future with significant recent advances in our understanding of the roles of PSCs and their interactions with immune and other pancreatic cells.

PSCs: key to CP fibrosis

Among all pancreatic parenchymal cells, PSCs comprise 4%-7%,[32] and have been clearly established over the last 20 years as the key executors of pancreatic fibrogenesis. Indeed, numerous in vitro and in vivo studies clearly demonstrate the central role of activated PSCs in CP-associated fibrosis. PSCs are activated by a variety of toxic factors or by inflammatory cytokines and chemokines produced in CP, resulting in PSC proliferation and transformation into myofibroblast-like cells[25] that produce the pancreatic fibrosis that characterizes CP. The intracellular signaling mechanisms regulating PSC activation include the mitogen-activated protein kinase (MAPK) pathway, which

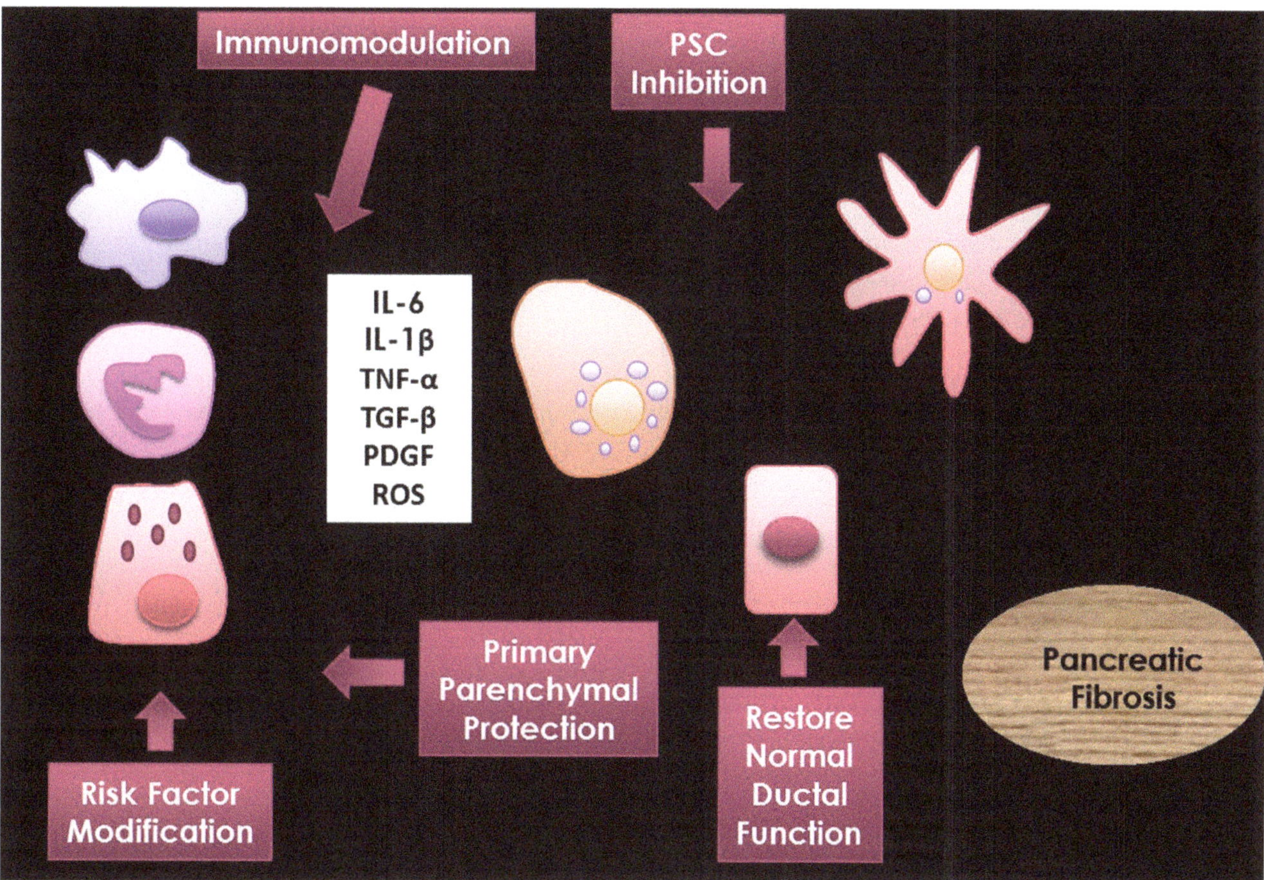

Figure 1. Potential therapeutic strategies for CP. The main areas that novel treatment strategies focus on are risk factor modification, the restoration of normal ductal function in circumstances where this may be altered (i.e., in CP with a predominant obstructive efferent duct etiology, primary parenchymal protection, immunomodulation), and pancreatic stellate cell (PSC) inhibition, applicable to all causes of CP. There is a significant overlap between strategies targeting the immune system and PSCs cells with agents often affecting both.

Table 1. Summary of the key pathoimmunological responses observed in CP

Key immunological changes in CP	Reference
↑ Myeloid cell pancreatic infiltrates, particularly macrophages	Treiber et al., 2011[27]
↑ Inflam. cytokines (IL-6, IL-1β, TNF-α, TGF-β, PDGF, ROS)	Mews et al., 2002[30]
↑ CD4+ and CD8+ T cell pancreas infiltrates	Hunger et al., 1997[28]
↑ Circulating memory T cells	Grundsten et al., 2005[29]
Changes in memory and regulatory T cell responses	Schmitz-Winnenthal et al., 2010[31]
↑ Activation of PSCs	Apte et al., 2005[25]

Changes predominantly are observed in macrophage and T cell infiltrates, an increase in inflammatory cytokines, and increased activation of quiescent PSCs. Increasing evidence exists demonstrating changes in the number and function of circulating memory and regulatory T cells.

plays a major role in ethanol- and acetaldehyde-dependent activation of PSCs, phosphatidylinositol-3-kinase, and protein kinase C.[33] The transition to the myofibroblast-like phenotype is associated with increased expression of specific smooth muscle genes such as α smooth muscle actin (*ACTA2*) and transgelin (*SM22α*) and of specific markers such as cytoglobin/PSC activation associated protein (Cygb/STAP) in fibrotic lesions of the pancreas.[34] PSCs can be activated directly by alcohol consumption[35] or by cytokines derived from the immigrating inflammatory cells.[36,37] Platelet-derived growth factor is the major promoter of PSC migration, whereas transforming growth factor A (TGFA) affects ECM production via a Smad-associated pathway. Upon phosphorylation by the TGFA receptor, Smad3 enters the nucleus to modulate the transcription of target genes.[38] Smad3 links TGFA signaling directly to the serum response factor (SRF)-associated regulatory network that controls the expression of smooth muscle-specific genes.[39]

Although the earliest studies tended to primarily focus on the role of PSCs in pathological fibrosis, recently the maintenance of homeostasis within the pancreas by PSCs has been further explored.[32] Roles in a number of physiological processes have been identified including the maintenance of normal ECM turnover, a role in cholecystokinin-mediated pancreatic exocrine secretion, recognition of pathogen-associated molecular patterns (PAMPs) via Toll-like receptors, a role in innate immunity by phagocytosing necrotic acinar cells and neutrophils, and the expression of stem cell markers with capacity to function as progenitor cells.[40]

It is generally agreed that the PSCs in CP are mainly derived from the resident cells with some contribution from bone marrow-derived pluripotent cells.[41] Increasing evidence highlights the role of PSCs in CP toward both exocrine and endocrine dysfunction. Increased PSC numbers have been detected in fibrotic areas around and within the islets of Langerhans in the pancreas of Goto-Kakizaki rats (a model of type 2 diabetes), and in vitro work has shown that PSCs inhibit insulin secretion by beta cells and cause apoptosis of those cells. Recent studies have reported that hyperglycemia aggravates the detrimental effects of PSCs on beta cell function,[42] and that in hyperglycemic mice, cerulein-induced CP is significantly aggravated when compared with normoglycemic mice.[43]

Utilizing the understanding gained from these studies about the role of PSCs in CP, many subsequent studies aimed at developing novel therapeutic approaches to minimize or reverse the fibrosis have been performed. These treatments have mostly been applied in established experimental models of pancreatic fibrosis, frequently utilizing histopathological assessment and assays of PSC activation. Improvements in methods to isolate PSCs have allowed previously difficult in vitro methods to be applied to assess drug efficacy. A variety of therapeutic strategies have been tested with promising results in a range of experimental CP models over the last 10 years: antioxidants,[44] inhibition of profibrogenic growth factors such as TGF-β,[45] peroxisome proliferator-activated receptor gamma (PPARγ) ligands such as thiazolidinediones,[46] protease inhibitors,[47] a prostacyclin analogue ONO-1301,[48] the flavonoid apigenin and its analogues,[49] inhibition of collagen synthesis by targeted treatment of PSCs with collagen small interfering RNA (siRNA),[50] an anthraquinone derivative Rhein,[51] and others (**Table 2**).

The models of CP used have included repetitive cerulein injections over 3 to 10 weeks. The most common model has the advantage of targeting the pancreas. Dibutyltin dichloride (DBTC) induces fibrosis in the pancreas and liver, chronic ethanol is administered with lipopolysaccharide (LPS), and combinations of these,[52] as well as transgenic animals (e.g., those expressing normal and mutated human cationic trypsinogen genes).[53] The above studies are encouraging as potential treatments for pancreatic fibrosis in CP, but the real challenge lies in translating these preclinical findings to the clinical setting. Among these studies, a variety of in vitro and in vivo techniques ranging using both mouse and human tissue have been employed, and some of the more promising treatments are appraised in more detail in the subsequent sections. Nevertheless, greater standardization is required in both preclinical models and clinical trial designs, the latter being especially underdeveloped for drug trials.

Primary parenchymal protection as a treatment strategy

The repetitive and/or continuous injury of the pancreatic parenchyma inflicted by toxic, metabolic, genetic, and other causes first and foremost damages the acinar cells making up the vast majority of the parenchyma, as well as the ductal cells.[54] Both cell types are injured by fatty acid ethyl esters, nonoxidative metabolites of ethanol, and fatty acids that are implicated in alcohol-associated and hyperlipidemic AP and CP.[55-58] Both induce cytosolic calcium overload that in turn induces mitochondrial calcium overload, compromising the ATP supply and inhibiting autophagy that would otherwise clear the associated premature intracellular digestive enzyme activation. The compromise in ATP production occurs through excessive mitochondrial matrix calcium concentrations that induce the mitochondrial permeability transition pore (MPTP), likely formed by the F_0F_1ATP synthase and regulated by cyclophilin D, allowing molecules <1,500 daltons to pass through the inner mitochondrial membrane.[59] Mitochondrial membrane potential is lost, ATP production is compromised, and cellular necrosis results, inducing the necroinflammatory sequences that drive AP and, likely with repetitive injury, CP. Similar events occur in hyperstimulation-induced AP and CP, exploited in the repetitive cerulein injection model of CP, which is the most widely used (**Table 2**). The severities of both experimental AP and CP are dependent on the toxin dose and the number of times repeated. Treatments that either inhibit calcium entry into pancreatic parenchymal cells or protect mitochondria have been shown to be highly effective in experimental AP[59,60] and could have a place in CP treatment. Inhibition of the principal store-operated calcium channel Orai1 has been shown to markedly reduce the severity of experimental AP, and inhibition of cyclophilin D can eliminate almost all pathological consequences in some models of experimental AP. The latter strategy is

Table 2. Summary of key molecular targets and putative treatments tested in experimental CP in the last 10 years

Target/Drug	Model of CP	Findings	*Reference*
TGF-β/adenoviral vector expressing	C57BL/6 mice cerulein for 3 wks	Reduced fibrosis and reduced activated PSCs	Nagashio et al., 2004[69]
AdTb-ExR/ halofuginone	C57BL/6 mice cerulein for 4/8 wks	Reduced fibrosis	Zion et al., 2009[45]
Protease inhibitors/ camostat mesilate	DBTC rat for 4 wks with treatment at 1 wk, cultured PSCs	Reduced fibrosis and PSC activation	Gibo et al., 2005[47]
PPAR-γ /thiazolidinediones	Immortalized rat PSCs	Reduced PSC activation	Jaster et al., 2005[46]
Mucolytic/bromhexine hydrochloride	12 human patients	Improvement in pain and exocrine function	Tsujimoto et al., 2005[106]
Curcumin	Cultured rat PSCs	Reduced activation and proliferation	Masamune et al., 2006[91]
Green tea	Isolated cultured rat PSCs	Inhibited PSC activation	Asaumi et al., 2006[84]
COX-2/rofecoxib	WBN/Kob rats	Reduction in macrophage infiltration and fibrosis	Reding et al., 2006[113]
MPTP/tocotrienol (Vit. E derivative)	Isolated rat PSCs	Induce activated PSC death	Rickmann et al., 2007[102]
Interferon-γ	Isolated rat PSCs	Reduce PSC activation	Fitzner et al., 2007[119]
Withdrawal of alcohol	Rats fed an alcohol diet for 10 wks then LPS for 3 wks	Improvement in fibrosis and decreased PSC apoptosis	Vonlaufen et al., 2010[120]
Rapamycin	DBTC & cerulein rats	Reduced fibrosis, preservation of normoglycemia	Mayer et al, 2012[61]
Collagen siRNA to PSC/VA-lip-siRNAgp46	DBTC & cerulein rats	Resolution of pancreatic fibrosis	Ishiwatari et al., 2013[50]
Rhein (anthraquinone deriv.)	C57BL/6 mice cerulein for 6 wks, Treatment given on induction and later at 4wks	Decreased PSC activation and fibrosis in both intervention groups	Tsang et al., 2013[51]
ROS/edaravone	DBTC rat for 4 weeks; treatment after 2 weeks	Reduced fibrosis, PSC activation, and cytokine expression	Zhou et al., 2013[44]
ONO-1301 (prostacyclin analogue)	DBTC rats, treatment initiation at 1 wk, sacrifice 2 & 3 wks	Decrease in inflam. infiltrate 2 wks & fibrosis 3 wks	Niina et al., 2014[48]
Apigenin (flavonoid)	C57BL/6 mice cerulein treatment initiation at 1 wk, sacrifice at 4 wks	Decreased fibrosis and PSC activation	Mrazick et al., 2015[49]
IL-4/IL-13	C57BL/6 cerulein, IL-4/IL-13 -/- mice, human tissue	Inhibition decreases alternatively activated macrophages and fibrosis	Xue et al., 2015[78]

Most studies have employed standard cerulein mouse models of CP with assays of pancreatic fibrosis and PSC activation most commonly used as endpoints to assess efficacy (studies in chronological order; DBTC = dibutyltin dichloride; MPTP = mitochondrial permeability transition pore; ROS = reactive oxygen species).

especially attractive as cyclophilin D knockout is compatible with viability in utero and only a modest murine phenotype, whereas constitutive Orai1 knockout is not viable in utero. There is evidence that primary parenchymal protection is a workable strategy from studies of rapamycin in rats administered DBTV and cerulein to induce CP,[61] which acts at least in part to protect the mitochondrial compartment.[62,63] Nevertheless the approach requires further preclinical validation and the development of agents that are safe and can be administered orally over prolonged periods, if not indefinitely.

Cytokine inhibition

Cytokines as signaling molecules play a major role in CP pathogenesis. While they may comprise a disparate group with many individual cytokines and are often pleiotropic, they remain key factors for cell-cell signaling and PSC activation and thus important potential targets for CP. Indeed, numerous strategies have been employed to target cytokine signaling and attempt to develop treatments that might improve CP outcomes.

Transforming growth factor-β (TGF-β) is thought to regulate the production, degradation, and accumulation of ECM proteins, and to play an important role in the fibroproliferative changes that follow tissue injury in many vital organs and tissues including the heart, lung, kidney, and liver.[64,65] The importance of TGF-β signaling in fibrosis formation is underlined by experiments in transgenic mice overexpressing TGF-β1 in the pancreas.[66,67] These animals show histological changes that resemble human CP, including destruction of the exocrine pancreas and progressive accumulation of ECM in the pancreas. Pharmacological TGF-β inhibition holds promise as a treatment strategy. Halofuginone, an analogue of the plant alkaloid febrifugine, was recently tested in a cerulein experimental CP mouse model.[45] Halofuginone was found to prevent cerulein-dependent increase in collagen synthesis, collagen cross-linking enzyme P4HA, Cygb/STAP, and tissue inhibitors of metalloproteinase 2, through inhibition of serum response factor and the downstream TGF-β signaling component of Smad3 phosphorylation. Furthermore, in vitro cultured PSC proliferation and TGF-β-dependent increases in Cygb/STAP and transgelin synthesis and metalloproteinase 2 activity were inhibited. However, few specific TGF-β receptor kinase inhibitors exist, and while compounds such as SB-431542 that are being developed for the treatment of neoplasia[68] are available, their potential applications in CP remain to be explored. Gene therapy has been assessed to specifically target TGF-β[69] and shall be discussed further in the next section.

Interferons (IFNs) are multifunctional cytokines that block viral infection, modulate immune and inflammatory responses, and inhibit cell proliferation.[70] IFN-α is an effective drug already established in clinical practice for the treatment of patients with chronic hepatitis B or C associated with liver fibrosis,[71,72] acting partly through an inhibitory effect on hepatic stellate cells.[73,74] However, conflicting evidence exists about their potential role in CP. IFN-γ but not IFN-α has been demonstrated to exert inhibitory effects on PSC proliferation and collagen synthesis in vitro using recombinant rat IFN on isolated rat PSCs, but IFN-γ has been shown to decrease glucose-stimulated insulin release from islet cells and thus potentially play a role in CP endocrine dysfunction.[75] IFN-α in combination with ribavirin has been associated with drug-induced acute pancreatitis,[76] so although IFNs may still be of potential use as novel treatments in the chronic form of the disease, further characterization of their molecular effects is required before proceeding with further drug development. Similarly, TNF-α and IL-6 are both upregulated in CP and may be involved in immune cell signaling as well as activation of quiescent PSCs,[25] but modulating strategies using experimental and clinical anti-TNF (infliximab, golimumab) or anti-IL-6 (tocilizumab) agents[77] remain to be explored in CP. The clinical use of licensed biologics has increased in many inflammatory and other diseases over the last two decades such that this type of drug accounts for a major share of all drugs administered. Repositioning of a licensed drug or biological response modifier has many attractions, not least that drug development expense is substantially reduced.

Recent evidence suggests that pharmacological inhibition of IL-4 and IL-13 may hold significant potential in CP treatment. A very detailed and wide-ranging study was undertaken utilizing in vitro, in vivo, and ex vivo approaches to assess both transgenic mouse models and human pancreatic tissue from CP patients; the authors focused on the interaction between alternatively activated macrophages (AAMs) and PSCs through IL-4/IL-13 signaling.[78] The investigators found that AAMs are dominant in mouse and human CP and are dependent on interleukin IL-4 and IL-13 signaling. Furthermore they observed that mice lacking IL-4Rα, myeloid-specific IL-4Rα, and IL-4/IL-13 were less susceptible to pancreatic fibrosis, with mouse and human PSCs being a source of IL-4/IL-13. Finally, and probably most importantly, they showed that pharmacologic inhibition of IL-4/IL-13 using IL-4/IL-13 blocking peptide halfway through the course of an established mouse CP model and in human ex vivo studies decreased pancreatic AAMs and fibrosis.[78] Thus, as one of the most thorough studies published in the CP literature to date, the strategy of IL-4/IL-13 inhibition holds promise as a novel treatment pipeline for CP and identifies other potential immune targets associated with AAMs that may also be considered for targeting. As an example of possibilities with this target, Regeneron has developed dupilumab, an inhibitor of IL-4Rα, which is at an advanced stage of development for atopic disease.[79] There are thus significant possibilities for targeting cytokines in the treatment of CP that remain to be explored both experimentally and clinically.[80]

Treatments based on natural compounds

Natural products have been a rich source of compounds for drug discovery, but their use has somewhat diminished, partly due to the technical barriers of screening natural products in high-throughput assays against molecular targets.[81] Recent strategies have often employed natural product screening that utilizes recent technical advances in genomic and metabolomics approaches to augment traditional methods of studying natural products with an appreciation of functional assays and phenotypic screens specific to the particular disease under consideration, with most applications in the fields of cancer and microbiology.[82,83] The use of natural products as a base to guide drug discovery for CP has been increasingly implemented over the last 10 years,[35,45,70] with a number of compounds showing promise in experimental CP models. Polyphenols extracted from green tea exert inhibitory effects on isolated rat PSC activation and may be able to prevent the pancreatic fibrosis of CP.[84] Likewise, curcumin (diferuloyl-methane), a natural product from the spice turmeric,[85] has a variety of biological activities including anti-inflammatory,[86,87] antioxidant,[88] antifibrotic,[89,90] and has previously been shown to inhibit activation of isolated PSCs in vitro.[91] Vitamin A (retinol) and its metabolites all-trans retinoic acid (ATRA) and 9-cis retinoic acid (9-RA) were found to significantly inhibit cultured PSC proliferation and activation.[92] While further studies to evaluate these compounds in vivo are awaited, a number of natural compounds have been explored in more detail in the setting of CP.

Apigenin (4',5,7-trihydroxyflavone) is a natural compound with low intrinsic toxicity found in various fruits, vegetables, herbs, and beverages such as chamomile tea.[93] A recent study reported that apigenin treatment in a standard cerulein model of experimental CP inhibited PSC proliferation, induced PSC apoptosis, and minimized parathyroid hormone related peptide (PTHrP)-mediated PSC response to injury.[49] Furthermore novel analogues of apigenin are under development with chemical modifications directed to build a focused library of *O*-alkylamino-tethered apigenin derivatives at 4'-*O* position of the ring C, with the aim of enhancing the potency and overall drug-like properties including aqueous solubility.[94]

Rhein is a natural anthraquinone derivative, also known chemically as 9,10-dihydro-4, 5-dihydroxy-9, 10-dioxo-2-anthracenecarboxylic acid, that can be extracted from roots of Polygonaceae (rhubarb).[51] This yellow crystalline rhubarb extract has been used as a mild laxative agent and an astringent since ancient times in China.[95] In recent decades, administration of rhein in the range of 25 to 100 mg/kg/day has been demonstrated to exert diverse pharmacological actions including antimicrobial,[96] anti-angiogenic,[97] and anticancer activities.[98] Rhein administered at 50 mg/kg/day halfway through the course of an experimental cerulein CP mouse model was able to reverse fibrotic outcomes, and when administered in vitro, it was found to attenuate PSC activation and suppress sonic hedgehog signaling.[51]

Recent evidence suggests that the MPTP, a gatekeeper for cell death pathways in the injured cell, may be a crucial target for drug discovery in AP.[59] However as indicated previously, its potential use in CP is yet to be fully explored. Tocotrienol (α, β, γ, δ) and tocopherol (α, β, γ, δ) stereoisomers represent the two naturally occurring subclasses of vitamin E compounds. Although the diet of millions of people includes tocotrienol-rich foods such as palm oil or rice bran, more than 95% of the scientific literature on vitamin E has focused exclusively on α-tocopherol.[99] Despite some previous concerns on their bioavailability, it is now clear that dietary tocotrienols are well absorbed, show measurable plasma levels,[100] and are readily distributed throughout the tissues.[101] Accumulating evidence suggests that tocotrienols display greater beneficial effects than α-tocopherol because of their prominent antineoplastic, neuroprotective, cardioprotective, and cholesterol-lowering properties.[99] A recent study using a tocotrienol-rich fraction (TRF) from palm oil found that TRF but not α-tocopherol reduced viability of activated PSCs (not quiescent PSCs or isolated acinar cells) in vitro through apoptosis and autophagy and caused a sustained mitochondrial membrane depolarization and extensive cytochrome c release that was completely abolished with the MPTP inhibitor cyclosporine A.[102]

Although the findings from drugs developed based on natural compounds on isolated PSCs show promise,[102] they require validation in experimental CP models as well as ultimately human CP. The main challenge remains in refining compounds with regard to specificity for cell type and action, and this should remain the main focus of ongoing research.

Gene therapy strategies

Gene therapy strategies provide a distinct advantage in terms of treatment specificity and have been utilized in various CP studies. While pharmacological inhibition of TGF-β inhibition has previously been considered, inhibition employing an adenoviral vector expressing the entire extracellular domain of type II human TGF-β receptor (AdTβ-ExR) on a cerulein mouse model of experimental CP has also been tested.[69] The study evaluated pancreatic fibrosis, PSC activation, and apoptosis and proliferation of acinar cells by histology and immunostaining and found that pancreatic fibrosis in AdTβ-ExR-injected mice was significantly attenuated with a reduction of activated PSCs and apoptotic acinar cells but no change in proliferation.[69] Targeted encephalin gene therapy has been shown to reduce pain in experimental CP[103] but is unlikely to modify disease progression. Further research indicates that gene therapy may hold potential promise specifically in CP patients carrying a CFTR mutation.[104] Exogenous gene delivery of aquaporin water channels into the parotid glands of primary Sjögren syndrome patients has been successfully applied to treat the dry mouth symptoms that form part of the condition.[105] As an aside, the changes of pancreatic ductal fluid and ion concentration in pancreatitis are very similar to the mechanisms visible in cystic fibrosis (CF).[104] Therefore, drugs that are effective in CF may have benefits for patients suffering with CP, such as bromhexine hydrochloride, a bronchial mucolytic, that when administered to 12 patients with alcoholic CP yielded improvements in symptoms and exocrine function.[106]

Clearly like many other conditions, while having the advantage of being specific in nature, adopting gene therapy as an approach in CP remains challenging. This strategy is open to various potential drawbacks that have been discussed in length in the recent literature. CP is a multifactorial disorder with a polygenic predisposition; long-term outcomes remain unclear posing a number of ethical issues; and risks may exist from induction of tumor growth, initiation of the endogenous immune response, and the use of viral vectors for gene transmission.[107]

A strategy that harnesses the benefits of specific genetic technologies and bypasses the problems that may be associated with viral adenovectors is the use of siRNA to target the degradation of relevant mRNAs key to CP pathogenesis. Previous studies have demonstrated that siRNA against collagen-specific chaperone protein gp46, encapsulated in vitamin A-coupled liposomes (VA-lip-siRNAgp46), resolved fibrosis in a model of liver cirrhosis.[108] Subsequently the treatment was assessed as a treatment for pancreatic fibrosis in experimental DBTC- and cerulein-induced CP in rats.[50] The experimenters were able to demonstrate specific uptake of VA-lipsiRNAgp46 by conjugation with 60-carboxyfluorescein (FAM) followed by immunofluorescence showing uptake through the retinol-binding protein receptor by activated PSCs in vitro. This was accompanied by successful knockdown of gp46 and suppression of collagen secretion. The technique allowed specific delivery of VA-lip-siRNAgp46 to PSCs in fibrotic areas in DBTC rats, with 10 systemic treatments resolving pancreatic fibrosis and suppressing tissue hydroxyproline levels in both models.[50] While full translation of such siRNA strategies to the clinical setting remains some distance away, this study provides the first key demonstration of successful targeting of an antifibrotic drug to cells known to be responsible for pancreatic fibrosis and creates hope that similar strategies may be employed, potentially with other similar or even contrasting drug targets, to alter the course of CP.

Other approaches

A number of other drugs and strategies have been recently explored as treatments for CP with some promising findings. Camostat mesilate (CM), an oral protease inhibitor, has been used clinically for the treatment of CP in Japan.[47] This is mainly based on the theoretical benefit of decreasing prematurely activated trypsinogen in the pancreas, which is a key feature of acute acinar cell injury from a variety of pancreatic toxins.[109] Interestingly, CM has been shown to attenuate DBTC-induced rat pancreatic fibrosis probably via inhibition of monocytes and PSC activity.[47] However, a recent study employing transgenic mice conditionally expressing an endogenously activated trypsinogen within pancreatic acinar cells demonstrated that trypsin-mediated injury was sufficient for AP, but was not sufficient to drive pancreatic fibrosis and CP in the absence of other factors, raising questions as to the utility of protease inhibition as a strategy in CP.[110]

Cyclooxygenase (COX) is an enzyme that produces prostaglandins such as prostacyclin and thromboxane. COX-2 is not expressed under normal conditions in most cells but is elevated during inflammation. Modulation of prostaglandins in CP has produced conflicting findings. Numerous chronic inflammatory diseases can be successfully suppressed by COX-2 inhibitors,[111] and COX-2 is elevated in CP.[112] A recent study assessed administration of the selective COX-2 inhibitor rofecoxib on an experimental model of CP (WBN/Kob rat) and found reductions in chronic inflammatory changes and fibrosis following treatment, and in vitro studies suggested that the migration of macrophages in CP conditions is COX-2 dependent.[113] This would suggest a beneficial effect for CP from the reduction of prostaglandins including prostacyclin, which is in line with other inflammatory conditions. However, understanding this treatment strategy remains complex as a further recent study using ONO-1301, a novel sustained-release prostacyclin analogue shown to have antifibrotic effects in other organs, improved fibrosis in a DBTC rat model of CP although in vitro studies showed no effect of ONO-1301 on PSCs.[48] Clearly, COX-2 inhibition will decrease levels of prostaglandins other than prostacyclin, such as thromboxane, and this may be responsible for an overriding beneficial effect observed for this treatment strategy. Overall, these studies highlight that further characterization of this mechanistic pathway in the setting of CP is required to guide better drug development.

Braganza and colleagues first proposed that CP arose as a result of oxidative stress and that a deficient free radical-quenching system combined with excess free radical production led to cellular injury.[114] Reactive oxygen species (ROS) are known to be involved in PSC activation[40] and theoretically play an important role in CP pathogenesis. Braganza et al. reasoned that exogenous supplementation with antioxidants or precursors for antioxidant pathways might help reduce ongoing acinar injury.[114] After a small randomized trial of selenium, β-carotene, vitamins C and E, and methionine-based antioxidant therapy reported reductions in the severity and frequency of episodes of pain in patients with recurrent and CP, a commercially available formulation was developed; however, antioxidant therapy for CP has not become accepted as standard therapy, with recent trials suggesting that administration of antioxidants to patients with CP does not improve quality of life,[115] and a recent Cochrane review suggesting they may have only a small beneficial effect on pain.[116]

Many lessons can be learnt from the antioxidant treatment pipeline that can be implemented for other future strategies that may involve targets and compounds previously outlined in this review. The timing of intervention in the pathological process of fibrogenesis remains crucial, and studies allowing cross-comparability of interventional time points in preclinical studies with human CP are further required. Trials must use standardized clearly defined criteria for diagnosis of CP and hence include the most appropriate patients in trials. The composition of test compounds must be refined and standardized with multiple constituent strategies causing inevitable difficulties in cross-comparison between studies. Finally, relevant disease outcome measures must be standardized, and caution must be exercised in interpreting subjective measures such as pain and quality of life scores, alongside objective measures such as endocrine and exocrine insufficiency.

Conclusion

Multiple novel treatment pipelines have been identified by preclinical studies in CP over the last decade (**Figure 2**), with recent investigation focused on parenchymal protection, immunomodulation, and PSC inhibition as strategies to reduce pancreatic injury and fibrosis[117] and reduce the symptomatic and long-term impacts of the disease. Ultimately, whether these promising preclinical findings can impact human CP will depend on translation through well-structured and coordinated clinical trials. To date, trials have not provided any disease course-altering specific treatments, with many promising compounds still to be tested. There remain many pharmacological challenges in human CP that must be overcome for effective translation of preclinical findings. Drug absorption in patients with CP might be affected by disease pathophysiology, with exocrine insufficiency associated with changes in gastrointestinal intraluminal pH, motility disorder, bacterial overgrowth, and changed pancreatic gland secretion, resulting in potential malabsorption.[118] Coupled with this, the lifestyle of CP patients may also contribute to these pharmacological challenges with many patients limiting their food intake due to pain caused by eating that will affect drug absorption and compliance, as well as alcohol and drug interactions known to influence pharmacokinetics.[118] Nevertheless, there is considerable hope that future research will provide successful treatments. These treatments will likely originate from preidentified or novel drug targets based on a thorough understanding of pathogenesis, accompanied by clever drug design sensitive to the challenging group of CP patients, supported by sufficiently large and well-conducted clinical trials, with focused research for improved bench-to-beside translation.

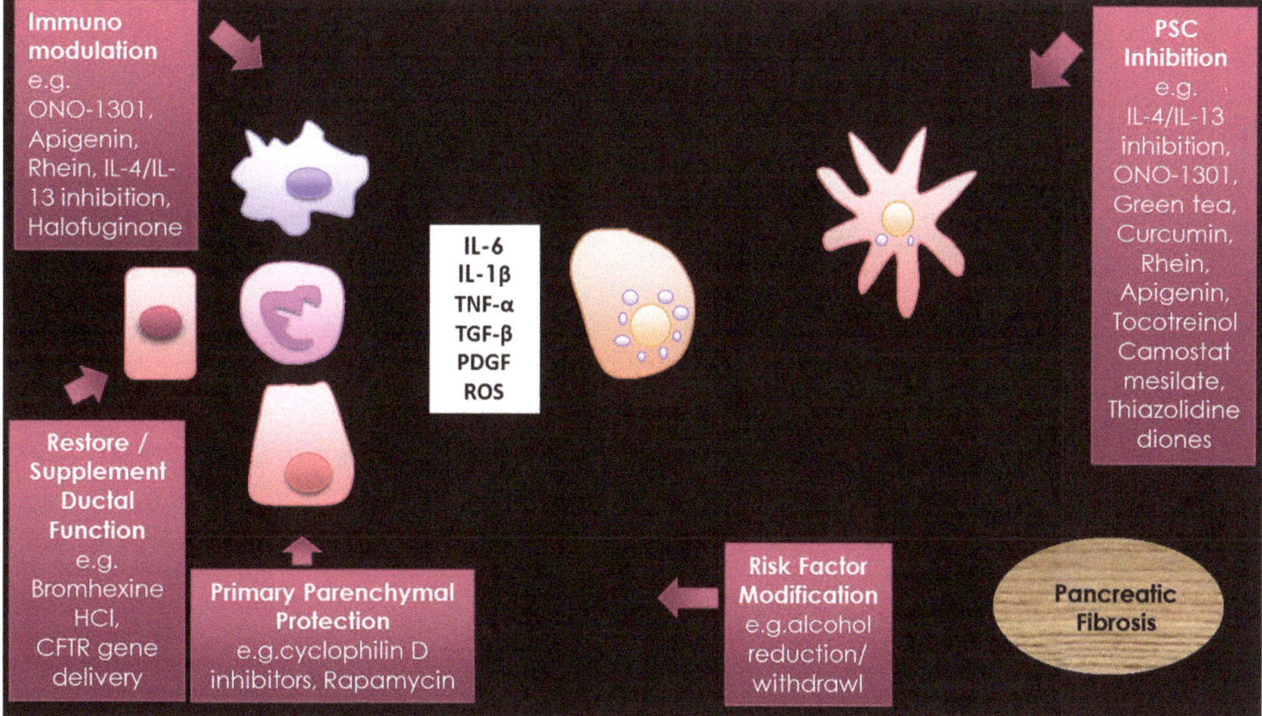

Figure 2. Summary of novel CP treatment pipelines. Numerous agents tested in the preclinical setting have been shown to be efficacious in improving experimental CP outcomes (predominantly PSC activation and histopathological evidence of pancreatic fibrosis), with many agents chiefly acting through modulation of either immune pathways, PSC activation, or both. Alcohol may exert its deleterious effects indirectly through repeated acinar cell injury or directly on PSCs. Recent evidence indicates an amplifying loop between alternatively activated macrophages and PSCs in CP through IL-4/IL-13 signaling, offering another therapeutic target.

Acknowledgement

We acknowledge funding support from CORE, the UK Medical Research Council, and the Biomedical Research Unit Funding scheme of the UK National Institute for Health Research. Robert Sutton is an NIHR Senior Investigator.

References

1. Muniraj T, Aslanian HR, Farrell J, Jamidar PA. Chronic pancreatitis, a comprehensive review and update. Part I: epidemiology, etiology, risk factors, genetics, pathophysiology, and clinical features. *Dis Mon.* 2014; 60: 530-550. PMID: 25510320.
2. Brock C, Nielsen LM, Lelic D, Drewes AM. Pathophysiology of chronic pancreatitis. *World J Gastroenterol.* 2013; 19: 7231-7240. PMID: 24259953.
3. Lévy P, Dominguez-Muñoz E, Imrie C, Löhr M, Maisonneuve P. Epidemiology of chronic pancreatitis: burden of the disease and consequences. *United European Gastroenterol J.* 2014; 2: 345-354. PMID: 25360312.
4. Lévy P, Milan C, Pignon JP, Baetz A, Bernades P. Mortality factors associated with chronic pancreatitis. Unidimensional and multidimensional analysis of a medical-surgical series of 240 patients. *Gastroenterology.* 1989; 96: 1165-1172. PMID: 2925060.
5. Pedrazzoli S, Pasquali C, Guzzinati S, Berselli M, Sperti C. Survival rates and cause of death in 174 patients with chronic pancreatitis. *J Gastrointest Surg.* 2008; 12: 1930-1937. PMID: 18766421.
6. Cote GA, Yadav D, Slivka A, Hawes RH, Anderson MA, Burton FR, et al. Alcohol and smoking as risk factors in an epidemiology study of patients with chronic pancreatitis. *Clin Gastroenterol Hepatol.* 2011; 9: 266-273; quiz e227. PMID: 21029787.
7. Whitcomb DC, Gorry MC, Preston RA, Furey W, Sossenheimer MJ, Ulrich CD, et al. Hereditary pancreatitis is caused by a mutation in the cationic trypsinogen gene. *Nat Genet.* 1996; 14: 141-145. PMID: 8841182.
8. Whitcomb DC, LaRusch J, Krasinskas AM, Klei L, Smith JP, Brand RE, et al. Common genetic variants in the CLDN2 and PRSS1-PRSS2 loci alter risk for alcohol-related and sporadic pancreatitis. *Nat Genet.* 2012; 44: 1349-1354. PMID: 23143602.
9. Trikudanathan G, Navaneethan U, Vege SS. Modern treatment of patients with chronic pancreatitis. *Gastroenterol Clin North Am.* 2012; 41: 63-76. PMID: 22341250.
10. Forsmark CE. Management of chronic pancreatitis. *Gastroenterology.* 2013; 144: 1282-1291.e3. PMID: 23622138.
11. Anderson MA, Akshintala V, Albers KM, Amann ST, Belfer I, Brand R, et al. Mechanism, assessment and management of pain in chronic pancreatitis: Recommendations of a multidisciplinary study group. *Pancreatology.* 2016; 16: 83-94. PMID: 26620965.
12. Everhart JE, Ruhl CE. Burden of digestive diseases in the United States Part III: Liver, biliary tract, and pancreas. *Gastroenterology.* 2009; 136: 1134-1144. PMID: 19245868.
13. Pelli H, Sand J, Laippala P, Nordback I. Long-term follow-up after the first episode of acute alcoholic pancreatitis: time course and risk factors for recurrence. *Scand J Gastroenterol.* 2000; 35: 552-555. PMID: 10868461.
14. Lankisch PG, Breuer N, Bruns A, Weber-Dany B, Lowenfels AB, Maisonneuve P. Natural history of acute pancreatitis: a long-term population-based study. *Am J Gastroenterol.* 2009; 104: 2797-2805; quiz 2806. PMID: 19603011.
15. Ammann RW, Muellhaupt B, Meyenberger C, Heitz PU. Alcoholic nonprogressive chronic pancreatitis: prospective long-term study of a large cohort with alcoholic acute pancreatitis (1976-1992). *Pancreas.* 1994; 9: 365-373. PMID: 8022760.
16. Nøjgaard C. Prognosis of acute and chronic pancreatitis - a 30-year follow-up of a Danish cohort. *Dan Med Bull.* 2010; 57: B4228. PMID: 21122467.
17. McKay CJ, Glen P, McMillan DC. Chronic inflammation and pancreatic cancer. *Best Pract Res Clin Gastroenterol.* 2008; 22: 65-73. PMID: 18206813.
18. Vitone LJ, Greenhalf W, Howes NR, Neoptolemos JP. Hereditary pancreatitis and secondary screening for early pancreatic cancer. *Rocz Akad Med Bialymst.* 2005; 50: 73-84. PMID: 16358943.
19. Whitcomb DC. Hereditary pancreatitis: new insights into acute and chronic pancreatitis. *Gut.* 1999; 45: 317-322. PMID: 10446089.
20. Schneider A, Whitcomb DC. Hereditary pancreatitis: a model for inflammatory diseases of the pancreas. *Best Pract Res Clin Gastroenterol.* 2002; 16: 347-363. PMID: 12079262.
21. Whitcomb DC. Mechanisms of disease: Advances in understanding the mechanisms leading to chronic pancreatitis. *Nat Clin Pract Gastroenterol Hepatol.* 2004; 1: 46-52. PMID: 16265044.
22. Witt H, Apte MV, Keim V, Wilson JS. Chronic pancreatitis: challenges and advances in pathogenesis, genetics, diagnosis, and therapy. *Gastroenterology.* 2007; 132: 1557-1573. PMID: 17466744.
23. Wilcox CM, Yadav D, Ye T, Gardner TB, Gelrud A, Sandhu BS, et al. Chronic pancreatitis pain pattern and severity are independent of abdominal imaging findings. *Clin Gastroenterol Hepatol.* 2015; 13: 552-560; quiz e28-e29. PMID: 25424572.
24. Omary MB, Lugea A, Lowe AW, Pandol SJ. The pancreatic stellate cell: a star on the rise in pancreatic diseases. *J Clin Invest.* 2007; 117: 50-59. PMID: 17200706.
25. Apte MV, Pirola RC, Wilson JS. Molecular mechanisms of alcoholic pancreatitis. *Dig Dis.* 2005; 23: 232-240. PMID: 16508287.
26. Schmid-Kotsas A, Gross HJ, Menke A, Weidenbach H, Adler G, Siech M, et al. Lipopolysaccharide-activated macrophages stimulate the synthesis of collagen type I and C-fibronectin in cultured pancreatic stellate cells. *Am J Pathol.* 1999; 155: 1749-1758. PMID: 10550331.
27. Treiber M, Neuhöfer P, Anetsberger E, Einwächter H, Lesina M, Rickmann M, et al. Myeloid, but not pancreatic, RelA/p65 is required for fibrosis in a mouse model of chronic pancreatitis. *Gastroenterology.* 2011; 141: 1473-1485. PMID: 21763242.
28. Hunger RE, Mueller C, Z'Graggen K, Friess H, Büchler MW. Cytotoxic cells are activated in cellular infiltrates

of alcoholic chronic pancreatitis. *Gastroenterology*. 1997; 112: 1656-1663. PMID: 9136845.

29. Grundsten M, Liu GZ, Permert J, Hjelmstrom P, Tsai JA. Increased central memory T cells in patients with chronic pancreatitis. *Pancreatology*. 2005; 5: 177-182. PMID: 15849488.
30. Mews P, Phillips P, Fahmy R, Korsten M, Pirola R, Wilson J, et al. Pancreatic stellate cells respond to inflammatory cytokines: potential role in chronic pancreatitis. *Gut*. 2002; 50: 535-541. PMID: 11889076.
31. Schmitz-Winnenthal H, Pietsch DH, Schimmack S, Bonertz A, Udonta F, Ge Y, et al. Chronic pancreatitis is associated with disease-specific regulatory T-cell responses. *Gastroenterology*. 2010; 138: 1178-1188. PMID: 19931255.
32. Apte MV, Pirola RC, Wilson JS. Pancreatic stellate cells: a starring role in normal and diseased pancreas. *Front Physiol*. 2012; 3: 344. PMID: 22973234.
33. McCarroll JA, Phillips PA, Park S, Doherty E, Pirola RC, Wilson JS, et al. Pancreatic stellate cell activation by ethanol and acetaldehyde: is it mediated by the mitogen-activated protein kinase signaling pathway? *Pancreas*. 2003; 27: 150-160. PMID: 12883264.
34. Nakatani K, Okuyama H, Shimahara Y, Saeki S, Kim DH, Nakajima Y, et al. Cytoglobin/STAP, its unique localization in splanchnic fibroblast-like cells and function in organ fibrogenesis. *Lab Invest*. 2004; 84: 91-101. PMID: 14647402.
35. Apte MV, Phillips PA, Fahmy RG, Darby SJ, Rodgers SC, McCaughan GW, et al. Does alcohol directly stimulate pancreatic fibrogenesis? Studies with rat pancreatic stellate cells. *Gastroenterology*. 2000; 118: 780-794. PMID: 10734030.
36. Luttenberger T, Schmid-Kotsas A, Menke A, Siech M, Beger H, Adler G, et al. Platelet-derived growth factors stimulate proliferation and extracellular matrix synthesis of pancreatic stellate cells: implications in pathogenesis of pancreas fibrosis. *Lab Invest*. 2000; 80: 47-55. PMID: 10653002.
37. Hirose H, Maruyama H, Kido K, Ito K, Koyama K, Tashiro Y, et al. Defective insulin and glucagon secretion in isolated perfused pancreata of diabetic WBN/Kob rats. *Pancreas*. 1995; 10: 71-77. PMID: 7899463.
38. Roberts AB, Russo A, Felici A, Flanders KC. Smad3: a key player in pathogenetic mechanisms dependent on TGF-beta. *Ann N Y Acad Sci*. 2003; 995: 1-10. PMID: 12814934.
39. Qiu P, Feng XH, Li L. Interaction of Smad3 and SRF-associated complex mediates TGF-beta1 signals to regulate SM22 transcription during myofibroblast differentiation. *J Mol Cell Cardiol*. 2003; 35: 1407-1420. PMID: 14654367.
40. Apte M, Pirola RC, Wilson JS. Pancreatic stellate cell: physiologic role, role in fibrosis and cancer. *Curr Opin Gastroenterol*. 2015; 31: 416-423. PMID: 26125317.
41. Ino K, Masuya M, Tawara I, Miyata E, Oda K, Nakamori Y, et al. Monocytes infiltrate the pancreas via the MCP-1/CCR2 pathway and differentiate into stellate cells. *PLoS One*. 2014; 9: e84889. PMID: 24416305.
42. Zha M, Xu W, Zhai Q, Li F, Chen B, Sun Z. High glucose aggravates the detrimental effects of pancreatic stellate cells on Beta-cell function. *Int J Endocrinol*. 2014; 2014: 165612. PMID: 25097548.
43. Zechner D, Knapp N, Bobrowski A, Radecke T, Genz B, Vollmar B. Diabetes increases pancreatic fibrosis during chronic inflammation. *Exp Biol Med (Maywood)*. 2014; 239: 670-676. PMID: 24719378.
44. Zhou CH, Lin L, Zhu XY, Wen T, Hu DM, Dong Y, et al. Protective effects of edaravone on experimental chronic pancreatitis induced by dibutyltin dichloride in rats. *Pancreatology*. 2013; 13: 125-132. PMID: 23561970.
45. Zion O, Genin O, Kawada N, Yoshizato K, Roffe S, Nagler A, et al. Inhibition of transforming growth factor beta signaling by halofuginone as a modality for pancreas fibrosis prevention. *Pancreas*. 2009; 38: 427-435. PMID: 19188864.
46. Jaster R, Lichte P, Fitzner B, Brock P, Glass A, Karopka T, et al. Peroxisome proliferator-activated receptor gamma overexpression inhibits pro-fibrogenic activities of immortalised rat pancreatic stellate cells. *J Cell Mol Med*. 2005; 9: 670-682. PMID: 16202214.
47. Gibo J, Ito T, Kawabe K, Hisano T, Inoue M, Fujimori N, et al. Camostat mesilate attenuates pancreatic fibrosis via inhibition of monocytes and pancreatic stellate cells activity. *Lab Invest*. 2005; 85: 75-89. PMID: 15531908.
48. Niina Y, Ito T, Oono T, Nakamura T, Fujimori N, Igarashi H, et al. A sustained prostacyclin analog, ONO-1301, attenuates pancreatic fibrosis in experimental chronic pancreatitis induced by dibutyltin dichloride in rats. *Pancreatology*. 2014; 14: 201-210. PMID: 24854616.
49. Mrazek AA, Porro LJ, Bhatia V, Falzon M, Spratt H, Zhou J, et al. Apigenin inhibits pancreatic stellate cell activity in pancreatitis. *J Surg Res* 196(1): 8-16, 2015. PMID: 25799526.
50. Ishiwatari H, Sato Y, Murase K, Yoneda A, Fujita R, Nishita H, et al. Treatment of pancreatic fibrosis with siRNA against a collagen-specific chaperone in vitamin A-coupled liposomes. *Gut*. 2013; 62: 1328-1339. PMID: 23172890.
51. Tsang SW, Zhang H, Lin C, Xiao H, Wong M, Shang H, et al. Rhein, a natural anthraquinone derivative, attenuates the activation of pancreatic stellate cells and ameliorates pancreatic fibrosis in mice with experimental chronic pancreatitis. *PLoS One*. 2013; 8: e82201. PMID: 24312641.
52. Lerch MM, Gorelick FS. Models of acute and chronic pancreatitis. *Gastroenterology*. 2013; 144: 1180-1193. PMID: 23622127.
53. Athwal T, Huang W, Mukherjee R, Latawiec D, Chvanov M, Clarke R, et al. Expression of human cationic trypsinogen (PRSS1) in murine acinar cells promotes pancreatitis and apoptotic cell death. *Cell Death Dis*. 2014; 5: e1165. PMID: 24722290.
54. Etemad B, Whitcomb DC. Chronic pancreatitis: diagnosis, classification, and new genetic developments. *Gastroenterology*. 2001; 120: 682-707. PMID: 11179244.
55. Criddle DN, Raraty MG, Neoptolemos JP, Tepikin AV, Petersen OH, Sutton R. Ethanol toxicity in pancreatic acinar cells: mediation by nonoxidative fatty acid metabolites. *Proc Natl Acad Sci U S A*. 2004; 101: 10738-10743. PMID: 15247419.
56. Criddle DN, Murphy J, Fistetto G, Barrow S, Tepikin AV, Neoptolemos JP, et al. Fatty acid ethyl esters cause pancreatic calcium toxicity via inositol trisphosphate receptors and loss of ATP synthesis. *Gastroenterology*. 2006; 130: 781-793. PMID: 16530519.

57. Huang W, Booth DM, Cane MC, Chvanov M, Javed MA, Elliott VL, et al. Fatty acid ethyl ester synthase inhibition ameliorates ethanol-induced Ca^{2+}-dependent mitochondrial dysfunction and acute pancreatitis. *Gut*. 2014; 63: 1313-1324. PMID: 24162590.
58. Maléth J, Balázs A, Pallagi P, Balla Z, Kui B, Katona M, et al. Alcohol disrupts levels and function of the cystic fibrosis transmembrane conductance regulator to promote development of pancreatitis. *Gastroenterology*. 2015; 148: 427-439. PMID: 25447846.
59. Mukherjee R, Mareninova OA, Odinokova IV, Huang W, Murphy J, Chvanov M, et al. Mechanism of mitochondrial permeability transition pore induction and damage in the pancreas: inhibition prevents acute pancreatitis by protecting production of ATP. *Gut*. 2016; 65: 1333-1146. PMID: 26071131.
60. Wen L, Voronina S, Javed MA, Awais M, Szatmary P, Latawiec D, et al. Inhibitors of ORAI1 prevent cytosolic calcium-associated injury of human pancreatic acinar cells and acute pancreatitis in 3 mouse models. *Gastroenterology*. 2015; 149: 481-492. PMID: 25917787.
61. Mayer JM, Kolodziej S, Jukka Laine V, Kahl S. Immunomodulation in a novel model of experimental chronic pancreatitis. *Minerva Gastroenterol Dietol*. 2012; 58: 347-354. PMID: 23207611.
62. Perluigi M, Di Domenico F, Butterfield DA. mTOR signaling in aging and neurodegeneration: At the crossroad between metabolism dysfunction and impairment of autophagy. *Neurobiol Dis*. 2015; 84: 39-49. PMID: 25796566.
63. Green DR, Galluzzi L, Kroemer G. Cell biology. Metabolic control of cell death. *Science*. 2014; 345: 1250256. PMID: 25237106.
64. Massague J. The transforming growth factor-beta family. *Annu Rev Cell Biol*. 1990; 6: 597-641. PMID: 2177343.
65. Broekelmann TJ, Limper AH, Colby TV, McDonald JA. Transforming growth factor beta 1 is present at sites of extracellular matrix gene expression in human pulmonary fibrosis. *Proc Natl Acad Sci U S A*. 1991; 88: 6642-6646. PMID: 1862087.
66. Lee MS, Gu D, Feng L, Curriden S, Arnush M, Krahl T, et al. Accumulation of extracellular matrix and developmental dysregulation in the pancreas by transgenic production of transforming growth factor-beta 1. *Am J Pathol*. 1995; 147: 42-52. PMID: 7604884.
67. Sanvito F, Nichols A, Herrera PL, Huarte J, Wohlwend A, Vassalli JD, et al. TGF-beta 1 overexpression in murine pancreas induces chronic pancreatitis and, together with TNF-alpha, triggers insulin-dependent diabetes. *Biochem Biophys Res Commun*. 1995; 217: 1279-1286. PMID: 8554587.
68. Halder SK, Beauchamp RD, Datta PK. A specific inhibitor of TGF-beta receptor kinase, SB-431542, as a potent antitumor agent for human cancers. *Neoplasia*. 2005; 7: 509-521. PMID: 15967103.
69. Nagashio Y, Ueno H, Imamura M, Asaumi H, Watanabe S, Yamaguchi T, et al. Inhibition of transforming growth factor beta decreases pancreatic fibrosis and protects the pancreas against chronic injury in mice. *Lab Invest*. 2004; 84: 1610-1618. PMID: 15502860.
70. Stark GR, Kerr IM, Williams BR, Silverman RH, Schreiber RD. How cells respond to interferons. *Annu Rev Biochem*. 1998; 67: 227-264. PMID: 9759489.
71. Nguyen MH, Wright TL. Therapeutic advances in the management of hepatitis B and hepatitis C. *Curr Opin Infect Dis*. 2001; 14: 593-601. PMID: 11964881.
72. Schuppan D, Krebs A, Bauer M, Hahn EG. Hepatitis C and liver fibrosis. *Cell Death Differ*. 2003; 10 Suppl 1: S59-S67. PMID: 12655347.
73. Shen H, Zhang M, Minuk GY, Gong Y. Different effects of rat interferon alpha, beta and gamma on rat hepatic stellate cell proliferation and activation. *BMC Cell Biol*. 2002; 3: 9. PMID: 11940252.
74. Baroni GS, D'Ambrosio L, Curto P, Casini A, Mancini R, Jezequel AM, et al. Interferon gamma decreases hepatic stellate cell activation and extracellular matrix deposition in rat liver fibrosis. *Hepatology*. 1996; 23: 1189-1199. PMID: 8621153.
75. Pavan Kumar P, Radhika G, Rao GV, Pradeep R, Subramanyam C, Talukdar R, et al. Interferon gamma and glycemic status in diabetes associated with chronic pancreatitis. *Pancreatology*. 2012; 12: 65-70. PMID: 22487478.
76. Eland IA, Rasch MC, Sturkenboom MJ, Bekkering FC, Brouwer JT, Delwaide J, et al. Acute pancreatitis attributed to the use of interferon alfa-2b. *Gastroenterology*. 2000; 119: 230-233. PMID: 10889173.
77. Scheller J, Garbers C, Rose-John S. Interleukin-6: from basic biology to selective blockade of pro-inflammatory activities. *Semin Immunol*. 2014; 26: 2-12. PMID: 24325804.
78. Xue J, Sharma V, Hsieh MH, Chawla A, Murali R, Pandol SJ, et al. Alternatively activated macrophages promote pancreatic fibrosis in chronic pancreatitis. *Nat Commun*. 2015; 6: 7158. PMID: 25981357.
79. Wenzel S, Castro M, Corren J, Maspero J, Wang L, Zhang B, et al. Dupilumab efficacy and safety in adults with uncontrolled persistent asthma despite use of medium-to-high-dose inhaled corticosteroids plus a long-acting beta2 agonist: a randomised double-blind placebo-controlled pivotal phase 2b dose-ranging trial. *Lancet*. 2016; 388: 31-44. PMID: 27130691.
80. Xue J, Sharma V, Habtezion A. Immune cells and immune-based therapy in pancreatitis. *Immunol Res*. 2014; 58: 378-386. PMID: 24710635.
81. Harvey AL, Edrada-Ebel R, Quinn RJ. The re-emergence of natural products for drug discovery in the genomics era. *Nat Rev Drug Discov*. 2015; 14: 111-129. PMID: 25614221.
82. Jones RJ, Gu D, Bjorklund CC, Kuiatse I, Remaley AT, Bashir T, et al. The novel anticancer agent JNJ-26854165 induces cell death through inhibition of cholesterol transport and degradation of ABCA1. *J Pharmacol Exp Ther*. 2013; 346: 381-392. PMID: 23820125.
83. Balakrishnan K, Gandhi V. Bcl-2 antagonists: a proof of concept for CLL therapy. *Invest New Drugs*. 2013; 31: 1384-1394. PMID: 23907405.
84. Asaumi H, Watanabe S, Taguchi M, Tashiro M, Nagashio Y, Nomiyama Y, et al. Green tea polyphenol (-)-epigallocatechin-3-gallate inhibits ethanol-induced activation of pancreatic stellate cells. *Eur J Clin Invest*. 2006; 36: 113-122. PMID: 16436093.

85. Govindarajan VS. Turmeric--chemistry, technology, and quality. *Crit Rev Food Sci Nutr*. 1980; 12: 199-301. PMID: 6993103.
86. Sugimoto K, Hanai H, Tozawa K, Aoshi T, Uchijima M, Nagata T, et al. Curcumin prevents and ameliorates trinitrobenzene sulfonic acid-induced colitis in mice. *Gastroenterology*. 2002; 123: 1912-1922. PMID: 12454848.
87. Gukovsky I, Reyes CN, Vaquero EC, Gukovskaya AS, Pandol SJ. Curcumin ameliorates ethanol and nonethanol experimental pancreatitis. *Am J Physiol Gastrointest Liver Physiol*. 2003; 284: G85-95. PMID: 12488237.
88. Rajakumar DV, Rao MN. Antioxidant properties of phenyl styryl ketones. *Free Radic Res*. 1995; 22: 309-317. PMID: 7633561.
89. Punithavathi D, Venkatesan N, Babu M. Curcumin inhibition of bleomycin-induced pulmonary fibrosis in rats. *Br J Pharmacol*. 2000; 131: 169-172. PMID: 10991907.
90. Kang HC, Nan JX, Park PH, Kim JY, Lee SH, Woo SW, et al. Curcumin inhibits collagen synthesis and hepatic stellate cell activation in-vivo and in-vitro. *J Pharm Pharmacol*. 2002; 54: 119-126. PMID: 11829122.
91. Masamune A, Suzuki N, Kikuta K, Satoh M, Satoh K, Shimosegawa T. Curcumin blocks activation of pancreatic stellate cells. *J Cell Biochem*. 2006; 97: 1080-1093. PMID: 16294327.
92. McCarroll JA, Phillips PA, Santucci N, Pirola RC, Wilson JS, Apte MV. Vitamin A inhibits pancreatic stellate cell activation: implications for treatment of pancreatic fibrosis. *Gut*. 2006; 55: 79-89. PMID: 16043492.
93. Shukla S, Gupta S. Apigenin: a promising molecule for cancer prevention. *Pharm Res*. 2010; 27: 962-978. PMID: 20306120.
94. Chen H, Mrazek AA, Wang X, Ding C, Ding Y, Porro LJ, et al. Design, synthesis, and characterization of novel apigenin analogues that suppress pancreatic stellate cell proliferation in vitro and associated pancreatic fibrosis in vivo. *Bioorg Med Chem*. 2014; 22: 3393-3404. PMID: 24837156.
95. Yang DY, Fushimi H, Cai SQ, Komatsu K. Molecular analysis of Rheum species used as Rhei Rhizoma based on the chloroplast matK gene sequence and its application for identification. *Biol Pharm Bull*. 2004; 27: 375-383. PMID: 14993806.
96. Wang J, Zhao H, Kong W, Jin C, Zhao Y, Qu Y, et al. Microcalorimetric assay on the antimicrobial property of five hydroxyanthraquinone derivatives in rhubarb (Rheum palmatum L.) to Bifidobacterium adolescentis. *Phytomedicine*. 2010; 17: 684-689. PMID: 19962872.
97. He ZH, Zhou R, He MF, Lau CB, Yue GG, Ge W, et al. Anti-angiogenic effect and mechanism of rhein from Rhizoma Rhei. *Phytomedicine* 18(6): 470-478, 2011. PMID: 21112197.
98. Yang X, Sun G, Yang C, Wang B. Novel rhein analogues as potential anticancer agents. *ChemMedChem*. 2011; 6: 2294-2301. PMID: 21954017.
99. Sen CK, Khanna S, Roy S. Tocotrienols: Vitamin E beyond tocopherols. *Life Sci*. 2006; 78: 2088-2098. PMID: 16458936.
100. Khosla P, Patel V, Whinter JM, Khanna S, Rakhkovskaya M, Roy S, et al. Postprandial levels of the natural vitamin E tocotrienol in human circulation. *Antioxid Redox Signal*. 2006; 8: 1059-1068. PMID: 16771695.
101. Patel V, Khanna S, Roy S, Ezziddin O, Sen CK. Natural vitamin E alpha-tocotrienol: retention in vital organs in response to long-term oral supplementation and withdrawal. *Free Radic Res*. 2006; 40: 763-771. PMID: 16984003.
102. Rickmann M, Vaquero EC, Malagelada JR, Molero X. Tocotrienols induce apoptosis and autophagy in rat pancreatic stellate cells through the mitochondrial death pathway. *Gastroenterology*. 2007; 132: 2518-2532. PMID: 17570223.
103. Westlund KN. Gene therapy for pancreatitis pain. *Gene Ther*. 2009; 16: 483-492. PMID: 19262610.
104. Balazs A, Hegyi P. Cystic fibrosis-style changes in the early phase of pancreatitis. *Clin Res Hepatol Gastroenterol*. 39 Suppl 1: S12-17, 2015. PMID: 26206571.
105. Yin H, Cabrera-Perez J, Lai Z, Michael D, Weller M, Swaim WD, et al. Association of bone morphogenetic protein 6 with exocrine gland dysfunction in patients with Sjögren's syndrome and in mice. *Arthritis Rheum*. 2013; 65: 3228-3238. PMID: 23982860.
106. Tsujimoto T, Tsuruzono T, Hoppo K, Matsumura Y, Yamao J, Fukui H. Effect of bromhexine hydrochloride therapy for alcoholic chronic pancreatitis. *Alcohol Clin Exp Res*. 2005; 29 12 Suppl: 272S-276S. PMID: 16385235.
107. Kaufmann KB, Buning H, Galy A, Schambach A, Grez M. Gene therapy on the move. *EMBO Mol Med*. 2013; 5: 1642-1661. PMID: 24106209.
108. Sato Y, Murase K, Kato J, Kobune M, Sato T, Kawano Y, et al. Resolution of liver cirrhosis using vitamin A-coupled liposomes to deliver siRNA against a collagen-specific chaperone. *Nat Biotechnol*. 2008; 26: 431-442. PMID: 18376398.
109. Rinderknecht H. Activation of pancreatic zymogens. Normal activation, premature intrapancreatic activation, protective mechanisms against inappropriate activation. *Dig Dis Sci*. 1986; 31: 314-321. PMID: 2936587.
110. Gaiser S, Daniluk J, Liu Y, Tsou L, Chu J, Lee W, et al. Intracellular activation of trypsinogen in transgenic mice induces acute but not chronic pancreatitis. *Gut*. 2011; 60: 1379-1388. PMID: 21471572.
111. Matheson AJ, Figgitt DP. Rofecoxib: a review of its use in the management of osteoarthritis, acute pain and rheumatoid arthritis. *Drugs*. 2001; 61: 833-865. PMID: 11398914.
112. Schlosser W, Schlosser S, Ramadani M, Gansauge F, Gansauge S, Beger HG. Cyclooxygenase-2 is overexpressed in chronic pancreatitis. *Pancreas*. 2002; 25: 26-30. PMID: 12131767.
113. Reding T, Bimmler D, Perren A, Sun LK, Fortunato F, Storni F, et al. A selective COX-2 inhibitor suppresses chronic pancreatitis in an animal model (WBN/Kob rats): significant reduction of macrophage infiltration and fibrosis. *Gut*. 2006; 55: 1165-1173. PMID: 16322109.
114. Uden S, Bilton D, Nathan L, Hunt LP, Main C, Braganza JM. Antioxidant therapy for recurrent pancreatitis: placebo-controlled trial. *Aliment Pharmacol Ther*. 1990; 4: 357-371. PMID: 2103755.
115. Siriwardena AK, Mason JM, Sheen AJ, Makin AJ, Shah NS. Antioxidant therapy does not reduce pain in patients with chronic pancreatitis: the ANTICIPATE study. *Gastroenterology*. 2012; 143: 655-663. PMID: 22683257.

116. Ahmed Ali U, Jens S, Busch OR, Keus F, van Goor H, Gooszen HG, et al. Antioxidants for pain in chronic pancreatitis. *Cochrane Database Syst Rev*. 2014; 8: CD008945. PMID: 25144441.
117. Zheng L, Xue J, Jaffee EM, Habtezion A. Role of immune cells and immune-based therapies in pancreatitis and pancreatic ductal adenocarcinoma. *Gastroenterology*. 2013; 144: 1230-1240. PMID: 23622132.
118. Olesen AE, Brokjaer A, Fisher IW, Larsen IM. Pharmacological challenges in chronic pancreatitis. *World J Gastroenterol*. 2013; 19: 7302-7307. PMID: 24259961.
119. Fitzner B, Brock P, Nechutova H, Glass A, Karopka T, Koczan D, et al. Inhibitory effects of interferon-gamma on activation of rat pancreatic stellate cells are mediated by STAT1 and involve down-regulation of CTGF expression. *Cell Signal*. 2007; 19: 782-790. PMID: 17116388.
120. Vonlaufen A, Phillips PA, Xu Z, Zhang X, Yang L, Pirola RC, et al. Withdrawal of alcohol promotes regression while continued alcohol intake promotes persistence of LPS-induced pancreatic injury in alcohol-fed rats. *Gut*. 2011; 60: 238-246. PMID: 20870739.

Autoimmune Pancreatitis

Section Editors: Suresh T. Chari and Philip A. Hart

Chapter 54

Evolution of the concept of autoimmune pancreatitis and its subtypes

Daniel Longnecker*

Department of Pathology, Geisel School of Medicine at Dartmouth, Lebanon, NH.

The concept, recognition, and characterization of autoimmune pancreatitis (AIP) have evolved in multiple centers and countries over the course of more than 50 years. The possibility that pancreatitis is sometimes caused by autoimmune mechanisms was considered as early as 1959, but the characteristic clinical, imaging, and histopathologic features for such patients were not recorded until the 1990s. Yoshida is credited with introducing the term "autoimmune pancreatitis" into the English literature in 1995, although "autoimmunpankreatitis" was mentioned in a German review by Putzke in 1979.[1-2] Acceptance of the term AIP and an increasing focus on the diagnosis, description, and treatment of the disease is evident in Ovid searches for "autoimmune pancreatitis" in sequential intervals. There were 192 papers published between 1996 and 2005, with the majority initially coming from Japan, and 888 papers from around the world between 2006 and June 2013. Putzke suggested AIP as a possible cause of chronic sclerosing pancreatitis, noting the prominence of interstitial lymphoplasmacytic infiltrates and perilobular, intralobular, and periductal fibrosis in some pancreases consistent with current histopathologic criteria for the diagnosis of AIP.[1] Yoshida mentioned 11 cases including 1 of their own and 10 others reported from 1961–1991.[2]

Thal et al. made an early reference to the possible autoimmune etiology of pancreatitis in 1959 when they reported antipancreatic antibodies in patients with chronic pancreatitis[3] and subsequently commented that "the finding of true auto-antibodies in this case raised the interesting possibility that his disease was either precipitated by or aggravated by an auto-immunizing mechanism".[4]

In 1961, Sarles described a group of patients as having "primary inflammatory sclerosis" of the pancreas.[5] The authors mentioned lymphoplasmacytic infiltrate, perilobular fibrosis, and lobular sclerosis in one pancreas and hypergammaglobulinemia in two patients. These findings are supportive of a diagnosis of AIP although the clinical and pathologic data are insufficient to allow a firm retrospective diagnosis of AIP for all patients in the group. The authors speculated, "It is thus possible to put forward the hypothesis that this type of pancreatitis is an inflammatory, noninfectious disease that is caused by phenomena of self-immunization".[5]

The dominant view regarding the pathogenesis of immune-mediated pancreatitis initially centered on humoral immunity. This view was partly based on studies in which animals were immunized with and developed antibodies against pancreas-derived fractions and subsequently developed pancreatic fibrosis.[6] Thal stated, "It is not yet clear whether these circulating antibodies are merely a side result of a more important reaction of the delayed hypersensitivity type occurring at the cellular level".[6] A central role for antibody-mediated injury was supported by a later study in which diffuse interstitial pancreatitis developed in mice treated with antiserum from guinea pigs immunized with pancreatic fractions.[7] More recently, Narula and colleagues noted that it is unclear whether autoantibodies that induce immunoglobulin G (IgG) and IgG4 elevations in AIP patients represent an epiphenomenon or play a role in disease pathogenesis.[8]

The central role of cell-mediated immunity in the pathogenesis of autoimmune diseases was initially recognized in 1974.[9] It was specifically supported as a possible mechanism in AIP by the demonstration of high numbers of T lymphocytes in pancreatic infiltrates in AIP[10-11] and experimentally by the induction of pancreatitis in rats by adoptive transfer of CD4(+) T cells sensitized to a pancreatic epitope.[12]

AIP is a rare disease with an estimated annual incidence of 0.82 per 100,000 in Japan.[13] The incidence in western nations is probably similarly low,[14-15] and most clinicians, radiologists, and pathologists likely see only occasional cases, slowing diagnosis. There is evidence that the incidence of AIP has dramatically risen in the past two decades, providing a basis for recent wider recognition of the disease.[16]

Because AIP may cause pancreatic enlargement that is often localized in the head or present with obstructive jaundice, many patients with these inflammatory masses

*Corresponding author. Email: daniel.s.longnecker@dartmouth.edu

have undergone pancreatectomies based on a preoperative clinical diagnosis of a pancreatic neoplasm and were postoperatively diagnosed with pancreatitis by the surgical pathologist. Experience with such cases is the basis for the histopathologic diagnosis of AIP. Retrospective studies indicate that 2.2%-2.6% of pancreatectomies were done because of mass-forming AIP.[17-20] Most of these data reflect a period before an emphasis on the clinical diagnosis of AIP, and this rate is expected to decrease with improved recognition.[21]

Heterogeneity in the pathology of AIP resection specimens has now resolved into the recognition of at least two AIP subtypes. Early descriptions focused on the prominence of mixed infiltrates of lymphocytes and plasma cells in some cases of chronic pancreatitis and led to the descriptive diagnosis "lymphoplasmacytic sclerosing pancreatitis" (LPSP), now often referred to as type 1 AIP.[22]

The 1997 paper by Ectors et al. identified a pattern of chronic pancreatitis in a group of resected pancreases from non-alcoholic patients that was clearly different than that seen in alcoholics.[10] The term "chronic non-alcoholic duct destructive pancreatitis" was coined. Some (4/12) of these patients had autoimmune disease manifestations in other organs. An autoimmune etiology was carefully considered, although the pancreatitis was ultimately classified as idiopathic. Ectors noted that intraductal aggregates of neutrophilic granulocytes were commonly associated with duct destructive lesions.[10] Later, the neutrophilic aggregates were called "granulocytic epithelial lesions (GEL), which are now recognized as a characteristic of type 2 AIP.[23-24] This pattern is also referred to as IDCP. The basis for this acronym is ambiguous, being defined variously as "idiopathic duct centric pancreatitis" and "idiopathic duct-centric chronic pancreatitis".[11,15,25-26]

Suda described early and late-stage AIP, with the latter based on prominent acinar cell loss.[27] All specimens were from pancreatic resection or biopsy and contained inflamed ducts. Although the late-stage patients (n = 11) were about 2.5 years older than the early stage group (n = 20) at disease onset, the age difference was not significant. The degree of lymphoplasmacytic infiltration was more variable, and venulitis was less frequent in the late-stage pancreases, but it is not obvious that they should be regarded as end stage. It is not known if end-stage AIP can be distinguished from the late state of chronic pancreatitis due to other etiologies.

The possible role of IgG4 in AIP pathogenesis and subsequent recognition of IgG4-associated systemic autoimmune disease has evolved.[28] As noted above, there is often concordant involvement of other organs in AIP patients.[2,10] There is evidence of autoimmune processes affecting other organs in a quarter to more than half of AIP patients in different series.

A variety of autoantibodies were detected in patients with AIP, and hypergammaglobulinemia was documented in some patients.[2,5] This led to the examination of immunoglobulin subclasses and recognition in 2001 that IgG4 was elevated in the serum of most Japanese patients with AIP.[28,29] Later, increased numbers of IgG4-positive plasma cells were demonstrated in a high fraction of pancreases with AIP, and similar elevations of IgG4-positive cells were identified in other involved organs.[28] This led to the proposal that AIP was part of an IgG4-associated systemic autoimmune disease (13, 15).[28,30] In a 2008 review, Kamisawa stated, "This disease includes AIP, sclerosing cholangitis, cholecystitis, sialadenitis, retroperitoneal fibrosis, tubulointerstitial nephritis, interstitial pneumonia, prostatitis, inflammatory pseudotumor and lymphadenopathy, all IgG4-related".[31] Almost all "autoimmune" disorders associated with AIP have now been proven to be manifestations of IgG4-related disease.

As the literature for AIP is reviewed, it is necessary to consider the content of each report. It is typical for series from Japan to be entirely or predominantly composed of type 1 AIP patients, which is the form seen in multi-organ IgG4-related disease. Accordingly, we find that as many as 95% of patients in Japanese series have elevated serum IgG4.[29] In contrast, the fraction of patients with elevated IgG4 in series from the US and Europe is 50%-76% depending in part on the cut-off level.[32-33] The lower frequency of serum IgG4 elevation may be due to the inclusion of type 2 AIP patients who typically do not have serum IgG4 elevations.[34] However, true seronegative type 1 AIP (i.e., with normal serum IgG4) is also well described; such patients do show abundant IgG4+ plasma cell infiltration despite normal serum IgG4 levels.[35]

Although most AIP can be classified by expert pathologists as type 1 or 2 based on resection specimen histopathology, a few cases are difficult to classify with the current criteria.[25,36] We do not know if these are simply examples of atypical type 1 or 2 AIP due to differences in stage or degree of involvement or whether they represent rarer disease subtypes. Recognition of rare subtypes of a rare disease will be difficult and may require new genetic or immunologic markers.

The concept of AIP and its subtypes has evolved as the understanding of this unique form of pancreatitis has improved. The following chapters further expand this discussion and focus on a variety of aspects of AIP, including the key diagnostic features, treatment, and long-term outcomes. Recent immunohistochemical and molecular studies have demonstrated differences in inflammatory mediators between type 1 and type 2 AIP that validate their distinction as was originally established on the basis of histologic and clinical data.[37]

Acknowledgement

This introduction is excerpted in part from a previously published chapter on a similar topic.[38]

The author thanks the current editors for substantive input during preparation of this updated overview.

References

1. Putzke HP. Morphology of acute and chronic pancreatitis. *Z Gesamte Inn Med.* 1979; 34(10): 266-271. PMID: 483921
2. Yoshida K, Toki F, Takeuchi T, Watanabe S, Shiratori K and Hayashi N. Chronic pancreatitis caused by an autoimmune abnormality. Proposal of the concept of autoimmune pancreatitis. *Dig Dis Sci.* 1995; 40(7): 1561-1568. PMID: 7628283
3. Thal AP, Murray MJ and Egner W. Isoantibody formation in chronic pancreatic disease. *Lancet.* 1959; 1(7083): 1128-1129. PMID: 13665981
4. Murray MJ and Thal AP. The clinical significance of circulating pancreatic antibodies. *Ann Intern Med.* 1960; 53: 548-555. PMID: 13727030
5. Sarles H, Sarles JC, Muratore R and Guien C. Chronic inflammatory sclerosis of the pancreas–an autonomous pancreatic disease? *Am J Dig Dis.* 1961; 6: 688-698. PMID: 13746542
6. Thal AP. The occurrence of pancreatic antibodies and the nature of the pancreatic antigen. *Surg Forum.* 1960; 11: 367-369. PMID: 13776154
7. Freytag G and Kloppel G. Experimental pancreatitis and inflammation of the islets after treatment with immune sera against extract of pancreas of varying degrees of purity. *Beitr Pathol Anat.* 1969; 139(2): 138-160. PMID: 4897405
8. Narula N, Vasudev M and Marshall JK. IgG4-related sclerosing disease: a novel mimic of inflammatory bowel disease. *Dig Dis Sci.* 2010; 55(11): 3047-3051. PMID: 20521111
9. Gonatas NK and Howard JC. Inhibition of experimental allergic encephalomyelitis in rats severely depleted of T cells. *Science.* 1974; 186(4166): 839-841. PMID: 4143378
10. Ectors N, Maillet B, Aerts R, Geboes K, Donner A, Borchard F, Lankisch P, Stolte M, Luttges J, Kremer B and Kloppel G. Non-alcoholic duct destructive chronic pancreatitis. *Gut.* 1997; 41(2): 263-268. PMID: 9301509
11. Notohara K, Burgart LJ, Yadav D, Chari S and Smyrk TC. Idiopathic chronic pancreatitis with periductal lymphoplasmacytic infiltration: clinicopathologic features of 35 cases. *Am J Surg Pathol.* 2003; 27(8): 1119-1127. PMID: 12883244
12. Davidson TS, Longnecker DS and Hickey WF. An experimental model of autoimmune pancreatitis in the rat. *Am J Pathol.* 2005; 166(3): 729-736. PMID: 15743785
13. Nishimori I, Tamakoshi A and Otsuki M. Research Committee on Intractable Diseases of the Pancreas, Ministry of Health, Labour, and Welfare of Japan. Prevalence of autoimmune pancreatitis in Japan from a nationwide survey in 2002. *J Gastroenterol.* 2007; 42(Suppl. 18): 6-8. PMID: 17520216
14. Pannala R and Chari ST. Autoimmune pancreatitis. *Curr Opin Gastroenterol.* 2008; 24(5): 591-596. PMID: 19122500
15. Sugumar A and Chari S. Autoimmune pancreatitis: an update. *Expert Rev Gastroenterol Hepatol.* 2009; 3(2): 197-204. PMID: 19351289
16. Kojima M, Sipos B, Klapper W, Frahm O, Knuth HC, Yanagisawa A, Zamboni G, Morohoshi T and Klöppel G. Autoimmune pancreatitis: frequency, IgG4 expression, and clonality of T and B cells. *Am J Surg Pathol.* 2007; 31(4): 521-528. PMID: 17414098
17. Abraham SC, Wilentz RE, Yeo CJ, Sohn TA, Cameron JL, Boitnott JK and Hruban RH. Pancreaticoduodenectomy (Whipple resections) in patients without malignancy: are they all 'chronic pancreatitis? *Am J Surg Pathol.* 2003; 27(1): 110-120. PMID: 12502933
18. Hardacre JM, Iacobuzio-Donahue CA, Sohn TA, Abraham SC, Yeo CJ, Lillemoe KD, Choti MA, Campbell KA, Schulick RD, Hruban RH, Cameron JL and Leach SD. Results of pancreaticoduodenectomy for lymphoplasmacytic sclerosing pancreatitis. *Ann Surg.* 2003; 237(6): 853-858. PMID: 12796582
19. van Heerde MJ, Biermann K, Zondervan PE, Kazemier G, van Eijck CH, Pek C, Kuipers EJ and van Buuren HR. Prevalence of autoimmune pancreatitis and other benign disorders in pancreatoduodenectomy for presumed malignancy of the pancreatic head. *Dig Dis Sci.* 2012; 57(9): 2458-2465. PMID: 22588243
20. Weber SM, Cubukcu-Dimopulo O, Palesty JA, Suriawinata A, Klimstra D, Brennan MF and Conlon K. Lymphoplasmacytic sclerosing pancreatitis: inflammatory mimic of pancreatic carcinoma. *J Gastrointest Surg.* 2003; 7(1): 129-137. PMID: 12559194
21. Hughes DB, Grobmyer SR and Brennan MF. Preventing pancreaticoduodenectomy for lymphoplasmacytic sclerosing pancreatitis: cost effectiveness of IgG4. *Pancreas.* 2004; 29(2): 167-168. PMID: 15257110
22. Kawaguchi K, Koike M, Tsuruta K, Okamoto A, Tabata I and Fujita N. Lymphoplasmacytic sclerosing pancreatitis with cholangitis: a variant of primary sclerosing cholangitis extensively involving pancreas. *Hum Pathol.* 1991; 22(4): 387-395. PMID: 2050373
23. Kloppel G, Detlefsen S, Chari ST, Longnecker DS and Zamboni G. Autoimmune pancreatitis: the clinicopathological characteristics of the subtype with granulocytic epithelial lesions. *J Gastroenterol.* 2010; 45(8): 787-793. PMID: 20549251
24. Zamboni G, Luttges J, Capelli P, Frulloni L, Cavallini G, Pederzoli P, Leins A, Longnecker D and Kloppel G. Histopathological features of diagnostic and clinical relevance in autoimmune pancreatitis: a study on 53 resection specimens and 9 biopsy specimens. *Virchows Arch.* 2004; 445(6): 552-563. PMID: 15517359
25. Chari ST, Kloeppel G, Zhang L, Notohara K, Lerch MM and Shimosegawa T. Autoimmune Pancreatitis International Cooperative Study Group (APICS). Histopathologic and clinical subtypes of autoimmune pancreatitis: the Honolulu consensus document. *Pancreas.* 2010; 39(5): 549-554. PMID: 20562576
26. Shimosegawa T and Kanno A. Autoimmune pancreatitis in Japan: overview and perspective. *J Gastroenterol.* 2009; 44(6): 503-517. PMID: 19377842
27. Suda K, Nishimori I, Takase M, Oi I and Ogawa M. Autoimmune pancreatitis can be classified into early and advanced stages. *Pancreas.* 2006; 33(4): 345-350. PMID: 17079937

28. Kamisawa T, Funata N, Hayashi Y, Eishi Y, Koike M, Tsuruta K, Okamoto A, Egawa N and Nakajima H. A new clinicopathological entity of IgG4-related autoimmune disease. *J Gastroenterol.* 2003; 38(10): 982-984. PMID: 14614606
29. Hamano H. High Serum IgG4 Concentrations in Patients with Sclerosing Pancreatitis. *N Engl J Med.* 2001; 344(10): 732-738. PMID: 11236777
30. Kamisawa T and Okamoto A. Autoimmune pancreatitis: proposal of IgG4-related sclerosing disease. *J Gastroenterol.* 2006; 41(7): 613-625. PMID: 16932997
31. Kamisawa T and Okamoto A. IgG4-related sclerosing disease. *World J Gastroenterol.* 2008; 14(25): 3948-3955. PMID: 18609677
32. Frulloni L, Scattolini C, Falconi M, Zamboni G, Capelli P, Manfredi R, Graziani R, D'Onofrio M, Katsotourchi AM, Amodio A, Benini L and Vantini I. Autoimmune pancreatitis: differences between the focal and diffuse forms in 87 patients. *Am J Gastroenterol.* 2009; 104(9): 2288-2294. PMID: 19568232
33. Ghazale A, Chari ST, Smyrk TC, Levy MJ, Topazian MD, Takahashi N, Clain JE, Pearson RK, Pelaez- Luna M, Petersen BT, Vege SS and Farnell MB. Value of serum IgG4 in the diagnosis of autoimmune pancreatitis and in distinguishing it from pancreatic cancer. *Am J Gastroenterol.* 2007; 102(8): 1646-1653. PMID: 17555461
34. Sah RP, Pannala R, Chari ST, Sugumar A, Clain JE, Levy MJ, Pearson RK, Smyrk TC, Petersen BT, Topazian MD, Takahashi N and Vege SS. Prevalence, diagnosis, and profile of autoimmune pancreatitis presenting with features of acute or chronic pancreatitis. *Clin Gastroenterol Hepatol.* 2010; 8(1): 91-96. PMID: 19800984
35. Balasubramanian G, Sugumar A, Smyrk TC, Takahashi N, Clain JE, Gleeson FC, Hart PA, Levy MJ, Pearson RK, Petersen BT, Topazian MD, Vege SS, and Chari, ST. Demystifying seronegative autoimmune pancreatitis. *Pancreatology.* 2012; 12(4): 289-294. PMID: 22898628
36. Zhang L, Chari S, Smyrk TC, Deshpande V, Kloppel G, Kojima M, Liu X, Longnecker DS, Mino- Kenudson M, Notohara K, Rodriguez-Justo M, Srivastava A, Zamboni G and Zen Y. Autoimmune pancreatitis (AIP) type 1 and type 2: an international consensus study on histopathologic diagnostic criteria. *Pancreas.* 2011; 40(8): 1172-1179. PMID: 21975436
37. Loos M, Lauffer F, Schlitter AM, Kleef J, Friess H, Klöppel G, Esposito I. Potential role of Th17 cells in the pathogenesis of type 2 autoimmune pancreatitis. *Virchows Arch.* 2015; 467(6): 641-648. PMID: 26427656
38. Longnecker DS. Background and Perspectives. Chapter 1. In: Levy MJ and Chari ST, eds. Autoimmune (IgG4-related) Pancreatitis and Cholangitis. New York, NY: Springer; 2013: 1-6.

Chapter 55

Diagnosis of autoimmune pancreatitis

Phil A. Hart* and Suresh T. Chari*

Division of Gastroenterology and Hepatology, Mayo Clinic, Rochester, Minnesota.

Introduction

When Yoshida et al. coined the term "autoimmune pancreatitis (AIP)" in 1995, they listed several serologic and imaging features that helped them recognize the entity.[1] These features formed the basis for the first diagnostic criteria proposed by the Japan Pancreas Society in 2002.[2] In these reports, hypergammaglobulinemia and nonspecific markers such as rheumatoid factor (RF) and antinuclear antibodies (ANAs) served as serologic markers of AIP. In 2001, Hamano et al. observed that elevated serum IgG4 levels were highly sensitive and specific for the diagnosis of AIP.[3] Even though this led to a rapid increase in the number of diagnosed patients, it soon became clear that this was an inadequate biomarker when used in isolation to diagnose AIP. As the larger spectrum of disease became apparent, the need for diagnostic criteria to distinguish AIP from other diseases including chronic pancreatitis, pancreatic cancer, and other systemic diseases was evident. Within a decade there were at least six versions of diagnostic criteria published by groups from Japan, Italy, the United States, and Korea.[4-9] Although the criteria were generally similar, there were major differences including the necessity of endoscopic retrograde cholangiopancreatography (ERCP) for diagnosis, the inclusion or exclusion of criteria for other organ involvement, and response to steroids. Unfortunately, these differences resulted in confusion among practicing clinicians and prevented the comparison of results between studies.

International Consensus Diagnostic Criteria

In 2011, a multinational group met to develop the International Consensus Diagnostic Criteria (ICDC) for AIP that would be meaningful for both clinical and research purposes.[10] The group achieved a consensus that recognizes our current understanding of AIP, permits flexibility in diagnostic evaluation (e.g., reliance on histology vs. pancreatography), and acknowledges the two AIP subtypes. Importantly, although the typical clinical presentation of patients with AIP is obstructive jaundice, occasionally with a mass, the criteria also permit diagnosis in those with less common disease presentations and indeterminate imaging findings. The cardinal clinical features of AIP in the ICDC are pancreatic parenchymal imaging, pancreatic ductal imaging (i.e., endoscopic retrograde pancreatography [ERP]), serum IgG4 level, other organ involvement, pancreas histology, and response to steroid treatment.

Diagnostic components of the ICDC

Historically, pancreatic imaging findings (both parenchymal and ductal) were considered as essential for diagnosing AIP. ERCP is not necessary for diagnosis using the ICDC; rather, parenchymal and ductal imaging are recognized as separate yet complementary criteria. The serum IgG4 level is appreciated as a more sensitive and specific disease marker than previously used serologies including total IgG, γ-globulin, and autoantibody (ANAs and RF) levels; therefore, it is the preferred serologic test (See **Chapter 4**, "Serologic Abnormalities in AIP"). AIP is now recognized as the pancreatic manifestation of a multiorgan syndrome called IgG4-related disease (IgG4-RD). As a result, the presence of other organs commonly associated with IgG4-RD (e.g., biliary strictures located proximal to the intrapancreatic portion of the common bile duct, retroperitoneal fibrosis, and sialadenitis) are supportive findings for AIP and referred to as other organ involvement (OOI) (See **Chapter 8**, "Extrapancreatic Features of Autoimmune Pancreatitis"). Pancreatic histology obtained by core tissue biopsy (or a resected pancreatic specimen) is uniquely recognized as the "gold standard" for AIP diagnosis (See **Chapter 3**, "Histology of AIP"). This distinction is made on the basis that pathologists are able to accurately diagnose AIP independently of other clinical information.[11] Finally, response to steroid treatment evidenced by resolution or marked improvement in radiographic features is recognized as an important criterion. Although not included in some of the initial diagnostic criteria schemes, it was later recognized that a significant proportion of patients

*Corresponding authors. Email: philip.hart@osumc.edu, chari.suresh@mayo.edu

Table 1. Level 1 and 2 criteria for type 1 AIP using the ICDC. Used with permission from Shimosegawa et al.[10]

Diagnosis	Primary Basis for Diagnosis	Imaging Evidence	Collateral Evidence
Definitive type 1 AIP	Histology	Typical/indeterminate	Histologically confmned LPSP (level 1 H)
	Imaging	Typical	Any non-D level 1/ level 2
		Indeterminate	Two or more from level 1 (+ level 2 D*)
	Response to steroid	Indeterminate	Level 1 S/OOI + Rt or level 1 D + level 2 S/OOI/H + Rt
Probable type 1 AIP		Indeterminate	Level 2 S/OOI/H + Rt

*Level 2 D is counted as level 1 in this setting. LPSP, lymphoplasmacytic sclerosing pancreatitis; OOI, other organ involvement.

who did not have characteristic imaging findings still responded to steroid therapy.

Use of the ICDC to diagnose AIP

The ICDC are organized to allow the user to diagnose AIP along several potential pathways including characteristic imaging, characteristic histology, or response to steroid therapy. However, it all starts with a review of pancreatic findings on cross-sectional imaging (CT or MRI). These are classified as typical of AIP (level 1) or atypical/ indeterminate for AIP (level 2). Next, available data supporting the diagnosis of AIP (i.e., collateral evidence) is considered in combination with imaging findings. Collateral evidence (i.e., pancreatic ductal imaging, serum IgG4, OOI, and response to treatment) is assigned one of two levels based on the strength of association with AIP (**Table 1**). To establish a definitive diagnosis of type 1 AIP, varying strengths of collateral evidence are needed depending on imaging findings (**Table 2**). For example, in patients with typical parenchymal imaging for AIP, which is a relatively specific finding, any level of nonpancreatic collateral evidence secures a definitive diagnosis. Conversely, stronger collateral evidence is required when imaging is indeterminate for AIP. Using these criteria several combinations can establish an AIP diagnosis, even without the need for histology or ERP.

One advantage of the ICDC is the recognition of the two AIP subtypes. Type 2 is generally characterized by the lack of serum IgG4 elevation and OOI and is occasionally associated with inflammatory bowel disease. However, this profile is also present in some patients with type 1 AIP, so histology is the only means of establishing a definitive diagnosis. While the ICDC are specific for AIP, a subset of subjects with unequivocal steroid-responsive pancreatic mass/enlargement who have no or minimal collateral evidence fail to meet the diagnostic criteria for a definitive AIP subtype. Such patients are classified as AIP-not otherwise specified (AIP-NOS). When inflammatory bowel disease is present, these patients are considered likely to have type 2 AIP and are classified as probable type 2 AIP.

A practical approach to using the ICDC

The complexity of the criteria used in the ICDC is necessary due to the protean disease presentations. Although it may initially appear too cumbersome for clinical use, a practical approach for using the ICDC is possible with thoughtful consideration. Because AIP is extremely rare, the responsibility of the clinician is primarily to exclude an alternative etiology (namely malignancy) rather than to establish an AIP diagnosis. Therefore, unless noninvasive studies (i.e., imaging and typical other organ involvement) are characteristic for AIP, some form of cytology obtained with or without core biopsy for histology is necessary in most cases. In the absence of convincing evidence for malignancy, additional testing can be pursued for cases in which AIP is suspected.

Our current approach for diagnosing AIP and distinguishing it from pancreatic cancer using the ICDC is shown in **Table 3**. The initial step is to determine the likelihood of AIP based on pancreatic parenchymal imaging. When typical imaging (e.g., diffuse pancreatic enlargement with delayed enhancement of the parenchyma, with or without a capsule sign) is present, any nonductal imaging collateral evidence (i.e., elevated serum IgG4 or OOI) will establish an AIP diagnosis. In these patients, a diagnostic steroid trial and core biopsy of the pancreas are not needed to support the diagnosis (although steroids are generally initiated for therapeutic purposes). On the other hand, if pancreatic imaging shows focal/segmental enlargement or has atypical features (e.g., low-density mass, pancreatic duct dilation, or distal atrophy) the subsequent evaluation is dictated by the amount and strength

Table 2. Diagnosis of definitive and probable type 1 AIP using the ICDC. Used with permission from Shimosegawa et al.[10]

	Criterion	Level 1	Level 2
P	Parenchymal imaging	Typical: Diffuse enlargement with delayed enhancement (sometimes associated with rim-like enhancement)	Indeterminate (including atypical†): Segmental/focal enlargement with delayed enhancement
D	Ductal imaging (ERP)	Long (>1/3 length of the main pancreatic duct) or multiple strictures without marked upstream dilatation	Segmental/focal narrowing without marked upstream dilatation (duct size, <5 mm)
S	Serology	IgG4, >2× upper limit of normal value a or b	IgG4, 1-2× upper limit of normal value
OOI	Other organ involvement	a. Histology of extrapancreatic organs Any three of the following: (1) Marked lymphoplasmacytic infiltration with fibrosis and without granulocytic infiltration (2) Storiform fibrosis (3) Obliterative phlebitis (4) Abundant (>10 cells/HPF) IgG4-positive cells b. Typical radiological evidence At least one of the following: (1) Segmental/multiple proximal (hilar/intrahepatic) or proximal and distal bile duct stricture (2) Retroperitoneal fibrosis	a. Histology of extrapancreatic organs including endoscopic biopsies of bile duct‡: Both of the following: (1) Marked lymphoplasrnacytic infiltration without granulocytic infiltration (2) Abundant (>10 cells/HPF) IgG4-positive cells b. Physical or radiological evidence At least one of the following: (1) Symmetrically enlarged salivary/lachrymal glands (2) Radiological evidence of renal involvement described in association with AIP
H	Histology of the pancreas	LPSP (core biopsy/resection) At least 3 of the following: (1) Periductal lymphoplasmacytic infiltrate without granulocytic infiltration (2) Obliterative phlebitis (3) Storiform fibrosis (4) Abundant (>10 cells/HPF) IgG4-positive cells	LPSP (core biopsy) Any 2 of the following: (1) Periductallymphoplasmacytic infiltrate without granulocytic infiltration (2) Obliterative phlebitis (3) Storiform fibrosis (4) Abundant (>10 cells/HPF) IgG4-positive cells
Response to steroid (Rt)*		Diagnostic steroid trial Rapid (≤2 wk) radiologically demonstrable resolution or marked improvement in pancreatic/extrapancreatic manifestations	

*Diagnostic steroid trial should be conducted carefully by pancreatologists with caveats (see text) only after negative workup for cancer including endoscopic ultrasound-guided fine needle aspiration.

†Atypical: Some AIP cases may show low-density mass, pancreatic ductal dilatation, or distal atrophy. Such atypical imaging findings in patients with obstructive jaundice and/or pancreatic mass are highly suggestive of pancreatic cancer. Such patients should be managed as pancreatic cancer unless there is strong collateral evidence for AIP, and a thorough workup for cancer is negative (see algorithm).

‡Endoscopic biopsy of duodenal papilla is a useful adjunctive method because ampulla often is involved pathologically in AIP.

of the collateral evidence. If there is strong collateral evidence (two of the following: pancreatic duct stricture without upstream dilation, serum IgG4 >2x upper limit of normal, or histologic demonstration of OOI or radiographic evidence of proximal biliary disease or retroperitoneal fibrosis), the diagnosis of AIP can be confirmed without additional measures. Conversely, if the collateral evidence is only modest, fine- needle aspiration (FNA) is recommended to rule out cancer, then steroid treatment trial is needed to secure the AIP diagnosis. Modest collateral evidence would be satisfied with the presence of one of the following: typical long or multiple pancreatic ductal strictures on ERP AND either serum IgG4 elevation or presence of OOI, serum IgG4 >2x upper limit of normal, or histologic documentation of OOI or radiographic evidence of proximal biliary disease or retroperitoneal fibrosis. It should be highlighted that diagnostic steroid trials are rarely needed and are not recommended unless cancer has been excluded by FNA of a mass lesion. Repeat imaging is recommended after 2 weeks of steroid treatment, and alternative etiologies should be considered if there is not significant improvement. Finally, regardless

Table 3. Our approach for determining the need for fine-needle aspiration (FNA) to rule out cancer, and additional measures to establish the diagnosis of type 1 AIP according to ICDC.

Parenchymal imaging	Strength of collateral evidence	FNA recommended	Steroid trial needed	Pancreas histology needed
Typical	Any	No	No	No
Indeterminate	Any two of level 1 evidence from Table 2	No	No	No
Focal enlargement/atypical	Any level 1 S/OOI or level 2 S/OOI/H evidence from Table 2	Yes	Yes	No
Typical or indeterminate	None	Yes	No	Yes

of the nature of pancreatic imaging features, if there is no supportive collateral evidence for AIP, an FNA is recommended to exclude cancer and a core biopsy of the pancreas is needed, to reach an AIP diagnosis.

Summary

AIP is an increasingly recognized clinical entity. Although elevated serum IgG4 is an important diagnostic clue, it is insufficient to independently establish a diagnosis, and other collateral evidence is needed. The ICDC are recently published diagnostic criteria that help both the clinician and researcher accurately identify those with AIP using one of several combinations of key diagnostic features (pancreatic parenchymal imaging, pancreatic ductal imaging [i.e., ERP], serum IgG4 level, other organ involvement, pancreas histology, and response to steroid treatment). Because AIP is rare, the clinician's diagnostic approach must primarily focus on the excluding malignancy and then on solidifying the AIP diagnosis.

References

1. Yoshida K, Toki F, Takeuchi T, Watanabe S, Shiratori K, and Hayashi N. Chronic pancreatitis caused by an autoimmune abnormality. Proposal of the concept of autoimmune pancreatitis. *Dig Dis Sci.* 2995; 40: 1561-1568. PMID: 7628283
2. Society MotCCfAPotJP. Diagnostic criteria for autoimmune pancreatitis by the Japan Pancreas Society. *J Jpn Pancreas Soc.* 2002; 17: 585-587.
3. Hamano H, Kawa S, Horiuchi A, Unno H, Furuya N, Akamatsu T, Fukushima M, Nikaido T, Nakayama K, Usuda N, and Kiyosawa K. High serum IgG4 concentrations in patients with sclerosing pancreatitis. *N Engl J Med.* 2001; 344: 732-738. PMID: 11236777
4. Chari ST, Smyrk TC, Levy MJ, Topazian MD, Takahashi N, Zhang L, Clain JE, Pearson RK, Petersen BT, Vege SS, and Farnell MB. Diagnosis of autoimmune pancreatitis: the Mayo Clinic experience. *Clin Gastroenterol Hepatol.* 2006; 4: 1010-1016; quiz 1934. PMID: 16843735
5. Chari ST, Takahashi N, Levy MJ, Smyrk TC, Clain JE, Pearson RK, Petersen BT, Topazian MA, and Vege SS. A diagnostic strategy to distinguish autoimmune pancreatitis from pancreatic cancer. *Clin Gastroenterol Hepatol.* 2009; 7: 1097-1103. PMID: 19410017
6. Frulloni L, Scattolini C, Falconi M, Zamboni G, Capelli P, Manfredi R, Graziani R, D'Onofrio M, Katsotourchi AM, Amodio A, Benini L, and Vantini I. Autoimmune pancreatitis: differences between the focal and diffuse forms in 87 patients. *Am J Gastroenterol.* 2009; 104: 2288-2294. PMID: 19568232
7. Kim KP, Kim MH, Kim JC, Lee SS, Seo DW, and Lee SK. Diagnostic criteria for autoimmune chronic pancreatitis revisited. *World J Gastroenterol.* 2006; 12: 2487-2496. PMID: 16688792
8. Otsuki M, Chung JB, Okazaki K, Kim MH, Kamisawa T, Kawa S, Park SW, Shimosegawa T, Lee K, Ito T, Nishimori I, Notohara K, Naruse S, Ko SB, and Kihara Y. Asian diagnostic criteria for autoimmune pancreatitis: consensus of the Japan-Korea Symposium on Autoimmune Pancreatitis. *J Gastroenterol.* 2008; 43: 403-408. PMID: 18600383
9. Pearson RK, Longnecker DS, Chari ST, Smyrk TC, Okazaki K, Frulloni L, and Cavallini G. Controversies in clinical pancreatology: autoimmune pancreatitis: does it exist? *Pancreas.* 2003; 27: 1-13. PMID: 12826899
10. Shimosegawa T, Chari ST, Frulloni L, Kamisawa T, Kawa S, Mino-Kenudson M, Kim MH, Kloppel G, Lerch MM, Lohr M, Notohara K, Okazaki K, Schneider A, and Zhang L. International consensus diagnostic criteria for autoimmune pancreatitis: guidelines of the International Association of Pancreatology. *Pancreas.* 2011; 40: 352-358. PMID: 21412117
11. Zhang L, Chari S, Smyrk TC, Deshpande V, Kloppel G, Kojima M, Liu X, Longnecker DS, Mino- Kenudson M, Notohara K, Rodriguez-Justo M, Srivastava A, Zamboni G, and Zen Y. Autoimmune pancreatitis (AIP) type 1 and type 2: an international consensus study on histopathologic diagnostic criteria. *Pancreas.* 2011; 40: 1172-1179. PMID: 21975436

Chapter 56

Histology of autoimmune pancreatitis

Kenji Notohara[1*] and Lizhi Zhang[2*]

[1]*Kurashiki Central Hospital, 1-1-1 Miwa, Kurashiki 710-8602, Japan;*
[2]*Department of Laboratory and Anatomic Pathology, Mayo Clinic, Rochester, Minnesota.*

Introduction

Chronic pancreatitis, as represented by alcoholic chronic pancreatitis, is a progressive fibroinflammatory disease of the pancreas wherein the pancreatic parenchyma is extensively and severely destroyed by fibrosis but inflammatory cell infiltration is usually mild. Dense inflammatory cell infiltration in established chronic pancreatitis is a rare but eye-catching finding and is usually seen in cases with tumefactive pancreatitis. Thus, such cases used to be sporadically reported as a distinctive type of pancreatitis and were pathologically designated as chronic inflammatory sclerosis, lymphoplasmacytic sclerosing pancreatitis (LPSP), and nonalcoholic duct destructive chronic pancreatitis.[1-3] After Yoshida et al. proposed the concept of autoimmune pancreatitis (AIP) in 1995, those pathological entities have come to be recognized as related conditions that represent the pathological features of AIP.[4]

Since 2003, some groups have argued that what had been diagnosed as AIP and its related pathological entities did not constitute a single entity but consisted of at least two different conditions. A group from Mayo Clinic conducted a retrospective study with resected pancreases diagnosed with pancreatitis and concluded that in addition to a group with an entity that corresponded to LPSP, there was another with idiopathic duct-centric chronic pancreatitis (IDCP).[5] Similar observations were also reported from Europe and Massachusetts General Hospital (MGH).[6,7] AIP with and without granulocytic epithelial lesions (GELs, a term used by the European group), and ductocentric and lobulocentric AIP (terms used by the MGH group) are considered to be identical or similar to IDCP and LPSP, respectively.

In 2001, Hamano et al. demonstrated that serum IgG4 values are elevated in AIP patients. Subsequent studies showed that affected pancreatic and nonpancreatic tissues in AIP are infiltrated by numerous IgG4-positive plasma cells.[8,9] These pivotal observations allowed the emergence of the new disease concept now called IgG4-related disease (IgG4- RD).[10-12] The number of IgG4-positive plasma cells was noted to be significantly higher in LPSP than in IDCP, leading to the realization that LPSP and IDCP are different entities, with LPSP encompassed in the spectrum of IgG4-RD.[13,14] Various clinical differences between LPSP and IDCP were also clarified.[15-17] At present, LPSP and IDCP are called type 1 and 2 AIP, respectively,[13] and separate criteria for the subtypes have been proposed in the International Consensus Diagnostic Criteria (ICDC) for AIP.[18]

The presence of numerous IgG4-positive plasma cells is a histological feature of type 1 AIP/LPSP. However, it is noteworthy that the distinction between types 1 and 2 AIP was clarified based on a histomorphological study.[5,7] An interobserver concordance study revealed that pathologists can distinguish these two entities based on histological findings even without IgG4 immunostaining.[19] In addition, the presence of numerous IgG4- positive cells is not specific to type 1 AIP and can be observed in other conditions such as pancreatic abscess and cancer.[14,20] Thus, for the pathological diagnosis of type 1 AIP, the morphological features are the most important and IgG4 immunostaining is only an adjunct to diagnosis, most useful in interpreting pancreatic biopsies.

In this chapter, the unique histological features of type 1 AIP are described, with the histological features of type 2 AIP outlined later.

Pathological characteristics of type 1 AIP (LPSP)

Macroscopically, the affected pancreas is usually enlarged. Lesions can be diffuse or focal, but focal lesions are particularly prone to resection because of the clinical difficulty in distinguishing them from pancreatic cancer. The pancreatic lobules are relatively well preserved (**Figure 1**), but focal destruction is not uncommon. The pancreatic duct system is open despite imaging findings suggestive of stenosis. The pancreatic parenchyma is often surrounded by a sheath of inflammation involving the peripheral parenchyma and peripancreatic adipose tissue. This feature corresponds to the radiological finding of a "capsule-like rim."

*Corresponding authors. Email: notohara@kchnet.or.jp, zhang.lizhi@mayo.edu

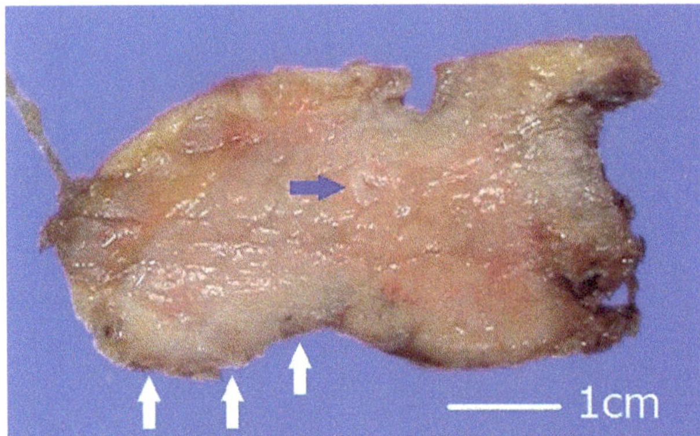

Figure 1. Macroscopic features of type 1 AIP. A portion of the pancreas is surrounded by a sheath of inflammation (white arrows). Pancreatic lobular structure is well preserved. The main pancreatic duct (blue arrow) is open and is involved by the fibroinflammatory legion ("thickened duct wall").

Type 1 AIP is histologically characterized by dense lymphoplasmacytic infiltration and fibrosis. Lymphoid follicles and eosinophils are common and sometimes prominent, but neutrophils are almost never observed. In addition to these relatively nonspecific findings that may be shared with other chronic inflammatory diseases, type 1 AIP shows the following unique histological features that distinguish it from other inflammatory lesions, including type 2 AIP.

Storiform fibrosis

Storiform fibrosis is a peculiar fibrosing lesion seen in almost all cases of type 1 AIP. It is not the uniform streaming pattern commonly seen in other chronic inflammatory diseases; rather, it is characterized by a haphazard and typically swirling pattern. Similar to granulation tissues changing into fibrosis over time, a series of histological differences in storiform fibrosis can be appreciated. In the early stage, a cellular component of small spindle cells, lymphocytes, and plasma cells predominates, with minimal collagen formation (**cell-rich type, Figure 2a**). Collagen formation then gradually proceeds, and the cell component decreases (**transitional type, Figure 2b**) until fibrotic foci consisting mostly of collagen with a scanty cell component finally develop (**fibrotic type, Figure 2c**). A mixture of various stages may be seen in a single case.

Ductal inflammation (periductal inflammation)

Collars with lymphoplasmacytic infiltration and/or fibrosis are seen around the pancreatic duct epithelium. Notably, neither inflammatory cell infiltration nor regressive/regenerative changes occur in the duct epithelium itself, thereby providing a useful clue to differentiation from type 2 AIP. With all of these histological features, ductal inflammation

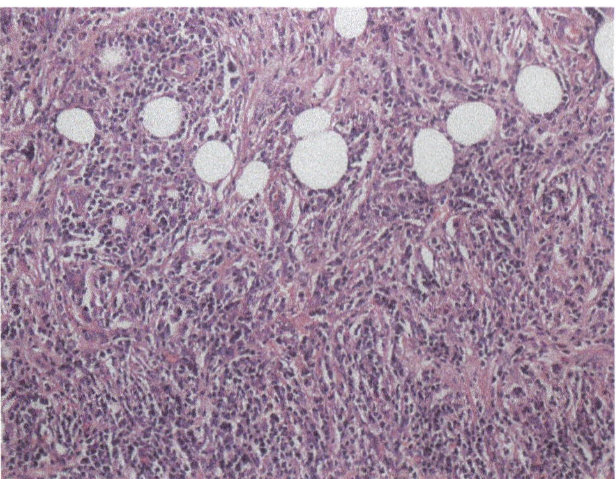

Figure 2a. Cell-rich- storiform fibrosis of type 1 AIP.

seen in type 1 AIP used to be called "periductal inflammation." Ductal inflammation is easily identified in the main and interlobular pancreatic ducts but also involves the intralobular pancreatic ducts. Two types of ductal inflammation can be recognized. The first pattern consists of a thin layer packed with lymphocytes and plasma cells just beneath the epithelium and an outer layer of fibrosis. The other pattern is composed of a thick inflammatory band with storiform fibrosis that surrounds the epithelium, giving the impression of a thickened pancreatic duct wall (**Figure 3**). The lumen of the ducts is narrowed and stellate-shaped due to compression by dense lymphoplasmacytic infiltration fibrosis. Because no structure corresponding to this kind of wall is originally present in the pancreatic ducts, it is attributed to the inflammation itself.

Lobular inflammation

Pancreatic lobules are almost always inflamed at least focally in type 1 AIP. With inflammation, the lobules are

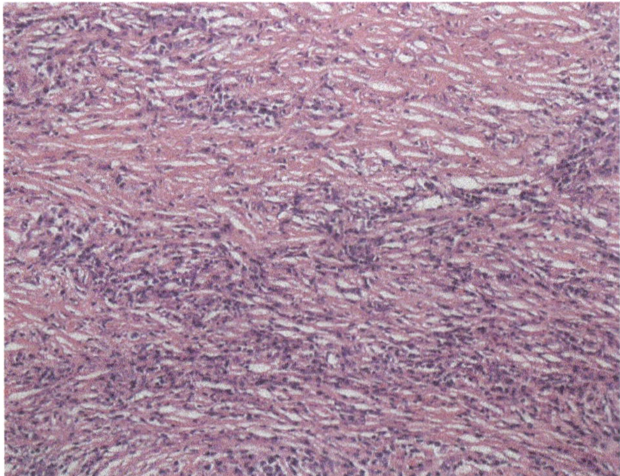

Figure 2b. Transitional storiform fibrosis of type 1 AIP.

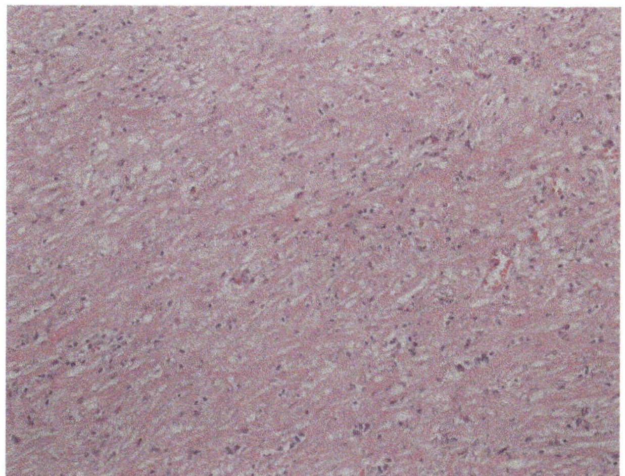

Figure 2c. Fibrotic storiform fibrosis of type 1 AIP.

infiltrated by lymphocytes and plasma cells with accompanying acinar cell loss. The interlobular spaces are fibrotic. Inflamed lobules maintain their original size and shape in type 1 AIP (**Figure 4**), which is in contrast to lobular atrophy seen in pancreatitis due to other etiologies. The lobules also occasionally become edematous. Lobular architecture is relatively well preserved, but focal destruction and replacement by fibrosis is not uncommon. In the latter scenario, areas of storiform fibrosis can be seen.

Inflammation involving peripancreatic adipose tissue in the pancreatic border

The inflammation seen at the pancreatic border is most marked in type 1 AIP, giving the appearance of a shell surrounding the pancreatic parenchyma (**Figure 5**). This finding corresponds to the radiological finding of a capsule-like rim. Inflammation in both the pancreatic parenchyma and peripancreatic adipose tissue is involved in the formation of this lesion, obscuring the border between the two tissues. Storiform fibrosis and obliterative phlebitis are most prominent in this lesion type. Inflammation occurs in the peripancreatic adipose tissue in type 1 AIP, and it spreads by enclosing individual adipocytes until fat lobules are entirely replaced by fibroinflammatory lesions. Fat necrosis is not typically seen in type 1 AIP.

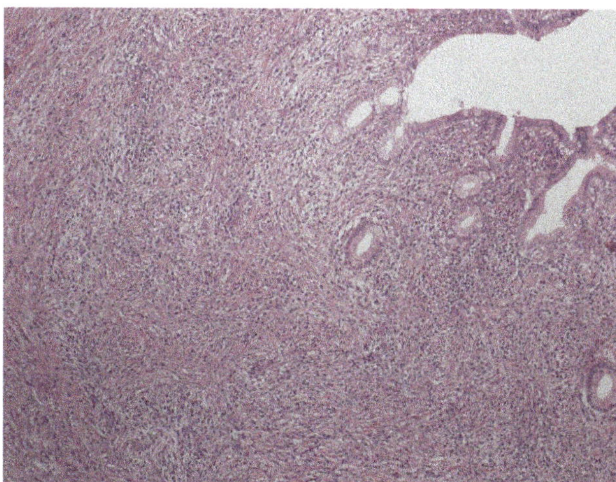

Figure 3. Ductal inflammation of type 1 AIP. A thick inflammatory band with storiform fibrosis surrounding the duct epithelium, giving the impression of a "thickened duct wall." Note that the duct epithelium is intact.

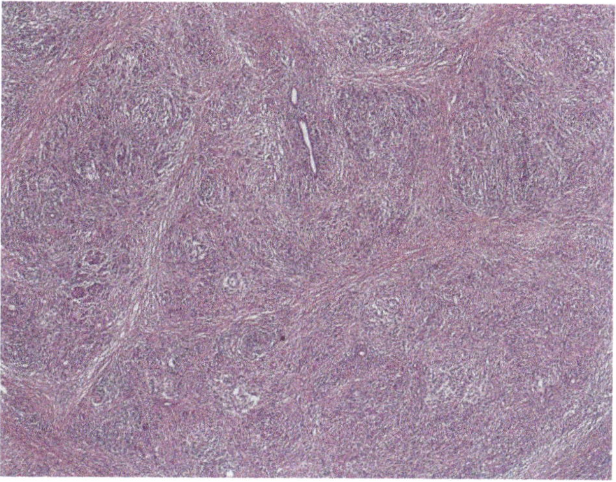

Figure 4. Lobular inflammation of type 1 AIP. The lobules maintain their original size and shape despite inflammation and acinar cell loss.

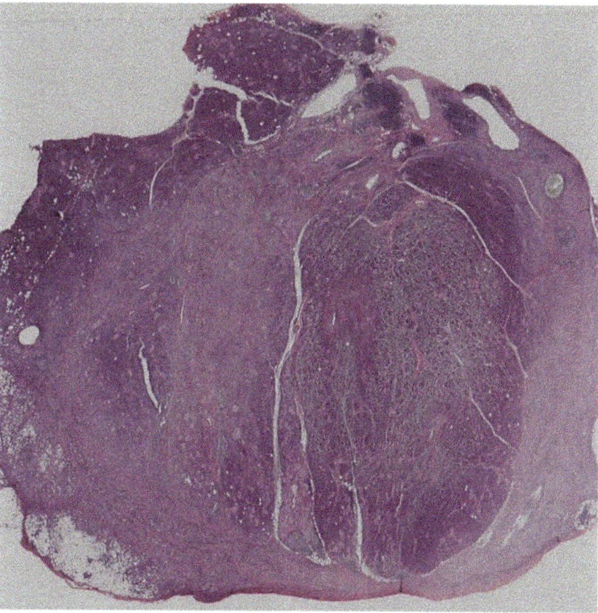

Figure 5a. Inflammation of type 1 AIP at the pancreatic border. The pancreatic parenchyma is surrounded by a cuff of the fibroinflammatory lesion.

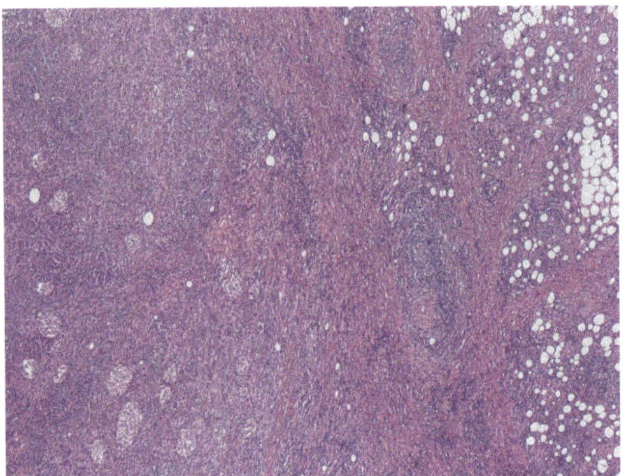

Figure 5b. Inflammation at the border involves both the pancreatic parenchyma (left) and peripancreatic adipose tissue (right).

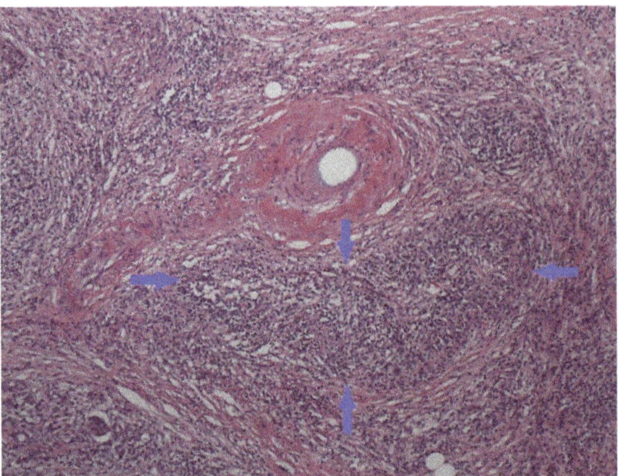

Figure 6. Obliterative phlebitis of type 1 AIP. The nodular inflammatory lesion (arrows) adjacent to an artery is a vein obliterated by the inflammation.

Obliterative phlebitis and other vascular lesions

Venule inflammation is another unique and common feature of type 1 AIP. It is characterized by lymphocyte and plasma cell infiltration from the venous wall to the lumen, culminating in venous obliteration. For this reason, this condition is called obliterative phlebitis. Similar inflammation may also be found in large veins such as the splenic and portal veins. In these instances the inflammation is limited to only a portion of the wall, and rarely results in obliteration.

In type 1 AIP all sizes of venules can be involved by obliterative phlebitis. A large number of relatively large (>100 μm in diameter) venules are affected, making obliterative phlebitis perceptible even on H& E-stained slides.[21] In the normal pancreas arteries and veins run in parallel; therefore, obliterative phlebitis can be suspected when there is no vein next to an artery and instead a nodular inflammatory lesion is present (**Figure 6**). Use of elastic stains, such as Verhoeff-van Gieson, is helpful for identifying and confirming the presence of obliterated veins, but care has to be taken to distinguish obliterative phlebitis in type 1 AIP from nonspecific fibrous venous occlusion due to venous wall damage or organized thrombosis as seen in chronic pancreatitis and pancreatic cancer.[21] In this regard, it should be emphasized that the histological picture seen in obliterative phlebitis is the same as that of the surrounding inflammatory lesions, and storiform fibrosis may also be found.

Arteries and arterioles are occasionally inflamed in type 1 AIP, with the adventitia and outer layer of the media usually involved. This finding can be designated as periarteritis/periarteriolitis in the same way as the lesions seen in the aorta and its branches (periaortitis/periarteritis) that are included in IgG4-related disease. In contrast to venous lesions, luminal occlusion is rare in arterial lesions. Because inflammation is marked around the arterioles in type 1 AIP, it is difficult to accurately evaluate the arterial lesions; for this reason, this finding has not been emphasized in previous pathological reports on type 1 AIP.

IgG4-positive plasma cells

Abundant IgG4-positive plasma cells are observed in type 1 AIP (**Figure 7**). In resected materials, the number of IgG4-positive plasma cells is usually >50 per high power field (hpf).[22] However, because it is difficult to satisfy this criterion in the biopsy diagnosis of type 1 AIP, the number of IgG4-positive plasma cells has been set at >10/hpf in the ICDC.[18]

The presence of >10 IgG4-positive plasma cells per hpf is not specific for type 1 AIP and can be satisfied in

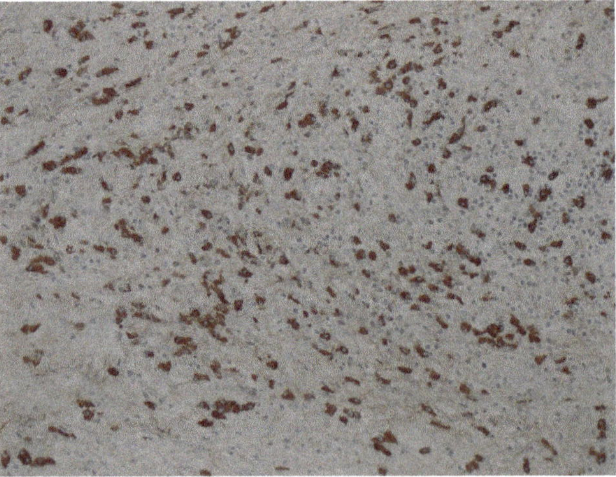

Figure 7. Abundant IgG4-positive plasma cells seen in type 1 AIP.

conditions with copious plasmacytic infiltration (e.g., pancreatic abscess or inflammation associated with pancreatic cancer).[14,20] In addition, more IgG4-positive plasma cells are present adjacent to lymphoid follicles. Therefore, a higher count of IgG4- positive plasma cells from those areas may be not representative. In this regard, evaluation of the IgG4/IgG-positive cell ratio is useful: the ratio is high (>40%) in type 1 AIP and low in the other pancreatic diseases.[23] However a minority of cases do not satisfy this criterion; the IgG4/IgG-positive cell ratio can be ≤40% in some type 1 AIP cases and >40% in a minority of patients with pancreatic cancer.

Thus, IgG4-immunostaining is only of limited value for the pathological diagnosis of type 1 AIP, and the importance of morphological features, notably storiform fibrosis and obliterative phlebitis, should be emphasized. The ICDC stands by this principle by specifying that a diagnosis of type 1 AIP can be established when at least three of the following histological features are satisfied: 1) periductal lymphoplasmacytic infiltrate without granulocytic infiltration, 2) obliterative phlebitis, 3) storiform fibrosis, or 4) abundant (>10/hpf) IgG4-positive cells.[18] The same policy has been also adopted in the consensus statement on the pathology of IgG4-related disease.[23]

Biopsy diagnosis of type 1 AIP

The distinction between AIP and pancreas cancer is vital but difficult in some cases, for example in lesions with focal pancreatic enlargement and/or negative serological tests. In these situations, pancreatic biopsies may be needed to reach an accurate diagnosis. This trend has been driven by technological advances in endoscopic ultrasound-guided fine needle aspiration (EUS-FNA) and EUS-guided Trucut biopsy (EUS-TCB).

As described earlier, the histological features of type 1 AIP are so characteristic that the diagnosis can be easily rendered based on study of the resected specimens. However, a biopsy diagnosis of type 1 AIP is challenging because diagnostic hallmarks such as storiform fibrosis, ductal inflammation, and obliterative phlebitis, are rarely obtained or are difficult to identify in tiny biopsy samples. Nevertheless, the histological diagnosis of type 1 AIP with EUS-TCB is promising and is reported to be effective in about half of patients.[24,25] Unfortunately, this procedure is only currently available in a small number of institutions. Compared to EUS-TCB, the diagnostic usefulness of EUS-FNA is limited because of the smaller amount of tissue obtained, but some groups have also found this procedure to be effective.[24-26]

In biopsy samples, a relatively high frequency of storiform fibrosis can be seen. Obliterative phlebitis can be occasionally identified, and elastic stains are of help in this regard. Immunostaining for IgG4 is mandatory, and as described in the ICDC, the presence of >10 positive plasma cells/hpf is a diagnostic standard. Infiltration of numerous neutrophils, proliferation of plump fibroblasts, and/or epithelioid granuloma formation makes the diagnosis of type 1 AIP less likely.

So far, EUS-FNA cytology is believed to be unsatisfactory for diagnosing AIP. However, it is a highly sensitive (80%-97%) and specific (82%-100%) test for diagnosing pancreatic cancer and can therefore play an important role in excluding this disease.

Type 1 AIP and neoplasms

IgG4-positive plasma cells may be numerous in and around cancers, and these patients may show elevated serum IgG4 levels.[14,27] Tissue IgG4 infiltration is usually focal in the lesions, rather than diffuse like in type 1 AIP, and it is not usually associated with a high IgG4/IgG-positive cell ratio.[22] Inflammation is commonly seen around pancreatic cancer. Histological features included in cancer-associated inflammation are proliferation of plump fibroblasts (desmoplastic reaction), neutrophilic infiltration, and inflammatory cell infiltration with prominent lobular edema, all of which are distinct from type 1 AIP.

Type 1 AIP may be associated with neoplastic diseases. On rare occasions, the histological features of type 1 AIP can be seen in the setting of pancreatic cancer.[28,29] IgG4-positive cells are numerous in these lesions, and even the IgG4/IgG-positive cell ratio is high. Such cases have been regarded as concomitant pancreatic cancer and type 1 AIP. From the clinical standpoint, metachronous association of pancreatic cancer after steroid treatment for type 1 AIP has been reported.[30] Extrahepatic bile duct neoplasms (a case with cancer in an early stage and another case with biliary intraepithelial neoplasia) have been reported in patients with both type 1 AIP and IgG4-related sclerosing cholangitis.[31,32] A case with concomitant intraductal papillary mucinous neoplasm (IPMN) and type 1 AIP was also described.[33] Finally, there is emerging evidence that the cancer risk may be higher in those with AIP.[34] The risk was particularly high in the first year after AIP diagnosis and did not recur in a small number of patients after cancer treatments, suggesting the possibility of a paraneoplastic syndrome.

Summary

Type 1 AIP is a unique form of chronic pancreatitis with distinct histomorphology that permits a histologic diagnosis of AIP without the need for other diagnostic criteria. It is characterized by nonspecific, dense lymphoplasmacytic inflammation. Additional features of storiform fibrosis and obliterative phlebitis are not shared with other chronic inflammatory diseases of the pancreas, helping distinguish type 1 AIP from other causes of pancreatic disease including type 2 AIP. Finally, an abundance of IgG4-positive plasma cells is a helpful clue to diagnosis when present, but this finding is not entirely specific and can also be seen in pancreatic cancer.

Acknowledgment

This work was supported in part by Health and Labour Sciences Research Grants (Intractable Diseases) from the Japanese Ministry of Health, Labour, and Welfare.

References

1. Ectors N, Maillet B, Aerts R, Geboes K, Donner A, Borchard F, Lankisch P, Stolte M, Lüttges J, Kremer B, and Klöppel G. Non-alcoholic duct destructive chronic pancreatitis. *Gut.* 1997; 41: 263-268. PMID: 9301509.
2. Kawaguchi K, Koike M, Tsuruta K, Okamoto A, Tabata I, and Fujita N. Lymphoplasmacytic sclerosing pancreatitis with cholangitis: a variant of primary sclerosing cholangitis extensively involving pancreas. *Hum Pathol.* 1991; 22: 387-395. PMID: 2050373.
3. Sarles H, Sarles JC, Muratore R, and Guien C. Chronic inflammatory sclerosis of the pancreas—an autonomous pancreatic disease? *Am J Dig Dis.* 1961; 6: 688-698. PMID: 13746542.
4. Yoshida K, Toki F, Takeuchi T, Watanabe S, Shiratori K, and Hayashi N. Chronic pancreatitis caused by an autoimmune abnormality. Proposal of the concept of autoimmune pancreatitis. *Dig Dis Sci.* 1995; 40: 1561-1568. PMID: 7628283.
5. Notohara K, Burgart LJ, Yadav D, Chari S, and Smyrk TC. Idiopathic chronic pancreatitis with periductal lymphoplasmacytic infiltration: clinicopathologic features of 35 cases. *Am J Surg Pathol.* 2003; 27: 1119-1127. PMID: 12883244.
6. Deshpande V, Chicano S, Finkelberg D, Selig MK, Mino-Kenudson M, Brugge WR, Colvin RB, and Lauwers GY. Autoimmune pancreatitis: a systemic immune complex mediated disease. *Am J Surg Pathol.* 2006; 30: 1537-1545. PMID: 17122509.
7. Zamboni G, Lüttges J, Capelli P, Frulloni L, Cavallini G, Pederzoli P, Leins A, Longnecker D, and Klöppel G. Histopathological features of diagnostic and clinical relevance in autoimmune pancreatitis: a study on 53 resection specimens and 9 biopsy specimens. *Virchows Arch.* 2004; 445: 552-563. PMID: 15517359.
8. Hamano H, Kawa S, Horiuchi A, Unno H, Furuya N, Akamatsu T, Fukushima M, Nikaido T, Nakayama K, Usuda N, and Kiyosawa K. High serum IgG4 concentrations in patients with sclerosing pancreatitis. *N Engl J Med.* 2001; 344: 732-738. PMID: 11236777.
9. Hamano H, Kawa S, Ochi Y, Unno H, Shiba N, Wajiki M, Nakazawa K, Shimojo H, and Kiyosawa K. Hydronephrosis associated with retroperitoneal fibrosis and sclerosing pancreatitis. *Lancet.* 2002; 359: 1403-1404. PMID: 11978339.
10. Kamisawa T, Funata N, Hayashi Y, Tsuruta K, Okamoto A, Amemiya K, Egawa N, and Nakajima H. Close relationship between autoimmune pancreatitis and multifocal fibrosclerosis. *Gut.* 2003; 52: 683-687. PMID: 12692053.
11. Stone JH, Khosroshahi A, Deshpande V, Chan JK, Heathcote JG, Aalberse R, Azumi A, Bloch DB, Brugge WR, Carruthers MN, Cheuk W, Cornell L, Castillo CF, Ferry JA, Forcione D, Klöppel G, Hamilos DL, Kamisawa T, Kasashima S, Kawa S, Kawano M, Masaki Y, Notohara K, Okazaki K, Ryu JK, Saeki T, Sahani D, Sato Y, Smyrk T, Stone JR, Takahira M, Umehara H, Webster G, Yamamoto M, Yi E, Yoshino T, Zamboni G, Zen Y, and Chari S. Recommendations for the nomenclature of IgG4-related disease and its individual organ system manifestations. *Arthritis Rheum.* 2012; 64: 3061-3067. PMID: 22736240.
12. Umehara H, Okazaki K, Masaki Y, Kawano M, Yamamoto M, Saeki T, Matsui S, Yoshino T, Nakamura S, Kawa S, Hamano H, Kamisawa T, Shimosegawa T, Shimatsu A, Nakamura S, Ito T, Notohara K, Sumida T, Tanaka Y, Mimori T, Chiba T, Mishima M, Hibi T, Tsubouchi H, Inui K, and Ohara H. Comprehensive diagnostic criteria for IgG4-related disease (IgG4-RD), 2011. *Mod Rheumatol.* 2012; 22: 21-30. PMID: 22218969.
13. Chari ST, Kloeppel G, Zhang L, Notohara K, Lerch MM, and Shimosegawa T. Autoimmune Pancreatitis International Cooperative Study Group (APICS). Histopathologic and clinical subtypes of autoimmune pancreatitis: the Honolulu consensus document. *Pancreas.* 2010; 39: 549-554. PMID: 20562576.
14. Zhang L, Notohara K, Levy MJ, Chari ST, and Smyrk TC. IgG4-positive plasma cell infiltration in the diagnosis of autoimmune pancreatitis. *Mod Pathol.* 2007; 20: 23-28. PMID: 16980948.
15. Kamisawa T, Chari ST, Giday SA, Kim MH, Chung JB, Lee KT, Werner J, Bergmann F, Lerch MM, Mayerle J, Pickartz T, Lohr M, Schneider A, Frulloni L, Webster GJ, Reddy DN, Liao WC, Wang HP, Okazaki K, Shimosegawa T, Kloeppel G, and Go VL. Clinical profile of autoimmune pancreatitis and its histological subtypes: an international multicenter survey. *Pancreas.* 2011; 40: 809-814. PMID: 21747310.
16. Sah RP, Chari ST, Pannala R, Sugumar A, Clain JE, Levy MJ, Pearson RK, Smyrk TC, Petersen BT, Topazian MD, Takahashi N, Farnell MB, and Vege SS. Differences in clinical profile and relapse rate of type 1 versus type 2 autoimmune pancreatitis. *Gastroenterology.* 2010; 139: 140-148. PMID: 20353791.
17. Song TJ, Kim JH, Kim MH, Jang JW, Park do H, Lee SS, Seo DW, Lee SK, and Yu E. Comparison of clinical findings between histologically confirmed type 1 and type 2 autoimmune pancreatitis. *J Gastroenterol Hepatol.* 2012; 27: 700-708. PMID: 21929653.
18. Shimosegawa T, Chari ST, Frulloni L, Kamisawa T, Kawa S, Mino-Kenudson M, Kim MH, Klöppel G, Lerch MM, Löhr M, Notohara K, Okazaki K, Schneider A, and Zhang L. International Association of Pancreatology. International

consensus diagnostic criteria for autoimmune pancreatitis: guidelines of the International Association of Pancreatology. *Pancreas.* 2011; 40: 352-358. PMID: 21412117.

19. Zhang L, Chari S, Smyrk TC, Deshpande V, Klöppel G, Kojima M, Liu X, Longnecker DS, Mino- Kenudson M, Notohara K, Rodriguez-Justo M, Srivastava A, Zamboni G, and Zen Y. Autoimmune pancreatitis (AIP) type 1 and type 2: an international consensus study on histopathologic diagnostic criteria. *Pancreas.* 2011; 40: 1172-1179. PMID: 21975436.
20. Suda K, Takase M, Fukumura Y, and Kashiwagi S. Pathology of autoimmune pancreatitis and tumor- forming pancreatitis. *J Gastroenterol.* 2007; 42 Suppl 18: 22-27. PMID: 17520219.
21. Miyabe K, Notohara K, Nakazawa T, Hayashi K, Naitoh I, Okumura F, Shimizu S, Yoshida M, Yamashita H, Takahashi S, Ohara H, and Joh T. Histological evaluation of obliterative phlebitis for the diagnosis of autoimmune pancreatitis. *J Gastroenterol.* 2014; 49: 715-726. PMID: 23645070.
22. Dhall D, Suriawinata AA, Tang LH, Shia J, and Klimstra DS. Use of immunohistochemistry for IgG4 in the distinction of autoimmune pancreatitis from peritumoral pancreatitis. *Hum Pathol.* 2010; 41: 643-652. PMID: 20149413.
23. Deshpande V, Zen Y, Chan JK, Yi EE, Sato Y, Yoshino T, Klöppel G, Heathcote JG, Khosroshahi A, Ferry JA, Aalberse RC, Bloch DB, Brugge WR, Bateman AC, Carruthers MN, Chari ST, Cheuk W, Cornell LD, Fernandez-Del Castillo C, Forcione DG, Hamilos DL, Kamisawa T, Kasashima S, Kawa S, Kawano M, Lauwers GY, Masaki Y, Nakanuma Y, Notohara K, Okazaki K, Ryu JK, Saeki T, Sahani DV, Smyrk TC, Stone JR, Takahira M, Webster GJ, Yamamoto M, Zamboni G, Umehara H, and Stone JH. Consensus statement on the pathology of IgG4-related disease. *Mod Pathol.* 2012; 25: 1181-1192. PMID: 22596100.
24. Levy MJ, Reddy RP, Wiersema MJ, Smyrk TC, Clain JE, Harewood GC, Pearson RK, Rajan E, Topazian MD, Yusuf TE, Chari ST, and Petersen BT. EUS-guided trucut biopsy in establishing autoimmune pancreatitis as the cause of obstructive jaundice. *Gastrointest Endosc.* 2005; 61: 467-472. PMID: 15758927.
25. Mizuno N, Bhatia V, Hosoda W, Sawaki A, Hoki N, Hara K, Takagi T, Ko SB, Yatabe Y, Goto H, and Yamao K. Histological diagnosis of autoimmune pancreatitis using EUS-guided trucut biopsy: a comparison study with EUS-FNA. *J Gastroenterol.* 2009; 44: 742-750. PMID: 19434362.
26. Kanno A, Ishida K, Hamada S, Fujishima F, Unno J, Kume K, Kikuta K, Hirota M, Masamune A, Satoh K, Notohara K, and Shimosegawa T. Diagnosis of autoimmune pancreatitis by EUS-FNA by using a 22-gauge needle based on the International Consensus Diagnostic Criteria. *Gastrointest Endosc.* 2012; 76: 594-602. PMID: 22898417.
27. Ghazale A, Chari ST, Smyrk TC, Levy MJ, Topazian MD, Takahashi N, Clain JE, Pearson RK, Pelaez- Luna M, Petersen BT, Vege SS, and Farnell MB. Value of serum IgG4 in the diagnosis of autoimmune pancreatitis and in distinguishing it from pancreatic cancer. *Am J Gastroenterol.* 2007; 102: 1646-1653. PMID: 17555461.
28. Motosugi U, Ichikawa T, Yamaguchi H, Nakazawa T, Katoh R, Itakura J, Fujii H, Sato T, Araki T, and Shimizu M. Small invasive ductal adenocarcinoma of the pancreas associated with lymphoplasmacytic sclerosing pancreatitis. *Pathol Int.* 2009; 59: 744-747. PMID: 19788620.
29. Witkiewicz AK, Kennedy EP, Kennyon L, Yeo CJ, and Hruban RH. Synchronous autoimmune pancreatitis and infiltrating pancreatic ductal adenocarcinoma: case report and review of the literature. *Hum Pathol.* 2008; 39: 1548-1551. PMID: 18619645.
30. Fukui T, Mitsuyama T, Takaoka M, Uchida K, Matsushita M, and Okazaki K. Pancreatic cancer associated with autoimmune pancreatitis in remission. *Intern Med.* 2008; 47: 151-155. PMID: 18239323.
31. Oh HC, Kim JG, Kim JW, Lee KS, Kim MK, Chi KC, Kim YS, and Kim KH. Early bile duct cancer in a background of sclerosing cholangitis and autoimmune pancreatitis. *Intern Med.* 2008; 47: 2025-2028. PMID: 19043254.
32. Ohtani H, Ishida H, Ito Y, Yamaguchi T, and Koizumi M. Autoimmune pancreatitis and biliary intraepithelial neoplasia of the common bile duct: a case with diagnostically challenging but pathogenetically significant association. *Pathol Int.* 2011; 61: 481-485. PMID: 21790863.
33. Naitoh I, Nakazawa T, Notohara K, Miyabe K, Hayashi K, Shimizu S, Kondo H, Yoshida M, Yamashita H, Umemura S, Ohara H, and Joh T. Intraductal papillary mucinous neoplasm associated with autoimmune pancreatitis. *Pancreas.* 2013; 42: 552-554. PMID: 23486370.
34. Shiokawa M, Kodama Y, Yoshimura K, Kawanami C, Mimura J, Yamashita Y, Asada M, Kikuyama M, Okabe Y, Inokuma T, Ohana M, Kokuryu H, Takeda K, Tsuji Y, Minami R, Sakuma Y, Kuriyama K, Ota Y, Tanabe W, Maruno T, Kurita A, Sawai Y, Uza N, Watanabe T, Haga H, and Chiba T. Risk of cancer in patients with autoimmune pancreatitis. *Am J Gastroenterol.* 2013; 108: 610-617. PMID: 23318486.

Chapter 57

Serologic abnormalities in autoimmune pancreatitis

Kazuichi Okazaki* and Kazushige Uchida

Department of Gastroenterology and Hepatology, Kansai Medical University, Osaka, Japan.

Introduction

In 1961, Sarles et al. published a case report of pancreatitis with hypergammaglobulinemia, which in retrospect appears to be identical to autoimmune pancreatitis (AIP).[1] In 1995, Yoshida et al. described such a case as AIP.[2] In 2001, Hamano et al. reported increased serum levels of IgG4 in AIP.[3] The histopathological findings of AIP include periductal localization of predominantly CD4-positive T cells, IgG4-positive plasma cells, storiform fibrosis with acinar cell atrophy frequently resulting in the stenosis of the main pancreatic duct, and obliterative fibrosis, resulting in so-called lymphoplasmacytic sclerosing pancreatitis (LPSP).[4-7] Although the infiltration of IgG4-positive cells and increased serum levels of IgG4 are characteristic, they are not specific for type 1 AIP, and the role of IgG4 in the development of AIP and IgG4-related disease remains unclear.[8-10]

Immunology of immunoglobulin subclasses

Generally, the amount of IgG4 does not vary with sex or age, and both IgG4 quantity and the IgG4/total IgG ratio tends to remain constant.[11] In normal subjects, IgG4 consists of 4%-6% of total IgG, and its level in serum can be elevated in several conditions such as allergic disease, parasite infection, and pemphigus vulgaris.[11] In type 1 AIP, total IgG, IgG1, IgG2, IgG4, and IgE are usually increased compared with healthy subjects, while IgM, IgA, and the ratios of IgG to IgM or IgA are decreased compared with normal subjects or those with other diseases[3,12] (**Table 1**). In AIP, all IgG subclasses are increased compared with other types of pancreatitis.

Although the association with IgE-mediated allergy and IgG4 antibodies is well known, the characteristics of IgG4 are less understood.[13] IgG4 antibodies participate in a continuous process referred to as Fab-arm exchange, which describes swapping a heavy chain and attached light chain (half-molecule) with a heavy-light chain pair from another molecule.[14] This produces asymmetric antibodies with two different antigen-combining sites. While these modified antibodies are heterobivalent, they behave as monovalent antibodies (**Figure 1A**).[14] Another aspect of IgG4 mimics IgG rheumatoid factor (RF) activity by interacting with IgG on a solid support (**Figure 1B**).[15] In contrast to conventional RF, which binds via its variable domains, IgG4's activity occurs in its constant domains but is inefficient in activating potentially dangerous effector systems due to its low affinity for C1q and the classical Fcγ-receptors.

Comparison of various markers in differentiating between AIP and pancreatic cancer showed that the best results are obtained using IgG4, which has 86% sensitivity, 96% specificity, and 91% accuracy (**Table 2**).[16] IgG4 was therefore adopted as the best marker in the diagnostic criteria of type 1 AIP.[16] However, serum IgG4 elevation or marked IgG4-bearing plasma cell infiltration has been reported in some patients with pancreatic cancer, suggesting that these features are not completely specific for AIP and cannot exclude the presence of pancreatic cancer.[17]

The complement system

Patients with active AIP occasionally have decreased complement (C3, C4) levels with elevated circulating immune complexes and serum IgG4 elevation.[3,18] However, a recent study showed that the classical pathway of complement activation through IgG1 may be involved in the development of AIP rather than mannose-binding lectin or alternative IgG4 pathways.[19] Moreover, IgG4 bound to other isotypes such as IgG1, IgG2, and IgG3 with an Fc-Fc interaction develop immune complexes in patients with AIP. In this setting, IgG4 may contribute to the clearance of immune complexes or termination of the inflammatory process by preventing the formation of large immune complexes by blocking the Fc-mediated effector functions of IgG1.[15] Compared with systemic lupus erythematosus (SLE), tubulointerstitial nephritis (TIN) is more often observed in renal lesions of IgG4-related

*Corresponding author. Email: okazaki@hirakata.kmu.ac.jp

Table 1. Serum immunoglobulin levels in patients with AIP.[3,12]

Author	Year		n	IgG	IgG1	IgG2	IgG3	IgG4 (/IgG)	IgM	IgA	IgE	IC (μg/mL)
Hamano et al.	2001	AIP	20	2,201	868	617	53	663 (30%)	91	226	176	30
		Control	20	1,341	664	592	34	51	142	247	79	
Taguchi et al.	2009	AIP	20	2,556	NT	NT	NT	762	85	213	NT	
		CP	21	1,245*	NT	NT	NT	NT	122	294	NT	

*Data from Roitt.[11]

AIP, autoimmune pancreatitis; CP, chronic pancreatitis; IC, immune complex; NT, not tested. All Ig values are in units of mg/dl.

disease. In TIN associated with AIP, immune complex (IgG and C3) deposition is more commonly observed in the tubular basement membrane rather than the in the glomerular basement membrane as typically seen in SLE.[20]

Autoantibodies

In addition to increased total IgG and IgG4, patients with IgG4-related disease often have detectable autoantibodies, albeit not organ specific.[5,6] Some patients with IgG4-related disease have nonspecific antibodies such as antinuclear antibody (ANA), but aside from overlapping symptoms, there is no clear association between IgG4-related disease and common autoimmune diseases such as Sjögren's syndrome and SLE. With regard to IgG4 function, it remains unclear if IgG4-related disease is a true autoimmune or allergic disease. However, the frequent coexistence of other organ involvement led to the concept that there may be common

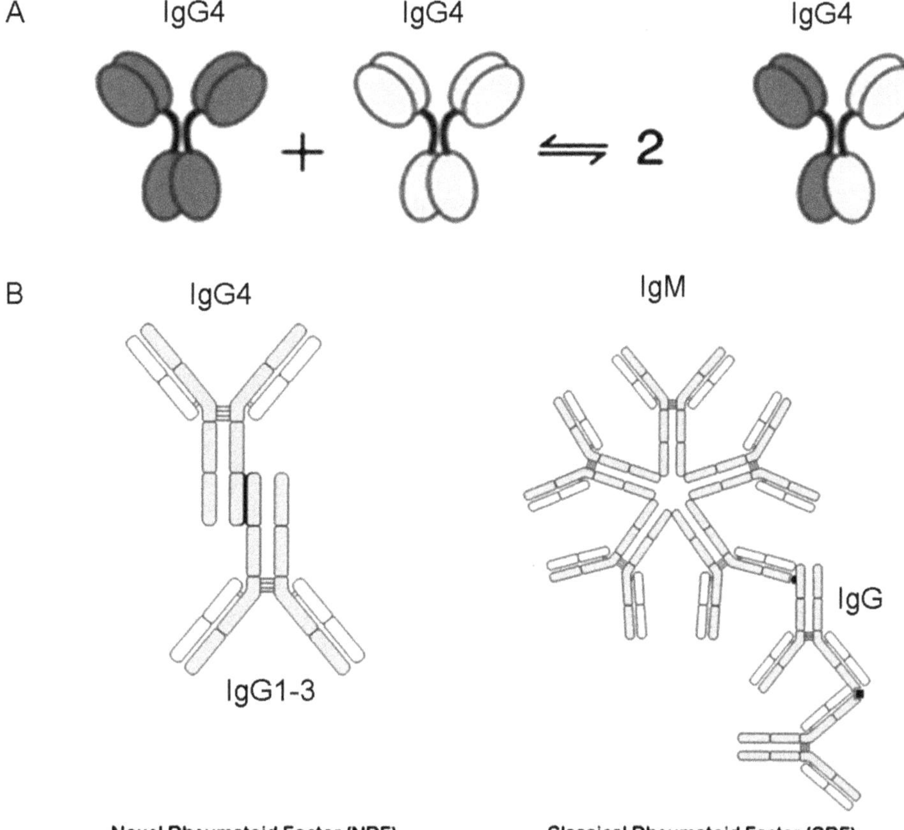

Figure 1. Characteristic forms of IgG4. A, Schematic representation of the generation of bispecific IgG4 antibodies by the exchange of half-molecules ("Fab-arm exchange") From van der Neut Kolfschoten et al.[14] with permission. IgG4 Fab arm exchange occurs by the exchange of a heavy-light chain pair (half-molecule) of one IgG4 molecule with that of another IgG4 molecule. The IgG4 molecule may thereby acquire two distinct Fab arms and become bispecific. The Fc structure remains essentially unchanged apart from potential changes due to differences in glycosylation or allotype. Fab arm exchange is proposed to be stochastic and dynamic. B, Left: IgG4 Fc interacts with Ig Fc. Right: IgM RF recognizes IgG in a "classical" Fab-Fc recognition. From Kawa et al.[15] with permission.

Table 2. Comparison of various markers in the differentiation of AIP and pancreatic cancer using identical sera.

	Sensitivity (AIP n = 100) (%)	Specificity (vs. PC n = 80) (%)	Accuracy (vs. PC)
IgG4	86	96	91
IgG	69	75	72
ANA (anti-nuclear antibody)	58	79	67
RF (rheumatoid factor)	23	94	54
IgG4+ANA	95	76	87
IgG+ANA	85	63	75
IgG4+IgG+ANA	95	63	81
IgG4+RF	90	90	90
IgG+RF	78	73	76
IgG4+IgG+RF	91	71	82
ANA+RF	69	60	78
IgG4+ANA+RF	97	73	86
IgG+ANA+RF	91	61	78
IgG4+IgG+ANA+RF	97	61	81

AIP autoimmune pancreatitis, *PC* pancreatic cancer.
Cited from with permission.[16]

target antigens in the involved organs such as the pancreas, salivary gland, biliary tract, lung, renal tubules, and others. Although the disease-specific antibodies have not been identified, several disease-related antibodies such as anti-lactoferrin (LF),[21,22] anti-carbonic anhydrase (CA)-II,[21-24] anti-CA-IV,[25] anti-pancreatic secretory trypsin inhibitor (PSTI),[26] anti-amylase-alpha,[27] anti-HSP-10,[28] and anti-plasminogen-binding protein (PBP) peptide autoantibodies[29] have been reported. Although patients have increased serum IgG4 levels, the major subclass of these autoantibodies is not necessarily IgG4, but IgG1.[26] CA-II,[21] CA-IV,[25] LF,[21] and PSTI[26] are often distributed in the ductal cells of several exocrine organs including the pancreas, salivary gland, biliary duct, and lung.[21,24] Although not all peptides have been systematically studied, immunization with CA-II or LF induces systemic lesions such as pancreatitis, sialadenitis, cholangitis, and interstitial nephritis in mice models, and these are similar to human IgG4-related diseases.[30,31] The high prevalence of these antibodies suggests that they are at least potential candidate target antigens in AIP.[21,22]

Molecular mimicry among microbes and target antigens may be a possible mechanism to overcome immune tolerance. This hypothesis is based on the concepts that infectious agents share one or more epitopes with self-components and that infectious agents cause bystander activation of immune cells with autoaggressive potential.[32-34] Guarneri and colleagues showed significant homology between human CA-II (a fundamental enzyme for bacterial survival and proliferation in the stomach) and alpha-CA of *Helicobacter pylori*.[32] Moreover, the homologous segments contain the binding motif of DRB1*0405, which confers increased risk for AIP development.[32] The PBP peptide identified in European patients with AIP shows homology with an amino acid sequence of PBP of *H. pylori* and with the ubiquitin-protein ligase E3 component n-recognin 2 (UBR2), an enzyme highly expressed in acinar cells of the pancreas.[29] These findings suggest that gastric *H. pylori* infection might trigger AIP in genetically predisposed subjects.[32-34]

Diabetes mellitus affects 43%-68% of patients with AIP, but autoantibodies against glutamic acid decarboxylase, beta cells, or tyrosine phosphatase-like protein-associated type 1 DM are rarely observed.[35] These findings suggest that islet cells are not likely targeted in the development of DM associated with AIP.

Summary

Although serum IgG4 elevation is a characteristic finding and useful to establish a diagnosis of type 1 AIP, it is not specific for this disorder. Importantly, it can be seen in other conditions with similar clinical presentations including pancreatic cancer. The role of IgG4 antibodies in the pathogeneses of AIP and IgG4-related disease remains unclear. Several autoantibodies have been identified in subjects with AIP, but additional studies are needed to clarify the significance of these findings in the pathophysiology of AIP.

Acknowledgment

This study was partly supported by a Grant-in-Aid for Scientific Research of Ministry of Culture and Science of Japan (23591017), Grants-in-Aid from the CREST Japan Science and Technology

Agency, and a Grant-in-Aid from the "Research for Intractable Disease" Program from the Ministry of Health, Labour, and Welfare of Japan.

References

1. Sarles H, Sarles JC, Muratore R, and Guien C. Chronic inflammatory sclerosis of the pancreas–an autonomous pancreatic disease? *Am J Dig Dis.* 1961; 6: 688-698. PMID: 13746542
2. Yoshida K, Toki F, Takeuchi T, Watanabe S, Shiratori K, and Hayashi N. Chronic pancreatitis caused by an autoimmune abnormality. Proposal of the concept of autoimmune pancreatitis. *Dig Dis Sci.* 1995; 40: 1561-1568. PMID: 7628283
3. Hamano H, Kawa S, Horiuchi A, Unno H, Furuya N, Akamatsu T, Fukushima M, Nikaido T, Nakayama K, Usuda N, and Kiyosawa K. High serum IgG4 concentrations in patients with sclerosing pancreatitis. *N Engl J Med.* 2001; 344: 732-738. PMID: 11236777
4. Kawaguchi K, Koike M, Tsuruta K, Okamoto A, Tabata I, and Fujita N. Lymphoplasmacytic sclerosing pancreatitis with cholangitis: a variant of primary sclerosing cholangitis extensively involving pancreas. *Hum Pathol.* 1991; 22: 387-395. PMID: 2050373
5. Okazaki K, Uchida K, Koyabu M, Miyoshi H, and Takaoka M. Recent advances in the concept and diagnosis of autoimmune pancreatitis and IgG4-related disease. *J Gastroenterol.* 2011; 46: 277-288. PMID: 21452084
6. Okazaki K, Uchida K, Ikeura T, and Takaoka M. Current concept and diagnosis of IgG4-related disease in the hepato-bilio-pancreatic system. *J Gastroenterol.* 2013; 48: 303-314. PMID: 23417598
7. Shimosegawa T, Chari ST, Frulloni L, Kamisawa T, Kawa S, Mino-Kenudson M, Kim MH, Klöppel G, Lerch MM, Löhr M, Notohara K, Okazaki K, Schneider A, and Zhang L; International Association of Pancreatology. International consensus diagnostic criteria for autoimmune pancreatitis: guidelines of the International Association of Pancreatology. *Pancreas.* 2011; 40: 352-358. PMID: 21412117
8. Kamisawa T, and Okamoto A. Autoimmune pancreatitis: proposal of IgG4-related sclerosing disease. *J Gastroenterol*; 41: 613-25, 2006. PMID: 16932997
9. Umehara H, Okazaki K, Masaki Y, Kawano M, Yamamoto M, Saeki T, Matsui S, Yoshino T, Nakamura S, Kawa S, Hamano H, Kamisawa T, Shimosegawa T, Shimatsu A, Nakamura S, Ito T, Notohara K, Sumida T, Tanaka Y, Mimori T, Chiba T, Mishima M, Hibi T, Tsubouchi H, Inui K, Ohara H. Comprehensive diagnostic criteria for IgG4-related disease (IgG4-RD), 2011. *Mod Rheumatol* 22: 21-30, 2012. PMID: 22620057
10. Umehara H, Okazaki K, Masaki Y, Kawano M, Yamamoto M, Saeki T, Matsui S, Sumida T, Mimori T, Tanaka Y, Tsubota K, Yoshino T, Kawa S, Suzuki R, Takegami T, Tomosugi N, Kurose N, Ishigaki Y, Azumi A, Kojima M, Nakamura S, and Inoue D. A novel clinical entity, IgG4-related disease (IgG4RD): general concept and details. *Mod Rheumatol.* 2012; 22: 1-14. PMID: 21881964
11. Roitt I. Antibodies. In: Roitt I, ed. *Roitt's essential immunology.* 9th ed. London: Blackwell Science; 1997.
12. Taguchi M, Kihara Y, Nagashio Y, Yamamoto M, Otsuki M, and Harada M. Decreased production of immunoglobulin M and A in autoimmune pancreatitis. *J Gastroenterol.* 2009; 44: 1133-1139. PMID: 19626266
13. Robinson DS, Larche M, and Durham SR. Tregs and allergic disease. *J Clin Invest.* 2004; 114: 1389-1397. PMID: 15545986
14. van der Neut Kolfschoten M, Schuurman J, Losen M, Bleeker WK, Martínez-Martínez P, Vermeulen E, den Bleker TH, Wiegman L, Vink T, Aarden LA, De Baets MH, van de Winkel JG, Aalberse RC, and Parren PW. Anti-inflammatory activity of human IgG4 antibodies by dynamic Fab arm exchange. *Science.* 2007; 317: 1554-1557. PMID: 17872445
15. Kawa S, Kitahara K, Hamano H, Ozaki Y, Arakura N, Yoshizawa K, Umemura T, Ota M, Mizoguchi S, Shimozuru Y, and Bahram S. A novel immunoglobulin-immunoglobulin interaction in autoimmunity. *PLoS One.* 2008; 3: e1637. PMID: 18297131
16. Kawa S, Okazaki K, Kamisawa T, Shimosegawa T, and Tanaka M. Working members of Research Committee for Intractable Pancreatic Disease and Japan Pancreas Society. Japanese consensus guidelines for management of autoimmune pancreatitis: II. Extrapancreatic lesions, differential diagnosis. *J Gastroenterol.* 2010; 45: 355-369. PMID: 20127119
17. Ghazale A, Chari ST, Smyrk TC, Levy MJ, Topazian MD, Takahashi N, Clain JE, Pearson RK, Pelaez- Luna M, Petersen BT, Vege SS, and Farnell MB. Value of serum IgG4 in the diagnosis of autoimmune pancreatitis and in distinguishing it from pancreatic cancer. *Am J Gastroenterol.* 2007; 102: 1646-1653. PMID: 17555461
18. Cornell LD, Chicano SL, Deshpande V, Collins AB, Selig MK, Lauwers GY, Barisoni L, and Colvin RB. Pseudotumors due to IgG4 immune-complex tubulointerstitial nephritis associated with autoimmune pancreatocentric disease. *Am J Surg Pathol.* 2007; 31: 1586-1597. PMID: 17895762
19. Muraki T, Hamano H, Ochi Y, Komatsu K, Komiyama Y, Arakura N, Yoshizawa K, Ota M, Kawa S, and Kiyosawa K. Autoimmune pancreatitis and complement activation system. *Pancreas.* 2006; 32: 16-21. PMID: 16340739
20. Uchiyama-Tanaka Y, Mori Y, Kimura T, Sonomura K, Umemura S, Kishimoto N, Nose A, Tokoro T, Kijima Y, Yamahara H, Nagata T, Masaki H, Umeda Y, Okazaki K, and Iwasaka T. Acute tubulointerstitial nephritis associated with autoimmune-related pancreatitis. *Am J Kidney Dis.* 2004; 43: e18-e25. PMID: 14981637
21. Okazaki K, Uchida K, Ohana M, Nakase H, Uose S, Inai M, Matsushima Y, Katamura K, Ohmori K, and Chiba T. Autoimmune-related pancreatitis is associated with autoantibodies and a Thl/Th2-type cellular immune response. *Gastroenterology.* 2000; 118: 573-581. PMID: 10702209
22. Uchida K, Okazaki K, Konishi Y, Ohana M, Takakuwa H, Hajiro K, and Chiba T. Clinical analysis of autoimmune-related pancreatitis. *Am J Gastroenterol.* 2000; 95: 2788-2794. PMID: 11051349

23. Aparisi L, Farre A, Gomez-Cambronero L, Martinez J, De Las Heras G, Corts J, Navarro S, Mora J, Lopez-Hoyos M, Sabater L, Ferrandez A, Bautista D, Perez-Mateo M, Mery S, and Sastre J. Antibodies to carbonic anhydrase and IgG4 levels in idiopathic chronic pancreatitis: relevance for diagnosis of autoimmune pancreatitis. *Gut.* 2005; 54: 703-709. PMID: 15831920
24. Nishi H, Tojo A, Onozato ML, Jimbo R, Nangaku M, Uozaki H, Hirano K, Isayama H, Omata M, Kaname S, and Fujita T. Anti-carbonic anhydrase II antibody in autoimmune pancreatitis and tubulointerstitial nephritis. *Nephrol Dial Transplant.* 2007; 22: 1273-1275. PMID: 17138573
25. Nishimori I, Miyaji E, Morimoto K, Nagao K, Kamada M, and Onishi S. Serum antibodies to carbonic anhydrase IV in patients with autoimmune pancreatitis. *Gut.* 2005; 54: 274-281. PMID: 15647194
26. Asada M, Nishio A, Uchida K, Kido M, Ueno S, Uza N, Kiriya K, Inoue S, Kitamura H, Ohashi S, Tamaki H, Fukui T, Matsuura M, Kawasaki K, Nishi T, Watanabe N, Nakase H, Chiba T, and Okazaki K. Identification of a novel autoantibody against pancreatic secretory trypsin inhibitor in patients with autoimmune pancreatitis. *Pancreas.* 2006; 33: 20-26. PMID: 16804408
27. Endo T, Takizawa S, Tanaka S, Takahashi M, Fujii H, Kamisawa T, and Kobayashi T. Amylase alpha-2A autoantibodies: novel marker of autoimmune pancreatitis and fulminant type 1 diabetes. *Diabetes.* 2009; 58: 732-737. PMID: 19001184
28. Takizawa S, Endo T, Wanjia X, Tanaka S, Takahashi M, and Kobayashi T. HSP 10 is a new autoantigen in both autoimmune pancreatitis and fulminant type 1 diabetes. *Biochem Biophys Res Commun.* 2009; 386: 192-196. PMID: 19520060
29. Frulloni L, Lunardi C, Simone R, Dolcino M, Scattolini C, Falconi M, Benini L, Vantini I, Corrocher R, and Puccetti A. Identification of a novel antibody associated with autoimmune pancreatitis. *N Engl J Med.* 2009; 361: 2135-2142. PMID: 19940298
30. Nishimori I, Bratanova T, Toshkov I, Caffrey T, Mogaki M, Shibata Y, and Hollingsworth MA. Induction of experimental autoimmune sialoadenitis by immunization of PL/J mice with carbonic anhydrase II. *J Immunol.* 1995; 154: 4865-4873. PMID: 7722336
31. Ueno Y, Ishii M, Takahashi S, Igarashi T, Toyota T, and LaRusso NF. Different susceptibility of mice to immune-mediated cholangitis induced by immunization with carbonic anhydrase II. *Lab Invest.* 1998; 78: 629-637. PMID: 9605187
32. Guarneri F, Guarneri C, and Benvenga S. Helicobacter pylori and autoimmune pancreatitis: role of carbonic anhydrase via molecular mimicry? *J Cell Mol Med.* 2005; 9: 741-744. PMID: 16202223
33. Kountouras J, Zavos C, and Chatzopoulos D. A concept on the role of Helicobacter pylori infection in autoimmune pancreatitis. *J Cell Mol Med.* 2005; 9: 196-207. PMID: 15784177
34. Kountouras J, Zavos C, Gavalas E, and Tzilves D. Challenge in the pathogenesis of autoimmune pancreatitis: potential role of helicobacter pylori infection via molecular mimicry. *Gastroenterology.* 2007; 133: 368-369. PMID: 17631165
35. Okazaki K. Autoimmune pancreatitis: etiology, pathogenesis, clinical findings and treatment. The Japanese experience. *JOP.* 2005; 6 Suppl 1: 89-96. PMID: 15650291
36. Aoki S, Nakazawa T, Ohara H, Sano H, Nakao H, Joh T, Murase T, Eimoto T, and Itoh M. Immunohistochemical study of autoimmune pancreatitis using anti-IgG4 antibody and patients' sera. *Histopathology.* 2005; 47: 147-158. PMID: 16045775
37. Uchida K, Okazaki K, Nishi T, Uose S, Nakase H, Ohana M, Matsushima Y, Omori K, and Chiba T. Experimental immune-mediated pancreatitis in neonatally thymectomized mice immunized with carbonic anhydrase II and lactoferrin. *Lab Invest.* 2002; 82: 411-424. PMID: 11950899

Chapter 58

CT and MR features of autoimmune pancreatitis

Naoki Takahashi*

Department of Radiology, Mayo Clinic, Rochester, MN.

Introduction

Patients with autoimmune pancreatitis (AIP) often present with vague abdominal pain, jaundice, or weight loss. Differentiating AIP from pancreatic cancer is important to avoid unnecessary surgery or invasive intervention. It is not difficult to make a correct diagnosis when computed tomography (CT) or magnetic resonance (MR) reveals characteristic imaging findings of AIP; however, differentiating AIP from pancreatic ductal adenocarcinoma on CT or MR can be very challenging at times. AIP is one of the most common benign conditions for which pancreatic resection is performed for suspected pancreatic ductal adenocarcinoma.[1,2] Combinations of ancillary findings may lead to the correct diagnosis; therefore, it is important to be familiar with the various imaging findings of AIP.

Features of AIP

Pancreatic parenchymal morphology

Diffuse parenchymal enlargement of the pancreas is the characteristic feature of AIP seen in 24%-73% of patients (**Figure 1**).[3-8] The pancreatic border becomes featureless with effacement of the lobular contour of the pancreas, resulting in the so-called "sausage shaped pancreas."[5] Focal, mass-like enlargement of the pancreas is seen in 18%-40% of patients with AIP.[5-7,8] Any portion of the pancreas can be involved, but involvement of the pancreatic head is more common.[6,9] The enlarged segment of the pancreas is typically isoattenuated compared to the nonenlarged segment of pancreatic parenchyma.[5] In a small number of cases, the focally enlarged segment forms a low-attenuation mass and may be indistinguishable from pancreatic cancer.[5,7,8,10] The demarcation between the normal parenchyma tends to be sharp in such cases.[10] Atrophy of the pancreas upstream to the focally involved area is uncommon in patients with AIP as opposed to patients with pancreatic ductal adenocarcinoma. The pancreas may exhibit a long segment of low attenuation without mass-like enlargement. Rarely, AIP may present as multiple low-attenuation lesions.[11] Finally, the pancreas may appear normal in size or atrophic in 9%-36% of patients.[3,6,7] A normal size pancreas may be observed in a milder form of disease, but the enhancement pattern is usually altered in such cases.[6] Pancreatic atrophy usually represents a late burnt-out phase of the disease or the posttreatment state.[5]

Capsule sign

A capsule-like rim (**Figure 1**) is a highly specific sign of AIP, and can been seen in 14%-48% of patients with AIP.[4,5-7] The capsule-like rim is low attenuation on contrast-enhanced CT, hypointense on both T1- and T2-weighted images, and shows delayed enhancement on MR. The rim may diffusely surround the entire pancreas or only focal regions.[6] The rim is thought to represent peripancreatic extension of the characteristic inflammatory cell infiltration.[4] This is contrary to the high-attenuation rim that can sometimes be seen in infiltrating pancreatic ductal adenocarcinoma.[12] The high-attenuation rim represents a normal parenchyma compressed by carcinoma.

Pancreatic parenchymal enhancement

The enhancement pattern of the pancreatic parenchyma should be carefully evaluated on CT or MR using a multiphasic technique because it often provides a helpful diagnostic clue. The involved segment(s) of the pancreas commonly demonstrate delayed enhancement in AIP.[4] CT attenuation of the pancreas in AIP is similar or higher than that of the liver and lower than that of spleen during the pancreatic phase, whereas it is similar or higher than that of the liver and higher than that of spleen in the hepatic phase on a biphasic CT scan.[9,13] One study quantitatively showed that the mean CT attenuation value of the pancreatic parenchyma in AIP was significantly lower than in normal controls during the pancreatic phase (AIP: 85 HU, normal pancreas: 104 HU; $P < .05$) but not significantly different in the hepatic phase (AIP: 96 HU, normal pancreas: 89 HU; $P < .6$).[14] Similar enhancement patterns were observed on MR.[15,16]

*Corresponding author. Email: takahashi.naoki@mayo.edu

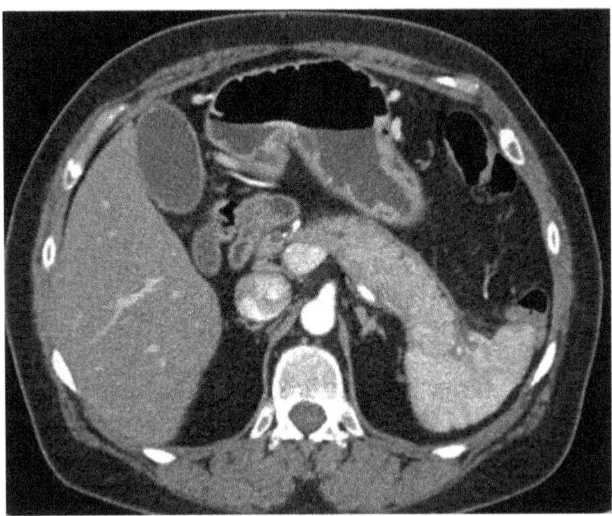

Figure 1. Abdomen CT with contrast demonstrating a diffusely enlarged, hypoattenuating pancreas with a capsule-like rim.

A similar enhancement pattern is also seen in patients with focal AIP: decreased and delayed enhancement during the pancreatic and hepatic phases, respectively. On the other hand, pancreatic ductal adenocarcinoma commonly shows decreased enhancement in the pancreatic phase with a minimal change in enhancement in the hepatic phase. Wakabayashi et al. evaluated the CT enhancement pattern in nine patients with focal AIP; they found that six lesions were hypoattenuating in the early phase, but all were homogeneously isoattenuating in the delayed phase.[8] Conversely, only 2 of 80 patients with pancreatic ductal adenocarcinoma had homogeneous enhancement in the delayed phase. A different study showed that the mean CT attenuation value of focal AIP was not significantly different in the pancreatic phase (AIP: 71 HU, carcinoma: 59 HU; $P = .06$), but was significantly higher than carcinoma in the hepatic phase (AIP: 90 HU, carcinoma: 64 HU; $P < .001$).[14] Delayed enhancement of the mass or focally enlarged segment, defined as a ≥15-HU increase from the pancreatic to hepatic phases, was found in 7 of the 13 (54%) patients with focal AIP and 5 of 33 (15%) patients with carcinoma ($P = .02$).[14]

MR features of AIP

On MR, the pancreas is diffusely hypointense on T1-weighted images and slightly hyperintense on T2-weighted images (**Figure 2**).[4,5,15,16] Enhancement characteristics on MR are similar to those seen on CT. Diffusion-weighted MR has been shown to be helpful in differentiating AIP from pancreatic cancer. Kamisawa et al. reported that apparent diffusion coefficient values were significantly lower in AIP ($1.01 - 0.11 \times 10^{-3}$ mm^2/s) than in pancreatic cancer ($1.25 - 0.11 \times 10^{-3}$ mm^2/s) and the normal pancreas ($1.49 - 0.16 \times 10^{-3}$ mm^2/s) ($P < .001$).[17] Taniguchi et al. showed that apparent diffusion coefficient values were significantly lower in AIP ($0.97 - 0.18 \times 10^{-3}$ mm^2/s) compared to other types of chronic pancreatitis ($1.45 - 0.10 \times 10^{-3}$ mm^2/s).[18] In addition, diffusion-weighted MR was helpful in reclassifying what appeared to be focal mass-forming AIP to diffuse AIP by showing diffusely decreased apparent diffusion coefficient values in the nonenlarged pancreatic segment.

Pancreatic ductal imaging

Diffuse or segmental narrowing of the main pancreatic duct (MPD) is the characteristic endoscopic retrograde pancreatocholangiography (ERCP) finding of AIP (see chapter T. Kamisawa, ERCP Features of Autoimmune Pancreatitis).[5,19] Diffuse narrowing of the duct is often difficult to differentiate from a normal-caliber duct on CT or MR. Segmental narrowing of the MPD may be seen as a poorly visualized segment on CT or MRCP compared to a normal- caliber pancreatic duct in uninvolved segments of the pancreas.[20,21] Mild pancreatic ductal dilation may be present upstream of the narrowed segment. The degree of MPD dilation is usually milder than that seen in cases of pancreatic ductal adenocarcinoma. A relatively specific MPD change of AIP is multifocal narrowing, and this may be depicted on CT or MRCP.[21,22] Although it is helpful if classic abnormalities are present, MRCP often does not provide adequate visualization of the MPD and is thus not considered as a satisfactory means of pancreatic ductal imaging in the current diagnostic criteria (see chapter P.A. Hart & S.T. Chari, Diagnosis of Autoimmune Pancreatitis). The duct-penetrating sign of a visible duct within a mass may be helpful in differentiating AIP from pancreatic cancer.[23,24] Secretin-stimulated MRCP may

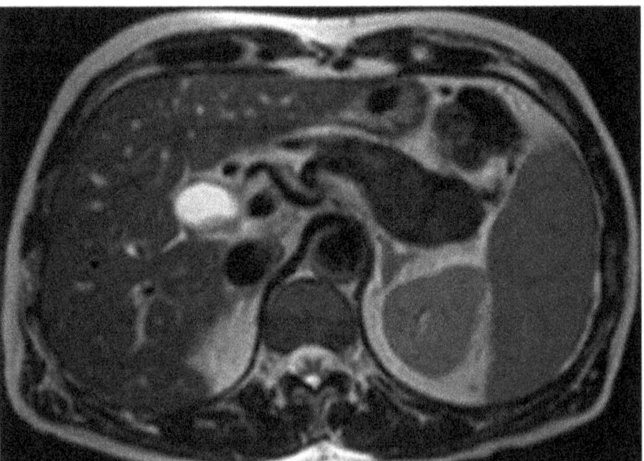

Figure 2. MRI abdomen (T2 weighted image) demonstrating diffuse pancreatic enlargement with a low T2 signal rim around the tail.

enhance detection of the pancreatic duct-penetrating sign.[22] Enhancement of the pancreatic duct wall may be present in patients with AIP on portal- or delayed-phase CT.[6,25]

Miscellaneous pancreatic findings

Pancreatic pseudocysts and/or calcifications are typically associated with alcohol-induced chronic pancreatitis.[8] However, calcifications and cysts are seen in 14%-32% and 10%-12% of patients with AIP, respectively,[6,7] especially in the late or postacute phase. Therefore, the presence of calcifications or cysts should not exclude the possibility of AIP.[26,27] Vessels are commonly involved by extension of peripancreatic soft tissue in patients with AIP (44%-68%). Involved veins are often narrowed, but occlusion may also occur.[6]

Extrapancreatic abdomen involvement

The most common site of extrapancreatic involvement is the biliary tree presenting as asymptomatic liver test abnormalities or jaundice.[7] On imaging, biliary involvement commonly appears as multifocal biliary strictures similar to primary sclerosing cholangitis. On CT or MR, the strictured bile duct commonly appears as diffuse or focal thickening of the wall. Rarely, it may form a mass that mimics cholangiocarcinoma. The kidneys are also commonly involved.[28] On CT or MR, renal lesions are commonly bilateral and multiple, predominantly involving the renal cortex (**Figure 3**). Renal parenchymal lesions can be classified as small peripheral cortical nodules, round or wedge-shaped lesions, or diffuse patchy involvement. Renal lesions may present as large, solitary masses that mimic primary renal neoplasm. Retroperitoneal fibrosis is seen in 10% of cases (**Figure 4**).

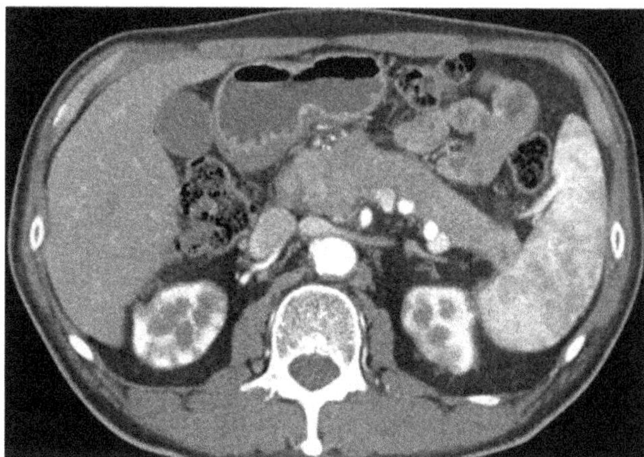

Figure 3. Abdomen CT with contrast demonstrating diffuse pancreatic enlargement with hypoattenuation. Multiple wedge-shaped low-attenuation lesions are present in the bilateral renal cortices.

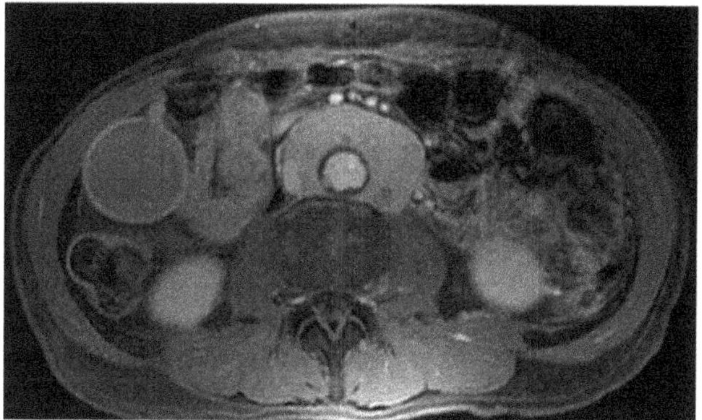

Figure 4. Gadolinium-enhanced abdomen MRI (T1-weighted image) demonstrating enhancing, soft tissue thickening surrounding the abdominal aorta, consistent with retroperitoneal fibrosis.

Differences between types 1 and 2 AIP

A recent study by Deshpande et al. showed that the pancreatic tail cut-off sign was only seen in type 2 AIP.[29,30] Other imaging features such as the type of pancreatic swelling, presence of capsule-like rim, and common bile duct strictures were not helpful in distinguishing the two types. An international multicenter survey showed that diffuse pancreas swelling was more common in type 1 compared to type 2 AIP (40% vs 25%).[30] The pattern of extrapancreatic organ involvement is distinct between the two types and helpful when present.[30] Biliary or renal involvement and retroperitoneal fibrosis are exclusively seen in type 1 AIP, whereas inflammatory bowel disease is commonly associated with type 2 AIP.[30]

Summary

Imaging features of CT and MR are critical for establishing the diagnosis of AIP and excluding other potential etiologies, especially pancreatic cancer. Classic imaging features that are relatively specific for AIP include diffuse pancreatic enlargement, the presence of a hypoattenuating capsule rim, and delayed parenchymal enhancement. Although not always present, findings of multifocal narrowing of the MPD or other organ involvement such as biliary strictures, renal involvement, and retroperitoneal fibrosis are helpful clues for AIP diagnosis. The imaging variants of AIP (focal and multifocal involvement) are sometimes indistinguishable from malignancy and require careful evaluation for collateral diagnostic evidence.

References

1. Hardacre JM, Iacobuzio-Donahue CA, Sohn TA, Abraham SC, Yeo CJ, Lillemoe KD, Choti MA, Campbell KA, Schulick RD, Hruban RH, Cameron JL, and Leach SD.

Results of pancreaticoduodenectomy for lymphoplasmacytic sclerosing pancreatitis. *Ann Surg.* 2003; 237: 853-858.

2. Yadav D, Notahara K, Smyrk TC, Clain JE, Pearson RK, Farnell MB, and Chari ST. Idiopathic tumefactive chronic pancreatitis: clinical profile, histology, and natural history after resection. *Clin Gastroenterol Hepatol.* 2003; 1: 129-135. PMID: 15017505
3. Church NI, Pereira SP, Deheragoda MG, Sandanayake N, Amin Z, Lees WR, Gillams A, Rodriguez-Justo M, Novelli M, Seward EW, Hatfield AR, and Webster GJ. Autoimmune pancreatitis: clinical and radiological features and objective response to steroid therapy in a UK series. *Am J Gastroenterol.* 2007; 102: 2417-2425. PMID: 17894845
4. Irie H, Honda H, Baba S, Kuroiwa T, Yoshimitsu K, Tajima T, Jimi M, Sumii T, and Masuda K. Autoimmune pancreatitis: CT and MR characteristics. *AJR Am J Roentgenol.* 1998; 170: 1323-1327. PMID: 9574610
5. Sahani DV, Kalva SP, Farrell J, Maher MM, Saini S, Mueller PR, Lauwers GY, Fernandez CD, Warshaw AL, and Simeone JF. Autoimmune pancreatitis: imaging features. *Radiology.* 2004; 233: 345-352. PMID: 15459324
6. Suzuki K, Itoh S, Nagasaka T, Ogawa H, Ota T, and Naganawa S. CT findings in autoimmune pancreatitis: assessment using multiphase contrast-enhanced multisection CT. *Clin Radiol.* 2010; 65: 735-743. PMID: 20696301
7. Takahashi N, Fletcher JG, Fidler JL, Hough DM, Kawashima A, and Chari ST. Dual-phase CT of autoimmune pancreatitis: a multireader study. *AJR Am J Roentgenol.* 2008; 190: 280-286. PMID: 18212210
8. Wakabayashi T, Kawaura Y, Satomura Y, Watanabe H, Motoo Y, Okai T, and Sawabu N. Clinical and imaging features of autoimmune pancreatitis with focal pancreatic swelling or mass formation: comparison with so-called tumor-forming pancreatitis and pancreatic carcinoma. *Am J Gastroenterol.* 2003; 98: 2679-2687. PMID: 14687817
9. Muhi A, Ichikawa T, Motosugi U, Sou H, Sano K, Tsukamoto T, Fatima Z, and Araki T. Mass-forming autoimmune pancreatitis and pancreatic carcinoma: differential diagnosis on the basis of computed tomography and magnetic resonance cholangiopancreatography, and diffusion-weighted imaging findings. *J Magn Reson Imaging.* 2012; 35: 827-836. PMID: 22069025
10. Van Hoe L, Gryspeerdt S, Ectors N, Van Steenbergen W, Aerts R, Baert AL, and Marchal G. Nonalcoholic duct-destructive chronic pancreatitis: imaging findings. *AJR Am J Roentgenol.* 1998; 170: 643-647. PMID: 9490945
11. Kajiwara M, Kojima M, Konishi M, Nakagohri T, Takahashi S, Gotohda N, Hasebe T, Ochiai A, and Kinoshita T. Autoimmune pancreatitis with multifocal lesions. *J Hepatobiliary Pancreat Surg.* 2008; 15: 449-452. PMID: 18670850
12. Choi YJ, Byun JH, Kim JY, Kim MH, Jang SJ, Ha HK, and Lee MG. Diffuse pancreatic ductal adenocarcinoma: characteristic imaging features. *European Journal of Radiology.* 2008; 67: 321-328. PMID: 17766075
13. Yang DH, Kim KW, Kim TK, Park SH, Kim SH, Kim MH, Lee SK, Kim AY, Kim PN, Ha HK, and Lee MG. Autoimmune pancreatitis: radiologic findings in 20 patients. *Abdom Imaging.* 2006; 31: 94-102. PMID: 16333694
14. Takahashi N, Fletcher JG, Hough DM, Fidler JL, Kawashima A, Mandrekar JN, and Chari ST. Autoimmune pancreatitis: differentiation from pancreatic carcinoma and normal pancreas on the basis of enhancement characteristics at dual-phase CT. *AJR Am J Roentgenol.* 2009; 193: 479-484. PMID: 19620446
15. Manfredi R, Frulloni L, Mantovani W, Bonatti M, Graziani R, and Pozzi Mucelli R. Autoimmune Pancreatitis: Pancreatic and Extrapancreatic MR Imaging-MR Cholangiopancreatography Findings at Diagnosis, after Steroid Therapy, and at Recurrence. *Radiology.* 2011; 260: 428-436. PMID: 21613442
16. Rehnitz C, Klauss M, Singer R, Ehehalt R, Werner J, Buchler MW, Kauczor HU, and Grenacher L. Morphologic patterns of autoimmune pancreatitis in CT and MRI. *Pancreatology: official journal of the International Association of Pancreatology.* 2011; 11: 240-251. PMID: 21625195
17. Kamisawa T, Takuma K, Anjiki H, Egawa N, Hata T, Kurata M, Honda G, Tsuruta K, Suzuki M, Kamata N, and Sasaki T. Differentiation of autoimmune pancreatitis from pancreatic cancer by diffusion- weighted MRI. *Am J Gastroenterol.* 2010; 105: 1870-1875. PMID: 20216538
18. Taniguchi T, Kobayashi H, Nishikawa K, Iida E, Michigami Y, Morimoto E, Yamashita R, Miyagi K, and Okamoto M. Diffusion-weighted magnetic resonance imaging in autoimmune pancreatitis. *Japanese journal of radiology.* 2009; 27: 138-142. PMID: 19412681
19. Horiuchi A, Kawa S, Hamano H, Hayama M, Ota H, and Kiyosawa K. ERCP features in 27 patients with autoimmune pancreatitis. *Gastrointest Endosc.* 2002; 55: 494-499. PMID: 11923760
20. Kamisawa T, Tu Y, Egawa N, Tsuruta K, Okamoto A, Kodama M, and Kamata N. Can MRCP replace ERCP for the diagnosis of autoimmune pancreatitis? *Abdom Imaging.* 2009; 34: 381-384. PMID: 18437450
21. Park SH, Kim MH, Kim SY, Kim HJ, Moon SH, Lee SS, Byun JH, Lee SK, Seo DW, and Lee MG. Magnetic resonance cholangiopancreatography for the diagnostic evaluation of autoimmune pancreatitis. *Pancreas.* 2010; 39: 1191-1198. PMID: 20467343
22. Sahani DV, Kalva SP, Farrell J, Maher MM, Saini S, Mueller PR, Lauwers GY, Fernandez CD, Warshaw AL, and Simeone JF. Autoimmune pancreatitis: imaging features. *Radiology.* 2004; 233: 345-352. PMID: 15459324
23. Ichikawa T, Sou H, Araki T, Arbab AS, Yoshikawa T, Ishigame K, Haradome H, and Hachiya J. Duct- penetrating sign at MRCP: usefulness for differentiating inflammatory pancreatic mass from pancreatic carcinomas. *Radiology.* 2001; 221: 107-116. PMID: 11568327
24. Muhi A, Ichikawa T, Motosugi U, Sou H, Sano K, Tsukamoto T, Fatima Z, and Araki T. Mass-forming autoimmune pancreatitis and pancreatic carcinoma: differential diagnosis on the basis of computed tomography and magnetic resonance cholangiopancreatography, and diffusion-weighted imaging findings. *Journal of Magnetic Resonance Imaging: JMRI.* 2012; 35: 827-836. PMID: 22069025
25. Kawai Y, Suzuki K, Itoh S, Takada A, Mori Y, and Naganawa S. Autoimmune pancreatitis: assessment of the enhanced duct sign on multiphase contrast-enhanced computed tomography. *European journal of radiology.* 2012; 81: 3055-3060. PMID: 22613506

26. Muraki T, Hamano H, Ochi Y, Arakura N, Takayama M, Komatsu K, Komiyama Y, Kawa S, Uehara T, and Kiyosawa K. Corticosteroid-responsive pancreatic cyst found in autoimmune pancreatitis. *J Gastroenterol.* 2005; 40: 761-766. PMID: 16082595
27. Nishimura T, Masaoka T, Suzuki H, Aiura K, Nagata H, and Ishii H. Autoimmune pancreatitis with pseudocysts. *J Gastroenterol.* 2004; 39: 1005-1010. PMID: 15549456
28. Takahashi N, Kawashima A, Fletcher JG, and Chari ST. Renal involvement in patients with autoimmune pancreatitis: CT and MR imaging findings. *Radiology.* 2007; 242: 791-801. PMID: 17229877
29. Deshpande V, Gupta R, Sainani N, Sahani DV, Virk R, Ferrone C, Khosroshahi A, Stone JH, and Lauwers GY. Subclassification of autoimmune pancreatitis: a histologic classification with clinical significance. *Am J Surg Pathol.* 2011; 35: 26-35. PMID: 21164284
30. Kamisawa T, Chari ST, Giday SA, Kim MH, Chung JB, Lee KT, Werner J, Bergmann F, Lerch MM, Mayerle J, Pickartz T, Lohr M, Schneider A, Frulloni L, Webster GJ, Reddy DN, Liao WC, Wang HP, Okazaki K, Shimosegawa T, Kloeppel G, and Go VL. Clinical profile of autoimmune pancreatitis and its histological subtypes: an international multicenter survey. *Pancreas.* 2011; 40: 809-814. PMID: 21747310

Chapter 59

ERCP features of autoimmune pancreatitis

Terumi Kamisawa*

Department of Internal Medicine, Tokyo Metropolitan Komagome Hospital.

Introduction

Autoimmune pancreatitis (AIP) is a newly recognized form of pancreatitis that can mimic malignancy.[1] Patients with AIP and pancreatic cancer share many clinical features such as a higher prevalence among elderly males, frequent presentation with painless jaundice, development of diabetes mellitus, and elevated levels of serum tumor markers. Radiologically, focal swelling of the pancreas, the "double-duct sign" (representing dilation of both the biliary and pancreatic ducts), and encasement of peripancreatic arteries and portal veins can be seen in both AIP and pancreatic cancer.[2-3] Because AIP responds dramatically to steroid therapy, differentiating between AIP and pancreatic cancer is of paramount importance to avoid unnecessary laparotomy or pancreatic resection. As definite serological markers for AIP are lacking, its diagnosis is currently based on a combination of clinical, laboratory, and imaging studies. Imaging of the pancreatic duct with endoscopic retrograde pancreatocholangiography (ERCP) plays an important role in diagnosing AIP.

Autoimmune pancreatitis and ERCP

The concept of AIP emerged from pancreatographic study of chronic pancreatitis. Four cases of peculiar pancreatitis showing diffuse irregular narrowing of the entire main pancreatic duct (MPD) on endoscopic retrograde pancreatography (ERP) were reported by Toki et al. of Tokyo Women's Medical University in 1992.[4] Yoshida et al., from the same group, proposed the concept of AIP on the basis of a case with diffuse irregular narrowing of the MPD on ERP that responded to steroids.[5] ERCP is basically required in the focal/segmental type AIP in the 2011 Japanese clinical diagnostic criteria for AIP.[6]

ERCP features suggesting autoimmune pancreatitis

Unlike obstruction or stenosis, narrowing of the MPD (in which the duct diameter is smaller than normal with irregular walls) that extends to a certain degree is seen in AIP patients. Typical AIP cases show narrowing extending over one-third of the entire length of the MPD. Typical AIP cases show narrowing extending over one-third of the entire length of the MPD (**Figure 1**).[7] In one study that compared ERCP findings of 48 AIP patients and 143 pancreatic cancer patients, the length of the narrowed portion of the MPD was significantly longer and the diameter of the upstream MPD was significantly smaller in AIP than in pancreatic cancer.[8]

Furthermore, pancreatographic findings such as a lack of MPD obstruction, skip lesions in the MPD (**Figure 2**), side branch derivation from the narrowed portion of the MPD (**Figure 2**), a >3-cm-long narrowed portion of the MPD, and maximal diameter of the upstream MPD <5 mm are highly suggestive of AIP rather than pancreatic cancer (**Table 1**).

Although stenosis of the lower bile duct is frequently detected on cholangiography in both AIP and pancreatic

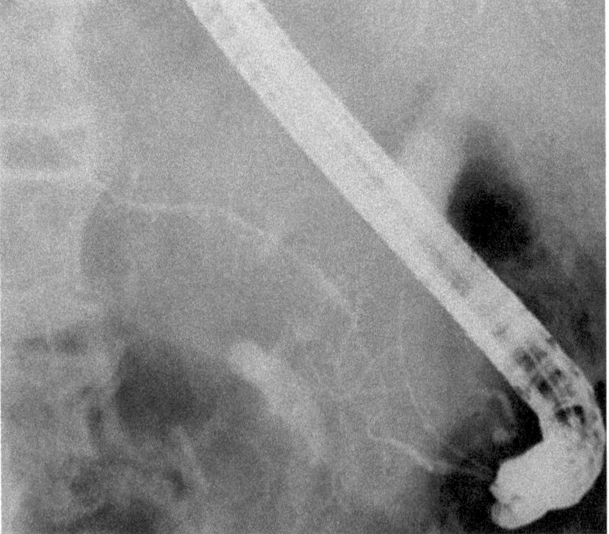

Figure 1. ERP demonstrating diffuse narrowing of the MPD in AIP.

*Corresponding author. Email: kamisawa@cick.jp

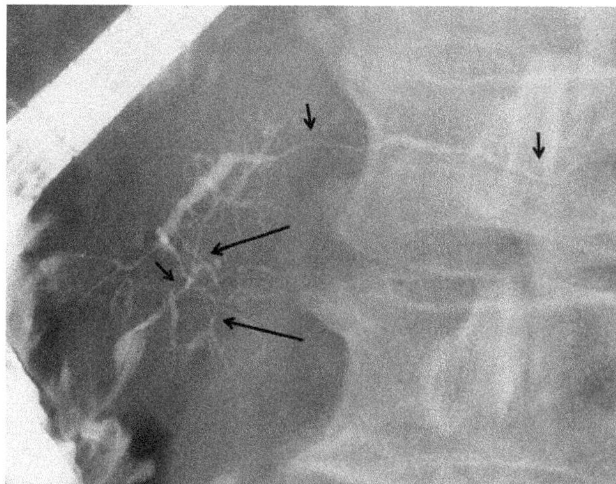

Figure 2. ERP demonstrating skipped, narrowed lesions of the MPD (short arrows). Many side branches were derived from the narrowed lesions (long arrows). Reproduced with permission from Sugumar et al.[12]

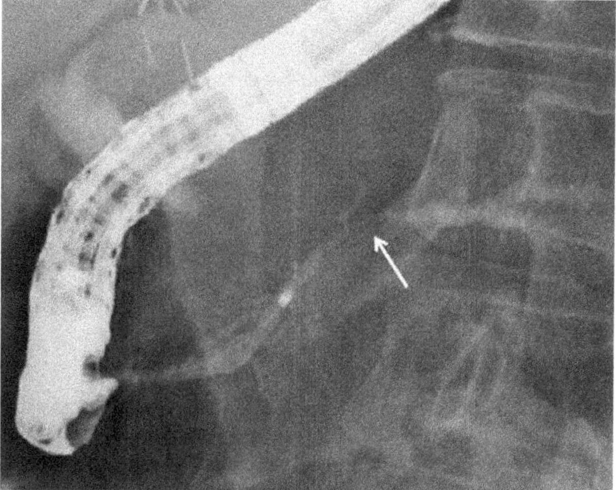

Figure 3. ERP demonstrating a short narrowing of the MPD (arrow) in AIP. The upstream dilatation is less prominent than in pancreatic cancer.

cancer, stenosis of the intrahepatic or hilar bile duct is only seen in AIP patients. Differentiating a short narrowing of the MPD in AIP from stenosis in patients with pancreatic cancer is difficult (**Figure 3**), and some cases of pancreatic cancer have pancreatographic findings similar to those of AIP.[9] According to an international multicenter study, the presence of single or multiple pancreatic duct strictures without upstream dilatation (<5 mm) offered the highest specificity for AIP (>90%).[10]

Histopathological examination of type 1 AIP shows lymphoplasmacytic sclerosing pancreatitis (LPSP), characterized by dense lymphoplasmacytic infiltration and fibrosis in the pancreas. Abundant lymphoplasmacytic cells infiltrate with fibrosis around interlobular pancreatic ducts including the MPD. Although periductal inflammation is usually extensive and distributed throughout the entire pancreas, the degree and extent of the inflammation differ from duct to duct. The infiltrate is primarily subepithelial, and inflammatory cells rarely infiltrate the epithelium. It encompasses the pancreatic ducts and narrows their lumens.[11-13] On the other hand, pancreatic cancer cells infiltrate scirrhously, destroying the epithelium of the pancreatic and bile ducts and frequently obstructing the MPD and branch pancreatic ducts. These histopathological differences around the ducts may account for the different pancreatographic findings between AIP and pancreatic cancer.

ERCP for diagnosing AIP: variable usage worldwide

There are several features specific to ERCP that appear potentially useful for differentiating AIP from pancreatic cancer. However, local expertise and patterns of practice in the use of various tests vary considerably worldwide. Although diagnostic ERP is frequently performed in Japan, western endoscopists generally avoid injecting the pancreatic duct in patients with obstructive jaundice for fear of inducing pancreatitis. Instead, AIP is often diagnosed without an ERP in western countries.[10,14]

According to the International Consensus Diagnostic Criteria, patients with diffuse pancreatic enlargement with elevated serum IgG4 levels can be diagnosed with AIP without pancreatography (See **Chapter 2**, "Diagnosis of

Table 1. Pancreatographic differences between AIP and pancreatic cancer.[8]

ERP feature	AIP (n = 48)	Pancreatic cancer (n = 143)	p-value
Obstruction of the MPD (+/-)	2/46 (4%)	98/45 (69%)	<.001
Skipped lesions of the MPD (+/-)	13/35 (27%)	0/143 (0%)	<.001
Side branch derivation from the narrowed MPD (+/-)	39/9 (81%)	10/35 (22%)	<.001
Length of the narrowed MPD (cm)	7.6 – 4.3	2.5 – 0.9	<.001
Length of the narrowed MPD >3 cm (+/-)	43/5 (90%)	12/33 (27%)	<.001
Diameter of upstream MPD (mm)	2.9 – 0.8	6.8 – 2.1	<.001
Diameter of upstream MPD <5 mm (+/-)	19/1 (95%)	12/33 (27%)	<.001

Autoimmune Pancreatitis").[15] However, based on the high specificity for AIP, the presence of a long (more than one-third of the MPD) or multiple strictures without marked upstream dilation is strong collateral evidence for diagnosing AIP in patients with atypical parenchymal imaging, such as segmental or focal pancreatic enlargement. Thus, ERP can be helpful in differentiating AIP from pancreatic cancer, and in these cases, brush cytology of the narrowed portion of the MPD is often performed.

Role of MRCP in diagnosing AIP

Magnetic resonance cholangiopancreatography (MRCP) has become a popular noninvasive method for obtaining high-quality images of the pancreaticobiliary tree and is replacing diagnostic ERCP for the diagnosis and follow-up of many pancreatobiliary diseases. However, because the narrowed portion of the MPD seen on ERCP in AIP can rarely be visualized on MRCP due to its inferior resolution, this modality cannot yet replace ERCP in AIP diagnosis. However, MRCP findings such as skipped narrowing of the MPD with a lack of upstream MPD dilatation suggest AIP. Furthermore, as the resolution allows full evaluation of the pancreatic and bile ducts after steroid therapy on MRCP, this approach is useful to determine the effect of steroid therapy and follow-up after steroid therapy.[8]

Summary

ERP can demonstrate findings specific for AIP including long or multiple strictures without marked upstream dilation of the MPD. These findings can be particularly useful for differentiating from pancreatic cancer in patients with atypical AIP features on parenchymal imaging. Although MRCP may be useful for evaluating the effect of steroid therapy, its sensitivity for detecting changes in the MPD is inadequate to replace ERP in patients with AIP.

References

1. Kamisawa T, Takuma K, Egawa N, Tsuruta K, and Sasaki T. Autoimmune pancreatitis and IgG4-related sclerosing disease. *Nat Rev Gastroenterol Hepatol.* 2010; 7: 401-409. PMID: 20548323
2. Kamisawa T, Egawa N, Nakajima H, Tsuruta K, Okamoto A, and Kamata N. Clinical difficulties in the differentiation of autoimmune pancreatitis and pancreatic carcinoma. *Am J Gastroenterol.* 2003; 98: 2694-2699. PMID: 14687819
3. Kamisawa T, Imai M, Yui Chen P, Tu Y, Egawa N, Tsuruta K, Okamoto A, Suzuki M, and Kamata N. Strategy for differentiating autoimmune pancreatitis from pancreatic cancer. *Pancreas.* 2008; 37: e62-67. PMID: 18815540
4. Toki F KT, Oi I, Nakasako T, Suzuki M, and Hanyu F. An unusual type of chronic pancreatitis showing diffuse irregular narrowing of the entire main pancreatic duct on ERCP - a report of four cases. *Endoscopy.* 1992; 24: 640.
5. Yoshida K, Toki F, Takeuchi T, Watanabe S, Shiratori K, and Hayashi N. Chronic pancreatitis caused by an autoimmune abnormality. Proposal of the concept of autoimmune pancreatitis. *Dig Dis Sci.* 1995; 40: 1561-1568. PMID: 7628283
6. Shimosegawa T; Working Group Members of the Japan Pancreas Society; Research Committee for Intractable Pancreatic Disease by the Ministry of Labor, Health and Welfare of Japan. The amendment of the Clinical Diagnostic Criteria in Japan (JPS2011) in response to the proposal of the International Consensus of Diagnostic Criteria (ICDC) for autoimmune pancreatitis. *Pancreas.* 2012; 41: 1341-1342. PMID: 23086247
7. Okazaki K, Kawa S, Kamisawa T, Ito T, Inui K, Irie H, Nishino T, Notohara K, Nishimori I, Tanaka S, Nishiyama T, Suda K, Shiratori K, Tanaka M, Shimosegawa T; Working Committee of the Japan Pancreas Society and the Research Committee for Intractable Pancreatic Disease supported by the Ministry of Health, Labour and Welfare of Japan. Amendment of the Japanese Consensus Guidelines for Autoimmune Pancreatitis, 2013 I. Concept and diagnosis of autoimmune pancreatitis. *J Gastroenterol.* 2014; 49: 567-588. PMID: 24639057
8. Takuma K, Kamisawa T, Tabata T, Inaba Y, Egawa N, and Igarashi Y. Utility of pancreatography for diagnosing autoimmune pancreatitis. *World J Gastroenterol.* 2011; 17: 2332-2337. PMID: 21633599
9. Nishino T, Oyama H, Toki F, and Shiratori K. Differentiation between autoimmune pancreatitis and pancreatic carcinoma based on endoscopic retrograde cholangiopancreatography findings. *J Gastroenterol.* 2010; 45: 988-996. PMID: 20396913
10. Sugumar A, Levy MJ, Kamisawa T, Webster GJ, Kim MH, Enders F, Amin Z, Baron TH, Chapman MH, Church NI, Clain JE, Egawa N, Johnson GJ, Okazaki K, Pearson RK, Pereira SP, Petersen BT, Read S, Sah RP, Sandanayake NS, Takahashi N, Topazian MD, Uchida K, Vege SS, and Chari ST. Endoscopic retrograde pancreatography criteria to diagnose autoimmune pancreatitis: an international multicentre study. *Gut.* 2011; 60: 666-670. PMID: 21131631
11. Chandan VS, Iacobuzio-Donahue C, and Abraham SC. Patchy distribution of pathologic abnormalities in autoimmune pancreatitis: implications for pre-operative diagnosis. *Am J Surg Pathol.* 2008; 32: 1762-1769. PMID: 18779731
12. Kamisawa T, Funata N, Hayashi Y, Tsuruta K, Okamoto A, Amemiya K, Egawa N, and Nakajima H. Close relationship between autoimmune pancreatitis and multifocal fibrosclerosis. *Gut.* 2003; 52: 683-687. PMID: 12692053
13. Kloppel G, Sipos B, Zamboni G, Kojima M, and Morohoshi T. Autoimmune pancreatitis: histo- and immunopathological features. *J Gastroenterol.* 2007; 42(Suppl 18): 28-31. PMID: 17520220
14. Chari ST, Takahashi N, Levy MJ, Smyrk TC, Clain JE, Pearson RK, Petersen BT, Topazian MA, and Vege SS. A diagnostic strategy to distinguish autoimmune pancreatitis from pancreatic cancer. *Clin Gastroenterol Hepatol.* 2009; 7: 1097-1103. PMID: 19410017
15. Shimosegawa T, Chari ST, Frulloni L, Kamisawa T, Kawa S, Mino-Kenudson M, Kim MH, Kloppel G, Lerch MM, Lohr M, Notohara K, Okazaki K, Schneider A, and Zhang L. International consensus diagnostic criteria for autoimmune pancreatitis: guidelines of the International Association of Pancreatology. *Pancreas.* 2011; 40: 352-358. PMID: 21412117

Chapter 60

Endoscopic ultrasound in the diagnosis of autoimmune pancreatitis

Larissa L. Fujii* and Michael J. Levy*

Division of Gastroenterology and Hepatology, Mayo Clinic, Rochester, MN.

Introduction

Autoimmune pancreatitis (AIP) has historically been considered a rare disorder but is increasingly recognized due to improved understanding of its diverse nature and the proper means of diagnosis. The current International Consensus Diagnostic Criteria (ICDC) for the diagnosis of AIP incorporate five cardinal features: imaging characteristics of the pancreas (parenchyma and duct), serology, other organ involvement, pancreatic histology, and response to steroids.[1] Imaging techniques recognized in the guidelines include computed tomography (CT), magnetic resonance imaging (MRI), magnetic resonance cholangiopancreatography (MRCP), and endoscopic retrograde cholangiopancreatography (ERCP). Endoscopic ultrasound (EUS) is notably absent from the diagnostic algorithms.

Even when AIP is strongly considered, the diagnosis often remains elusive.[2-4] Despite the use of existing diagnostic algorithms, there is often a significant delay in diagnosis, which can result in unnecessary interventions including pancreatic resection. In addition, some patients remain undiagnosed, leading to diagnostic steroid trials that risk patient safety and often contribute to further diagnostic confusion. With these uncertainties, further refinement of the current ICDC may be beneficial for some cases.

There are emerging data suggesting the potential utility of EUS in diagnosing AIP.[5-9] EUS not only has the ability to provide high-definition imaging of the pancreas, it can also be used to acquire tissue through either fine-needle aspiration (FNA) or trucut biopsy (TCB). These characteristics make it one of the most useful techniques in the diagnosis of pancreatic cancer and chronic pancreatitis.[10-13] Therefore, EUS has the potential to play a role in the both diagnosing AIP and excluding other pancreatic diseases.

EUS imaging features

Standard EUS imaging

There are no pathognomonic EUS imaging findings of AIP. The "classic" appearance is a diffusely enlarged "sausage-shaped" gland with a hypoechoic, patchy, heterogeneous parenchyma (**Figure 1**).[5,14,15] In our experience, when a patient has all of these classic features, which are observed in up to 57% of cases, there is a high probability of AIP.[5,15] However, patients often do not have all of the features, limiting the diagnosis of AIP using EUS (**Figures 2 & 3**). Another pancreatic finding on EUS is a focal solitary mass (**Figure 4**). The hypoechoic lesion is commonly located in the head of the pancreas, resulting in obstructive jaundice. The mass may appear to invade adjacent vessels, cause upstream dilation of the main pancreatic duct (MPD), and be associated with enlarged peripancreatic lymph nodes, mimicking locally advanced pancreatic cancer (**Figure 5**).[5,14,15] In areas of pancreatic involvement, the MPD may be narrowed with duct wall thickening.[14] EUS features of the pancreatic parenchyma may overlap with some characteristics seen in chronic pancreatitis, including the presence of hyperechoic foci, hyperechoic strands, and lobularity (**Figure 6**). In a case series of patients given steroid therapy, the parenchymal enlargement, lobularity, and

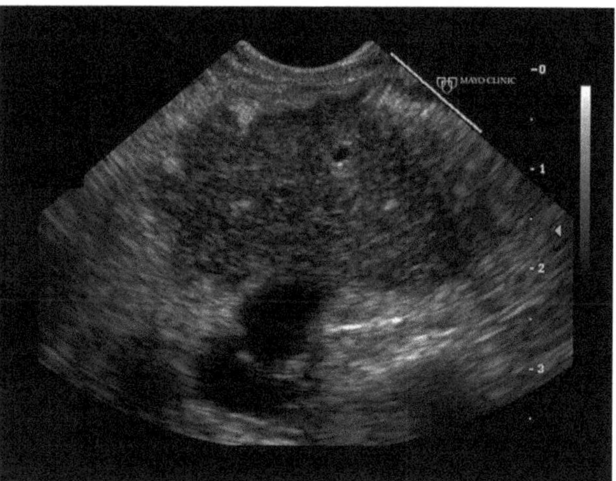

Figure 1. Classic EUS appearance of AIP including diffuse, sausage-shaped pancreatic enlargement with hypoechoic, coarse, patchy, heterogeneous parenchyma.

*Corresponding authors. Email: fujii.larissa@mayo.edu, levy.michael@mayo.edu

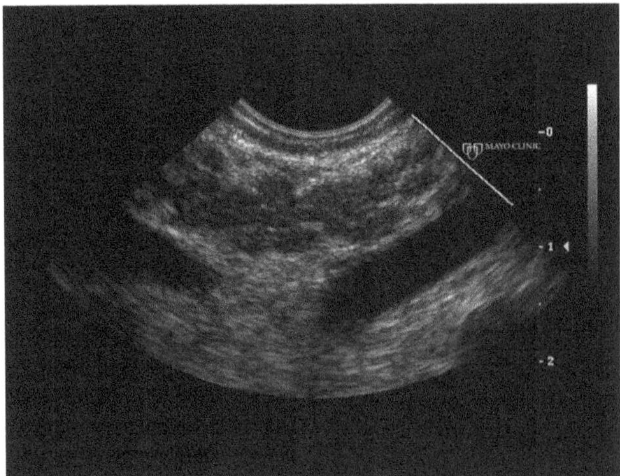

Figure 2. EUS reveals a hypoechoic, coarse, pancreas in which the features are patchy and heterogeneous, but there is no diffusely enlarged gland.

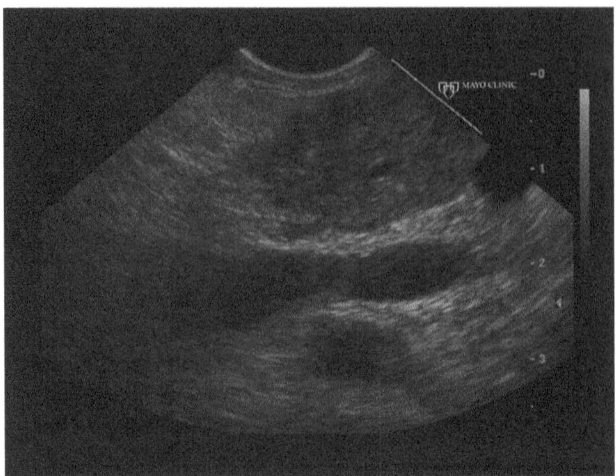

Figure 3. EUS appearance of a hypoechoic, diffusely enlarged, sausage-shaped gland without coarse and heterogeneous features.

lobular outer margins improved with steroid treatment, but the hyperechoic foci and strands remained.[16] Finally, EUS may demonstrate a normal- appearing pancreas.

As the biliary tree is the most common extrapancreatic organ involved in AIP, the extrahepatic duct may be abnormal on EUS. In a study of 37 patients with AIP, 38% had ultrasonographic findings of the extrahepatic bile duct and gallbladder wall thickening. There were two types of bile duct wall thickening including a "three-layer type" with a high-low-high echo appearance and a "parenchymal-echo type" with a thickened wall throughout the entire bile lumen and a parenchymal echo present within the bile duct itself.[17] In one series, a similar appearance to the "three-layer type" with a regular homogeneous thickening with a hyper-hypo-hyperechoic series of layers of the ductal wall ("sandwich pattern") was seen on EUS in addition to bile duct dilatation.[15] This EUS appearance is different than what is often seen with pancreaticobiliary malignancies, which may be more irregular.

It is important to distinguish focal AIP from the dreaded pancreatic cancer. Hoki et al. compared EUS findings in patients who were diagnosed with AIP and resected pancreatic cancer.[18] They found that diffuse hypoechoic areas, diffuse enlargement of the pancreas, bile duct wall thickening, and peripancreatic hypoechoic margins were more commonly seen in patients ultimately diagnosed with AIP compared with those determined to have pancreatic cancer. On the other hand, focal hyperechoic areas and focal enlargement were more common in the latter group. Although all comparisons reached statistical significance, each characteristic (other than peripancreatic hypoechoic margins) was seen in both diseases. In addition, the frequencies of lymph node enlargement were similar in AIP and pancreatic cancer.

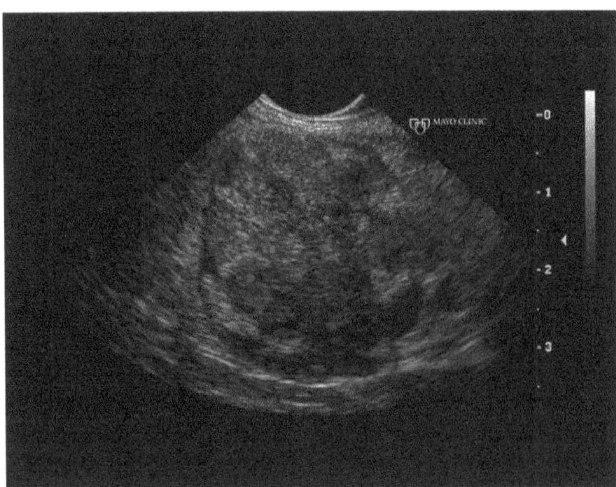

Figure 4. EUS finding of a mass-like lesion in a patient with AIP.

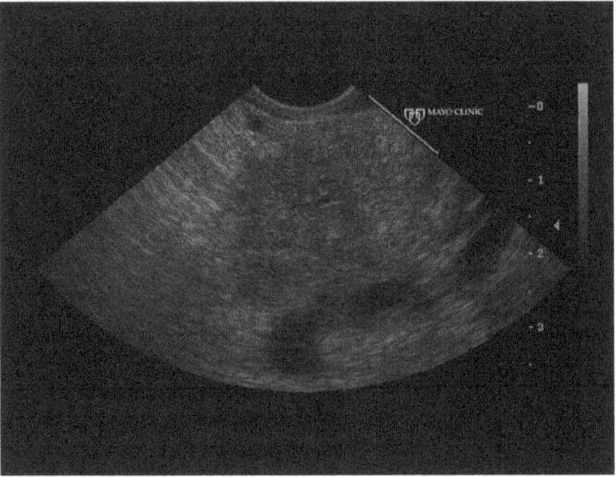

Figure 5. EUS finding of a mass-like lesion in a patient with AIP that may be confused with an "unresectable" pancreatic ductal adenocarcinoma.

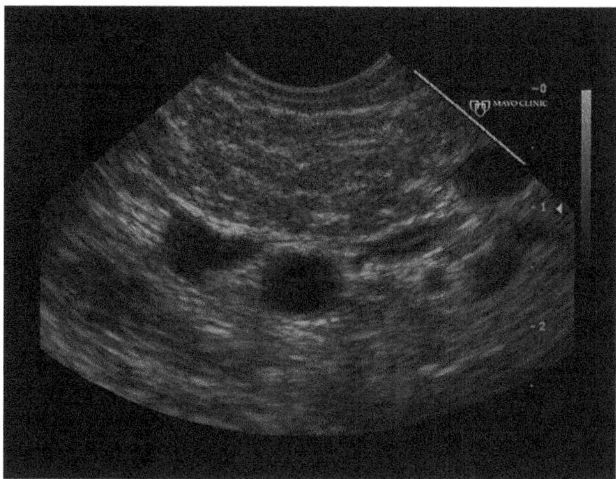

Figure 6. EUS features of nonspecific chronic pancreatitis in a patient with AIP.

To our knowledge, there are no studies that have directly compared EUS to other imaging modalities such as CT, MRI, or ERCP for the diagnosis of AIP. Therefore, it is unclear if EUS has additive value to the other imaging techniques. However, a cohort of 48 patients seen at Mayo Clinic Rochester with a diagnosis of AIP based on the HISORt criteria (Histology, Imaging, Serology, Other organ involvement, and Response to steroid therapy) underwent EUS with TCB.[7,19,20] The diagnosis of AIP was strongly suspected in 14 patients prior to EUS based on their clinical, laboratory, and imaging findings. In 22 patients, the diagnosis was considered as a part of a broader differential prior to EUS, and in the remaining 12 patients, EUS appearance alone led to the initial suspicion of AIP. This suggests that EUS imaging alone may increase the diagnostic accuracy of AIP in patients in whom other imaging modalities did not provide a definitive diagnosis.

Image-enhancing EUS techniques

With the lack of pathognomonic features and diverse spectrum of EUS imaging findings in patients with AIP, several image-enhancing techniques have been evaluated to improve diagnostic accuracy. Each of these complementary imaging methods is in the experimental phase and cannot be recommended for routine use in the diagnostic algorithm for AIP until further studies determine their roles.

One image-enhancing technique is EUS elastography, which distinguishes tissues based on their stiffness by measuring tissue strain while slightly compressing an area that encompasses both the abnormal and normal tissue.[21] Five patients with focal AIP were found to have a homogeneous stiff (blue) pattern in the mass and throughout the entire pancreas, which differed from cancerous or normal pancreas in which the pancreatic parenchyma was predominately of intermediate stiffness (green).[22]

Contrast-enhanced EUS requires intravenously administered ultrasound contrast agents (e.g., Sonovue [sulfur hexafluoride MBs; Bracco Interventional BV, Amsterdam, the Netherlands], Levovist [Bayer AG, Leverkusen, Germany], or Sonazoid [perfluorobutane; GE Healthcare, Little Chalfont, Buckinghamsire, UK]) to produce microbubbles that allow visualization of the vascular pattern within the pancreatic mass lesion.[21] In an cohort of 10 patients who received Sonovue contrast and EUS imaging in the bicolor Doppler mode, AIP was associated with hypervascularity within the mass-like lesion and the surrounding pancreatic parenchyma as compared to pancreatic cancer where the mass was hypovascular in comparison to the surrounding pancreatic tissue.[23]

Contrast-enhanced harmonic EUS is similar to the technique described above but uses a dedicated contrast harmonic mode rather than Doppler imaging. The use of contrast harmonic-enhanced imaging decreases Doppler-associated artifacts, including ballooning and overpainting.[21] In one study, 8 patients with focal AIP and 22 patients with pancreatic cancer were given Sonazoid ultrasonographic contrast and analyzed using a radial echoendoscope with conventional tissue harmonic echo (for standard harmonic imaging) and extended pure harmonic detection (for contrast-enhanced harmonic imaging).[24] The ultra-sonographic contrast uptake and distribution was isoehanced and homogeneous in all eight patients with AIP compared to only one patient with pancreatic cancer. The majority of patients with pancreatic cancer had hypoenhanced uptake in a heterogeneous pattern. Furthermore, the optimal maximum intensity gain cutoff value to differentiate between AIP and pancreatic cancer with a 100% specificity and sensitivity using a receiver operator characteristic (ROC) curve was 12.5. All of the results mentioned above must be interpreted with caution; additional studies are required to confirm the utility of the image-enhancing techniques in differentiating between AIP and pancreatic cancer.

EUS-guided tissue acquisition

FNA

EUS imaging itself has not proven to be useful when used in isolation to diagnose AIP. Although the role of EUS-guided tissue acquisition has not been extensively studied, pancreatic histology is recognized as an important diagnostic criterion in the ICDC. Despite a few reports on the ability to diagnose AIP using only FNA, there are no broadly accepted consensus cytological diagnostic criteria for AIP, and most pathologists are reluctant to rely solely on FNA specimens.[25-28] FNA commonly yields small specimen samples with minimal tissue architecture, making its interpretation challenging. Even EUS-guided FNA using a 19-gauge needle for histologic review was only able to achieve an AIP diagnosis in 43% of patients.[29]

Due to the inability to obtain adequate core specimens using standard FNA needles, some advocate for the use of less rigorous or incomplete pathology criteria for the cytologic diagnosis of AIP. For example, less stringent criteria may rely on the presence of a lymphoplasmacytic infiltrate alone without the requirement to find infiltrate in a periductal location or the degree of preservation of ductules, venules, or arterioles required within the specimen.[25,26,28] Although lowering the pathologic criteria requirements may improve diagnostic sensitivity, it would be at the expense of decreasing the specificity of FNA for AIP. This is particularly problematic for differentiating AIP from pancreatic cancer, which is often associated with a lymphoplasmacytic infiltration.

Some suggest that the benefit of EUS-guided FNA relies on its ability to exclude pancreatic cancer rather than diagnose AIP.[9,30,31] However, assuming that a negative EUS FNA of a pancreas mass equates to exclusion of an underlying malignancy can be dangerous given the 10%-40% false-negative FNA rate for cancer.[32-36]

Trucut biopsy

To overcome the limitations of FNA needles, larger caliber cutting biopsy needles have been developed that acquire samples with preserved tissue architecture, allowing for histologic examination.[37-44] An EUS TCB device (QuickCore, Wilson-Cook, Winston- Salem, NC) uses a 19-gauge needle with a tissue tray and sliding sheath that is designed to capture a core tissue sample. This device has been shown to be useful for diagnosing neoplasms that are often difficult to diagnose based on cytopathology alone, including stromal tumors and lymphoma when immunohistochemical analysis is useful and well- differentiated desmoplastic tumors that make aspiration difficult.[45-52] Furthermore, with larger specimen size and the ability to preserve tissue architecture, TCB has been shown to help differentiate between AIP, chronic pancreatitis, and pancreatic cancer.[4,53]

We looked at the previous Mayo Clinic experience regarding the diagnostic sensitivity and safety of EUS TCB in patients with a final diagnosis of AIP based on the HISORt criteria (unpublished data). The cohort comprised 48 patients (38 male, mean age 59.7 years) in whom a mean of 2.9 EUS TCB (range 1-7) were performed. Histologic examination of the EUS TCB specimens provided a diagnosis in 35 (73%) patients. The diagnostic sensitivity varied among the five endosonographers (from 33%-90%). Nondiagnostic cases were found to have chronic pancreatitis (n = 8), nonspecific histology (n = 2), or a failed tissue acquisition (n = 3). Complications included mild transient abdominal pain (n = 3) and self- limited intraprocedural bleeding (n = 1). It is unclear if TCB and/or FNA can be attributed to these complications. No patient required hospitalization or therapeutic intervention. Of note, the serum IgG4 level was >2× the upper limit of normal in just 23% of patients. None of the patients with an EUS TCB diagnosis of AIP required surgical intervention for diagnosis. Over a mean follow-up of 2.6 years, no false-negative diagnoses of pancreatic cancer were identified. Prior to EUS, the diagnosis of AIP was strongly suspected in 14 patients as a result of their clinical, laboratory, and/or imaging findings. For 22 patients, the diagnosis was considered pre-EUS as part of a broader differential. Our data suggest the potential utility of EUS imaging to lead to the initial suspicion of AIP in 12 patients, thereby initiating pancreatic TCB and subsequent clinical evaluation of AIP. More recently, we examined the use of EUS TCB in pediatric patients with a suspected diagnosis of AIP.[54] The diagnostic yield of EUS TBC in this patient population was 87%.

EUS TCB appears to be safe and may provide sufficient material to aid in the diagnosis of AIP, thereby guiding treatment and avoiding surgical intervention. Some suggest the use of EUS TCB as a "rescue" technique to obtain adequate tissue samples if EUS FNA failed.[7,28] The current ICDC guidelines recommend a pancreatic core biopsy in patients presenting with a focal mass and/or obstructive jaundice if cancer has been excluded and the diagnosis remains elusive.[1]

ProCore biopsy

The ProCore needle (Cook Medical Inc., Bloomington, IN) has a lateral bevel that may occasionally provide a sufficient specimen to allow histologic analysis and diagnosis of AIP. However, studies on the use of the ProCore needle in the diagnosis of AIP are lacking, and in our experience, it is inferior to EUS TCB in this setting.

Summary

Although personal opinion and limited data suggest that EUS imaging alone may improve the diagnosis of AIP, there are few studies to substantiate this view. Despite early promise, the utility and role of elastography, contrast-enhanced EUS, and harmonic imaging in patients with AIP remain to be determined. The lack of pathognomonic EUS imaging characteristics and the diverse spectrum of both the clinical presentation and pancreatic findings of AIP emphasize the need for a safe and reliable way to acquire tissue specimens, particularly in cases with atypical features.

While FNA cytologic samples can be examined for the presence of lymphocytes and plasma cells, other disorders may have a similar appearance. This limits the specificity of FNA and risks inappropriate management of patients who may have unrecognized pancreatic cancer. Therefore, until data suggests otherwise, it is not recommended to rely on FNA to diagnose AIP. Instead, core biopsies using EUS TCB should be used for histologic examination and IgG4 immunostaining. We perform EUS TCB in patients with an AIP-compatible clinical presentation but in whom the diagnosis remains uncertain and when the findings are likely to alter management. By performing EUS TCB, pancreatic cancer may be excluded, and unnecessary surgical intervention can be averted. Unfortunately, it may not be possible to obtain pancreatic core biopsies in all patients with an indeterminate diagnosis due to technical, anatomical, or personnel limitations. In such patients, it is even more critical to consider all possible diagnostic components of the ICDC to attempt to establish a diagnosis without histological evaluation. Further study is needed to determine the diagnostic yields of EUS imaging alone, newer imaging- enhancing techniques, and FNA or TCB for AIP.

References

1. Shimosegawa T, Chari ST, Frulloni L, Kamisawa T, Kawa S, Mino-Kenudson M, Kim MH, Kloppel G, Lerch MM, Lohr M, Notohara K, Okazaki K, Schneider A, and Zhang L. International consensus diagnostic criteria for autoimmune pancreatitis: guidelines of the International Association of Pancreatology. *Pancreas*. 2011; 40: 352-358. PMID: 21412117
2. Kamisawa T, Egawa N, Nakajima H, Tsuruta K, Okamoto A, and Kamata N. Clinical difficulties in the differentiation of autoimmune pancreatitis and pancreatic carcinoma. *Am J Gastroenterol*. 2003; 98: 2694-2699. PMID: 14687819
3. Taniguchi T, Tanio H, Seko S, Nishida O, Inoue F, Okamoto M, Ishigami S, and Kobayashi H. Autoimmune pancreatitis detected as a mass in the head of the pancreas without hypergammaglobulinemia, which relapsed after surgery: case report and review of the literature. *Dig Dis Sci*. 2003; 48: 1465-1471. PMID: 12924637
4. Yadav D, Notahara K, Smyrk TC, Clain JE, Pearson RK, Farnell MB, and Chari ST. Idiopathic tumefactive chronic pancreatitis: clinical profile, histology, and natural history after resection. *Clin Gastroenterol Hepatol*. 2003; 1: 129-135. PMID: 15017505
5. Farrell JJ, Garber J, Sahani D, and Brugge WR. EUS findings in patients with autoimmune pancreatitis. *Gastrointest Endosc*. 2004; 60: 927-936. PMID: 15605008
6. Finkelberg DL, Sahani D, Deshpande V, and Brugge WR. Autoimmune pancreatitis. *N Engl J Med*. 2006; 355: 2670-2676. PMID: 17182992
7. Levy MJ, Reddy RP, Wiersema MJ, Smyrk TC, Clain JE, Harewood GC, Pearson RK, Rajan E, Topazian MD, Yusuf TE, Chari ST, and Petersen BT. EUS-guided trucut biopsy in establishing auto-immune pancreatitis as the cause of obstructive jaundice. *Gastrointest Endosc*. 2005; 61: 467-472. PMID: 15758927
8. Levy MJ, Wiersema MJ, and Chari ST. Chronic pancreatitis: focal pancreatitis or cancer? Is there a role for FNA/biopsy? Autoimmune pancreatitis. *Endoscopy*. 2006; 38 Suppl 1: S30-S35. PMID: 16802220
9. Moon SH and Kim MH. The role of endoscopy in the diagnosis of autoimmune pancreatitis. *Gastrointest Endosc*. 2012; 76: 645-656. PMID: 24079796
10. Catanzaro A, Richardson S, Veloso H, Isenberg GA, Wong RC, Sivak MV Jr, and Chak A. Long-term follow-up of patients with clinically indeterminate suspicion of pancreatic cancer and normal EUS. *Gastrointest Endosc*. 2003; 58: 836-840. PMID: 14652549
11. Chang DK, Nguyen NQ, Merrett ND, Dixson H, Leong RW, and Biankin AV. Role of endoscopic ultrasound in pancreatic cancer. *Expert Rev Gastroenterol Hepatol*. 2009; 3: 293-303. PMID: 19485810
12. Kahl S, Glasbrenner B, Leodolter A, Pross M, Schulz HU, and Malfertheiner P. EUS in the diagnosis of early chronic pancreatitis: a prospective follow-up study. *Gastrointest Endosc*. 2002; 55: 507-511. PMID: 11923762
13. Klapman JB, Chang KJ, Lee JG, and Nguyen P. Negative predictive value of endoscopic ultrasound in a large series of patients with a clinical suspicion of pancreatic cancer. *Am J Gastroenterol*. 2005; 100: 2658-2661. PMID: 16393216
14. Buscarini E, Lisi SD, Arcidiacono PG, Petrone MC, Fuini A, Conigliaro R, Manfredi G, Manta R, Reggio D, and Angelis CD. Endoscopic ultrasonography findings in autoimmune pancreatitis. *World J Gastroenterol*. 2011; 17: 2080-2085. PMID: 21547126
15. De Lisi S, Buscarini E, Arcidiacono PG, Petrone M, Menozzi F, Testoni PA, and Zambelli A. Endoscopic ultrasonography findings in autoimmune pancreatitis: be aware of the ambiguous features and look for the pivotal ones. *JOP*. 2010; 11: 78-84. PMID: 20065561
16. Okabe Y, Ishida Y, Kaji R, Sugiyama G, Yasumoto M, Naito Y, Toyonaga A, Tsuruta O, and Sata M. Endoscopic ultrasonographic study of autoimmune pancreatitis and the effect of steroid therapy. *J Hepatobiliary Pancreat Sci*. 2012; 19: 266-273. PMID: 21671062
17. Koyama R, Imamura T, Okuda C, Sakamoto N, Honjo H, and Takeuchi K. Ultrasonographic imaging of bile duct lesions in autoimmune pancreatitis. *Pancreas*. 2008; 37: 259-264. PMID: 18815546
18. Hoki N, Mizuno N, Sawaki A, Tajika M, Takayama R, Shimizu Y, Bhatia V, and Yamao K. Diagnosis of autoimmune pancreatitis using endoscopic ultrasonography. *J Gastroenterol*. 2009; 44: 154-159. PMID: 19214678
19. Chari ST, Smyrk TC, Levy MJ, Topazian MD, Takahashi N, Zhang L, Clain JE, Pearson RK, Petersen BT, Vege SS, and Farnell MB. Diagnosis of autoimmune pancreatitis: the Mayo Clinic experience. *Clin Gastroenterol Hepatol*. 2006; 4: 1010-1016; quiz 1934. PMID: 16843735
20. Levy MJ, Smyrk TC, Takahashi N, Zhang L, and Chari ST. Idiopathic duct-centric pancreatitis: disease description and

endoscopic ultrasonography-guided trucut biopsy diagnosis. *Pancreatology*. 2011; 11: 76-80. PMID: 21525775

21. Fusaroli P, Saftoiu A, Mancino MG, Caletti G, and Eloubeidi MA. Techniques of image enhancement in EUS (with videos). *Gastrointest Endosc*. 2011; 74: 645-655. PMID: 21679945
22. Dietrich CF, Hirche TO, Ott M, and Ignee A. Real-time tissue elastography in the diagnosis of autoimmune pancreatitis. *Endoscopy*. 2009; 41: 718-720. PMID: 19618344
23. Hocke M, Ignee A, and Dietrich CF. Contrast-enhanced endoscopic ultrasound in the diagnosis of autoimmune pancreatitis. *Endoscopy*. 2011; 43: 163-165. PMID: 22139794
24. Imazu H, Kanazawa K, Mori N, Ikeda K, Kakutani H, Sumiyama K, Hino S, Ang TL, Omar S, and Tajiri H. Novel quantitative perfusion analysis with contrast-enhanced harmonic EUS for differentiation of autoimmune pancreatitis from pancreatic carcinoma. *Scand J Gastroenterol*. 2012; 47: 853-860. PMID: 22507131
25. Chari ST, Kloeppel G, Zhang L, Notohara K, Lerch MM, and Shimosegawa T. Histopathologic and clinical subtypes of autoimmune pancreatitis: the Honolulu consensus document. *Pancreas*. 2010; 39: 549-554. PMID: 21242705
26. Deshpande V, Mino-Kenudson M, Brugge WR, Pitman MB, Fernandez-del Castillo C, Warshaw AL, and Lauwers GY. Endoscopic ultrasound guided fine needle aspiration biopsy of autoimmune pancreatitis: diagnostic criteria and pitfalls. *Am J Surg Pathol*. 2005; 29: 1464-1471. PMID: 16224213
27. Kanno A, Ishida K, Hamada S, Fujishima F, Unno J, Kume K, Kikuta K, Hirota M, Masamune A, Satoh K, Notohara K, and Shimosegawa T. Diagnosis of autoimmune pancreatitis by EUS-FNA by using a 22-gauge needle based on the International Consensus Diagnostic Criteria. *Gastrointest Endosc*. 2012; 76: 594-602. PMID: 22898417
28. Mizuno N, Bhatia V, Hosoda W, Sawaki A, Hoki N, Hara K, Takagi T, Ko SB, Yatabe Y, Goto H, and Yamao K. Histological diagnosis of autoimmune pancreatitis using EUS-guided trucut biopsy: a comparison study with EUS-FNA. *J Gastroenterol*. 2009; 44: 742-750. PMID: 19434362
29. Iwashita T, Yasuda I, Doi S, Ando N, Nakashima M, Adachi S, Hirose Y, Mukai T, Iwata K, Tomita E, Itoi T, and Moriwaki H. Use of samples from endoscopic ultrasound-guided 19-gauge fine-needle aspiration in diagnosis of autoimmune pancreatitis. *Clin Gastroenterol Hepatol*. 2012; 10: 316-322. PMID: 22019795
30. Naitoh I, Nakazawa T, Hayashi K, Okumura F, Miyabe K, Shimizu S, Kondo H, Yoshida M, Yamashita H, Ohara H, and Joh T. Clinical differences between mass-forming autoimmune pancreatitis and pancreatic cancer. *Scand J Gastroenterol*. 2012; 47: 607-613. PMID: 22416894
31. Takuma K, Kamisawa T, Gopalakrishna R, Hara S, Tabata T, Inaba Y, Egawa N, and Igarashi Y. Strategy to differentiate autoimmune pancreatitis from pancreas cancer. *World J Gastroenterol*. 2012; 18: 1015-1020. PMID: 22416175
32. Chen J, Yang R, Lu Y, Xia Y, and Zhou H. Diagnostic accuracy of endoscopic ultrasound-guided fine-needle aspiration for solid pancreatic lesion: a systematic review. *J Cancer Res Clin Oncol*. 2012; 138: 1433-1441. PMID: 22752601
33. Eloubeidi MA and Tamhane A. EUS-guided FNA of solid pancreatic masses: a learning curve with 300 consecutive procedures. *Gastrointest Endosc*. 2005; 61: 700-708. PMID: 15855975
34. Mitsuhashi T, Ghafari S, Chang CY, and Gu M. Endoscopic ultrasound-guided fine needle aspiration of the pancreas: cytomorphological evaluation with emphasis on adequacy assessment, diagnostic criteria and contamination from the gastrointestinal tract. *Cytopathology*. 2006; 17: 34-41. PMID: 16417563
35. Turner BG, Cizginer S, Agarwal D, Yang J, Pitman MB, and Brugge WR. Diagnosis of pancreatic neoplasia with EUS and FNA: a report of accuracy. *Gastrointest Endosc*. 2010; 71: 91-98. PMID: 19846087
36. Voss M, Hammel P, Molas G, Palazzo L, Dancour A, O'Toole D, Terris B, Degott C, Bernades P, and Ruszniewski P. Value of endoscopic ultrasound guided fine needle aspiration biopsy in the diagnosis of solid pancreatic masses. *Gut*. 2000; 46: 244-249. PMID: 10644320
37. Ball AB, Fisher C, Pittam M, Watkins RM, and Westbury G. Diagnosis of soft tissue tumours by Tru-Cut biopsy. *Br J Surg*. 1990; 77: 756-758. PMID: 2383749
38. Brandt KR, Charboneau JW, Stephens DH, Welch TJ, and Goellner JR. CT- and US-guided biopsy of the pancreas. *Radiology*. 1993; 187: 99-104. PMID: 8451443
39. Harrison BD, Thorpe RS, Kitchener PG, McCann BG, and Pilling JR. Percutaneous Trucut lung biopsy in the diagnosis of localised pulmonary lesions. *Thorax*. 1984; 39: 493-499. PMID: 6463928
40. Ingram DM, Sheiner HJ, and Shilkin KB. Operative biopsy of the pancreas using the Trucut needle. *Aust N Z J Surg*. 1978; 48: 203-206. PMID: 280329
41. Kovalik EC, Schwab SJ, Gunnells JC, Bowie D, and Smith SR. No change in complication rate using spring-loaded gun compared to traditional percutaneous renal allograft biopsy techniques. *Clin Nephrol*. 1996; 45: 383-385. PMID: 8793230
42. Lavelle MA and O'Toole A. Trucut biopsy of the prostate. *Br J Urol*. 1994; 73: 600. PMID: 8012797
43. Piccinino F, Sagnelli E, Pasquale G, and Giusti G. Complications following percutaneous liver biopsy. A multicentre retrospective study on 68,276 biopsies. *J Hepatol*. 1986; 2: 165-173. PMID: 3958472
44. Welch TJ, Sheedy PF, 2nd, Johnson CD, Johnson CM, and Stephens DH. CT-guided biopsy: prospective analysis of 1,000 procedures. *Radiology*. 1989; 171: 493-496. PMID: 2704815
45. DeWitt J, Emerson RE, Sherman S, Al-Haddad M, McHenry L, Cote GA, and Leblanc JK. Endoscopic ultrasound-guided Trucut biopsy of gastrointestinal mesenchymal tumor. *Surg Endosc*. 2011; 25: 2192-2202. PMID: 21184105
46. Gines A, Wiersema MJ, Clain JE, Pochron NL, Rajan E, and Levy MJ. Prospective study of a Trucut needle for performing EUS-guided biopsy with EUS-guided FNA rescue. *Gastrointest Endosc*. 2005; 62: 597-601. PMID: 16185976
47. Lee JH, Choi KD, Kim MY, Choi KS, Kim do H, Park YS, Kim KC, Song HJ, Lee GH, Jung HY, Yook JH, Kim BS, Kang YK, and Kim JH. Clinical impact of EUS-guided

Trucut biopsy results on decision making for patients with gastric subepithelial tumors ≥2 cm in diameter. *Gastrointest Endosc*. 2011; 74: 1010-1018. PMID: 21889136

48. Levy MJ, Jondal ML, Clain J, and Wiersema MJ. Preliminary experience with an EUS-guided trucut biopsy needle compared with EUS-guided FNA. *Gastrointest Endosc*. 2003; 57: 101-106. PMID: 12518144
49. Levy MJ, Smyrk TC, Reddy RP, Clain JE, Harewood GC, Kendrick ML, Pearson RK, Petersen BT, Rajan E, Topazian MD, Wang KK, Wiersema MJ, Yusuf TE, and Chari ST. Endoscopic ultrasound- guided trucut biopsy of the cyst wall for diagnosing cystic pancreatic tumors. *Clin Gastroenterol Hepatol*. 2005; 3: 974-979. PMID: 16234042
50. Levy MJ and Wiersema MJ. EUS-guided Trucut biopsy. *Gastrointest Endosc*. 2005; 62: 417-426. PMID: 16111962
51. Saftoiu A, Vilmann P, Guldhammer Skov B, and Georgescu CV. Endoscopic ultrasound (EUS)-guided Trucut biopsy adds significant information to EUS-guided fine-needle aspiration in selected patients: a prospective study. *Scand J Gastroenterol*. 2007; 42: 117-125. PMID: 17190771
52. Wiersema MJ, Levy MJ, Harewood GC, Vazquez-Sequeiros E, Jondal ML, and Wiersema LM. Initial experience with EUS-guided trucut needle biopsies of perigastric organs. *Gastrointest Endosc*. 2002; 56: 275-278. PMID: 12145612
53. Suda K, Takase M, Fukumura Y, Ogura K, Ueda A, Matsuda T, and Suzuki F. Histopathologic characteristics of autoimmune pancreatitis based on comparison with chronic pancreatitis. *Pancreas*. 2005; 30: 355-358. PMID: 15841047
54. Fujii LL, Chari ST, El-Youssef M, Takahashi N, Topazian MD, Zhang L, and Levy MJ. Pediatric pancreatic EUS-guided trucut biopsy for evaluation of autoimmune pancreatitis. *Gastrointest Endosc*. 2013; 77: 824-828. PMID: 23433594

Chapter 61

Extrapancreatic features of autoimmune pancreatitis (IgG4-related disease)

John H. Stone*

Rheumatology Unit, Massachusetts General Hospital, Boston, Massachusetts.

Introduction

IgG4-related disease (IgG4-RD) was identified and recognized as a multiorgan disease during the first decade of this century. The disease is characterized by histopathology and immunohistochemical staining patterns that are consistent across many organ systems.[1] It is easier to indicate which organs are not affected than to list all of the systems influenced by this condition. To date, it has been rare to find confirmed cases of IgG4-RD affecting the brain parenchyma, muscle tissue, synovium, or bone marrow; however, virtually every other organ is now known to be affected by IgG4-RD, and some are affected more than others.

IgG4-RD was first identified in the pancreas. During the 1990s, the concept of "autoimmune pancreatitis" (AIP) began to emerge from a variety of other names for a condition associated with sclerosing inflammation in that organ.[2] "Sclerosing pancreatitis" was linked to elevated serum concentrations of IgG4 in 2001.[3] IgG4-RD was recognized as a systemic condition in 2003, when a variety of extrapancreatic lesions were observed to occur in patients with AIP.[4,5]

IgG4-RD is now known to affect the pancreas, biliary tree, salivary glands, periorbital tissues (e.g., the lacrimal gland and retro-orbital space), kidneys, lungs, lymph nodes, meninges, aorta, breast, prostate, thyroid gland, pericardium, and skin (**Table 1**).[6-23] The general pathology findings in any organ include a lymphoplasmacytic infiltrate, fibrosis that typically has a storiform pattern, obliterative phlebitis, modest tissue eosinophilia, and the tendency to form tumefactive lesions.[24] This chapter is devoted to a review of the extrapancreatic features of IgG4-RD that can be seen in those with type 1 AIP.

Nomenclature

The Organizing Committee of the 2011 Boston International Symposium on IgG4-RD recommended names for the individual organ system manifestations of this disease.[25] These are shown in **Table 2**. The nomenclature system reinforces the concept that the same fundamental pathophysiologic processes are operative across organ systems, regardless of whether the role of IgG4 is primary or secondary. Individual organ involvement is referred to in a style that employs "*IgG4-related-*" as a prefix. As examples, the most common form of kidney involvement in IgG4-RD is termed IgG4-related tubulointerstitial nephritis, and eye manifestations of this condition are collectively regarded as IgG4-related ophthalmic disease.

Systemic Features

IgG4-RD typically has an indolent presentation. Features of the disease generally manifest after months or even years. In addition, constitutional symptoms are subtle or absent in the majority of patients, who often feel relatively well even in the setting of multiorgan disease. Others, however, have anorexia and weight loss that become substantial over time. A minority of patients have more explosive presentations characterized by constitutional symptoms, fevers, and acute-phase reactant elevations.

Tumefactive lesions (pseudotumors)

Patients with IgG4-RD are often initially suspected or even misdiagnosed as having a malignancy because of the disease's predilection for causing mass-forming lesions within organs. Many patients are subjected to pancreatic resection out of concern for pancreatic cancer. In addition, pseudotumors are commonly reported in the orbital region, salivary glands, lung, kidney, lymph nodes, retroperitoneum, and other organs.[15,23,26] Many have an indolent course, but local tissue destruction including the erosion of bone and aortic aneurysms or dissections have been reported.[20,27-31] Diffuse infiltrative lesions also occur in organs such as the meninges, skin, or aorta.

Inflammatory pseudotumors have been described in IgG4-RD involving the lung and central nervous

*Corresponding author. Email: jhstone@partners.org

Table 1. Clinical Manifestations of IgG4-RD by Organ System.

Organ System	Clinical Feature
Eyes	Chronic sclerosing dacryoadenitis Orbital pseudotumor Extension of pseudotumor along trigeminal nervetrun Orbital myositis Scleritis
Ears	Destructive disease of middle ear
Nose	Eosinophilic angiocentric fibrosis
Salivary glands	Chronic sclerosing sialadenitis (submandibular & parotid glands)
Lymph nodes	Generalized or localized lymphadenopathy
Thyroid gland	Fibrosing variant of Hashimoto's thyroiditis, Riedel's thyroiditis
Lungs and airways	Pulmonary nodules, ground-glass opacities, alveolar/ interstitial inflammation, bronchovascular bundle thickening, pleural thickening, large airway disease leading to tracheobronchial stenosis
Heart	Pericarditis (sometimes with constriction)
Aorta	Thoracic aortitis, abdominal aortitis, inflammatory aortic aneurysms, aortic dissection
Retroperitoneum	Retroperitoneal fibrosis
Pancreas	Type 1 autoimmune pancreatitis
Biliary tree	Sclerosing cholangitis mimicking primary sclerosing cholangitis
Skin	Erythematous or flesh-colored papules or plaques on the face or head
Central nervous system	Hypopituitarism, hypertrophic pachymeningitis
Peripheral nervous system	Perineural inflammation
Other	Prostatism, sclerosing mesenteritis, fibrosing mediastinitis

Table 2. Preferred Nomenclature for Individual Organ Manifestations of IgG4-RD.

Organ System/Tissue	Preferred Name
Pancreas	Type 1 autoimmune pancreatitis (lgG4- related pancreatitis)
Eye	IgG4-related ophthalmic disease is the general term for the peri-ocular manifestations of this disease. There are several subsets, outlined below.
Lacrimal glands	IgG4-related dacryoadenitis
Orbital soft tissue (orbital inflammatory pseudotumor)	IgG4-related orbital inflammation (or IgG4- related orbital inflammatory pseudotumor)
Extra-ocular muscle disease	IgG4-related orbital myositis
Orbit with involvement of multiple anatomic structures	IgG4-related pan-orbital inflammation (includes lacrimal gland disease, extra-ocular muscle involvement, and other potential intra-orbital complications)
Salivary glands (parotid and submandibular glands)	IgG4-related sialadenitis or, more specifically, IgG4-related parotitis or IgG4- related submandibular gland disease
Pachymeninges	IgG4-related pachymeningitis
Hypophysis	IgG4-related hypophysitis
Thyroid (Riedel's thyroiditis)	IgG4-related thyroiditis
Aorta	IgG4-related aortitis/periaortitis
Arteries	IgG4-related periarteritis
Mediastinum	IgG4-related mediastinitis
Retroperitoneum	IgG4-related retroperitoneal fibrosis
Mesentery	IgG4-related mesenteritis
Skin	IgG4-related skin disease
Lymph node	IgG4-related lymphadenopathy
Bile ducts	IgG4-related sclerosing cholangitis
Gallbladder	IgG4-related cholecystitis
Liver	IgG4-related hepatopathy (refers to liver involvement that is distinct from biliary tract involvement)
Lung	IgG4-related lung disease
Pleura	IgG4-related pleuritis

Table 2. Continued

Organ System/Tissue	Preferred Name
Pericardium	IgG4-related pericarditis
Kidney	IgG4-related kidney disease. The specific renal complications should be termed tubulointerstitial nephritis secondary toIgG4- RD and membranous glomerulonephritis secondary to IgG4-RD. Involvement of the renal pelvis should be termed IgG4-related renal pyelitis.
Breast	IgG4-related mastitis
Prostate	IgG4-related prostatitis

system,[14,15,23,32] as well as in the orbit,[33] salivary gland,[34] paraspinal regions,[35] and other tissues and organs. Because of the tendency of IgG4-RD to cause tumefactive lesions, immunostaining should be performed on all pseudotumors with significant infiltrates of plasma cells and fibrosis.[36]

Multifocal fibrosclerosis

A condition known as multifocal fibrosclerosis was first identified in the 1960s.[37] Most cases of multifocal fibrosclerosis, often characterized by the simultaneous occurrence of other fibrotic syndromes such as Riedel's thyroiditis, hypertrophic pachymeningitis,[38,39] retroperitoneal fibrosis, fibrosing mediastinitis,[9] sclerosing mesenteritis,[40] and orbital pseudotumor, are probably explained by IgG4-RD.

Allergic disease

Allergic or atopic manifestations occur in approximately 50% of patients with IgG4-RD. Such patients often have longstanding histories of allergic rhinitis, sinusitis, asthma, and other clinical features of this nature. Many patients have substantial elevations of serum IgE or peripheral eosinophilias that sometimes approach 25% of the total white blood cell count. Mild to moderate eosinophil infiltration is also typical of tissue lesions.[24]

Eosinophilic angiocentric fibrosis

One subset of IgG4-RD associated with striking allergic features is eosinophilic angiocentric fibrosis (EAF), an uncommon tumefactive lesion of the orbit and upper respiratory tract.[41,42] The histopathology of this condition is characterized by an overabundance of eosinophils, as well as an admixture of lymphocytes and plasma cells. Small-caliber arterioles in EAF demonstrate "onion-skinning" – concentric layers of fibrosis – of the blood vessels. Patients with EAF share the broader tendency of IgG4-RD to form tumefactive lesions within involved organs.

Lymphadenopathy

Lymphadenopathy in IgG4-RD generally takes two forms. First, generalized lymphadenopathy can be the major or sole component of the clinical presentation. Patients with IgG4-related lymphadenopathy of this nature are often constitutionally well, at least for prolonged periods. Second, involvement of lymph nodes as localized disease adjacent to a specific organ affected by IgG4-RD (e.g., the pancreas) is common.

Patients with IgG4-related lymphadenopathy often undergo serial lymph node biopsies to exclude lymphoma, sarcoidosis, multicentric Castleman's disease, or disseminated malignancies. Rendering the diagnosis of IgG4-RD purely on the basis of lymph node pathology is difficult because the histology of lymph nodes in this setting is remarkably variable.[16] Clinicians must seek evidence of disease in other organ systems typically affected by IgG4-RD to be confident of the diagnosis. Increased numbers of $IgG4^+$ plasma cells, of course, are universal, but the storiform fibrosis so common in other types of IgG4-RD organ involvement is unusual in IgG4-related lymphadenopathy. Lymph node biopsies in most cases are reported as "reactive follicular hyperplasia," and specific stains for IgG4 are not generally performed because the diagnosis is not considered.

Specific Organ Involvement by Body Region

The discussion of specific organ involvement is divided by the different major body regions: the head and neck, chest, abdomen/retroperitoneum, and miscellaneous.

Head & neck

Meninges

A study of 15 cases of idiopathic hypertrophic pachymeningitis found that IgG4-RD, linked to four (27%) of the cases, was the most common disease association.[17] Other causes in that series were granulomatosis with polyangiitis (three cases) and miscellaneous other diagnoses including sarcoidosis, lymphoma, giant cell arteritis, and rheumatoid arthritis. This study confirmed an earlier one that demonstrated IgG4-RD to be the cause of 5 out of 10 cases of idiopathic lymphoplasmacytic meningeal inflammation.[39]

Pituitary gland

The presence of IgG4-RD in other organs and elevated serum IgG4 concentrations are common features of IgG4-related hypophysitis and often constitute a major clue to the diagnosis of IgG4-related hypophysitis. The radiologic findings in this entity include a pituitary mass or thickened pituitary stalk. Most IgG4-RD patients with hypophysitis are middle-aged males who present with various degrees of anterior or posterior hypopituitarism. IgG4-RD must be differentiated from sarcoidosis, granulomatosis with polyangiitis (formerly Wegener's), histiocytosis, and lymphoma as causes of hypophysitis. Both glucocorticoid therapy and rituximab can resolve imaging abnormalities and clinical signs of pituitary insufficiency.

Salivary glands

"Küttner's tumor," another disorder originally described in the 1890s,[43] consists of a tumorous swelling of the submandibular glands (**Figure 1**). Bilateral submandibular gland swelling in the absence of stones within Wharton's duct is commonly associated with IgG4-RD.[6,44] In contrast to Sjögren's syndrome (SjS) in which the degree of parotid enlargement is often dramatically out of proportion to that of the submandibular glands, the opposite pattern is more typical of IgG4-related sialadenitis. Submandibular gland disease often occurs in IgG4-RD in the absence of any clinical evidence of parotid gland enlargement, but parotid disease in IgG4-RD is also described **(Figure 2)**. Salivary gland involvement consists of firm, nodular swelling that is generally symmetrical and associated with pain, tenderness, and decreased saliva production. The sublingual glands can also be affected by IgG4-RD (**Figure 2**).

The triad of swelling in the submandibular, parotid, and lacrimal glands, first described in 1892, was termed "Mikulicz disease" for more than 100 years.[45,46,68] For decades, Mikulicz disease was believed to be a variant of SjS,[47,48] and patients with IgG4-RD continue to be misdiagnosed with SjS. IgG4-RD can be clearly differentiated from SjS on the basis of clinical, serological, and pathological findings.[49]

Minor salivary glands of the lip may be affected, as demonstrated by lip biopsy.[50] Minor salivary gland disease can be present even when the glands are macroscopically normal. The sensitivity and specificity of minor salivary gland biopsy in patients with IgG4-RD have not been well defined.

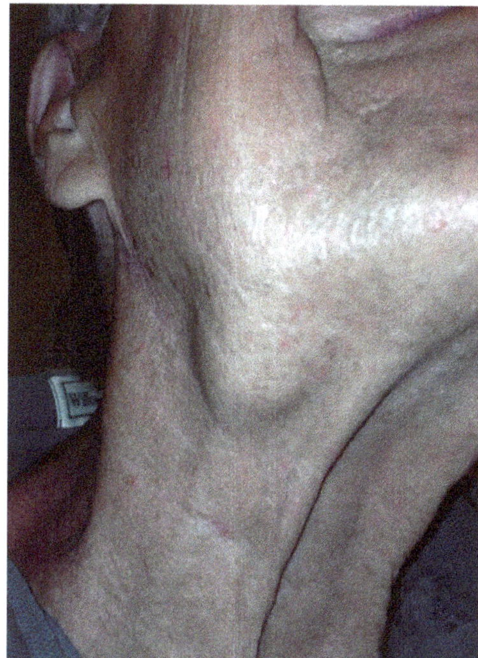

Figure 1. Submandibular gland involvement. Submandibular gland enlargement occurring during a flare of IgG4-related disease in a patient with a history of IgG4-related sclerosing cholangitis.

Ophthalmic disease

The orbital tissues are perhaps the most commonly affected region of the body in IgG4- RD. IgG4-RD accounts for a substantial percentage – at least 25% – of the cases of "idiopathic" orbital inflammation, a differential diagnosis that includes lymphoma, granulomatosis with polyangiitis, Graves' orbitopathy, and other conditions.[61]

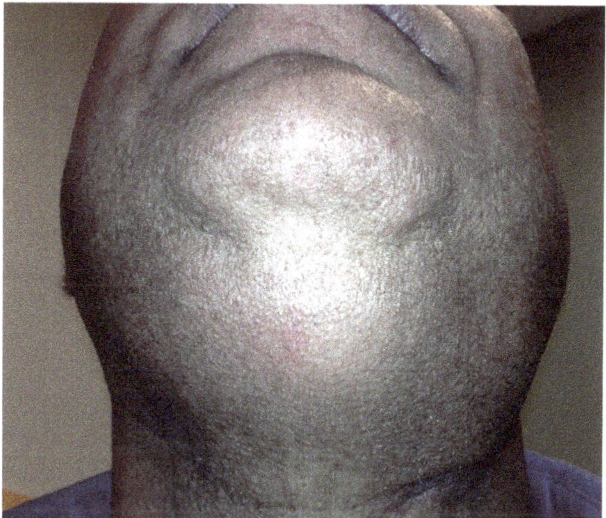

Figure 2. Parotid and sublingual gland disease. Parotid and sublingual gland enlargement. The sublingual glands have herniated through the floor of the mouth.

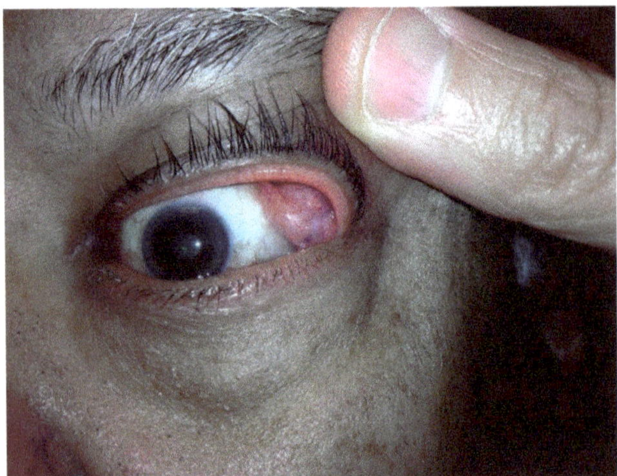

Figure 3. Dacryoadenitis. Lacrimal gland swelling in a patient with IgG4-RD.

The ocular structures affected by IgG4-RD include the lacrimal glands (dacryoadenitis) (**Figure 3**), nasolacrimal duct, and retro-bulbar region that is frequently involved by orbital pseudotumor (**Figure 4**), and the extraocular muscles (a condition often termed "orbital myositis").[13,52-54,72] As noted, many cases of IgG4-related dacryoadenitis are accompanied by salivary gland disease. In some patients with IgG4-related ophthalmic disease, the process extends beyond the orbit and tracks along the course of the trigeminal nerve.[52,55]

Thyroid gland

Riedel's thyroiditis has been identified as a manifestation of IgG4-RD.[11] Although thyroid gland biopsies from patients with advanced disease simply demonstrate glandular fibrosis, biopsies taken early in the disease course demonstrate the classic pathologic hallmarks of IgG4-RD. The fibrosing variant of Hashimoto's thyroiditis also appears to be part of the IgG4-RD spectrum, at least in a percentage of cases.[56] Finally, it has been postulated that classic Hashimoto's thyroiditis, distinct from the fibrosing variant discussed above, also falls within the IgG4-RD spectrum and might account for the high frequency of hypothyroidism in AIP. This putative "IgG4-related thyroiditis" is said to have a lower likelihood of antithyroid autoantibodies compared with Hashimoto's thyroiditis, a low likelihood of diffuse goiter, and a favorable response to glucocorticoid treatment. However, relatively few such cases have been examined histopathologically, and this hypothesis remains controversial and unconfirmed.

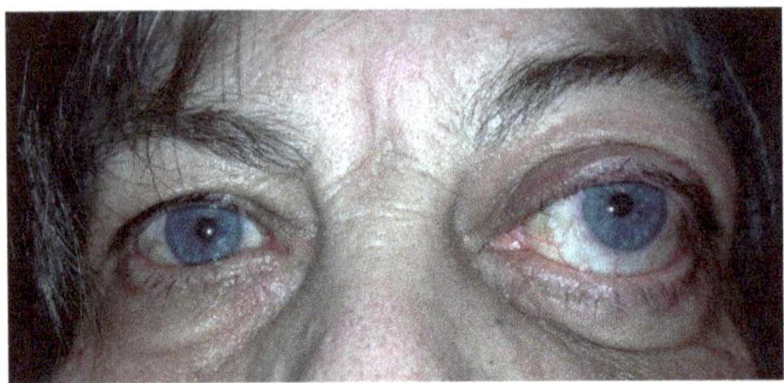

Figure 4. Orbital pseudotumor. Left eye proptosis caused by an orbital pseudotumor that spared the lacrimal gland.

Chest

Lung

Pulmonary involvement in IgG4-RD is protean in its scope, and understanding of the nature and extent of lung and airway disease continues to evolve. At least six major patterns of IgG4-related pulmonary disease are described on the basis of radiological and histological findings[15,57-59]: 1) nodules, 2) thickening of the bronchovascular bundle (**Figure 5**), 3) alveolar interstitial disease (with honeycombing, bronchiectasis, and diffuse ground-glass opacities), 4) rounded ground-glass opacities, 5) pleural lesions associated with severely thickened visceral or parietal pleura with diffuse sclerosing inflammation, and 6) airway lesions leading to narrowing.

Some patients with IgG4-related lung disease experience cough, hemoptysis, dyspnea, pleural effusion, or chest discomfort.[15,57,59] In others, however, the presence of lung disease is asymptomatic and discovered only incidentally upon imaging.

Thoracic aorta

IgG4-RD appears to account for at least 10% of cases of inflammatory aortitis involving the thoracic aorta.[60] The

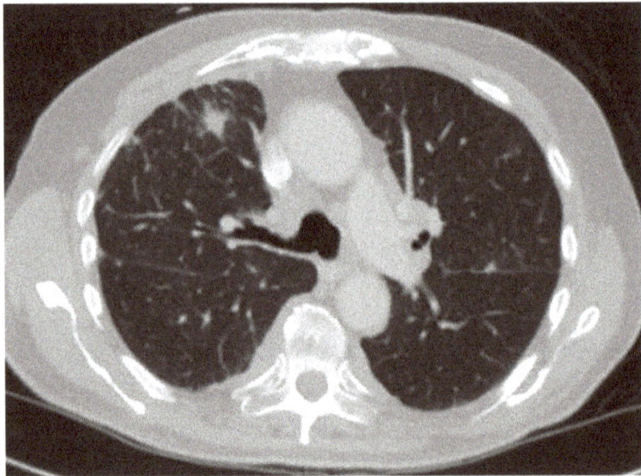

Figure 5. Pulmonary involvement in IgG4-RD. This computed tomographic scan of the chest shows thickening of the bronchial wall and a pulmonary nodule in the anterior right upper lobe.

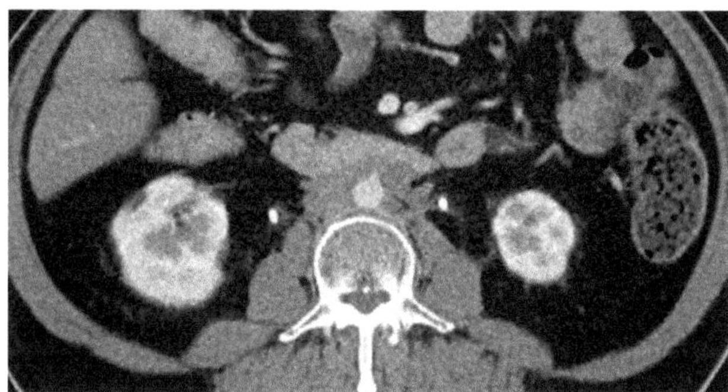

Figure 6. Retroperitoneal fibrosis. Computed tomographic scan of the abdomen reveals an inflammatory mass surrounding the abdominal aorta.

lymphoplasmacytic aortitis associated with IgG4-RD must be distinguished from the granulomatous inflammation that accompanies a somewhat larger subset of cases diagnosed as giant cell aortitis. The entity referred to by the descriptive pathologic term "chronic sclerosing aortitis" probably represents IgG4-RD in the great majority of cases. The term "isolated aortitis" should generally be regarded as unsatisfactory without thorough attempts at differentiating IgG4-related aortitis from giant cell aortitis and other causes of aortic inflammation.

Retroperitoneum & abdomen

Manifestations of IgG4-RD within many of the abdominal organs are addressed in detail in other sections of this publication; namely, those associated with pancreatic, biliary, liver, or gallbladder disease (See **Chapter 5**, "CT and MR features of autoimmune pancreatitis"; **Chapter 6**, "ERCP features of autoimmune pancreatitis"). This section, therefore, focuses on retroperitoneal organs.

Chronic periaortitis

Chronic periaortitis is now regarded as the umbrella term for inflammation in the retroperitoneum and periaortic regions that includes such entities as retroperitoneal fibrosis, inflammatory abdominal aortic aneurysm, and perianeurysmal fibrosis.[61] IgG4- RD is now known to cause well over half of the cases previously regarded as "idiopathic" retroperitoneal fibrosis (**Figure 6**).[62,63] When detected early, biopsies from patients with retroperitoneal fibrosis exhibit histopathological and immunohistochemical features that are diagnostic of IgG4-RD.[63] In contrast, biopsies performed in patients at a later phase of disease simply show fibrosis because they represent a more advanced IgG4-RD stage in which the fibrotic features have become predominant. Nevertheless, the storiform morphology of the fibrosis can still be highly suggestive of IgG4-RD. In such cases, the IgG4/total IgG ratio within tissue rather than the number of IgG4-positive plasma cells/ high-power field is often a key to recognizing IgG4-related retroperitoneal fibrosis.[62]

The first study to connect retroperitoneal fibrosis and the entity now termed IgG4-RD was that of Hamano et al.,[7] who described three patients with retroperitoneal fibrosis and elevated serum IgG4 concentrations. Zen et al. reported that 10 of 17 retroperitoneal fibrosis patients had both elevated serum IgG4 concentrations and histopathological features typical of IgG4-RD.[63]

Moreover, IgG4-related retroperitoneal fibrosis has an overwhelming tendency to occur in males. This was confirmed by Khosroshahi et al.,[62] who identified the histopathological and immunohistochemistry signature of IgG4-RD in the biopsies of 13 of 23 cases of "idiopathic" retroperitoneal fibrosis.

Inflammatory abdominal aortic aneurysm is also associated with IgG4-RD.[19,31] Patients with inflammatory abdominal aortic aneurysms have clinical, demographic, and radiologic features that are distinct from those of patients with classic atherosclerotic aortic aneurysms.

Kidney

The radiologic appearance of the kidneys in IgG4-related renal disease can take several forms. Diffuse enlargement accompanied by parenchymal hypodensities may occur. Focal tumefactive lesions may also develop, mimicking renal cell carcinoma.[14] More than one such lesion within any kidney can occur. A thickening of the renal pelvis has also been described.[64,70] Finally, following a period of IgG4-related renal disease, pronounced atrophy of the kidneys can ensue. This atrophy can occur even in patients whose disease has appeared to respond to therapy with glucocorticoids.[65]

The most common histopathological correlate of these radiologic findings is tubulointerstitial nephritis (TIN), which consists of patchy or diffuse tubulointerstitial lymphoplasmacytic infiltrates within a fibrotic interstitium.[66] The clinical manifestations of IgG4-related TIN include proteinuria, hematuria, and decreased kidney function, sometimes culminating in end-stage renal disease.[67,68]

Patients with IgG4-related renal disease are typically hypocomplementemic and often profoundly so.[69] The basis for this phenomenon remains incompletely defined because the IgG4 molecule itself does not avidly activate complement. Nevertheless, renal biopsies in IgG4-related TIN demonstrate immune complexes that consist in part of IgG4.[14] The TIN associated with IgG4-RD can be differentiated histopathologically and immunohistochemically from other causes of TIN.[64,70] The great majority of patients with IgG4-related renal disease also have disease in other organs.[65]

A second form of renal disease – membranous glomerulonephritis (MGN) – has also been described in IgG4-RD, although this lesion is decidedly less common than TIN.[65,71] Nephrotic-range proteinuria can occur in IgG4-related MGN. This condition is distinct from idiopathic MGN, even though the autoantibody associated with the latter disorder is also principally of the IgG4 subclass. MGN associated with IgG4-RD is probably secondary to immune complex deposition rather than to the usual destructive inflammatory process that characterizes other organ involvement by this condition.

Miscellaneous organ involvement

Miscellaneous organs in which the typical histopathological features of IgG4-RD have been reported include the skin,[18] prostate gland,[22,72,73] and pericardium.[21] In all of these reports, the patients' clinical features were also associated with disease in more classic IgG4-RD organs. The true frequency with which IgG4-RD affects these organs is not known because the presence of disease there can be extremely subtle. In the skin, for example, IgG4-RD causes flesh-colored or erythematous papules that are often asymptomatic. Similarly, symptoms of prostatism in middle-aged to elderly males are likely to be diagnosed as benign prostatic hypertrophy. Conversely, IgG4-related prostate disease is known to cause symptoms of "benign prostatic hypertrophy" in men in their 30s.

Summary

Type 1 AIP is the pancreatic manifestation of a systemic disease referred to as IgG4-RD. The current diagnostic criteria for AIP recognize typical other organ involvement including proximal biliary strictures, retroperitoneal fibrosis, symmetric enlargement of salivary/lacrimal glands, and renal disease. However, manifestations can involve essentially any organ. Histology is important for identifying diagnostic features of IgG4-RD and excluding malignancy in those with mass-forming lesions.

References

1. Stone JH, Zen Y, and Deshpande, V. IgG4-related disease. *N Engl J Med.* 2012; 366: 539-51. PMID: 22316447
2. Yoshida K, Toki F, Takeuchi T, Watanabe S, Shiratori K, and Hayashi N. Chronic pancreatitis caused by an autoimmune abnormality. Proposal of the concept of autoimmune pancreatitis. *Dig Dis Sci.* 1995; 40: 1561-1568. PMID: 7628283
3. Hamano H, Kawa S, Horiuchi A, Unno H, Furuya N, Akamatsu T, et al. High serum IgG4 concentrations in patients with sclerosing pancreatitis. *N Engl J Med.* 2001; 344: 732-738. PMID: 11450670
4. Kamisawa T, Funata N, Hayashi Y, Eishi Y, Koike M, Tsuruta K, Okamoto A, Egawa N, and Nakajima H. A new clinicopathological entity of IgG4-related autoimmune disease. *J Gastroenterol.* 2003; 38: 982-984. PMID: 14614606
5. Kamisawa T, and Okamoto A. Autoimmune pancreatitis: proposal of IgG4-related sclerosing disease. *J Gastroenterol.* 2006; 41: 613-625. PMID: 16932997
6. Geyer JT, Ferry JA, Harris NL, Stone JH, Zukerberg LR, Lauwers GY, et al. Chronic sclerosing sialadenitis (Küttner tumor) is an IgG4-associated disease. *Am J Surg Pathol.* 2010; 34: 202-210. PMID: 20061932
7. Hamano H, Kawa S, Ochi Y, Unno H, Shiba N, Wajiki M, et al. Hydronephrosis associated with retroperitoneal fibrosis and sclerosing pancreatitis. *Lancet.* 2002; 359: 1403-1404. PMID: 11978339
8. Fukukura Y, Fujiyoshi F, Nakamura F, Hamada H, and Nakajo M. Autoimmune pancreatitis associated with idiopathic retroperitoneal fibrosis. *AJR Am J Roentgenol.* 2003; 181: 993-995. PMID: 16936451
9. Taniguchi T, Kobayashi H, Fukui S, Ogura K, Saiga T, and Okamoto M. A case of multifocal fibrosclerosis involving posterior mediastinal fibrosis, retroperitoneal fibrosis, and a left seminal vesicle with elevated serum IgG4. *Hum Pathol.* 2006; 37: 1237-1239. PMID: 16938531
10. Kamisawa T, Okamoto A, and Funata N. Clinicopathological features of autoimmune pancreatitis in relation to elevation of serum IgG4. *Pancreas.* 2005; 31: 28-31. PMID: 15968244
11. Dahlgren M, Khosroshahi A, Nielsen GP, Deshpande V, and Stone JH. Riedel's thyroiditis and multifocal fibrosclerosis are part of the IgG4-related systemic disease spectrum. *Arthritis Care Res (Hoboken).* 2010; 62: 1312-1318. PMID: 20506114
12. Stone JH, Caruso PA, and Deshpande V. Case records of the Massachusetts General Hospital. Case 24-2009. A 26-year-old woman with painful swelling of the neck. *N Engl J Med.* 2009; 361: 511-518. PMID: 19641208
13. Wallace ZS, Khosroshahi A, Jakobiec FA, Deshpande V, Hatton MP, Ritter J, et al. IgG4-related systemic disease as a cause of "idiopathic" orbital inflammation, including orbital myositis and trigeminal nerve involvement. *Surv Ophthalmol.* 2012; 57: 26-33. PMID: 22018678
14. Cornell LD, Chicano SL, Deshpande V, Collins AB, Selig MK, Lauwers GY, et al. Pseudotumors due to IgG4 immune-complex tubulointerstitial nephritis associated with autoimmune pancreatocentric disease. *Am J Surg Pathol.* 2007; 31: 1586-1597. PMID: 17895762
15. Zen Y, Kitagawa S, Minato H, Kurumaya H, Katayanagi K, Masuda S, et al. IgG4-positive plasma cells in inflammatory pseudotumor (plasma cell granuloma) of the lung. *Hum Pathol.* 2005; 36: 710-717. PMID: 16084938
16. Sato Y, and Yoshino T. IgG4-related lymphadenopathy. *Int J Rheumatol.* 2012; 2012: 572539. PMID: 22719769
17. Wallace ZS, Carruthers MN, Khosroshahi A, Carruthers R, Shingare S, Despande V, and Stone JH. IgG4- related disease and hypertrophic pachymeningitis. *Medicine (Baltimore).* 2013; 92: 206-216. PMID: 23793110

18. Khosroshahi A, Carruthers MD, Deshpande V, Leb L, Reed J, and Stone JH. Cutaneous IgG4-related disease. *Am J Med.* 2011; 124: e7-e8.
19. Kasashima S, Zen Y, Kawashima A, Endo M, Matsumoto Y, and Kasashima F. A new clinicopathological entity of IgG4-related inflammatory abdominal aortic aneurysm. *J Vasc Surg.* 2009; 49: 1264-1271. PMID: 19217746
20. Stone JH, Khosroshahi A, Hilgenberg A, Spooner A, Isselbacher EM, and Stone JR. IgG4-related systemic disease and lymphoplasmacytic aortitis. *Arthritis Rheum.* 2009; 60: 3139-3145. PMID: 19790067
21. Sugimoto T, Morita Y, Isshiki K, Yamamoto T, Uzu T, Kashiwagi A, et al. Constrictive pericarditis as an emerging manifestation of hyper-IgG4 disease. *Int J Cardiol.* 2008; 130: e100-e101. PMID: 17727980
22. Hamed G, Tsushima K, Yasuo M, Kubo K, Yamazaki S, Kawa S, et al. Inflammatory lesions of the lung, submandibular gland, bile duct and prostate in a patient with IgG4-associated multifocal systemic fibrosclerosis. *Respirology.* 2007; 12: 455-457. PMID: 17539856
23. Zen Y, Kasahara Y, Horita K, Miyayama S, Miura S, Kitagawa S, et al. Inflammatory pseudotumor of the breast in a patient with a high serum IgG4 level: histologic similarity to sclerosing pancreatitis. *Am J Surg Pathol.* 2005; 29: 275-278. PMID: 15644785
24. Deshpande V, Zen Y, Chan JK, Yi EE, Sato Y, Yoshino T, et al. Consensus statement on the pathology of IgG4-related disease. *Mod Pathol.* 2012; 25: 1181-1192. PMID: 22596100
25. Stone JH, Khosroshahi A, Deshpande V, Chan JKC, Heathcote JG, Aalberse R, et al. Recommendations for the nomenclature of IgG4-related disease and its individual organ system manifestations. *Arthritis Rheum.* 2012; 64: 3061-3067. PMID: 22736240
26. Khosroshahi A, and Stone JH. A clinical overview of IgG4-related systemic disease. *Curr Opin Rheumatol.* 2011; 23: 57-66. PMID: 21124086
27. Khosroshahi A, Stone JR, Pratt DS, Deshpande V, and Stone JH. Painless jaundice with serial multi-organ dysfunction. *Lancet.* 2009; 373: 1494. PMID: 19394539
28. Narain S, Wallace ZS, Deshpande V, Carruthers R, Liebsch N, and Stone JH. IgG4-related systemic disease (IgG4-RD): an emerging condition and novel cause of saddle-nose deformity. (Submitted).
29. Schiffenbauer AI, Wahl C, Pittaluga S, Jaffe ES, Hoffman R, Khosroshahi A, et al. IgG4-related disease masquerading as recurrent mastoiditis. *Laryngoscope.* 2012; 122: 681-684. PMID: 22252885
30. Cheuk W, and Chan JK. IgG4-related sclerosing disease: a critical appraisal of an evolving clinicopathologic entity. *Adv Anat Pathol.* 2010; 17: 303-332. PMID: 20733352
31. Stone JH, Patel V, Oliveira G, and Stone JR. Case records of the Massachusetts General Hospital. Case 38-2012. A 60-year-old man with abdominal pain and multiple aortic aneurysms. *N Engl J Med.* 2012; 367: 2335-2346. PMID: 23234517
32. Lui PC, Fan YS, Wong SS, Chan AN, Wong G, Chau TK, et al. Inflammatory pseudotumors of the central nervous system. *Hum Pathol.* 2009; 40: 1611-1617. PMID: 19656549
33. Kishi K, Fujii T, Kohno T, and Yoshimura K. Inflammatory pseudotumour affecting the lung and orbit. *Respirology.* 2009; 14: 449-451. PMID: 19353778
34. Yamamoto H, Yamaguchi H, Aishima S, Oda Y, Kohashi K, Oshiro Y, et al. Inflammatory myofibroblastic tumor versus IgG4-related sclerosing disease and inflammatory pseudotumor: a comparative clinicopathologic study. *Am J Surg Pathol.* 2009; 33: 1330-1340. PMID: 19718789
35. Cheuk W, Tam FK, Chan AN, Luk IS, Yuen AP, Chan WK, et al. Idiopathic cervical fibrosis: A new member of IgG4-related sclerosing diseases. *Am J Surg Pathol.* 2010; 34: 1678-1685. PMID: 20871392
36. Umehara H, Okazaki K, Masaki Y, Kawano M, Yamamoto M, Saeki T, et al. A novel clinical entity, IgG4-related disease (IgG4-RD): general concepts and details. *Mod Rheumatol.* 2012; 22: 1-14. PMID: 21881964
37. Comings DE, Skubi KB, Van Eyes J, and Motulsky AG. Familial multifocal fibrosclerosis. Findings suggesting that retroperitoneal fibrosis, mediastinal fibrosis, sclerosing cholangitis, Riedel's thyroiditis, and pseudotumor of the orbit may be different manifestations of a single disease. *Ann Intern Med.* 1967; 66: 884-892. PMID: 6025229
38. Chan SK, Cheuk W, Chan KT, and Chan JK. IgG4-related sclerosing pachymeningitis: a previously unrecognized form of central nervous system involvement in IgG4-related sclerosing disease. *Am J Surg Pathol.* 2009; 33: 1249-1252. PMID: 19561447
39. Lindstrom KM, Cousar JB, and Lopes MB. IgG4-related meningeal disease: clinico-pathological features and proposal for diagnostic criteria. *Acta Neuropathol.* 2010; 120: 765-776. PMID: 20844883
40. Chen TS, and Montgomery EA. Are tumefactive lesions classified as sclerosing mesenteritis a subset of IgG4-related sclerosing disorders? *J Clin Pathol.* 2008; 61: 1093-1097. PMID: 18682417
41. Roberts PF, and McCann BG. Eosinophilic angiocentric fibrosis of the upper respiratory tract: a mucosal variant of granuloma faciale? A report of three cases. *Histopathology.* 1985; 9: 1217-1225. PMID: 4085985
42. Deshpande V, Khosroshahi A, Nielsen GP, Hamilos DL, and Stone JH. Eosinophilic angiocentric fibrosis is a form of IgG4-related systemic disease. *Am J Surg Pathol.* 2011; 35: 701-706. PMID: 21502911
43. Küttner H. Über entzündliche tumoren der submaaxillärspeicheldrüse. *Beitr Klin Chir.* 1896; 15: 815-834.
44. Chow TL, Chan TT, Choi CY, and Lam SH. Kuttner's tumour (chronic sclerosing sialadenitis) of the submandibular gland: a clinical perspective. *Hong Kong Med J.* 2008; 14: 46-49. PMID: 18239243
45. Mikulicz J. Über eine eigenartige symmetrische erkränkung der Thränen- und Mundspeicheldrüsen. In: Billroth T, editor. *Beiträge zur chirurgie festschrift gewidmet.* Stuttgart, Germany: Ferdinand Enke; 1892: 610-630.
46. Mikulicz J. Concerning a peculiar symmetrical disease of the lacrimal and salivary glands. *Modern Classics.* 2: 165-186, 1937-1938.
47. Morgan WS, and Castleman B. A clinicopathologic study of Mikulicz's disease. *Am J Pathol.* 1953; 29: 471-503. PMID: 13040489

48. Morgan WS. The probable systemic nature of Mikulicz's disease and its relation to Sjögren's syndrome. *N Engl J Med.* 1954; 251: 5-10. PMID: 13176645
49. Yamamoto M, Takahashi H, Ohara M, Suzuki C, Naishiro Y, Yamamoto H, et al. A new conceptualization for Mikulicz's disease as an IgG4-related plasmacytic disease. *Mod Rheumatol.* 2006; 16: 335-340. PMID: 17164992
50. Baer AN, Gourin CG, Westra WH, Cox DP, Greenspan JS, and Daniels TE. Rare diagnosis of IgG4-related systemic disease by lip biopsy in an international Sjögren syndrome registry. *Oral Surg Oral Med Oral Pathol Oral Radiol.* 2013; 115: e34-e39. PMID: 23146570
51. Takahira M, Ozawa Y, Kawano M, Zen Y, Hamaoka S, Yamada K, et al. Clinical Aspects of IgG4- Related Orbital Inflammation in a Case Series of Ocular Adnexal Lymphoproliferative Disorders. *Int J Rheumatol.* 2012; 2012: 635473. PMID: 22548072
52. Wallace ZS, Deshpande V, Stone JH. Ophthalmic manifestations of IgG4-related disease: Single-center experience and review of the literature. (Submitted). PMID:
53. Sato Y, Ohshima K, Ichimura K, Sato M, Yamadori I, Tanaka T, et al. Ocular adnexal IgG4-related disease has uniform clinicopathology. *Pathol Int.* 58(8): 465-70, 2008. PMID: 18705764
54. Cheuk W, Yuen HK, and Chan JK. Chronic sclerosing dacryoadenitis: part of the spectrum of IgG4-related sclerosing disease? *Am J Surg Pathol.* 2007; 31: 643-645. PMID: 17414116
55. Katsura M, Morita A, Horiuchi H, Ohtomo K, and Machida T. IgG4-related inflammatory pseudotumor of the trigeminal nerve: another component of igg4-related sclerosing disease? *AJNR Am J Neuroradiol.* 2011; 32: E150-E152. PMID: 20864523
56. Deshpande V, Khosroshahi A, Nielsen GP, and Stone JH. Fibrosing variant of Hashimoto's thyroiditis is a IgG4-related disease. *J Clin Pathol.* 2012; 65: 725-728. PMID: 22659333
57. Zen Y, Inoue D, Kitao A, Onodera M, Abo H, Miyayama S, et al. IgG4-related lung and pleural disease: a clinicopathologic study of 21 cases. *Am J Surg Pathol.* 2009; 33: 1886-1893. PMID: 19898222
58. Taniguchi T, Ko M, Seko S, Nishida O, Inoue F, Kobayashi H, et al. Interstitial pneumonia associated with autoimmune pancreatitis. *Gut.* 2004; 53: 770. PMID: 15082601
59. Shrestha B, Sekiguchi H, Colby TV, Graziano P, Aubry MC, Smyrk TC, et al. Distinctive pulmonary histopathology with increased IgG4-positive plasma cells in patients with autoimmune pancreatitis: report of 6 and 12 cases with similar histopathology. *Am J Surg Pathol.* 2009; 33: 1450-1462. PMID: 19623032
60. Stone JH, Khosroshahi A, Deshpande V, and Stone JR. IgG4-related systemic disease accounts for a significant proportion of thoracic lymphoplasmacytic aortitis cases. *Arthritis Care Res (Hoboken).* 2010; 62: 316-322. PMID: 20391477
61. Palmisano A, and Vaglio A. Chronic periaortitis: a fibro-inflammatory disorder. *Best Pract Res Clin Rheumatol.* 2009; 23: 339-353. PMID: 19508942
62. Khosroshahi A, Carruthers M, Stone JH, Shingare S, Sainani N, and Deshpande V. Re-thinking Ormond's Disease: A study of "idiopathic" and secondary cases of retroperitoneal fibrosis in the era of IgG4-related disease. *Medicine (Baltimore).* 2013; 92: 82-91. PMID: 23429355
63. Zen Y, Onodera M, Inoue D, Kitao A, Matsui O, Nohara T, et al. Retroperitoneal fibrosis: a clinicopathologic study with respect to immunoglobulin G4. *Am J Surg Pathol.* 2009; 33: 1833-1839. PMID: 19950407
64. Raissian Y, Nasr SH, Larsen CP, Colvin RB, Smyrk TC, Takahashi N, et al. Diagnosis of IgG4-related tubulointerstitial nephritis. *J Am Soc Nephrol.* 2011; 22: 1343-1352. PMID: 21719792
65. Saeki T, Kawano M, Mizushima I, Yamamota M, Wada Y, Nakashima H, et al. The clinical course of patients with IgG4-related kidney disease. *Kidney Int.* 2013; 84: 826-833. PMID: 23698232
66. Saeki T, Nishi S, I to T, Yamazaki H, Miyamura S, Emura I, et al. Renal lesions in IgG4-related systemic disease. *Intern Med.* 2007; 46: 1365-1371. PMID: 17827834
67. Takeda S, Haratake J, Kasai T, Takaeda C, Takazakura E. IgG4-associated idiopathic tubulointerstitial nephritis complicating autoimmune pancreatitis. *Nephrol Dial Transplant.* 19(2): 474-6, 2004. PMID: 14736977
68. Watson SJ, Jenkins DA, and Bellamy CO. Nephropathy in IgG4-related systemic disease. *Am J Surg Pathol.* 2006; 30: 1472-1477. PMID: 17063091
69. Saeki T, Nishi S, Imai N, Ito T, Yamazaki H, Kawano M, et al. Clinicopathological characteristics of patients with IgG4-related tubulointerstitial nephritis. *Kidney Int.* 2010; 78: 1016-1023. PMID: 23698232
70. Nishi S, Imai N, Yoshida K, Ito Y, and Saeki T. Clinicopathological findings of immunoglobulin G4- related kidney disease. *Clin Exp Nephrol.* 2011; 15: 810-819. PMID: 21870078
71. Alexander MP, Larsen CP, Gibson IW, Nasr SH, Sethi S, Fidler ME, et al. Membranous glomerulonephritis in IgG4-related disease. *Kidney Int.* 2013; 83: 455-462. PMID: 23254897
72. Yoshimura Y, Takeda S, Ieki Y, et al. IgG4-associated prostatitis complicating autoimmune pancreatitis. *Intern Med.* 45: 897-901, 2006. PMID: 16946571
73. Uehara T, Hamano H, Kawakami M, et al. Autoimmune pancreatitis-associated prostatitis: distinct clinicopathological entity. *Pathol Int.* 58: 118-125, 2008. PMID: 18199162

Chapter 62

Steroid therapy in the management of autoimmune pancreatitis

Tae Jun Song* and Myung-Hwan Kim*

Department of Internal Medicine, University of Ulsan College of Medicine, Asan Medical Center, Seoul, South Korea.

Introduction

Although there are no prospective randomized studies on steroid use in autoimmune pancreatitis (AIP), it is evident that this disease is exquisitely responsive to steroid therapy regardless of the subtype.[1] As a result, steroid therapy has become the standard therapy for AIP.[2] Spontaneous resolution of symptoms and radiological abnormalities has been reported in some patients.[3] However, the use of steroids may bring about remission consistently and more quickly. In a recent large retrospective study in Japan, the remission rate was significantly higher in the group with steroid therapy compared to those without steroid therapy.[2] Likewise, significantly fewer patients who received steroid therapy experienced a relapse compared to those who received only supportive care.[2] Hirano et al. reported that unfavorable events related to AIP including obstructive jaundice due to a bile duct stricture or pancreatic pseudocyst and other extrapancreatic manifestations were significantly lower in patients receiving steroid therapy compared to those who received only supportive care.[4] In addition, a recent study concluded that early therapeutic intervention has been clinically and histopathologically demonstrated to be important for the preservation of gland function.[5]

In the following review, we discuss steroid therapy for type 1 AIP.

Definition of Treatment Outcomes

Remission

The treatment goal of AIP is to achieve and maintain remission. So far, there is no generally accepted consensus on the specific parameters that define remission, including specific radiological, biochemical, or serological variables; neither is there consensus concerning the extent to which the outcome should be interpreted as remission. Because remission is also related to the timing of the steroid tapering after the initial high-dose administration, some patients may be undertreated. Differences in definitions of remission may account, at least in part, for the variability in the reported frequency of disease remission for patients on steroid and the relapse rates among different studies.[6] Thus, clearly defining remission is an important cornerstone in discussions on treatment and relapse.

Remission may be defined as the resolution or normalization of symptoms, biochemical abnormalities, radiological abnormalities, and pancreas/extrapancreatic organ histology.[7] In a practical setting, the end point of treatment is often symptomatic remission along with radiological remission because histological remission is difficult to confirm.[7] After steroid therapy, persistently elevated serum IgG4 levels may be observed in patients without symptoms or residual radiological abnormalities.[8] However, it is unclear as to whether this represents subclinical disease activity.

Relapse

In practice, relapse is generally defined as the recurrence of radiological manifestations of AIP with or without symptoms in the pancreas or extrapancreatic organs after remission has been achieved.[7] It should be discerned from failed weaning of the steroid, which is defined by a flare of disease activity during the initial steroid course.[9] Isolated elevation of serum IgG4, without symptoms or radiological abnormalities is usually not regarded as relapse.

Similar to remission, the definition of relapse is not uniform among studies. Because the lack of consensus on the definition of relapse may be related to the different relapse rates among studies, a consensus definition of relapse is important.[9]

Treatment

Indication for steroid therapy

In the initial inflammatory phase of AIP, the aim of treatment is to alleviate symptoms and improve radiological and

*Corresponding authors: Email: mhkim@amc.seoul.kr, medi01@naver.com

biochemical abnormalities.[10] In general, the indications for steroid therapy in type 1 AIP include symptoms such as obstructive jaundice or abdominal pain and the presence of symptomatic extrapancreatic lesions.[11,12]

A major determinant of treatment responsiveness may be the degree of fibrosis within the pancreas.[13] Similar to other autoimmune diseases, which are characterized by an active phase and then an inactive burnt-out phase, it is generally agreed that steroids should be offered to AIP patients with active disease.[14] There does not appear to be a role for steroids in patients who present in the postacute phase with pancreatic atrophy.

Steroid regimen

Current practice in the treatment of type 1 AIP is shown in **Figure 1**. To date, although the International Consensus Diagnostic Criteria defines the starting dose of steroid for induction of remission as 0.6-1 mg/kg per day, a steroid regimen for type 1 AIP has not been standardized, and there is no consensus on the duration of induction, tapering schedule, or optimal dose and duration of maintenance therapy.[15] In the clinical setting, most clinicians in Japan, Korea, and the United States use 30-40 mg of prednisolone (or prednisone) daily as an induction therapy.[2,9,16,17] Some European doctors use an initial prednisolone dose of 60 mg per day.[18]

Different patterns of steroid tapering have been proposed by medical centers around the world. In the United States, in which a relatively short overall course of initial steroid therapy with selective maintenance therapy is used, the starting dose of prednisolone is 40 mg per day for 4 weeks, after which the dose is tapered by 5 mg per week with an attempt to completely withdraw the steroid without an extended tapering period or maintenance therapy (i.e., 4 weeks of induction therapy plus 8 weeks of tapering).[17] In Japan, the initial daily dose of prednisolone (0.6 mg/kg) is given for 2-4 weeks and then reduced by 5 mg every 1-2 weeks. After reaching the prednisolone dose of 15 mg, the dose is reduced more slowly, by 2.5-5 mg every 2-8 weeks, until a maintenance dose of 2.5-5 mg per day is reached.[2,11] In Korea, remission is usually achieved on a regimen of prednisolone 30 mg per day for 1-2 months, followed by gradual tapering of 5-10 mg per month to

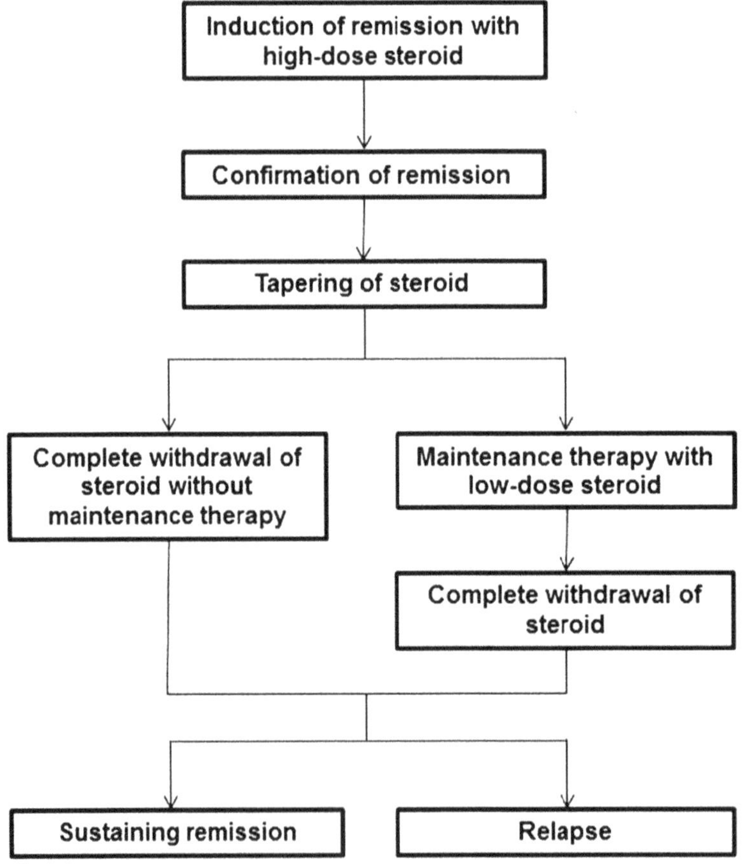

Figure 1. Current principles in steroid treatment of type 1 autoimmune pancreatitis.

the maintenance dose of 5 mg per day, which is continued for several months and then completely stopped. The goal of tapering is not to achieve remission but to avoid possible cortisol deficiency resulting from the suppression of the hypothalamic-pituitary-adrenal axis while maintaining sustained remission. Therefore, induction of remission should be confirmed before steroid tapering is begun.

From our experience, resolution of pancreatic abnormalities is achieved relatively quickly, whereas extrapancreatic lesions such as retroperitoneal fibrosis or proximal bile duct stricture and ductal wall thickening take more time. In some patients, complete resolution of these abnormalities may take several months. However, the duration of induction therapy with high-dose steroids does not exceed 1 month in the United States and Japan.[2,17] After only a month of steroids, a considerable portion of the abnormalities might still remain. In this situation, remaining abnormalities represent persistent disease activity rather than a true disease relapse. Therefore, the duration of the initial induction therapy with high-dose steroid may need to be tailored to each patient according to the disease activity of the specific organs involved.

Maintenance therapy

Maintenance therapy is used to prevent disease relapse while maintaining remission. The Japanese guidelines for AIP suggest that maintenance therapy with low-dose steroids (2.5-5 mg/day) should be administered to all patients, with the aim of stopping steroid therapy within 3 years.[11] According to the study by Kamisawa et al., patients with maintenance steroid therapy are less likely to relapse, and most relapses are in the first 3 years following initial diagnosis.[2] Therefore, medical centers in Japan routinely use a prolonged maintenance therapy for up to 3 years based on the logic that most relapses occur within that timeframe. However, low-dose steroids (2.5-5 mg/day) may be insufficient to prevent relapses because it is only a physiological dose. Additional outcome data are needed to establish the risk-benefit before endorsing this practice.

Unlike the Japanese practice of using maintenance therapy in most patients, maintenance therapy in the United States is used only in those patients who relapse after an initial course of steroids.[19,20] The rationale against the universal use of maintenance steroids is that nearly half of patients did not relapse even after a short-course of steroid therapy.[10]

Unfortunately, the different approaches to patient selection for maintenance therapy have not been directly compared. It remains to be proven whether maintenance therapy should be used for all patients or restricted to those who relapse or those who are likely to relapse after an initial steroid course.

Steroid-related side effects

The exact rates of steroid therapy side effects in AIP have not been established.[10] A recent multicenter study on steroid therapy for AIP reported several cases of glucose intolerance, osteoporosis (10/459), spinal compression fracture (5/459), avascular necrosis of the femoral head (3/459), and pneumonia (3/459).[2] In general, cosmetic changes including moon face, dorsal hump formation, abdominal striae, weight gain, acne, and alopecia are relatively common after long-term steroid therapy.[21] Aggravated glycemic control and labile hypertension can also occur. Serious side effects requiring steroid discontinuation include osteoporosis with compression fracture, avascular necrosis, steroid-induced psychosis, and opportunistic infections.[2,4] Patients on long-term steroid therapy, especially those with individual risk factors, including the use of other medications or comorbidities, should be closely monitored for side effects of long-term steroid use.

Treatment of Relapse

Patients may experience AIP relapse, either during maintenance steroid therapy or after complete discontinuation of the steroid.[7] Most patients with disease relapse need a full course of therapy similar to the initial therapy, but isolated serological relapse can be observed without a specific therapy.[12]

There are currently three options for managing patients suffering from a relapse of type 1 AIP (**Figure 2**).[19] The remission rates achieved using steroids at disease relapse remain very high and are similar to those achieved at the time of initial disease presentation.[10,22] For patients who relapse, steroids are often given at a higher induction dose that is tapered more gradually, and maintenance therapy is often more prolonged.[7,23] Unfortunately, it is uncertain as to how long steroid treatment should be continued in patients with relapsing AIP.

Summary

There is a variety of steroid treatment regimens that differ according to the dose and duration of induction therapy and whether or not maintenance therapy is administered. These regimens are based on institutional experiences, are not standardized, and have not been systematically compared. Developing a consensus regarding definitions of remission and the optimal treatment regimen including the need for and duration of maintenance treatment may help to increase the complete remission rate and lower relapse rates.

Additional studies are needed to advance our understanding of the role of steroids in the optimal management of AIP.

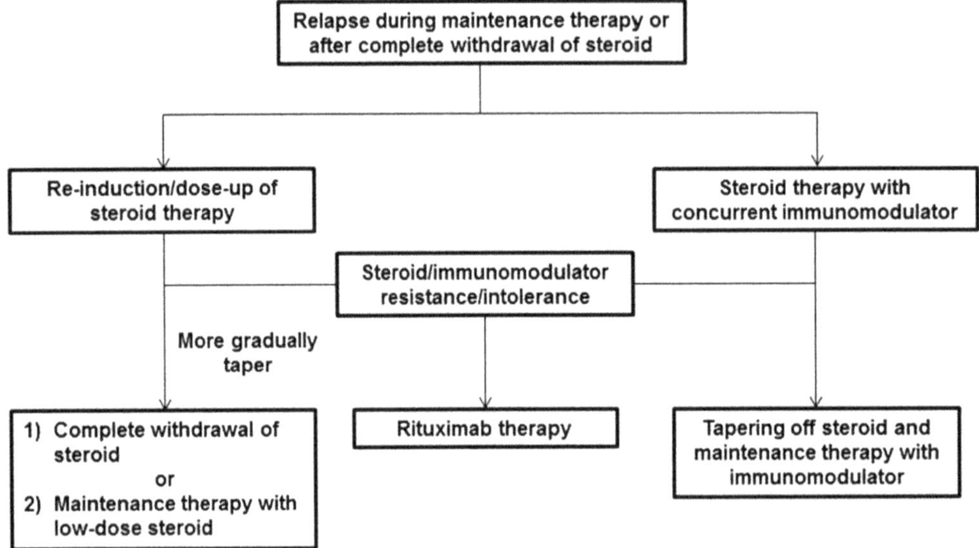

Figure 2. The current algorithm for treatment of relapsed type 1 AIP.

References

1. Song TJ, Kim JH, Kim MH, Jang JW, Park do H, Lee SS, Seo DW, Lee SK, and Yu E. Comparison of clinical findings between histologically confirmed type 1 and type 2 autoimmune pancreatitis. *J Gastroenterol Hepatol.* 2012; 27: 700-708. PMID: 21929653
2. Kamisawa T, Shimosegawa T, Okazaki K, Nishino T, Watanabe H, Kanno A, Okumura F, Nishikawa T, Kobayashi K, Ichiya T, Takatori H, Yamakita K, Kubota K, Hamano H, Okamura K, Hirano K, Ito T, Ko SB, and Omata M. Standard steroid treatment for autoimmune pancreatitis. *Gut.* 2009; 58: 1504-1507. PMID: 19398440
3. Kamisawa T, Yoshiike M, Egawa N, Nakajima H, Tsuruta K, and Okamoto A. Treating patients with autoimmune pancreatitis: results from a long-term follow-up study. *Pancreatology.* 2005; 5: 234-238. PMID: 15855821
4. Hirano K, Tada M, Isayama H, Yagioka H, Sasaki T, Kogure H, Nakai Y, Sasahira N, Tsujino T, Yoshida H, Kawabe T, and Omata M. Long-term prognosis of autoimmune pancreatitis with and without corticosteroid treatment. *Gut.* 2007; 56: 1719-1724. PMID: 22249131
5. Shimizu Y, Yamamoto M, Naishiro Y, Sudoh G, Ishigami K, Yajima H, Tabeya T, Matsui M, Suzuki C, Takahashi H, Seki N, Himi T, Yamashita K, Noguchi H, Hasegawa T, Suzuki Y, Honda S, Abe T, Imai K, and Shinomura Y. Necessity of early intervention for IgG4-related disease-delayed treatment induces fibrosis progression. *Rheumatology.* 2013; 52: 679-683. PMID: 23258649
6. Kalaitzakis E, and Webster GJ. Review article: autoimmune pancreatitis - management of an emerging disease. *Aliment Pharmacol Ther.* 2011; 33: 291-303. PMID: 21138452
7. Moon SH, Kim MH, and Park do H. Treatment and relapse of autoimmune pancreatitis. *Gut Liver.* 2008; 2: 1-7. PMID: 20485603
8. Sah RP, and Chari ST. Serologic issues in IgG4-related systemic disease and autoimmune pancreatitis. *Curr Opin Rheumatol.* 2011; 23: 108-113. PMID: 21124093
9. Sandanayake NS, Church NI, Chapman MH, Johnson GJ, Dhar DK, Amin Z, Deheragoda MG, Novelli M, Winstanley A, Rodriguez-Justo M, Hatfield AR, Pereira SP, and Webster GJ. Presentation and management of post-treatment relapse in autoimmune pancreatitis/immunoglobulin G4-associated cholangitis. *Clin Gastroenterol Hepatol.* 2009; 7: 1089-1096. PMID: 19345283
10. Pannala R, and Chari ST. Corticosteroid treatment for autoimmune pancreatitis. *Gut.* 2009; 58: 1438-1439. PMID: 19834112
11. Kamisawa T, Okazaki K, Kawa S, Shimosegawa T, and Tanaka M. Japanese consensus guidelines for management of autoimmune pancreatitis: III. Treatment and prognosis of AIP. *J Gastroenterol.* 2010; 45: 471-477. PMID: 20213336
12. Sugumar A, and Chari ST. Diagnosis and treatment of autoimmune pancreatitis. *Curr Opin Gastroenterol.* 2010; 26: 513-518. PMID: 20693897
13. Stone JH, Zen Y, and Deshpande V. IgG4-related disease. *N Engl J Med.* 2012; 366: 539-551. PMID: 24111912
14. Sah RP, and Chari ST. Autoimmune pancreatitis: an update on classification, diagnosis, natural history and management. *Curr Gastroenterol Rep.* 2012; 14: 95-105. PMID: 22350841
15. Shimosegawa T, Chari ST, Frulloni L, Kamisawa T, Kawa S, Mino-Kenudson M, Kim MH, Klöppel G, Lerch MM, Löhr M, Notohara K, Okazaki K, Schneider A, and Zhang L. International consensus diagnostic criteria for autoimmune pancreatitis: guidelines of the International Association of Pancreatology. *Pancreas.* 2011; 40: 352-358. PMID: 21412117
16. Moon SH, Kim MH, Park DH, Hwang CY, Park SJ, Lee SS, Seo DW, and Lee SK. Is a 2-week steroid trial after initial negative investigation for malignancy useful in

differentiating autoimmune pancreatitis from pancreatic cancer? A prospective outcome study. *Gut.* 2008; 57: 1704-1712. PMID: 18583399

17. Sah RP, Chari ST, Pannala R, Sugumar A, Clain JE, Levy MJ, Pearson RK, Smyrk TC, Petersen BT, Topazian MD, Takahashi N, Farnell MB, and Vege SS. Differences in clinical profile and relapse rate of type 1 versus type 2 autoimmune pancreatitis. *Gastroenterology.* 2010; 139: 140-148. PMID: 20353791
18. Frulloni L, Scattolini C, Falconi M, Zamboni G, Capelli P, Manfredi R, Graziani R, D'Onofrio M, Katsotourchi AM, Amodio A, Benini L, and Vantini I. Autoimmune pancreatitis: differences between the focal and diffuse forms in 87 patients. *Am J Gastroenterol.* 2009; 104: 2288-2294. PMID: 19568232
19. Hart PA, Topazian MD, Witzig TE, Clain JE, Gleeson FC, Klebig RR, Levy MJ, Pearson RK, Petersen BT, Smyrk TC, Sugumar A, Takahashi N, Vege SS, and Chari ST. Treatment of relapsing autoimmune pancreatitis with immunomodulators and rituximab: the Mayo Clinic experience. *Gut.* 2013; 62: 1607-1615. PMID: 22936672
20. Raina A, Yadav D, Krasinskas AM, McGrath KM, Khalid A, Sanders M, Whitcomb DC, and Slivka A. Evaluation and management of autoimmune pancreatitis: experience at a large US center. *Am J Gastroenterol.* 2009; 104: 2295-2306. PMID: 19532132
21. Manns MP, Czaja AJ, Gorham JD, Krawitt EL, Mieli-Vergani G, Vergani D, and Vierling JM. Diagnosis and management of autoimmune hepatitis. *Hepatology.* 2010; 51: 2193-2213. PMID: 20513004
22. Hart PA, Kamisawa T, Brugge WR, Chung JB, Culver EL, Czakó L, Frulloni L, Go VL, Gress TM, Kim MH, Kawa S, Lee KT, Lerch MM, Liao WC, Löhr M, Okazaki K, Ryu JK, Schleinitz N, Shimizu K, Shimosegawa T, Soetikno R, Webster G, Yadav D, Zen Y, and Chari ST. Long-term outcomes of autoimmune pancreatitis: a multicentre, international analysis. *Gut.* 2013; 62: 1771-1776. PMID: 23232048
23. Okazaki K, Kawa S, Kamisawa T, Ito T, Inui K, Irie H, Irisawa A, Kubo K, Notohara K, Hasebe O, Fujinaga Y, Ohara H, Tanaka S, Nishino T, Nishimori I, Nishiyama T, Suda K, Shiratori K, Shimosegawa T, and Tanaka M. Japanese clinical guidelines for autoimmune pancreatitis. *Pancreas.* 2009; 38: 849-866. PMID: 19745774

Chapter 63

Immunomodulators and rituximab in the management of autoimmune pancreatitis

Phil A. Hart* and Suresh T. Chari*

Gastroenterology and Hepatology, Mayo Clinic, Rochester, Minnesota.

Introduction

Autoimmune pancreatitis (AIP) is a unique form of chronic pancreatitis that is characterized by a dramatic response to steroid therapy. The remission rate for induction treatment with steroids is essentially 100%, and steroids remain highly effective when used to treat relapses. Unfortunately, an important subset of patients has difficult to treat disease on the basis of inability to tolerate steroids or the development of frequent relapses requiring prolonged treatment with high-dose steroids. Steroid-sparing immunomodulators such as azathioprine and mycophenolate mofetil were primarily introduced in an effort to manage these patients. More recently, the monoclonal anti-CD20 antibody rituximab has also been used in these patients including those who were resistant or intolerant to immunomodulators. Available data suggests there may be a role for these steroid-sparing treatments, but further studies are awaited to more accurately define the benefit of these agents for maintenance of disease remission.

Treatment of Disease Relapse

Approximately half of patients with type 1 AIP relapse within the first 3 years following AIP diagnosis. Although this risk may be decreased by providing long-term, low-dose steroids, relapses still occur in almost one-quarter of subjects on low-dose maintennace steroids.[1] The organs most frequently affected by disease relapses are the pancreas and biliary tract and can cause significant morbidity. Relapses can be treated with one of four strategies: 1) tapered high-dose steroids without maintenance treatment, 2) tapered high-dose steroids with maintenance low-dose steroids, 3) tapered high-dose steroids with a maintenance steroid-sparing immunomodulator, or 4) rituximab monotherapy. Fortunately, when steroids are used to treat disease relapse, remission is successfully reinduced in >95% of patients.[2] However, some patients are either unable to successfully wean from steroids without precipitating disease recurrence or have frequent relapses that require chronic, high-dose steroid exposure. A small proportion of patients are unable to tolerate induction treatment with high-dose steroids due to short-term severe adverse effects (e.g., severe hyperglycemia or emotional/mental instability). These subsets of difficult-to-treat patients are most likely to benefit from steroid-sparing immunomodulators or rituximab.

Steroid-sparing immunomodulators

Immunomodulators were initially considered as a steroid-sparing alternative to long-term steroid use for maintaining disease remission. Because patients tend to present with AIP later in life, it is felt that these subjects may also be more susceptible to complications from chronic steroid use. Four case series were published in the late 2000s describing the effectiveness of immunomodulators in AIP.[3-6] In each study, the clinical response to initial treatment with immunomodulators was consistently high (**Table 1**). Almost all patients were able to achieve clinical remission, and only a small number relapsed, typically following discontinuation of the immunomodulator. However, in these studies, a variety of agents was used (azathioprine, mycophenolate mofetil, and methotrexate), the sample sizes were small, and median follow-up times were relatively brief.

More recently, we evaluated our experience treating 41 AIP subjects with immunomodulators at the Mayo Clinic.[2] Azathioprine (dosed at 2 mg/kg/day) was the most commonly used immunomodulator, followed by 6-mercaptopurine (1 mg/kg/day) and mycophenolate mofetil (750-1,000 mg twice daily). Relapse-free survival was similar between those patients who were treated with steroids alone compared to steroids and an immunomodulator at the time of their first disease relapse (**Figure 1**). Although there was a trend toward longer remission in those who received immunomodulators, this did not achieve statistical significance.

*Corresponding authors. Email: philip.hart@osumc.edu, chari.suresh@mayo.edu

Table 1. Data published prior to 2010 regarding the use of immunomodulators in the treatment of AIP.

Author, Country	n	Achieved steroid- free remission (*n*)	Disease relapses (*n*)	Median follow-up, (range)	Drugs used (*n*)	Comments
Ghazale et al.,[4] United States	7	7/7	2*	6 mos, (2–19)	AZA (4), MMF (2), CTX (1)	* Both relapses occurred while patients were taking low-dose AZA
Sandanayake et al.,[6] UK	10	7/8*	0	4 mos, (1–36)	AZA	* Two patients started on AZA and steroids did not have follow-up
Raina et al.,[5] United States	10	10/10	1*	NR	AZA (9), MTX (1)	* Two additional patients later had relapses <2 months after AZA discontinuation
Frulloni et al.,[3] Italy	6	6/6	0	17 mos (6–36)	AZA (4), MTX (2)	

AZA, azathioprine; CTX, cyclophosphamide; MMF, mycophenolate mofetil, NR, not reported.

Importantly, a significant number of patients either developed immunomodulator resistance (i.e., relapse while on the immunomodulator or inability to wean prednisone) or did not tolerate the treatment's side effects. During the study period, 17 patients were either resistant ($n = 15$) or intolerant to steroids ($n = 2$) to immunomodulator treatment. Also, 9 (22%) patients required drug discontinuation due to side effects including nausea/ vomiting, drug-induced liver injury, myelosuppression, and bacteremia. Many of these patients were able to tolerate substitution with either another thiopurine or mycophenolate mofetil. Steroid-sparing immunomodulators may have a modest benefit in some patients, but there remains a group of refractory patients who cannot be satisfactorily maintained in remission with immunomodulators.

Rituximab

An important breakthrough occurred when rituximab, a monoclonal anti-CD20 antibody, was demonstrated to successfully treat a patient with refractory AIP.[8] This complicated patient had recurrent intrahepatic biliary disease, was unable to tolerate steroids (due to a serious infection), and subsequently developed a relapse during treatment with a thiopurine. The observation was made that there

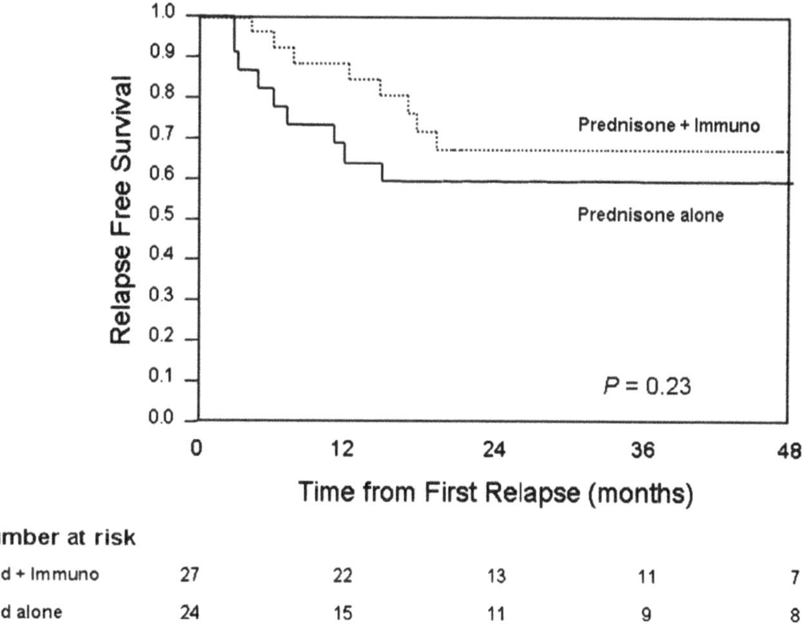

Figure 1. Relapse-free survival following treatment of initial disease relapse with either tapered prednisone alone, or tapered prednisone plus an immunomodulator for maintenance treatment. Used with permission from Hart et al.[7]

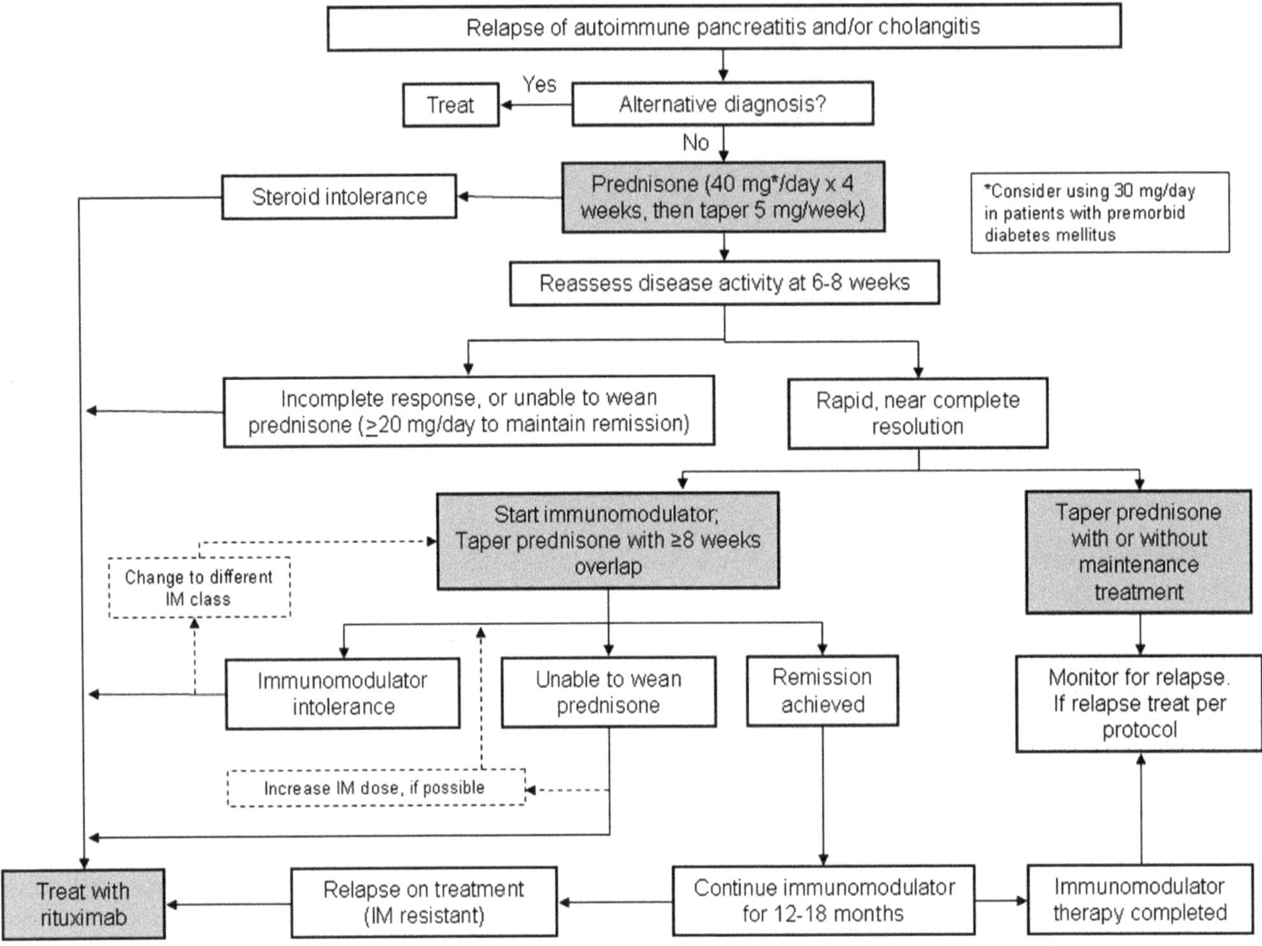

Figure 2. Algorithm for managing AIP relapses. Used with permission from Hart et al.[7]

were abundant CD-20-positive lymphocytes on a pancreas biopsy, analogous to the findings seen in orbital pseudolymphoma (a disease known to respond to rituximab).[9] After a series of four infusions, the patient exhibited an impressive clinical and radiographic response.

Since the initial report, we have continued to use rituximab in these difficult-to-treat patients by providing a series of infusions over 2 years. The protocol consists of administering 375 mg/m^2 (body surface area) intravenously weekly for 4 weeks, followed by eight additional maintenance infusions every 3 months (a protocol that is similar to B-cell lymphoma treatment). We reported that 10 out of 12 patients who had completed at least the 4 induction infusions achieved a convincing symptomatic, biochemical, and radiographic remission.[7] One patient had a partial response and was later found to have an alternative, but concurrent diagnosis to explain his lack of response. None of the patients relapsed during rituximab treatment. One subject did develop a pancreatic relapse more than 2 years after discontinuing rituximab, which remained responsive to readministration of rituximab.

Rituximab has also been shown to be effective in subjects with IgG4-related disease without pancreatic-predominant disease. Khosroshahi et al. reported their experience treating 10 patients, the majority of whom had systemic IgG4-related disease manifestations such as salivary gland involvement, orbital disease, or lymphadenopathy (n = 2 had biliary and/or pancreatic involvement).[10] The rituximab protocol used in this study consisted of two infusions of 1,000 mg administered intravenously on days 0 and 14, with no maintenance infusions (a protocol that is similar to treatment of rheumatologic conditions). Nine of these 10 patients had clinical improvement within 1 month of treatment; however, 4 patients required retreatment within 6 months due to disease relapse. A recent a phase I/II open-label study of 28 patients with IgG4-related disease using the two-dose (1000 mg each) protocol confirmed the utility of rituximab in inducing remission as a single agent.[11]

Although it has been shown to be effective as a first-line agent, due to cost and limited experience, we have reserved its use for difficult-to-treat patients. Also, the optimal dosing regimen and durability of this response is unknown.

Treatment-related complications

Because steroids are excellent at controlling disease and inexpensive, any alternative treatment must be effective and offer a more favorable side effect profile. Due to the rarity of AIP, there are no large studies describing long-term side effects of immunomodulators. However, these agents have been well studied in rheumatologic and inflammatory gastrointestinal conditions (e.g., inflammatory bowel disease and autoimmune hepatitis). Common side effects of azathioprine (and 6-mercaptopurine) include nausea, myelosuppression, hepatotoxicity, increased risk of infections, and acute pancreatitis.[12] Mycophenolate mofetil can also lead to a variety of side effects including headache, diarrhea, edema, leukopenia, and increased risk of infections.[13] When taken for many years, these medications also increase the risk of lymphoma and nonmelanoma skin cancers.[13,14] As previously discussed, almost a quarter of patients in the Mayo Clinic immunomodulator study who were started on an immunomodulator discontinued the drug due to intolerable side effects, so vigilance for the development of complications is warranted.

Likewise, data regarding the use of rituximab in AIP are too limited to provide a meaningful assessment of any disease-specific side effects; however, these risks have been extensively investigated in the treatment of lymphoma and rheumatoid arthritis. Rituximab was generally safe and well-tolerated in those studies. The most common complication is a cytokine-mediated infusion reaction consisting of flu-like symptoms. This develops in 10% of subjects during the initial infusion and resolves with cessation of the infusion and supportive measures.[15] True allergic reactions with hypotension and bronchospasm are exceedingly uncommon. Reactivation of chronic hepatitis B and C can occur, so hepatitis serologies should be checked prior to treatment.[15] Other rare but possible late adverse events include interstitial pneumonitis, delayed-onset neutropenia, and progressive multifocal leukoencephalopathy.[16]

Summary

Although AIP disease activity is generally well-controlled with intermittent high-dose or chronic low-dose steroids, there is a subset of difficult to treat patients who require an alternative treatment strategy. Rituximab is highly effective for both remission induction and maintenance; however, it is generally reserved for refractory patients due to its high cost. For those who develop frequent relapses or are unable to be weaned from steroids, we generally administer azathioprine or another steroid-sparing immunomodulator. In patients who are either unable to tolerate the immunomodulator or relapse during immunomodulator treatment, there are no other options aside from rituximab treatment. Our current algorithm for managing relapsing AIP is shown in **Figure 2**. This treatment approach is based on observational data and clinical experience. More rigorous, controlled trials investigating different means of maintaining disease remission in AIP are needed to refine this treatment strategy.

References

1. Kamisawa T, Shimosegawa T, Okazaki K, Nishino T, Watanabe H, Kanno A, Okumura F, Nishikawa T, Kobayashi K, Ichiya T, Takatori H, Yamakita K, Kubota K, Hamano H, Okamura K, Hirano K, Ito T, Ko SB, and Omata M. Standard steroid treatment for autoimmune pancreatitis. *Gut*. 2009; 58: 1504-1507. PMID: 19398440
2. Hart PA, Kamisawa T, Brugge WR, Chung JB, Culver EL, Czakó L, Frulloni L, Go VL, Gress TM, Kim MH, Kawa S, Lee KT, Lerch MM, Liao WC, Löhr M, Okazaki K, Ryu JK, Schleinitz N, Shimizu K, Shimosegawa T, Soetikno R, Webster G, Yadav D, Zen Y, and Chari ST. Long-term outcomes of autoimmune pancreatitis: a multicentre, international analysis. *Gut*. 2013; 62: 1771-1776. PMID: 23232048
3. Frulloni L, Scattolini C, Falconi M, Zamboni G, Capelli P, Manfredi R, Graziani R, D'Onofrio M, Katsotourchi AM, Amodio A, Benini L, and Vantini I. Autoimmune pancreatitis: differences between the focal and diffuse forms in 87 patients. *Am J Gastroenterol*. 2009; 104: 2288-2294. PMID: 19568232
4. Ghazale A, Chari ST, Zhang L, Smyrk TC, Takahashi N, Levy MJ, Topazian MD, Clain JE, Pearson RK, Petersen BT, Vege SS, Lindor K, and Farnell MB. Immunoglobulin G4-associated cholangitis: clinical profile and response to therapy. *Gastroenterology*. 2008; 134: 706-715. PMID: 18222442
5. Raina A, Yadav D, Krasinskas AM, McGrath KM, Khalid A, Sanders M, Whitcomb DC, and Slivka A. Evaluation and management of autoimmune pancreatitis: experience at a large US center. *Am J Gastroenterol*. 2009; 104: 2295-2306. PMID: 19532132
6. Sandanayake NS, Church NI, Chapman MH, Johnson GJ, Dhar DK, Amin Z, Deheragoda MG, Novelli M, Winstanley A, Rodriguez-Justo M, Hatfield AR, Pereira SP, and Webster GJ. Presentation and management of post-treatment relapse in autoimmune pancreatitis/immunoglobulin G4-associated cholangitis. *Clin Gastroenterol Hepatol*. 2009; 7: 1089-1096. PMID: 19345283
7. Hart PA, Topazian MD, Witzig TE, Clain JE, Gleeson FC, Klebig RR, Levy MJ, Pearson RK, Petersen BT, Smyrk TC, Sugumar A, Takahashi N, Vege SS, and Chari ST. Treatment of relapsing autoimmune pancreatitis with immunomodulators and rituximab: the Mayo Clinic experience. *Gut*. 2013; 62: 1607-1615. PMID: 22936672
8. Topazian M, Witzig TE, Smyrk TC, Pulido JS, Levy MJ, Kamath PS, and Chari ST. Rituximab therapy for refractory biliary strictures in immunoglobulin G4-associated cholangitis. *Clin Gastroenterol Hepatol*. 2008; 6: 364-366. PMID: 18328441
9. Witzig TE, Inwards DJ, Habermann TM, Dogan A, Kurtin PJ, Gross JB, Jr., Ananthamurthy A, Ristow KM, and Garity

JA. Treatment of benign orbital pseudolymphomas with the monoclonal anti-CD20 antibody rituximab. *Mayo Clin Proc.* 2007; 82: 692-699. PMID: 17550749

10. Khosroshahi A, Carruthers MN, Deshpande V, Unizony S, Bloch DB, and Stone JH. Rituximab for the treatment of IgG4-related disease: lessons from 10 consecutive patients. *Medicine.* 2012; 91: 57-66. PMID: 22210556
11. Carruthers MN, Topazian MD, Khosroshahi A, Witzig TE, Wallace ZS, Hart PA, Deshpande V, Smyrk TC, Chari S, and Stone JH. Rituximab for IgG4-related disease: a prospective, open-label trial. *Ann Rheum Dis.* 2015; 74: 1171-1177. PMID: 25667206.
12. Su C, and Lichtenstein GR. Treatment of inflammatory bowel disease with azathioprine and 6-mercaptopurine. *Gastroenterol Clin North Am.* 2004; 33: 209-234, viii. PMID: 15177535
13. Wang K, Zhang H, Li Y, Wei Q, Li H, Yang Y, and Lu Y. Safety of mycophenolate mofetil versus azathioprine in renal transplantation: a systematic review. *Transplant Proc.* 2004; 36: 2068-2070. PMID: 15518748
14. Peyrin-Biroulet L, Khosrotehrani K, Carrat F, Bouvier AM, Chevaux JB, Simon T, Carbonnel F, Colombel JF, Dupas JL, Godeberge P, Hugot JP, LØmann M, Nahon S, Sabate JM, Tucat G, and Beaugerie L. Increased risk for nonmelanoma skin cancers in patients who receive thiopurines for inflammatory bowel disease. *Gastroenterology.* 2011; 141: 1621-1628. PMID: 21708105
15. Kimby E. Tolerability and safety of rituximab (MabThera). *Cancer Treat Rev.* 2005; 31: 456-473. PMID: 16054760
16. Ram R, Ben-Bassat I, Shpilberg O, Polliack A, and Raanani P. The late adverse events of rituximab therapy–rare but there! *Leuk Lymphoma.* 2009; 50: 1083-1095. PMID: 19399690

Chapter 64

Prognosis and long-term outcomes of autoimmune pancreatitis

Shigeyuki Kawa[1*], Masahiro Maruyama[2*], and Takayuki Watanabe[3*]

[1]*Center for Health, Safety and Environmental Management, Shinshu University;*
[2/3]*Department of Gastroenterology, Shinshu University School of Medicine, 3-1-1 Asahi, Matsumoto 390-8621, Japan.*

Introduction

Autoimmune pancreatitis (AIP) is characterized by pancreatic swelling and irregular narrowing of the main pancreatic duct (MPD), which often mimic pancreatic cancer.[1-4] AIP was recently classified into two types based on pathological differences: type 1 for lymphoplasmacytic sclerosing pancreatitis (LPSP) and type 2 for idiopathic duct centric chronic pancreatitis (IDCP) or AIP with granulocytic epithelial lesion (GEL).[5] Type 1 AIP is closely associated with increased levels of IgG4 antibodies in the serum and affected tissues.[5-8] Although the long-term prognosis and outcomes of type 1 AIP are relatively well described, they are less understood in type 2 AIP. Accordingly, the following discussion primarily refers to type 1 AIP; what is understood regarding type 2, which is almost exclusively found in Western countries, is discussed at the end.[9,10]

Long-term Prognosis and Outcome of type 1 AIP

Most patients with type 1 AIP (referred to as "AIP" in this section) respond favorably to corticosteroid therapy, which results in the amelioration of symptomatic, radiographic, serologic, and pathologic findings. It is possible for patients to have a spontaneous recovery. However, during long-term follow-up, some patients with AIP are noted to progress to the advanced stage of pancreatic stone formation after recurrence, which may be similar to the findings of chronic pancreatitis (**Figure 1**).[11-13] In addition, a possible association with malignant conditions such as pancreatic cancer or other malignancies has been reported.[14-20]

Progression to chronic pancreatitis

AIP is characterized by high serum IgG4 concentration, IgG4-positive plasma cell infiltration in affected pancreatic tissue, and a favorable response to corticosteroid therapy. Imaging analyses by ultrasonography (US), computed tomography (CT), and endoscopic retrograde cholangiopancreatography (ERCP) show sonolucent (i.e., hypoechoic) swelling and irregular narrowing of the MPD, both of which are due to lymphoplasmacytic inflammation in the acute stage. In 1995, Yoshida et al. first proposed the concept of AIP, which was considered to be free from calcification and to rarely progress to ordinary chronic pancreatitis.[21] Although most patients have a favorable response to corticosteroid therapy, some develop pancreatic atrophy and stone formation with irregular MPD dilatation.[12,13] These imaging findings mimic those of chronic pancreatitis, suggesting that AIP may progress into chronic pancreatitis in some cases.

If this is the case, ordinary chronic pancreatitis could also include the advanced stage of AIP. This is supported by the observation that serum IgG4 remains elevated in over 60% of patients after clinical improvement.[22] To clarify whether ordinary chronic pancreatitis includes the advanced stage of AIP, we measured serum levels of IgG4 in 175 patients with chronic pancreatitis who had been diagnosed before 1995 when the concept of AIP was first proposed. High serum IgG4 concentrations were found in 7.4% of patients with ordinary chronic pancreatitis, suggesting that the advanced stage of AIP may result in the development of ordinary chronic pancreatitis.[23] Similarly, serum IgG4 was elevated in 11.9% of sera from Korean patients with ordinary chronic pancreatitis.[24] A French study showed that more than one-third of AIP patients developed pancreatic imaging abnormalities (e.g., atrophy, calcification, and/or duct irregularities) and functional insufficiency within 3 years of diagnosis.[10] Finally, one autopsy case of AIP showed similar pathological findings to chronic pancreatitis instead of the typical AIP findings of abundant lymphoplasmacytic infiltration, IgG4-bearing plasma cell infiltration, and obstructive phlebitis.[25]

*Corresponding authors. Email: skawapc@shinshu-u.ac.jp, masa10_hiro15@yahoo.co.jp, wat1400@shinshu-u.ac.jp

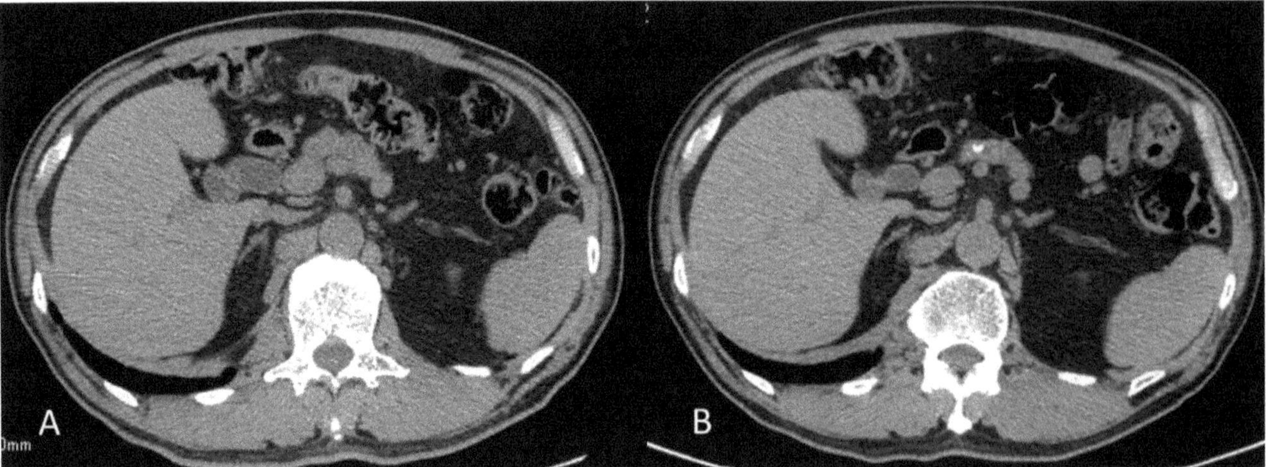

Figure 1. CT scan of a patient with AIP demonstrating the development of a pancreatic stone. There were no calcifications at disease onset (A), but a pancreatic stone was visible 14 months later (B).

Pancreatic stone formation

Features of chronic pancreatitis include clinical findings of exocrine or endocrine dysfunction; imaging findings of pancreatic calcifications in the parenchyma or duct and irregular MPD dilatation; and pathological findings of acinar or ductal cell loss, fibrosis, and stone formation. Of all these, pancreatic stone formation is a representative imaging finding that correlates particularly well with functional and pathological abnormalities.

The reported prevalence of pancreatic stone formation in AIP has been variable. Increased or de novo stone formation, including small calculi, was seen in 28 of 69 (41%) patients followed for at least 3 years at our institution (Shinshu University Hospital). Multivariate analysis identified narrowing of both Wirsung's and Santorini's ducts at diagnosis as an independent risk factor for pancreatic stone formation, which presumably led to pancreatic juice stasis and stone development.[12] A long-term follow up study showed that 16 of 73 (22%) AIP patients progressed to chronic pancreatitis that fulfilled the revised Japanese clinical diagnostic criteria for chronic pancreatitis in the chronic stage.[11] However, other studies have indicated a lower prevalence of pancreatic stone formation during long-term follow-up.[26,27] A recent multicenter, international analysis estimated that pancreatic stones occurred in only 7% of subjects with follow-up imaging permitting evaluation for stone disease.[9] Further studies are needed to explain these discrepancies and to understand if stone formation can be prevented.

Disease relapse

AIP is a chronic disease that can have a relapsing clinical course. To illustrate the frequency and distribution of disease relapses, we reviewed the medical charts of 84 patients with AIP who were followed up for more than 1 year at Shinshu University Hospital. Twenty-eight of the 84 (33%) patients experienced a total of 60 recurrences, including AIP (*n*=26), sclerosing cholangitis (*n*=18), lacrimal and salivary gland lesions (*n*=5), and retroperitoneal fibrosis (*n*=4). Seventy-two percent of the recurrences occurred in the maintenance stage of corticosteroid therapy. Although no markers at diagnosis significantly predicted recurrence, IgG and immune complexes tended to be elevated in the relapse group compared to the nonrelapse group. During clinical follow-up, the development of pancreatic stones was more frequent in the relapse group (14 patients, 50%) than in the nonrelapse group (13 patients, 23%). Collectively, one-third of patients with AIP developed a pancreatic stone. Close observation with activity markers during follow-up and early intervention with corticosteroid therapy may help to prevent recurrence in such cases.[28]

Published series have reported similar relapse rates in AIP ranging from 30% to 50%.[13,29-33] Patients with relapse generally experienced 1 or 2 episodes, although some experienced many relapses. Corticosteroid therapy was reported to significantly increase the remission rate and reduce the relapse rate.[30,32] Thus, corticosteroid therapy is currently considered the standard treatment for inducing remission in AIP.[33] Although spontaneous remission occurs in some patients with AIP, these patients are usually good candidates for corticosteroid therapy.[29-32,34] According to the Japanese Consensus Guidelines for Management of AIP, the indications for corticosteroid therapy in AIP patients are symptoms such as obstructive jaundice, abdominal pain, back pain, and symptomatic extrapancreatic lesions.[35] In principle, corticosteroid therapy should be administered for all patients diagnosed with AIP.[35]

Because AIP is the pancreatic manifestation of IgG4-related disease (IgG4-RD), other manifestations of this condition can be seen at disease relapse.[36,37] In addition to pancreatic lesions, other common manifestations include sclerosing cholangitis, lacrimal/salivary gland lesions, retroperitoneal fibrosis, and interstitial pneumonitis.[9,31] These lesions also respond well to corticosteroid therapy. In our study population, the first, second, and third recurrences occurred at medians of 33, 66, and 122 months following steroid therapy, and 72% of recurrences occurred during the maintenance therapy stage. Other studies have shown that relapse generally occurs within the first 3 years following diagnosis.[32] In those who relapsed, 56% did so within 1 year, and 92% relapsed within 3 years from the start of steroid treatment.[30] Although relapse in our study occurred mostly during the maintenance stage of corticosteroid therapy, the relapse rate of patients with AIP on maintenance treatment was 23%, which was significantly lower than patients who stopped maintenance treatment (34%).[30] According to the Japanese Consensus Guidelines for Management of AIP, maintenance therapy (2.5-5 mg/day) is recommended to prevent recurrence, and stopping of maintenance therapy should be planned within at least 3 years in cases with serologic and radiologic improvement.[35]

Previous studies indicated that various factors at diagnosis, including involvement of proximal biliary tract, diffuse pancreatic swelling, jaundice, IgG4, immune complex, soluble interleukin-2 receptor, and complement are predictive factors of relapse.[23,26,29,31,32] Specific human-leukocyte antigens (HLAs) were reported to predict the recurrence of AIP, and substitution of aspartic acid at position 57 of *HLA DQβ1* purportedly affects AIP recurrence.[36] We reported that serum elevations of IgG4 and immune complex preceded the clinical manifestations of recurrence.[3] Accordingly, serial measurements of IgG, IgG4, and immune complex in the follow-up period may be useful to predict recurrence.[3,23,34]

Relapse after surgical resection of the pancreas

Detlefsen et al. recently reported that 21 of 51 (41.2%) AIP patients who underwent surgical resection of the pancreas experienced recurrence during long-term follow-up; the sites of recurrence were the pancreas (n=8) and extrapancreatic bile ducts (n=7).[39] The recurrence rate and sites were similar to those of the nonresection group. Their results are in contrast to a previous study, which described a decreased risk of relapse in those undergoing surgical resection.[40]

Pancreatic function

Pancreatic exocrine function

AIP is associated with exocrine dysfunction in 83%-88% of cases during the acute inflammatory stage.[34,35,41,42] Exocrine dysfunction resolves in most patients following corticosteroid treatment and during the chronic stage. However, exocrine dysfunction persists or may develop during long-term follow-up in some patients, which may be associated with the transition to chronic pancreatitis.[27]

Pancreatic endocrine function

Diabetes mellitus occurs in 42%-78% of cases during the acute stage of AIP.[34,41-44] Similar to exocrine dysfunction, endocrine dysfunction, especially diabetes mellitus, is often ameliorated after corticosteroid therapy.[27,29,43,45] Miyamoto et al. reported amelioration of diabetes mellitus in 10 of 16 (63%) AIP patients 3 years after corticosteroid therapy, indicating that it is often an effective treatment for diabetes in AIP.[45] However, corticosteroid therapy sometimes causes deterioration of glycemic control, especially in aged patients, and thus requires cautious administration.[44] Ito et al. reported that 10 of 50 AIP patients who received insulin treatment experienced hypoglycemic attacks, suggesting the need for vigilance when insulin therapy is administered.[45] One- third of AIP patients with diabetes mellitus suffered from diabetes at the onset of AIP; they frequently had a family history of diabetes mellitus and had poor nutritional status. Half of AIP patients are diagnosed with diabetes mellitus at AIP onset, but only 10% experienced persistent diabetes mellitus after corticosteroid therapy.[43,45]

AIP and Complications of Pancreatic Cancer and other Malignancies

Chronic pancreatitis has been regarded as a risk factor for pancreatic cancer.[46] If AIP can progress to chronic pancreatitis, it also may be complicated with pancreatic cancer. A Japanese survey indicated that the average life expectancies of male and female patients with chronic pancreatitis were 11 and 17 years shorter than those of the general population, respectively. The major cause of the death was malignancy, indicating that the standard death rates for bile duct and pancreatic cancer were very high (3.44 and 7.84, respectively). It is possible that immunodeficiency due to corticosteroid therapy and chronic pancreas inflammation may contribute to the occurrence of malignancy.

There have been a few previous reports of AIP complicated with pancreatic cancer.[14-17,19,20] Characteristic features of pancreatic cancer complicated with AIP are more frequent occurrence at the body and tail regions compared with ordinary pancreatic cancer,[35] and earlier occurrence after AIP diagnosis compared with chronic pancreatitis. These results raise the possibility that AIP may contribute to the occurrence of pancreatic cancer; however, these cases are highly subject to selection bias.

Because AIP predominantly occurs in elderly patients, deficiency of the immunosurveillance system may be associated with its pathogenesis, which in turn may be associated with various malignancies other than pancreatic cancer.[18] In addition to AIP, IgG4-RD was reported to be highly complicated with malignancies.[48] We identified a close association between IgG4-RD and malignancy formation within 12 years after diagnosis, particularly during the first year. An active IgG4-RD state is presumed to be a strong risk factor for malignancy development.[20] In clinical follow-up for AIP and IgG4-RD, caution is recommended to monitor for malignancy; however, further studies are needed to clarify the true risk and determine the most appropriate methods of cancer surveillance.

Long-Term Prognosis and Outcome of Type 2 AIP

The long-term prognosis and outcome of type 2 AIP have not been fully clarified. The two subtypes can be definitively distinguished based on their histology (See **Chapter 3**, "Histology of Autoimmune Pancreatitis"). Type 2 AIP patients are younger than those with type 1 AIP, do not show the male sex bias seen in type 1 AIP, and are unlikely to have elevation of serum IgG4 or other organ involvement.[5] A multicenter international analysis showed that the average ages at diagnosis were 61.4 and 39.9 years for types 1 and 2 AIP, respectively, and the corresponding proportions of males were 77% and 55%. In addition, type 2 AIP represented a smaller proportion of AIP in Asian countries compared with European and North American countries.[9]

During the acute stage, imaging findings of type 2 AIP appear similar to those of type 1, including pancreatic swelling and irregular narrowing of the MPD. Similar to type 1 AIP, those with type 2 AIP respond favorably to corticosteroid therapy. However, the recurrence rate of type 2 AIP is significantly lower, and the site of type 2 AIP recurrence is limited to the pancreas. Few pancreatic stones are found in type 2 AIP during follow-up, suggesting that it is uncommon for type 2 AIP to progress to an advanced stage.[9] However, another study indicated that the outcome of patients with type 2 AIP is not different from that of patients with type 1 AIP, except for diabetes, which is significantly higher in type 1 AIP.[10] Further studies are therefore needed to better define the long-term prognosis and outcomes of type 2 AIP.

Summary

Type 1 AIP is a chronic, relapsing disease. Although the acute inflammatory phase is very responsive to corticosteroid therapy, several potential long-term complications can develop. Endocrine and exocrine pancreatic dysfunction are more typical during the acute phase; they may resolve with corticosteroid therapy but occur later when the pancreas has atrophied. Disease relapses are common and can develop in the pancreas, biliary tree, or other distant sites associated with IgG4-RD. Careful observation of prodromal symptoms and activity markers during follow-up, as well as early intervention with corticosteroid therapy, may help to limit morbidity from disease relapses. Pancreatic duct stones can develop and are more likely in those with relapsing disease. There is a theoretical increased risk for developing pancreatic cancer, but the actual risk is not fully understood. In contrast, disease relapse and other long-term complications in type 2 AIP are uncommon.

Acknowledgements

We would like to thank Drs. Takashi Muraki, Tetsuya Ito, Keita Kanai, Takaya Oguchi, Hideaki Hamano, and Norikazu Arakura for their clinical assistance and contributions to this work.

References

1. Chari ST, Takahashi N, Levy MJ, Smyrk TC, Clain JE, Pearson RK, Petersen BT, Topazian MA, and Vege SS. A diagnostic strategy to distinguish autoimmune pancreatitis from pancreatic cancer. *Clin Gastroenterol Hepatol.* 2009; 7: 1097-1103. PMID: 194100172
2. Kawa S, Fujinaga Y, Ota M, Hamano H, and Bahram S. Autoimmune Pancreatitis and Diagnostic Criteria. *Curr Immunol Rev.* 2011; 7: 144-161.
3. Kawa S, and Hamano H. Clinical features of autoimmune pancreatitis. *J Gastroenterol.* 2007; 42 Suppl 18: 9-14. PMID: 17520217
4. Kawa S, Hamano H, and Kiyosawa K. Pancreatitis. In: Rose N, MacKay I, eds. *The Autoimmune Diseases.* 4th ed. St. Louis, MO: Academic Press; 2006: 779-786.
5. Sugumar A, Kloppel G, and Chari ST. Autoimmune pancreatitis: pathologic subtypes and their implications for its diagnosis. *Am J Gastroenterol.* 2009; 104: 2308-2310. PMID: 19727085
6. Hamano H, Kawa S, Horiuchi A, Unno H, Furuya N, Akamatsu T, Fukushima M, Nikaido T, Nakayama K, Usuda N, and Kiyosawa K. High serum IgG4 concentrations in patients with sclerosing pancreatitis. *N Engl J Med.* 2001; 344: 732-738. PMID: 11236777
7. Hamano H, Kawa S, Ochi Y, Unno H, Shiba N, Wajiki M, Nakazawa K, Shimojo H, and Kiyosawa K. Hydronephrosis associated with retroperitoneal fibrosis and sclerosing pancreatitis. *Lancet.* 2002; 359: 1403-1404. PMID: 11978339
8. Zen Y, Bogdanos DP, and Kawa S. Type 1 autoimmune pancreatitis. *Orphanet J Rare Dis.* 2011; 6: 82. PMID: 22151922
9. Hart PA, Kamisawa T, Brugge WR, Chung JB, Culver EL, Czako L, Frulloni L, Go VL, Gress TM, Kim MH, Kawa S, Lee KT, Lerch MM, Liao WC, Lohr M, Okazaki K, Ryu JK, Schleinitz N, Shimizu K, Shimosegawa T, Soetikno R, Webster G, Yadav D, Zen Y, and Chari ST. Long-term

outcomes of autoimmune pancreatitis: a multicentre, international analysis. *Gut.* 2013; 61: 1771-1776. PMID: 23232048
10. Maire F, Le Baleur Y, Rebours V, Vullierme MP, Couvelard A, Voitot H, Sauvanet A, Hentic O, Levy P, Ruszniewski P, and Hammel P. Outcome of patients with type 1 or 2 autoimmune pancreatitis. *Am J Gastroenterol.* 2011; 106: 151-156. PMID: 20736934
11. Maruyama M, Arakura N, Ozaki Y, Watanabe T, Ito T, Yoneda S, Maruyama M, Muraki T, Hamano H, Matsumoto A, and Kawa S. Type 1 autoimmune pancreatitis can transform into chronic pancreatitis: a long-term follow-up study of 73 Japanese patients. *Int Rheumatol.* 2013; 2013(8): 272595. PMID: 23762066
12. Maruyama M, Arakura N, Ozaki Y, Watanabe T, Ito T, Yoneda S, Muraki T, Hamano H, Matsumoto A, and Kawa S. Risk factors for pancreatic stone formation in autoimmune pancreatitis over a long-term course. *J Gastroenterol.* 2012; 47: 553-560. PMID: 22183858
13. Takayama M, Hamano H, Ochi Y, Saegusa H, Komatsu K, Muraki T, Arakura N, Imai Y, Hasebe O, and Kawa S. Recurrent attacks of autoimmune pancreatitis result in pancreatic stone formation. *Am J Gastroenterol.* 2004; 99: 932-937. PMID: 15128363
14. Fukui T, Mitsuyama T, Takaoka M, Uchida K, Matsushita M, and Okazaki K. Pancreatic cancer associated with autoimmune pancreatitis in remission. *Intern Med.* 2008; 47: 151-155. PMID: 18239323
15. Ghazale A, and Chari S. Is autoimmune pancreatitis a risk factor for pancreatic cancer? *Pancreas.* 2007; 35: 376. PMID: 18090248
16. Inoue H, Miyatani H, Sawada Y, and Yoshida Y. A case of pancreas cancer with autoimmune pancreatitis. *Pancreas.* 2006; 33: 208-209. PMID: 16868495
17. Motosugi U, Ichikawa T, Yamaguchi H, Nakazawa T, Katoh R, Itakura J, Fujii H, Sato T, Araki T, and Shimizu M. Small invasive ductal adenocarcinoma of the pancreas associated with lymphoplasmacytic sclerosing pancreatitis. *Pathol Int.* 2009; 59: 744-747. PMID: 19788620
18. Shiokawa M, Kodama Y, Yoshimura K, Kawanami C, Mimura J, Yamashita Y, Asada M, Kikuyama M, Okabe Y, Inokuma T, Ohana M, Kokuryu H, Takeda K, Tsuji Y, Minami R, Sakuma Y, Kuriyama K, Ota Y, Tanabe W, Maruno T, Kurita A, Sawai Y, Uza N, Watanabe T, Haga H, and Chiba T. Risk of cancer in patients with autoimmune pancreatitis. *Am J Gastroenterol.* 2013; 108: 610-617. PMID: 23318486
19. Witkiewicz AK, Kennedy EP, Kennyon L, Yeo CJ, and Hruban RH. Synchronous autoimmune pancreatitis and infiltrating pancreatic ductal adenocarcinoma: case report and review of the literature. *Hum Pathol.* 2008; 39: 1548-1551. PMID: 18619645
20. Asano J, Watanabe T, Oguchi T, Kanai K, Maruyama M, Ito T, Muraki T, Hamano H, Arakura N, Matsumoto A, Kawa S. Association Between Immunoglobulin G4-related Disease and Malignancy within 12 Years after Diagnosis: An Analysis after Longterm Followup. *J Rheumatol.* 2015; 42: 2135-2142. PMID: 26472416
21. Yoshida K, Toki F, Takeuchi T, Watanabe S, Shiratori K, and Hayashi N. Chronic pancreatitis caused by an autoimmune abnormality. Proposal of the concept of autoimmune pancreatitis. *Dig Dis Sci.* 1995; 40: 1561-1568. PMID: 7628283
22. Kawa S, Hamano H, and Kiyosawa K. High serum IgG4 concentrations in patients with sclerosing pancreatitis. Reply. *N Engl J Med.* 2001; 345: 148-148. PMID: 11236777
23. Kawa S, Hamano H, Ozaki Y, Ito T, Kodama R, Chou Y, Takayama M, and Arakura N. Long-term follow-up of autoimmune pancreatitis: characteristics of chronic disease and recurrence. *Clin Gastroenterol Hepatol.* 2009; 7: S18-S22. PMID: 19896092
24. Choi EK, Kim MH, Lee TY, Kwon S, Oh HC, Hwang CY, Seo DW, Lee SS, and Lee SK. The sensitivity and specificity of serum immunoglobulin G and immunoglobulin G4 levels in the diagnosis of autoimmune chronic pancreatitis: Korean experience. *Pancreas.* 2007; 35: 156-161. PMID: 17632322
25. Kitano Y, Matsumoto K, Chisaka K, Imazawa M, Takahashi K, Nakade Y, Okada M, Aso K, Yokoyama K, Yamamoto M, Yoshie M, Ogawa K, and Haneda M. An autopsy case of autoimmune pancreatitis. *JOP.* 2007; 8: 621-627. PMID: 17873471
26. Takuma K, Kamisawa T, Tabata T, Inaba Y, Egawa N, and Igarashi Y. Short-term and long-term outcomes of autoimmune pancreatitis. *Eur J Gastroenterol Hepatol.* 2011; 23: 146-152. PMID: 21287714
27. Uchida K, Yazumi S, Nishio A, Kusuda T, Koyabu M, Fukata M, Miyoshi H, Sakaguchi Y, Fukui T, Matsushita M, Takaoka M, and Okazaki K. Long-term outcome of autoimmune pancreatitis. *J Gastroenterol.* 2009; 44: 726-732. PMID: 19396390
28. Kawa S, Ito T, Watanabe T, Maruyama M, Yoneda S, Maruyama M, Kodama R, Ozaki Y, Muraki T, Hamano H, and Arakura N. Frequency and prevention of autoimmune pancreatitis relapse in a Japanese population. *4th AOPA & KPBA.* Jeju, 2011: 27-33.
29. Hirano K, Tada M, Isayama H, Yagioka H, Sasaki T, Kogure H, Nakai Y, Sasahira N, Tsujino T, Yoshida H, Kawabe T, and Omata M. Long-term prognosis of autoimmune pancreatitis with and without corticosteroid treatment. *Gut.* 2007; 56: 1719-1724. PMID: 17525092
30. Kamisawa T, Shimosegawa T, Okazaki K, Nishino T, Watanabe H, Kanno A, Okumura F, Nishikawa T, Kobayashi K, Ichiya T, Takatori H, Yamakita K, Kubota K, Hamano H, Okamura K, Hirano K, Ito T, Ko SB, and Omata M. Standard steroid treatment for autoimmune pancreatitis. *Gut.* 2009; 58: 1504-1507. PMID: 19398440
31. Kim HM, Chung MJ, and Chung JB. Remission and relapse of autoimmune pancreatitis: focusing on corticosteroid treatment. *Pancreas.* 2010; 39: 555-560. PMID: 20182397
32. Kubota K, Watanabe S, Uchiyama T, Kato S, Sekino Y, Suzuki K, Mawatari H, Iida H, Endo H, Fujita K, Yoneda M, Takahashi H, Kirikoshi H, Kobayashi N, Saito S, Sugimori K, Hisatomi K, Matsuhashi N, Sato H, Tanida E, Sakaguchi T, Fujisawa N, and Nakajima A. Factors predictive of relapse and spontaneous remission of autoimmune pancreatitis patients treated/not treated with corticosteroids. *J Gastroenterol.* 2011; 46: 834-842. PMID: 21491208

33. Wakabayashi T, Kawaura Y, Satomura Y, Watanabe H, Motoo Y, and Sawabu N. Long-term prognosis of duct-narrowing chronic pancreatitis: strategy for steroid treatment. *Pancreas.* 2005; 30: 31-39. PMID: 15632697
34. Ito T, Nishimori I, Inoue N, Kawabe K, Gibo J, Arita Y, Okazaki K, Takayanagi R, and Otsuki M. Treatment for autoimmune pancreatitis: consensus on the treatment for patients with autoimmune pancreatitis in Japan. *J Gastroenterol.* 2007; 42 Suppl 18: 50-58. PMID: 17520224
35. Kamisawa T, Okazaki K, Kawa S, Shimosegawa T, and Tanaka M. Japanese consensus guidelines for management of autoimmune pancreatitis: III. Treatment and prognosis of AIP. *J Gastroenterol.* 2010; 45: 471-477. PMID: 20213336
36. Kawa S, and Sugai S. History of Autoimmune Pancreatitis and Mikulicz's Disease. *Curr Immunol Rev.* 2011; 7: 137-143.
37. Stone JH, Zen Y, and Deshpande V. IgG4-related disease. *N Engl J Med.* 2012; 366: 539-551. PMID: 22316447
38. Park do H, Kim MH, Oh HB, Kwon OJ, Choi YJ, Lee SS, Lee TY, Seo DW, and Lee SK. Substitution of aspartic acid at position 57 of the DQbeta1 affects relapse of autoimmune pancreatitis. *Gastroenterology.* 2008; 134: 440-446. PMID: 18155707
39. Detlefsen S, Zamboni G, Frulloni L, Feyerabend B, Braun F, Gerke O, Schlitter AM, Esposito I, and Kloppel G. Clinical features and relapse rates after surgery in type 1 autoimmune pancreatitis differ from type 2: a study of 114 surgically treated European patients. *Pancreatology.* 2012; 12: 276-283. PMID: 22687385
40. Sah RP, Chari ST, Pannala R, Sugumar A, Clain JE, Levy MJ, Pearson RK, Smyrk TC, Petersen BT, Topazian MD, Takahashi N, Farnell MB, and Vege SS. Differences in clinical profile and relapse rate of type 1 vs type 2 autoimmune pancreatitis. *Gastroenterology.* 2010; 139: 140-148. PMID: 20353791
41. Ito T, Kawabe K, Arita Y, Hisano T, Igarashi H, Funakoshi A, Sumii T, Yamanaka T, and Takayanagi R. Evaluation of pancreatic endocrine and exocrine function in patients with autoimmune pancreatitis. *Pancreas.* 2007; 34: 254-259. PMID: 17312466
42. Kamisawa T, Egawa N, Inokuma S, Tsuruta K, Okamoto A, Kamata N, Nakamura T, and Matsukawa M. Pancreatic endocrine and exocrine function and salivary gland function in autoimmune pancreatitis before and after steroid therapy. *Pancreas.* 2003; 27: 235-238. PMID: 14508128
43. Nishino T, Toki F, Oyama H, Shimizu K, and Shiratori K. Long-term outcome of autoimmune pancreatitis after oral prednisolone therapy. *Intern Med.* 2006; 45: 497-501. PMID: 16702740
44. Nishimori I, Tamakoshi A, Kawa S, Tanaka S, Takeuchi K, Kamisawa T, Saisho H, Hirano K, Okamura K, Yanagawa N, and Otsuki M. Influence of steroid therapy on the course of diabetes mellitus in patients with autoimmune pancreatitis: findings from a nationwide survey in Japan. *Pancreas.* 2006; 32: 244-248. PMID: 16628078
45. Miyamoto Y, Kamisawa T, Tabata T, Hara S, Kuruma S, Chiba K, Inaba Y, Kuwata G, Fujiwara T, Egashira H, Koizumi K, Sekiya R, Fujiwara J, Arakawa T, Momma K, and Asano T. Short and long-term outcomes of diabetes mellitus in patients with autoimmune pancreatitis after steroid therapy. *Gut Liver.* 2012; 6: 501-504. PMID: 23170157
46. Ito T, Nakamura T, Fujimori N, Niina Y, Igarashi H, Oono T, Uchida M, Kawabe K, Takayanagi R, Nishimori I, Otsuki M, and Shimosegawa T. Characteristics of pancreatic diabetes in patients with autoimmune pancreatitis. *J Dig Dis.* 2011; 12: 210-216. PMID: 21615876
47. Lowenfels AB, Maisonneuve P, Cavallini G, Ammann RW, Lankisch PG, Andersen JR, Dimagno EP, Andren-Sandberg A, and Domellof L. Pancreatitis and the risk of pancreatic cancer. International Pancreatitis Study Group. *N Engl J Med.* 1993; 328: 1433-1437. PMID: 8479461
48. Yamamoto M, Takahashi H, Tabeya T, Suzuki C, Naishiro Y, Ishigami K, Yajima H, Shimizu Y, Obara M, Yamamoto H, Himi T, Imai K, and Shinomura Y. Risk of malignancies in IgG4-related disease. *Mod Rheumatol.* 2012; 22: 414-418. PMID: 21894525

Chapter 65

Type 2 autoimmune pancreatitis

Günter Klöppel*

Department of Pathology, Technical University Munich, Germany.

Introduction

Autoimmune pancreatitis (AIP) encompasses at least two entities: one is related to a systemic disease referred to as IgG4-related disease (type 1 AIP), and the other is an isolated pancreatic disorder (type 2 AIP). Importantly, histology can generally separate these two diseases. The following discussion describes characteristics of type 2 AIP.

Histopathology of type 2 AIP

The pancreas of a patient with type 2 AIP is often only focally involved. The region that seems to be most often affected is the pancreatic head including the pancreatic portion of the distal bile duct. As in type 1 AIP, the outstanding histologic feature is a periductal lymphoplasmacytic infiltrate usually affecting some or all of the medium-sized ducts (**Figure 1**). It is often accompanied by a collar-like periductal fibrosis, with narrowing of the affected duct. The lymphoplasmacytic infiltrate may extend from the periductal area to the acinar tissue. In addition, there is a perilobular fibrosis, occasionally of the storiform-type. These histological changes can also be found in type 1 AIP but are usually less pronounced in type 2. Conversely, the finding of the so-called granulocytic epithelial lesion (GEL) is specific to AIP 2.[1] This lesion is characterized by focal disruption and destruction of the duct epithelium due to invasion by neutrophilic granulocytes. GELs affect medium-sized and small ducts (**Figure 2**) and may also be recognized in the acinar tissue. In the ducts, they often cause destruction and obliteration of the duct lumen. The number of GELs and their severities differ from patient to patient. If a GEL is included in a biopsy specimen from the pancreas, it is diagnostic for type 2 AIP.[2] Another less specific criterion for the diagnosis of type 2 AIP is absent or scant (<10 cells/high-powered field [hpf]) IgG4-positive plasma cells in the inflamed pancreatic tissue (**Figure 3**).[2,3]

Differential diagnosis of type 1 versus type 2 AIP

Macroscopically, the subtypes of AIP are indistinguishable. In approximately 80% of cases, they present as a tumorous mass in the head of the pancreas mimicking ductal adenocarcinoma.[1,4] Inflammatory infiltration of the pancreas head and wall of the extrahepatic bile duct can cause narrowing of the distal bile duct and main pancreatic duct (MPD). Pseudocysts and calculi are uncommon in both types of AIP.[1,5]

The histopathologies of the two types of AIP differ. Type 2 AIP is characterized by the presence of GELs, which are absent in type 1 AIP.[1,5] The second distinctive feature is the absence or small number (<10 cells/hpf) of immunostained IgG4-positive plasma cells in type 2 AIP, in contrast with the abundant (>10 cells/hpf) IgG4-positive plasma cells in type 1 AIP. Other features that are not specific but usually more pronounced in type 1 AIP

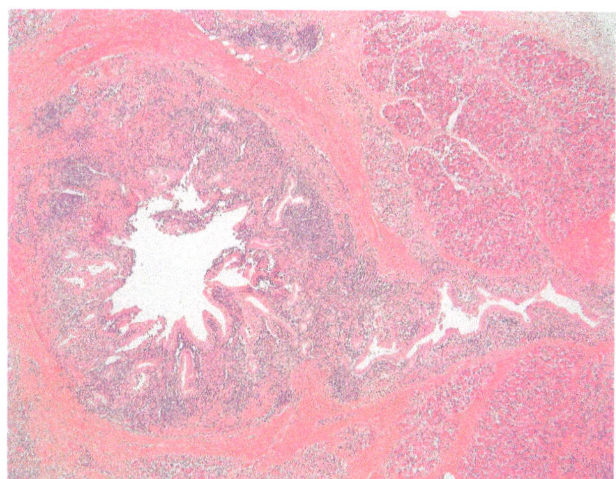

Figure 1. Resected pancreatic specimen from a patient with type 2 AIP demonstrates an intense periductal lymphoplasmacellular infiltrate and fibrosis extending into the surrounding interlobular tissue. The epithelium of the large duct is focally destroyed by granulocytic infiltrates.

*Corresponding author. Email: guenter.kloeppel@alumni.uni-kiel.de

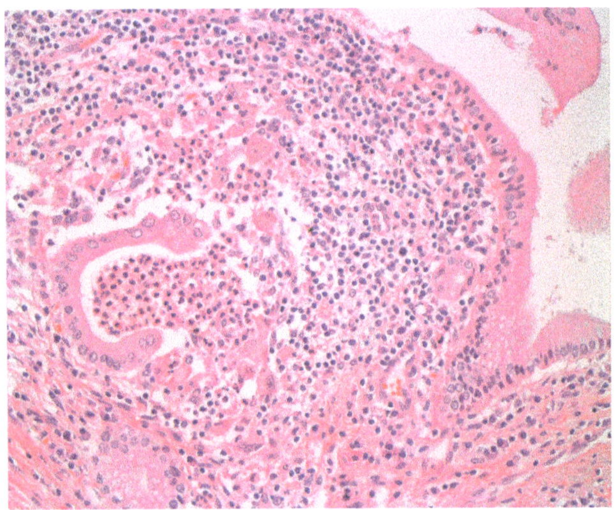

Figure 2. A small pancreatic duct is seen next to a large duct containing a GEL, which causes duct disruption.

are: 1) the presence of an intense lymphoplasmacytic infiltration not only around ducts, but also in the acinar tissue; 2) swirling (storiform) fibrosis centered around ducts and extending into the lobules; and 3) vasculitis with lymphoplasmacytic infiltration surrounding and obliterating the veins (phlebitis) and, to a lesser extent, arteries (arteritis). Immunostaining for CD3-, CD4-, and CD8-positive lymphocytes; CD79a-positive plasma cells; and CD68-positive macrophages often reveals a higher number of these cells in type 1 AIP compared to type 2 AIP.[3,6]

Extrapancreatic disease in type 2 AIP

Patients with type 2 AIP usually do not have immune-mediated diseases that are observed in about 20% to 40% of patients with IgG4-related disease.[7–9] Instead they commonly suffer from chronic inflammatory bowel diseases such as ulcerative colitis or Crohn's disease.[1,9] Moreover, these patients mostly fail to exhibit elevated IgG4 serum levels and increased numbers of IgG4-positive plasma cells.

Epidemiology of type 2 AIP

The subtypes of AIP differ in their clinical features such as sex and mean age at diagnosis.[7] Type 2 AIP is associated with an equal sex distribution and a mean age (45-48 years) that is considerably lower than that seen in type 1 AIP, which peaks between 60 and 65 years.[1,5,9] It is interesting to note that the relative frequencies of the two AIP types in Europe and the U.S. seem to differ from those in East Asia. In Europe, each subtype can be expected in about 40%-60% of cases (in biopsy series they amount to 38% and 45%, respectively), whereas type 2 AIP seems to be rare in East Asia.[10]

Clinical features and laboratory data of type 1 versus type 2 AIP

Symptomatically, AIP patients are indistinguishable. Many patients complain of abdominal pain, although the frequency and intensity of pain attacks tend to be lower in patients with type 1 AIP.[9] Other frequent symptoms are jaundice and weight loss. Corticosteroid treatment resolves strictures of the extrahepatic bile ducts and MPD, as well as the pancreatic mass and focal lesions in the lungs, kidneys, and retroperitoneal inflammatory pseudotumors. These improvements can already be observed after 1 to 2 weeks of steroid therapy.[11,12]

Long-term follow-up in patients with AIP after pancreatic resection revealed that disease recurrence is often observed in type 1 AIP, while it is very rare in type 2 AIP.[1,5,7] Another interesting question is whether pancreatic ductal adenocarcinoma (PDAC), which has recently been described in association with AIP, has a predilection for one of the two AIP types. So far, it seems that PDAC is more commonly associated with type 1 AIP.[13,14]

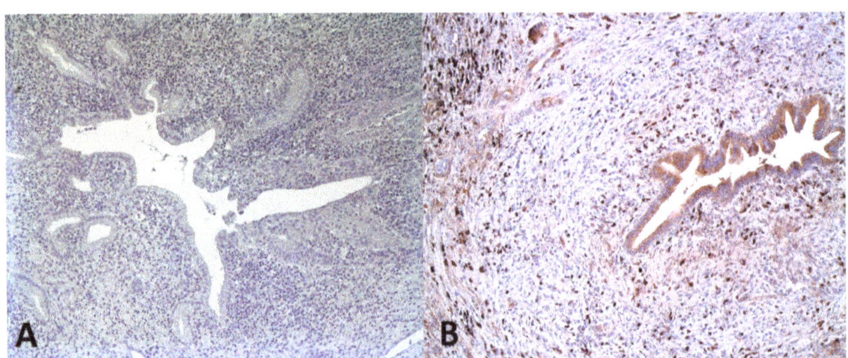

Figure 3. IgG4 immunostaining. There are no positive plasma cells in type 2 AIP (A) but abundant IgG4-positive plasma cells in type 1 AIP (B).

Among the autoantibodies that may be detected are antigens from the pancreatic ducts and acini such as lactoferrin, carbonic anhydrase type II, SPINK1, and trypsinogen.[15,16] Other autoantibodies associated with AIP are antinuclear antibody, rheumatoid factor, and antismooth muscle antibody.

Pathogenesis

The pathogenesis of AIP is still not known, but several findings common to both types of AIP are suggestive of an immune-related etiopathogenesis. This assumption is based on the general histopathological features of both AIP types, their frequent association with immune-related disorders such as the systemic manifestations of IgG4-related disease on one hand and idiopathic inflammatory bowel diseases on the other, and the response to steroid treatment. Whether the demonstrated circulating autoantibodies against carbonic anhydrase II, lactoferrin, and nuclear and smooth muscle antigens, as well as SPINK1, are found in the same frequencies in type 1 and 2 AIP is unknown.

A clear difference between the AIP subtypes concerns the number of IgG4-positive plasma cells in the pancreatic tissue, a finding that often correlates with patients' serum IgG4 levels. It was recently found that renal tissue from AIP patients with tubulointerstitial nephritis contained granular deposits in the tubular basement membranes that were positive for IgG4 and complement C3, and occasionally IgG1, IgG2, and IgG3.[17] In a similar study on pancreatic tissue and bile duct tissue from six GEL-negative AIP patients, double immunofluorescence microscopy revealed deposits of IgG, IgG4, and C3c (but not C1q, IgA, and IgM); these deposits colocalized with basement membrane-associated collagen IV of ducts and acini.[18] On the basis of these findings, it may be hypothesized that IgG4 could play a role in the deposition of immune complexes at pancreatic structures that seem to be the target of the AIP fibroinflammatory process. To clarify whether this hypothesis is only valid in IgG4-positive patients with type 1 AIP, a patient was included in the study whose clinical features were indistinguishable from those of the other six patients of the series but whose immunohistochemical staining was more consistent with type 2 AIP (very low numbers of IgG4-positive plasma cells in the pancreatic tissue). This patient did not have any IgG4-positive deposits at the basement membranes of the ducts and acini but remained positive for C3c and IgG. If this unique finding is confirmed in future studies, it would imply that in type 2 AIP, the mechanisms leading to the changes in the ducts and acini and the fibrosis are independent of the effects of IgG4. This then raises the question as to whether the increased number of IgG4 plasma cells, high IgG4 serum levels, and IgG4 tissue depositions play a primary and active role in the pathogenesis of AIP or if they are secondary phenomena.

Summary

AIP has two distinct subtypes that are primarily defined by their pathologic features. The subtypes have different clinical profiles, disease manifestations, and clinical outcomes. Type 2 AIP is histologically defined by the presence of GELs and a lack of abundant IgG4-positive plasma cells. Patients with type 2 AIP tend to be younger at the time of diagnosis, and the sex distribution is more equal than in type 1 AIP. While type 1 is recognized as part of systemic IgG4-related disease, type 2 AIP is an isolated pancreatic disorder. Aside from the frequent association with inflammatory bowel disease, no other organs are characteristically involved. The disease manifestations of type 2 AIP are extremely sensitive to steroid therapy, and disease relapses are exceedingly uncommon.

References

1. Zamboni G, Lüttges J, Capelli P, Frulloni L, Cavallini G, Pederzoli P, Leins A, Longnecker D, and Klöppel G. Histopathological features of diagnostic and clinical relevance in autoimmune pancreatitis: a study on 53 resection specimens and 9 biopsy specimens. *Virchows Arch.* 2004; 445: 552-563. PMID: 15517359
2. Detlefsen S, Mohr Drewes A, Vyberg M, and Klöppel G. Diagnosis of autoimmune pancreatitis by core needle biopsy: application of six microscopic criteria. *Virchows Arch.* 2009; 454: 531-539. PMID: 19238431
3. Zhang L, Notohara K, Levy MJ, Chari ST, and Smyrk C. IgG4-positive plasma cell infiltration in the diagnosis of autoimmune pancreatitis. *Mod Pathol.* 2007; 20: 23-28. PMID: 16980948
4. Notohara K, Burgart LJ, Yadav D, Chari S, and Smyrk TC. Idiopathic chronic pancreatitis with periductal lymphoplasmacytic infiltration: clinicopathologic features of 35 cases. *Am J Surg Pathol.* 2003; 27: 1119-1127. PMID: 12883244
5. Chari ST, and Murray JA. Autoimmune pancreatitis, part II: relapse. *Gastroenterology.* 2008; 134: 625-628. PMID: 18242227
6. Kojima M, Sipos B, Klapper W, Frahm O, Knuth HC, Yanagisawa A, Zamboni G, Morohoshi T, and Klöppel G. Autoimmune pancreatitis: frequency, IgG4 expression, and clonality of T and B cells. *Am J Surg Pathol.* 2007; 31: 521-528. PMID: 17414098
7. Detlefsen S, Zamboni G, Frulloni L, Feyerabend B, Braun F, Gerke O, Schlitter AM, Esposito I, Klöppel G. Clinical features and relapse rates after surgery in type 1 autoimmune pancreatitis differ from type 2: a study of 114 surgically treated European patients. *Pancreatology.* 2012; 12: 276-283. PMID: 22687385
8. Kamisawa T, and Okamoto A. Autoimmune pancreatitis: proposal of IgG4-related sclerosing disease. *J Gastroenterol.* 2006; 41: 613-625. PMID: 16932997
9. Kamisawa T, Chari ST, Giday SA, Kim M-H, Chung JB, Lee KT, Werner J, Bergmann F, Lerch MM, Mayerle J, Pickartz T, Löhr M, Schneider A, Frulloni L, Webster GJM, Reddy DN, Liao WC, Wang HP, Okazaki K, Shimosegawa T, Klöppel

G, and Go VLW. Clinical profile of autoimmune pancreatitis and its histological subtypes: an international multicenter survey. *Pancreas*. 2011; 40: 809-814. PMID: 21747310
10. Klöppel G, Detlefsen S, Chari ST, Longnecker DS, and Zamboni G. Autoimmune pancreatitis: the clinicopathological characteristics of the subtype with granulocytic epithelial lesions. *J Gastroenterol*. 2010; 45: 787-793. PMID: 20549251
11. Ito T, Nishimori I, Inoue N, Kawabe K, Gibo J, Arita Y, Okazaki K, Takayanagi R, and Otsuki M. Treatment for autoimmune pancreatitis: consensus on the treatment for patients with autoimmune pancreatitis in Japan. *J Gastroenterol*. 2007; 42 Suppl 18: 50-58. PMID: 17520224
12. Saito T, Tanaka S, Yoshida H, Imamura T, Ukegawa J, Seki T, Ikegami A, Yamamura F, Mikami T, Aoyagi Y, Niikawa J, and Mitamura K. A case of autoimmune pancreatitis responding to steroid therapy. Evidence of histologic recovery. *Pancreatology*. 2002; 2: 550-556. PMID: 12435868
13. Inoue H, Miyatani H, Sawada Y, and Yoshida Y. A case of pancreas cancer with autoimmune pancreatitis. *Pancreas*. 2006; 33: 208-209. PMID: 16868495
14. Witkiewicz AK, Kennedy EP, Kennyon L, Yeo CJ, and Hruban RH. Synchronous autoimmune pancreatitis and infiltrating pancreatic ductal adenocarcinoma: case report and review of the literature. *Hum Pathol*. 2008; 39: 1548-1551. PMID: 18619645
15. Löhr JM, Faissner R, Koczan D, Bewerunge P, Bassi C, Brors B, Eils R, Frulloni L, Funk A, Halangk W, Jesnowski R, Kaderali L, Kleef J, Krüger B, Lerch M, Lösel R, Magnani M, Neumaier M, Nittka S, Sahin- Tóth M, Sänger J, Serafini S, Schnölzer M, Thierse HJ, Wandschneider S, Zamboni G, and Klöppel G. Autoantibodies against the exocrine pancreas in autoimmune pancreatitis: gene and protein expression profiling and immunoassays identify pancreatic enzymes as a major target of the inflammatory process. *Am J Gastroenterol*. 2010; 105: 2060-2071. PMID: 20407433
16. Taniguchi T, Okazaki K, Okamoto M, Seko S, Tanaka J, Uchida K, Nagashima K, Kurose T, Yamada Y, Chiba T, and Seino Y. High prevalence of autoantibodies against carbonic anhydrase II and lactoferrin in type 1 diabetes: concept of autoimmune exocrinopathy and endocrinopathy of the pancreas. *Pancreas*. 2003; 27: 26-30. PMID: 12826902
17. Deshpande V, Chicano S, Finkelberg D, Selig MK, Mino-Kenudson M, Brugge WR, Colvin RB, and Lauwers GY. Autoimmune pancreatitis: a systemic immune complex mediated disease. *Am J Surg Pathol*. 2006; 30: 1537-1545. PMID: 17122509
18. Detlefsen S; Bräsen JH, Zamboni G, Capelli P, and Klöppel G. Deposition of complement C3c, immunoglobulin (Ig)G4 and IgG at the basement membrane of pancreatic ducts and acini in autoimmune pancreatitis. *Histopathology*. 2010; 57: 825-835. PMID: 21166697

INDEX

In page numbers *t* denotes table and *f* denotes figure.

www.ingramcontent.com/pod-product-compliance
Lightning Source LLC
Chambersburg PA
CBHW040142200326
41458CB00025B/6349

* 9 7 8 1 6 0 7 8 5 3 6 9 5 *